VISUALIZING
NUTRITION
EVERYDAY CHOICES

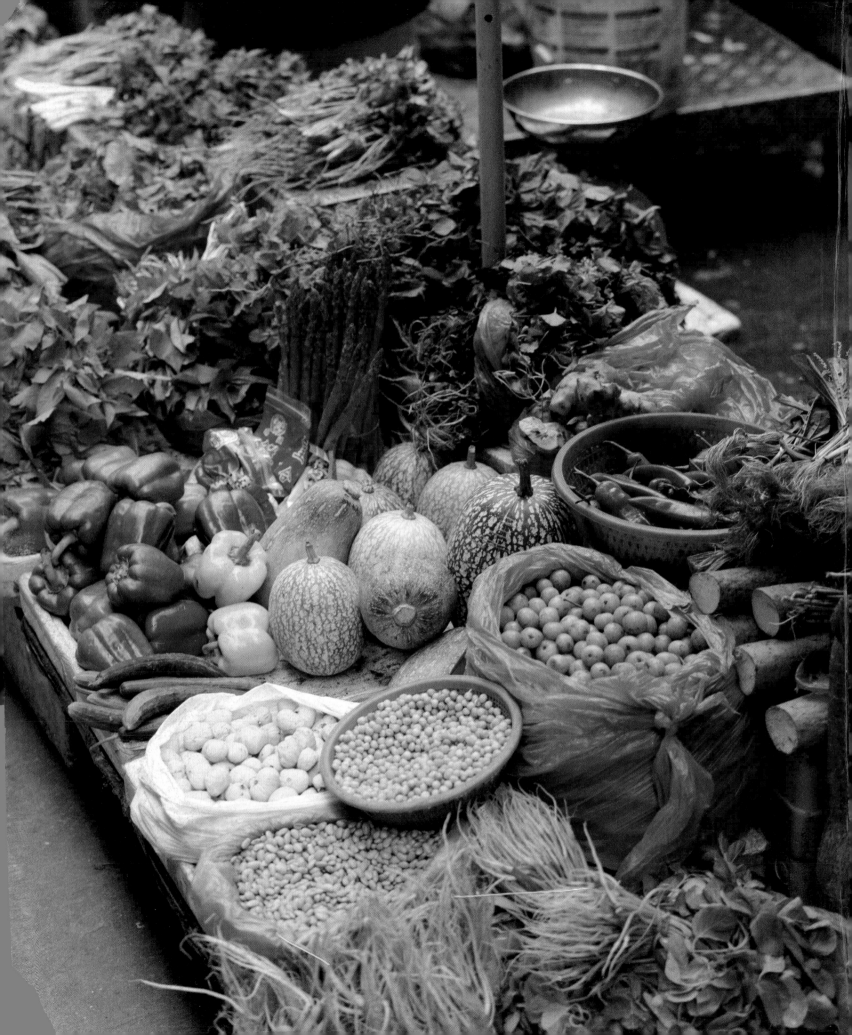

VISUALIZING
NUTRITION
EVERYDAY CHOICES

— Second Edition —

MARY B. GROSVENOR, MS, RD

LORI A. SMOLIN, PHD

UNIVERSITY OF CONNECTICUT

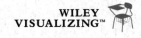

WILEY
VISUALIZING™

WILEY

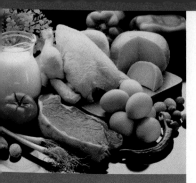
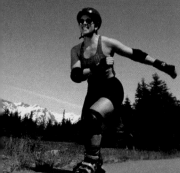
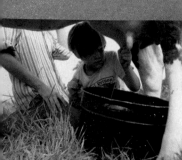
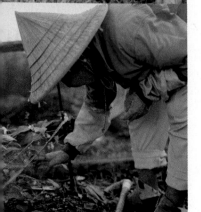

VICE PRESIDENT AND EXECUTIVE PUBLISHER   Kaye Pace
ACQUISITION EDITOR   Kevin Witt
PROJECT EDITOR   Lorraina Raccuia
ASSISTANT CONTENT EDITOR   Lauren Morris
EDITORIAL ASSISTANT   Christina Picciano
SENIOR PRODUCTION EDITOR   Elizabeth Swain
MARKETING MANAGER   Clay Stone
INTERIOR AND COVER DESIGNER   Harry Nolan
PHOTO DEPARTMENT MANAGER   Hilary Newman
ILLUSTRATION EDITOR   Sandra Rigby
SENIOR MEDIA EDITOR   Linda Muriello
MEDIA SPECIALIST   Svetlana Barskaya
PRODUCTION SERVICES   Furino Production

COVER CREDITS:
(Top, center photo): Masterfile
(Bottom inset photos, left to right): Cheryl Power/Photo Researchers, Inc.; Masterfile; Peter Reali/Getty Images, Inc.; Marc Romanelli/Getty Images, Inc.; spxChrome/iStockphoto

This book was set in Times Roman by Prepare, and printed and bound by Quad Graphics/Dubuque. The cover was printed by Quad Graphics/Dubuque

This book is printed on acid-free paper. ∞

Founded in 1807, John Wiley & Sons, Inc. has been a valued source of knowledge and understanding for more than 200 years, helping people around the world meet their needs and fulfill their aspirations. Our company is built on a foundation of principles that include responsibility to the communities we serve and where we live and work. In 2008, we launched a Corporate Citizenship Initiative, a global effort to address the environmental, social, economic, and ethical challenges we face in our business. Among the issues we are addressing are carbon impact, paper specifications and procurement, ethical conduct within our business and among our vendors, and community and charitable support. For more information, please visit our website: *www.wiley.com/go/citizenship*.

Evaluation copies are provided to qualified academics and professionals for review purposes only, for use in their courses during the next academic year. These copies are licensed and may not be sold or transferred to a third party. Upon completion of the review period, please return the evaluation copy to Wiley. Return instructions and a free-of-charge return shipping label are available at www.wiley.com/go/returnlabel. If you have chosen to adopt this textbook for use in your course, please accept this book as your complimentary desk copy. Outside of the United States, please contact your local representative.

Library of Congress Cataloging-in-Publication Data

Grosvenor, Mary B.
Visualizing nutrition: everyday choices / Mary B. Grosvenor, Lori A. Smolin. – 2nd ed.
    p. cm.
    Includes bibliographical references and index.
    ISBN 978-1-118-01380-9 (pbk.) – ISBN 978-1-118-12922-7 (Binder-ready version)
1. Nutrition–Textbooks. I. Smolin, Lori A. II. Title.
    QP141.G767 2011
    612.3–dc23

                                                                            2011032990

Printed in the United States of America
10 9 8 7 6 5 4 3 2 1

How Is Wiley Visualizing Different?

Wiley Visualizing is based on decades of research on the use of visuals in learning (Mayer, 2005)[1]. The visuals teach key concepts and are pedagogically designed to **explain, present, and organize** new information. The figures are tightly integrated with accompanying text; the visuals are conceived with the text in ways that clarify and reinforce major concepts, while allowing students to understand the details. This commitment to distinctive and consistent visual pedagogy sets Wiley Visualizing apart from other textbooks.

Wiley Visualizing texts offer an array of remarkable photographs, maps, media, and film from photo collections around the world, including that of National Geographic. Visualizing images are not decorative, which can often be distracting to students, but purposeful and the primary driver of the content. These authentic materials immerse the student in real-life issues and experiences and support thinking, comprehension, and application.

Together these elements deliver a level of rigor in ways that maximize student learning and involvement. Wiley Visualizing has proven to increase student learning through its unique combination of text, photographs, and illustrations, with online video, animations, simulations, and assessments.

1. Visual Pedagogy. Using the Cognitive Theory of Multimedia Learning, which is backed up by hundreds of empirical research studies, Wiley's authors create visualizations for their texts that specifically support students' thinking and learning. For example, visuals help students identify important topics, organize new information, and integrate new material with prior knowledge.

2. Authentic Situations and Problems. *Visualizing Nutrition: Everyday Choices, 2e* benefits from National Geographic's more than century-long recording of the world. Through this resource, it offers an array of remarkable photographs, maps, and media. These materials immerse the student in real-life issues related to nutrition and thereby enhance interest, learning, and retention (Donovan & Bransford, 2005)[2].

3. Designed with Interactive Multimedia. *Visualizing Nutrition: Everyday Choices, 2e* is tightly integrated with WileyPLUS, our online learning environment that provides interactive multimedia activities in which learners can actively engage with the materials. The combination of textbook and *WileyPLUS* provides learners with multiple entry points to the content, giving them greater opportunity to explore concepts and assess their understanding as they progress through the course. *WileyPLUS* is a key component of the Wiley Visualizing learning and problem-solving experience. This sets Wiley Visualizing apart from other textbooks whose online component is mere drill-and-practice.

Wiley Visualizing and *WileyPLUS* are designed to be a natural extension of how we learn

To understand why the Visualizing approach is effective, it is first helpful to understand how we learn.

1. Our brain processes information using two main channels: visual and verbal. Our *working memory* holds information that our minds process as we learn. This "mental workbench" helps us with decisions, problem-solving, and making sense of words and pictures by building verbal and visual models of the information.

2. When the verbal and visual models of corresponding information are integrated in working memory, we form more comprehensive, lasting, mental models.

3. When we link these integrated mental models to our prior knowledge, stored in our *long-term memory*, we build even stronger mental models. When an integrated (visual plus verbal) mental model is formed and stored in long-term memory, real learning begins.

The effort our brains put forth to make sense of instructional information is called *cognitive load*. There are two kinds of cognitive load: productive cognitive load, such as when we're engaged in learning or exert positive effort to create mental models; and unproductive cognitive load, which occurs when the brain is trying to make sense of needlessly complex content or when information is not presented well. The learning process can be impaired when the information to be processed exceeds the capacity of working memory. Well-designed visuals and text with effective pedagogical guidance can reduce the unproductive cognitive load in our working memory.

---

[1] Mayer, R.E. (Ed) (2005). *The Cambridge Handbook of Multimedia Learning*. Cambridge University Press.
[2] Donovan, M.S., & Bransford, J. (Eds.) (2005). *How Students Learn: Science in the Classroom*.
The National Academy Press. Available at http://www.nap.edu/openbook.php?record_id=11102&page=1

Wiley Visualizing is designed for engaging and effective learning

The visuals and text in *Visualizing Nutrition: Everyday Choices, 2e* are integrated to present complex processes in clear steps, organize information and integrate related pieces of information with one another. This approach minimizes unproductive cognitive load and helps students engage with the content. When students are engaged, they are reading and learning; this leads to both greater acquisition of knowledge and academic success. Examples of this integration of textual concepts with visual elements include the following:

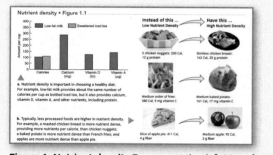

Figure 1: Nutrient density To augment the definition of nutrient density, which appears in the text, this 2-part figure integrates a graphical depiction of the concept of nutrient density with a photographic illustration. The arrows visually guide students to the more nutrient dense choice while captions add specific information about the nutrient density of each food.

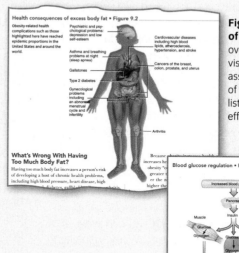

Figure 2: Health consequences of excess body fat This visual overview enhances learning by visually relating the health conditions associated with obesity to the area of the body affected. Organizing the list of health conditions and their effects reduces cognitive load.

Figure 3: Cellular respiration (process diagram) Visually ordering the steps in this process diagram makes metabolism easier to understand. Analogous metabolism process illustrations appear throughout the book to review, reinforce, and build student's metabolism knowledge.

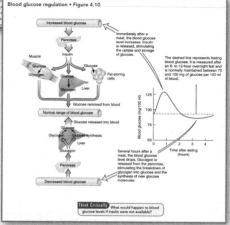

Figure 4: Blood glucose regulation Physically integrating textual elements with the visual elements, as shown here, eliminates split attention (when we must divide our attention between several sources of different information).

Research shows that well-designed visuals, integrated with comprehensive text, can improve the efficiency with which a learner processes information. In this regard, SEG Research, an independent research firm, conducted a national, multisite study evaluating the effectiveness of Wiley Visualizing. Its findings indicate that students using Wiley Visualizing products (both print and multimedia) were more engaged in the course, exhibited greater retention throughout the course, and made significantly greater gains in content area knowledge and skills, as compared to students in similar classes that did not use Wiley Visualizing.[3]

The use of *WileyPLUS* can also increase learning. According to a white paper titled "Leveraging Blended Learning for More Effective Course Management and Enhanced Student Outcomes" by Peggy Wyllie of Evince Market Research & Communications, studies show that effective use of online resources can increase learning outcomes. Pairing supportive online resources with face-to-face instruction can help students to learn and reflect on material, and deploying multimodal learning methods can help students to engage with the material and retain their acquired knowledge. *WileyPLUS* provides students with an environment that stimulates active learning and enables them to optimize the time they spend on their coursework. Continual assessment/remediation is also key to helping students stay on track. The *WileyPLUS* system facilitates instructors' course planning, organization, and delivery and provides a range of flexible tools for easy design and deployment of activities and tracking of student progress for each learning objective.

[3] SEG Research (2009). Improving Student-Learning with Graphically-Enhanced Textbooks: A Study of the Effectiveness of the Wiley Visualizing Series

How Are the Wiley Visualizing Chapters Organized?

Student engagement is more than just catching their interest with exciting videos or interesting animations—engagement means keeping students motivated to keep going. It is easy to get bored or lose focus when presented with large amounts of information, and it is easy to lose motivation when the relevance of the information is unclear. The design of *WileyPLUS* is based on cognitive science, instructional design, and extensive research into user experience. It transforms learning into an interactive, engaging, and outcomes-oriented experience for students.

Wiley Visualizing and *WileyPLUS* work together to reorganize course content into manageable learning objectives and learning modules and relates it to everyday life. Each module has a clear instructional objective, one or more examples, and an opportunity for assessment. These modules are the building blocks of each Wiley Visualizing title.

Each Wiley Visualizing chapter engages students from the start

Chapter-opening text and visuals introduce the subject and connect the student with the material that follows.

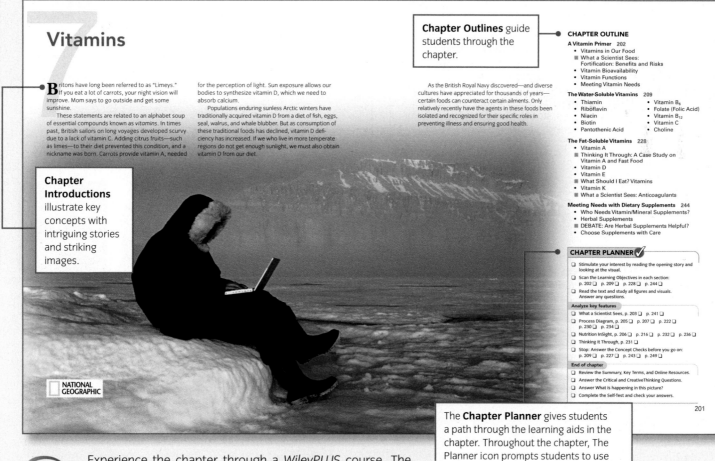

Chapter Introductions illustrate key concepts with intriguing stories and striking images.

Chapter Outlines guide students through the chapter.

The **Chapter Planner** gives students a path through the learning aids in the chapter. Throughout the chapter, The Planner icon prompts students to use the learning aids and to set priorities as they study.

Experience the chapter through a *WileyPLUS* course. The content through *WileyPLUS* transports the student into a rich world of online experience that can be personalized, customized, and extended. Students can create a personal study plan to help prioritize which concepts to learn first and to focus on weak points.

Wiley Visualizing media engages students in the chapter

Wiley Visualizing in *WileyPLUS* gives students a variety of approaches—text, visuals, illustrations, interactions, and assessments—that work together to provide a guided path through the content. But this path isn't static: It can be personalized, customized, and extended to suit individual needs, and so it offers students flexibility as to how they want to study and learn.

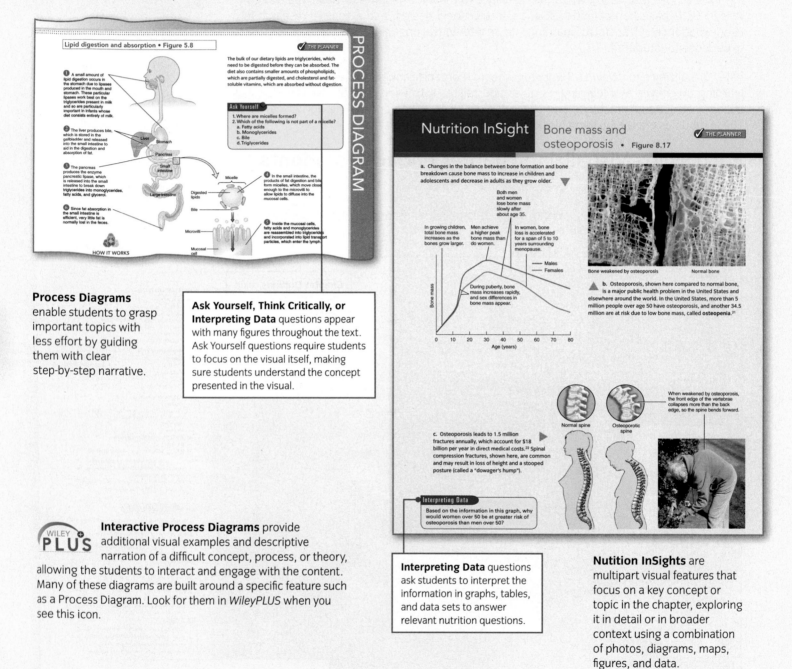

Process Diagrams enable students to grasp important topics with less effort by guiding them with clear step-by-step narrative.

Ask Yourself, Think Critically, or Interpreting Data questions appear with many figures throughout the text. Ask Yourself questions require students to focus on the visual itself, making sure students understand the concept presented in the visual.

Interactive Process Diagrams provide additional visual examples and descriptive narration of a difficult concept, process, or theory, allowing the students to interact and engage with the content. Many of these diagrams are built around a specific feature such as a Process Diagram. Look for them in *WileyPLUS* when you see this icon.

Interpreting Data questions ask students to interpret the information in graphs, tables, and data sets to answer relevant nutrition questions.

Nutrition InSights are multipart visual features that focus on a key concept or topic in the chapter, exploring it in detail or in broader context using a combination of photos, diagrams, maps, figures, and data.

What a Scientist Sees highlights a concept or phenomenon that is of concern to nutrition scientists. Photos and figures are used to improve students' understanding of the nutrition perspective and apply their observational skills to answer questions.

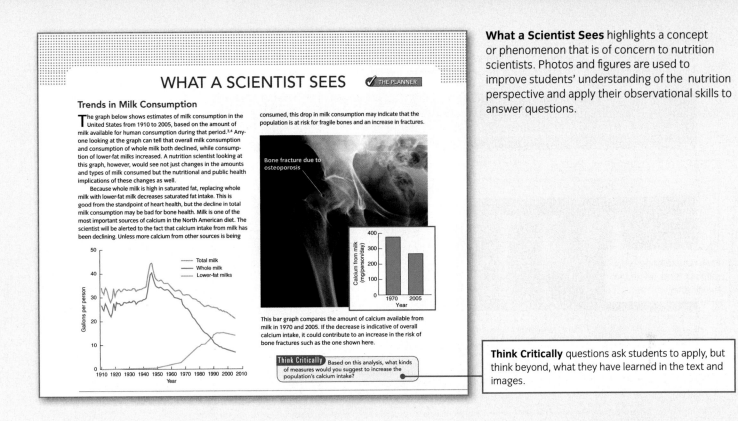

WHAT A SCIENTIST SEES ✓ THE PLANNER

Trends in Milk Consumption

The graph below shows estimates of milk consumption in the United States from 1910 to 2005, based on the amount of milk available for human consumption during that period.[3,4] Anyone looking at the graph can tell that overall milk consumption and consumption of whole milk both declined, while consumption of lower-fat milks increased. A nutrition scientist looking at this graph, however, would see not just changes in the amounts and types of milk consumed but the nutritional and public health implications of these changes as well.

Because whole milk is high in saturated fat, replacing whole milk with lower-fat milk decreases saturated fat intake. This is good from the standpoint of heart health, but the decline in total milk consumption may be bad for bone health. Milk is one of the most important sources of calcium in the North American diet. The scientist will be alerted to the fact that calcium intake from milk has been declining. Unless more calcium from other sources is being consumed, this drop in milk consumption may indicate that the population is at risk for fragile bones and an increase in fractures.

Bone fracture due to osteoporosis

This bar graph compares the amount of calcium available from milk in 1970 and 2005. If the decrease is indicative of overall calcium intake, it could contribute to an increase in the risk of bone fractures such as the one shown here.

Think Critically Based on this analysis, what kinds of measures would you suggest to increase the population's calcium intake?

Think Critically questions ask students to apply, but think beyond, what they have learned in the text and images.

What Should I Eat? provides simple, usable tips that help students translate the nutrition recommendations discussed in each chapter into healthy food choices.

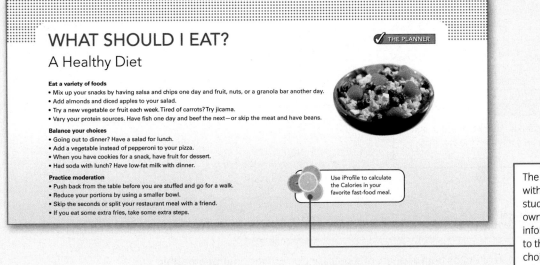

WHAT SHOULD I EAT? ✓ THE PLANNER
A Healthy Diet

Eat a variety of foods
- Mix up your snacks by having salsa and chips one day and fruit, nuts, or a granola bar another day.
- Add almonds and diced apples to your salad.
- Try a new vegetable or fruit each week. Tired of carrots? Try jicama.
- Vary your protein sources. Have fish one day and beef the next—or skip the meat and have beans.

Balance your choices
- Going out to dinner? Have a salad for lunch.
- Add a vegetable instead of pepperoni to your pizza.
- When you have cookies for a snack, have fruit for dessert.
- Had soda with lunch? Have low-fat milk with dinner.

Practice moderation
- Push back from the table before you are stuffed and go for a walk.
- Reduce your portions by using a smaller bowl.
- Skip the seconds or split your restaurant meal with a friend.
- If you eat some extra fries, take some extra steps.

Use iProfile to calculate the Calories in your favorite fast-food meal.

The **iProfile icon** appears with suggestions to help students analyze their own diets and apply the information they are learning to their own everyday food choices.

Debate is an essay that explores both sides of a controversial nutrition topic. Students synthesize the material for greater understanding.

Debate Energy Drinks for Athletic Performance?

The Issue: Energy drinks are sold alongside sports drinks, and manufacturers of these beverages often sponsor athletes and athletic events. Should they be used as ergogenic aids? Is drinking them a safe way to improve your game?

Each debate brings up a relevant issue related to the chapter.

The popularity of energy drinks with names like Red Bull, Monster, and Full Throttle has soared over the past decade. They promise to keep you alert to study, work, drive, party all night, and perhaps excel at your next athletic competition. The main ingredients in these drinks are sugar and caffeine. Glucose is an important fuel for exercise, and caffeine is known to enhance endurance, so these drinks may seem like an ideal ergogenic aid.

A traditional sports drink, like Gatorade, contains about 28 g of sugar in 16 ounces; a typical energy drink provides twice this much (55 to 60 g, or about 14 teaspoons). Since carbohydrate fuels activity, it may seem that the additional sugar would provide energy for prolonged exercise. But more is not always better during activity. The double load of sugar cannot be absorbed quickly, and unabsorbed sugar in the stomach can cause GI distress and also slow fluid absorption.

The caffeine content of energy drinks ranges from 50 to about 500 mg per can or bottle. Caffeine is an effective ergogenic aid that enhances endurance when consumed before or during exercise.[44] But too much caffeine, referred to as *caffeine intoxication*, causes

nervousness, anxiety, restlessness, insomnia, gastrointestinal upset, tremors, increased blood pressure, and rapid heartbeat. A number of cases of caffeine-associated death, seizure, and cardiac arrest have occurred after consumption of energy drinks.[45-47] Even if the caffeine in an energy drink increases endurance, depending on when it is consumed, it can affect timing and coordination and hurt overall performance. Caffeine is also a diuretic; at the levels contained in these drinks, it may contribute to dehydration, particularly in first-time users.[48] The FDA limits the amount of caffeine in soft drinks to 0.02% (about 71 mg in 12 oz), but energy drinks are considered dietary supplements, so the caffeine content is not regulated.

Energy drinks often also contain other ingredients that promise to improve performance, such as B vitamins, taurine, guarana, and ginseng. B vitamins are needed to produce ATP, so they are marketed to enhance energy production from sugar. But unless you are deficient in these vitamins, drinking them in an energy drink will not enhance your ATP production. Taurine is an amino acid that may reduce the amount of muscle damage and improve exercise performance and capacity, but not all research supports these claims.[47] Guarana is an herbal ingredient that contains caffeine as well as small amounts of the stimulants theobromine and theophylline. The extra caffeine from guarana (not included in the caffeine listed for these beverages) may contribute to caffeine toxicity. Ginseng is also claimed to have performance-enhancing effects, but these effects have not been demonstrated scientifically.[46,49] In general, the amounts of these ingredients are too small to have much effect, and the safety of consuming them in combination with caffeine prior to or during exercise has yet to be established.[46]

So should you down an energy drink before your next competition? They do provide a caffeine boost, but is it so much caffeine that you risk dehydration, high blood pressure, and heart problems? Energy drinks provide sugar to fuel activity, but will they upset your stomach? What about the herbal ingredients—do they offer a benefit you are looking for?

Think critically: Use the table below to assess the advantages and disadvantages of consuming an 8-oz can of Red Bull versus a 12-oz can of Coca-Cola Classic before your 30-minute run.

Think Critically questions at the end of each debate ask students to integrate and evaluate the information presented.

Caffeine content				
Beverage	Serving (fluid ounces)	Caffeine (mg)	Sugar (g)	Energy (calories)
Coffee	8	100–200	0	0
Espresso with sugar	1.5	100	15–30	60–120
Coca-Cola Classic	12	35	39	140
Mountain Dew	12	54	46	170
Monster	16	160	54	200
Jolt Cola	8	80	30	120
Arizona Caution Extreme Energy Shot	8	100	33	130
Red Bull	8	80	28	110
Rockstar	16	160	62	280
Monster	8	80	27	100
Full Throttle	16	160	57	220

Tables, graphs, and photos focus student attention and add additional information and are often the focus of think critically questions.

NATIONAL GEOGRAPHIC **Video** See this in your Wiley*PLUS* course.

A rich collection of videos from a variety of sources, including **National Geographic videos** from their award-winning collection, help students think critically and solve real-life nutrition problems. Each video is linked to the text, and questions allow students to solve problems online. Videos are also available as lecture launcher PowerPoint presentations designed for in-class viewing and can be easily integrated into existing presentations.

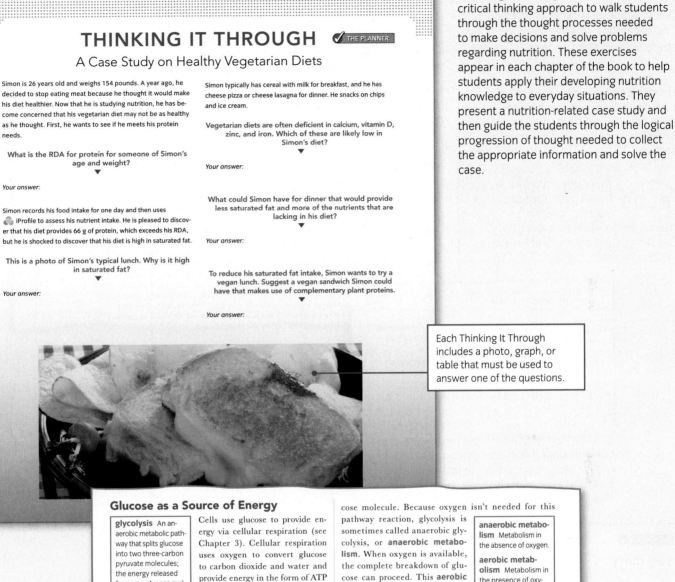

THINKING IT THROUGH ✓ THE PLANNER

A Case Study on Healthy Vegetarian Diets

Simon is 26 years old and weighs 154 pounds. A year ago, he decided to stop eating meat because he thought it would make his diet healthier. Now that he is studying nutrition, he has become concerned that his vegetarian diet may not be as healthy as he thought. First, he wants to see if he meets his protein needs.

What is the RDA for protein for someone of Simon's age and weight?
▼

Your answer:

Simon records his food intake for one day and then uses 🌐 iProfile to assess his nutrient intake. He is pleased to discover that his diet provides 66 g of protein, which exceeds his RDA, but he is shocked to discover that his diet is high in saturated fat.

This is a photo of Simon's typical lunch. Why is it high in saturated fat?
▼

Your answer:

Simon typically has cereal with milk for breakfast, and he has cheese pizza or cheese lasagna for dinner. He snacks on chips and ice cream.

Vegetarian diets are often deficient in calcium, vitamin D, zinc, and iron. Which of these are likely low in Simon's diet?
▼

Your answer:

What could Simon have for dinner that would provide less saturated fat and more of the nutrients that are lacking in his diet?
▼

Your answer:

To reduce his saturated fat intake, Simon wants to try a vegan lunch. Suggest a vegan sandwich Simon could have that makes use of complementary plant proteins.
▼

Your answer:

Thinking It Through exercises use a critical thinking approach to walk students through the thought processes needed to make decisions and solve problems regarding nutrition. These exercises appear in each chapter of the book to help students apply their developing nutrition knowledge to everyday situations. They present a nutrition-related case study and then guide the students through the logical progression of thought needed to collect the appropriate information and solve the case.

Each Thinking It Through includes a photo, graph, or table that must be used to answer one of the questions.

Glucose as a Source of Energy

glycolysis An anaerobic metabolic pathway that splits glucose into two three-carbon pyruvate molecules; the energy released from one glucose molecule is used to make two molecules of ATP.

Cells use glucose to provide energy via cellular respiration (see Chapter 3). Cellular respiration uses oxygen to convert glucose to carbon dioxide and water and provide energy in the form of ATP (**Figure 4.11**).

The first step in cellular respiration is **glycolysis** (*glyco* = "glucose," *lysis* = "to break down"). Glycolysis can rapidly produce two molecules of ATP from each glucose molecule. Because oxygen isn't needed for this pathway reaction, glycolysis is sometimes called anaerobic glycolysis, or **anaerobic metabolism**. When oxygen is available, the complete breakdown of glucose can proceed. This **aerobic metabolism** produces about 36 molecules of ATP for each glucose molecule, 18 times more ATP than is generated by anaerobic glycolysis.

anaerobic metabolism Metabolism in the absence of oxygen.

aerobic metabolism Metabolism in the presence of oxygen. It can completely break down glucose to yield carbon dioxide, water, and energy in the form of ATP.

Margin Gossary Terms (in green boldface) define important terms in each chapter. Other important terms appear in **black boldface** and are defined in the text.

Student understanding is assessed at different levels

Wiley Visualizing with *WileyPLUS* offers students lots of practice material for assessing their understanding of each study objective. Students know exactly what they are getting out of each study session through immediate feedback and coaching.

Learning Objectives at the start of each section indicate in behavioral terms the concepts that students are expected to master while reading the section.

 Every content resource is related to a specific learning objective so that students will easily discover relevant content organized in a more meaningful way.

Carbohydrates in Our Food

LEARNING OBJECTIVES

1. **Distinguish** refined carbohydrates from unrefined carbohydrates.
2. **Compare** whole grains to enriched grains.
3. **Explain** how added refined sugars and naturally occurring sugars differ from each other.

Our hunter-gatherer ancestors ate very differently from the way we eat. Their diet consisted almost entirely of **unrefined foods**—foods eaten either just as they are found in nature or with only minimal processing, such as cooking. Today we still consume some unrefined sources of carbohydrate, but many of the foods we consume are made with refined grains and contain

refined Refers to foods that have gone processing

foods high in refined carbohydrates, such as candies, cookies, and sweetened beverages.

What Is a Whole Grain?

When you eat a bowl of oatmeal or a slice of whole-wheat toast, you are consuming a **whole-grain product**. Whole-grain products include the entire kernel of the grain: the **germ**, the **bran**, and the **endosperm** (Figure 4.2a). Refined grain products, such as white bread, include just the endosperm. The bran and germ are discarded during refining, and along with them the fiber and some vitamins and minerals are lost. To make up some of these losses, refined grains sold in the United States are required to be enriched. **Enrichment**, which is a type of **fortification**, adds back some, but not all, of the nutrients lost in processing (Figure 4.2)

enrichment The addition of specific amounts of thiamin, riboflavin, niacin, and iron to refined grains. Since 1998, folic acid has also been added to enriched grains.

fortification The

CONCEPT CHECK STOP

1. **What** is the difference between a whole-grain product and a product made with a refined grain?

2. **How** do the nutrients in enriched grains compare to those in whole grains?

3. **Why** are foods high in added refined sugars said to contribute empty calories?

Concept Check questions at the end of each section allow students to test their comprehension of the learning objectives.

 At the end of each learning objective module, students can assess their progress with independent practice opportunities and quizzes. This feature gives them the ability to gauge their comprehension and grasp of the material. Practice tests and quizzes help students self-monitor and prepare for graded course assessments

---

THE PLANNER ✓

Summary

1 Proteins in Our Food 168

• Dietary protein comes from both animal and plant sources. Animal sources of protein are generally good sources of iron, zinc, and calcium but are high in saturated fat and cholesterol. Plant sources of protein, such as the nuts, peas, and beans shown in the photo, are higher in unsaturated fat, fiber, and phytochemicals.

Plant proteins • Figure 6.1b

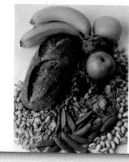

2 The Structure of Amino Acids and Proteins 169

• **Amino acids** are the building blocks from which proteins are made. Each amino acid contains an amino group, an acid group, and a unique side chain. The amino acids that the body is unable to make in sufficient amounts are called **essential amino acids** and must be consumed in the diet.

• Proteins are made by linking amino acids by **peptide bonds**, as shown here, to form **polypeptides**. Polypeptide chains fold to create unique three-dimensional protein structures. The shape of a protein determines its function.

Amino acid and protein structure • Figure 6.2c

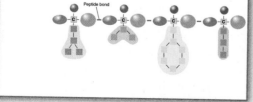

The **Summary** revisits each major section, with informative images taken from the chapter. These visuals reinforce important elements. The glossary terms are featured here, in boldface, and are also included in the alphabetical **KEY TERMS** list. Students are thus able to study vocabulary words in the context of related concepts.

Online Resources

- For more information on diabetes, go to http://diabetes.niddk.nih.gov.

- For more information on how beverages affect our calorie intake, go to www.cdc.gov/healthyweight/healthy_eating/drinks.html.

- For more information on choosing whole grains, go to www.mayoclinic.com/health/whole-grains/NU00204.

- For more information on the 2010 Dietary Guidelines, go to www.health.gov/dietaryguidelines/.

- Visit your *WileyPLUS* site for videos, animations, podcasts, self-study, and other media that will aid you in studying and understanding this chapter.

Online Resources highlight a few relevant Web sites where students can go to get additional information on topics covered in the chapter.

Critical and Creative Thinking Questions challenge students to think more broadly about chapter concepts. The level of these questions ranges from simple to advanced; they encourage students to think critically and develop an analytical understanding of the nutrition concepts discussed in the chapter. Some of these exercises feature clinical applications and therefore also help reinforce the importance of nutrition in health promotion and disease prevention. Some of these can be done as collaborative learning exercises that encourage students to work together and learn from each other to solve a problem.

Critical and Creative Thinking Questions

1. Record everything you eat for three days. Use iProfile to calculate your fiber intake. How does it compare with the recommendations? How could you increase your fiber intake?

2. For each high-carbohydrate food on your food record, indicate whether it is refined or unrefined. Suggest some changes that would increase your intake of unrefined carbohydrates. List some foods in your diet that are high in added sugars. Suggest some changes that would reduce your intake of these sugars.

3. Adam is 19 and plays basketball. Recently, he has been thirsty all the time, and he needs to get up several times a night to urinate. He has lost 10 pounds and is so tired that he has been missing basketball practice. What type of diabetes is most likely affecting Adam? How does it need to be managed? Why is it important to keep blood sugar levels within the normal range in both type 1 and type 2 diabetes?

4. Are carbohydrates good for you? Explain why or why not.

5. Imagine that you have gained 20 pounds over the past 5 years, and you decide to use a low-carbohydrate diet to return to a healthy weight. You are happy with your initial weight loss but begin to have headaches and bad breath. What is causing these symptoms, and why?

6. This is the label from a hot breakfast cereal. How much fiber and sugars does it provide? Is it a whole-grain product? What does this label tell you about the amount of added sugar it contains? Would you recommend this product to a friend? Why or why not?

Nutrition Facts
Serving Size 1 packet (43g)
Servings Per Container 10

Amount Per Serving	Cereal
Calories	160
Calories from Fat	15

	% Daily Value**
Total Fat 1.5g	2%
Saturated Fat 0g	0%
Trans Fat 0g	
Cholesterol 0mg	0%
Sodium 230mg	10%
Total Carbohydrate 33g	11%
Dietary Fiber 3g	12%
Soluble Fiber 1g	
Sugars 13g	
Protein 4g	

INGREDIENTS: WHOLE GRAIN ROLLED OATS (WITH OAT BRAN), SUGAR, SALT, NATURAL AND ARTIFICIAL FLAVORS, CALCIUM CARBONATE (A SOURCE OF CALCIUM), GUAR GUM, CARAMEL COLOR, VITAMIN A PALMITATE, NIACINAMIDE*, REDUCED IRON, PYRIDOXINE HYDROCHLORIDE*, RIBOFLAVIN*, THIAMIN MONONITRATE*, FOLIC ACID*. *ONE OF THE B VITAMINS.

WILEY PLUS Students can explore module topics further with customizable question sets that put the learning path in the hands of the instructor and student, promoting greater retention. The *WileyPLUS* Gradebook provides instant access to reports on trends in class performance, student use of course materials, and progress toward learning objectives. Class section results can also be seen in graph form, making it easy to see how an individual is progressing in comparison to the rest of the class section. Students can also see their own progress instantly for each assignment listed according to the built-in calendar.

What is happening in this picture?

These children, who live in Russia, are being exposed to UV radiation to prevent vitamin D deficiency.

Think Critically

1. Why does this treatment help them meet their need for vitamin D?
2. Why are children in Russia at risk for vitamin D deficiency?
3. What else could be done to ensure that they get adequate amounts of vitamin D?

What is happening in this picture? presents an uncaptioned photograph, relevant to a chapter topic, and illustrates a situation students are not likely to have encountered previously. The photograph is paired with Think Critically questions that ask the students to analyze and interpret what they can observe in the photo based on what they have learned.

Visual end-of-chapter **Self-Tests** pose questions that ask students to demonstrate their understanding of key concepts. The inclusion of graphs, diagrams, and other images taken from the text, encourage students to actively and visually engage with the material.

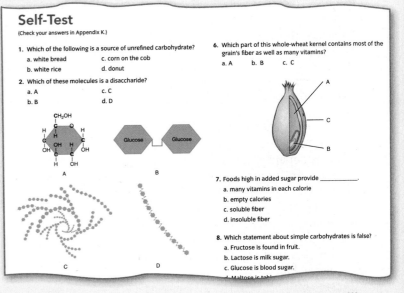

Self-Test

(Check your answers in Appendix K.)

1. Which of the following is a source of unrefined carbohydrate?
   a. white bread
   b. white rice
   c. corn on the cob
   d. donut

2. Which of these molecules is a disaccharide?
   a. A
   b. B
   c. C
   d. D

6. Which part of this whole-wheat kernel contains most of the grain's fiber as well as many vitamins?
   a. A
   b. B
   c. C

7. Foods high in added sugar provide _____.
   a. many vitamins in each calorie
   b. empty calories
   c. soluble fiber
   d. insoluble fiber

8. Which statement about simple carbohydrates is false?
   a. Fructose is found in fruit.
   b. Lactose is milk sugar.
   c. Glucose is blood sugar.
   d. Maltose is table...

Why Visualizing Nutrition?

What is the organization of this book?

Visualizing Nutrition: Everyday Choices, 2e provides the rigor needed in the study of science while integrating photography and illustrations into the learning process. Information that would be buried in the text of other books is presented within the context of colorful illustrations and vibrant photographs. The images grab students' attention and, along with the text, tell the absorbing story of nutrition. The text captures the interest of college students from every background and engages them by demonstrating the applications of the science of nutrition to everyday choices.

This book is intended to serve as an introductory text for undergraduate students. The accessible format of *Visualizing Nutrition: Everyday Choices, 2e*, which assumes that readers have little prior knowledge of nutrition, allows students to easily make the connection between their individual experience with food and nutrition concepts and the science of nutrition. The text uses a critical thinking approach to teaching human nutrition, bringing nutrition out of the classroom by asking students to apply the logic of science to their own nutrition concerns. *Visualizing Nutrition: Everyday Choices, 2e* educates students about the functions and sources of individual nutrients and also focuses on the total diet, so students understand that no one food choice determines the healthfulness of their overall dietary pattern. The examples and exercises throughout the book allow students to think critically while exploring the similarities and differences in the diets and health concerns of the diverse ethnic and cultural mix of the population of the United States and the rest of the world. The text presents information using a clear, concise writing style and addresses the most recent advances in nutrition science. Each chapter extensively references the most current literature. In addition to supplying unique photographs, the National Geographic Society has performed the invaluable service of fact-checking *Visualizing Nutrition: Everyday Choices, 2e*. They have verified every fact in the book with two outside sources, to ensure that the text is accurate and up-to-date.

Visualizing Nutrition: Everyday Choices, 2e is unique in its integrated approach to the presentation of nutrition science. While the chapter organization follows the traditional format of nutrition books, this book integrates metabolism and health and disease information throughout the text. To make the study of metabolism more accessible, *Visualizing Nutrition: Everyday Choices, 2e* provides a simple overview of metabolism in Chapter 3 and then builds on this base with more complex discussions in subsequent chapters. In Chapter 4, the discussion of carbohydrate metabolism presents the basics of intermediary metabolism. Chapters 5 through 10, which cover lipids, proteins, micronutrients, energy balance, and exercise, review and add to this information. The integration throughout the text of discussions of nutrition, health, and disease serves to consistently engage student interest. By incorporating this information, students can see that a nutrient's function in metabolism is related to its role in health and disease. This integration continuously reinforces the applicability of nutrition science to students' lives and helps them appreciate how and why their food choices affect their health.

- The first two chapters of this book introduce nutrition science. **Chapter 1, "Nutrition: Everyday Choices,"** begins by discussing the U.S. diet—how it has changed and how healthy it is—and emphasizing the fact that food choices affect current and future health. This chapter provides an overview of the nutrients and their roles in the body and defines the basic principles of balance, variety, and moderation that are key to a healthy diet. It also introduces the scientific method and the steps students need to follow to sort accurate from inaccurate nutrition information. **Chapter 2, "Guidelines for a Healthy Diet,"** begins with a history of nutrition recommendations and a discussion of how valuable these recommendations are for assessing the nutritional health of populations and individuals. It then takes the science out of the laboratory and shows how advances in nutrition knowledge have been used to develop the Dietary Reference Intakes (DRIs), the 2010 *Dietary Guidelines for Americans*, and tools for diet planning, including the new 2011 MyPlate food guidance system, food labels, and exchange lists.

- **Chapter 3, "Digestion: From Meals to Molecules,"** provides the background students need to understand how nutrients are used by their bodies. It discusses how food is digested, how nutrients from foods are absorbed into the body and transported to the cells where metabolism occurs, and how wastes are removed. This chapter provides an overview of metabolism that serves as a launching pad for the more in-depth metabolism information presented in subsequent chapters.

- Chapters 4, 5, and 6 feature the energy-yielding nutrients carbohydrates, lipids, and proteins. Each of these chapters begins with a discussion of the respective macronutrient in the food we eat. The body of each chapter then illustrates the digestion and absorption of these nutrients, their functions, and the impact of each on health and particular disease states. Each chapter ends with a discussion of how to choose a diet that meets recommendations. Emphasis is placed on the types and proportions of these nutrients that are optimal for health. **Chapter 4, "Carbohydrates: Sugars, Starches, and Fibers,"** discusses the health impact of refined grains and added sugar versus whole grains and foods that naturally contain sugars. **Chapter 5, "Lipids: Fats, Phospholipids, and Sterols,"** points out that Americans are not eating too much fat but are often choosing the wrong types of fat for a healthy diet. **Chapter 6, "Proteins and Amino Acids,"** discusses animal and plant sources of protein and points out that both can meet protein needs, but these protein sources contain different combinations of nutrients. In addition to discussing how to meet protein needs, this chapter includes information on how to plan a healthy vegetarian diet.

- The next two chapters present the micronutrients and water. **Chapter 7, "Vitamins,"** begins with a general overview of vitamins: where vitamins are found in the diet, factors affecting their bioavailability, and how they function. The chapter then discusses each of the vitamins individually, providing information on sources in the diet, functions in the body, impact on health, recommended intakes, and potential for toxicity. The chapter ends with a discussion of dietary supplements, who might benefit from using them, and risks associated with their use. **Chapter 8, "Water and Minerals,"** addresses water, a nutrient often overlooked, and the major and trace minerals. The chapter presents information on the sources of these nutrients in the diet and discusses their functions in the body, relationships to health and disease, and recommended intakes. A discussion of hypertension illustrates the importance of certain minerals in blood pressure regulation and the impact of the total diet on healthy blood pressure. A discussion of nutrients and bone health includes a section on the relationship between nutrition and the development of osteoporosis. Sections on trace minerals engage students with discussions of health concerns related to both deficiencies and excesses.

- **Chapter 9, "Energy Balance and Weight Management,"** begins with a discussion of the obesity epidemic and the effect of excess body fat on health. The chapter explains energy balance, illustrates the impact of small changes in diet and behavior on long-term weight management, and presents up-to-date information on how body weight is regulated and the role of genetic versus lifestyle factors in determining body fatness. The chapter includes recommendations for healthy body weight and composition and equations for determining energy needs. It also discusses weight-loss options that range from simple energy restriction to potentially risky surgical approaches. The chapter ends with a comprehensive discussion of eating disorders and their causes, consequences, and treatment.

- **Chapter 10, "Nutrition, Fitness, and Physical Activity,"** discusses the relationships among physical activity, nutrition, and health and includes the most up-to-date activity recommendations including those from the 2010 Dietary Guidelines. It emphasizes the importance of exercise for health maintenance as well as the impact nutrition can have on exercise performance. Because nutrients fuel activity, this chapter serves as a review of metabolism. By this point in the text, students have studied all the essential nutrients, so this chapter includes a discussion of the macronutrients and micronutrients needed for ATP production. A discussion of ergogenic aids for competitive athletes directs students to do a risk–benefit analysis of these products before deciding whether to use them.

- **Chapter 11, "Nutrition During Pregnancy and Infancy,"** addresses the role of nutrition in human development and discusses the nutritional needs of women during pregnancy and lactation as well as the nutritional needs of infants. The chapter also discusses the benefits and risks of breast versus bottle feeding.

- **Chapter 12, "Nutrition from 1 to 100,"** travels through the life cycle, discussing the energy and nutrient needs of growing children, adolescents, adults, and older adults. The chapter discusses the importance of learning healthy eating habits early in life, particularly in relation to the rising rates of obesity and other chronic diseases in today's youth. The chapter then addresses how nutrition affects aging and how aging affects nutrition. It presents the interrelationships between aging and nutritional status and the impact medications and chronic disease can have on nutritional status. The chapter ends with a discussion of alcohol: how it affects metabolism and impacts health at all stages of life.

- **Chapter 13, "How Safe Is Our Food Supply?"** discusses the risks and benefits associated with the U.S. food supply and includes information on the impact of microbial hazards, chemical toxins, food additives, irradiation, and food packaging. It addresses the directives of the Food Safety Initiative and the Food Safety Modernization Act, including the use of HACCP (Hazard Analysis Critical Control Point) to ensure safe food and advances in technology that help identify the sources of food-borne illness. The chapter ends with a discussion of biotechnology, including an explanation of how plants are genetically modified and the potential benefits and risks associated with this expanding technology.

- **Chapter 14, "Feeding the World,"** discusses the coexistence of hunger and malnutrition along with obesity in both developed and developing nations. It examines the causes of world hunger and potential solutions that can affect the amounts and types of food that are available.

New To This Edition

This second edition of *Visualizing Nutrition: Everyday Choices* includes the most recent nutrition recommendations, some new features, and improved illustrations and critical thinking pedagogy.

- Dietary Guidelines for Americans 2010: The new recommendations of the 2010 Dietary Guidelines have been described in Chapter 2 and addressed in all applicable subsequent chapters.

- MyPlate: The USDAs new 2011 guide to making healthy food choices is introduced in Chapter 2. Illustrations and discussions of the MyPlate recommendations and how to apply them are included in chapters throughout the book.

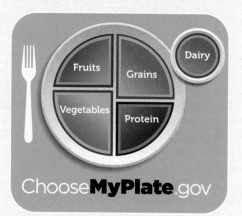

- Updated 2011 Dietary Reference Intake values for vitamin D and calcium: These are introduced in Chapters 7 and 8 and applied where applicable in the chapters where recommendations for infants, children, teens, and older adults are addressed.

- Debate: This new feature helps students understand that there are not always clear answers to nutrition questions and allows them to see both sides of controversial topics and think critically about these issues. Debates address topics such as "How involved should the government be in your food choices?", "Should you be gluten free?", "Should you avoid high-fructose corn syrup?", and "Is surgery a good solution to obesity?".

- Improved layout and labeling of illustrations: In this new edition the authors rethought the layout, labels, arrow placement, and font size of many of the illustrations to make them easier to understand and more informative.

- New visuals with Critical and Creative Thinking Questions: Graphs, charts, and illustrations have been included with Critical and Creative Thinking Questions, adding a visual component to the thought processes.

- Thinking it Through: These critical thinking case studies use a logical step by step progression of information and questions to help students think through nutrition problems. Topics include Using Food Labels to Make Healthy Choices, Improving Heart Health, and Genetics, Lifestyle, and Body Weight.

- Online Resources: This end of chapter feature provides students with a few reliable Web sites that they can visit to find additional information relevant to the chapter.

- New Pedagogy: The following types of questions appear with visuals throughout the book and answers are provided at the end of the book:

- Ask Yourself: These fill-in, multiple-choice, or short answer closed-ended questions require students to answer, focusing on the visual itself and are meant to make sure students understand the concept presented in the visual.

- Think Critically: These thought-provoking questions ask students to apply what they have learned in order to interpret, explain, or think beyond what they observe in the image. Think critically questions are always included with What A Scientist Sees, Debates, and What is Happening In this Picture?

- Interpreting Data: These fill-in, multiple-choice, or short answer closed-ended questions ask students to reach conclusions based on data in the figures they are studying.

How Does Wiley Visualizing Support Instructors?

Wiley Visualizing Site

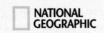

The Wiley Visualizing site hosts a wealth of information for instructors using Wiley Visualizing, including ways to maximize the visual approach in the classroom and a white paper titled "How Visuals Can Help Students Learn," by Matt Leavitt, instructional design consultant. Visit Wiley Visualizing at www.wiley.com/college/visualizing.

Wiley Custom Select

Wiley Custom Select gives you the freedom to build your course materials exactly the way you want them, offering your students a cost-efficient alternative to traditional texts. In a simple three-step process create a solution containing the content you want, in the sequence you want, delivered how you want. Visit Wiley Custom Select at http://customselect.wiley.com.

PowerPoint Presentations

(available in *WileyPLUS* and on the book companion site)

A complete set of highly visual PowerPoint presentations—one per chapter—by Cheryl Neudauer, Minneapolis Community and Technical College, is available online and in WileyPLUS to enhance classroom presentations. Tailored to the text's topical coverage and learning objectives, these presentations are designed to convey key text concepts, illustrated by embedded text art. Lecture Launcher PowerPoints also offer embedded links to videos to help introduce classroom discussions with short, engaging video clips.

Test Bank

(available in *WileyPLUS* and on the book companion site)

The visuals from the textbook are also included in the Test Bank by Melanie Burns, Eastern Illinois University. The Test Bank has approximately 75 test items, many of which incorporate visuals from the book. The test items include multiple-choice and essay questions testing a variety of comprehension levels. The test bank is available online in MS Word files, as a Computerized Test Bank, and within *WileyPLUS*. The easy-to-use test-generation program fully supports graphics, print tests, student answer sheets, and answer keys. The software's advanced features allow you to produce an exam to your exact specifications.

Instructor's Manual

(available in *WileyPLUS* and on the book companion site)

The Instructor's Manual includes creative ideas for in-class activities.

Guidance is also provided on how to maximize the effectiveness of visuals in the classroom.

1. **Use visuals during class discussions or presentations.** Point out important information as the students look at the visuals, to help them integrate separate visual and verbal mental models.
2. **Use visuals for assignments and to assess learning.** For example, learners could be asked to identify samples of concepts portrayed in visuals.
3. **Use visuals to encourage group activities.** Students can study together, make sense of, discuss, hypothesize, or make decisions about the content. Students can work together to interpret and describe a visual or use the visual to solve problems and conduct related research.
4. **Use visuals during reviews**. Students can review key vocabulary, concepts, principles, processes, and relationships displayed visually. This recall helps link prior knowledge to new information in working memory, building integrated mental models.
5. **Use visuals for assignments and to assess learning.** For example, learners could be asked to identify samples of concepts portrayed in visuals.
6. **Use visuals to apply facts or concepts to realistic situations or examples**. For example, a familiar image, such as a hungry child with a bloated belly, can illustrate key information about the nutritional impact of famine, linking this new concept to prior knowledge.

Nutrition Visual Library

All photographs, figures, maps, and other visuals from the text are online and in WileyPLUS and can be used as you wish in the classroom. These online electronic files allow you to easily incorporate images into your PowerPoint presentations as you choose, or to create your own handouts.

Book Companion Site

All instructor resources (the Test Bank, Instructor's Manual, PowerPoint presentations, and all textbook illustrations and photos in jpeg format) are housed on the book companion site (www.wiley.com/college/grosvenor). Student resources include self quizzes and flashcards.

Wiley Faculty Network

The Wiley Faculty Network (WFN) is a global community of faculty, connected by a passion for teaching and a drive to learn, share, and collaborate. Their mission is to promote the effective use of technology and enrich the teaching experience. Connect with the Wiley Faculty Network to collaborate with your colleagues, find a mentor, attend virtual and live events, and view a wealth of resources all designed to help you grow as an educator. Visit the Wiley Faculty Network at www.wherefacultyconnect.com.

How Has Wiley Visualizing Been Shaped by Contributors?

Wiley Visualizing and the *WileyPLUS* learning environment would not have come about without lots of people, each of whom played a part in sharing their research and contributing to this new approach.

Academic Research Consultants

Richard Mayer, Professor of Psychology, UC Santa Barbara. His Cognitive Theory of Multimedia Learning provided the basis on which we designed our program. He continues to provide guidance to our author and editorial teams on how to develop and implement strong, pedagogically effective visuals and use them in the classroom.

Jan L. Plass, Professor of Educational Communication and Technology in the Steinhardt School of Culture, Education, and Human Development at New York University. He co-directs the NYU Games for Learning Institute and is the founding director of the CREATE Consortium for Research and Evaluation of Advanced Technology in Education.

Matthew Leavitt, Instructional Design Consultant, advises the Wiley Visualizing team on the effective design and use of visuals in instruction and has made virtual and live presentations to university faculty around the country regarding effective design and use of instructional visuals.

Independent Research Studies

SEG Research, an independent research and assessment firm, conducted a national, multisite effectiveness study of students enrolled in entry-level college courses. The study was designed to evaluate the effectiveness of Wiley Visualizing. You can view the full research paper at www.wiley.com/college/visualizing/huffman/efficacy.html.

Instructor and Student Contributions

Throughout the process of developing the concept of guided visual pedagogy for Wiley Visualizing, we benefited from the comments and constructive criticism provided by the instructors and colleagues listed below. We offer our sincere appreciation to these individuals for their helpful reviews and general feedback:

Wiley Visualizing Reviewers, Focus Group Participants, and Survey Respondents

Melinda Anderson, Tennessee Tech University
Tracy Bonoffski, University of North Carolina
Dale Brigham, University of Missouri
Tracey Brigman, University of Georgia
Linda Brothers, Indiana University- Purdue University Indianapolis
Erin Caudill, Southeast Community College
Melissa Chabot, University at Buffalo
Wen-Hsing Cheng, University of Maryland
Anne Cioffi, Hudson Valley Community College
James Collins, University of Florida
Jill Comess, Norfolk State University
Danielle Gandolpho, Delgado Community College
Barbara Goldman, Palm Beach State College
Aleida Gordon, California State Polytechnic University, Pomona
Margaret Gunther, Palomar Community College
Melissa Gutschall, Radford University
Cindy Handley, Seward Community College
Charlene Harkins, University of Minnesota
Judy Kaufman, Monroe Community College
Youjin Kim, Florida State University
Betty Kenyon, Western Nebraska Community College

Sarah Leupen, University of Maryland
Darlene Levinson, Oakland Community College
Lourdes Lore, Henry Ford Community College
Sharon Lytle, Carl Sandburg College
Mara Manis, Hillsborough Community College
Shireen Merrill, Pensacola State College
Elaine Mostow, Bergen Community College
Owen Murphy, University of Colorado
Deborah Murray, Ohio University
Cheryl Neudauer, Minneapolis Community and Technical College
Steven Nizielski, Grand Valley State University
Susan O'Neill-Cook, Ferris State University
Anna Page, Johnson County Community College
John Perozich, Franciscan University of Steubenville
Anne Rogan, State University of New York- Cobleskill
Janice Rueda, Wayne State University
Susan Shaw, Los Angeles Mission College
Jamie Sheppard, Highline Community College
Ingrid Skoog, Oregon State University
Priya Venkatesan, Pasadena City College
Cindy Waters, Upper Iowa University

Students and Class Testers

To make certain that Visualizing Nutrition Second Edition met the needs of current students, we asked several instructors to class-test a chapter. The feedback that we received from students and instructors confirmed our belief that the Visualizing approach taken in this book is highly effective in helping students to learn. We wish to thank the following instructors and their students who provided us with helpful feedback and suggestions:

Anne Alexander, Radford University
Charalee Allen, Cincinnati State Technical Community College
Karen Arbuckle, Cossatot Community College of the University of Arkansas
Cathy Armacost, Spokane Community College
Garry Auld, Colorado State University
Kathy Beberniss, Missouri State University
Marian Benz, Milwaukee Area Technical College
Jennifer Bess, Hillsborough Community College
Judah Boulet, Merrimack College
Brenda Bertrand, East Carolina University
Dale Brigham, University of Missouri, Columbia
Tracey Brigman, University of Georgia
Linda Brothers, Indiana University- Purdue University Indianapolis
Kenneth Broughton, University of Wyoming
Lora Brown, Brigham Young University, Provo
Jay Burgess, Purdue University
Ricarda Cerda, Fresno City College
Susan Chou, American River College
Janet Colson, Middle Tennessee State University
Harlan Dean, University of Massachusetts, Boston
Nancy DiMarco, Texas Woman's University, Denton
Juliet D'Souza, Highland Community College
Sara Ducey, Montgomery College, Rockville
Jim Egeberg, Inver Hills Community College
Heather Payne Emerson, Murray State University
Candace Fox, Mount Vernon Nazarene University
Bernard Frye, University of Texas, Arlington
Karen Gabrielsen, Everett Community College
Stephanie Gall, Avista Hospital

Aleida Gordon, California State Polytechnic University, Pomona
Andrea Grim, Idaho State University
Charlene Harkins, University of Minnesota, Duluth
Tersea Heisey, Lehigh Carbon Community College
Beckee Hobson, College of the Sequoias
Dave Holben, Ohio University
Laura Horn, Cincinnati State Technical Community College
Owen Kelly, Texas Woman's University, Denton
Elizabeth Ann Kenyon, Western Nebraska Community College
Sarah Leupen, University of Maryland Baltimore County
Jana Kicklighter, Georgia State University
Mara Manis, Hillsborough Community College
Dorothy Chen Maynard, California State University, San Bernardino
Lisa Moran, Jefferson Community and Technical College
Holly Morris, Lehigh Carbon Community College
Deborah Murray, Ohio University
Lia Nightingale, Palmer College of Chiropractic
Steve Nizielski, Grand Valley State University
Milli Owens, College of the Sequoias
Peter Pribis, Andrews University
Beth Rice, Murray State University
Heather Rothenberg, Mission College
Louise Schneider, Loma Linda University
Leigh Sears, Hope College
Susan Shaw, Los Angeles Mission College
Sarah Short, Syracuse University
Terry Shaw, Austin Community College
Crystal Sims, Cossatot Community College of the University of Arkansas
Laura Taylor, University of Wisconsin, Milwaukee
Kathy Timmons, Murray State University
Allisha Weeden, Idaho State University
Donna Pauline Williams, Brigham Young University, Provo
Brenda Wingard-Haynes, Milwaukee Area Technical College
Cynthia Wright, Southern Utah University
Linda Wright, Dixie State College of Utah
Linda Wright, University of Wisconsin, Milwaukee
Lisa Zucker, Front Range Community College

Special Thanks

Special thanks to Peter Ambrose for providing a fresh eye by writing the chapter introductions for this project. We appreciate his "non-nutritionist" view of the science we know too well. His ability to help us organize and articulate our thoughts throughout the text is greatly appreciated.

Our appreciation goes to the professors who have written quizzes for the *WileyPLUS* course: Jeremy Akers, James Madison University, Melanie Burns, Eastern Illinois University, Charlene Harkins, University of Minnesota-Duluth, Judy Kaufman, Monroe Community College, Holly Morris, Lehigh Carbon Community College, Cheryl Neudauer, Minneapolis Community and Technical College, Cindy Wright, Southern Utah University, and Priya Venkatesan, Pasadena City College.

Sincere thanks also to Elizabeth Quintana, West Virginia University, who helped us develop the MyPlate Interactivity.

We are extremely grateful to the many members of the editorial and production staff at John Wiley and Sons who guided us through the challenging steps of developing this book. Their tireless enthusiasm, professional assistance, and endless patience smoothed the path as we found our way. We thank in particular Executive Editor Bonnie Roesch, who expertly launched and directed our process; Editor Kevin Witt, took up the mantle and lent us his unflagging support and tireless effort to ensure the book's success; and Micheline Frederick, Senior Production Manager, who stepped in whenever we needed expert advice. Our sincere thanks also go to Kaye Pace, Vice President and Executive Publisher, who oversaw the entire project; Clay Stone, Executive Marketing Managers, who, together with Christine Kushner adeptly represent the Visualizing imprint. We appreciate the expertise of Hilary Newman, Photo Research Department Manager, in managing and researching our photo program; and of Sandra Rigby, Senior Illustration Editor, for her creativity and management of the extensive illustration program. We also wish to thank those who worked on the wide assortment of media resources: Senior Media Editor Linda Muriello and Media Specialist Svetlana Barskaya. We are grateful to Christina Picciano, editorial assistant, Helen McInnis, editor, and Lauren Morris Content Editor, for helping to bring this project to fruition. And last but not least to Project Editor, Lorraina Raccuia, for her continuous and tireless support through all aspects of developing and writing this text and its ancillary materials.

Next, we would like to offer our thanks to Furino Production—particularly Jeanine Furino, whose dedication and desire for perfection can be seen throughout this book. The careful and professional approach of Jeanine and her staff was critical to the successful production of this edition.

We thank Stacey Gold and Mimi Dornack, research editors and account executives as the National Geographic Society photos.

We thank Richard Easby, Supervising Editor, National Geographic School Division and his team of fact-checkers and proofreaders. We appreciate their contributions and support.

Nutrition Advisory Board

About the Authors

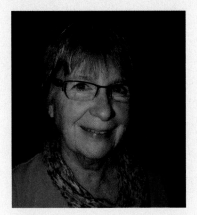

Mary B. Grosvenor holds a bachelor of arts in English and a master of science in Nutrition Science, affording her an ideal background for nutrition writing. She is a registered dietitian and has worked in clinical as well as research nutrition, in hospitals and communities large and small in the western United States. She teaches at the community college level and has published articles in peer-reviewed journals in nutritional assessment and nutrition and cancer. Her training and experience provide practical insights into the application and presentation of the science in this text.

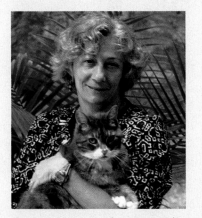

Lori A. Smolin received a bachelor of science degree from Cornell University, where she studied human nutrition and food science. She received a doctorate from the University of Wisconsin at Madison, where her doctoral research focused on B vitamins, homocysteine accumulation, and genetic defects in homocysteine metabolism. She completed postdoctoral training both at the Harbor–UCLA Medical Center, where she studied human obesity, and at the University of California—San Diego, where she studied genetic defects in amino acid metabolism. She has published articles in these areas in peer-reviewed journals. Dr. Smolin is currently at the University of Connecticut, where she has taught both in the Department of Nutritional Science and in the Department of Molecular and Cell Biology. Courses she has taught include introductory nutrition, life cycle nutrition, food preparation, nutritional biochemistry, general biochemistry, and introductory biology.

Dedication

To my sons, David and John, and my husband, Peter. In the beginning, their contribution was support and patience with my long hours but over the years it has grown to include editing and writing as well. Thanks for keeping my projects, and me, on track.

(from Mary Grosvenor)

To my sons, Zachary and Max, who have grown up along with my textbooks, helping me to keep a healthy perspective on the important things in life. To my husband, David, who has continuously provided his love and support and is always there to assist with the computer and technological issues that arise when writing in the electronic age.

(from Lori Smolin)

Contents in Brief

Contents

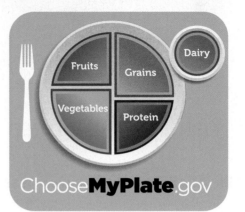

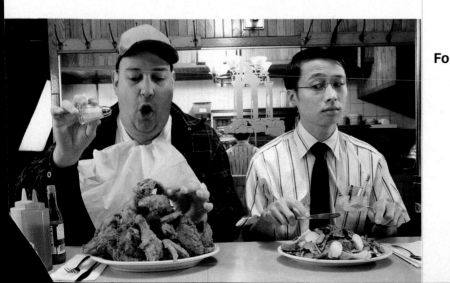

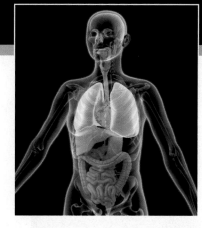

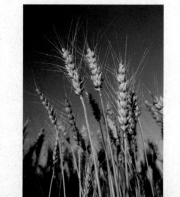

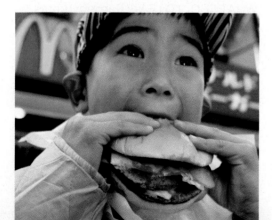

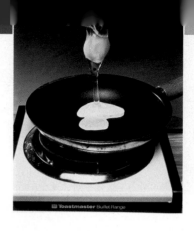

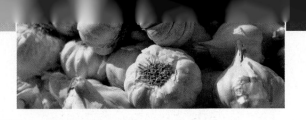

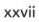

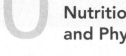

9 Energy Balance and Weight Management 308

10 Nutrition, Fitness, and Physical Activity 352

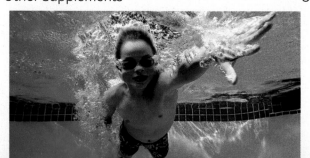

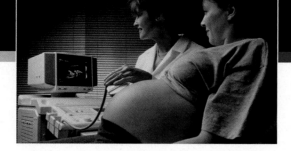

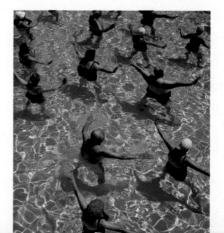

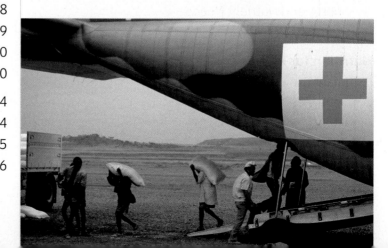

Multipart visual presentations that focus on a key concept or topic in the chapter.

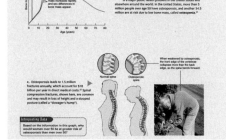

A series or combination of drawings and photos that describe and depict a complex process.

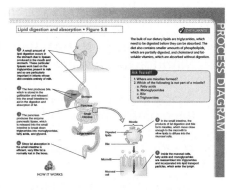

Second Edition

VISUALIZING
NUTRITION
EVERYDAY CHOICES

1 Nutrition: Everyday Choices

How do you choose what to eat? For most of the world's population, the answer is simple: You eat what you can grow, raise, catch, kill, or afford. Fundamentally, subsistence is the principal motivator of food consumption: If you don't eat, you die. Historically, the game or crops people could kill or cultivate successfully became staples of their diet. As agriculture and food production became more sophisticated, a greater array of food choices became available. Colonization and exploitation of native peoples introduced new foods to the colonizers: Corn became part of the diet of European settlers in North America, for instance, and the potato was brought to the Old World from the New. Today, in a cosmopolitan, global society, one may literally choose from the world's dinner table.

The implications of food choices are significant not only because what you eat affects your health but also because what you like affects what you choose to eat.

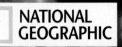

Hundreds of millions of people enjoy eating insects, raw fish, horses, and even dogs, while hundreds of millions of others abhor pork, beef, shellfish, dairy products, and even chocolate! Most of us enjoy the sweet and avoid the bitter, yet some of us choose the zip of the bitter or the bite of the zesty.

Because the nutrients in the food we eat form and maintain the structure of our bodies, we really are what we eat. The challenge is to find a satisfying balance between what we like and what optimizes our health.

The choice is ours.

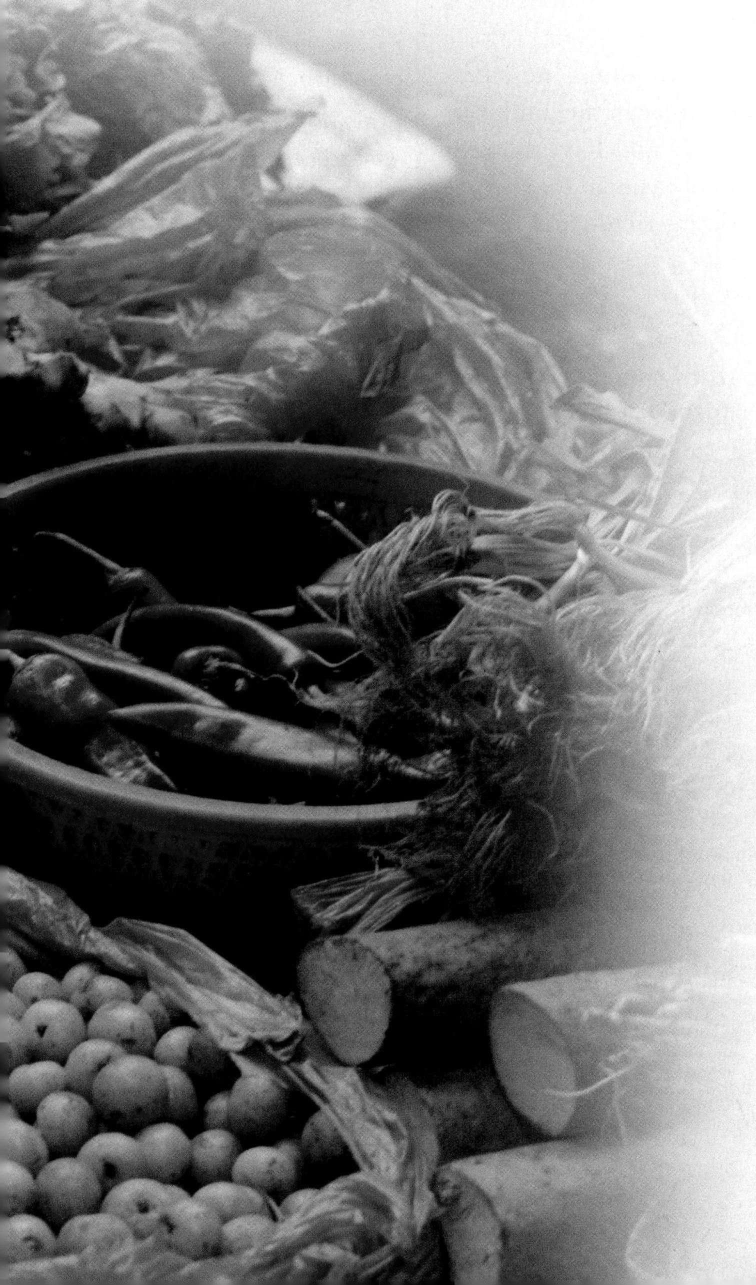

CHAPTER PLANNER ✓

- ❏ Stimulate your interest by reading the opening story and looking at the visual.
- ❏ Scan the Learning Objectives in each section:
  p. 4 ❏   p. 8 ❏   p. 11 ❏   p. 13 ❏   p. 16 ❏
- ❏ Read the text and study all figures and visuals. Answer any questions.

Analyze key features

- ❏ Nutrition InSight, p. 6 ❏   p. 10 ❏
- ❏ Thinking It Through, p. 14 ❏
- ❏ Process Diagram, p. 17 ❏
- ❏ What a Scientist Sees, p. 20 ❏
- ❏ Stop: Answer the Concept Checks before you go on:
  p. 7 ❏   p. 11 ❏   p. 13 ❏   p. 16 ❏   p. 24 ❏

End of chapter

- ❏ Review the Summary, Key Terms, and Online Resources.
- ❏ Answer the Critical and Creative Thinking Questions.
- ❏ Answer What is happening in this picture?
- ❏ Complete the Self-Test and check your answers.

Food Choices and Nutrient Intake

LEARNING OBJECTIVES

1. **Define** nutrient density.
2. **Compare** fortified foods and dietary supplements.
3. **Distinguish** essential nutrients from phytochemicals.
4. **Identify** the factors that determine food choices.

What are you going to eat today? Will breakfast be a vegetable omelet or a bowl of sugar-coated cereal? How about lunch—a burger or a turkey sandwich? The foods we choose determine the **nutrients** we consume. To stay healthy, humans need more than 40 **essential nutrients**. Because the foods we eat vary from day to day, so do the amounts and types of nutrients and the number of **calories** we consume.

> **nutrient** A substance in food that provides energy and structure to the body and regulates body processes.

nutrient-dense foods. Foods with a high **nutrient density** contain more nutrients per calorie than do foods with a lower nutrient density (**Figure 1.1**). If a large proportion of your diet consists of foods that are low in nutrient density, such as soft drinks, chips, and candy, you could have a hard time meeting your nutrient needs without exceeding your calorie needs. By choosing nutrient-dense foods, you can meet all your nutrient needs and have calories left over for occasional treats that are lower in nutrients and higher in calories.

> **essential nutrient** A nutrient that must be consumed in the diet because it cannot be made by the body or cannot be made in sufficient quantities to maintain body functions.
>
> **calorie** A unit of measure used to express the amount of energy provided by food.
>
> **nutrient density** A measure of the nutrients provided by a food relative to its calorie content.

Nutrients from Foods, Fortified Foods, and Supplements

Any food you eat adds some nutrients to your diet, but to make your diet healthy, it is important to choose

Nutrient density • Figure 1.1

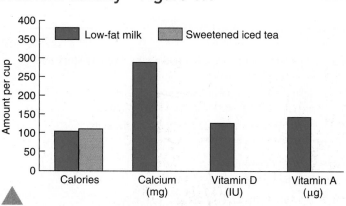

a. Nutrient density is important in choosing a healthy diet. For example, low-fat milk provides about the same number of calories per cup as bottled iced tea, but it also provides calcium, vitamin D, vitamin A, and other nutrients, including protein.

b. Typically, less processed foods are higher in nutrient density. For example, a roasted chicken breast is more nutrient dense, providing more nutrients per calorie, than chicken nuggets; a baked potato is more nutrient dense than French fries; and apples are more nutrient dense than apple pie.

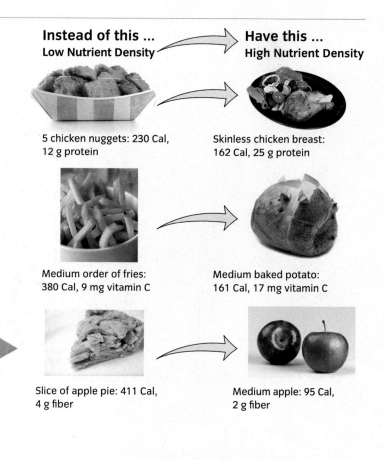

Instead of this ...
Low Nutrient Density

Have this ...
High Nutrient Density

5 chicken nuggets: 230 Cal, 12 g protein

Skinless chicken breast: 162 Cal, 25 g protein

Medium order of fries: 380 Cal, 9 mg vitamin C

Medium baked potato: 161 Cal, 17 mg vitamin C

Slice of apple pie: 411 Cal, 4 g fiber

Medium apple: 95 Cal, 2 g fiber

In addition to nutrients that occur naturally in foods, we obtain nutrients from fortified foods. The **fortification** of foods was begun to help eliminate nutrient deficiencies in the population, with the federal government mandating that certain nutrients be added to certain foods. Foods such as milk with added vitamin D and grain products with added B vitamins and iron are examples of this mandated fortification that have been part of the U.S. food supply for decades.

fortification The addition of nutrients to foods.

Recently, however, voluntary fortification of foods has become common practice. Vitamins and minerals are routinely added to breakfast cereals and a variety of snack foods. The amounts and types of nutrients added to these voluntarily fortified foods are at the discretion of the manufacturer. These added nutrients contribute to the diet but are not necessarily designed to address deficiencies and may increase the likelihood of consuming an excess of some nutrients.

Dietary supplements are another source of nutrients; about half of U.S. adults take some sort of daily dietary supplement. Supplements provide nutrients but do not offer all the benefits of food (see Chapters 2 and 7).

dietary supplement A product sold to supplement the diet; may include nutrients (vitamins, minerals, amino acids, fatty acids), enzymes, herbs, or other substances.

Food Provides More Than Nutrients

In addition to nutrients, food contains substances that, though not essential to life, can be beneficial for health. In plants, these health-promoting substances are called **phytochemicals** (**Figure 1.2**). Although fewer such substances have been identified in animal foods, animal foods also contain substances with health-promoting properties. These are called **zoochemicals**.

phytochemical A substance found in plant foods that is not an essential nutrient but may have health-promoting properties.

Foods that are high in phytochemicals • Figure 1.2

Fruits, vegetables, and whole grains provide a variety of phytochemicals, such as those highlighted here. Supplements of individual phytochemicals are available, but there is little evidence that they provide the health benefits obtained from foods that are high in phytochemicals.[1]

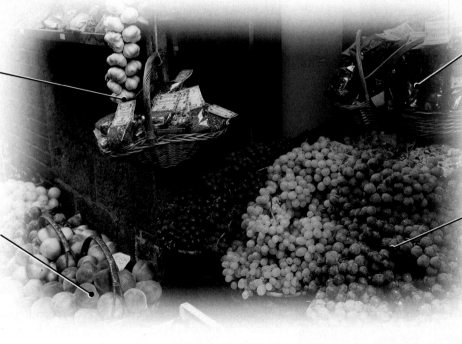

Garlic, broccoli, and onions provide sulfur-containing phytochemicals that help protect us from some forms of cancer by inactivating carcinogens or stimulating the body's natural defenses.[2,3]

Yellow-orange fruits and vegetables, such as peaches, apricots, carrots, and cantaloupe, as well as leafy greens, are rich in carotenoids, which are phytochemicals that may prevent oxygen from damaging our cells.[7]

Soybeans are a source of phytoestrogens, hormone-like compounds found in plants that may reduce the risk of certain types of cancer and cause small reductions in blood cholesterol.[4,5,6]

Purple grapes, berries, and onions provide red, purple, and pale yellow pigments called flavonoids, which prevent oxygen damage and may reduce the risk of cancer and heart disease.[8,9]

Functional foods provide benefits beyond their nutrients Table 1.1	
Food	**Potential health benefit**
Blueberries	May reduce the risk of heart disease and cancer.[9,10]
Breakfast cereal with added flaxseed	Helps reduce blood cholesterol levels and the overall risk of heart disease.[11]
Chocolate	May help reduce blood pressure and other risk factors for heart disease.[12]
Garlic	Helps reduce blood cholesterol levels and the overall risk of heart disease.[13]
Kale	May reduce the risk of age-related blindness (macular degeneration).[14]
Margarine with added plant sterols	Reduces blood cholesterol levels.[15]
Nuts	May reduce the risk of heart disease.[16]
Oatmeal	Helps reduce blood cholesterol.[17]
Orange juice with added calcium	Helps prevent osteoporosis.
Salmon	Reduces the risk of heart disease.[18]
Tea, green and black	May reduce the risk of certain types of cancer.[19]
Whole-grain bread	Helps reduce the risk of cancer, heart disease, obesity, and diabetes.[20]

functional food A food that has health-promoting properties beyond basic nutritional functions.

Some foods, because of the complex mixtures of nutrients and other chemicals they contain, provide health benefits that extend beyond basic nutrition. Such foods have been termed **functional foods**. The simplest functional foods are unmodified whole foods, such as broccoli and fish, that naturally contain substances that promote health and protect against disease, but some foods fortified with nutrients or enhanced with phytochemicals or other substances are also classified as functional foods (**Table 1.1**). These modified foods, such as water with

Nutrition InSight Food choices • Figure 1.3

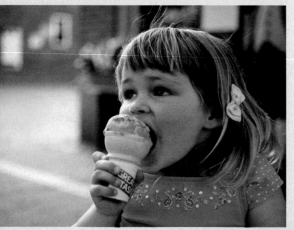

We use food as reward and punishment. A well-behaved child may be rewarded with an ice cream cone, while a child who misbehaves may be sent to bed without dessert. We also use food to commemorate milestones such as birthdays and anniversaries.

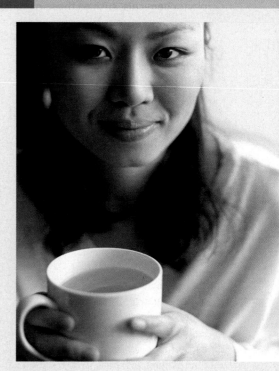

Food can provide comfort and security. "Comfort foods" such as hot tea, chicken soup, and chocolate help us to feel better when we are sick, cold, tired, or lonely.

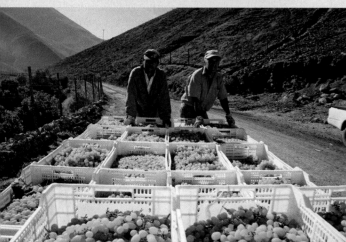

We can choose only from foods that are available to us. What is available is affected by season, geography, economics, health, and living conditions. In many parts of the world, food choices are limited to foods produced locally, but in more developed regions, many nonnative and seasonal foods, such as these grapes, are available year-round because they can be stored and shipped from distant locations.

added vitamins, oatmeal with added soy protein, and orange juice with added calcium, have also been called **designer foods** or **nutraceuticals**. As food manufacturers cash in on the concept that "health sells," the line between what is a dietary supplement and what is a food has become blurred.

What Determines Food Choices?

Do you eat oranges to boost your vitamin C intake or ice cream to add a little calcium to your diet? Probably not. We need these nutrients to survive, but we generally choose foods for reasons other than the nutrients they contain. Sometimes we choose a food simply because it is put in front of us; often our choices also depend on what we have learned to eat, what is socially acceptable in our cultural heritage or religion, what we think is healthy, or what our personal convictions—such as environmental consciousness or vegetarianism—demand. Tradition and values may dictate what foods we consider appropriate,

but individual preferences for taste, smell, appearance, and texture affect which foods we actually consume. All these factors are involved in food choices because food does more than meet our physiological requirements. It also provides sensory pleasure and helps meet our social and emotional needs (**Figure 1.3**).

CONCEPT CHECK   STOP

1. **Which** has a higher nutrient density: a soda or a glass of milk?
2. **Why** are foods fortified?
3. **Why** is it better to meet your vitamin C needs by eating an orange than by taking a dietary supplement?
4. **What** factors determine which foods you eat at a family picnic?

WILEY PLUS   Video   ✓ THE PLANNER

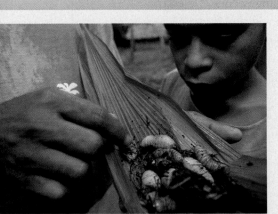

Food preferences and eating habits are learned as part of an individual's family, cultural, national, and social background. In many parts of the world, insects, such as these palm beetle larvae, are considered a delicacy, but in U.S. culture, insects are considered food contaminants, and most people would refuse to eat them.

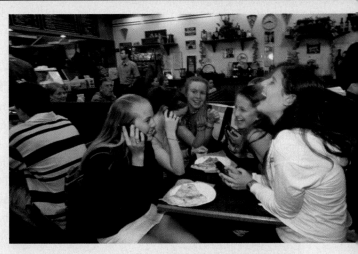

For an adolescent, stopping for pizza after school may be part of being accepted by his or her peers. Food is the centerpiece of everyday social interactions. We meet friends for dinner or a cup of coffee. The family dinner table is a focal point for communication, where experiences of the day are shared.

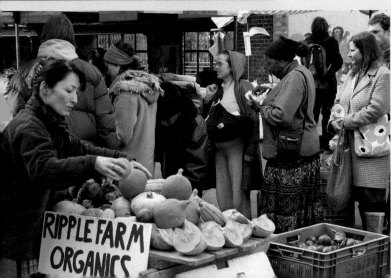

Often people's attitudes about what foods they think are good for them or are good for the environment affect what they choose. For example, you may choose organic produce because you are concerned about exposure to pesticides or green tea to increase your intake of cancer-fighting antioxidants.

Nutrients and Their Functions

LEARNING OBJECTIVES

1. **List** the six classes of nutrients.
2. **Discuss** the three functions of nutrients in the body.

There are six classes of nutrients: carbohydrates, lipids, proteins, water, vitamins, and minerals. Carbohydrates, lipids, proteins, and water are considered **macronutrients** because they are needed in large amounts. Vitamins and minerals are referred to as **micronutrients** because they are needed in small amounts. Together, the macronutrients and micronutrients in our diet provide us with energy, contribute to the structure of our bodies, and regulate the biological processes that go on inside us. Each nutrient provides one or more of these functions, but all nutrients together are needed to provide for growth, maintain and repair the body, and support reproduction.

The Six Classes of Nutrients

Carbohydrates, lipids, and proteins are all **organic compounds** that provide energy to the body (**Figure 1.4**).

> **organic compound** A substance that contains carbon bonded to hydrogen.
>
> **carbohydrates** A class of nutrients that includes sugars, starches, and fibers. Chemically, they all contain carbon, along with hydrogen and oxygen, in the same proportions as in water (H_2O).

Although we tend to think of each of them as a single nutrient, there are actually many different types of molecules in each of these classes. **Carbohydrates** include starches, sugars, and **fiber** (**Figure 1.4a**). Several types of **lipids** play important roles in nutrition (**Figure 1.4b**). The most familiar of these are **cholesterol**, **saturated fats**, and **unsaturated fats**. There are thousands of different **proteins** in our bodies and our diets. All proteins are made up of units called **amino acids** that are linked together in different combinations to form different proteins (**Figure 1.4c**).

Water, unlike the other classes of nutrients, is only a single substance. Water makes up about 60% of an adult's body weight. Because we can't store water, the water the body loses must constantly be replaced by water obtained from the diet. In the body, water acts as a lubricant, a transport fluid, and a regulator of body temperature.

Vitamins are organic molecules that are needed in small amounts to maintain health. There are 13 vitamins, which perform a variety of unique functions in the body, such as regulating energy metabolism, maintaining vision, protecting cell membranes, and helping blood to clot. **Minerals** are **elements** that are essential nutrients needed in small amounts to provide a variety of diverse functions in the body. For example, iron is an element needed for the transport of oxygen in the blood, calcium is an element important in keeping bones strong. We consume vitamins and minerals in almost all the foods we eat. Some are natural sources: Oranges contain vitamin C, milk provides calcium, and carrots give us vitamin A. Other foods are fortified with vitamins and minerals; fortified breakfast cereals often have 100% of the recommended intake of many vitamins and minerals. Dietary supplements are another source of vitamins and minerals for some people.

> **fiber** A type of carbohydrate that cannot be broken down by human digestive enzymes.
>
> **lipids** A class of nutrients that is commonly called fats. Chemically, they contain carbon, hydrogen, and oxygen, and most of them do not dissolve in water.
>
> **cholesterol** A type of lipid that is found in the diet and in the blood. High blood levels increase the risk of heart disease.
>
> **saturated fat** A type of lipid that is most abundant in solid animal fats and is associated with an increased risk of heart disease.
>
> **unsaturated fat** A type of lipid that is most abundant in plant oils and is associated with a reduced risk of heart disease.
>
> **protein** A class of nutrients that includes molecules made up of one or more intertwining chains of amino acids.

What Nutrients Do

Carbohydrates, lipids, and proteins are often referred to as **energy-yielding nutrients**; they provide energy that can be measured in calories. The calories people talk about and see listed on food labels are actually **kilocalories** (abbreviated kcalorie or kcal), units of 1000 calories. When spelled with a capital *C*, Calorie means kilocalorie. Carbohydrates provide 4 Calories/gram; they are the most immediate source of energy for the body. Lipids also help fuel our activities

a. Some high-carbohydrate foods, such as rice, pasta, and bread, contain mostly starch; some, such as berries, kidney beans, and broccoli, are high in fiber; and others, such as cookies, cakes, and carbonated beverages, are high in added sugar. High-fiber, low-sugar foods have a higher nutrient density than do low-fiber, high-sugar foods.

b. High-fat plant foods such as vegetable oils, avocados, olives, and nuts have no cholesterol and are high in unsaturated fat, so they don't increase the risk of heart disease. High-fat animal foods such as cream, butter, meat, and whole milk are high in saturated fat and cholesterol; a diet high in these increases the risk of heart disease.

c. The proteins we obtain from animal foods, such as meat, fish, and eggs, better match our amino acid needs than do most individual plant proteins, such as those found in grains, nuts, and beans. However, when plant sources of protein are combined, they can provide all the amino acids we need.

◀ **Energy**
Whether riding a bike through the fall foliage, walking to the mailbox, or gardening, physical activity is fueled by the energy in the food we eat.

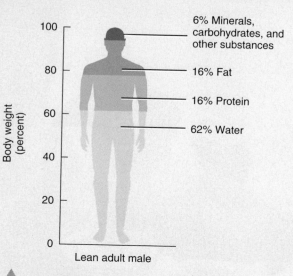

- 6% Minerals, carbohydrates, and other substances
- 16% Fat
- 16% Protein
- 62% Water

Body weight (percent)

Lean adult male

▲ **Structure**
Proteins, lipids, carbohydrates, minerals, and water all contribute to the shape and structure of our bodies.

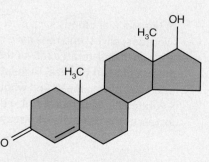

▲ **Regulation**
Lipids, such as the hormone testosterone, illustrated here, help regulate body processes. Testosterone is made from cholesterol. In men, it stimulates sperm production and the development of secondary sex characteristics, such as body and facial hair, a deep voice, and increased muscle mass.

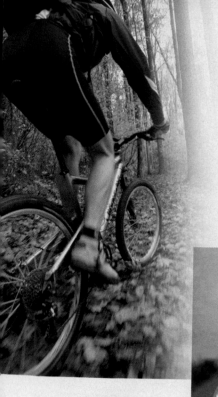

Regulation ▶
Water helps regulate body temperature. When body temperature increases, sweat is produced, cooling the body as it evaporates from the skin.

and are the major form of stored energy in the body. One gram of fat provides 9 Calories. Protein can supply 4 Calories/gram but is not the body's first choice for meeting energy needs because protein has other roles that take priority. Alcohol, although it is not a nutrient because it is not needed for life, provides about 7 Calories/gram. Water, vitamins, and minerals do not provide energy (calories).

With the exception of vitamins, all the classes of nutrients are involved in forming and maintaining the body's structure. Fat deposited under the skin contributes to our body shape, for instance, and proteins form the ligaments and tendons that hold our bones together and attach our muscles to our bones. Minerals harden bone. Protein and water make up the structure of the muscles, which help define our body contours, and protein and carbohydrates form the cartilage that cushions our joints. On a smaller scale, lipids, proteins, and water form the structure of individual cells. Lipids and proteins make up the membranes that surround each cell, and water and dissolved substances fill the cells and the spaces around them.

All six classes of nutrients play important roles in regulating body processes. Keeping body temperature, blood pressure, blood sugar level, and hundreds of other parameters relatively constant involves thousands of chemical reactions and physiological processes. Proteins, vitamins, and minerals are regulatory nutrients that help control how quickly chemical reactions take place throughout the body. Lipids and proteins are needed to make regulatory molecules called **hormones** that stimulate or inhibit various body processes.

Figure 1.5 illustrates some of the ways in which various nutrients are involved in providing energy, forming body structures, and regulating physiological processes.

| CONCEPT CHECK | STOP |

1. **Which** classes of nutrients provide energy?
2. **What** three nutrient functions help ensure normal growth, maintenance of body structure and functions, and reproduction?

Nutrition in Health and Disease

LEARNING OBJECTIVES

1. **Describe** the different types of malnutrition.
2. **Explain** ways in which nutrient intake can affect health in both the short term and the long term.
3. **Discuss** how the genes you inherit affect the impact your diet has on your health.

What we eat has an enormous impact on how healthy we are now and how likely we are to develop chronic diseases such as heart disease, obesity, and diabetes. Consuming either too much or too little of one or more nutrients or energy will result in **malnutrition**. Malnutrition can affect your health not just today but 20, 30, or 40 years from now. The impact of your diet on your health is also affected by your genetic background.

malnutrition A condition resulting from an energy or nutrient intake either above or below that which is optimal.

Undernutrition and Overnutrition

Undernutrition occurs when intake doesn't meet the body's needs (**Figure 1.6**). The more severe the deficiency, the more dramatic the symptoms. Some nutrient deficiencies occur quickly. Dehydration, a deficiency of water, can cause symptoms in a matter of hours. Drinking water can relieve the headache, fatigue, and dizziness caused by dehydration almost as rapidly as these symptoms appeared. Other nutritional deficiencies may take much longer to become evident. Symptoms of scurvy, a disease caused by a deficiency of vitamin C, appear after months of deficient intake; **osteoporosis**, a condition in which the bones become weak and break easily, occurs after years of consuming a calcium-deficient diet.

Undernutrition • Figure 1.6

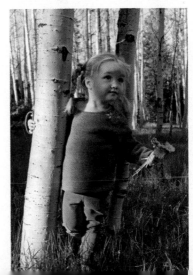

a. Even though this child looks normal and healthy, she has low iron stores. If the iron content of her diet is not increased, she will eventually develop iron deficiency anemia. Mild nutrient deficiencies like hers may go unnoticed because the symptoms either are not immediately apparent or are nonspecific. Two common nonspecific symptoms of iron depletion are fatigue and decreased ability to fight infection.

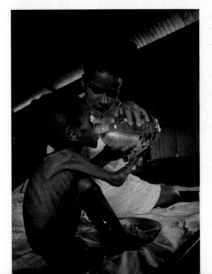

b. The symptoms of starvation, the most obvious form of undernutrition, occur gradually over time when the energy provided by the diet is too low to meet the body's needs. Body tissues are broken down to provide the energy to support vital functions, resulting in loss of body fat and wasting of muscles.

We typically think of malnutrition as undernutrition, but **overnutrition**, an excess intake of nutrients or calories, is also a concern. An overdose of iron can cause liver failure, for example, and too much vitamin B_6 can cause nerve damage. These nutrient toxicities usually result from taking large doses of vitamin and mineral supplements, because foods generally do not contain high enough concentrations of nutrients to be toxic. However, chronic overconsumption of calories and certain nutrients from foods can also cause health problems. The typical U.S. diet, which provides more calories than are needed, has resulted in an epidemic of obesity in which more than 68% of adults are overweight or obese (**Figure 1.7a**).[21] Diets that are high in sodium contribute to high blood pressure; an excess intake of saturated fat contributes to heart disease; and a dietary pattern that is high in red meat and saturated fat and low in fruits, vegetables, and fiber may increase the risk of certain cancers.[22] It has been estimated that about 15% of all deaths in the United States can be attributed to poor diet and sedentary lifestyle (**Figure 1.7b**).[23]

Diet-Gene Interactions

Diet affects your health, but diet alone does not determine whether you will develop a particular disease. Each of us inherits a unique combination of **genes**. Some of these genes affect your risk of developing chronic diseases, such as heart disease, cancer, high blood pressure, and diabetes, but their impact is affected by what you eat (**Figure 1.8**). Your genetic makeup determines the impact a certain nutrient will have on you. For example, some people inherit a combination of genes that

> **genes** Units of a larger molecule called DNA that are responsible for inherited traits.

Overnutrition • Figure 1.7

a. Obesity is a form of overnutrition that occurs when energy intake surpasses energy expenditure over a long period, causing the accumulation of an excessive amount of body fat. Adults are not the only ones who are getting fatter. An estimated 17% of U.S. children and adolescents, ages 2 to 19 years, are obese.[24]

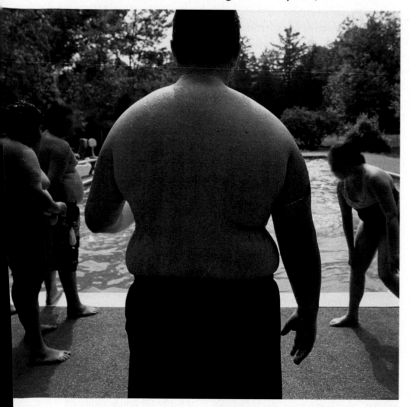

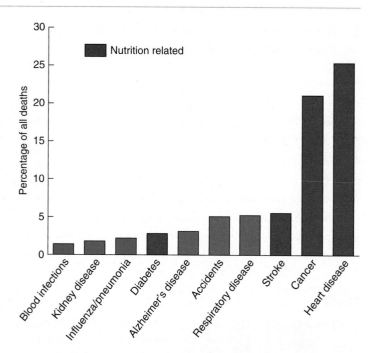

b. The top three causes of death in the United States are nutrition related.[25] They are all thought to be exacerbated by obesity.

Interpreting Data

Based on this graph showing leading causes of death in the United States, about what percentage of all deaths are due to nutrition-related diseases?

a. 5%   b. 10%   c. 50%   d. 90%

Nutritional genomics • Figure 1.8

Your actual risk of disease results from the interplay between the genes you inherit and the diet and lifestyle choices you make.

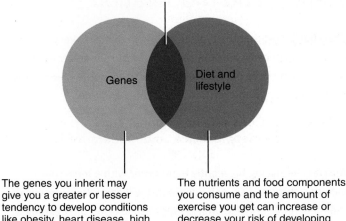

Genes

Diet and lifestyle

The genes you inherit may give you a greater or lesser tendency to develop conditions like obesity, heart disease, high blood pressure, or diabetes.

The nutrients and food components you consume and the amount of exercise you get can increase or decrease your risk of developing nutrition-related diseases.

Think Critically Can you become obese even if both of your parents are thin?

results in a tendency to have high blood pressure. When these individuals consume even an average amount of sodium, their blood pressure increases (discussed further in Chapter 8). Others inherit genes that allow them to consume more sodium without much of a rise in blood pressure. Those whose genes dictate a significant rise in blood pressure with a high-sodium diet can reduce their blood pressure, and the complications associated with high blood pressure, by eating a diet that is low in sodium.

Our increasing understanding of human genetics has given rise to the discipline of **nutritional genomics** or **nutrigenomics**, which explores the interaction between genetic variation and nutrition.[26] Research in this area has led to the development of the concept of "personalized nutrition," the idea that a diet based on the genes an individual has inherited can be used to prevent, moderate, or cure chronic disease. Although today we do not know enough to take a sample of your DNA and use it to tell you what to eat to optimize your health, we do know that certain dietary patterns can reduce the risk of many chronic diseases.

> **nutritional genomics** or **nutrigenomics** The study of how diet affects our genes and how individual genetic variation can affect the impact of nutrients or other food components on health.

CONCEPT CHECK STOP

1. **What** causes malnutrition?
2. **How** can your diet today affect your health 20 years from now?
3. **Why** might the diet that optimizes health be different for different people?

Choosing a Healthy Diet

LEARNING OBJECTIVES

1. **Explain** why it is important to eat a variety of foods.

2. **Describe** how you can sometimes eat foods that are low in nutrient density and still have a healthy diet.

3. **Discuss** how dietary moderation can reduce the risk of chronic disease.

A healthy diet is one that provides the right number of calories to keep your weight in the desirable range; the proper balance of carbohydrates, proteins, and fat; plenty of water; and sufficient but not excessive amounts of vitamins and minerals. Such a healthy diet is rich in whole grains, fruits, and vegetables; high in fiber; moderate in fat, sugar, and sodium; and low in unhealthy fats (saturated fat, cholesterol, and *trans* fat). In short, a healthy diet is based on variety,

THINKING IT THROUGH

A Case Study on Variety, Balance, and Moderation

For many college students, their freshman year is the first time they are making all their own food choices, and they don't always make the best ones. Learning to apply the principles of variety, balance, and moderation can help improve these choices.

Amad loves fast food. He grabs a doughnut for breakfast, a burger and fries for lunch, and either tacos or pizza for dinner. He has gained a few pounds and is worried that he will become a victim of the "freshman 15"—the 15 or so pounds gained in the first year away from home.

What's wrong with Amad's diet?

▼

Answer: Amad's diet needs more balance. An occasional fast-food meal is fine, but eating these foods every day results in a diet that is high in calories and low in some vitamins and minerals. Amad needs to balance his fast-food choices with lower-calorie meals that are higher in nutrient density. For example, if he plans to eat a doughnut for breakfast, he could balance this with a more nutrient-dense lunch, such as a sandwich on whole-grain bread with turkey, lettuce, tomatoes, and peppers. If his dinner is a high-calorie fast-food meal, he could balance this with a bowl of cereal with fruit for breakfast.

What about Helen? She isn't gaining weight but has a boring diet. Every day she eats cereal for breakfast, a peanut butter sandwich for lunch, and chicken, broccoli, and rice for dinner.

What's wrong with Helen's diet?

▼

Your answer:

Chris has heard that the typical American diet isn't very healthy—especially his daily pattern of a burger and fries for dinner. So, to improve his diet, he decides to try some Chinese food. He orders orange chicken with vegetables and rice.

How does Chris's Chinese dinner stack up in terms of variety, balance, and moderation?

▼

Answer: Replacing his nightly hamburger with a meal that includes chicken, rice, and vegetables will add variety. However, the meal really only includes about a tablespoon of vegetables and the chicken is breaded and fried, making it high in calories and fat, so the overall meal doesn't help keep his diet moderate. To balance his overall diet Chris would need to include more vegetables and fruits at other meals.

Marty knows that legumes are a healthy choice, so she decides to try some Mexican food. She orders the beef and bean burrito platter shown here.

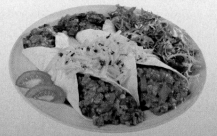

How does Marty's meal stack up in terms of variety, balance, and moderation?

▼

Your answer:

(Check your answers in Appendix J.)

---

balance, and moderation (see *Thinking It Through: A Case Study on Variety, Balance, and Moderation*).

Eat a Variety of Foods

In nutrition, choosing a variety of foods is important because no single food can provide all the nutrients the body needs for optimal health. *Variety* means choosing foods from different food groups—vegetables, grains, fruits, dairy products, and high-protein foods. Some of these foods

are rich in vitamins and phytochemicals, others are rich in protein and minerals, and all are important.

Variety also means choosing diverse foods from within each food group. Different vegetables provide different nutrients. Potatoes, for example, are the only vegetable in many Americans' diets. Potatoes provide vitamin C but are low in vitamin A. If potatoes are your only vegetable, it is unlikely that you will meet your nutrient needs. If instead you have a salad, potatoes, and broccoli, you will be getting plenty of vitamins C and A, as well as many other vitamins and minerals. Making varied choices both from the different food groups and from within each food group is also important because nutrients and other food components interact. Such interactions may be positive, enhancing nutrient utilization, or negative, inhibiting nutrient availability. Variety averages out these interactions. Some foods may also contain toxic substances. Eating a variety of foods reduces the risk that you will consume enough of any one toxin to be harmful. For example, tuna may contain traces of mercury, but as long as you don't eat tuna too often, you are unlikely to consume a toxic amount.

Variety involves choosing different foods not only each day but also each week and throughout the year. If you had apples and grapes today, for example, have blueberries and cantaloupe tomorrow. If you can't find tasty tomatoes in December, replace them with a winter vegetable such as squash.

Balance Your Choices

Choosing a healthy diet is a balancing act. Healthy eating doesn't mean giving up your favorite foods. There is no such thing as a good food or a bad food—only healthy diets and unhealthy diets. Any food can be part of a healthy diet, as long as your diet throughout the day or week provides enough of all the nutrients you need without excesses of any. When you choose a food that is lacking in fiber, for example, balance it with one that provides lots of fiber. When you choose a food that is very high in fat, balance that choice with a low-fat one.

A balanced diet also balances the calories you take in with the calories you burn in your daily activities so that your body weight stays in the healthy range (**Figure 1.9**).

Balance calories in with calories out • Figure 1.9

To keep your weight stable, you need to burn the same number of calories as you consume. Extra calories consumed during the day can be balanced by increasing the calories you burn in physical activity.

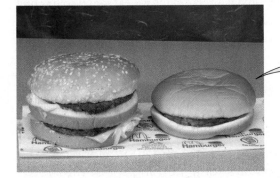

If you have a Big Mac for lunch instead of a smaller plain burger, you will have to increase your energy expenditure by 300 Calories.

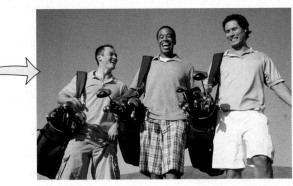

You could do this by playing golf for about an hour, carrying your own clubs.

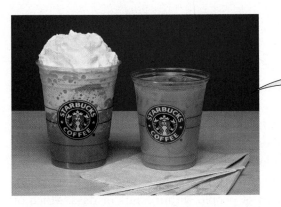

If you have a grande Mocha Frappuccino instead of a regular iced coffee, you will have to increase your energy expenditure by 370 Calories.

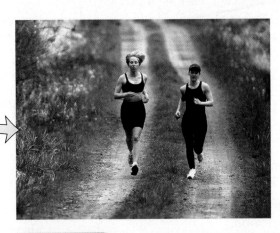

You could do this by jogging for about 30 minutes.

Ask Yourself

If you add a daily grande Mocha Frappuccino to your usual diet and do not increase your activity, what will happen to your weight?

WHAT SHOULD I EAT?
A Healthy Diet

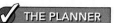
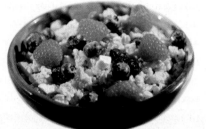

Eat a variety of foods
- Mix up your snacks by having salsa and chips one day and fruit, nuts, or a granola bar another day.
- Add almonds and diced apples to your salad.
- Try a new vegetable or fruit each week. Tired of carrots? Try jicama.
- Vary your protein sources. Have fish one day and beef the next—or skip the meat and have beans.

Balance your choices
- Going out to dinner? Have a salad for lunch.
- Add a vegetable instead of pepperoni to your pizza.
- When you have cookies for a snack, have fruit for dessert.
- Had soda with lunch? Have low-fat milk with dinner.

Practice moderation
- Push back from the table before you are stuffed and go for a walk.
- Reduce your portions by using a smaller bowl.
- Skip the seconds or split your restaurant meal with a friend.
- If you eat some extra fries, take some extra steps.

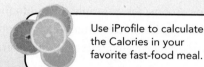

Use iProfile to calculate the Calories in your favorite fast-food meal.

Practice Moderation

Moderation means not overdoing it—not having too many calories, too much fat, too much sugar, too much salt, or too much alcohol. Choosing moderately will help you maintain a healthy weight and prevent some of the chronic diseases, such as heart disease and cancer, that are on the rise in the U.S. population (see *What Should I Eat?*).

The fact that more than 68% of adult Americans are overweight or obese demonstrates that we have not been practicing moderation when it comes to calorie intake.[21] One of the main culprits is likely the size of our food portions. The sandwiches, soft drinks, and French fry orders served in fast-food restaurants today are two to five times larger than what they were 40 years ago. The sizes of the snacks and meals we eat at home have also increased. As these portion sizes have grown, so has the amount we eat—and so has our weight.[27] Moderation makes it easier to balance your diet and allows you to enjoy a greater variety of foods.

CONCEPT CHECK | STOP

1. **Why** is variety in a diet important?

2. **How** might you balance the 400-Calorie cinnamon roll you had for a morning snack with your lunch choice?

3. **What** is the connection between obesity and moderation in a diet?

Evaluating Nutrition Information
LEARNING OBJECTIVES

1. **Explain** the scientific method and give an example of how it is used in nutrition.

2. **Discuss** three different types of experiments used to study nutrition.

3. **Describe** the components of a sound scientific experiment.

4. **Distinguish** between reliable and unreliable nutrition information.

We are bombarded with nutrition information almost every day. The evening news, the morning papers, and the World Wide Web continually offer us tantalizing tidbits of nutrition advice. Food and nutrition information that used to take professionals years to disseminate now travels with lightning speed, reaching millions of people within hours or days. Much of this information is reliable, but some can be misleading. In order to choose a healthy diet, we need to be able to sort out the useful material in this flood of information.

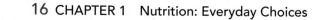

The Science Behind Nutrition

Like all other sciences, the science of nutrition is constantly evolving. As new discoveries provide clues to the right combination of nutrients needed for optimal health, new nutritional principles and recommendations are developed. Sometimes established beliefs and concepts give way to new information. Understanding the process of science can help consumers understand the nutrition information they encounter.

The systematic, unbiased approach that allows any science to acquire new knowledge and correct and update previous knowledge is the **scientific method**. The scientific method involves making observations of natural events, formulating **hypotheses** to explain these events, designing and performing experiments to test these hypotheses, and developing **theories** that explain the observed phenomenon based on the results of many studies (**Figure 1.10**). In nutrition, the scientific method is used to develop nutrient recommendations, understand the functions of nutrients, and learn about the role of nutrition in promoting health and preventing disease.

> **hypothesis** A proposed explanation for an observation or a scientific problem that can be tested through experimentation.
>
> **theory** A formal explanation of an observed phenomenon made after a hypothesis has been tested and supported through extensive experimentation.

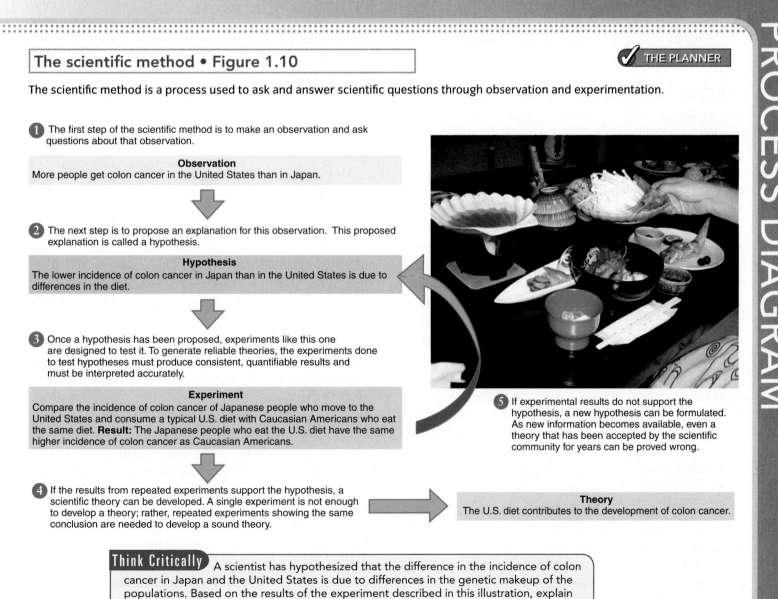

The scientific method • Figure 1.10

THE PLANNER

The scientific method is a process used to ask and answer scientific questions through observation and experimentation.

1 The first step of the scientific method is to make an observation and ask questions about that observation.

Observation
More people get colon cancer in the United States than in Japan.

2 The next step is to propose an explanation for this observation. This proposed explanation is called a hypothesis.

Hypothesis
The lower incidence of colon cancer in Japan than in the United States is due to differences in the diet.

3 Once a hypothesis has been proposed, experiments like this one are designed to test it. To generate reliable theories, the experiments done to test hypotheses must produce consistent, quantifiable results and must be interpreted accurately.

Experiment
Compare the incidence of colon cancer of Japanese people who move to the United States and consume a typical U.S. diet with Caucasian Americans who eat the same diet. **Result:** The Japanese people who eat the U.S. diet have the same higher incidence of colon cancer as Caucasian Americans.

4 If the results from repeated experiments support the hypothesis, a scientific theory can be developed. A single experiment is not enough to develop a theory; rather, repeated experiments showing the same conclusion are needed to develop a sound theory.

5 If experimental results do not support the hypothesis, a new hypothesis can be formulated. As new information becomes available, even a theory that has been accepted by the scientific community for years can be proved wrong.

Theory
The U.S. diet contributes to the development of colon cancer.

Think Critically A scientist has hypothesized that the difference in the incidence of colon cancer in Japan and the United States is due to differences in the genetic makeup of the populations. Based on the results of the experiment described in this illustration, explain why this hypothesis is not supported.

PROCESS DIAGRAM

How Scientists Study Nutrition

Many different types of experiments are used to expand our knowledge of nutrition. Some make observations about relationships between diet and health; these are based on the science of **epidemiology**. Other types of experiments evaluate the affect of a particular dietary change on health. Some of these experiments study humans, others use animals; some look at whole populations, others study just a few individuals; and some use just cells or molecules (**Figure 1.11**). For any nutrition study to provide reliable information, it must collect quantifiable data from the right experimental population, use proper experimental controls, and interpret the data accurately.

epidemiology The branch of science that studies health and disease trends and patterns in populations.

Reliable data can be quantified, meaning that they include parameters that can be measured reliably and repeatedly, such as body weight or blood pressure. Individual testimonies or opinions alone are not quantifiable, objective measures.

For an experiment to answer the right question, scientists must study the appropriate group of people. For an experiment to determine whether a treatment does or does not have an effect, it must include enough subjects. For example, if a dietary supplement claims to increase bone strength in older women, it must be tested in older women and include enough subjects to demonstrate that the supplement causes the effect to occur more frequently than it would by chance. The number of subjects needed depends on how likely an effect is to occur without the treatment. For example, if weight training for four weeks without a muscle-building supplement causes an increase in muscle mass, a large number of experimental subjects may be needed to demonstrate that there is a greater increase in muscle mass when the supplement is taken. Results from studies with only a few subjects may not be able to distinguish effects that occur due to chance and should therefore be interpreted with caution.

In order to know whether what is being tested has an effect, one must compare it with something. A **control group** acts as a standard of comparison for the factor, or

control group In a scientific experiment, the group of participants used as a basis of comparison. They are similar to the participants in the experimental group but do not receive the treatment being tested.

variable, being studied. A control group is treated in the same way as the **experimental group** except that the control group does not receive the treatment being tested. For example, in a study examining the effect of a dietary supplement on muscle strength, the control group would consist of individuals of similar age, gender, and ability, eating similar diets and following similar workout regimens as individuals in the experimental group. Instead of the supplement, the control subjects would consume a **placebo**, a fake product that is identical in appearance to the dietary supplement.

experimental group In a scientific experiment, the group of participants who undergo the treatment being tested.

When an experiment has been completed, the results must be interpreted. Accurate interpretation is just as important as conducting a study carefully. If a study conducted on a large group of young women indicates that a change in diet reduces breast cancer risk later in life, the results of that study cannot be used to claim that the same effect will occur if older women make a similar dietary change. Likewise, if the study looks only at the connection between a change in diet and breast cancer, the findings can't be used to claim a reduced risk for other cancers.

One way to ensure that the results of experiments are interpreted correctly is to have them reviewed by experts in the field who did not take part in the study being evaluated. Such a **peer-review process** is used in determining whether experimental results should be published in scientific journals. The reviewing scientists must agree that the experiments were conducted properly and that the results were interpreted appropriately. Nutrition articles that have undergone peer review can be found in many journals, including *The American Journal of Clinical Nutrition*, *The Journal of Nutrition*, *The Journal of the American Dietetic Association*, *The New England Journal of Medicine*, and *The International Journal of Sport Nutrition*. Newsletters from reputable institutions, such as the *Tufts Health and Nutrition Letter* and the *Harvard Health Letter*, are also reliable sources of nutrition and health information. The information in these newsletters comes from peer-reviewed articles but is written for a consumer audience.

Recommendations and policies regarding nutrition and health care are made by compiling the evidence from the wealth of well-controlled, peer-reviewed studies that are available. This is referred to as **evidence-based practice**.

Types of nutrition studies • Figure 1.11

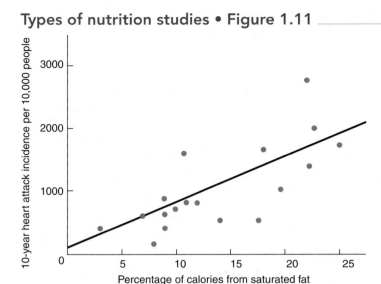

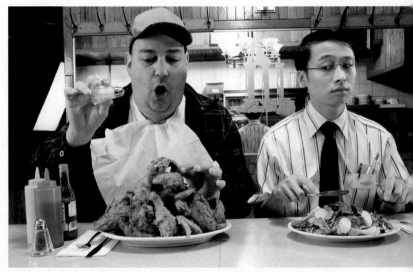

a. Epidemiological studies

Epidemiological studies of populations around the world explore the impact of nutrition on health. If you were to measure saturated fat intake and the incidence of heart attacks in populations around the world, you might get a graph that looks like this one. It indicates that a high percentage of calories from saturated fat in a population is associated with an increased incidence of heart attacks. However, epidemiology does not determine cause-and-effect relationships—it just identifies patterns. Therefore, it cannot determine whether the higher incidence of heart attacks is caused by the high intake of saturated fat.

b. Clinical trials

The observations and hypotheses that arise from epidemiology can be tested using clinical trials. Nutrition clinical trials are studies that explore the health effects of altering people's diets—for instance, the possible effects of eliminating meat on blood cholesterol levels.

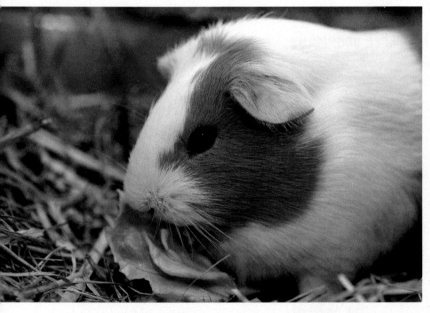

c. Animal studies

Ideally, studies of human nutrition should be done with human subjects. However, because studying humans is costly, time-consuming, inconvenient for the subjects, and in some cases impossible for ethical reasons, many studies are done using animals. Guinea pigs are a good model for studying heart disease, but even the best animal model is not the same as a human, and care must be taken when extrapolating animal results to humans.

d. Biochemistry and molecular biology

Laboratory-based techniques can be used to study nutrient functions in the body. For example, biochemistry can be used to study the chemical reactions that provide energy or synthesize molecules, such as cholesterol, and molecular biology can be used to study how nutrients regulate our genes.

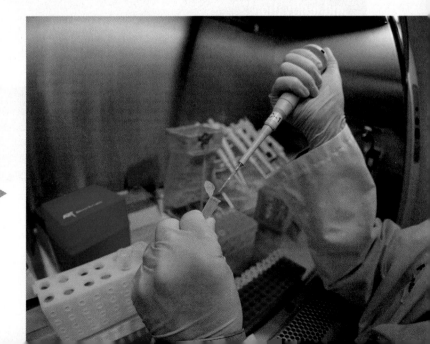

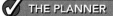

Behind the Claims

This product must be amazing! It will increase your muscle strength, decrease your body fat, and boost your drive and motivation. This is what consumers see. The claims sound great, but a scientist looking at the same ad may have some concerns.

First of all, the claims about muscle strength and motivation are testimonials based on individuals' feelings and impressions, and these are not objective measures.

A scientist would also question whether the research evidence supports the claim that the product increases lean body mass and decreases body fat. The study measured the amount of lean tissue and fat tissue in weightlifters before and four weeks after they began consuming the POWER BOOST drink. The measures used provide quantifiable, repeatable data. The results report a gain of 5.2 lb of lean tissue and a loss of 4.5 lb of fat tissue in weight lifters taking POWER BOOST. This looks convincing, but the results for the control group are not reported in the ad. When the results for the experimental group are compared to those for the control group, a different picture emerges. This comparison (see graph) shows that the control group gained almost as much lean mass and lost slightly more fat mass than the group taking POWER BOOST.

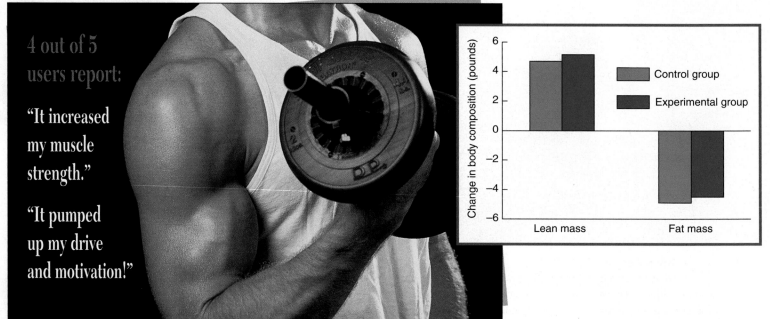

POWER BOOST

BOOST your STRENGTH • POWER up your DRIVE • MAXIMIZE your MASS

4 out of 5 users report:

"It increased my muscle strength."

"It pumped up my drive and motivation!"

POWER BOOST

Years of research were needed to develop this special nutritional formulation. Just mix with water and drink one shake with every meal or snack.

In a university study, 25 experienced weight lifters consumed one POWER BOOST shake at meals and snacks, 5 times a day for 4 weeks.

Lean body mass and fat mass were measured by underwater weighing before the study began and after 4 weeks of training while taking POWER BOOST.

RESULTS
The weight lifters gained an average of 5.2 lbs of lean muscle and lost 4.5 pounds of unwanted fat.

Think Critically Based on the information in the graph, explain why you would or would not recommend this product.

Judging for Yourself

Not everything you hear is accurate. Because much of the nutrition information we encounter is intended to sell products, that information may be embellished to make it more appealing. Understanding the principles scientists use to perform nutrition studies can help consumers judge the nutrition information they encounter in their daily lives (see *What a Scientist Sees*). Some things that may tip you off to misinformation are claims that sound too good to be true, information from unreliable sources, information intended to sell a product, and information that is new or untested.

Let's now look at questions that can help you evaluate any piece of nutrition information you encounter.

Does it make sense? Some claims are too outrageous to be true. For example, if a product claims to increase your muscle size without any exercise or decrease your weight without a change in diet, common sense should tell you that the claim is too good to be true. In contrast, an article that tells you that adding exercise to your daily routine will help you lose weight and increase your stamina is not so outrageous.

What's the source? If a claim seems reasonable, find out where it came from. Personal testimonies are not a reliable source (**Figure 1.12**), but government recommendations regarding healthy dietary practices and information disseminated by universities generally are. Government recommendations are developed by committees of scientists who interpret the latest well-conducted research studies and use their conclusions to develop recommendations for the population as a whole. The information is designed to improve the health of the population

Individual testimonies are not proof • Figure 1.12

Weight-loss product advertisements commonly show before-and-after photos of people who have successfully lost weight using the product. The success of such individuals is not a guarantee that the product they used will produce the same results for you or anyone else. These individuals' results are not compared to those for a control group or subjected to scientific evaluation. Therefore, it cannot be assumed that similar results will occur in other people.

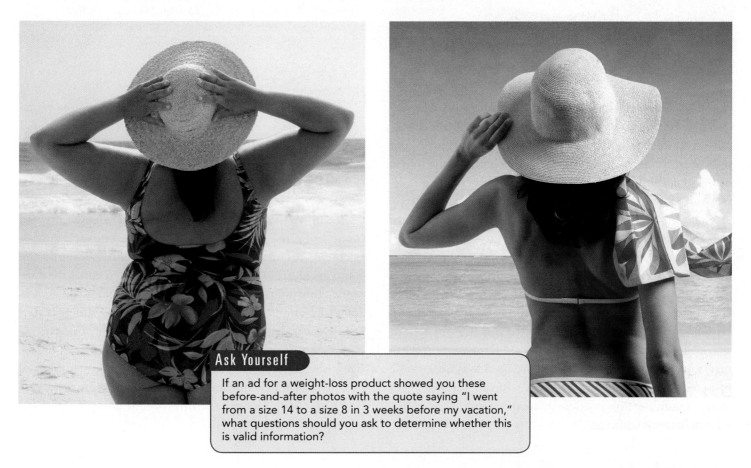

Ask Yourself

If an ad for a weight-loss product showed you these before-and-after photos with the quote saying "I went from a size 14 to a size 8 in 3 weeks before my vacation," what questions should you ask to determine whether this is valid information?

The Issue: Poor dietary habits in the United States have resulted in a largely unfit, unhealthy nation. Should we as individuals take responsibility for our diet and health, or should the government intervene?

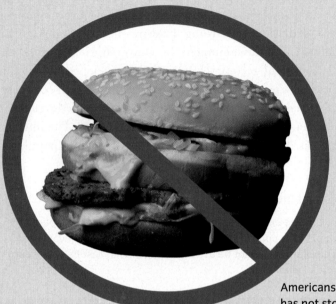

Americans want the personal freedom to choose what they eat, but that has not stopped people from blaming fast-food for their health problems.

The typical U.S. diet is not as healthy as it could be. Our lack of discretion has contributed to our high rates of obesity, diabetes, high blood pressure, and heart disease.[22] This is not only the concern of the individuals whose lives it affects but also the government. The dollar cost to our health care system is huge; half of the $147 billion per year the United States spends on obesity comes from government-funded Medicare and Medicaid. Government concern is not just financial. The fact that almost one in four applicants to the military is rejected for being overweight is suggested to be a threat to national security and military readiness.[28]

So, who is responsible for our unhealthy diet, and who should be responsible for changing what we eat? Proponents of more government involvement in our food choices suggest that our food environment is the cause of our unhealthy eating habits. Obesity expert Kelly Brownell believes that environment plays a more powerful role in determining food choices than does personal irresponsibility.[29] Brownell and other proponents of government intervention argue that the government should treat our noxious food environment like any other public

(See *Debate: How involved should the government be in your food choices?*). Information that comes from universities is supported by research studies that are well scrutinized and published in peer-reviewed journals. Many universities also provide information that targets the general public. Not-for-profit organizations such as the American Dietetic Association and the American Medical Association are also reliable sources of nutrition information.

If you are looking at an article in print or posted on a Web site, checking the author's credentials can help you evaluate the credibility of the information. Where does the author work? Does this person have a degree in nutrition or medicine? Although "nutritionists" and "nutrition counselors" may provide accurate information, these terms are not legally defined and are used by a wide range of people, from college professors with doctoral degrees from reputable universities to health food store clerks with no formal training.

One reliable source of nutrition information is registered dietitians (RDs). An RD is a nutrition professional who has earned a four-year college degree in a nutrition-related field and has met established criteria for certification to provide nutrition education and counseling.

Is it selling something? If a person or company will profit from the information presented, be wary. Advertisements are designed to increase product sales, and the company stands to profit if you believe the claims that are made. Information presented in newspapers and magazines and on television may also be biased or exaggerated because it is designed to help sell magazines or boost ratings, not necessarily to promote health and well-being. Even a well-designed, carefully executed study published in a peer-reviewed journal can be a source of misinformation if its results have been interpreted incorrectly or exaggerated (**Figure 1.13**).

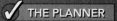

health threat and develop programs to keep us safe and healthy. Just as government regulations help to ensure that our food is not contaminated with harmful bacteria, laws could ensure that what you order at a restaurant will not contribute to heart disease or cancer. Unfortunately, unlike bacteria, individual foods are difficult to classify as healthy or unhealthy. Almost all food has some nutritional benefits, and the arguments as to what is a "junk food" and what we should add or subtract from our diets are ongoing. However, many people believe there are things that could be done to ensure healthier choices.

One option to encourage healthier choices suggested by proponents of government intervention is to tax junk food, making it more expensive, and increase subsidies for fruits and vegetables, making them less expensive. Other suggestions include zoning restrictions to keep fast-food restaurants away from schools and child-care facilities and limitations on the types of foods that can be advertised on children's television. All these ideas have pros and cons, and none will absolve individuals of the responsibility for getting more exercise and making healthier food choices.

Opponents of government involvement believe it is an infringement on personal freedom and suggest that individuals need to take responsibility for their actions. They propose that the food industry work with the public to make healthier food more available and affordable. Many food companies have already responded to the need for a better diet; General Mills and Kellogg's offer whole-grain cereals. And the giant food retailer Wal-Mart has announced a major campaign to make healthy food more affordable.

Our current food environment makes unhealthy eating easy. Opportunities for fatty, salty, and sweet foods are available 24/7, and the portions offered are often massive. To preserve our public health, the United States needs to change the way it eats. This change could be driven by government regulations and taxes, it could come from changes in the food industry, or it could come from individuals taking more responsibility for their choices and their health. A synergy of policy intervention, industry cooperation, and personal efforts is likely needed to solve the crisis.

Think critically: If someone eats fast-food daily and becomes obese, is that person to blame for eating the food, or is the restaurant to blame for not informing the person of the health risks?

Results may be misinterpreted in order to sell products • Figure 1.13

These rats, which were given large doses of vitamin E, lived longer than rats that consumed less vitamin E. Does this mean that dietary supplements of vitamin E will increase longevity in people? Not necessarily. The results of animal studies can't always be extrapolated to humans, but they are often the basis of claims in ads for dietary supplements.

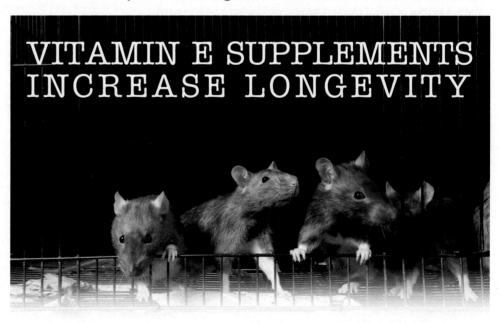

VITAMIN E SUPPLEMENTS INCREASE LONGEVITY

Has it stood the test of time? Often the results of new scientific studies are on the news the same day they are presented at a meeting or published in a peer-reviewed journal. However, a single study cannot serve as a basis for a reliable theory. Results need to be reproduced and supported numerous times before they can be used as a foundation for nutrition recommendations.

Headlines based on a single study should therefore be viewed skeptically. The information may be accurate, but there is no way to know because there has not been enough time to repeat the work and reaffirm the conclusions. If, for example, someone has found the secret to easy weight loss, you will undoubtedly encounter this information again at some later time if the finding is valid. If the finding is not valid, it will fade away with all the other weight-loss concoctions that have come and gone.

CONCEPT CHECK   STOP

1. **What** is the difference between a hypothesis and a theory?

2. **How** is epidemiology used to study nutrition?

3. **Why** are control groups important in any scientific experiment?

4. **Why** is information in advertisements likely to be exaggerated or inaccurate?

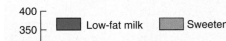 THE PLANNER

Summary

1 Food Choices and Nutrient Intake   4

- The foods you choose determine which **nutrients** you consume. Choosing foods that are high in **nutrient density** allows you to obtain more nutrients in fewer calories, as shown in this graph. Fortified foods, or foods to which nutrients have been added, and **dietary supplements** can also contribute nutrients to the diet.

Nutrient density • Figure 1.1a

[Bar graph: "Amount per cup" (y-axis, 0 to 400) vs. categories Calories, Calcium (mg), Vitamin D (IU), Vitamin A (µg). Legend: Low-fat milk, Sweetened iced tea]

- Food contains not only nutrients but also nonnutritive substances, such as **phytochemicals**, that may provide additional health benefits. Foods that provide health benefits beyond basic nutrition are called **functional foods**. Some foods are naturally functional and others are made functional through fortification.

- The food choices we make are affected by many factors other than nutrition, including food availability; what we learn to eat from family, culture, and traditions; personal tastes; and what we think we should eat to maintain health.

2 Nutrients and Their Functions   8

- Nutrients are grouped into six classes. **Carbohydrates**, **lipids**, **proteins**, and water are referred to as **macronutrients** because they are needed in large amounts. **Vitamins** and **minerals** are **micronutrients** because they are needed in small amounts to maintain health.

- Carbohydrates, lipids, and proteins are nutrients that provide energy, typically measured in **calories**. Lipids, proteins, carbohydrates, minerals, and water perform structural roles, as shown, forming and maintaining the structure of our bodies. All six classes of nutrients help regulate body processes. The energy, structure, and regulation provided by nutrients are needed for growth, maintenance and repair of the body, and reproduction.

Nutrient functions • Figure 1.5b

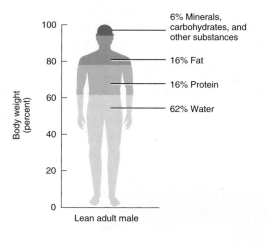

- 6% Minerals, carbohydrates, and other substances
- 16% Fat
- 16% Protein
- 62% Water

Lean adult male

3 Nutrition in Health and Disease 11

- Your diet affects your health. The foods you choose contain the nutrients needed to keep you alive and healthy and prevent **malnutrition**. **Undernutrition** results from consuming too few calories and/or too few nutrients. **Overnutrition** can result from a toxic dose of a nutrient or from a chronic excess of nutrients or calories, which over time contributes to chronic diseases, such as those shown in this graph.

Overnutrition • Figure 1.7

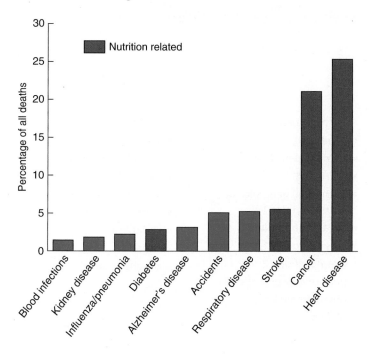

Nutrition related

Percentage of all deaths

Blood infections, Kidney disease, Influenza/pneumonia, Diabetes, Alzheimer's disease, Accidents, Respiratory disease, Stroke, Cancer, Heart disease

- The diet you consume can affect your genetic predisposition for developing a variety of chronic diseases.

4 Choosing a Healthy Diet 13

- A healthy diet includes a variety of nutrient-dense foods from the different food groups as well as a variety of foods from within each group. Variety is important because different foods provide different nutrients and health-promoting substances as well as a variety of tastes.

- Balance means mixing and matching foods and meals in order to obtain enough of the nutrients you need and not too much of the ones that can potentially harm your health. Extra calories you consume during the day can be balanced by increasing the calories you burn in physical activity, as shown.

Balance calories in with calories out • Figure 1.9

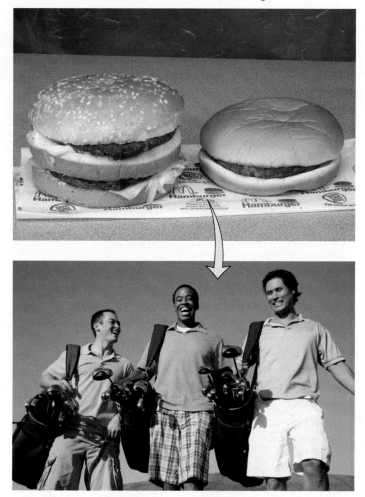

- Moderation means not ingesting too many calories or too much fat, sugar, salt, or alcohol. Eating moderate portions helps you maintain a healthy weight and helps prevent chronic diseases such as heart disease and cancer.

5 Evaluating Nutrition Information   16

• Nutrition uses the **scientific method** to study the relationships among food, nutrients, and health. The scientific method, illustrated here, involves observing and questioning natural events, formulating **hypotheses** to explain these events, designing and performing experiments to test the hypotheses, and developing **theories** that explain the observed phenomena based on the experimental results.

• To be valid, a nutrition experiment must provide quantifiable measurements, study the right type and number of subjects, and use appropriate **control groups**. When a study has been completed, the results must be interpreted fairly and accurately. The **peer-review process** ensures that studies published in professional journals adhere to a high standard of experimental design and interpretation of results.

• Not all the nutrition information we encounter is accurate. The first step in deciding whether a nutritional claim is valid is to ask whether the claim makes sense. If it sounds too good to be true, it probably is. It is also important to determine whether the information came from a reliable source, whether it is trying to sell a product, and whether it has been confirmed by multiple studies.

The scientific method • Figure 1.10

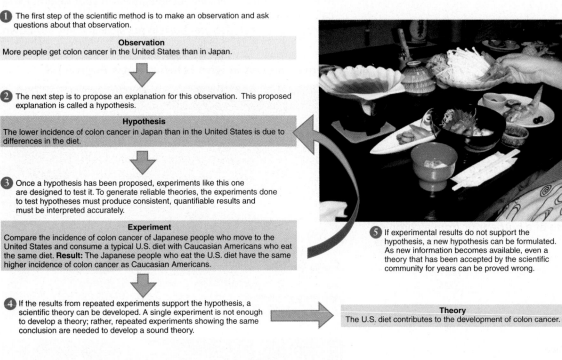

1 The first step of the scientific method is to make an observation and ask questions about that observation.

Observation
More people get colon cancer in the United States than in Japan.

2 The next step is to propose an explanation for this observation. This proposed explanation is called a hypothesis.

Hypothesis
The lower incidence of colon cancer in Japan than in the United States is due to differences in the diet.

3 Once a hypothesis has been proposed, experiments like this one are designed to test it. To generate reliable theories, the experiments done to test hypotheses must produce consistent, quantifiable results and must be interpreted accurately.

Experiment
Compare the incidence of colon cancer of Japanese people who move to the United States and consume a typical U.S. diet with Caucasian Americans who eat the same diet. **Result:** The Japanese people who eat the U.S. diet have the same higher incidence of colon cancer as Caucasian Americans.

4 If the results from repeated experiments support the hypothesis, a scientific theory can be developed. A single experiment is not enough to develop a theory; rather, repeated experiments showing the same conclusion are needed to develop a sound theory.

5 If experimental results do not support the hypothesis, a new hypothesis can be formulated. As new information becomes available, even a theory that has been accepted by the scientific community for years can be proved wrong.

Theory
The U.S. diet contributes to the development of colon cancer.

Key Terms

- amino acid 8
- calorie 4
- carbohydrates 8
- cholesterol 8
- control group 18
- designer food or nutraceutical 7
- dietary supplement 5
- element 8
- energy-yielding nutrient 8
- epidemiology 18
- essential nutrient 4

- evidence-based practice 18
- experimental group 18
- fiber 8
- fortification 5
- functional food 6
- genes 12
- hormone 11
- hypothesis 17
- kilocalorie 8
- lipids 8
- macronutrient 8
- malnutrition 11

- micronutrient 8
- mineral 8
- nutrient density 4
- nutrient 4
- nutritional genomics or nutrigenomics 13
- organic compound 8
- osteoporosis 11
- overnutrition 12
- peer-review process 18
- phytochemical 5
- placebo 18

- protein 8
- saturated fat 8
- scientific method 17
- theory 17
- undernutrition 11
- unsaturated fat 8
- variable 18
- vitamin 8
- zoochemical 5

Online Resources

- To learn more about healthy food choices, go to www.nutrition.gov and click on Shopping, Cooking, and Meal Planning.

- To learn more about nutrients in health and disease, go to www.mayohealth.org.

- To learn more about choosing a healthy diet, go to www.cdc.gov/healthyweight/healthy_eating/index.html.

- To learn more about evidence-based nutrition information, go to www.adaevidencelibrary.com/default.cfm?library=EBG.

- Visit your *WileyPLUS* site for videos, animations, podcasts, self-study, and other media that will aid you in studying and understanding this chapter.

Critical and Creative Thinking Questions

1. Zach eats in the dorm cafeteria. He has a banana and a glass of orange juice for breakfast and potatoes or corn for dinner every day, but he doesn't eat any other fruits or vegetables. How could his choices be improved? Why is such an improvement important?

2. A typical fast-food meal consists of a cheeseburger, French fries, and a soft drink. Use iProfile or the *Nutrient Composition of Foods* booklet to calculate the calories in this meal. How long would a person of your gender, height, and weight need to jog to burn off the calories in this meal?

3. A NASA space probe finds life on a distant planet. An analysis of the food supply for these organisms reveals three classes of nutrients, which NASA names vital A, nutrion, and essential S. The table below shows the amounts of these nutrients in the food supply and the amounts in the organisms' bodies. Based on these data, predict whether each nutrient provides energy, structure, or regulation for these organisms. Explain your answers.

4. Which type of malnutrition—overnutrition or undernutrition—is most common in the United States today? Why?

5. A nutrition student observes that people who skip breakfast tend to be overweight more often than people who eat breakfast every day. He hypothesizes that people who skip breakfast get hungry later in the day and overeat, actually consuming more total calories in a day than people who eat breakfast. Propose an experiment that might be used to test this hypothesis.

6. Look up an advertisement for a dietary supplement on the Internet. What nutrients does the supplement contain? Does it contain substances that are not nutrients? Do you think this dietary supplement is worth the money? Why or why not?

Nutrient class	Amount in the food supply	Amount in the body
Vital A	65%	Less than 1%
Nutrion	15%	45%
Essential S	Less than 1%	Less than 1%

What is happening in this picture?

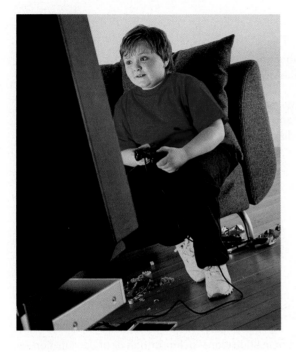

Instead of playing basketball and hide-and-seek like American kids a generation ago, this boy is sitting in front of the television snacking and playing video games.

Think Critically

1. What impact do you think this lifestyle change has had on the balance between food intake and activity?
2. How have video games impacted the incidence of childhood obesity?
3. Do you think active video games (such as Wii games) will help American children increase their activity level?

Self-Test

(Check your answers in Appendix K.)

1. True or false: If you choose a high-fat, high-salt fast-food lunch, your nutrient intake for the day cannot meet the recommendations for a healthy diet.

   a. True   b. False

2. Which of these foods has the lowest nutrient density?

   a. an orange   c. whole-wheat bread

   b. strawberry yogurt   d. orange soda

3. This graph indicates that _____.

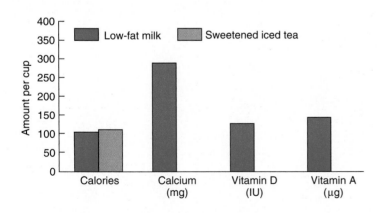

a. low-fat milk contains more calcium per calorie than iced tea

b. low-fat milk is a poor source of calcium

c. iced tea is more nutrient dense than milk

d. low-fat milk has less vitamin D per calorie than iced tea

4. Which group consists only of nutrients that are classified as energy-yielding nutrients?

   a. vitamins and minerals

   b. carbohydrates, lipids, and proteins

   c. lipids, carbohydrates, proteins, and water

   d. carbohydrates and vitamins

5. Which group consists only of nutrients that are considered micronutrients?

   a. protein and water

   b. carbohydrates, lipids, and proteins

   c. vitamins and minerals

   d. minerals and water

6. Which nutrient class provides the most calories per gram?

   a. carbohydrates   c. lipids

   b. proteins   d. vitamins

7. Based on this illustration, which nutrient class makes up the greatest proportion of body weight?

   a. protein

   b. carbohydrate

   c. fat

   d. water

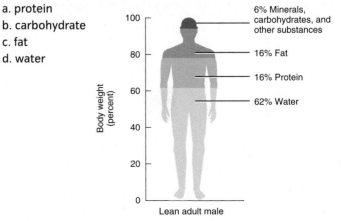

8. Which of these statements about essential nutrients is false?

   a. If you do not get enough of them in your diet, your body will synthesize enough to meet its needs.

   b. If you do not get enough of them in your diet, deficiency symptoms will eventually appear.

   c. Some of them provide energy.

   d. Some of them provide structure.

9. Why it is better to obtain your vitamins and minerals from foods than from dietary supplements?

   a. Dietary supplements are more likely to contain toxic amounts of nutrients.

   b. Foods provide a greater variety of phytochemicals and zoochemicals.

   c. Foods provide pleasurable tastes and aromas.

   d. All of the above are correct.

10. Which of these factors can limit the availability of food?

    a. socioeconomic status

    b. health status

    c. living conditions

    d. All of the above are correct.

11. A diet that follows the principles of variety, balance, and moderation _____.

    a. can include all kinds of foods

    b. includes only foods that have high nutrient density

    c. includes exactly the right amount of each nutrient each day

    d. includes only unprocessed foods

12. Which of these sources would be most likely to exaggerate the beneficial effects of a dietary supplement?

    a. a government publication

    b. a dietitian's recommendations

    c. a pamphlet published by the supplement manufacturer

    d. a peer-reviewed article in a scientific journal

13. When the scientific method is used, a hypothesis is first proposed and then tested through experimentation. Which of the following hypotheses can be tested by means of experiments that use a quantifiable measure?

    a. Iron supplements increase feelings of vitality.

    b. A high vitamin E intake makes you feel younger.

    c. Eating an apple a day will lower blood cholesterol.

    d. B vitamin supplements give you an energy boost.

14. The information in this graph was collected in an epidemiological study. Which of the following statements is true?*

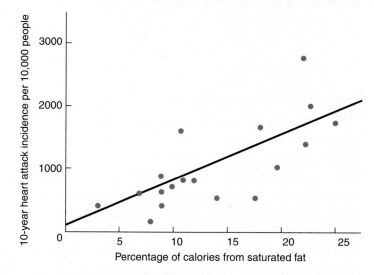

    a. A diet that is high in saturated fat causes heart disease.

    b. A higher incidence of heart attacks is associated with a higher intake of saturated fat.

    c. People who lower their intake of saturated fat will have fewer heart attacks.

    d. Moving to a country with less heart disease will lower your intake of saturated fat.

15. In a scientific experiment, a group that is identical to the experimental group in every way except that its members do not receive the treatment being tested is called _____.

    a. a control group

    b. a placebo

    c. a variable

    d. an alternative group

THE PLANNER ✓

Review your Chapter Planner on the chapter opener and check off your completed work.

Guidelines for a Healthy Diet

"What you don't know could kill you" may have been the first nutrition recommendation. To swallow the wrong berry or gulp down water from a suspect source could have been fatal to early humans. Such lessons served as anecdotal guideposts to survival. As societies developed, dietary cautions turned into taboos, sometimes laws, and ultimately, nutrition recommendations.

Governments have been providing what we would call modern nutrition information for the past 150 years. As the Industrial Revolution swept through Great Britain, urban populations—and poverty and hunger—swelled. To ensure a healthy workforce, the British government developed minimum dietary guidelines utilizing the cheapest foods. It wasn't until World War I that the British Royal Society determined that a healthy workforce required a healthy diet—not necessarily the cheapest. So fruits, vegetables, and milk became elements of nutritional guidance. Since then, virtually every nation has sought to establish dietary standards for its citizens.

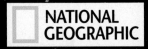

Today, modern public health agencies provide valuable information regarding healthy food choices. However, this information isn't always understood or used properly. As portion sizes grow, so do waistlines—and the attendant health concerns. "What you don't know could kill you" remains as vital an admonition today as it was 40,000 years ago.

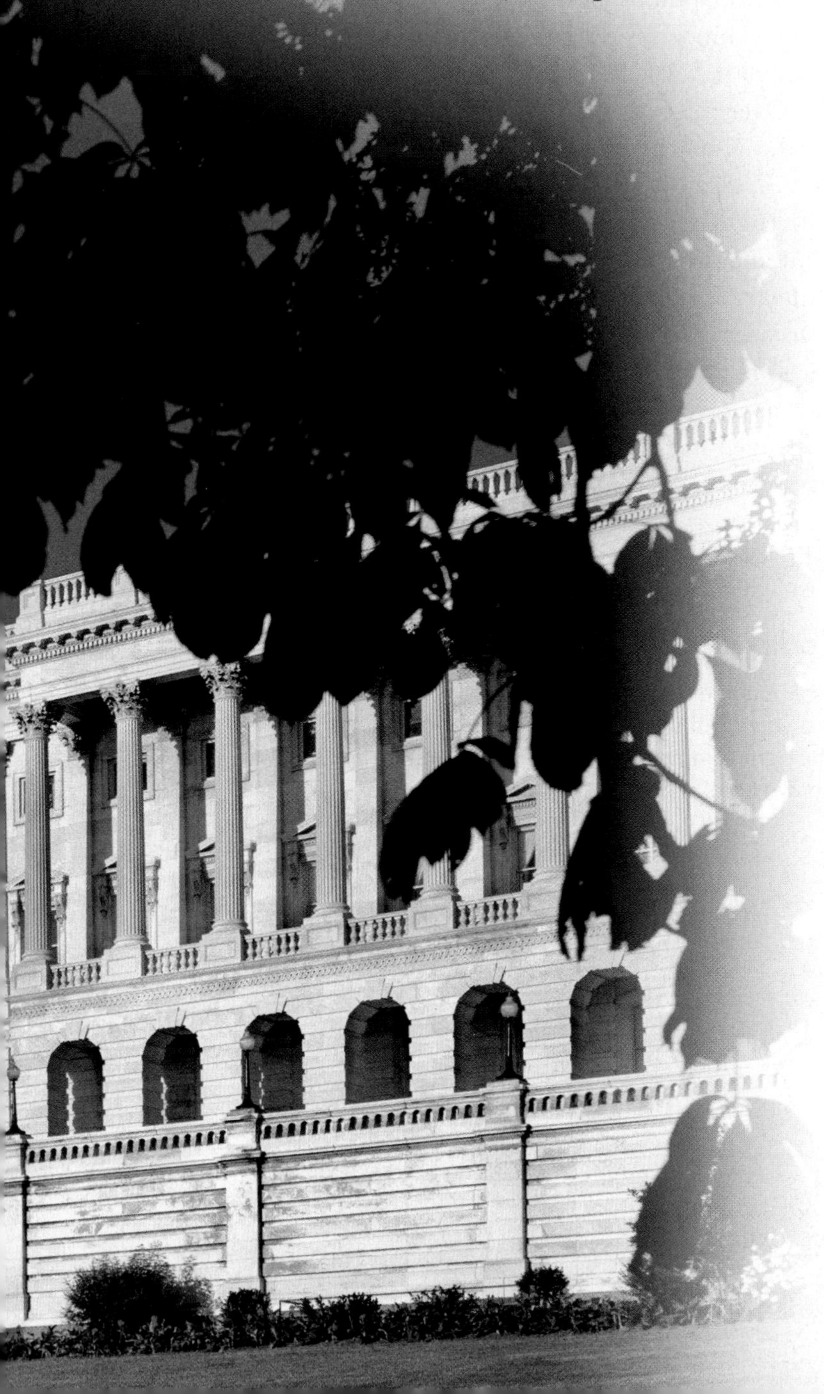

CHAPTER OUTLINE

CHAPTER PLANNER ✔

- ❑ Stimulate your interest by reading the introduction and looking at the visual.
- ❑ Scan the Learning Objectives in each section:
  p. 32 ❑   p. 38 ❑   p. 40 ❑   p. 49 ❑
- ❑ Read the text and study all figures and visuals. Answer any questions.

Analyze key features

- ❑ What a Scientist Sees, p. 33 ❑
- ❑ Process Diagram, p. 34 ❑
- ❑ Nutrition InSight, p. 42 ❑   p. 45 ❑   p. 50 ❑
- ❑ Thinking It Through, p. 52 ❑
- ❑ Stop: Answer the Concept Checks before you go on:
  p. 36 ❑   p. 39 ❑   p. 49 ❑   p. 55 ❑

End of chapter

- ❑ Review the Summary, Key Terms, and Online Resources.
- ❑ Answer the Critical and Creative Thinking Questions.
- ❑ Answer What is happening in this picture?
- ❑ Complete the Self-Test and check your answers.

Nutrition Recommendations

LEARNING OBJECTIVES

1. **Explain** the purpose of government nutrition recommendations.
2. **Discuss** how U.S. nutrition recommendations have changed over the past 100 years.
3. **Describe** how nutrition recommendations are used to evaluate nutritional status and set public health policy.

W hat should we be eating if we want to satisfy our nutrient needs? Our taste buds, food marketers and advertisers, and magazine and newspaper headlines all influence our choices. These choices may not always be healthy ones, however. Our taste buds respond to flavor and sensation, not necessarily to sensible nutrition; manufacturers want to sell products; and magazines want to sell subscriptions. Government recommendations, on the other hand, are designed with individual health as well as public health in mind. They can be used to plan diets and to evaluate what we are eating, both as individuals and as a nation.

Past and Present U.S. Recommendations

The federal government has been in the business of making nutritional recommendations for over 100 years. These recommendations have changed over time as our food intake patterns have changed and our knowledge of what constitutes a healthy diet has evolved.

The first dietary recommendations in the United States, published in 1894 by the U.S. Department of Agriculture (USDA), suggested amounts of protein, carbohydrate, fat, and "mineral matter" needed to keep Americans healthy.[1] At the time, specific vitamins and minerals essential for health had not been identified; nevertheless, this work set the stage for the development of the first **food guides**. Food guides are used to translate nutrient-intake recommendations into food choices (**Figure 2.1**). The food guide *How to Select Foods*, released in 1917, made recommendations based on five food groups: meat and milk, cereals, vegetables and fruit, fats and fatty foods, and sugars and sugary foods.

In the early 1940s, as the United States entered World War II, the Food and Nutrition Board was established to advise the Army and other federal agencies regarding problems related to food and the nutritional health of the armed forces and the general population. The Food and Nutrition Board developed the first set of recommendations for specific amounts of nutrients. These came to be known as the Recommended Dietary Allowances (RDAs). The original RDAs made recommendations on amounts of energy and on specific nutrients that were most likely to be deficient in people's diets—protein, iron, calcium, vitamins A and D, thiamin, riboflavin, niacin, and vitamin C. Recommended intakes were based on amounts that would prevent nutrient deficiencies.

Over the years since those first standards were developed, dietary habits and disease patterns have changed, and dietary recommendations have had to change along with them. Overt nutrient deficiencies are now rare in the United States, but the incidence of chronic diseases, such as heart disease, diabetes, osteoporosis, and obesity, has increased. To combat these more recent health concerns, recommendations are now intended to promote health as well as prevent deficiencies. The original RDAs have been expanded into the Dietary Reference Intakes, which address problems of excess as well as deficiency. The *Dietary Guidelines for Americans*, introduced in 1980 to make diet and lifestyle recommendations that promote health and

Today's Food Guide • Figure 2.1

How food guides present recommendations has changed over the years, but the basic message has stayed the same: Choose the right combinations of foods to promote health. MyPlate, shown here, is the latest food guide.

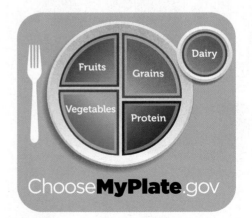

WHAT A SCIENTIST SEES

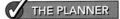

Trends in Milk Consumption

The graph below shows estimates of milk consumption in the United States from 1910 to 2005, based on the amount of milk available for human consumption during that period.[3,4] Anyone looking at the graph can tell that overall milk consumption and consumption of whole milk both declined, while consumption of lower-fat milks increased. A nutrition scientist looking at this graph, however, would see not just changes in the amounts and types of milk consumed but the nutritional and public health implications of these changes as well.

Because whole milk is high in saturated fat, replacing whole milk with lower-fat milk decreases saturated fat intake. This is good from the standpoint of heart health, but the decline in total milk consumption may be bad for bone health. Milk is one of the most important sources of calcium in the North American diet. The scientist will be alerted to the fact that calcium intake from milk has been declining. Unless more calcium from other sources is being consumed, this drop in milk consumption may indicate that the population is at risk for fragile bones and an increase in fractures.

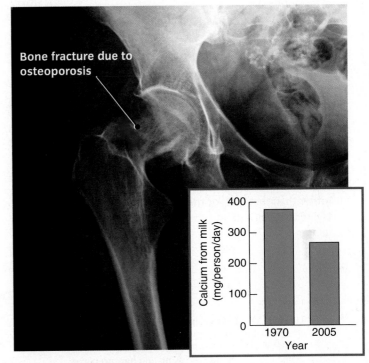

Bone fracture due to osteoporosis

This bar graph compares the amount of calcium available from milk in 1970 and 2005. If the decrease is indicative of overall calcium intake, it could contribute to an increase in the risk of bone fractures such as the one shown here.

Think Critically Based on this analysis, what kinds of measures would you suggest to increase the population's calcium intake?

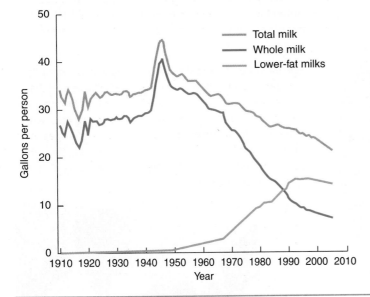

---

reduce the risks of obesity and chronic disease, have been revised every 5 years.[2] Early food guides have evolved into *MyPlate*, which suggests amounts and types of food from five food groups to meet the recommendations of the Dietary Guidelines (see Figure 2.1). In addition, standardized food labels have been developed to help consumers choose foods that meet these recommendations.

How We Use Nutrition Recommendations

Nutrition recommendations are developed to address the nutritional concerns of the population and help individuals meet their nutrient needs. These recommendations can also be used to evaluate the nutrient intake of populations and of individuals within populations (see *What a Scientist Sees*). Determining what people eat and how their nutrient intake compares to nutrition recommendations is important for assessing their **nutritional status**.

When evaluating the nutritional status of a population, food intake can be assessed by having individuals track their food intake or by using information about the amounts and types of food available to the population to identify trends in the diet.

> **nutritional status**
> An individual's health, as it is influenced by the intake and utilization of nutrients.

Assessing nutritional status • Figure 2.2

A complete assessment of an individual's nutritional status includes a diet analysis, a physical exam, a medical history, and an evaluation of nutrient levels in the body. An interpretation of this information can determine whether an individual is well nourished, malnourished, or at risk of malnutrition.

1 **Determine typical food intake.** People's typical food intake can be evaluated by having them record their food as they consume it or recall what they have eaten during the past day or so. Because food intake varies from day to day, to obtain a realistic picture, an individual's intake should be monitored for more than one day. An accurate food record includes the amounts of all foods and beverages consumed, along with descriptions of cooking methods and brand names of products. It is often difficult to obtain an accurate record because people may change what they are eating rather than record it, or they may forget what they ate when trying to recall it.

2 **Analyze nutrient intake.** A quick diet analysis can be done by comparing an individual's food intake to the recommendations of a food guide. A more thorough analysis can be done by using a computer program that compares nutrient intake to recommendations. In this example, which shows only a few nutrients, intake of vitamin A, iron, and calcium is below the recommended amounts, and intake of vitamin C and saturated fat is above the recommended amounts.

Nutrient	Percent of recommendation 0% 50% 100%
Vitamin A	75%
Vitamin C	115%
Iron	54%
Calcium	75%
Saturated fat	134%

FOOD DIARY

Record all the food and beverages you eat. Include the food, how it was prepared, the amount you ate and the brand name. Don't forget to list all fats used in cooking and all spreads and sauces added.

Time	Food	Kind and how prepared	Amount
7:00 A.M.	Eggs	scrambled	2
	Butter	in eggs	1 tsp.
	toast	whole wheat	2 slices
	Butter	on toast	2 tsp.
	Milk	non-fat	8 oz.
	Orange juice	from frozen concentrate	8 oz.
12:00 P.M.	Big Mac	McDonald's	1

3 **Evaluate physical health.** A physical examination can detect signs of nutrient deficiencies or excesses. Measures of body dimensions such as height and weight can be monitored over time or compared with standards for a given population. Drastic changes in measurements or measurements that are significantly above or below the standards could indicate nutritional deficiency or excess.

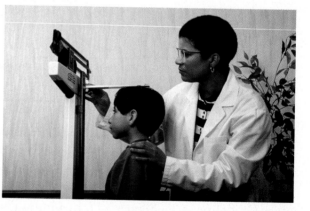

When food intake data are evaluated in conjunction with information about the health and nutritional status of individuals in the population (**Figure 2.2**), relationships between dietary intake and health and disease can be identified. This is important for developing public health measures that address nutritional problems. For example, population surveys such as the National Health and Nutrition Examination Survey (NHANES) helped public health officials recognize that low iron levels are a problem for many people, including young women, preschool children, and elderly people. This information led to the fortification of grain products with iron beginning in the 1940s.

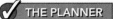

4 **Consider medical history and lifestyle.** Personal and family medical histories are important because genetic risk factors affect an individual's risk of developing a nutrition-related disease. For example, if you have high cholesterol and your father died of a heart attack at age 50, you have a higher-than-average risk of developing heart disease. Lifestyle factors such as physical activity level and eating habits can add to or reduce your inherited risk.

5 **Assess with laboratory tests.** Measures of nutrients, their by-products, or their functions in the blood, urine, and body cells can help detect nutrient deficiencies and excesses or the risk of nutrition-related chronic diseases (see Appendix B). For instance, levels of iron-carrying proteins in the blood can be used to determine whether a person has iron-deficiency anemia, and levels of blood cholesterol such as those shown here can provide information about an individual's risk of heart disease.

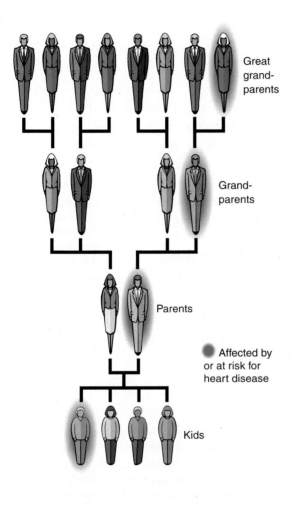

Great grand-parents

Grand-parents

Parents

● Affected by or at risk for heart disease

Kids

Blood Lipid Panel

Test	Result	Healthy range
Cholesterol, total	185 mg/dL	<200
Triglycerides	56 mg/dL	<150
HDL cholesterol	59 mg/dL	>40
LDL cholesterol, calculated	90 mg/dL	<100

Think Critically If a medical history reveals that one of your parents has had a heart attack, what other components of nutrition assessment would help you to determine your overall risk for heart disease? Why?

Recent NHANES data have also shown that the number of calories Americans consume per day has increased over the past few decades and that the incidence of obesity has increased dramatically during the same period. This has led public health experts to develop programs to improve both the diet and the fitness of Americans.

The information obtained from population health and nutrition surveys is also used to determine whether the nation is meeting health and nutrition goals, such as those established by *Healthy People*. This set of health-promotion and disease-prevention objectives is revised every 10 years, with the goal of increasing the quality and length of healthy lives for the population as a whole and eliminating health disparities among different segments of the population. The latest version of these objectives has been released as *Healthy People 2020*. The long-term goal is to create a social climate in which everyone has a chance to live long, healthy lives (see Appendix D).[5]

CONCEPT CHECK STOP

1. **How** do nutrition recommendations benefit individual and public health?
2. **Why** do the current DRIs focus on preventing chronic disease?
3. **What** factors are considered in evaluating nutritional status?

Dietary Reference Intakes (DRIs)

LEARNING OBJECTIVES

1. **Summarize** the purpose of the DRIs.
2. **Describe** the four sets of DRI values used in recommending nutrient intake.
3. **List** the factors that are considered when estimating an individual's energy needs (EERs).
4. **Define** the concept of the Acceptable Macronutrient Distribution Ranges (AMDRs).

he **Dietary Reference Intakes (DRIs)** are recommendations for the amounts of energy, nutrients, and other food components that healthy people should consume in order to stay healthy, reduce the risk of chronic disease, and prevent deficiencies.[6] The DRIs can be used to evaluate whether a person's diet provides all the essential nutrients in adequate amounts. They include several types of recommendations that address both nutrient intake and energy intake and include values that are appropriate for people of different genders and stages of life (**Figure 2.3**).

Recommendations for Nutrient Intake

The DRI recommendations for nutrient intake include four sets of values. The **Estimated Average Requirements (EARs)** are

> **Estimated Average Requirements (EARs)** Nutrient intakes estimated to meet the needs of 50% of the healthy individuals in a given gender and life-stage group.

DRIs for all population groups • Figure 2.3

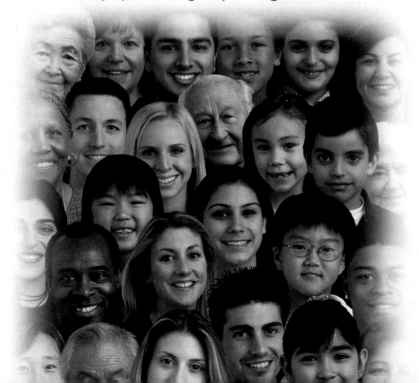

Because gender and life stage affect nutrient needs, Dietary Reference Intake values have been set for each gender and for various life-stage groups. These values take into account the physiological differences that affect the nutrient needs of men and women, infants, children, adolescents, adults, older adults, and pregnant and lactating women.

The EAR and RDA for a nutrient are determined by measuring the amount of the nutrient required by different individuals in a population group and plotting all the values. The resulting plot is a bell-shaped curve; a few individuals in the group need only a small amount of the nutrient, a few need a large amount, and the majority need an amount that falls between the extremes.

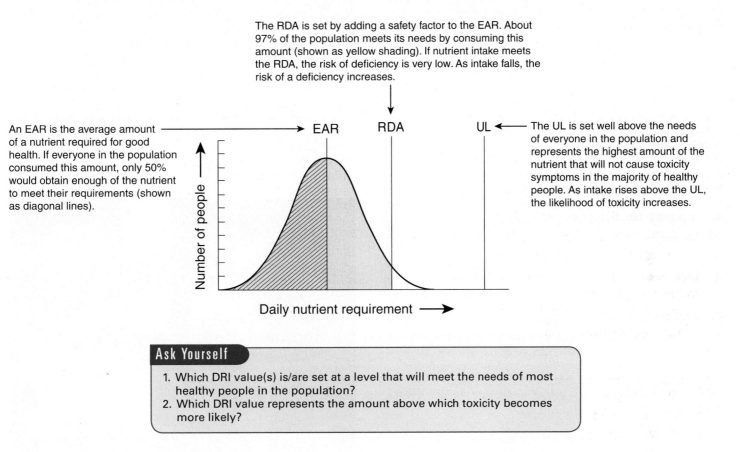

The RDA is set by adding a safety factor to the EAR. About 97% of the population meets its needs by consuming this amount (shown as yellow shading). If nutrient intake meets the RDA, the risk of deficiency is very low. As intake falls, the risk of a deficiency increases.

An EAR is the average amount of a nutrient required for good health. If everyone in the population consumed this amount, only 50% would obtain enough of the nutrient to meet their requirements (shown as diagonal lines).

The UL is set well above the needs of everyone in the population and represents the highest amount of the nutrient that will not cause toxicity symptoms in the majority of healthy people. As intake rises above the UL, the likelihood of toxicity increases.

Ask Yourself

1. Which DRI value(s) is/are set at a level that will meet the needs of most healthy people in the population?
2. Which DRI value represents the amount above which toxicity becomes more likely?

average amounts of nutrients or other dietary components required by healthy individuals in a population (**Figure 2.4**). They are used to assess the adequacy of a population's food supply or typical nutrient intake and are not appropriate for evaluating an individual's intake. The **Recommended Dietary Allowances (RDAs)** are set higher than the EARs and represent amounts of nutrients and other dietary components that will meet the needs of most healthy people (see Figure 2.4). When there aren't enough data about nutrient requirements to establish RDAs, **Adequate Intakes (AIs)**

Recommended Dietary Allowances (RDAs) Nutrient intakes that are sufficient to meet the needs of almost all healthy people in a specific gender and life-stage group.

are set, based on what healthy people typically eat. RDA or AI values can be used as goals for individual intake and to plan and evaluate individual diets (see Appendix A and the inside covers). They are meant to represent the amounts that most healthy people should consume, on average, over several days or even weeks, not each and every day. Because they are set high enough to meet the needs of almost all healthy people, intake below the RDA or AI does not necessarily mean that an individual is deficient, but the risk of deficiency is greater than if the individual consumed the recommended amount.

Adequate Intakes (AIs) Nutrient intakes that should be used as a goal when no RDA exists. AI values are an approximation of the nutrient intake that sustains health.

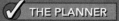
The Issue: Some foods, such as protein bars and energy drinks, are fortified with large amounts of nutrients. These foods add nutrients to the diet, but if eaten in large quantities or in combination with other highly fortified foods, they may pose a risk of toxicity. Are they a safe, healthy addition to your diet?

An orange, a tomato, a slice of bread, and a piece of grilled salmon—these are foods that are part of a healthy diet. What about an energy drink with 23 added vitamins and minerals, a protein bar with 100% of your daily vitamin requirements, soft drinks with Echinacea and green tea extract, fruit juice with added phytochemicals, and bottled water fortified with vitamin C? Are these products foods, or are they supplements?

One could argue that fortified protein bars and juices are foods, not supplements, because they provide calories like traditional foods, and the substances added to them, such as vitamin C, fish oil, or phytochemicals, are also naturally found in food. On the other hand, by definition, a supplement is a product intended to add nutrients or other substances to the diet, which these products certainly do. Does it matter if these supplemental substances come in a food or in a pill? Opponents of these foods would argue that it does because our decisions about eating foods are different than our decisions about supplements. Typically, we consider the dose when taking a supplement pill. But we eat to satisfy our sensory desires, fill our stomachs, and quench our thirsts. We don't think about whether the food or beverage might provide toxic amounts of nutrients.

In traditional foods, the amounts of nutrients are small, and the way they are combined limits absorption, making the risk of consuming a toxic amount of a nutrient almost nonexistent. In contrast, it is not difficult to swallow a very high dose of one or more nutrients from an excess of supplement pills or excessive servings of super-fortified foods. For example, if you drank your recommended 2 to 3 liters of fluid as water fortified with vitamin C, niacin, vitamin E, and vitamins B_6 and B_{12}, you would exceed the UL for these vitamins. Then if you also consume 2 cups of fortified breakfast cereal and 2 protein bars during the day, your risk of toxicity increases even more. The government labels these fortified products as foods, and we eat them like foods, but they may have the same toxicity risks as supplements.

Advocates of super-fortified foods point out that they add health-promoting substances to the diet. But do super-fortified foods provide the benefits that the original food would have? In some cases they do. For example, if you are getting your calcium from orange juice, studies show that you are getting just about as much calcium as you would from milk.[7] On the other hand, fish oil consumed in capsules does not have all the heart-health benefits of fish oil consumed in a piece of fish.[8]

So, are these products foods, or are they supplements? It is a fine line. Whether they are helpful or harmful depends on what is in them and how much you consume. Should the government get involved in regulating the amounts of nutrients that can be added to all foods? These answers depend on your view of the government's role in food regulation. Should we be gobbling them down without a thought? Probably not.

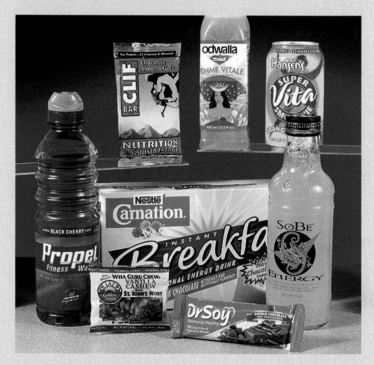

Think critically: Should foods fortified to levels above the RDA for one or more nutrients carry a consumer warning to avoid overconsumption?

> **Tolerable Upper Intake Levels (ULs)** Maximum daily intake levels that are unlikely to pose risks of adverse health effects to almost all individuals in a given gender and life-stage group.

The fourth set of values, **Tolerable Upper Intake Levels (ULs)**, specifies the maximum amount of a nutrient that most people can consume on a daily basis without some adverse effect (see Figure 2.4). For most nutrients, it is difficult to exceed the UL by consuming food. Most foods do not contain enough of any one nutrient to cause toxicity; however, some dietary supplements and fortified foods may (see *Debate: Super-Fortified Foods: Are They a Healthy Addition to Your Diet?*). For some nutrients, the UL is set for total intake from all sources, including food, fortified foods, and dietary supplements. For other nutrients, the UL refers to intake from supplements alone or from supplements and fortified foods. For many nutrients, there is no UL because too little information is available to determine it.

The right amount of energy from the right sources • Figure 2.5

a. Based on the EER calculation, a 19-year-old girl who is 5'4" tall, weighs 127 pounds, and gets no exercise needs about 1940 Calories a day. If she adds an hour of moderate activity to her daily routine, her EER will increase to by 460 Calories. She would need to eat an additional 460 Calories more per day to maintain her current weight.[6]

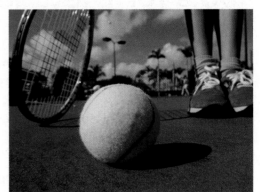

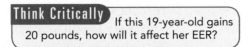

Think Critically If this 19-year-old gains 20 pounds, how will it affect her EER?

b. A healthy diet can include different proportions of carbohydrate, protein, and fat. These two plates show very different food combinations. Although only the meal on the left provides proportions of carbohydrate, protein, and fat that fall within the AMDRs, the meal on the right can still be part of a healthy diet if other meals are lower in protein and fat and higher in carbohydrate.

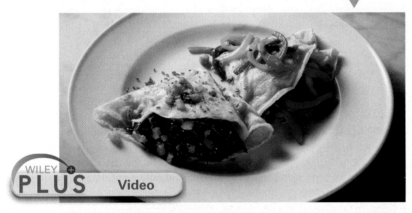

WILEY PLUS Video

This meal contains approximately 480 Calories, of which about 55% is from carbohydrate, 20% is from protein, and 25% is from fat.

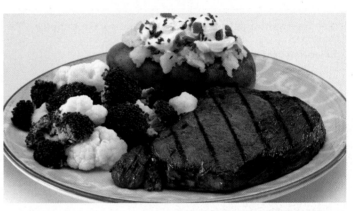

This meal contains approximately 740 Calories, of which about 30% is from carbohydrate, 35% is from protein, and 35% is from fat.

Recommendations for Energy Intake

The DRIs make two types of recommendations about energy intake. The first, called **Estimated Energy Requirements (EERs)**, provides an estimate of how many calories are needed to keep body weight stable. EER calculations take into account a person's age, gender, weight, height, and level of physical activity (see Appendix A). A change in any of these variables changes the person's energy needs (**Figure 2.5a**).

The second type of energy recommendation, called **Acceptable Macronutrient Distribution Ranges (AMDRs)**, makes recommendations about the proportions of calories that should come from carbohydrate, fat, and protein in a healthy diet. AMDRs are ranges—10 to 35% of calories from protein, 45 to 65% of calories from carbohydrate, and 20 to 35% of calories from fat—not exact values. This is because a wide range of macronutrient distributions is associated with health. AMDRs are intended to promote diets that minimize disease risk and allow flexibility in food intake patterns (**Figure 2.5b**).

Estimated Energy Requirements (EERs) Average energy intake values predicted to maintain body weight in healthy individuals.

Acceptable Macronutrient Distribution Ranges (AMDRs) Healthy ranges of intake for carbohydrate, fat, and protein, expressed as percentages of total energy intake.

CONCEPT CHECK STOP

1. **What** are RDAs and AIs used for?
2. **How** might you use ULs?
3. **What** are the five variables that affect your energy needs?
4. **Why** are AMDR values given as ranges rather than as single numbers?

Tools for Diet Planning

LEARNING OBJECTIVES

1. **Discuss** how following the recommendations of the Dietary Guidelines can help prevent chronic disease.
2. **Explain** how the Dietary Guidelines and My-Plate are related.
3. **Determine** your Daily Food Plan.
4. **Identify** foods that are high in empty calories.

he DRIs tell you how much of each nutrient you need, but they do not help you choose foods that will meet these needs. To help consumers choose diets that will meet their needs, the U.S. government has developed the *Dietary Guidelines for Americans* and *MyPlate*. The Dietary Guidelines are a set of diet and lifestyle recommendations designed to promote health and reduce the risk of overweight, obesity, and chronic diseases in the U.S. population.[2] **MyPlate** is the USDA's most recent food guide. It divides foods into groups, based on the nutrients they supply most abundantly,

---

Key Recommendation of the 2010 Dietary Guidelines[2]   Table 2.1

Balancing calories to manage weight

- Prevent and/or reduce overweight and obesity through improved eating and physical activity behaviors.
- Control total calorie intake to manage body weight. For people who are overweight or obese, this means consuming fewer calories from foods and beverages.
- Increase physical activity and reduce time spent in sedentary behaviors.
- Maintain appropriate calorie balance during each stage of life—childhood, adolescence, adulthood, pregnancy and breastfeeding, and older age.

Foods and nutrients to increase. Individuals should meet the following recommendations as part of a healthy eating pattern while staying within their calorie needs:

- Increase vegetable and fruit intake.
- Eat a variety of vegetables, especially dark-green and red and orange vegetables and beans and peas.
- Consume at least half of all grains as whole grains. Increase whole-grain intake by replacing refined grains with whole grains.
- Increase intake of fat-free or low-fat milk and milk products, such as milk, yogurt, cheese, or fortified soy beverages.
- Choose a variety of protein foods, including seafood, lean meat and poultry, eggs, beans and peas, soy products, and unsalted nuts and seeds.
- Increase the amount and variety of seafood consumed by choosing seafood in place of some meat and poultry.
- Replace protein foods that are higher in solid fats with choices that are lower in solid fats and calories and/or are sources of oils.
- Use oils to replace solid fats where possible.
- Choose foods that provide more potassium, dietary fiber, calcium, and vitamin D, which are nutrients of concern in U.S. diets. These foods include vegetables, fruits, whole grains, and milk and milk products.

Foods and food components to reduce

- Reduce daily sodium intake to less than 2300 milligrams (mg) and further reduce intake to 1500 mg among persons who are 51 and older and those of any age who are African American or have hypertension, diabetes, or chronic kidney disease. The 1500 mg recommendation applies to about half of the U.S. population, including children, and the majority of adults.
- Consume less than 10% of calories from saturated fatty acids by replacing them with monounsaturated and polyunsaturated fatty acids.
- Consume less than 300 mg per day of dietary cholesterol.
- Keep *trans* fatty acid consumption as low as possible by limiting foods that contain synthetic sources of *trans* fats, such as partially hydrogenated oils, and by limiting other solid fats.
- Reduce intake of calories from solid fats and added sugars.
- Limit consumption of foods that contain refined grains, especially refined grain foods that contain solid fats, added sugars, and sodium.
- If alcohol is consumed, consume it in moderation—up to one drink per day for women and two drinks per day for men—and only by adults of legal drinking age.

Building healthy eating patterns

- Select an eating pattern that meets nutrient needs over time at an appropriate calorie level.
- Account for all foods and beverages consumed and assess how they fit within a total healthy eating pattern.
- Follow food safety recommendations when preparing and eating foods to reduce the risk of food-borne illnesses.

---

and illustrates the appropriate proportions of foods from each food group that make up a healthy diet.

Recommendations of the *Dietary Guidelines for Americans*

The 2010 **Dietary Guidelines for Americans** provide evidence-based nutritional guidance to promote health and reduce the prevalence of overweight and obesity and the risk of chronic disease. The recommendations of this 7th edition of the *Dietary Guidelines for Americans* focus on balancing calorie intake with physical activity and consuming nutrient-dense foods and beverages (**Table 2.1**). These recommendations are designed for Americans 2 years of age and older. Additional recommendations target specific subpopulations (see Appendix D). Adopting the recommendations in the Dietary Guidelines will help Americans live healthier lives, which will lower health-care costs and help to strengthen America's long-term economic competitiveness and overall productivity.

Balancing calories to manage weight More Americans are overweight than ever before, and the numbers continue to grow. To address this problem, the 2010 Dietary Guidelines emphasize balancing the calories consumed in food and beverages with the calories expended through physical activity in order to achieve and maintain a healthy weight. Weight maintenance requires consuming the same number of calories as you burn; this means that if you eat more, you need to exercise more (see Chapter 9). Losing weight requires consuming fewer calories than you burn. This can be accomplished by reducing energy intake and increasing energy expenditure through exercise (**Figure 2.6**). The Dietary Guidelines recommend enjoying your food but eating less.

Foods and nutrients to increase The Dietary Guidelines recommend that we increase our vegetable and fruit intake to at least 2½ cups per day and improve our choices by selecting more fruits than fruit juices and eating a variety of vegetables, especially dark-green and red and orange

Healthy weight and exercise recommendations • Figure 2.6

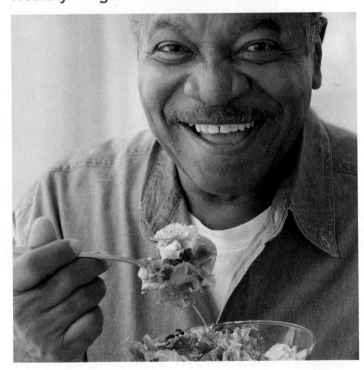

▲ **a.** To promote a healthy weight, the 2010 *Dietary Guidelines for Americans* recommend limiting portion sizes and reducing consumption of added sugars, solid fats, and alcohol, which provide calories but few essential nutrients. There is no optimal proportion of macronutrients that can facilitate weight loss or assist with maintaining weight loss; the critical issue is whether the eating pattern provides the number of calories needed to maintain or lose weight over time.

b. The Dietary Guidelines suggest that most Americans are in calorie imbalance, consuming more calories than they expend. To achieve calorie balance, adults should increase their weekly amount of aerobic physical activity gradually over time and decrease calorie intake to a point where they can achieve a healthy weight. To promote health and reduce disease risk, a minimum of 150 minutes of moderate exercise is recommended each week. Some adults will need a higher level of physical activity than others (the equivalent of more than 300 minutes of moderate-intensity activity) to ▼ achieve and maintain a healthy body weight.

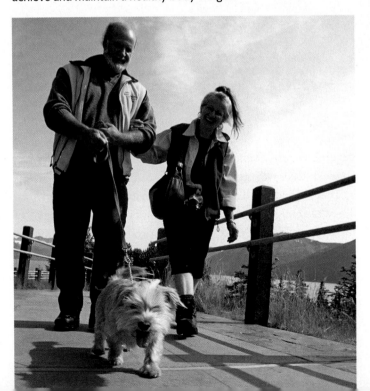

a. The current U.S. dietary pattern is not as healthy as it could be. The graph shown here compares the usual U.S. intake of selected foods and nutrients as a percentage of the recommended goal or limit.

b. The Dietary Guidelines for Americans suggest that there are many ways to choose a healthy diet, including the USDA Food Patterns, the DASH Eating Plan, and Mediterranean-style eating patterns. These patterns all focus on similar types of foods. (See Appendix D for more information.)

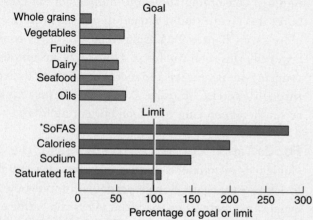

Percentage of goal or limit

*Calories from solid fats and added sugars

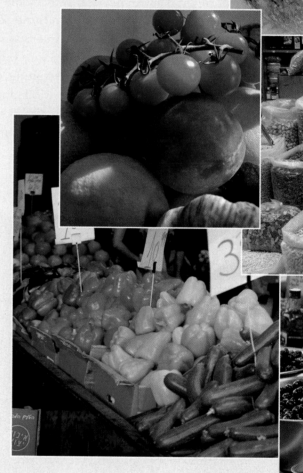

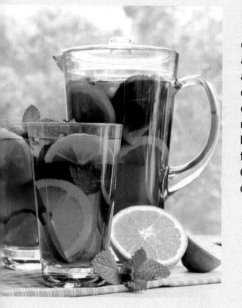

c. It is important to consider beverages as part of any healthy dietary pattern. Currently, American adults ages 19 years and older consume an average of about 400 Calories per day from beverages. Many of the most commonly consumed beverages, including regular sodas, fruit drinks, and alcoholic beverages, contain calories but provide few essential nutrients. The Dietary Guidelines recommend replacing sugary drinks with water.

vegetables and beans and peas. The Dietary Guidelines suggest that we replace refined grains with whole grains so that at least half of our grain servings are whole grains. They also suggest that Americans increase their intake of fat-free or low-fat milk and milk products, while limiting consumption of high-fat dairy products such as cheese. This pattern of fruit, vegetable, grain, and dairy consumption will increase our intake of potassium, dietary fiber, calcium, and vitamin D, which are nutrients of concern in American diets.

Protein choices should include a variety of protein foods, such as lean meat, poultry, seafood, eggs, beans and peas, soy products, and unsalted nuts and seeds. We should increase the variety and amount of seafood by choosing it in place of meat and poultry. The Dietary Guidelines also recommend that we use oils in place of solid fats when possible.

Foods and food components to reduce The Dietary Guidelines recommend reducing intake of

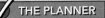

USDA Food Patterns

Food group	Amount/day
Vegetables	2.5 cups
Fruit and juices	2.0 cups
Grains	6.0 ounces
Dairy products	3.0 cups
Protein foods	5.5 ounces
Oils	27 grams
Solid fats	16 grams
Added sugars	32 grams

The USDA Food Patterns suggest amounts of foods from different food groups and subgroups for different calories levels (2000 Calories shown here). The USDA Food Patterns and their vegetarian variations (see Appendix D and Chapter 6) were developed to help individuals follow the Dietary Guidelines recommendations and are the basis for the MyPlate recommendations.

The DASH Eating Plan

Food group	#Servings
Grains	6–8/day
Vegetables	4–5/day
Fruits	4–5/day
Fat-free or low-fat milk and milk products	2–3/day
Lean meats, poultry, and fish	6 or less/day
Nuts, seeds, and legumes	4–5/week
Fat and oils	2–3/day
Sweets and added sugars	5 or less/week

The DASH Eating Plan focuses on increasing foods rich in potassium, calcium, magnesium, protein, and fiber. It is plentiful in fruits and vegetables, whole grains, low-fat dairy, fish, poultry, seeds, and nuts. It was first developed for lowering blood pressure and is discussed further in Chapter 8.

Traditional Mediterranean eating patterns are based on fruits, vegetables, grains, olive oil, beans, nuts, legumes, and seeds. They include moderate portions of cheese and yogurt. Fish and seafood are consumed at least twice a week; poultry and eggs every few days; and red meat and sweets less often. The incidence of chronic diseases such as heart disease is low in populations consuming this diet (see Chapter 5).

Mediterranean Eating Pattern

Foods	How often
Fruits, vegetables, grains (mostly whole), olive oil, nuts, legumes and seeds, herbs and spices	Every meal
Fish and seafood	At least twice a week
Cheese and yogurt	Moderate portions daily or weekly
Poultry and eggs	Moderate portions every 2 days or weekly
Meats and sweets	Less often

saturated fat, *trans* fat, and cholesterol—the types of lipids that increase the risk of heart disease (see Chapter 5). In order to prevent high blood pressure, the Dietary Guidelines recommend limiting sodium intake to less than 2300 mg/day. Those who are 51 and older, and those of any age who are African American or have hypertension, diabetes, or chronic kidney disease should limit sodium to less than 1500 mg/day. They also recommend that Americans reduce their intake of solid fats, added sugars, and refined grains, and consume alcohol only in moderation.

Building healthy eating patterns There is no single diet that defines healthy. Rather, there are a variety of healthy eating patterns that can accommodate differences in cultural, ethnic, traditional, and personal preferences and differences in food cost and availability (**Figure 2.7**). All these patterns are abundant in nutrient-dense foods, including vegetables, fruits, and whole grains; include moderate amounts of a variety of high-protein foods; and are low in full-fat dairy products. Healthy eating patterns include more oils than solid fats and limit added sugars and sodium. The Dietary Guidelines for Americans discuss three healthy eating patterns. There are also other dietary patterns that promote health. The Healthy Eating Pyramid in Figure 2.8 is a healthy dietary pattern developed by the Harvard School of Public Health (**Figure 2.8**).

A fundamental premise of the Dietary Guidelines is that nutrients should come primarily from foods; supplements and fortified foods may be advantageous in specific situations to increase intake of a specific vitamin or mineral. Fortification can provide a food-based means for increasing the intake of particular nutrients.

Paying attention to food safety is also part of healthful eating. Currently, food-borne illness affects about 48 million individuals in the United States every year and leads to 128,000 hospitalizations and 3000 deaths (see Chapter 13).[9] Consumers can prevent food-borne illness at home by washing hands, rinsing vegetables and fruits, preventing cross-contamination, cooking foods to safe internal temperatures, and storing foods safely.

MyPlate: Putting the Guidelines into Practice

MyPlate can be used to plan a diet based on the recommendations of the Dietary Guidelines. The plate icon illustrates the proportions of food recommended from each of five food groups: Fruits, vegetables, grains, protein foods, and dairy. Half of your plate should be fruits and vegetables, about a quarter grains and about a quarter protein foods. Dairy should accompany meals as shown by the glass to the side (**Figure 2.9a**).

The Healthy Eating Pyramid • Figure 2.8

The Healthy Eating Pyramid emphasizes that a healthy diet is based on whole grains, fruits, vegetables, and oils. This dietary pattern places red meat, refined grains, and potatoes in the "eat sparingly" tip of the pyramid, along with sugary soft drinks, butter, and salt.

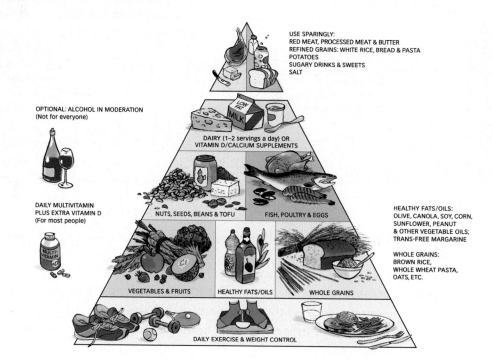

a. The MyPlate icon shows what a balanced meal should look like. Shown here next to the icon are some key messages from the Dietary Guidelines to help consumers balance calories and increase the nutrient density of their diet.

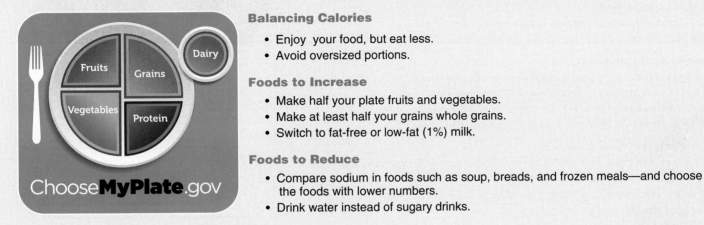

Balancing Calories

- Enjoy your food, but eat less.
- Avoid oversized portions.

Foods to Increase

- Make half your plate fruits and vegetables.
- Make at least half your grains whole grains.
- Switch to fat-free or low-fat (1%) milk.

Foods to Reduce

- Compare sodium in foods such as soup, breads, and frozen meals—and choose the foods with lower numbers.
- Drink water instead of sugary drinks.

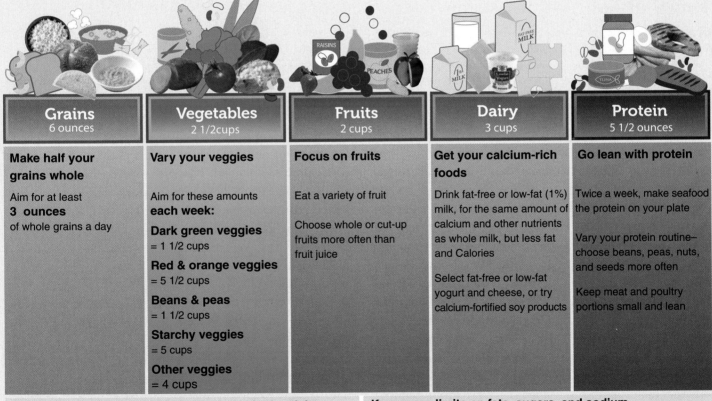

Grains 6 ounces	Vegetables 2 1/2cups	Fruits 2 cups	Dairy 3 cups	Protein 5 1/2 ounces
Make half your grains whole Aim for at least **3 ounces** of whole grains a day	**Vary your veggies** Aim for these amounts **each week:** **Dark green veggies** = 1 1/2 cups **Red & orange veggies** = 5 1/2 cups **Beans & peas** = 1 1/2 cups **Starchy veggies** = 5 cups **Other veggies** = 4 cups	**Focus on fruits** Eat a variety of fruit Choose whole or cut-up fruits more often than fruit juice	**Get your calcium-rich foods** Drink fat-free or low-fat (1%) milk, for the same amount of calcium and other nutrients as whole milk, but less fat and Calories Select fat-free or low-fat yogurt and cheese, or try calcium-fortified soy products	**Go lean with protein** Twice a week, make seafood the protein on your plate Vary your protein routine– choose beans, peas, nuts, and seeds more often Keep meat and poultry portions small and lean

Find your balance between food and physical activity
Be physically active for at least **150 minutes** each week.

Know your limits on fats, sugars, and sodium
Your allowance for oils is **6 teaspoons** a day. Limit calories from solid fats and added sugars to **260 Calories** a day. Reduce sodium intake to less than **2300 mg** a day.

b. You can obtain your own personalized food plan by looking up the USDA Food Plan that meets your calorie needs using Appendix D or by going to the Web site www.ChooseMyPlate.gov, clicking on "Get a Personalized Plan." The MyPlate Daily Food Plan shown here is for a person who needs 2000 Calories per day.

WHAT SHOULD I EAT?
To Fill My Plate

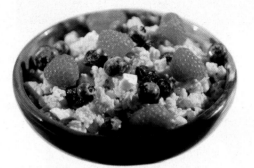

Balance calories to maintain weight
- Choose low-calorie snacks such as vegetables and fruits.
- Walk an extra 1000 steps; the more you exercise, the easier it is to keep your weight at a healthy level.
- Ride your bike to work or when running errands.
- Watch your portions. When you eat out, split an entrée with a friend.

Increase foods that promote health
- Have strawberries rather than strawberry shortcake for dessert.
- Make sure your breakfast cereal is a whole-grain cereal.
- Be colorful by adding some red and orange vegetables to your salad.
- Toss some shrimp on the grill to increase your seafood intake.

Limit nutrients that increase health risks
- Choose lean meat, fish, and low-fat dairy products in order to limit saturated fat.
- Have water and skip sugary soft drinks.
- Pass on the salt; instead, try lemon juice or some basil and oregano.
- If you drink alcohol, stop after one drink.

Use iProfile to look up the saturated fat and sugar content in your breakfast cereal.

MyPlate messages MyPlate emphasizes the importance of proportionality, variety, moderation, and nutrient density in a healthy diet (see *What Should I Eat?*). Proportionality means eating more of some types of foods than others. The MyPlate icon shows how much of your plate should be filled with foods from various food groups.

Variety is important for a healthy diet because no one food or food group provides all the nutrients and food components the body needs. A variety of foods should be selected from within each food group. The vegetables food group includes choices from 5 subgroups: dark green vegetables such as broccoli, collard greens, and kale; red and orange vegetables such as carrots, sweet potatoes, and red peppers; starchy vegetables such as corn, green peas, and potatoes; other vegetables such as cabbage, asparagus, and artichokes; and beans and peas such as lentils, chickpeas, and black beans. Beans and peas are good sources of the nutrients found in both vegetables and protein foods so they can be counted in either food group. Protein foods include meat, poultry, seafood, beans and peas, eggs, processed soy products, nuts, and seeds. Grains include whole grains such as whole-wheat bread, oatmeal, and brown rice as well as refined grains such as white bread, white rice, and white pasta (see Chapter 4). Fruits include fresh, canned, or dried fruit and 100%

fruit juice. Dairy includes all fluid milk products and many foods made from milk such as cheese, yogurt, and pudding, as well as calcium-fortified soy products.

Moderation involves limiting portion sizes and choosing nutrient-dense foods to balance calories consumed with calories expended. Tips such as make half your grains whole, choose whole or cut-up fruits more often than juice, select fat-free or low-fat dairy products, keep meat and poultry portions small and lean, and many more found on the MyPlate web site, are designed to help consumers make wise choices.

A Daily Food Plan Your Daily Food Plan tells you how much food to eat from each food group (**Figure 2.9b**). The amounts from the grains group are expressed in ounces. An ounce of grains is 1 cup of cold cereal, 1/2 cup of cooked cereal or grains, or a slice of bread. So if you have 2 cups of cereal and 2 slices of toast at breakfast, you have already consumed 4 ounces of grains for the day (two-thirds of the total for a 2000-Calorie diet). The amounts recommended for protein foods are also expressed in ounces. One ounce is equivalent to an ounce of cooked meat, poultry, or fish; one egg; 1 tablespoon of peanut butter; 1/4 cup of cooked dry beans; or 1/4 cup of nuts or seeds. The amounts recommended for fruits, vegetables, and dairy are given in cups.

It is easy to see where some foods in your diet fit on MyPlate. For example, a chicken breast is 3 ounces from the protein group; a scoop of rice is 2 ounces from the grains group. It is more difficult to see how much mixed foods such as pizza, stews, and casseroles contribute to each food group. To fit these on your plate individual ingredients must be considered. For example, a slice of pizza provides 1 ounce of grains, 1/8 cup of vegetables, and 1/2 cup of dairy. Having meat on your pizza adds about 1/4 ounce from the protein group (**Figure 2.10**).

How meals fit • Figure 2.10

This lunch, which is part of a 2000-Calorie menu, includes about a third of the amounts of grains, protein foods, and dairy recommended for the day, a quarter of the fruit, and half the oils, but only a small proportion of the vegetables recommended. The lettuce and celery fit into to the "other vegetables" category so other choices should come from dark green, red and orange, and starchy vegetables as well as beans and peas. To find out what counts as an ounce or a cup go to each food group at www.ChooseMyPlate.gov.

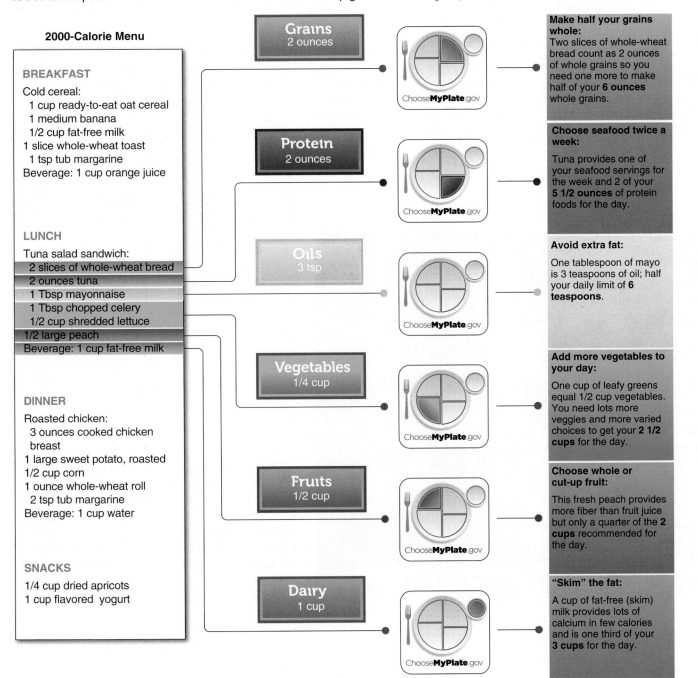

2000-Calorie Menu

BREAKFAST
Cold cereal:
 1 cup ready-to-eat oat cereal
 1 medium banana
 1/2 cup fat-free milk
1 slice whole-wheat toast
1 tsp tub margarine
Beverage: 1 cup orange juice

LUNCH
Tuna salad sandwich:
 2 slices of whole-wheat bread
 2 ounces tuna
 1 Tbsp mayonnaise
 1 Tbsp chopped celery
 1/2 cup shredded lettuce
 1/2 large peach
 Beverage: 1 cup fat-free milk

DINNER
Roasted chicken:
 3 ounces cooked chicken breast
1 large sweet potato, roasted
1/2 cup corn
1 ounce whole-wheat roll
 2 tsp tub margarine
Beverage: 1 cup water

SNACKS
1/4 cup dried apricots
1 cup flavored yogurt

Grains 2 ounces

Protein 2 ounces

Oils 3 tsp

Vegetables 1/4 cup

Fruits 1/2 cup

Dairy 1 cup

Make half your grains whole: Two slices of whole-wheat bread count as 2 ounces of whole grains so you need one more to make half of your **6 ounces** whole grains.

Choose seafood twice a week: Tuna provides one of your seafood servings for the week and 2 of your **5 1/2 ounces** of protein foods for the day.

Avoid extra fat: One tablespoon of mayo is 3 teaspoons of oil; half your daily limit of **6 teaspoons**.

Add more vegetables to your day: One cup of leafy greens equal 1/2 cup vegetables. You need lots more veggies and more varied choices to get your **2 1/2 cups** for the day.

Choose whole or cut-up fruit: This fresh peach provides more fiber than fruit juice but only a quarter of the **2 cups** recommended for the day.

"Skim" the fat: A cup of fat-free (skim) milk provides lots of calcium in few calories and is one third of your **3 cups** for the day.

A Daily Food Plan also includes recommendations about the amounts of oils (in teaspoons) that should be included in your diet (see Figure 2.9b and Figure 2.10). Oils are fats that are liquid at room temperature; they come from plants and fish. They are rich in unsaturated fats, which help protect against heart disease. Solid fats are fats that are solid at room temperature, such as butter and shortening. They provide saturated and *trans* fat and should be limited in the diet.

A MyPlate Daily Food Plan recommends at least 150 minutes of activity each week to help balance food and physical activity and includes a calorie limit for **empty calories** from solid fats and added sugars. It is important to limit empty calories because consuming too many means you can't meet your nutrient needs without exceeding you calorie needs. (**Figure 2.11**).

> **empty calories**
> Calories from solid fats and/or added sugars, which add calories to the food but few nutrients.

Empty calorie allowance • Figure 2.11

a. If you are at a healthy weight and you choose nutrient-dense foods, you can satisfy all your nutrient needs with fewer calories than you need to maintain your weight. The "extra" calories needed to maintain your weight can come from additional nutrient-dense choices or from foods such as candy, soda, or butter that are high in added sugar or solid fats.

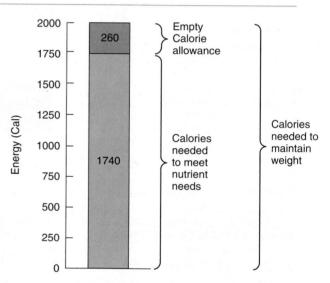

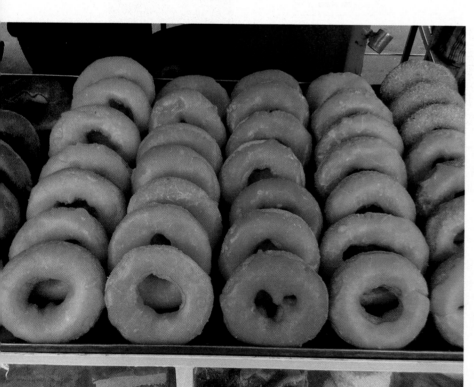

b. Some empty calories come from foods that belong to a food group but contain added sugars and solid fats. These donuts, for example, are in the grains group, but about half of their calories are empty calories from solid fat and sugar. Some foods, such as butter, table sugar, soft drinks, and candy, don't belong in any food group, because all their calories are empty. Oils are healthy fats so, they are not considered empty calories.

One way to see how your daily intake matches the My-Plate recommendations is to use the interactive tools on the MyPlate Web site to help track your progress toward choosing a healthy diet.

Exchange Lists

The **Exchange Lists** are a set of food-group recommendations developed in the 1950s to plan diets for people with diabetes. Since then, their use has been expanded to planning diets for anyone who has to monitor calorie intake. They group foods based on the amounts of energy, carbohydrate, protein, and fat they provide per serving. Foods in the same exchange list each contain approximately the same amounts of energy, carbohydrate, protein, and fat. Therefore, any one of the foods on a list can be exchanged with any other food on the list without altering the calories or amounts of carbohydrate, protein, or fat in the diet. The food groupings of the Exchange Lists differ from the MyPlate food groups because the lists are designed to meet energy and macronutrient criteria, whereas the My-Plate groups are designed to be good sources of nutrients regardless of their energy content. For example, a potato is included in the starch exchange list because it contains about the same amount of energy, carbohydrate, protein, and fat as breads and grains, but in MyPlate a potato is in the vegetable group because it is a good source of vitamins, minerals, and fiber. The Exchange Lists provide a useful tool whether you are controlling calorie intake for purposes of weight loss or carbohydrate intake for purposes of diabetes management. Appendix E provides more information about the Exchange Lists.

CONCEPT CHECK STOP

1. **How** can the recommendations of the Dietary Guidelines help Americans manage body weight?
2. **What** does the MyPlate graphic tell you about a healthy diet?
3. **How** many ounces from the grains group are recommended each day for you?
4. **Which** contains more empty calories—a bowl of oatmeal or a bowl of Froot Loops?

Food and Supplement Labels

LEARNING OBJECTIVES

1. **Discuss** how the information on food labels can help you choose a healthy diet.
2. **Determine** whether a food is high or low in fiber, saturated fat, and cholesterol.
3. **Explain** how the order of ingredients on a food label is determined.
4. **Explain** the types of claims that are common on dietary supplement labels.

T he Dietary Guidelines and MyPlate recommend appropriate amounts of nutritious foods, but sometimes it is difficult to tell how nutritious a particular food is. How do you know whether your frozen entrée is a good source of vitamin C, how much fiber your breakfast cereal provides, or how much calcium is in your daily vitamin/mineral supplement? You can find this information on food and supplement labels.

Food Labels

Food labels are designed to help consumers make informed food choices by providing information about the

a. Food labels must appear on all packaged foods except those produced by small businesses and those in packages too small to accommodate the information. This label from a macaroni-and-cheese package illustrates how the Nutrition Facts panel and the ingredient list can help you evaluate the nutritional contribution this food will make to your diet.

Standard serving sizes are required to allow consumers to compare products. For example, the number of Calories in one serving of this macaroni and cheese can be compared to the number of Calories in one serving of packaged rice because the values for both are for a standard 1-cup serving.

Food labels must list the "% Daily Value" for total fat, saturated fat, cholesterol, sodium, total carbohydrate, and dietary fiber, as well as for vitamins A and C, calcium, and iron. A % Daily Value of 5% or less is considered low, and a value of 20% or more is considered high.

The label provides information about the amounts of nutrients whose intake should be limited—total fat, saturated fat, *trans* fat, cholesterol, and sodium.

The label provides information about the amounts of nutrients that tend to be low in the American diet—fiber, vitamins A and C, calcium, and iron.

The footnote gives the Daily Values for 2,000 and 2,500 Calorie diets to illustrate that for some nutrients the Daily Value increases with increasing caloric intake.

The ingredients are listed in descending order by weight, from the most abundant to the least abundant. The wheat flour in the macaroni is the most abundant ingredient in this product.

Interpreting Data

This label shows 30 mg of cholesterol per serving. How much cholesterol would you consume if you ate the whole box? What percentage of the Daily Value would that represent?

Nutrition Facts

Serving Size 1 cup (228g)
Servings Per Container 2

Amount Per Serving

Calories 250   **Calories from Fat** 110

	% Daily Value*
Total Fat 12g	18%
Saturated Fat 3g	15%
Trans Fat 1.5g	
Cholesterol 30mg	10%
Sodium 470mg	20%
Total Carbohydrate 31g	10%
Dietary Fiber 0g	0%
Sugars 5g	
Protein 5g	
Vitamin A	4%
Vitamin C	2%
Calcium	20%
Iron	4%

* Percent Daily Values are based on a 2,000 calorie diet. Your daily values may be higher or lower depending on your calorie needs:

	Calories:	2,000	2,500
Total Fat	Less than	65g	80g
Sat. Fat	Less than	20g	25g
Cholesterol	Less than	300mg	300mg
Sodium	Less than	2,400mg	2,400mg
Total Carbohydrate		300g	375g
Dietary Fiber		25g	30g

Ingredients:
Enriched macaroni product (wheat flour, niacin, ferrous sulfate [iron], thiamine mononitrate, riboflavin, folic acid); cheese sauce mix (whey, modified food starch, milk fat, salt, milk protein concentrate, contains less tha 2% of sodium tripolyphosphate, cellulose gel, cellulose gum, citric acid, sodium phosphate, lactic acid, calcium phosphate, milk, yellow 5, yellow 6, enzymes, cheese culture)

Labels must contain basic product information, such as the name of the product, the weight or volume of the contents, and the name and place of business of the manufacturer, packager, or distributor.

nutrient composition of a food and how that food fits into the overall diet (**Figure 2.12**).[10] Knowing how to interpret the information on these labels can help you choose a healthy diet. This doesn't mean that you can never choose high-calorie, low-nutrient-density foods but rather that you should balance your choices. It is your total diet—not each choice—that counts.

Nutrition Facts All food labels must contain a **Nutrition Facts** panel (see Figure 2.12a).[10,13] This section of the label presents information about the amounts of

specific nutrients in a standard serving. The serving size on the label is followed by the number of servings per container, the total Calories, and the Calories from fat in each serving. If a person eats twice the standard serving, he or she is consuming twice the number of Calories listed.

The next section of the Nutrition Facts panel lists the amounts of nutrients contained in a serving and, for most, the amount they provide as a percentage of the **Daily Value**. The % Daily Value is the amount of a nutrient in a food as a percentage of the Daily Value recommended for

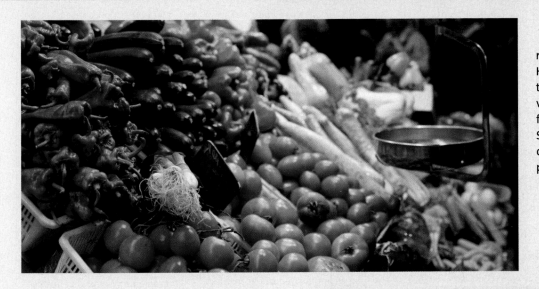

b. Raw fruits, vegetables, fish, meat, and poultry are not required to carry individual labels. However, grocery stores are asked to provide nutrition information voluntarily for the raw foods most frequently purchased in the United States. The information can appear on large placards or in consumer pamphlets or brochures.

c. Food served in restaurants, delicatessens, and bakeries is not required to carry labels unless the food is from a food establishment that has 20 or more locations. These food chains must list calorie content information for standard menu items and provide other nutrient information upon request.[11] In any restaurant nutrition information must be available upon request when a claim is made about a menu item's nutritional content or health benefits, such as "low-fat" or "heart healthy."[12]

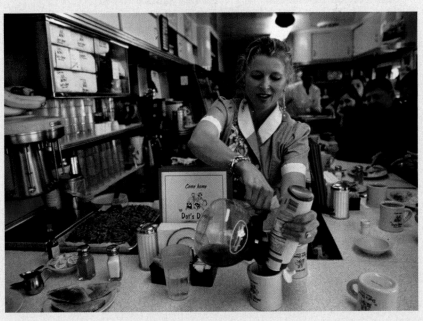

Daily Value A reference value for the intake of nutrients used on food labels to help consumers see how a given food fits into their overall diet.

a 2000-Calorie diet. For example, if a food provides 10% of the Daily Value for vitamin C, it provides 10% of the recommended daily intake for vitamin C in a 2000-Calorie diet (see Appendix F). Because a Daily Value is a single standard for all consumers, it may overestimate the amount of a nutrient needed for some population groups, but it does not underestimate the requirement for any group except pregnant and lactating women.

Ingredient List Do you want to know exactly what goes into your food? The ingredient list is the place to look. The ingredient list presents the contents of the product in order of their prominence by weight. This information can be very helpful to consumers who are allergic to nuts, trying to avoid animal products, or just curious about what is in the food they eat.

An ingredient list is required on all products containing more than one ingredient and optional on products that contain a single ingredient. Food additives, including food colors and flavorings, must be listed among the ingredients.

Food and Supplement Labels **51**

THINKING IT THROUGH ✓ THE PLANNER

A Case Study Using Food Labels to Make Healthy Choices

Scott is trying to improve his nutritional health. He has visited the MyPlate Web site and now knows how much food he should choose from each food group, but he sometimes has trouble making decisions when shopping for food.

For breakfast he likes hot or cold cereal. Whether he eats oatmeal or granola, it is a serving from the grains group.

Use the labels shown below to determine which contains more saturated fat and sugars.

▼

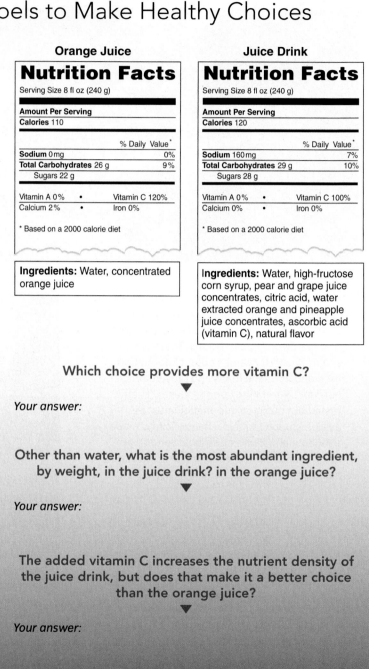

Old Fashioned Oats

Nutrition Facts
Serving Size ½ cup (40g) dry
Servings Per Container about 13

Amount Per Serving	Dry	Cereal with ½ cup Skim Milk
Calories	150	190
Calories from Fat	25	30

	% Daily Value**	
Total Fat 3g	5%	5%
Saturated Fat 0.5g	3%	3%
Trans Fat 0g		
Cholesterol 0mg	0%	0%
Sodium 0mg	0%	3%
Total Carbohydrate 27g	9%	11%
Dietary Fiber 4g	16%	16%
Sugars 0g		
Protein 5g		

Natural Granola

Nutrition Facts
Serving Size ½ cup (51g)
Servings Per Container about 16

Amount Per Serving	
Calories	230
Calories from Fat	80

	% Daily Value*
Total Fat 9g	13%
Saturated Fat 3.5g	18%
Trans Fat 1g	
Cholesterol 0mg	0%
Sodium 20mg	1%
Total Carbohydrate 34g	11%
Dietary Fiber 3g	13%
Sugars 16g	
Protein 5g	

Your answer:

Scott usually has an inexpensive juice drink with his breakfast. He is not sure whether or not this is nutritionally the same as the more expensive orange juice.

How much of the sugar in the orange juice is added?

▼

The only ingredients in the ingredient list are water and concentrated orange juice. This tells Scott that no sugar has been added. The 22 grams of sugars listed in the Nutrition Facts panel all come from the sugar found naturally in oranges.

Orange Juice

Nutrition Facts
Serving Size 8 fl oz (240 g)

Amount Per Serving	
Calories 110	

	% Daily Value*
Sodium 0mg	0%
Total Carbohydrates 26 g	9%
Sugars 22 g	

Vitamin A 0%	•	Vitamin C 120%
Calcium 2%	•	Iron 0%

* Based on a 2000 calorie diet

Ingredients: Water, concentrated orange juice

Juice Drink

Nutrition Facts
Serving Size 8 fl oz (240 g)

Amount Per Serving	
Calories 120	

	% Daily Value*
Sodium 160mg	7%
Total Carbohydrates 29 g	10%
Sugars 28 g	

Vitamin A 0%	•	Vitamin C 100%
Calcium 0%	•	Iron 0%

* Based on a 2000 calorie diet

Ingredients: Water, high-fructose corn syrup, pear and grape juice concentrates, citric acid, water extracted orange and pineapple juice concentrates, ascorbic acid (vitamin C), natural flavor

Which choice provides more vitamin C?

▼

Your answer:

Other than water, what is the most abundant ingredient, by weight, in the juice drink? in the orange juice?

▼

Your answer:

The added vitamin C increases the nutrient density of the juice drink, but does that make it a better choice than the orange juice?

▼

Your answer:

(Check your answers in Appendix J.)

Nutrient content and health claims Looking for low-fat or high-fiber foods (see *Thinking It Through: A Case Study Using Food Labels to Make Healthy Choices*)? You may not even need to look at the Nutrition Facts panel. Food labels often contain **nutrient content claims**. These are statements that highlight specific characteristics of a product that might be of interest to consumers, such as "fat free" or "low sodium." Standard definitions for these descriptors have been established by the Food and Drug Administration (FDA) (**Table 2.2** and Appendix F).

Because of the importance of certain types of foods and dietary components in disease prevention, food labels are permitted to include a number of **health claims**. Health claims refer to a relationship between a nutrient, food, food component, or dietary supplement and reduced risk of a disease or health-related condition. All health claims are reviewed by the FDA. To carry a health claim, a food must be a naturally good source of one of six nutrients (vitamin A, vitamin C, protein, calcium, iron, or fiber) and must not contain more than 20% of the Daily Value for fat, saturated fat, cholesterol, or sodium. Approved health claims are supported by

Nutrient content claims[13] Table 2.2	
Claim	**Description**
Free	Used on products that contain no amount of or only a trivial amount of fat, saturated fat, cholesterol, sodium, sugars, or calories. For example, "sugar free" and "fat free" both mean < 0.5 g per serving. Synonyms for *free* include *without*, *no*, and *zero*.
Low	Used for foods that can be eaten frequently without exceeding the Daily Value for fat, saturated fat, cholesterol, sodium, or calories. Specific definitions have been established for each of these nutrients. For example, *low-fat* means that the food contains ≤ 3 g of fat per serving, and *low cholesterol* means that the food contains ≤ 20 mg of cholesterol per serving. Synonyms for *low* include *little*, *few*, and *low source of*.
Lean and extra lean	Used to describe the fat content of meat, poultry, seafood, and game meats. *Lean* means that the food contains < 10 g fat, ≤ 4.5 g saturated fat, and < 95 mg of cholesterol per serving and per 100 g. *Extra lean* is defined as containing < 5 g fat, < 2 g saturated fat, and < 95 mg of cholesterol per serving and per 100 g.
High	Used for foods that contain 20% or more of the Daily Value for a particular nutrient. Synonyms for *high* include *rich in* and *excellent source of*.
Good source	Used for foods that contain 10 to 19% of the Daily Value for a particular nutrient per serving.
Reduced	Used on nutritionally altered products that contain 25% less of a nutrient or energy than the regular or reference product.
Less	Used on foods, whether altered or not, that contain 25% less of a nutrient or energy than the reference food. For example, pretzels may claim to have "less fat" than potato chips. *Fewer* may be used as a synonym for *less*.
Light	Used in different ways. First, it can be used on a nutritionally altered product that contains one-third fewer calories or half the fat of a reference food. Second, it can be used when the sodium content of a low-calorie, low-fat food has been reduced by 50%. The term *light* can be used to describe properties such as texture and color, as long as the label explains the intent—for example, "light and fluffy."
More	Used when a serving of food, whether altered or not, contains a nutrient in an amount that is at least 10% of the Daily Value more than the reference food. Synonyms for *more* are *fortified*, *enriched*, and *added*.
Healthy	Used to describe foods that are low in fat and saturated fat, contain limited amounts of sodium and cholesterol, and provide at least 10% of the Daily Value for vitamins A or C, or iron, calcium, protein, or fiber.
Fresh	Used on foods that are raw and have never been frozen or heated and contain no preservatives.

strong scientific evidence (**Figure 2.13** and Appendix F). Health claims for which there is emerging but not well-established evidence are called **qualified health claims**, and such a claim must be accompanied by an explanatory statement to avoid misleading consumers.

Dietary Supplement Labels

Products ranging from multivitamin pills to protein powders and herbal elixirs can all be defined as **dietary supplements**. These products are considered foods, not drugs, and therefore are regulated by the laws that govern food safety and labeling. To help consumers understand what they are choosing when they purchase these products, dietary supplements are required to carry a **Supplement Facts** panel similar to the Nutrition Facts panel found on food labels (**Figure 2.14**).[14]

> **dietary supplement** A product sold to supplement the diet; may include nutrients, enzymes, herbs, or other substances.

Labels on dietary supplements may also include nutrient content claims and FDA-approved health claims similar to those on food labels. For example, a product can claim to be an excellent source of a particular nutrient. To make this claim, one serving of the product must contain at least 20% of the Daily Value for that nutrient. A label may say "high potency" if one serving provides 100% or more of the Daily Value for the nutrient it contains. For multinutrient products, "high potency" means that a serving provides more than 100% of the Daily Value for two-thirds of the vitamins and minerals present.

Dietary supplement labels may also carry **structure/function claims**, which describe the role of a dietary ingredient in maintaining normal structure, function, or general well-being. For example, a structure/function claim about calcium may state that "calcium builds strong bones"; one about fiber may say "fiber maintains bowel regularity." These statements can be misleading. For example, the health claim "lowers cholesterol" requires FDA approval, but the structure/function claim "helps maintain normal cholesterol levels" does not. It would not be unreasonable for consumers with high cholesterol to conclude that a product that "helps maintain normal cholesterol levels" would help lower their elevated blood cholesterol level to within the normal range.

Health claims • Figure 2.13

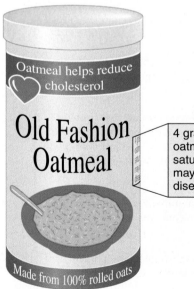

Oatmeal contains enough soluble fiber to be permitted to include this health claim about the relationship between soluble fiber and the risk of heart disease. Other health claims you may see on food labels are listed below and included in Appendix F.[13]

- Calcium intake and the risk of osteoporosis
- Calcium and vitamin D intake and the risk of osteoporosis
- Sodium intake and the risk of high blood pressure
- Saturated fat and cholesterol intake and the risk of heart disease
- Fiber-containing fruit, vegetable, and grain intake and the risk of heart disease and cancer
- Fruit and vegetable intake and the risk of cancer
- Dietary fat and the risk of cancer
- Whole-grain foods and the risk of heart disease and certain cancers

(Figure labels: Oatmeal helps reduce cholesterol. Old Fashion Oatmeal. Made from 100% rolled oats. 4 grams of soluble fiber from oatmeal daily in a diet low in saturated fat and cholesterol may reduce the risk of heart disease)

Dietary supplement label • Figure 2.14

Unlike food labels, dietary supplement labels must provide directions for use and must provide information about ingredients that are not nutrients and for which Daily Values have not been established. For such ingredients, it is difficult to tell from the label whether the amount included in a serving is helpful, is harmful, or has no effect at all.

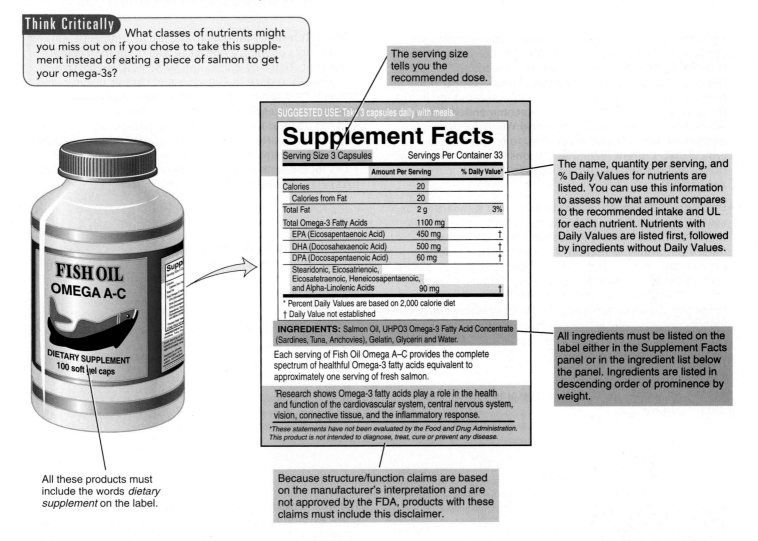

Think Critically What classes of nutrients might you miss out on if you chose to take this supplement instead of eating a piece of salmon to get your omega-3s?

The serving size tells you the recommended dose.

SUGGESTED USE: Take 3 capsules daily with meals.

Supplement Facts

Serving Size 3 Capsules   Servings Per Container 33

	Amount Per Serving	% Daily Value*
Calories	20	
Calories from Fat	20	
Total Fat	2 g	3%
Total Omega-3 Fatty Acids	1100 mg	
EPA (Eicosapentaenoic Acid)	450 mg	†
DHA (Docosahexaenoic Acid)	500 mg	†
DPA (Docosapentaenoic Acid)	60 mg	†
Stearidonic, Eicosatrienoic, Eicosatetraenoic, Heneicosapentaenoic, and Alpha-Linolenic Acids	90 mg	†

* Percent Daily Values are based on 2,000 calorie diet
† Daily Value not established

INGREDIENTS: Salmon Oil, UHPO3 Omega-3 Fatty Acid Concentrate (Sardines, Tuna, Anchovies), Gelatin, Glycerin and Water.

Each serving of Fish Oil Omega A–C provides the complete spectrum of healthful Omega-3 fatty acids equivalent to approximately one serving of fresh salmon.

'Research shows Omega-3 fatty acids play a role in the health and function of the cardiovascular system, central nervous system, vision, connective tissue, and the inflammatory response.

These statements have not been evaluated by the Food and Drug Administration. This product is not intended to diagnose, treat, cure or prevent any disease.

FISH OIL OMEGA A-C

DIETARY SUPPLEMENT
100 soft gel caps

The name, quantity per serving, and % Daily Values for nutrients are listed. You can use this information to assess how that amount compares to the recommended intake and UL for each nutrient. Nutrients with Daily Values are listed first, followed by ingredients without Daily Values.

All ingredients must be listed on the label either in the Supplement Facts panel or in the ingredient list below the panel. Ingredients are listed in descending order of prominence by weight.

All these products must include the words *dietary supplement* on the label.

Because structure/function claims are based on the manufacturer's interpretation and are not approved by the FDA, products with these claims must include this disclaimer.

Manufacturers must notify the FDA when including a structure/function claim on a dietary supplement label and are responsible for ensuring the accuracy and truthfulness of these claims. Structure/function claims are not approved by the FDA. For this reason, the law says that if a dietary supplement label includes such a claim, it must state in a disclaimer that the FDA has not evaluated the claim. The disclaimer must also state that the dietary supplement product is not intended to "diagnose, treat, cure, or prevent any disease" because only a drug can legally make such a claim (see Figure 2.14). Structure/function claims may also appear on food labels, but the FDA does not require conventional food manufactures to notify the FDA about their structure/function claims, and disclaimers are not required.

CONCEPT CHECK   STOP

1. **Why** are serving sizes standardized on food labels?
2. **What** food label information helps you find foods that are low in saturated fat and cholesterol?
3. **Where** should you look to see if a food contains nuts?
4. **How** do structure/function claims differ from health claims?

Summary

1 Nutrition Recommendations 32

- Nutrition recommendations are designed to encourage consumption of a diet that promotes health and prevents disease. Some of the earliest nutrition recommendations in the United States were in the form of **food guides**, which translate nutrient intake recommendations into food intake recommendations. The first set of Recommended Dietary Allowances, developed during World War II, focused on energy and the nutrients most likely to be deficient in a typical diet. Current recommendations focus on promoting health and preventing chronic disease as well as nutrient deficiencies.

- Dietary recommendations can be used as a standard for assessing the **nutritional status** of individuals and of populations. Records of dietary intake, such as the one shown here, along with information obtained from a physical examination, a medical history, and laboratory tests, can be used to assess an individual's nutritional status. Collecting information about the food intake and health of individuals in the population or surveying the foods available can help identify potential and actual nutrient deficiencies and excesses within a population and help policymakers improve nutrition recommendations.

Assessing nutritional status: Determine typical food intake • Figure 2.2

FOOD DIARY

Record all the food and beverages you eat. Include the food, how it was prepared, the amount you ate and the brand name. Don't forget to list all fats used in cooking and all spreads and sauces added.

Time	Food	Kind and how prepared	Amount
7:00 AM.	Eggs	scrambled	2
	Butter	in eggs	1 tsp.
	toast	whole wheat	2 slices
	Butter	on toast	2 tsp.
	Milk	non-fat	8 oz
	Orange juice	from frozen concentrate	8 oz.
12:00 P.M.	Big Mac	McDonald's	1

2 Dietary Reference Intakes (DRIs) 36

- **Dietary Reference Intakes (DRIs)** are recommendations for the amounts of energy, nutrients, and other food components that should be consumed by healthy people to promote health, reduce the incidence of chronic disease, and prevent deficiencies. **Estimated Average Requirements (EARs)** are average requirements, as seen in the illustration, and can be used to evaluate the adequacy of a population's nutrient intake. **Recommended Dietary Allowances (RDAs)** and **Adequate Intakes (AIs)** can be used by individuals as goals for nutrient intake, and **Tolerable Upper Intake Levels (ULs)** indicate safe upper intake limits.

Understanding EARs, RDAs, and ULs • Figure 2.4

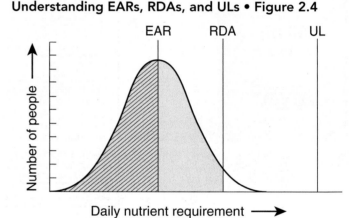

- The DRIs make two types of energy-intake recommendations. **Estimated Energy Requirements (EERs)** provide an estimate of how many calories are needed to maintain body weight. **Acceptable Macronutrient Distribution Ranges (AMDRs)** make recommendations about the proportion of energy that should come from carbohydrate, fat, and protein in a healthy diet.

- The *Dietary Guidelines for Americans* are a set of diet and lifestyle recommendations designed to promote health and reduce the risk of overweight and obesity and chronic disease in the U.S. population. They emphasize balancing the calories consumed in food and beverages with the calories expended through physical activity in order to achieve and maintain a healthy weight. To accomplish this, they recommend that Americans increase their activity level and choose a healthy eating pattern. Healthy eating patterns are higher in fruits, vegetables, whole grains, low-fat dairy products, and seafood than current American diets, and they are lower in saturated fat, *trans* fat, cholesterol, salt, and added sugar.

- **MyPlate**, shown here, is the USDA's current food guide. It shows the proportions of foods from five food groups that make up a healthy diet and recommends amounts of food from each group based on individual energy needs. It also makes recommendations about the amounts of oils and the number of **empty calories** that can be included in an individual's diet. MyPlate stresses using variety, proportionality, and moderation in choosing a healthy diet and promotes the physical activity recommendations included in the Dietary Guidelines.

MyPlate recommendations • Figure 2.9

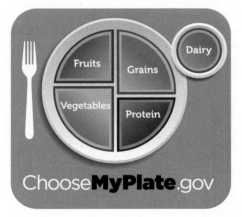

- **Exchange Lists** are a food group system used to plan individual diets that provide specific amounts of energy, carbohydrate, protein, and fat.

- Standardized food labels are designed to help consumers make healthy food choices by providing information about the nutrient composition of foods and about how a food fits into the overall diet. The **Nutrition Facts** panel, as illustrated here, presents information about the amounts of various nutrients in a standard serving. For most nutrients, the amount is also given as a percentage of the **Daily Value**. A food label's ingredient list states the contents of the product, in order of prominence by weight. Food labels often include FDA-defined **nutrient content claims**, such as "low fat" or "high fiber," and **health claims**, which refer to a relationship between a nutrient, food, food component, or dietary supplement and the risk of a particular disease or health-related condition. All health claims are reviewed by the FDA and permitted only when they are supported by scientific evidence, but the level of scientific support for such claims varies.

Food labels • Figure 2.12

Nutrition Facts	
Serving Size 1 cup (228g)	
Servings Per Container 2	
Amount Per Serving	
Calories 250	**Calories from Fat** 110
	% Daily Value*
Total Fat 12g	18%
Saturated Fat 3g	15%
Trans Fat 1.5g	
Cholesterol 30mg	10%
Sodium 470mg	20%
Total Carbohydrate 31g	10%
Dietary Fiber 0g	0%
Sugars 5g	
Protein 5g	
Vitamin A	4%
Vitamin C	2%
Calcium	20%
Iron	4%

- A **Supplement Facts** panel appears on the label of every dietary supplement. Because **structure/function claims** are not FDA approved, when they appear on supplement labels, they must be accompanied by a disclaimer.

Key Terms

- Acceptable Macronutrient Distribution Ranges (AMDRs) 39
- Adequate Intakes (AIs) 37
- Daily Value 50
- dietary supplement 54
- *Dietary Guidelines for Americans* 41
- Dietary Reference Intakes (DRIs) 36
- empty calories 48

- Estimated Average Requirements (EARs) 36
- Estimated Energy Requirements (EERs) 39
- Exchange Lists 49
- food guide 32
- health claim 53
- *Healthy People* 35
- *MyPlate* 40

- nutrient content claim 52
- Nutrition Facts 50
- nutritional status 33
- qualified health claim 54
- Recommended Dietary Allowances (RDAs) 37
- structure/function claim 54
- Supplement Facts 54
- Tolerable Upper Intake Levels (ULs) 38

Online Resources

- To view copies of the Dietary Reference Intakes reports, go to the National Academies Press site, at www.nap.edu, and search for "Dietary Reference Intakes."

- For additional information on the 2010 Dietary Guidelines, go to www.dietaryguidelines.gov.

- To learn more about MyPlate, go to www.ChooseMyPlate.gov.

- For information on Healthy People 2020, go to www.healthy-people.gov/2020/.

- For more information about the labeling of food and supplements, go to the FDA at www.fda.gov/Food/default.htm and click on "Labeling & Nutrition" or "Dietary Supplements."

- Visit your *WileyPLUS* site for videos, animations, podcasts, self-study, and other media that will aid you in studying and understanding this chapter.

Critical and Creative Thinking Questions

1. Keep a food diary of everything you eat for a day. Go to www.ChooseMyPlate.gov and look up the Daily Food Plan for a person of your age, gender, and activity level. Now click on "Plan a Healthy Menu" and use the Menu Planner to compare your intake with your Daily Food Plan.

2. Gina is a college sophomore on a tight budget. An analysis of her diet shows that she consumes less than the RDA for vitamin C and more than the RDA for thiamin. Does she have a vitamin C deficiency? Is she at risk of thiamin toxicity? What other factors need to be considered before you can draw any conclusions about her nutritional status?

3. Maryellen is trying to increase her intake of calcium and vitamin D by taking a dietary supplement. How can she determine whether it contains enough of these nutrients to meet her needs but not so much that it will cause toxicity? If the product claims to build strong bones, does this mean that Maryellen will never get osteoporosis? Why or why not?

4. Select three packaged foods that have food labels. What is the percentage of calories from fat in each product? How many grams of carbohydrate, fat, and fiber are in a serving of each? How does each product fit into your daily diet with regard to total carbohydrate recommended? total fat? dietary fiber? If you consumed a serving of each of these three foods, how much more saturated fat could you consume during the day without exceeding the Daily Value? How much more total carbohydrate and fiber should you consume that day to meet Daily Value recommendation for a 2000-Calorie diet?

5. Red meat is an excellent source of iron. The graph below estimates red meat consumption in the United States over the past 40 years. What can be concluded about the iron intake of the U.S. population during this period? How might the change in intake affect the health of the population?

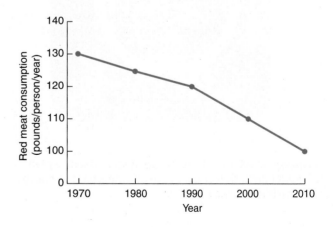

6. The Dietary Guidelines recommend reducing serving sizes to keep weight in a healthy range, limiting salt intake to prevent high blood pressure, limiting dietary cholesterol and saturated fat to reduce the risk of heart disease, and limiting added sugar to increase the nutrient density of the diet. Suggest some changes that the food industry could implement to support these nutrition recommendations.

What is happening in this picture?

When ordering from this menu, you need to check more than the price. The higher numbers below the prices show the number of Calories in each sandwich.

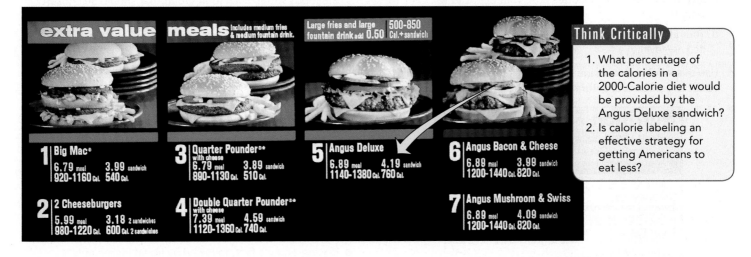

Think Critically

1. What percentage of the calories in a 2000-Calorie diet would be provided by the Angus Deluxe sandwich?
2. Is calorie labeling an effective strategy for getting Americans to eat less?

Self-Test

(Check your answers in Appendix K.)

1. Which DRI standards can be used as goals for individual intake?

   a. AIs
   b. RDAs
   c. EARs
   d. A and B only

2. Based on this graph, showing one day's intake of selected nutrients, which of these statements about this person's nutrient intake is true?

Nutrient	Percent of recommendation
	0% 50% 100%
Vitamin A	75%
Vitamin C	115%
Iron	54%
Calcium	75%
Saturated fat	134%

   a. She has an iron deficiency.
   b. She consumes the recommended amount of vitamin A.
   c. If she consumes this amount of iron every day, she is at risk for iron deficiency.
   d. She has osteoporosis.

3. Which DRI standard can help you determine whether a supplement contains a toxic level of a nutrient?

   a. RDA
   b. AI
   c. EAR
   d. UL

4. In this figure, which letter labels the DRI standard that represents the average needs of the population?

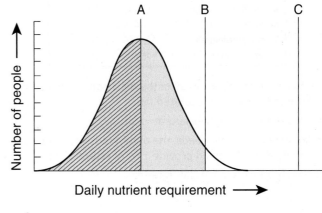

   a. A
   b. B
   c. C
   d. None of the above is correct.

5. Which of the following statements is false?

   a. An EER value gives the amount of energy needed to maintain body weight.

   b. Your EER stays the same when you gain weight.

   c. If you consume more calories than your EER, you will gain weight.

   d. Your EER depends on your age, gender, weight, height, and activity level.

6. Use this label to determine which of the following statements about the amount of saturated fat in this product is true.

Nutrition Facts

Serving Size 1 cup (228g)
Servings Per Container 2

Amount Per Serving	
Calories 250	**Calories from Fat** 110

	% Daily Value*
Total Fat 12g	18%
Saturated Fat 3g	15%
Trans Fat 1.5g	
Cholesterol 30mg	10%
Sodium 470mg	20%
Total Carbohydrate 31g	10%
Dietary Fiber 0g	0%
Sugars 5g	
Protein 5g	

Vitamin A	4%
Vitamin C	2%
Calcium	20%
Iron	4%

* Percent Daily Values are based on a 2,000 calorie diet. Your daily values may be higher or lower depending on your calorie needs:

	Calories:	2,000	2,500
Total Fat	Less than	65g	80g
Sat. Fat	Less than	20g	25g
Cholesterol	Less than	300mg	300mg
Sodium	Less than	2,400mg	2,400mg
Total Carbohydrate		300g	375g
Dietary Fiber		25g	30g

   a. This product contains 15% of the maximum daily recommended amount of saturated fat.

   b. This product is high in saturated fat.

   c. To meet nutritional needs, the other foods you consume during the day should provide 17 g of saturated fat.

   d. This product is low in saturated fat.

7. The MyPlate icon is designed to illustrate _____.

   a. the proportions of food from each group that make up a healthy diet

   b. the importance of meat in a healthy meal

   c. the foods within each food group that should be chosen more often than others

   d. that exercise is important for a healthy lifestyle

8. Which of these foods is highest in empty calories?

   a. an apple

   b. a tablespoon of olive oil

   c. a slice of whole-wheat bread

   d. a donut

9. In which order are the ingredients listed on a food label?

   a. alphabetical

   b. from largest proportion to smallest, by volume

   c. from largest proportion to smallest, by weight

   d. dry ingredients first, followed by liquid ingredients

10. Which of the following statements is an invalid interpretation of this graph showing trends in milk consumption?

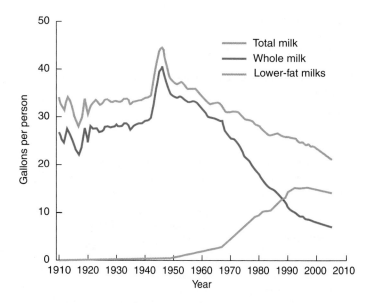

   a. People drank more milk in 1950 than in 2000.

   b. People drank more low-fat milk in 2000 than in 1950.

   c. Children drank less milk in 2000 than in 1950.

   d. Total consumption of whole milk declined between 1950 and 2000.

11. The Dietary Guidelines stress the importance of _____.

    a. choosing nutrient-dense foods

    b. balancing food intake with physical activity

    c. limiting nutrients that are associated with an increased risk of chronic disease

    d. handling food safely to prevent food-borne illness

    e. All of the above

12. Which of the following is used to assess nutritional status?

    a. nutritional analysis of the diet

    b. measurements of body dimensions

    c. medical history and physical examination

    d. laboratory tests

    e. All of the above are used.

13. Which of the following is a structure/function claim?

    a. Fiber maintains bowel regularity.

    b. Soluble fiber helps reduce the risk of heart disease.

    c. Calcium helps reduce the risk of osteoporosis.

    d. Diets that are low in sodium can reduce the risk of high blood pressure.

14. *Nutritional status* refers to _____.

    a. how healthy a person's diet is relative to that of his or her peer group

    b. the measure of a person's health in terms of his or her intake and utilization of nutrients

    c. a person's blood values relative to normal levels

    d. the quality of foods a family is able to afford

15. Which of the following is *not* a food group in MyPlate?

    a. dairy

    b. protein foods

    c. vegetables

    d. fats and sweets

THE PLANNER ✓

Review your Chapter Planner on the chapter opener and check off your completed work.

Digestion: From Meals to Molecules

The human body has been compared to a car: We fill the tank of our car with gasoline to get down the highway; we fill our body with food to get on with life. In both "machines," combustion with oxygen releases energy.

Our bodies are machine-like in another way as well: They are virtually identical to one another. Like cars, we look different on the outside but are basically the same on the inside. The processes that drive us—like the internal combustion engine, no matter where it's manufactured—are more similar than different because they are based on the same fundamental chemical reactions.

Despite the similarities, however, there are differences between human bodies and machines. An automobile cannot use gasoline to heal itself or to grow, as we do with nutrients. Although a gas tank and a stomach both store fuel, gasoline travels unchanged through the fuel line to the engine, whereas in humans the digestive system must break down the fuel into smaller units *before* it can be used by the body. Gas-powered cars are fueled only by gasoline, but the human digestive system must process fuel from many sources for use by the "high-performance machine" that is the human body.

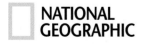

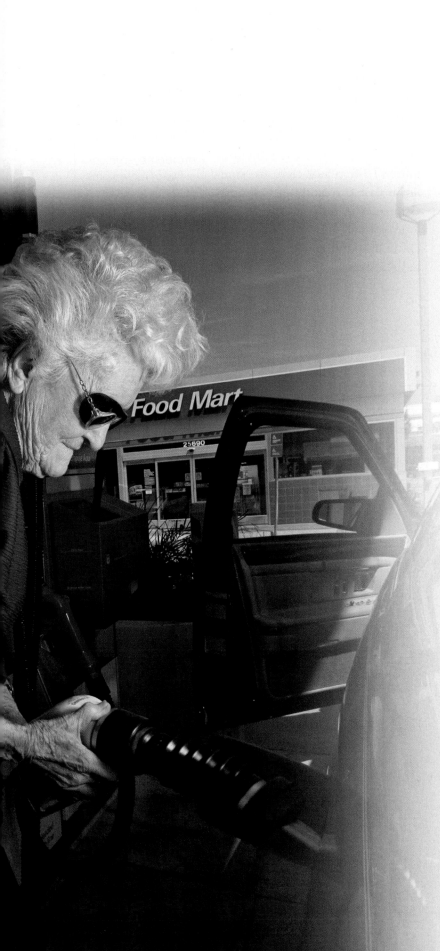

CHAPTER OUTLINE

CHAPTER PLANNER ✓

- ❏ Stimulate your interest by reading the opening story and looking at the visual.
- ❏ Scan the Learning Objectives in each section:
  p. 64 ❏ p. 68 ❏ p. 70 ❏ p. 79 ❏ p. 85 ❏ p. 90 ❏
- ❏ Read the text and study all figures and visuals. Answer any questions.

Analyze key features

- ❏ Process Diagram, p. 64 ❏ p. 74 ❏ p. 76 ❏ p. 86 ❏ p. 90 ❏
- ❏ Nutrition InSight, p. 75 ❏   p. 83 ❏
- ❏ What a Scientist Sees, p. 78 ❏
- ❏ Thinking It Through, p. 84 ❏
- ❏ Stop: Answer the Concept Checks before you go on:
  p. 67 ❏ p. 70 ❏ p. 78 ❏ p. 85 ❏ p. 89 ❏ p. 91 ❏

End of chapter

- ❏ Review the Summary, Key Terms, and Online Resources.
- ❏ Answer the Critical and Creative Thinking Questions.
- ❏ Answer What is happening in this picture?
- ❏ Complete the Self-Test and check your answers.

The Organization of Life

LEARNING OBJECTIVES

1. **Describe** the organization of living things, from atoms to organisms.

2. **Name** the organ systems that work with the digestive system to deliver nutrients and eliminate wastes.

atter, be it a meal you are about to eat or the plate you are about to eat it from, is made up of **atoms** (**Figure 3.1**). Atoms combine to form **molecules**, which can have different properties from those of the atoms they contain. In any living system, the molecules are organized into **cells**, the smallest units of life. Cells that are similar in structure and function form **tissues**. The human body contains four types of tissue: muscle, nerve, epithelial, and connective. These tissues are organized in varying

atom The smallest unit of an element that retains the properties of the element.

molecule A group of two or more atoms of the same or different elements bonded together.

cell The basic structural and functional unit of living things.

PROCESS DIAGRAM

From atoms to organisms • Figure 3.1

The organization of life begins with atoms that form molecules, which are then organized into cells to form tissues, organs, and whole organisms.

Atoms

1 Atoms linked by chemical bonds form molecules.

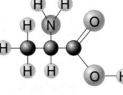

Molecule

2 Molecules form the structures that make up cells. Each cell is bounded by a membrane. In multicellular organisms, cells are usually specialized to perform specific functions.

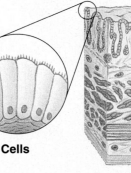

Cells

Tissues

3 Groups of similar cells form tissues. The tissue layers shown here make up the stomach wall.

organ A discrete structure composed of more than one tissue that performs a specialized function.

combinations to form **organs**. In most cases, an organ does not function alone but is part of an **organ system**. Moreover, an organ may be part of more than one organ system. For example, the pancreas is part of the endocrine system and also part of the digestive system.

The body's 11 organ systems interact to perform all the functions necessary for life (**Table 3.1** on page 66). For example, the digestive system, which is the primary organ system responsible for moving nutrients into the body, is assisted by the endocrine system, which secretes **hormones** that help regulate how much we eat and how quickly food and nutrients travel through the digestive system. The digestive system is also aided by the nervous system, which sends nerve signals that help control the passage of food through the digestive tract; by the cardiovascular system, which transports nutrients to individual cells in the body; and by the urinary, respiratory, and integumentary systems, which eliminate wastes generated in the body.

hormone A chemical messenger that is produced in one location in the body, is released into the blood, and travels to other locations, where it elicits responses.

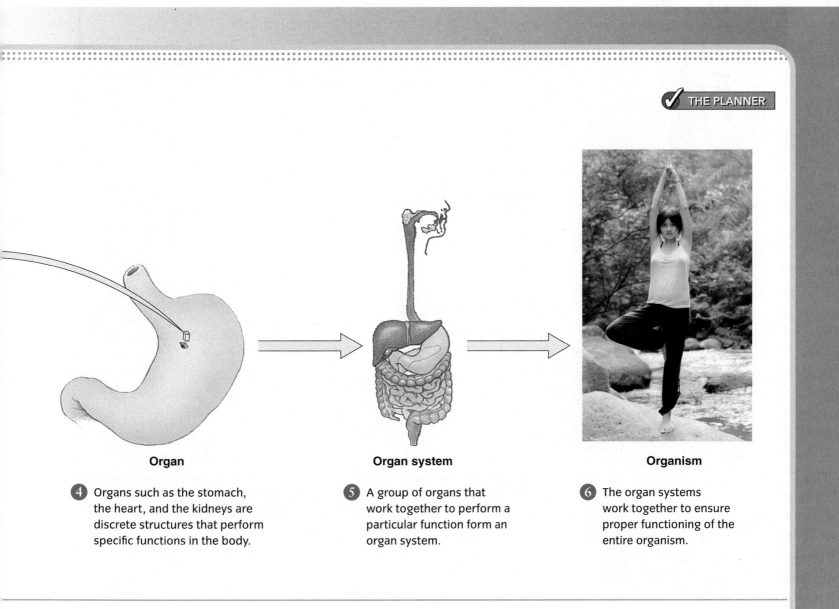

THE PLANNER

Organ

④ Organs such as the stomach, the heart, and the kidneys are discrete structures that perform specific functions in the body.

Organ system

⑤ A group of organs that work together to perform a particular function form an organ system.

Organism

⑥ The organ systems work together to ensure proper functioning of the entire organism.

The major organ systems of the human body   Table 3.1

Organ system	What it includes	What it does
Nervous	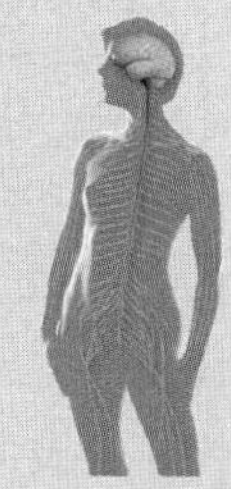 Nerves, sense organs, brain, and spinal cord	Responds to stimuli from external and internal environments; conducts impulses to activate muscles and glands; integrates activities of other systems.
Respiratory	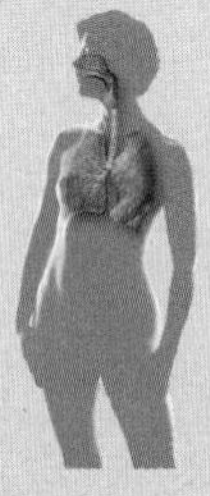 Lungs, trachea, and air passageways	Supplies the blood with oxygen and removes carbon dioxide.
Urinary	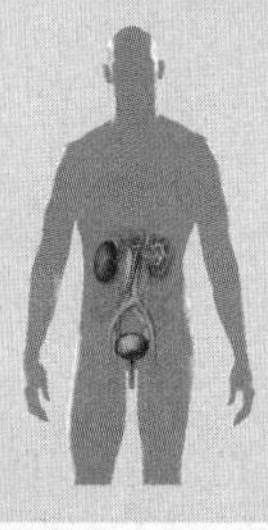 Kidneys and associated structures	Eliminates wastes and regulates the balance of water, electrolytes, and acid in the blood.
Reproductive	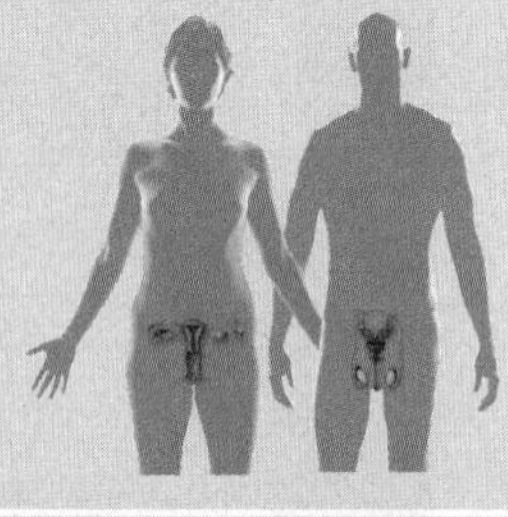 Testes, ovaries, and associated structures	Produces offspring.
Cardiovascular/circulatory	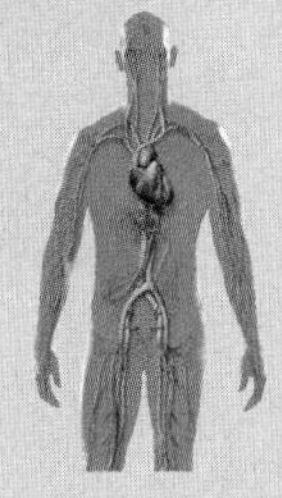 Heart and blood vessels	Transports blood, which carries oxygen, nutrients, and wastes.
Lymphatic/immune	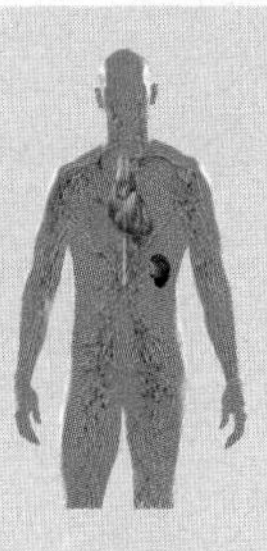 Lymph and lymph structures, white blood cells	Defends against foreign invaders; picks up fluid leaked from blood vessels; transports fat-soluble nutrients.

(Continued) **Table 3.1**

Organ system		What it includes	What it does
Muscular		Skeletal muscles	Provides movement and structure.
Skeletal		Bones and joints	Protects and supports the body, provides a framework for the muscles to use for movement.
Endocrine		Pituitary, adrenal, thyroid, pancreas, and other ductless glands	Secretes hormones that regulate processes such as growth, reproduction, and nutrient use.
Integumentary		Skin, hair, nails, and sweat glands	Covers and protects the body; helps control body temperature.
Digestive		Mouth, esophagus, stomach, intestines, pancreas, liver, and gallbladder	Ingests and digests food; absorbs nutrients into the blood; eliminates nonabsorbed food wastes.

CONCEPT CHECK   STOP

1. **How** are atoms, molecules, and cells related to one another?

2. **How** do the endocrine and nervous systems interact with the digestive system?

The Digestive System

LEARNING OBJECTIVES

1. **Define** digestion and absorption.
2. **List** the organs that make up the digestive system.
3. **Describe** the tissues that make up the wall of the gastrointestinal tract.
4. **Explain** the roles of mucus, enzymes, nerves, and hormones in digestion.

he digestive system is the organ system that is primarily responsible for **digestion** and for the **absorption** of nutrients into the body. When you eat a taco, for example, the tortilla, meat, cheese, lettuce, and tomato are broken apart, releasing the nutrients and other food components they contain. Water, vitamins, and minerals are taken into the body without being broken into smaller units, but proteins, carbohydrates, and

> **digestion** The process by which food is broken down into components small enough to be absorbed into the body.
>
> **absorption** The process of taking substances from the gastrointestinal tract into the interior of the body.

fats must be digested further. Proteins are broken down into amino acids, most of the carbohydrate is broken down into sugars, and most fats are digested to produce molecules with long carbon chains called **fatty acids**. The sugars, amino acids, and fatty acids can then be absorbed into the body. The fiber in whole grains, fruits, and vegetables cannot be digested and therefore is not absorbed into the body. It and other unabsorbed substances pass through the digestive tract and are eliminated in **feces**.

> **feces** Body waste, including unabsorbed food residue, bacteria, mucus, and dead cells, which is eliminated from the gastrointestinal tract by way of the anus.

Structure of the digestive system • Figure 3.2

a. The digestive system consists of the organs of the digestive tract—mouth, pharynx, esophagus, stomach, small intestine, and large intestine—plus four accessory organs—salivary glands, liver, gallbladder, and pancreas.

Ask Yourself

Bile is made in the _____ and stored in the _____. It is released into the _____, where it is important for the digestion and absorption of _____.

Mouth: Chews food and mixes it with saliva

Salivary glands: Produce saliva, which contains a starch-digesting enzyme

Pharynx: Swallows chewed food mixed with saliva

Esophagus: Moves food to the stomach

Stomach: Churns and mixes food; secretes acid and a protein-digesting enzyme

Liver: Makes bile, which aids in digestion and absorption of fat

Pancreas: Releases bicarbonate to neutralize intestinal contents; produces enzymes that digest carbohydrate, protein, and fat

Gallbladder: Stores bile and releases it into the small intestine when needed

Small intestine: Absorbs nutrients into blood or lymph; most digestion occurs here

Large intestine: Absorbs water and some vitamins and minerals; home to intestinal bacteria; passes waste material

Colon

Rectum

Anus: Opens to allow waste to leave the body

Organs of the Digestive System

The digestive system is composed of the **gastrointestinal tract** and accessory organs (**Figure 3.2a**). The gastrointestinal tract is a hollow tube, about 30 feet long, that runs from the mouth to the anus. It is also called the gut, GI tract, alimentary canal, or digestive tract. The inside of the tube is the **lumen** (**Figure 3.2b**). Food in the lumen is not technically inside the body because it has not been absorbed. When you swallow something that cannot be digested, such as a whole sesame seed or an unpopped kernel of popcorn, it passes through your digestive tract and exits in the feces, without ever entering your blood or cells. Only after substances have been absorbed into the cells that line the intestine can they be said to be inside the body.

The lumen is lined with a layer of **mucosal cells** called the **mucosa**. Because mucosal cells are in direct contact with churning food and harsh digestive secretions, they live only about two to five days. The dead cells are sloughed off into the lumen, where some components are digested and absorbed and the rest are eliminated in feces. New mucosal cells are formed continuously to replace those that die. To allow for this rapid replacement, the mucosa has high nutrient requirements and is one of the first parts of the body to be affected by nutrient deficiencies.

The time it takes food to travel the length of the GI tract from mouth to anus is called the **transit time**. The shorter the transit time, the more rapidly material is passing through the digestive tract. In a healthy adult, transit time is 24 to 72 hours, depending on the composition of the individual's diet and his or her level of physical activity, emotional state, health status, and use of medications.

Digestive System Secretions

Digestion is aided by substances secreted into the digestive tract from cells in the mucosa and from a number of accessory organs. One of these substances is **mucus**, which moistens, lubricates, and protects the digestive

> **mucus** A viscous fluid secreted by glands in the digestive tract and other parts of the body. It lubricates, moistens, and protects cells from harsh environments.

Contraction of the layers of smooth muscle—over which we do not have voluntary control—helps mix food, break it into small particles, and propel it through the digestive tract.

This external layer of connective tissue provides support and protection.

b. This cross section through the wall of the small intestine reveals the four tissue layers that make up the wall of the gastrointestinal tract.

The mucosa, which lines the GI tract, is a type of epithelial tissue. Nutrients must pass through these mucosal cells before they can reach the blood or lymph.

Lumen

This layer of connective tissue contains nerves and blood vessels. It provides support, nourishes the mucosa, and sends the nerve signals that control secretions and muscle contractions.

Think Critically
Why is food in the lumen still outside the body?

Enzyme activity • Figure 3.3

Enzymes are needed to break down different food components. The enzyme shown here, called an *amylase*, breaks large carbohydrate molecules, such as those in bread, into smaller ones. Amylases have no effect on fat, whereas enzymes called *lipases* digest fat and have no effect on carbohydrate.

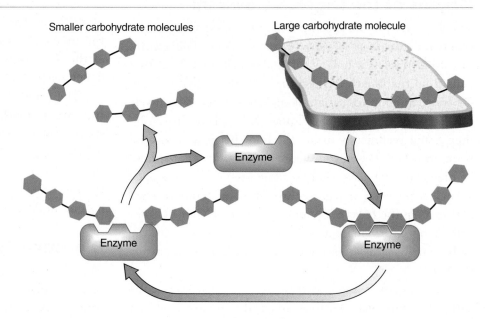

Smaller carbohydrate molecules

Large carbohydrate molecule

Enzyme

Enzyme

Enzyme

---

enzyme A protein molecule that accelerates the rate of a chemical reaction without itself being changed.

tract. **Enzymes** are also present in digestive system secretions. They accelerate the chemical reactions that break down food into units small enough to be absorbed (**Figure 3.3**).

The gastrointestinal tract is part of the endocrine system as well as the digestive system. It releases hormones that help prepare different parts of the gut for the arrival of food and thus regulate digestion and the rate at which food moves through the digestive system. Some hormonal signals slow digestion, whereas others facilitate it. For example, when the nutrients from your lunch reach your small intestine, they trigger the release of hormones that

signal the pancreas and gallbladder to secrete digestive substances into the small intestine.

CONCEPT CHECK STOP

1. **What** happens during digestion and absorption?

2. **Which** organs make up the gastrointestinal tract?

3. **What** are mucosal cells?

4. **How** are enzymes important for digestion and absorption?

Digestion and Absorption of Nutrients

LEARNING OBJECTIVES

1. **Describe** what happens in each of the organs of the gastrointestinal tract.

2. **Discuss** factors that influence how quickly food moves through the GI tract.

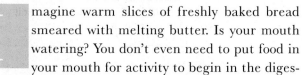

3. **Explain** how the structure of the small intestine aids in its function.

4. **Distinguish** passive diffusion from active transport.

I magine warm slices of freshly baked bread smeared with melting butter. Is your mouth watering? You don't even need to put food in your mouth for activity to begin in the digestive tract. Sensory input alone—the sight of the bread

being lifted out of the oven, the smell of the bread, the clatter of the butter knife—may make your mouth water and your stomach begin to secrete digestive substances. This response occurs when the nervous system signals the digestive system to ready itself for a meal. In order for food to be used by the body, however, you need to do more than smell your meal. The food must be consumed and digested, and the nutrients must be absorbed and transported to the body's cells. This involves the combined functions of all the organs of the digestive system, as well as the help of some other organ systems.

The Mouth

Digestion involves chemical and mechanical processes, both of which begin in the mouth. The presence of food in the mouth stimulates the flow of saliva from the salivary glands. Saliva moistens the food and carries dissolved food molecules to the taste buds, most of which are located on the tongue. Signals from the taste buds, along with the aroma of food, allow us to enjoy the taste of the food we eat. Saliva contains the enzyme **salivary amylase**, which begins the chemical digestion of food by breaking starch molecules into shorter sugar chains (see Figure 3.3). Saliva also helps protect against tooth decay because it washes away food particles and contains substances that inhibit the growth of bacteria that cause tooth decay.

> **saliva** A watery fluid that is produced and secreted into the mouth by the salivary glands. It contains lubricants, enzymes, and other substances.

Chewing food begins the mechanical aspect of digestion. Adult humans have 32 teeth, which are specialized for biting, tearing, grinding, and crushing foods. Chewing breaks food into small pieces. This makes the food easier to swallow and increases the surface area in contact with digestive juices. The tongue helps mix food with saliva and aids chewing by constantly repositioning food between the teeth. Chewing also breaks up fiber, which traps nutrients. If the fiber is not broken up, some of the nutrients in the food cannot be absorbed. For example, if the fibrous skin of a raisin is not broken open by the teeth, the nutrients inside the raisin remain inaccessible, and the raisin travels, undigested, through the intestines for elimination in the feces.

The Pharynx

The **pharynx**, the part of the gastrointestinal tract that is responsible for swallowing, is also part of the respiratory tract. Food passes through the pharynx on its way to the stomach, and air passes through the pharynx on its way to and from the lungs. As we prepare to swallow, the tongue moves the **bolus** of chewed food mixed with saliva to the back of the mouth. During swallowing, the air passages are blocked by a valvelike flap of tissue called the **epiglottis** so that food goes to the esophagus and not to the lungs (**Figure 3.4a**). Sometimes eating too quickly or talking while eating interferes with the movement of the epiglottis, and food passes into an upper air passageway. This food can usually be dislodged with a cough, but if it becomes stuck and causes choking, it may need to be forced out by means of the Heimlich maneuver (**Figure 3.4b**).

> **epiglottis** A piece of elastic connective tissue that covers the opening to the lungs during swallowing.

Swallowing and choking • Figure 3.4

a. When a bolus of food is swallowed, it normally pushes the epiglottis down over the opening to the passageway that leads to the lungs.

b. If food becomes lodged in the passageway leading to the lungs, it can block the flow of air. The Heimlich maneuver, which involves a series of thrusts directed upward from under the diaphragm (the muscle separating the chest and abdominal cavities), forces air out of the lungs, blowing the lodged food out of the air passageway.

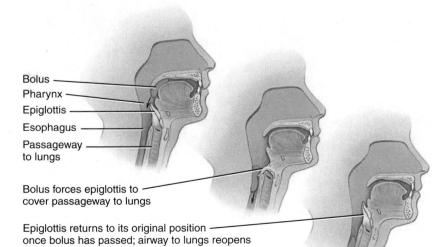

Bolus
Pharynx
Epiglottis
Esophagus
Passageway to lungs

Bolus forces epiglottis to cover passageway to lungs

Epiglottis returns to its original position once bolus has passed; airway to lungs reopens

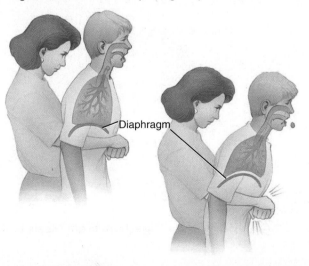

Diaphragm

The Esophagus

The esophagus connects the pharynx with the stomach. In the esophagus, the bolus of food is moved along by rhythmic contractions of the smooth muscles, an action called

> **peristalsis** Coordinated muscular contractions that move material through the GI tract.

peristalsis (**Figure 3.5**). The contractions of peristalsis are strong enough so that even if you ate while standing on your head, food would reach your stomach. This contractile movement, which is controlled automatically by the nervous system, occurs throughout the gastrointestinal tract, pushing the bolus along from the pharynx through the large intestine.

To leave the esophagus and enter the stomach, food must pass through a **sphincter**, a muscle that encircles the tube of the digestive tract and acts as a valve. When the sphincter contracts, the valve is closed; when it relaxes, the valve is open (see Figure 3.5). The sphincter, located between the esophagus and the stomach, prevents food from moving from the stomach back into the esophagus, but occasionally stomach contents do move in this direction. This is what occurs with heartburn (as discussed later in this chapter): Some of the acidic stomach contents leak up through this sphincter into the esophagus, causing a burning sensation.

Food also moves from the stomach into the esophagus during vomiting. Vomiting is initiated by a complex series of signals from the brain that cause the sphincter to relax and the muscles to contract, forcing the stomach contents upward, out of the stomach and toward the mouth.

Moving food through the GI tract • Figure 3.5

The food we swallow doesn't just fall down the esophagus and into the stomach. It is pushed along by muscular contractions and enters the stomach in response to the opening and closing of the sphincter, located where the esophagus meets the stomach.

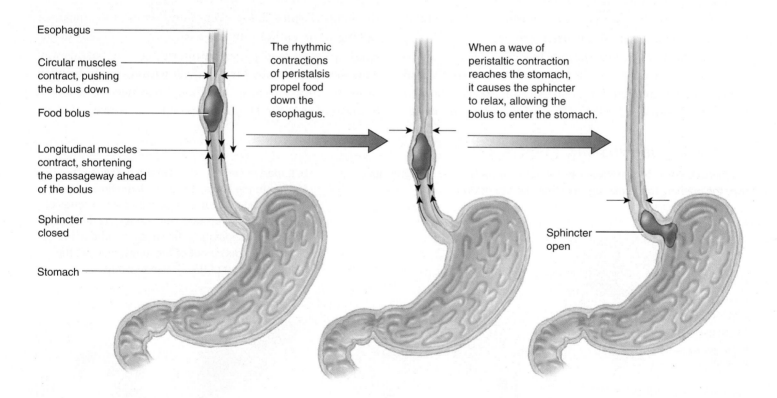

Esophagus

Circular muscles contract, pushing the bolus down

Food bolus

Longitudinal muscles contract, shortening the passageway ahead of the bolus

Sphincter closed

Stomach

The rhythmic contractions of peristalsis propel food down the esophagus.

When a wave of peristaltic contraction reaches the stomach, it causes the sphincter to relax, allowing the bolus to enter the stomach.

Sphincter open

Stomach structure and function • Figure 3.6

a. Most of the gastrointestinal tract is surrounded by two layers of smooth muscle, one that is longitudinal and one that is circular, but the stomach contains a third smooth muscle layer running diagonally. The presence of this diagonal layer allows for the powerful contractions that churn and mix the stomach contents. The sphincter at the bottom of the stomach controls the flow of chyme into the small intestine.

b. The lining of the stomach is covered with gastric pits. Inside these pits are the gastric glands, made up of different types of cells that produce the mucus, hydrochloric acid, and the inactive form of pepsin contained in gastric juice.

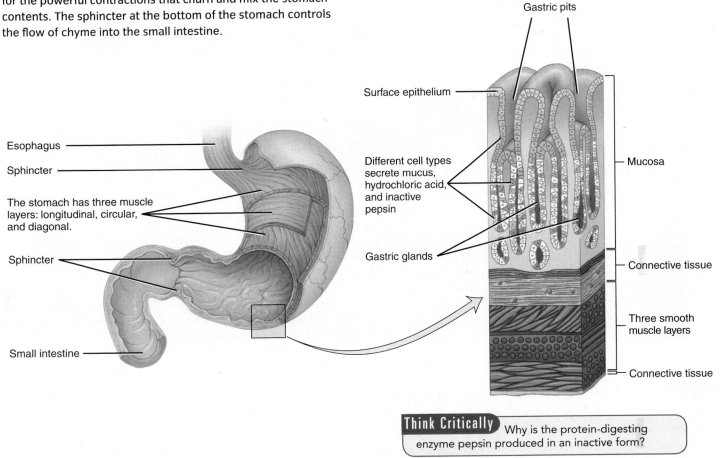

Gastric pits

Surface epithelium

Different cell types secrete mucus, hydrochloric acid, and inactive pepsin

Gastric glands

Esophagus

Sphincter

The stomach has three muscle layers: longitudinal, circular, and diagonal.

Sphincter

Small intestine

Mucosa

Connective tissue

Three smooth muscle layers

Connective tissue

Think Critically Why is the protein-digesting enzyme pepsin produced in an inactive form?

The Stomach

The stomach is an expanded portion of the gastrointestinal tract that serves as a temporary storage place for food. Here the bolus is mashed and mixed with highly acidic stomach secretions to form a semiliquid food mass called **chyme**. The mixing of food in the stomach is aided by an extra layer of smooth muscle in the stomach wall (**Figure 3.6a**). Some digestion takes place in the stomach, but, with the exception of some water, alcohol, and a few drugs, such as aspirin and acetaminophen (Tylenol), very little absorption occurs here.

Gastric juice Chemical digestion in the stomach is caused by **gastric juice** produced by gastric glands in

pits that dot the stomach lining (**Figure 3.6b**). Gastric juice is a mixture of water, mucus, hydrochloric acid, and an inactive form of the protein-digesting enzyme **pepsin**. This enzyme is secreted in an inactive form so that it will not damage the gastric glands that produce it. The hydrochloric acid in gastric juice kills most of the bacteria present in food. It also stops the activity of the carbohydrate-digesting enzyme salivary amylase and helps begin the digestion of protein by activating pepsin and unfolding proteins. A thick layer of mucus prevents the protein that makes up the stomach wall from being damaged by the hydrochloric acid and pepsin in gastric juice.

The regulation of stomach motility and secretion • Figure 3.7

Stomach activity is affected by food that has not yet reached the stomach, by food that is in the stomach, and by food that has left the stomach.

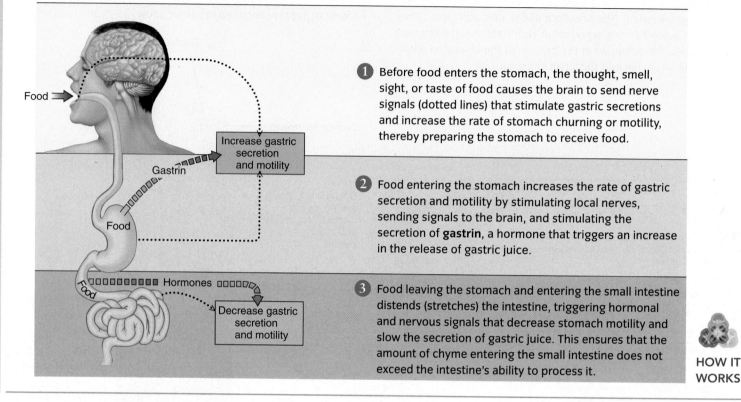

1 Before food enters the stomach, the thought, smell, sight, or taste of food causes the brain to send nerve signals (dotted lines) that stimulate gastric secretions and increase the rate of stomach churning or motility, thereby preparing the stomach to receive food.

2 Food entering the stomach increases the rate of gastric secretion and motility by stimulating local nerves, sending signals to the brain, and stimulating the secretion of **gastrin**, a hormone that triggers an increase in the release of gastric juice.

3 Food leaving the stomach and entering the small intestine distends (stretches) the intestine, triggering hormonal and nervous signals that decrease stomach motility and slow the secretion of gastric juice. This ensures that the amount of chyme entering the small intestine does not exceed the intestine's ability to process it.

HOW IT WORKS

Regulation of stomach activity How much your stomach churns, how much gastric juice is released, and how fast material empties out of the stomach are regulated by signals from both nerves and hormones. These signals originate from three sites—the brain, the stomach, and the small intestine (**Figure 3.7**).

As chyme moves out of the stomach, signals sent by the small intestine help regulate the rate at which the stomach empties. The small intestine stretches as it fills with chyme; this distension inhibits the stomach from emptying. Chyme normally empties from the stomach within two to six hours, but this rate varies with the size and composition of the meal that has been consumed. A large meal takes longer to leave the stomach than does a small meal. Liquids empty quickly, but solids linger until they are well mixed with gastric juice and are liquefied; hence, solids leave the stomach more slowly than liquids.

The nutritional composition of a meal also affects how long it stays in the stomach. A meal that consists primarily of starch or sugar leaves quickly, but a meal that is high in fiber or protein takes longer to leave the stomach. A high-fat meal stays in the stomach the longest. Because the nutrient composition of a meal affects how quickly it leaves your stomach, it affects how soon after eating you will feel hungry again (**Figure 3.8**).

Hunger and meal composition • Figure 3.8

What you choose for breakfast can affect how soon you become hungry for lunch. A small, carbohydrate-rich meal of dry toast and coffee will leave your stomach far more quickly than a larger meal containing more protein, fiber, and fat, such as a vegetable-and-cheese omelet with whole-wheat toast and butter.

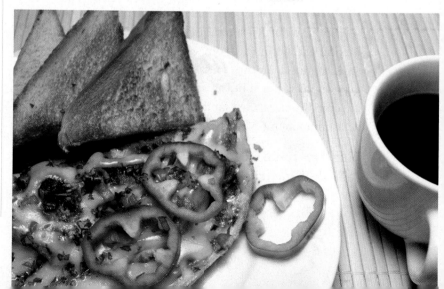

The Small Intestine

The small intestine is a narrow tube about 20 feet long. Here the chyme is propelled along by peristalsis and mixed by rhythmic constrictions called **segmentation** that slosh the material back and forth. The small intestine is the main site for the chemical digestion of food, completing the process that the mouth and stomach have started. It is also the primary site for the absorption of water, vitamins, minerals, and the products of carbohydrate, fat, and protein digestion.

The small intestine has a number of unique structural features that contribute to its digestive function and enhance the amount of surface area available for absorption (**Figure 3.9**). Together these features provide a surface area that is about the size of a tennis court (about 2700 ft^2).

Secretions that aid digestion In the small intestine, secretions from the pancreas, the gallbladder, and the small intestine itself aid digestion. The pancreas secretes **pancreatic juice**, which contains **bicarbonate**, and digestive enzymes. Bicarbonate, which is a base, neutralizes the acid in the chyme, making the environment in the small intestine neutral or slightly basic rather than acidic, as in the stomach. This neutrality allows enzymes from the pancreas and small intestine to function.

Nutrition InSight   The structure of the small intestine • Figure 3.9

THE PLANNER

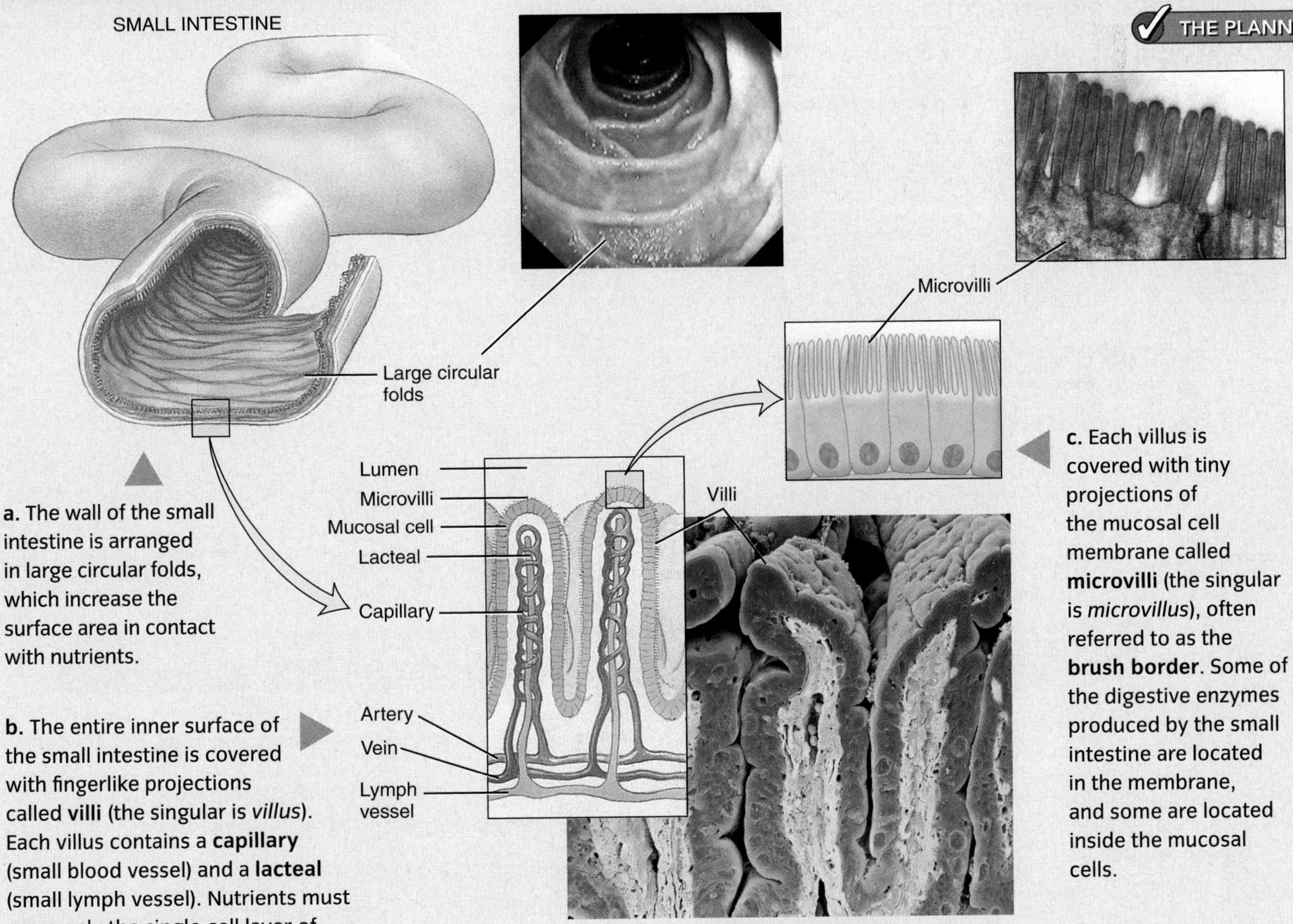

SMALL INTESTINE

Large circular folds

Microvilli

a. The wall of the small intestine is arranged in large circular folds, which increase the surface area in contact with nutrients.

b. The entire inner surface of the small intestine is covered with fingerlike projections called **villi** (the singular is *villus*). Each villus contains a **capillary** (small blood vessel) and a **lacteal** (small lymph vessel). Nutrients must cross only the single-cell layer of the mucosa to reach the blood or lymph for delivery to the tissues of the body.

Lumen
Microvilli
Mucosal cell
Lacteal
Capillary
Villi
Artery
Vein
Lymph vessel

c. Each villus is covered with tiny projections of the mucosal cell membrane called **microvilli** (the singular is *microvillus*), often referred to as the **brush border**. Some of the digestive enzymes produced by the small intestine are located in the membrane, and some are located inside the mucosal cells.

Ask Yourself

What are the three structural features of the small intestine that increase its surface area?

Pancreatic amylase is an enzyme that continues the job of breaking down starches into sugars that was started in the mouth by salivary amylase. Pancreatic **proteases** (protein-digesting enzymes), such as trypsin and chymotrypsin, break protein into shorter and shorter chains of amino acids, and fat-digesting enzymes called **lipases** break down fats into fatty acids. The pancreatic proteases, like the pepsin produced by the stomach, are released in an inactive form so that they will not digest the glands that produce them. Intestinal digestive enzymes, found in the cell membranes or inside the cells lining the small intestine, aid the digestion of double sugars (those that contain two sugar units) into single sugar units and the digestion of short amino acid chains into single amino acids. The sugars from carbohydrate digestion and the amino acids from protein digestion pass into the blood and are delivered to the liver (**Figure 3.10**).

The gallbladder stores and secretes **bile**, a substance that is produced in the liver and is necessary for the digestion and absorption of fat. Bile that is secreted into the small intestine mixes with fat and divides it into small globules,

> **bile** A digestive fluid made in the liver and stored in the gallbladder that is released into the small intestine, where it aids in fat digestion and absorption.

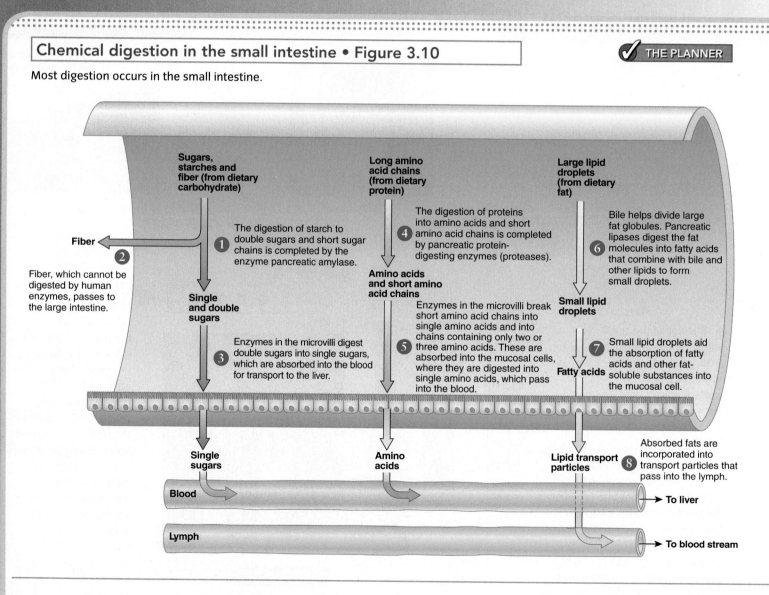

PROCESS DIAGRAM

Chemical digestion in the small intestine • Figure 3.10   ✓ THE PLANNER

Most digestion occurs in the small intestine.

Sugars, starches and fiber (from dietary carbohydrate)

Fiber

2 Fiber, which cannot be digested by human enzymes, passes to the large intestine.

1 The digestion of starch to double sugars and short sugar chains is completed by the enzyme pancreatic amylase.

Single and double sugars

3 Enzymes in the microvilli digest double sugars into single sugars, which are absorbed into the blood for transport to the liver.

Long amino acid chains (from dietary protein)

4 The digestion of proteins into amino acids and short amino acid chains is completed by pancreatic protein-digesting enzymes (proteases).

Amino acids and short amino acid chains

5 Enzymes in the microvilli break short amino acid chains into single amino acids and into chains containing only two or three amino acids. These are absorbed into the mucosal cells, where they are digested into single amino acids, which pass into the blood.

Large lipid droplets (from dietary fat)

6 Bile helps divide large fat globules. Pancreatic lipases digest the fat molecules into fatty acids that combine with bile and other lipids to form small droplets.

Small lipid droplets

7 Small lipid droplets aid the absorption of fatty acids and other fat-soluble substances into the mucosal cell.

Fatty acids

Single sugars

Amino acids

Lipid transport particles

8 Absorbed fats are incorporated into transport particles that pass into the lymph.

Blood

Lymph

→ **To liver**

→ **To blood stream**

Absorption mechanisms • Figure 3.11

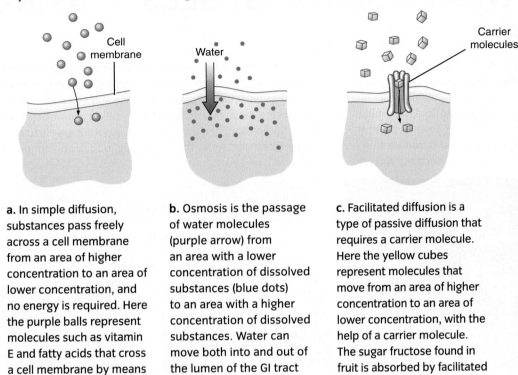

a. In simple diffusion, substances pass freely across a cell membrane from an area of higher concentration to an area of lower concentration, and no energy is required. Here the purple balls represent molecules such as vitamin E and fatty acids that cross a cell membrane by means of simple diffusion.

b. Osmosis is the passage of water molecules (purple arrow) from an area with a lower concentration of dissolved substances (blue dots) to an area with a higher concentration of dissolved substances. Water can move both into and out of the lumen of the GI tract by osmosis.

c. Facilitated diffusion is a type of passive diffusion that requires a carrier molecule. Here the yellow cubes represent molecules that move from an area of higher concentration to an area of lower concentration, with the help of a carrier molecule. The sugar fructose found in fruit is absorbed by facilitated diffusion.

d. Active transport requires energy and a carrier molecule. The red pyramids represent molecules that are transported from an area of lower concentration to an area of higher concentration. Active transport allows amino acids to be absorbed even when they are present in higher concentrations in the mucosal cell than in the lumen.

Ask Yourself

1. Which absorption mechanism(s) can only move nutrients from an area with a higher concentration of that nutrient to an area with a lower concentration?
2. Which absorption mechanism(s) require(s) a carrier molecule?
3. Which absorption mechanism(s) require(s) energy?

allowing lipases to access and digest the fat molecules more efficiently. The bile and digested fats then form small droplets that facilitate the absorption of fat into the mucosal cells. Once inside the mucosal cells, the products of fat digestion are incorporated into transport particles. These are absorbed into the lymph before passing into the blood (see Figure 3.10).

Absorption The small intestine is the main site for the absorption of nutrients. To be absorbed, nutrients must pass from the lumen of the GI tract into the mucosal cells lining the tract and then into either the blood or the lymph. Several different mechanisms are involved (**Figure 3.11**). Some rely on **diffusion**, which is the net movement of substances from an area of higher concentration to an area of lower concentration. **Simple diffusion**, in which material moves freely across a cell membrane; **osmosis**, which is the diffusion of water; and **facilitated diffusion**, in which a carrier molecule is needed for the substance to cross a cell membrane,

depend on diffusion and are passive, requiring no energy. **Active transport** requires energy and a carrier molecule. This process can transport material from an area of lower concentration to one of higher concentration.

The Large Intestine

Materials not absorbed in the small intestine pass through a sphincter between the small intestine and the large intestine. This sphincter prevents material from the large intestine from re-entering the small intestine.

The large intestine is about 5 feet long and is divided into the colon, which makes up the majority of the large intestine, and the rectum, the last 8 inches. The large intestine opens to the exterior of

simple diffusion The unassisted diffusion of a substance across a cell membrane.

osmosis The unassisted diffusion of water across a cell membrane.

facilitated diffusion Assisted diffusion of a substance across a cell membrane.

active transport The transport of substances across a cell membrane with the aid of a carrier molecule and the expenditure of energy.

WHAT A SCIENTIST SEES

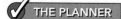

Bacteria on the Menu

The human gut is home to 300 to 500 species of bacteria. The right mix of bacteria is important for immune function, proper growth and development of colon cells, and optimal intestinal motility and transit time.[1] Having healthy microflora can inhibit the growth of harmful bacteria and has been shown to prevent the diarrhea associated with antibiotic use and to reduce the duration of diarrhea resulting from intestinal infections and other causes.[2,3] There is also evidence that having healthy microflora may relieve constipation, reduce allergy symptoms, and modify the risk of inflammatory bowel disease and colon cancer.[4,5,6] Consuming these beneficial bacteria, called **probiotics**, is one way of promoting healthy microflora. Another way is to consume **prebiotics**, substances that serve as a food supply for beneficial bacteria.

Think Critically Why might consuming a prebiotic increase the numbers of beneficial bacteria in the gut?

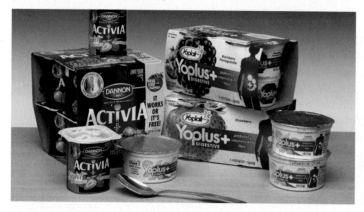

a. Ads claim that eating these specialized probiotic yogurts will help regulate the digestive system. Consumers see these products as a tasty way to help regulate digestion. Scientists recognize that these products as well as most other yogurts contain active cultures of beneficial bacteria, including *Lactobacillus* and *Bifidobacterium*.

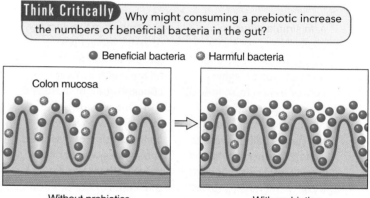

● Beneficial bacteria   ● Harmful bacteria

Colon mucosa

Without probiotics   With probiotics

b. When beneficial bacteria are consumed in adequate amounts, they live temporarily in the colon, where they inhibit the growth of harmful bacteria and confer other health benefits on the host. However, the bacteria must be consumed frequently because they are flushed out in the feces.

---

the body at the anus. Although most nutrient absorption occurs in the small intestine, water and some vitamins and minerals are also absorbed in the colon.

Peristalsis occurs more slowly in the large intestine than in the small intestine. Water, nutrients, and fecal matter may spend 24 hours in the large intestine, in contrast to the 3 to 5 hours it takes these materials to move through the small intestine. This slow movement favors the growth of bacteria. These bacteria, called the **intestinal microflora**, are permanent, beneficial residents of this part of the gastrointestinal tract (see *What a Scientist Sees*). They break down unabsorbed portions of food, such as fiber, producing nutrients that can be used by the microflora or, in some cases, absorbed into the body. For example, the microflora synthesize small amounts of certain B vitamins and vitamin K, some of which can be absorbed. As the microflora break down material in the colon, they produce gas, which causes flatulence. In a healthy adult, between 200 and 2000 ml of gas is produced in the intestine each day.

Material that is not absorbed in the colon passes into the rectum, where it is stored temporarily and then evacuated through the anus as feces. The feces are a mixture of undigested, unabsorbed matter, dead cells, secretions from the GI tract, water, and bacteria. The amount of bacteria varies but can make up more than half the weight of the feces. The amount of water in the feces is affected by fiber and fluid intake. Because fiber retains water, when adequate fiber and fluids are consumed, feces have a higher water content and are more easily passed.

CONCEPT CHECK

1. **What** are the functions of the stomach?

2. **How** does food move through the GI tract?

3. **How** do the villi and microvilli aid absorption?

4. **Why** is active transport needed for the complete absorption of some nutrients?

Digestion in Health and Disease

LEARNING OBJECTIVES

1. **Explain** how the gastrointestinal tract protects us from infection.

2. **Describe** the causes of food allergies.

3. **Discuss** the causes and consequences of ulcers, heartburn, and GERD.

4. **Explain** how dental problems and gallstones might affect food intake.

he health of the GI tract is essential to our overall health. The gut acts as a defense against invasion by disease-causing organisms and other contaminants and allows us to obtain nutrients efficiently. Food allergies, which can be life-threatening, have their origins in the GI tract, but most common gastrointestinal problems are minor and do not affect long-term health.

The Digestive System and Disease Prevention

Food almost always contains bacteria and other contaminants, but it rarely makes us sick. This is because the mucosa of the GI tract contains tissue that is part of the immune system (**Figure 3.12a**). This tissue prevents disease-causing bacteria and toxins from taking over the GI tract and invading the body.

If an invading substance, or **antigen**, enters the lumen or is absorbed into the mucosa, the immune system can use a number of weapons to destroy it. These include various types of white blood cells, which circulate in the blood and reside in the mucosa of the gastrointestinal tract. They can quickly destroy most antigens that enter the body through the mucosa.

When an antigen is present, **phagocytes** are the first type of white blood cell to come to the body's defense (**Figure 3.12b**). If the invader is not eliminated by the phagocytes, more specific white blood cells called **lymphocytes** join the battle. Some lymphocytes destroy specific antigens by binding to them. This type of lymphocyte helps eliminate cancer cells, foreign tissue, and cells that have been infected by viruses and bacteria. Other lymphocytes produce and secrete protein molecules called **antibodies**. Antibodies bind to antigens and help destroy them. Each antibody is designed to fight off only one type of antigen. Once antibodies to a specific antigen have been made, the immune system remembers and is ready to fight that antigen any time it enters the body again.

> **antigen** A foreign substance that, when introduced into the body, stimulates an immune response.
>
> **antibody** A protein, released by a type of lymphocyte, that interacts with and deactivates specific antigens.

Immune function in the small intestine • Figure 3.12

a. The darkly stained areas shown here are called Peyer's patches. They are made up of immune system tissue and are embedded throughout the mucosa of the small intestine. Peyer's patches contain cells that participate in the immune system's efforts to prevent harmful organisms or materials present in the GI tract from making us ill.

b. The cells shown here in pink *are phagocytes*, which can engulf and destroy invading substances. The cells shown in green *are lymphocytes*, which are specific with regard to which invaders they can attack. Some lymphocytes directly kill invaders, while others secrete antibodies that help destroy antigens.

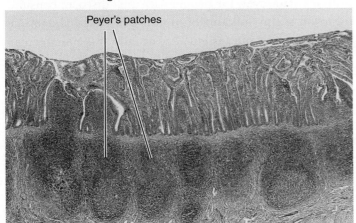

Peyer's patches

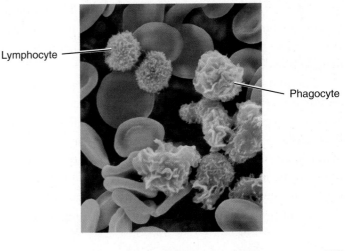

Lymphocyte

Phagocyte

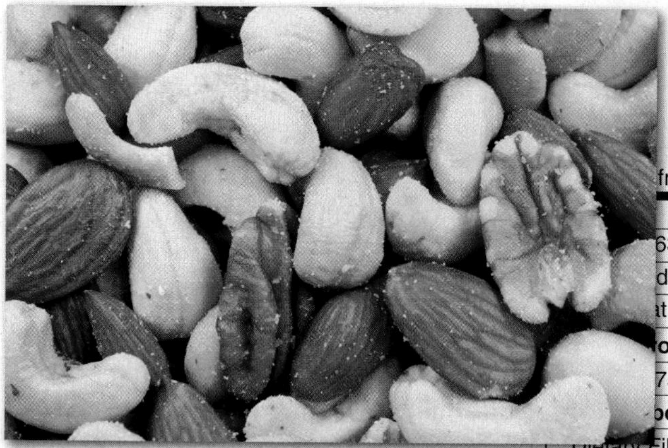

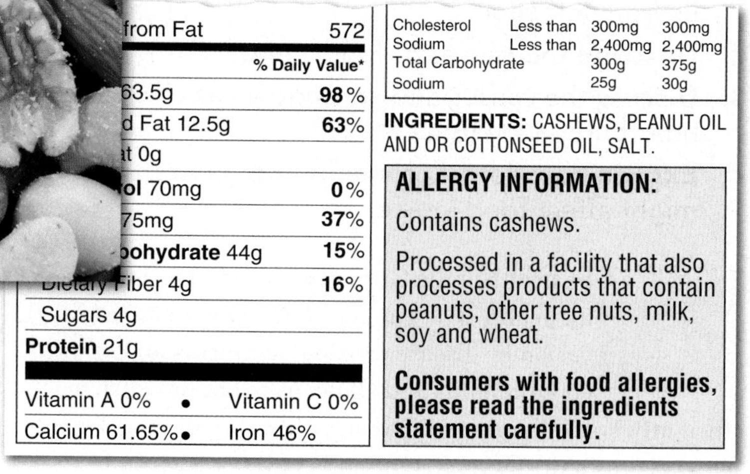

Food allergies affect about 2% of adults and 4 to 8% of children and are responsible for 150 deaths in the United States each year.[7] To protect consumers, food manufacturers are required to clearly state on the label whether a product contains any of the eight major ingredients that are most likely to cause allergic reactions: peanuts, tree nuts, milk, eggs, fish, shellfish, soy, and wheat.

			from Fat	572
				% Daily Value*
	63.5g			98%
d Fat 12.5g				63%
t 0g				
ol 70mg				0%
75mg				37%
ohydrate 44g				15%
Dietary Fiber 4g				16%
Sugars 4g				
Protein 21g				
Vitamin A 0%	•	Vitamin C 0%		
Calcium 61.65%	•	Iron 46%		

Cholesterol	Less than	300mg	300mg
Sodium	Less than	2,400mg	2,400mg
Total Carbohydrate		300g	375g
Sodium		25g	30g

INGREDIENTS: CASHEWS, PEANUT OIL AND OR COTTONSEED OIL, SALT.

ALLERGY INFORMATION:

Contains cashews.

Processed in a facility that also processes products that contain peanuts, other tree nuts, milk, soy and wheat.

Consumers with food allergies, please read the ingredients statement carefully.

If harmful organisms infect the GI tract, the body may help out the immune system by using diarrhea or vomiting to flush them out.

Food allergies

Our immune system protects us from many invaders without our being aware of it. Unfortunately, the response of the immune system to a foreign substance is also to blame for allergic reactions. An allergic reaction occurs when the immune system produces antibodies to a substance, called an **allergen**, that is present in our diet or environment. **Food allergies** occur when the body sees proteins present in food as foreign substances and therefore initiates an immune response. The immune response causes symptoms that range from hives to life-threatening reactions such as breathing difficulties or a drop in blood pressure.

> **allergen** A substance that causes an allergic reaction.

The first time a food is consumed, it does not trigger an allergic reaction, but in a susceptible person, this first exposure begins the process. As the food is digested, tiny fragments of undigested protein trigger the production of antibodies. When the food protein is eaten again, it binds to the antibodies, signaling the release of chemicals that cause redness, swelling, and other allergy symptoms. When the protein enters the mouth, the allergic person may experience an itching or tingling sensation on the tongue or lips. As the protein travels down to the stomach and intestines, the allergic response may lead to vomiting and cramps. After the protein fragments are absorbed and travel through the blood, they may cause a drop in blood pressure, hives, and breathing difficulties.

The best way to avoid allergy symptoms is to avoid foods to which you are allergic (**Figure 3.13**).

Celiac disease

Celiac disease is a condition in which the protein gluten, found in wheat, barley, and rye, triggers an immune system response that damages or destroys the villi of the small intestine. For most of us the gluten in our foods is digested and absorbed like other proteins. However, for people with this disease, consuming even a tiny amount of gluten can cause abdominal pain, diarrhea, and fatigue. Eventually this damage can lead to malnutrition, weight loss, anemia, osteoporosis, intestinal cancer, and other chronic illnesses.[8,9] Celiac disease, also called gluten intolerance, celiac sprue, nontropical sprue, and gluten-sensitive enteropathy, is an inherited condition that affects an estimated 1 in 133 people in the population. Although gluten intolerance is currently a trendy condition (See *Debate: Should You Be Gluten Free?*), the disease can be diagnosed only by a blood test or an intestinal biopsy. For people with celiac disease,

The Issue: Gluten-free diets are essential for people with celiac disease, but a gluten-free diet has also been promoted for weight loss and to treat a host of other ailments. Is gluten free a healthy alternative for everyone?

You see the term "gluten free" on breakfast cereals, cake mixes, pastas, soups, and a host of other products. Celebrities are touting the benefits of going gluten free. Chelsea Clinton even had her wedding cake baked without gluten. The increase in the number of gluten-free foods over the past few years is partly due to greater awareness and better diagnosis of celiac disease; however, a switch to gluten-free products has also been promoted as a healthier way of eating for everyone. Advocates claim that a gluten-free diet will promote weight loss and help those suffering with joint pain, rheumatoid arthritis, osteoporosis, anemia, and diabetes. They contend that individuals with these symptoms have undiagnosed celiac disease. Although a small number of people may benefit from a gluten-free diet because they have celiac disease but no obvious symptoms, eating a gluten-free diet is unlikely to cure these conditions in people who do not have celiac disease.

What about going gluten free for weight loss? Gluten-free foods are not any lower in calories than other foods, but eliminating everything that contains gluten from your diet—most types of cereal, bread, pasta, cakes, and cookies—will help cut calories. Gluten-free foods are also not nutritionally superior to other foods, but if you are trying to lose weight, carefully choosing everything you put in your mouth will force you to plan your diet carefully and may help with weight loss.

Is a gluten-free diet harmful? Eliminating gluten involves carefully checking each ingredient in the foods you eat to eliminate products made not only from wheat, which is the major grain in the American diet, but also from barley and rye as well as the myriad of foods that have wheat added as a thickener (see the figure). The major problem with a gluten-free diet is that it eliminates most flours, breads, pasta, and breakfast cereals, which are important sources of B vitamins and iron. This creates a risk for nutrient deficiencies. A gluten-free diet is not harmful as long as it provides enough of all the nutrients typically consumed in gluten-containing foods. People diagnosed with celiac disease generally work with a dietitian to make sure they have a well-balanced, varied diet that meets all their nutrient needs. People eating a gluten-free diet for other reasons generally do not.

So, although there is no research to support the benefits of eliminating gluten if you do not have celiac disease, anything that makes you consider your diet carefully is a good thing. Individuals with gluten sensitivity are benefiting from the gluten-free craze because it has increased the availability and quality of gluten-free foods, improved the labeling of gluten-free products, and heightened awareness of celiac disease. Proponents think a gluten-free diet will improve everyone's health. Skeptics consider gluten-free another trend like the low-carb fad of a few years back.

Think critically: Neither potatoes nor onions contain gluten. If you had celiac disease, based on the ingredients shown here, which would be a safer choice: the French fries or the onion rings?

French Fries

INGREDIENTS: POTATOES, VEGETABLE OIL (PALM, SUNFLOWER, SOYBEAN, AND/OR CANOLA), SALT, DEXTROSE, DISODIUM DIHYDROGEN PYROPHOSPHATE, ANNATTO (VEGETABLE COLOR).

Onion Rings

INGREDIENTS: ONIONS, BLEACHED WHEAT FLOUR, SOYBEAN OIL AND/OR CANOLA OIL, YELLOW CORN FLOUR, SUGAR, SALT, SOY FLOUR, WHEY, DEXTROSE, LEAVENING (MONOCALCIUM PHOSPHATE, SODIUM BICARBONATE), YEAST, POLYSORBATE 80, CALCIUM PROPIONATE (PRESERVATIVE).

consuming a diet that eliminates gluten provides relief from symptoms. This means eliminating products made from wheat, barley, or rye, including most breads, crackers, pastas, cereals, cakes, and cookies. It also requires eliminating foods ranging from packaged gravies to soy sauce that are processed with these grains.

Digestive System Problems and Discomforts

Almost everyone experiences digestive system problems from time to time. These problems often cause discomfort and frequently limit the types of foods a person can consume (**Figure 3.14a**). They also can interfere with nutrient digestion and absorption. Problems may occur anywhere in the digestive tract, from the mouth to the anus, and can affect the accessory organs that provide the secretions that are essential for proper GI function.

Heartburn and GERD
Heartburn occurs when the acidic contents of the stomach leak back into the esophagus (**Figure 3.14b**). The medical term for the leakage of stomach contents into the esophagus is *gastroesophageal reflux*. Occasional heartburn is common, but if it occurs more than twice a week, it may indicate a condition called **gastroesophageal reflux disease (GERD)**. If left untreated, GERD can eventually lead to more serious health problems, such as esophageal bleeding, ulcers, and cancer.

> **heartburn** A burning sensation in the chest or throat caused when acidic stomach contents leak back into the esophagus.
>
> **gastroesophageal reflux disease (GERD)** A chronic condition in which acidic stomach contents leak into the esophagus, causing pain and damaging the esophagus.

The discomforts of heartburn and GERD can be avoided by limiting the amounts and types of foods consumed. Eating small meals and consuming beverages between rather than with meals prevents heartburn by reducing the volume of material in the stomach. Avoiding fatty and fried foods, chocolate, peppermint, and caffeinated beverages, which increase stomach acidity or slow stomach emptying, can help minimize symptoms. Remaining upright after eating, wearing loose clothing, avoiding smoking and alcohol, and losing weight may also help prevent heartburn. For many people, medications that neutralize acid or reduce acid secretion are needed to manage symptoms.

Peptic ulcers
Peptic ulcers occur when the mucus barrier protecting the stomach, esophagus, or upper small intestine is penetrated and the acid and pepsin in digestive secretions damage the gastrointestinal lining (**Figure 3.14c**). Mild ulcers cause abdominal pain; more severe ulcers can cause life-threatening bleeding.

> **peptic ulcer** An open sore in the lining of the stomach, esophagus, or upper small intestine.

Peptic ulcers can result from GERD or from misuse of medications such as aspirin or nonsteroidal anti-inflammatory drugs (such as Motrin and Advil) but are more often caused by infection with the bacterium *Helicobacter pylori* (*H. pylori*). These bacteria burrow into the mucus and destroy the protective mucosal layer.[10] Over half of the world's population is infected with *H. pylori*, but not everyone who is infected develops ulcers.[11] *H. pylori* infection can be treated using antibiotics.

Gallstones
Clumps of solid material that accumulate in either the gallbladder or the bile duct are referred to as **gallstones** (**Figure 3.14d**). They can cause pain when the gallbladder contracts in response to fat in the intestine. Gallstones can interfere with bile secretion and reduce fat absorption. They are usually treated by removing the gallbladder. After the gallbladder has been removed, bile, which is produced in the liver, drips directly into the intestine as it is produced rather than being stored and squeezed out in larger amounts when fat enters the intestine.

Diarrhea and constipation
Diarrhea and constipation are common discomforts that are related to problems in the intestines. **Diarrhea** refers to frequent, watery stools. It occurs when material moves through the colon too quickly for sufficient water to be absorbed or when water is drawn into the lumen from cells lining the intestinal tract.

Diarrhea can be caused by bacterial or viral infections, irritants that inflame the lining of the GI tract, the passage of undigested food into the large intestine, medications, and chronic intestinal diseases. Diarrhea causes loss of fluids and minerals. Severe diarrhea lasting more than a day or two can be life-threatening.

Constipation refers to hard, dry stools that are difficult to pass; it occurs when the water content of the stool is too

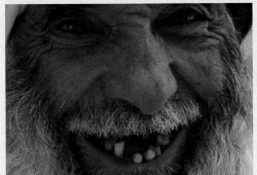

a. Tooth loss and dental pain can make chewing difficult. This may limit the intake of certain foods and reduce nutrient absorption because poorly chewed food may not be completely digested. Tooth decay and gum disease are more likely when saliva production is reduced. Reduced saliva production is a side effect of many medications and can cause changes in taste and difficulty swallowing.

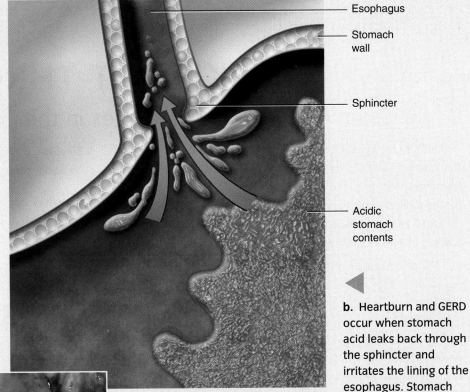

Esophagus

Stomach wall

Sphincter

Acidic stomach contents

b. Heartburn and GERD occur when stomach acid leaks back through the sphincter and irritates the lining of the esophagus. Stomach contents also pass through this sphincter during vomiting. Vomiting may be caused by an illness, a food allergy, medication, an eating disorder, or pregnancy.

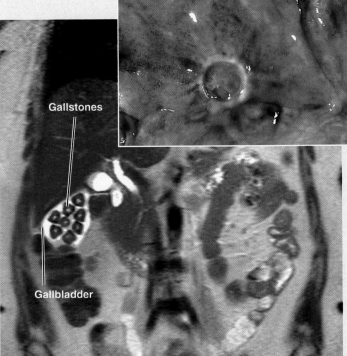

Gallstones

Gallbladder

c. Peptic ulcers occur when the mucosa is destroyed, exposing underlying tissues to gastric juices. Damage that reaches the nerve layer causes pain, and bleeding can occur if blood vessels are damaged. If the wall of the stomach or esophagus is perforated because of an ulcer, a serious abdominal infection can occur.

e. Constipation, in which the feces are hard and dry, is often due to a diet that is too low in fiber and fluids. It increases pressure in the colon and can lead to outpouches in the colon wall, shown here, called diverticula (discussed further in Chapter 4).

Colon wall

Diverticula

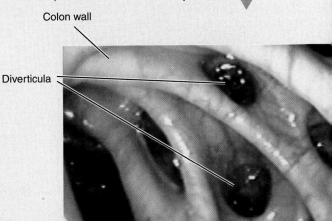

d. Gallstones, visible in this image of the abdomen, are deposits of cholesterol, bile pigments, and calcium that can be in the gallbladder or the bile duct. They can block bile from entering the small intestine, causing pain when the gallbladder contracts and reducing fat digestion and absorption.

low (**Figure 3.14e**). Constipation can be caused by a diet containing insufficient fluid or fiber, lack of exercise, a weakening of the muscles of the large intestine, and a variety of medications. It can be prevented by drinking plenty of fluids, consuming a high-fiber diet, and getting enough exercise (see *Thinking It Through* and *What Should I Eat?*).

THINKING IT THROUGH ✓ THE PLANNER

A Case Study on How Changes in the GI Tract Affect Health

Changes in the digestive system affect how our bodies process the food we eat. For each patient described here, think about how digestion and absorption are affected and the consequences for the patient's nutritional health.

A 50-year-old man is taking medication that reduces the amount of saliva he produces.

What effect might this have on his nutrition and health?
▼

Your answer:

An 80-year-old woman wearing dentures that don't fit well likes raw carrots and still eats them but can't chew them thoroughly.

How might this affect the digestion and absorption of nutrients contained in the carrots?
▼

Your answer:

A 47-year-old woman undergoes treatment for colon cancer, which requires that most of her large intestine be surgically removed.

How does this change affect the amount of fluid she needs to consume?
▼

Your answer:

A 56-year-old man has gallstones, which cause pain when his gallbladder contracts.

What type of foods should he avoid and why?
▼

Your answer:

A 50-year-old man has a deficiency of pancreatic enzymes.

How would this affect nutrient digestion?
▼

Your answer:

A 40-year-old woman weighing 300 pounds has undergone a surgical procedure called gastric banding to help her lose weight. The diagram shows how her stomach was altered.

Why can't she eat as much food as before? Will the procedure affect nutrient absorption?
▼

Your answer:

(Check your answers in Appendix J.)

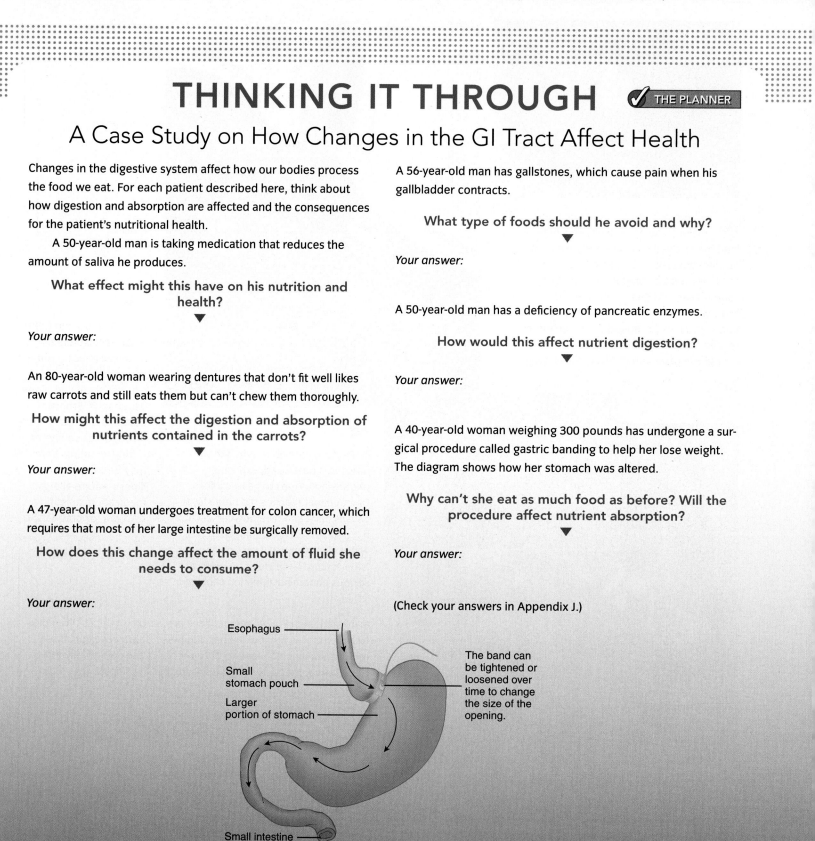

Esophagus

Small stomach pouch

Larger portion of stomach

The band can be tightened or loosened over time to change the size of the opening.

Small intestine

WHAT SHOULD I EAT?
For Digestive Health

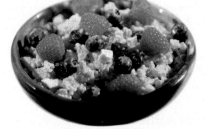

✓ THE PLANNER

Reduce your risk of adverse reactions
- Read food labels to avoid foods that you are allergic to.
- Chew each bite thoroughly to maximize digestion and avoid choking.
- Don't talk with food in your mouth.
- Learn the Heimlich maneuver: You could save a life.

Reduce the chances of heartburn
- Eat enough to satisfy your hunger but not so much that you are stuffed.
- Wait 10 minutes between your first and second courses to see how full you feel.
- Stay upright after you eat; don't flop on the couch in front of the television.

Avoid constipation by consuming enough fiber and fluid
- Choose whole-grain cereals such as oatmeal or raisin bran.
- Double your servings of vegetables at dinner.
- Eat two pieces of fruit with your lunch.
- Choose whole-grain bread.
- Have one or two beverages with or before each meal.

Use iProfile to find the fiber content of your favorite fruits and vegetables.

CONCEPT CHECK 🛑 STOP

1. **Why** is the immune function of the GI tract so important?
2. **How** can food allergy symptoms be prevented?
3. **When** can antibiotics be used to treat ulcers?
4. **What** foods should be avoided by people with heartburn? by people with gallstones?

Delivering Nutrients and Eliminating Wastes

LEARNING OBJECTIVES

1. **Trace** the path of blood circulation.
2. **Discuss** how blood flow is affected by eating and activity.
3. **Explain** the functions of the lymphatic system.
4. **List** four ways in which waste products are eliminated from the body.

After food has been digested and the nutrients have been absorbed, the nutrients must be delivered to the cells. This delivery is handled by the **cardiovascular system**, which consists of the heart and blood vessels. Amino acids from protein, single sugars from carbohydrate, and the water-soluble products of fat digestion

> **capillary** A small, thin-walled blood vessel through which blood and the body's cells exchange gases and nutrients.

are absorbed into **capillaries** in the villi of the small intestine and transported via the blood to the liver (see Figure 3.9b). The products of digestion that are not water soluble, such as cholesterol and large fatty acids, are absorbed into **lacteals**, which are part of the **lymphatic system**, before entering the blood.

>
> **lacteal** A lymph vessel in the villi of the small intestine that picks up particles containing the products of fat digestion.

The Cardiovascular System

The cardiovascular system circulates blood throughout the body. Blood carries nutrients and oxygen to the cells of all the organs and tissues of the body and removes carbon dioxide and other waste products from these cells. Blood also carries other substances, such as hormones, from one part of the body to another.

Blood circulation • Figure 3.15

Blood pumped to the lungs picks up oxygen and delivers nutrients. Blood pumped to the rest of the body delivers oxygen and nutrients.

1 Oxygen-poor blood that reaches the heart from the rest of the body is pumped through the arteries to the capillaries of the lungs.

2 In the capillaries of the lungs, oxygen from inhaled air is picked up by the blood, and carbon dioxide is released into the lungs and exhaled.

3 Oxygen-rich blood returns to the heart from the lungs via veins.

4 Oxygen-rich blood is pumped out of the heart into the arteries that lead to the rest of the body.

5 In the capillaries of the body, nutrients and oxygen move from the blood to the body's tissues, and carbon dioxide and other waste products move from the tissues to the blood, to be carried away.

6 Oxygen-poor blood returns to the heart via veins.

Think Critically Why is the cardiovascular system important in nutrition?

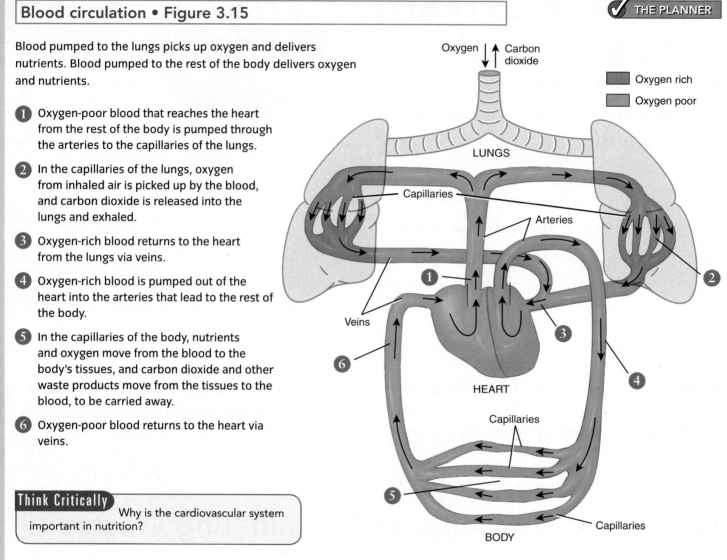

Oxygen ↓ ↑ Carbon dioxide

■ Oxygen rich
■ Oxygen poor

LUNGS
Capillaries
Arteries
Veins
HEART
Capillaries
BODY
Capillaries

The heart and blood vessels The heart is the workhorse of the cardiovascular system. It is a muscular pump with two circulatory loops—one that carries blood to and from the lungs and one that carries blood to and from the rest of the body (**Figure 3.15**).

The blood vessels that transport blood and dissolved substances toward the heart are called **veins**, and those that transport blood and dissolved substances away from the heart are called **arteries**. As arteries carry blood away from the heart, they branch many times to form smaller and smaller blood vessels. The smallest arteries are called **arterioles**. Arterioles branch to form capillaries. Blood from capillaries then flows into the smallest veins, the **venules**, which converge to form larger and larger veins for returning blood to the heart.

The exchange of nutrients and gases occurs across the thin walls of the capillaries. In most body tissues, oxygen and nutrients carried by the blood pass from the capillaries into the cells, and carbon dioxide and other waste products pass from the cells into the capillaries. In the capillaries of the lungs, blood releases carbon dioxide to be exhaled and picks up oxygen to be delivered to the cells. In the capillaries of the GI tract, blood delivers oxygen and picks up water-soluble nutrients absorbed from the diet.

The amount of blood, and hence the amounts of nutrients and oxygen, delivered to a specific organ or tissue depends on the need. When you are resting, about 25% of your blood goes to your digestive system, about 20% to your skeletal muscles, and the rest to the heart, kidneys, brain, skin, and other organs.[12] This distribution changes when you eat or exercise. When you have eaten a large meal, a greater proportion of your blood goes to your digestive system to provide the oxygen and nutrients needed by the GI muscles and glands for digestion of the meal and absorption of nutrients. When you are exercising strenuously, about 70% of your blood is directed to your skeletal muscles to deliver nutrients and oxygen and remove carbon dioxide and other waste products (**Figure 3.16**).

Blood flow at rest and during exercise • Figure 3.16

a. At rest between meals, the amount of blood directed to the abdomen, which includes the organs, muscles, and glands of the digestive system, is similar to the amount that goes to the skeletal muscles.[12]

b. During exercise, the demands of the muscles take priority, and only a small proportion of the blood is directed to the abdomen.[12] This is why you may get cramps if you exercise right after eating a big meal: Your body cannot direct enough blood to the intestines and the muscles at the same time. The muscles win out, and food remains in your intestines, often causing cramps.

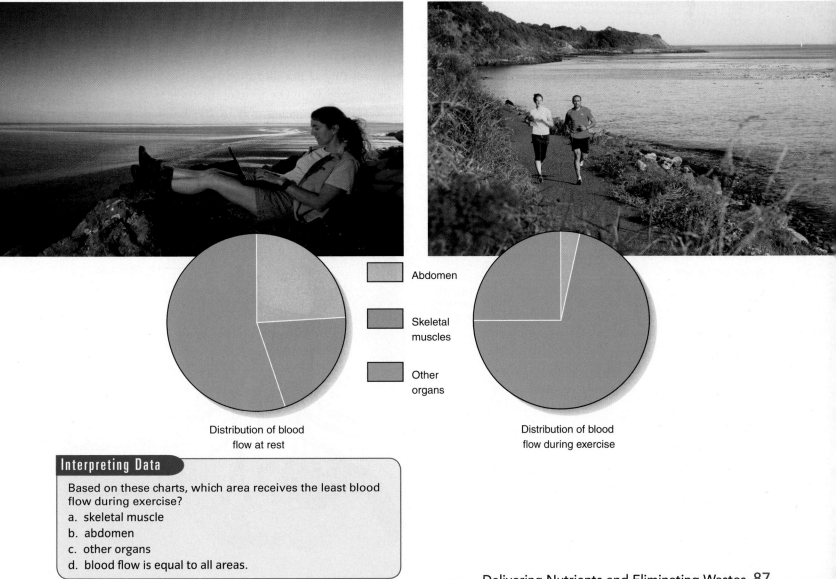

Abdomen

Skeletal muscles

Other organs

Distribution of blood flow at rest

Distribution of blood flow during exercise

Interpreting Data

Based on these charts, which area receives the least blood flow during exercise?

a. skeletal muscle

b. abdomen

c. other organs

d. blood flow is equal to all areas.

Delivering nutrients to the liver Water-soluble molecules in the small intestine, including amino acids, sugars, water-soluble vitamins, and the water-soluble products of fat digestion, cross the mucosal cells of the villi and enter the capillaries (see Figure 3.10). Once in the capillaries, these molecules are carried to the liver via the **hepatic portal vein** (Figure 3.17).

The liver acts as a gatekeeper between the body and substances absorbed from the intestine. Some nutrients are stored in the liver, some are changed into different forms, and others are allowed to pass through unchanged. The liver determines whether individual nutrients are stored or delivered immediately to the cells, depending on the body's needs. The liver is also important in the synthesis and breakdown of amino acids, proteins, and lipids. It modifies the products of protein breakdown to form molecules that can be safely transported to the kidney for excretion. The liver also contains enzyme systems that protect the body from toxins absorbed by the gastrointestinal tract.

The Lymphatic System

The lymphatic system consists of a network of tubules (lymph vessels) and lymph organs that contain infection-fighting cells. Fluid that collects in tissues and between cells drains into the lymphatic system. This prevents the fluid from accumulating and causing swelling.

The lymphatic system is an important part of the immune system. Fluid collected in the lymph vessels is filtered past a collection of infection-fighting cells before being returned to the blood. If the fluid contains antigen, an immune response is triggered. White blood cells and antibodies produced by this response enter the blood and help destroy the foreign substance.

In the small intestine, the lymph vessels aid in the absorption and transport of fat-soluble substances such as cholesterol, fatty acids, and fat-soluble vitamins. These pass from the intestinal mucosa into the lacteals located in the villi (see Figure 3.9b). The lacteals drain into larger lymph vessels. Lymph vessels from the intestine and most other organs drain into the thoracic duct, which empties into the blood near the neck. Therefore, substances absorbed into the lymphatic system do not pass through the liver before entering the general blood circulation.

Elimination of Wastes

Material that is not absorbed from the gut into the body is eliminated from the gastrointestinal tract in the feces. Wastes that are generated in the body, such as carbon dioxide, minerals, and nitrogen-containing wastes, must

Hepatic portal circulation • Figure 3.17

The hepatic portal circulation delivers nutrients to the liver. Water-soluble substances absorbed into the capillaries of the villi move into venules, which merge to form larger veins that eventually form the hepatic portal vein.

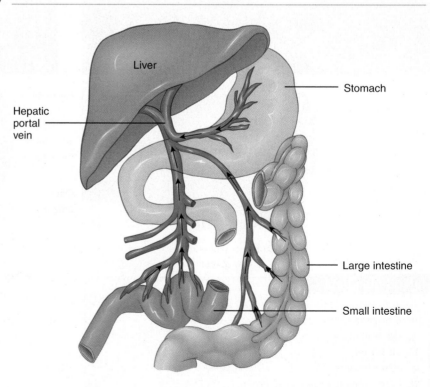

Liver

Stomach

Hepatic portal vein

Large intestine

Small intestine

Organ systems involved in elimination of wastes • Figure 3.18

The nutrients taken in by the digestive system and the oxygen taken in by the respiratory system are both distributed to all the cells in the body by the cardiovascular system. Unabsorbed materials are eliminated in the feces. Metabolic wastes are transferred to the outside environment by the skin and the urinary and respiratory systems.

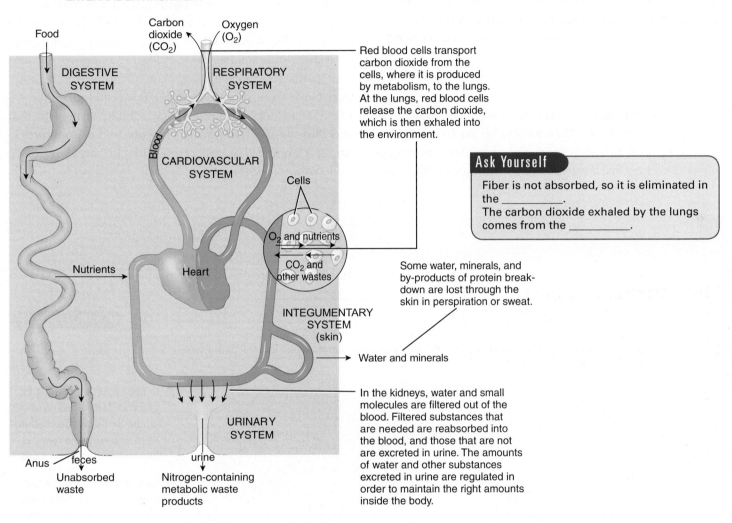

EXTERNAL ENVIRONMENT

Red blood cells transport carbon dioxide from the cells, where it is produced by metabolism, to the lungs. At the lungs, red blood cells release the carbon dioxide, which is then exhaled into the environment.

Ask Yourself

Fiber is not absorbed, so it is eliminated in the _____.
The carbon dioxide exhaled by the lungs comes from the _____.

Some water, minerals, and by-products of protein breakdown are lost through the skin in perspiration or sweat.

In the kidneys, water and small molecules are filtered out of the blood. Filtered substances that are needed are reabsorbed into the blood, and those that are not are excreted in urine. The amounts of water and other substances excreted in urine are regulated in order to maintain the right amounts inside the body.

also be eliminated. The same highway of blood vessels that picks up absorbed nutrients and oxygen helps remove wastes from the body. Carbon dioxide and some water are lost via the lungs, and water, minerals, and nitrogen-containing wastes are lost through the skin, but the kidney is the primary site for the excretion of metabolic wastes. Water, minerals, and the nitrogen-containing by-products of protein breakdown are filtered out of the blood by the kidneys and excreted in urine. **Figure 3.18** illustrates how the circulatory system is involved in both the delivery of nutrients and oxygen and the elimination of wastes.

CONCEPT CHECK

1. **Where** does blood go after it leaves the lungs?

2. **Why** is it not a good idea to exercise after eating a large meal?

3. **What** is the role of the lymphatic system in nutrient absorption?

4. **What** wastes are excreted by the kidneys? by the lungs?

An Overview of Metabolism

LEARNING OBJECTIVES

1. **Discuss** the two general ways in which nutrients can be used after they have been absorbed.
2. **Describe** what happens in cellular respiration.
3. **List** the types of molecules that can be made from glucose, from fatty acids, and from amino acids.

 nce they are inside the body's cells, nutrients are used either for energy or to synthesize all the structural and regulatory molecules needed for growth and maintenance. Together, the chemical reactions that break down molecules to provide energy and those that synthesize larger molecules are referred to as **metabolism**. Many of the reactions of metabolism occur in series known as **metabolic pathways**. Molecules that enter these pathways are modified at each step, with the help of enzymes. Some of the pathways use energy to build body structures, and others break large molecules into smaller ones, releasing energy. Reactions that synthesize molecules occur in different cellular compartments from those that break down molecules for energy. For example, ribosomes are cellular structures that specialize in the synthesis of proteins, and **mitochondria** are cell organs that are responsible for breaking down molecules to release energy.

PROCESS DIAGRAM

Producing ATP • Figure 3.19

✓ THE PLANNER

Cellular respiration uses oxygen to convert glucose, fatty acids, and amino acids into carbon dioxide, water, and energy, in the form of ATP.

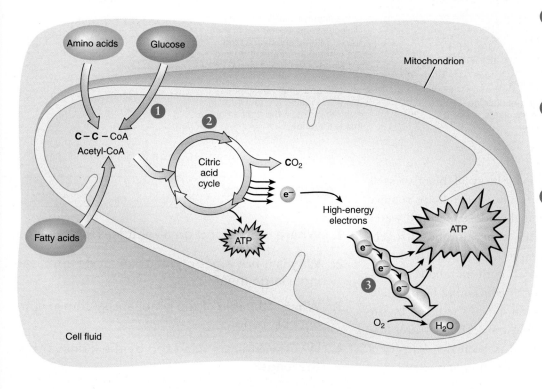

1. In the presence of oxygen, glucose, fatty acids, and amino acids can be metabolized to produce a two-carbon molecule (acetyl-CoA).

2. Each acetyl-CoA molecule enters a circular pathway, called the citric acid cycle, that produces two molecules of carbon dioxide (CO_2).

3. In the final step of this metabolic pathway, most of the energy released from the glucose, fatty acid, or amino acid molecules is used to produce ATP, and oxygen combines with electrons and hydrogen to form water.

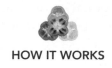

HOW IT WORKS

Releasing Energy

In the mitochondria, the sugar glucose, fatty acids, and amino acids derived from carbohydrates, fats, and proteins, respectively, are broken down in the presence of oxygen to produce carbon dioxide and water and release energy. This process, called **cellular respiration**, is like cell breathing: Oxygen goes into the cell, and carbon dioxide comes out. The energy released by cellular respiration is used to make a molecule called **adenosine triphosphate (ATP)** (**Figure 3.19**). ATP can be thought of as the cell's energy currency. The chemical bonds of ATP are very high in energy, and when they break, the energy is released and can be used either to power body processes, such as muscle contraction or the transport of molecules across membranes, or to synthesize new molecules needed to maintain and repair body tissues.

> **adenosine triphosphate (ATP)** A high-energy molecule that the body uses to power activities that require energy.

Synthesizing New Molecules

Glucose, fatty acids, and amino acids that are not broken down for energy are used, with the input of energy from ATP, to synthesize structural, regulatory, or storage molecules. Glucose molecules are used to synthesize the glucose-storage molecule glycogen and, in some cases, fatty acids. Fatty acids are used to make body fat, cell membranes, and regulatory molecules, and amino acids are used to synthesize the various proteins that the body needs and, when necessary, to make glucose. Excess amino acids can also be converted into fatty acids and stored as body fat.

CONCEPT CHECK STOP

1. **How** are nutrients used to produce ATP?
2. **Why** can cellular respiration be thought of as cell breathing?
3. **What** types of molecules can be made from amino acids?

THE PLANNER ✓

Summary

1 The Organization of Life 64

- Our bodies and the foods we eat are all made from the same building blocks—**atoms**. Atoms are linked together by chemical bonds to form **molecules**. Molecules can form **cells**, as shown. Cells with similar structures and functions are organized into **tissues**, and tissues are organized into the **organs** and **organ systems** that make up an organism. The body organ systems work together; for example, the passage of food through the digestive system and the secretion of digestive substances are regulated by the nervous and endocrine systems.

From atoms to organisms: Cells • Figure 3.1

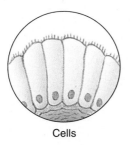

Cells

2 The Digestive System 68

- The digestive system has two major functions: **digestion** and **absorption**. Digestion breaks down food and nutrients into units that are small enough to be absorbed. Absorption transports nutrients into the body. The main component of the digestive system, illustrated here, is the **gastrointestinal tract**, which consists of a hollow tube that begins at the mouth and continues through the pharynx, esophagus, stomach, small intestine, and large intestine, ending at the anus.

Structure of the digestive system • Figure 3.2a

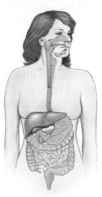

- The digestion of food and absorption of nutrients are aided by the secretion of **mucus** and **enzymes**.

3 Digestion and Absorption of Nutrients 70

- The processes involved in digestion begin in response to the smell or sight of food and continue as food enters the digestive tract at the mouth, where it is broken down into smaller pieces by the teeth and mixed with **saliva** to form a **bolus**. Carbohydrate digestion is begun in the mouth by **salivary amylase**. From the mouth, the **bolus** passes through the **pharynx** and into the esophagus. The rhythmic contractions of **peristalsis** propel it down the esophagus to the stomach.

- The stomach is a temporary storage site for food. The muscles of the stomach mix the food into a semiliquid mass called **chyme**, and **gastric juice**, which contains hydrochloric acid and **pepsin**, begins the digestion of protein. The rate at which the stomach empties varies with the amount and composition of food consumed and is regulated by nervous and hormonal signals.

- The small intestine is the primary site for nutrient digestion and absorption. The circular folds, **villi**, shown here, and microvilli of the small intestine, ensure a large absorptive surface area. In the small intestine, **bicarbonate** from the pancreas neutralizes stomach acid, and pancreatic and intestinal enzymes digest carbohydrate, fat, and protein. The digestion and absorption of fat in the small intestine are aided by **bile** from the gallbladder.

The structure of the small intestine • Figure 3.9b

Lumen
Microvilli
Mucosal cell
Lacteal
Capillary
Villi
Artery
Vein
Lymph vessel

- The absorption of food across the intestinal **mucosa** occurs by means of several different transport mechanisms. **Simple diffusion**, **osmosis**, and **facilitated diffusion** do not require energy, but **active transport** does.

- Components of **chyme** that are not absorbed in the small intestine pass on to the large intestine, where some water and nutrients are absorbed. The large intestine is populated by **intestinal microflora** that digest some of the unabsorbed materials, such as fiber, producing small amounts of nutrients and gas. The remaining unabsorbed materials are eliminated in the **feces**.

4 Digestion in Health and Disease 79

- Immune system cells and tissues located in the gastrointestinal tract help prevent disease-causing organisms or chemicals from entering the body. An **antigen** entering the digestive tract is attacked first by **phagocytes**. If it is not eliminated by the phagocytes, **lymphocytes** respond specifically to the antigen by producing **antibodies**. The immune system protects us from disease but can also cause **food allergies**.

- Diseases or discomforts at any point in the digestive system can interfere with food intake, digestion, or nutrient absorption. Common problems include dental problems, reduced saliva production, **heartburn**, **GERD**, **peptic ulcers** (such as the one shown here), **gallstones**, vomiting, **diarrhea**, and **constipation**.

Digestive disorders • Figure 3.14c

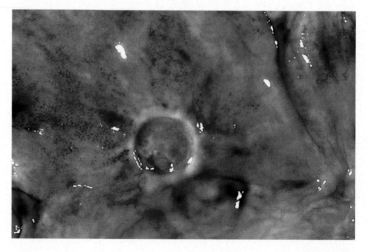

5 Delivering Nutrients and Eliminating Wastes 85

- Absorbed nutrients are delivered to the cells by the **cardiovascular system**. The heart pumps blood to the lungs to pick up oxygen and release carbon dioxide. From the lungs, blood returns to the heart and is then pumped to the rest of the body to deliver oxygen and nutrients and remove carbon dioxide and other wastes before returning to the heart. Exchange of nutrients and gases occurs at the **capillaries**.

- The products of carbohydrate and protein digestion and the water-soluble products of fat digestion enter capillaries in the intestinal **villi** and are transported to the liver via the **hepatic portal vein**, as illustrated here. The liver removes the absorbed substances for storage, converts them into other forms, or allows them to pass unaltered. The liver also protects the body from toxic substances that may have been absorbed.

Hepatic portal circulation • Figure 3.17

Liver

Hepatic portal vein

Stomach

Large intestine

Small intestine

- The fat-soluble products of digestion enter **lacteals** in the intestinal villi. Lacteals join larger lymph vessels. The nutrients absorbed via the **lymphatic system** enter the blood without first passing through the liver.

- Unabsorbed materials are eliminated in the feces. The waste products of metabolism are excreted by the lungs, skin, and kidneys.

6 An Overview of Metabolism 90

- In the cells, glucose, **fatty acids**, and amino acids absorbed from the diet can be broken down by means of **cellular respiration**, as shown here, to provide energy in the form of **ATP**.

Producing ATP • Figure 3.19

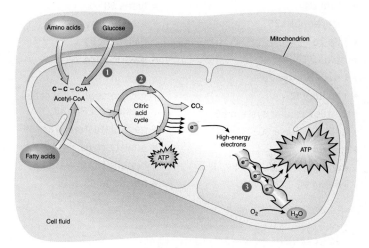

Amino acids Glucose

Mitochondrion

C – C – CoA
Acetyl-CoA

Citric acid cycle

CO_2

e⁻

High-energy electrons

Fatty acids

ATP

ATP

O_2 H_2O

Cell fluid

- In the presence of ATP, glucose, fatty acids, and amino acids can be used either to synthesize structural or regulatory molecules or to synthesize energy-storage molecules.

Key Terms

- absorption 68
- active transport 77
- adenosine triphosphate (ATP) 91
- allergen 80
- antibody 79
- antigen 79
- arteriole 86
- artery 86
- atom 64
- bicarbonate 75
- bile 76
- bolus 71
- brush border 75
- capillary 85
- cardiovascular system 85
- celiac disease 80
- cell 64
- cellular respiration 91
- chyme 73
- constipation 82
- diarrhea 82
- diffusion 77
- digestion 68
- enzyme 70
- epiglottis 71
- facilitated diffusion 77
- fatty acid 68
- feces 68
- food allergy 80
- gallstone 82
- gastric juice 73
- gastrin 74
- gastroesophageal reflux disease (GERD) 82
- gastrointestinal tract 69
- heartburn 82
- hepatic portal vein 88
- hormone 65
- intestinal microflora 78
- lacteal 85
- lipase 76
- lumen 69
- lymphatic system 85
- lymphocyte 79
- metabolic pathway 90
- metabolism 90
- microvillus 75
- mitochondrion 90
- molecule 64
- mucosa 69
- mucosal cells 69
- mucus 69
- organ 65
- organ system 65
- osmosis 77
- pancreatic amylase 76
- pancreatic juice 75
- pepsin 73
- peptic ulcer 82
- peristalsis 72
- phagocyte 79
- pharynx 71
- prebiotic 78
- probiotic 78
- protease 76
- saliva 71
- salivary amylase 71
- segmentation 75
- simple diffusion 77
- sphincter 72
- tissue 64
- transit time 69
- vein 86
- venule 86
- villi 75

Online Resources

- For more information on how the digestive system works, go to http://digestive.niddk.nih.gov/ddiseases/pubs/yrdd/.

- For more information on gluten, go to www.csaceliacs.org/AboutCSA.php.

- For more information on food, nutrition, and metabolism, go to http://health.nih.gov/category/FoodNutritionandMetabolism.

- Visit your *WileyPLUS* site for videos, animations, podcasts, self-study, and other media that will aid you in studying and understanding this chapter.

Critical and Creative Thinking Questions

1. For lunch, Joe, a college freshman, has a smoothie made with blended fruit and juice. His friend has a burger, fries, and a milk shake. Whose stomach will empty faster? Why?

2. Your grandmother's favorite snack is a crisp fresh apple, but she has difficulty chewing because of tooth loss and dental pain. How might you modify her snack to make it easier for her to eat?

3. Starting in the esophagus, trace the path of food through the digestive system. At each organ, indicate anatomical adaptations of the general GI tract tube structure that enable the functions of that organ. For example, how does the structure of the small intestine aid absorption?

4. After reading about the benefits of a high-fiber diet, 20-year-old Jeff decides to increase his fiber intake by eating more whole-grain products, beans, and fresh fruits and vegetables. Look at the graph and decide which bar (A or B) represents his daily stool weight after a week on his new diet. How might his higher fiber intake affect the amount of intestinal gas produced? Why?

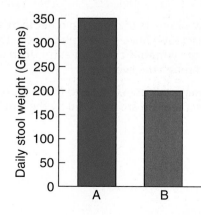

5. Water is absorbed from the small intestine and colon by osmosis. What might happen to the body's water balance if a large number of small, unabsorbed molecules end up in the colon?

6. What path does an amino acid follow from absorption to delivery to a cell? Compare this path with the path followed by a large fatty acid.

What is happening in this picture?

This man's digestive tract was damaged during surgery, so he cannot absorb nutrients. Doctors are ensuring that he is being nourished by infusing a nutrient solution into his blood through a process called total parenteral nutrition (TPN).

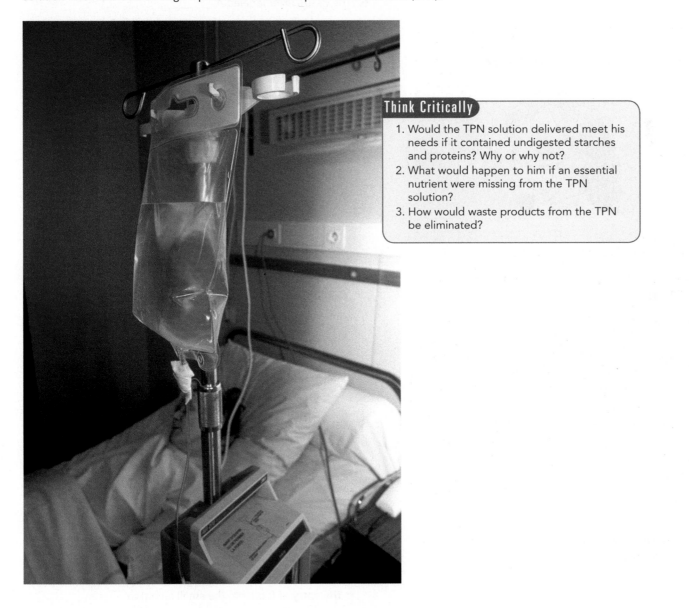

Think Critically

1. Would the TPN solution delivered meet his needs if it contained undigested starches and proteins? Why or why not?
2. What would happen to him if an essential nutrient were missing from the TPN solution?
3. How would waste products from the TPN be eliminated?

Self-Test

(Check your answers in Appendix K.)

1. Which of the following is the smallest unit of life?

   a. atom
   b. molecule
   c. cell
   d. tissue
   e. organism

2. Which of the following statements about saliva is false?

   a. It lubricates the mouth.
   b. It helps protect the teeth from decay.
   c. It moistens food so that it can be tasted and swallowed.
   d. It contains the enzyme salivary amylase.
   e. It contains the protein-digesting enzyme pepsin.

Use the diagram to answer questions 3 and 4.

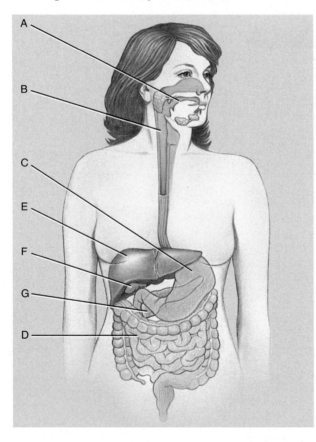

3. Which letter in this illustration points to the organ in which carbohydrate digestion begins?

   a. A
   b. B
   c. C
   d. D
   e. E

4. Which letter in this illustration points to the organ in which bile is stored?

   a. A
   b. C
   c. E
   d. F
   e. G

5. The secretion of digestive juices does not begin until food enters the mouth.

   a. True
   b. False

6. The tissue layer labeled A _____.

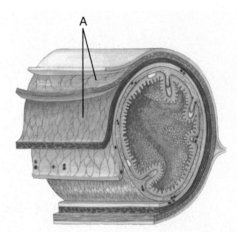

   a. secretes mucus
   b. contains nerves and blood vessels
   c. mixes and propels food through the GI tract
   d. provides external support to the gut

7. The _____ prevents food from entering the passageway to the lungs during swallowing.

   a. gallbladder
   b. pancreas
   c. epiglottis
   d. tongue

8. The rhythmic contractions that propel food through the GI tract are called _____.

   a. peristalsis
   b. enzymatic digestion
   c. swallowing
   d. gastroesophageal reflux
   e. chewing

9. Which of the following is most likely to inhibit stomach secretions and stomach motility?

   a. the release of gastrin
   b. the smell of freshly baked cookies
   c. the entry of food into the small intestine
   d. the entry of food into the stomach

10. The diffusion of water across a membrane is called
_____.

    a. simple diffusion   c. facilitated diffusion

    b. osmosis   d. active transport

11. Which of the following is not true of the microvilli?

    a. They help increase the surface area available for
       absorption.

    b. They contain digestive enzymes.

    c. Each contains a capillary and a lacteal.

    d. They are referred to as the brush border.

12. Which of the numbers on this illustration label blood that is
    rich in oxygen?

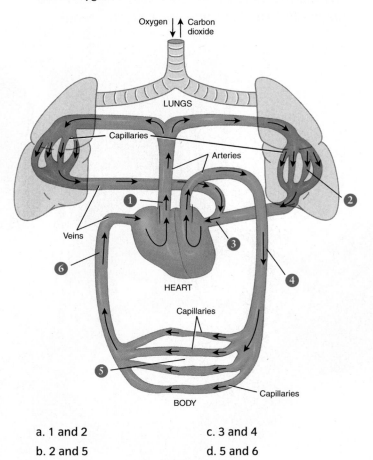

    a. 1 and 2   c. 3 and 4

    b. 2 and 5   d. 5 and 6

13. This diagram could represent all the following except
    _____.

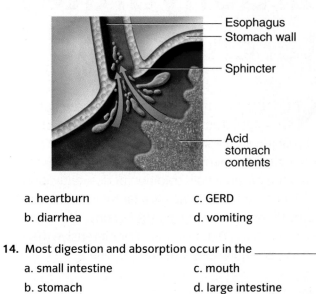

    a. heartburn   c. GERD

    b. diarrhea   d. vomiting

14. Most digestion and absorption occur in the _____.

    a. small intestine   c. mouth

    b. stomach   d. large intestine

15. All absorbed nutrients go directly to the liver.

    a. True   b. False

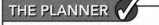
THE PLANNER ✓

Review your Chapter Planner on the chapter opener and
check off your completed work.

4

Carbohydrates: Sugars, Starches, and Fibers

"No one who can rise before dawn three hundred sixty days a year fails to make his family rich." Malcolm Gladwell cites this proverb as a principle of the connection between the stereotypical Asian work ethic and the millennia-old tradition of rice cultivation in China.[1] The production of rice is a far more demanding endeavor than the growing of other grains: Working in a rice field is 10 to 20 times more labor intensive than working on an equivalent-size corn or wheat field.

Every culture relies on carbohydrate-rich grains as a readily available, inexpensive source of calories, and grains occupy a prominent place in everyday life. The Chinese word for rice also means *food*, and the Japanese word for cooked rice means *meal*; bread is the "staff of life," and "breaking bread together" is a universal sign of friendship.

Westerners have a love-hate relationship with carbohydrates. We're told to "carbo-load" before serious

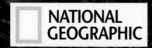

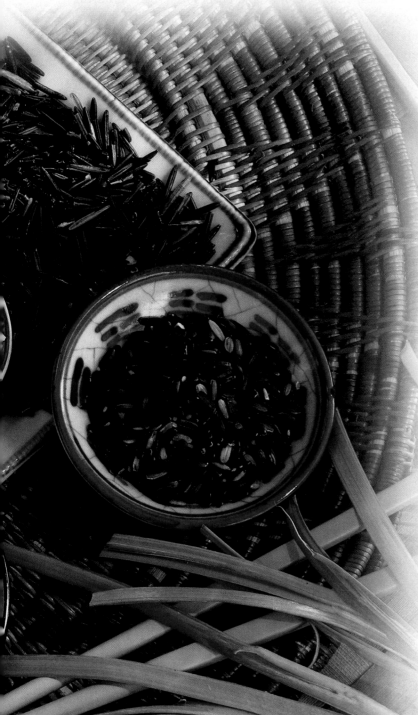

exercise, like a marathon, yet we're admonished by health and fitness authorities to moderate our intake of carbohydrate-rich foods. Many of us fear carbohydrates as a cause of unwanted weight gain and other health problems.

Should we manage our carbs as wisely—and diligently—as a rice farmer tends a paddy?

CHAPTER PLANNER ✓

- ❏ Stimulate your interest by reading the introduction and looking at the visual.
- ❏ Scan the Learning Objectives in each section:
  p. 100 ❏   p. 102 ❏   p. 105 ❏   p. 113 ❏   p. 122 ❏
- ❏ Read the text and study all figures and visuals. Answer any questions.

Analyze key features

- ❏ Nutrition InSight, p. 102 ❏   p. 107 ❏
- ❏ Process Diagram, p. 105 ❏   p. 111 ❏
- ❏ What a Scientist Sees, p. 108 ❏
- ❏ Thinking It Through, p. 123 ❏
- ❏ Stop: Answer the Concept Checks before you go on:
  p. 101 ❏   p. 104 ❏   p. 109 ❏   p. 112 ❏   p. 121 ❏
  p. 126 ❏

End of chapter

- ❏ Review the Summary, Key Terms, and Online Resources.
- ❏ Answer the Critical and Creative Thinking Questions.
- ❏ Answer What is happening in this picture?
- ❏ Complete the Self-Test and check your answers.

Carbohydrates in Our Food

LEARNING OBJECTIVES

1. **Distinguish** refined carbohydrates from unrefined carbohydrates.

2. **Compare** whole grains to enriched grains.

3. **Explain** how added refined sugars and naturally occurring sugars differ from each other.

ur hunter-gatherer ancestors ate very differently from the way we eat. Their diet consisted almost entirely of **unrefined foods**— foods eaten either just as they are found in nature or with only minimal processing, such as cooking. Today we still consume some unrefined sources of carbohydrate, but many of the foods we consume are made with **refined** grains and contain added refined sugar (**Figure 4.1**).

> **refined** Refers to foods that have undergone processing to remove the coarse parts of the original food.

The increased consumption of refined carbohydrates that has occurred around the world over the past few decades has been implicated as one of the causes of the current obesity epidemic and the rising incidence of chronic diseases. Recommendations for a healthy diet suggest that we select more unrefined sources of carbohydrates, including whole grains, vegetables, and fruits, and that we limit foods high in refined carbohydrates, such as candies, cookies, and sweetened beverages.

What Is a Whole Grain?

When you eat a bowl of oatmeal or a slice of whole-wheat toast, you are consuming a **whole-grain product**. Whole-grain products include the entire kernel of the grain: the **germ**, the **bran**, and the **endosperm** (**Figure 4.2a**). Refined grain products, such as white bread, include just the endosperm. The bran and germ are discarded during refining, and along with them the fiber and some vitamins and minerals are lost. To make up some of these losses, refined grains sold in the United States are required to be enriched. **Enrichment**, which is a type of **fortification**, adds back some, but not all, of the nutrients lost in processing (**Figure 4.2b**). For example, thiamin and iron are lost when grains are milled, and they are later added back to even higher levels through enrichment. Vitamin E and vitamin B_6 are also removed by milling, but they are not added back. Therefore, foods made with refined grains contain more of some nutrients and less of others than foods made from whole grains.

> **enrichment** The addition of specific amounts of thiamin, riboflavin, niacin, and iron to refined grains. Since 1998, folic acid has also been added to enriched grains.
>
> **fortification** The addition of nutrients to foods.

Unrefined and refined foods • Figure 4.1

Corn is an unrefined source of carbohydrate, but it can be refined through grinding, cooking, extruding, and drying to eventually end up as cornflakes in your cereal bowl. The sugar you sprinkle on cornflakes is also a refined carbohydrate; it has been refined from sugar cane or sugar beets.

Unrefined

Refined

Unrefined

Refined

Ask Yourself

Which is less refined: canned peaches or fresh peaches? Whole-wheat bread or white bread? Granola cereal or oatmeal?

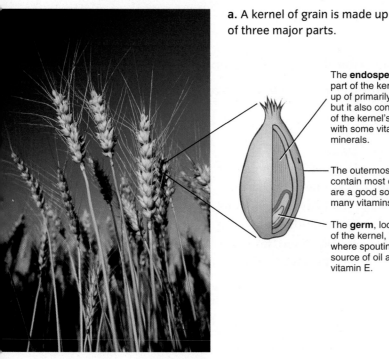

a. A kernel of grain is made up of three major parts.

The **endosperm** is the largest part of the kernel. It is made up of primarily starch, but it also contains most of the kernel's protein, along with some vitamins and minerals.

The outermost **bran** layers contain most of the fiber and are a good source of many vitamins and minerals.

The **germ**, located at the base of the kernel, is the embryo where spouting occurs. It is a source of oil and is rich in vitamin E.

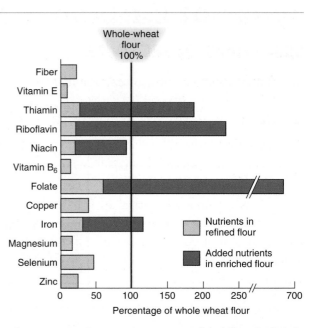

b. The amounts of many nutrients in refined flour (yellow bars) are much lower than the amounts originally present in the whole grain (100% line). In enriched flour, thiamin, riboflavin, niacin, iron, and folate have been added back in amounts that equal or exceed the original levels (red bars).

What Is Added Refined Sugar?

Refined sugars added to food during processing or at the table account for about 16% of the calories consumed in the typical American diet.[2] Refined sugars are nutritionally and chemically identical to sugars that occur naturally in foods. When separated from their plant sources, however, refined sugars no longer contain the fiber, vitamins, minerals, and other substances found in the original plant. Therefore, added refined sugars contribute empty calories to the diet. Foods that naturally contain sugars, such as fruits and milk, provide vitamins, minerals, and phytochemicals, along with the calories from the sugar, making them higher in nutrient density (**Figure 4.3**).

CONCEPT CHECK

1. **What** is the difference between a whole-grain product and a product made with a refined grain?

2. **How** do the nutrients in enriched grains compare to those in whole grains?

3. **Why** are foods high in added refined sugars said to contribute empty calories?

Nutrient density • Figure 4.3

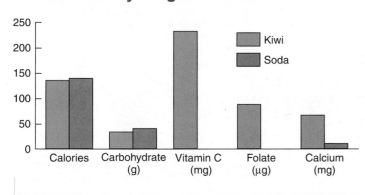

A 12-ounce can of soda contains about 140 Calories from sugar but almost no other nutrients. Three medium kiwis also provide about 140 Calories, along with plenty of other nutrients, including vitamin C, folate, and calcium, making the kiwis more nutrient dense than the soda.

Types of Carbohydrates

LEARNING OBJECTIVES

1. **Name** the basic unit of carbohydrate.

2. **Classify** carbohydrates as simple or complex.

3. **Describe** the types of complex carbohydrates.

4. **Distinguish** soluble fiber from insoluble fiber.

Chemically, carbohydrates are a group of compounds made up of one or more **sugar units** that contain carbon (*carbo*) as well as hydrogen and oxygen in the same two-to-one proportion found

> **sugar unit** A sugar molecule that cannot be broken down to yield other sugars.
>
> **monosaccharide** A carbohydrate made up of a single sugar unit.

in water (*hydrate*, H_2O). Carbohydrates made up of only one sugar unit are called **monosaccharides**, those made up of two sugar units are called **disaccharides**, and those made up of more than two sugar units are called **polysaccharides**.

> **disaccharide** A carbohydrate made up of two sugar units.
>
> **polysaccharide** A carbohydrate made up of many sugar units linked together.

Nutrition InSight — Carbohydrate structures and sources • Figure 4.4

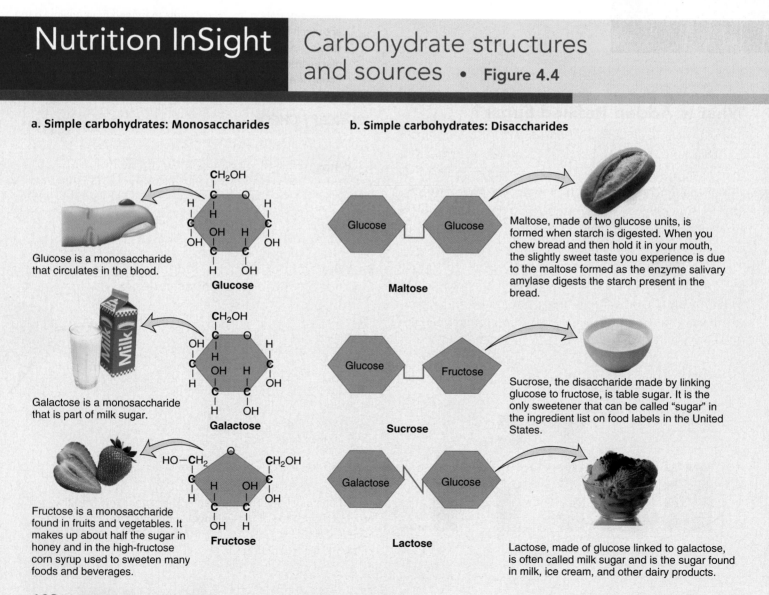

a. Simple carbohydrates: Monosaccharides

Glucose is a monosaccharide that circulates in the blood.

Glucose

Galactose is a monosaccharide that is part of milk sugar.

Galactose

Fructose is a monosaccharide found in fruits and vegetables. It makes up about half the sugar in honey and in the high-fructose corn syrup used to sweeten many foods and beverages.

Fructose

b. Simple carbohydrates: Disaccharides

Glucose — Glucose

Maltose

Maltose, made of two glucose units, is formed when starch is digested. When you chew bread and then hold it in your mouth, the slightly sweet taste you experience is due to the maltose formed as the enzyme salivary amylase digests the starch present in the bread.

Glucose — Fructose

Sucrose

Sucrose, the disaccharide made by linking glucose to fructose, is table sugar. It is the only sweetener that can be called "sugar" in the ingredient list on food labels in the United States.

Galactose — Glucose

Lactose

Lactose, made of glucose linked to galactose, is often called milk sugar and is the sugar found in milk, ice cream, and other dairy products.

Simple Carbohydrates

Monosaccharides and disaccharides are classified as **simple carbohydrates**. The three most common monosaccharides in the diet are **glucose**, **fructose**, and **galactose**. Each contains 6 carbon, 12 hydrogen, and 6 oxygen atoms ($C_6H_{12}O_6$), but these three sugars differ in the arrangement of these atoms (**Figure 4.4a**). Glucose, often called *blood sugar*, is the most important carbohydrate fuel for the human body.

The most common disaccharides in our diet are **maltose**, **sucrose**, and **lactose** (**Figure 4.4b**).

glucose A 6-carbon monosaccharide that is the primary form of carbohydrate used to provide energy in the body.

glycogen The storage form of carbohydrate in animals, made up of many glucose molecules linked together in a highly branched structure.

Complex Carbohydrates

Complex carbohydrates are polysaccharides; they are generally not sweet tasting the way simple carbohydrates are. They include **glycogen** in animals and starches and fibers in plants (**Figure 4.4c**). Glycogen is the storage form of glucose in humans and other animals. It is found in the liver and muscles, but we don't consume it in our diet because the glycogen in animal muscles is broken down soon after the animal is slaughtered.

Starch is made up of glucose molecules linked together in either straight or branched chains (see Figure 4.4c). It is the storage form of carbohydrate in plants and provides energy for plant growth

starch A carbohydrate found in plants, made up of many glucose molecules linked in straight or branched chains.

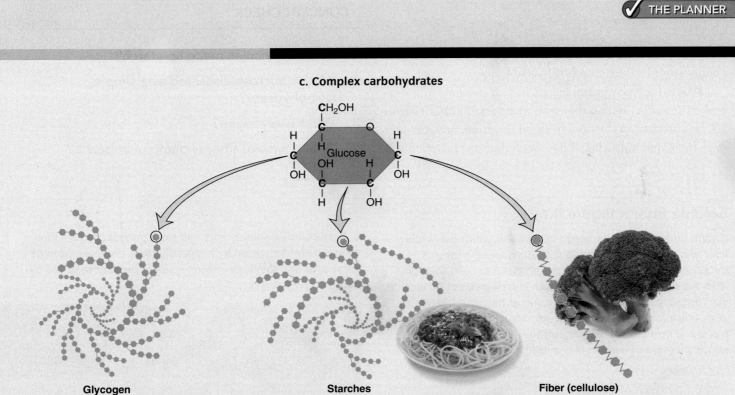

c. Complex carbohydrates

Glucose

Glycogen

The polysaccharide glycogen is made of highly branched chains of glucose. This branched structure allows glycogen, which is found in muscle and liver, to be broken down quickly when the body needs glucose.

Starches

Different types of starch consist of either straight chains or branched chains of glucose. We consume a mixture of starches in grain products, legumes, and other starchy vegetables.

Fiber (cellulose)

Most fiber is made of either straight or branched chains of monosaccharides, but the bonds that link the sugar units cannot be broken by human digestive enzymes. For example, **cellulose**, shown here, is a fiber made up of straight chains of glucose molecules. It is found in wheat bran and broccoli.

Think Critically How do the bonds that link the glucose units in a molecule of starch differ from those in a molecule of cellulose fiber?

Photosynthesis • Figure 4.5

Glucose is produced in plants through the process of **photosynthesis**, which uses energy from the sun to convert carbon dioxide and water to glucose. Plants most often convert glucose to starch. When a human eats plants, digestion converts the starch back to glucose.

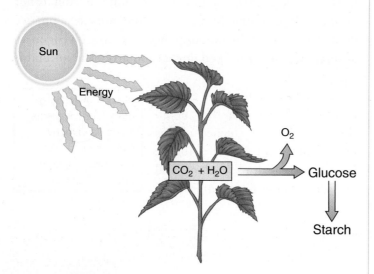

and reproduction. When we eat plants, we consume the energy stored in the starch (**Figure 4.5**).

Fiber is a type of complex carbohydrate that cannot be broken down by human digestive enzymes. Thus fiber cannot be absorbed in the human small intestine, and it passes into the large intestine. Fiber includes several chemical substances, some of which are soluble in water. **Soluble fiber**, found around and inside plant cells, dissolves in water to form viscous solutions. Although human enzymes can't digest soluble fiber, bacteria in the large intestine can break it down. Foods that contain soluble fiber include oats, apples, beans, and seaweed (**Figure 4.6**).

Fiber that does not dissolve in water is called **insoluble fiber**. Insoluble fiber comes primarily from structural parts of plants, such as cell walls. This type of fiber adds bulk to fecal matter because it passes, unchanged, through the gastrointestinal tract. Food sources of insoluble fiber include wheat and rye bran, broccoli, and celery.

soluble fiber Fiber that dissolves in water or absorbs water and can be broken down by intestinal microflora. It includes pectins, gums, and some hemicelluloses.

insoluble fiber Fiber that does not dissolve in water and cannot be broken down by bacteria in the large intestine. It includes cellulose, some hemicelluloses, and lignin.

CONCEPT CHECK

1. **What** molecules make up starch?

2. **Why is** sucrose classified as a simple carbohydrate?

3. **What** is glycogen?

4. **Which** type of fiber is plentiful in beans?

Soluble fiber • Figure 4.6

a. Jams and jellies are thickened with pectin, which is a soluble fiber found in fruits and vegetables. Gums are also used as thickeners because they combine with water to keep solutions from separating. Gums you might see in an ingredient list include gum arabic, gum karaya, guar gum, locust bean gum, xanthan gum, and gum tragacanth, which are extracted from shrubs, trees, and seedpods, and agar, carrageenan, and alginates, which are gums derived from seaweed.

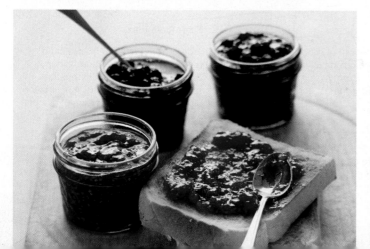

b. Beans contain soluble fiber and small polysaccharides that cannot be broken down by human digestive enzymes. Both of these pass into the large intestine, where they are digested by bacteria creating gas.

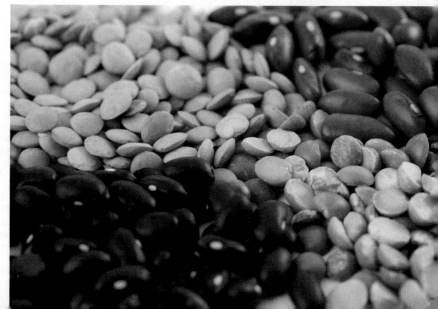

Carbohydrate Digestion and Absorption

LEARNING OBJECTIVES

1. **Describe** the steps of carbohydrate digestion.
2. **Explain** what is meant by lactose intolerance.
3. **Discuss** how indigestible carbohydrates affect the colon and feces.
4. **Draw** a graph that compares blood glucose levels after eating soda and after eating beans.

D isaccharides and complex carbohydrates must be digested to monosaccharides before they can be absorbed into the body. Carbohydrates that cannot be completely digested cannot be absorbed but still have an impact on the gastrointestinal tract and overall health. Once absorbed, carbohydrates travel in the blood to the liver.

Carbohydrate Digestion

Carbohydrate digestion begins in the mouth, but most digestion occurs in the small intestine (**Figure 4.7**). Carbohydrate that cannot be digested passes into the colon. Some of this is broken down by bacteria. Material that cannot be absorbed is excreted in the feces.

Carbohydrate digestion • Figure 4.7

THE PLANNER

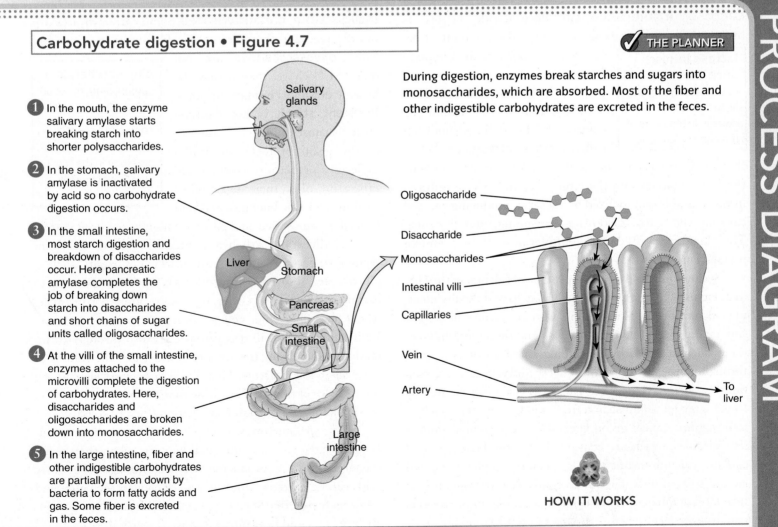

PROCESS DIAGRAM

During digestion, enzymes break starches and sugars into monosaccharides, which are absorbed. Most of the fiber and other indigestible carbohydrates are excreted in the feces.

❶ In the mouth, the enzyme salivary amylase starts breaking starch into shorter polysaccharides.

❷ In the stomach, salivary amylase is inactivated by acid so no carbohydrate digestion occurs.

❸ In the small intestine, most starch digestion and breakdown of disaccharides occur. Here pancreatic amylase completes the job of breaking down starch into disaccharides and short chains of sugar units called oligosaccharides.

❹ At the villi of the small intestine, enzymes attached to the microvilli complete the digestion of carbohydrates. Here, disaccharides and oligosaccharides are broken down into monosaccharides.

❺ In the large intestine, fiber and other indigestible carbohydrates are partially broken down by bacteria to form fatty acids and gas. Some fiber is excreted in the feces.

Salivary glands

Liver
Stomach
Pancreas
Small intestine

Large intestine

Oligosaccharide
Disaccharide
Monosaccharides
Intestinal villi
Capillaries
Vein
Artery
To liver

HOW IT WORKS

Lactose intolerance • Figure 4.8

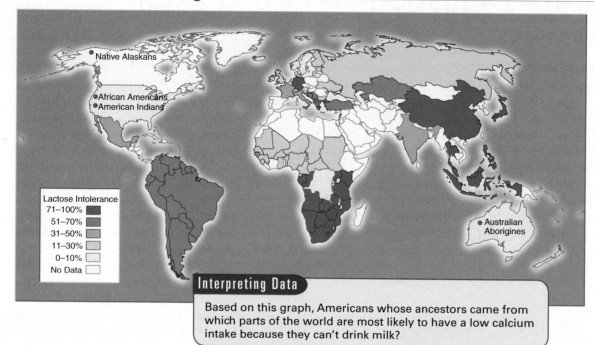

Lactose Intolerance
- 71–100%
- 51–70%
- 31–50%
- 11–30%
- 0–10%
- No Data

Native Alaskans

African Americans
American Indians

Australian Aborigines

This map illustrates the dramatic variation in the incidence of lactose intolerance around the world. In the United States, between 30 and 50 million people are lactose intolerant; it is more common in some ethnic and racial populations than in others. Up to 80% of African Americans, 80 to 100% of Native Americans, and 90 to 100% of Asian Americans are lactose intolerant, but only about 15% of Caucasian Americans are.[3]

Interpreting Data

Based on this graph, Americans whose ancestors came from which parts of the world are most likely to have a low calcium intake because they can't drink milk?

Lactose intolerance The disaccharide lactose is broken down by the enzyme lactase in the small intestine.

> **lactose intolerance** The inability to completely digest lactose due to a reduction in the levels of the enzyme lactase.

We are all born with adequate levels of lactase, but in many people, levels decline so much with age that lactose cannot be completely digested, a condition called **lactose intolerance**. When these individuals consume milk and other dairy products, the lactose passes into the large intestine, where it draws in water and is metabolized by bacteria, producing gas and causing abdominal distension, cramping, and diarrhea. The incidence of lactose intolerance varies among populations (**Figure 4.8**).

Because milk is the primary source of calcium in the U.S. diet, lactose-intolerant individuals may have difficulty meeting calcium needs. Many people who are lactose intolerant can handle small amounts of lactose and therefore can meet their calcium needs by consuming small portions of milk throughout the day and eating cheese and yogurt, which contain less lactose than milk. Those who cannot tolerate any lactose can get their calcium from nondairy sources, such as tofu, legumes, dark green vegetables, and canned salmon and sardines, which are consumed with the bones, as well as from calcium-fortified foods, calcium supplements, and lactase-treated milk (such as Lactaid). Another option is to take lactase tablets with or before consuming milk products to digest the lactose before it passes into the large intestine.

Indigestible carbohydrates Some carbohydrates are not digested and therefore not readily absorbed. Fiber and some **oligosaccharides** are not digested because they cannot be broken down by human enzymes. **Resistant starch** is not digested either because the natural structure of the grain protects the starch molecules or because cooking and processing alter their digestibility. Legumes, unripe bananas, and cold cooked potatoes, rice, and pasta are high in resistant starch.

> **oligosaccharide** A carbohydrate made up of 3 to 10 sugar units.
>
> **resistant starch** Starch that escapes digestion in the small intestine of healthy people.

As indigestible carbohydrates pass through the gastrointestinal tract, they slow the rate at which nutrients, such as glucose, are absorbed (**Figure 4.9a**). Fiber can also bind to certain minerals, preventing their absorption. For instance, wheat bran fiber binds zinc, calcium, magnesium, and iron. Indigestible carbohydrates also speed transit through the intestine by increasing the amount of water and the volume of material in the intestine. This stimulates peristalsis, causing the muscles of the large intestine to work more and function better, helping to prevent constipation (**Figure 4.9b**).

Some carbohydrates that are not digested by human enzymes are digested by intestinal bacteria when they reach the large intestine, producing fatty acids and gas. The fatty acids can be used as a fuel source for cells in the colon and other body tissues; they may play a role in regulating cellular processes and preventing disease (**Figure 4.9c**).

a. The bulk and volume of a fiber-rich meal dilutes the gastrointestinal contents. This dilution slows the digestion of food and absorption of nutrients (green dots), causing a delay and a blunting of the rise in blood glucose that occurs after a meal (see graph). With a low-fiber meal, nutrients are more concentrated; digestion and absorption occur more rapidly, causing a quicker, sharper rise in blood glucose. ▼

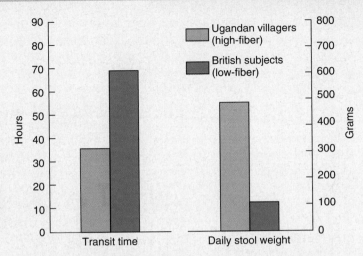

b. Ugandan villagers consume a diet high in fiber, but British subjects living in Uganda consume a more refined, low-fiber diet. Stool weights are greater and transit times shorter for Ugandan villagers, than for British subjects.[4]

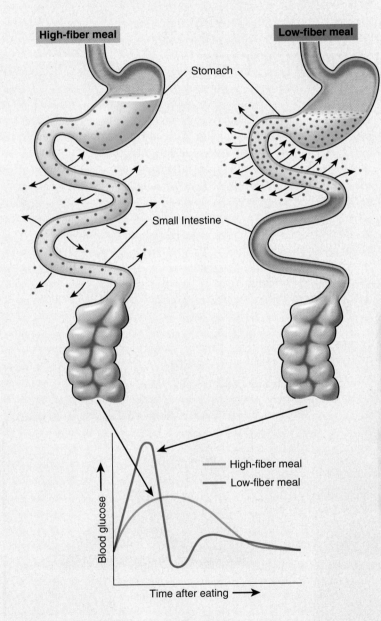

High-fiber meal

Low-fiber meal

Stomach

Small Intestine

Blood glucose

High-fiber meal
Low-fiber meal

Time after eating →

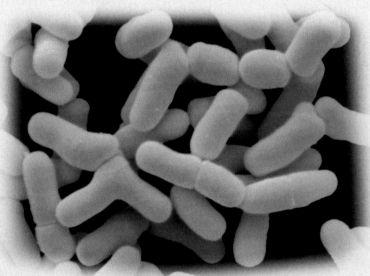

c. Indigestible carbohydrates are a food source for the bacteria in the colon. When bacteria break down these carbohydrates, fatty acids are formed. The acidic conditions inhibit the growth of undesirable bacteria and favor the growth of healthy ones, such as the *Bifidobacteria* shown here. These bacteria and their metabolic by-products may help prevent and treat diarrhea due to inflammation in the bowel and protect against colon cancer.[5]

Ask Yourself

Why does glucose rise more slowly after a high-fiber meal than after a low-fiber meal?

Carbohydrate Absorption

After a meal, the monosaccharides from carbohydrate digestion enter the portal circulation and travel to the liver. Glucose can be used to provide energy, stored as liver glycogen, or delivered via the general blood circulation to other body tissues, causing blood glucose levels to rise.

Glycemic response is a measure of how quickly and how high blood glucose levels rise after carbohydrate is consumed. Glycemic response is affected by how long it takes a food to leave

glycemic response
The rate, magnitude, and duration of the rise in blood glucose that occurs after food is consumed.

WHAT A SCIENTIST SEES

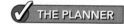 THE PLANNER

Glycemic Index

Potatoes are a source of unrefined carbohydrate, but scientists know that the effect potatoes have on blood glucose is very different from the effect beans have. Beans are also a source of unrefined carbohydrate, but they are much higher in fiber and protein, both of which slow digestion and absorption and therefore reduce the glycemic response.

The glycemic response of beans versus potatoes is shown here graphically, but it can also be expressed using the **glycemic index**, which is a ranking of how a food affects blood glucose relative to the effect of an equivalent amount of carbohydrate from a reference food, such as white bread or pure glucose. For example, on a glycemic index scale on which white bread is 100, potatoes are 90 and kidney beans are about 25. This means that blood glucose levels do not increase as much after eating beans as they do after eating white bread or potatoes.

A shortcoming of the glycemic index is that it is measured using a set amount of carbohydrate in a food (usually 50 grams),

not the typical serving of food that we eat. For example, it takes over 4 cups of strawberries to supply 50 g of carbohydrate, but people typically eat only about 1 cup. **Glycemic load** compares the effect of typical portions of food on blood glucose so it is a more practical way to assess the effect of a food on blood glucose levels.

A shortcoming of both the glycemic index and glycemic load is that they are determined for individual foods rather than for meals, which contain mixtures of foods. We typically eat meals, so knowing the glycemic index or load of a single food doesn't tell us much about the rise in blood glucose that will occur after eating a meal.

Think Critically How would the graph of blood glucose levels after eating meat and potatoes differ from the graph that would result after eating potatoes alone?

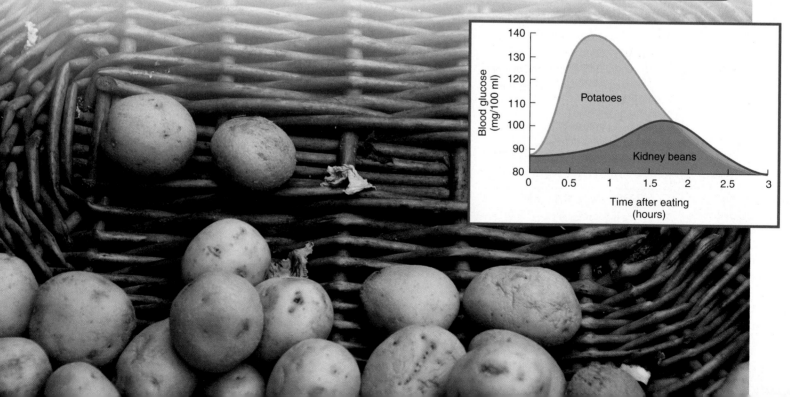

the stomach and by how fast it is digested and the glucose absorbed.

Refined sugars and starches generally cause a greater glycemic response than unrefined carbohydrates because sugars and starches consumed alone leave the stomach quickly and are rapidly digested and absorbed. For example, when you drink a bottle of sugary soda, your blood glucose increases within minutes. Because fiber takes longer to leave the stomach and slows absorption in the small intestine, a fiber-containing food such as oatmeal would take longer to leave your stomach and therefore cause a lower glycemic response (see *What a Scientist Sees*). When carbohydrate, fat, and protein are consumed together, stomach emptying is slowed, delaying both digestion and absorption of carbohydrate, so blood glucose rises more slowly than when carbohydrate is consumed alone. For instance, after a meal of chicken, brown rice, and green beans, which contains carbohydrate, fat, protein, and fiber, blood glucose doesn't begin to rise for 30 to 60 minutes.

CONCEPT CHECK STOP

1. **What** steps are involved in starch digestion?

2. **How** does lactose in the colon cause gas and diarrhea?

3. **Why** do indigestible carbohydrates affect the type of bacteria in the colon?

4. **How** does fiber affect the rate at which blood glucose rises after a meal?

Carbohydrate Functions

LEARNING OBJECTIVES

1. **Name** the main function of carbohydrate in the body.

2. **Contrast** the roles of insulin and glucagon in blood glucose regulation.

3. **Compare** anaerobic and aerobic metabolism.

4. **Discuss** what happens to protein and fat metabolism when dietary carbohydrate is insufficient.

The main function of carbohydrates is to provide energy, but carbohydrates also play other roles in the body. For example, nerve tissue needs the sugar galactose, and in breast-feeding women, galactose combines with glucose to produce the milk sugar lactose. The monosaccharides ribose and deoxyribose play nonenergy roles as components of RNA and DNA, respectively, the two molecules that contain a cell's genetic information. Ribose is also a component of the B vitamin riboflavin. Oligosaccharides are associated with cell membranes, where they help signal information about cells, and large polysaccharides found in connective tissue provide cushioning and lubrication.

Getting Enough Glucose to Cells

Glucose is an important fuel for body cells. Many body cells can use energy sources other than glucose, but brain cells, red blood cells, and a few others must have glucose to stay alive. In order to provide a steady supply of glucose, the concentration of glucose in the blood is regulated by the liver and by hormones secreted by the pancreas. The rise in blood glucose levels after eating stimulates the pancreas to secrete the hormone **insulin**, which allows glucose to be taken into body cells, causing blood glucose levels to drop. Once inside cells, glucose can be used immediately to provide energy or converted into energy-storage molecules for future use.

insulin A hormone made in the pancreas that allows glucose to enter cells and stimulates the synthesis of protein, fat, and liver and muscle glycogen.

In both muscle cells and liver cells, insulin promotes the conversion of glucose into glycogen for storage. In the liver and in fat-storing cells, it promotes the conversion of glucose to fat for storage (**Figure 4.10**).

A few hours after eating, blood glucose levels—and consequently the amount of glucose available to the cells—begin to decrease. This triggers the pancreas to secrete the hormone **glucagon** (see Figure 4.10). Glucagon raises blood glucose by signaling liver cells to break down glycogen into glucose, which is released into the blood. At the same time, glucagon signals the liver to synthesize new glucose molecules, which are also released into the blood, bringing blood glucose levels back to normal.

glucagon A hormone made in the pancreas that raises blood glucose levels by stimulating the breakdown of liver glycogen and the synthesis of glucose.

Blood glucose regulation • Figure 4.10

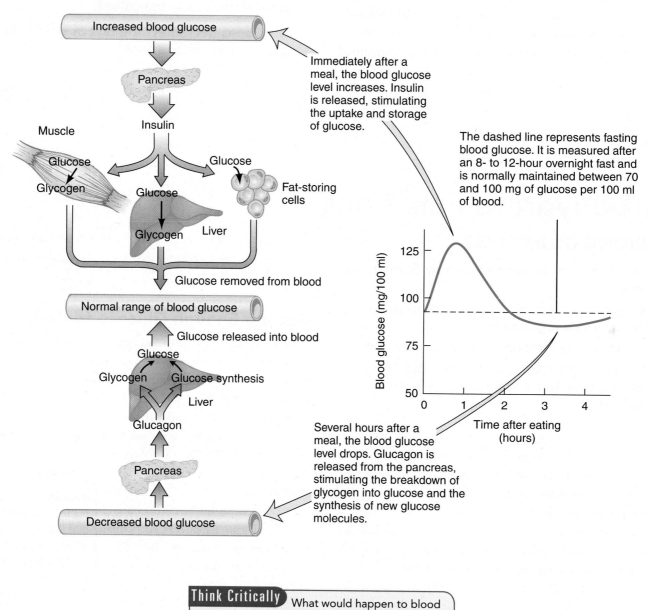

The dashed line represents fasting blood glucose. It is measured after an 8- to 12-hour overnight fast and is normally maintained between 70 and 100 mg of glucose per 100 ml of blood.

Immediately after a meal, the blood glucose level increases. Insulin is released, stimulating the uptake and storage of glucose.

Several hours after a meal, the blood glucose level drops. Glucagon is released from the pancreas, stimulating the breakdown of glycogen into glucose and the synthesis of new glucose molecules.

Think Critically What would happen to blood glucose levels if insulin were not available?

Cellular respiration • Figure 4.11

Inside body cells, the reactions of cellular respiration split the bonds between carbon atoms in glucose, releasing energy that is used to synthesize ATP. ATP is used to power the energy-requiring processes in the body.

1 Glycolysis, which takes place in the cell fluid, splits glucose, a six-carbon molecule, into two three-carbon molecules (pyruvate). This step releases high-energy electrons (purple balls) and produces a small amount of ATP. Pyruvate is then either broken down to produce more ATP or used to remake glucose.

2 Pyruvate can be used to produce more ATP when oxygen is available. In the mitochondria, pyruvate is broken down, releasing carbon dioxide and high-energy electrons and forming acetyl-CoA (2 carbons), which continues through aerobic metabolism.

3 Acetyl-CoA enters the citric acid cycle, where carbon dioxide and high-energy electrons are released and where a small amount of ATP is produced.

4 Most ATP is produced in the final step of aerobic metabolism. Here the energy in the high-energy electrons released in previous steps is transferred to ATP, and the electrons are combined with oxygen and hydrogen to form water.

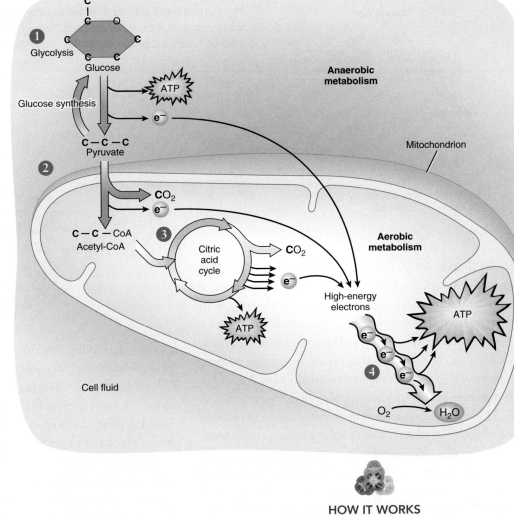

HOW IT WORKS

Glucose as a Source of Energy

glycolysis An anaerobic metabolic pathway that splits glucose into two three-carbon pyruvate molecules; the energy released from one glucose molecule is used to make two molecules of ATP.

Cells use glucose to provide energy via cellular respiration (see Chapter 3). Cellular respiration uses oxygen to convert glucose to carbon dioxide and water and provide energy in the form of ATP (**Figure 4.11**).

The first step in cellular respiration is **glycolysis** (*glyco* = "glucose," *lysis* = "to break down"). Glycolysis can rapidly produce two molecules of ATP from each glu-cose molecule. Because oxygen isn't needed for this pathway reaction, glycolysis is sometimes called anaerobic glycolysis, or **anaerobic metabolism**. When oxygen is available, the complete breakdown of glucose can proceed. This **aerobic metabolism** produces about 36 molecules of ATP for each glucose molecule, 18 times more ATP than is generated by anaerobic glycolysis.

anaerobic metabolism Metabolism in the absence of oxygen.

aerobic metabolism Metabolism in the presence of oxygen. It can completely break down glucose to yield carbon dioxide, water, and energy in the form of ATP.

Carbohydrate Functions **111**

Ketone formation • Figure 4.12

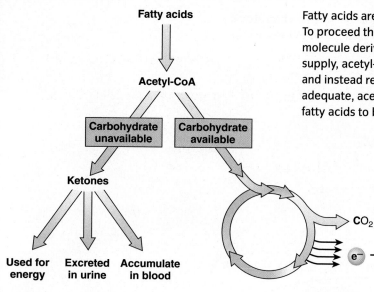

Fatty acids

↓

Acetyl-CoA

| Carbohydrate unavailable | Carbohydrate available |

Ketones

Used for energy | Excreted in urine | Accumulate in blood

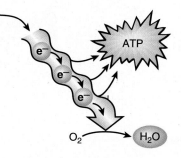

CO_2

e^-

ATP

O_2 → H_2O

Fatty acids are broken down into two-carbon units that form acetyl-CoA. To proceed through aerobic metabolism, acetyl-CoA must combine with a molecule derived primarily from carbohydrate. When carbohydrate is in short supply, acetyl-CoA molecules cannot proceed through aerobic metabolism and instead react with each other to form ketones. When carbohydrate is adequate, acetyl-CoA can proceed through aerobic metabolism, allowing the fatty acids to be completely broken down to yield ATP.

Carbohydrate and protein breakdown Glucose is an essential fuel for brain cells and red blood cells. If adequate amounts of glucose are not available, it can be synthesized from three-carbon molecules (see Figure 4.11, step 1 on previous page). Fatty acids cannot be used to make glucose because the reactions that break them down produce two-carbon, rather than three-carbon, molecules. Amino acids from protein breakdown can supply the three-carbon molecules. However, because protein is not stored in the body, this use of amino acids takes away functioning body proteins. Body proteins that are broken down to make glucose are no longer available to do their job, whether that job is to speed up a chemical reaction or contract a muscle. Sufficient dietary carbohydrate ensures that protein is not utilized in this way; carbohydrate is therefore said to *spare* protein.

Carbohydrate and fat breakdown Most of the energy stored in the body is stored as fat. In order to fully access the energy from fatty acids, carbohydrate is required. If carbohydrate is not available, such as during starvation or when consuming a low-carbohydrate diet, molecules called **ketones** or **ketone bodies** are formed (**Figure 4.12**). The heart, muscle, and kidney can use ketones for energy. After about three days of fasting, even the brain adapts and can obtain about half of its energy from ketones. The use of ketones for energy helps spare

ketone or **ketone body** An acidic molecule formed when there is not sufficient carbohydrate to break down acetyl-CoA.

glucose and decreases the amount of protein that must be broken down to synthesize glucose.

Ketones not used for energy can be excreted in the urine. However, when high levels of ketones build up in the blood, a condition known as **ketosis**, they can increase the blood's acidity so much that normal body processes are disrupted. Mild ketosis can occur during starvation or when consuming a low-carbohydrate weight-loss diet and can cause symptoms such as reduced appetite, headaches, dry mouth, and odd-smelling breath. Severe ketosis can occur with untreated diabetes and can cause coma and even death.

ketosis High levels of ketones in the blood.

CONCEPT CHECK STOP

1. **Why** is it important to keep blood glucose levels in the normal range?
2. **How** does insulin affect blood glucose levels?
3. **What** process breaks down glucose in the presence of oxygen to yield ATP?
4. **Why** is carbohydrate said to spare protein?

Carbohydrates in Health and Disease

LEARNING OBJECTIVES

1. **Define** diabetes and explain its health consequences.

2. **Describe** how carbohydrates contribute to the development of dental caries.

3. **Discuss** the role of carbohydrates in weight control.

4. **Explain** how fiber may help protect health.

 re carbohydrates good for you or bad for you? On the one hand, they have been blamed for everything from diabetes to obesity. On the other hand, U.S. guidelines for a healthy diet recommend that people base their diet on carbohydrate-rich foods in order to reduce disease risk. This incongruity relates to the health effects of different types of dietary carbohydrates: Diets high in unrefined carbohydrates from whole grains, fruits, and vegetables are associated with a lower incidence of a variety of chronic diseases, whereas diets high in refined carbohydrates, such as refined grains and foods high in added sugars, may increase chronic disease risk.

Diabetes

Diabetes mellitus, commonly referred to simply as diabetes, is a disease characterized by high blood glucose levels (**Figure 4.13**). Uncontrolled diabetes damages the heart, blood vessels, kidneys, eyes, and nerves. It is the leading cause of adult blindness and accounts for over 40% of new cases of kidney failure and more than 60% of nontraumatic lower-limb amputations. In the United States, nearly 26 million people have diabetes, and 7 million of these people have not been diagnosed.[6]

> **diabetes mellitus**
> A disease characterized by elevated blood glucose due to either insufficient production of insulin or decreased sensitivity of cells to insulin.

Blood glucose levels in diabetes • Figure 4.13

Normal blood glucose is less than 100 mg/100 ml blood after an 8-hour fast; a fasting blood level from 100 to 125 mg/100 ml is defined as prediabetes; a fasting level of 126 mg/100 ml or above is defined as diabetes. Two hours after consuming 75 g of glucose, normal blood levels are less than 140 mg/100 ml; prediabetes levels are from 140 to 199 mg/100 ml; diabetes levels are 200 mg/100 ml or greater.

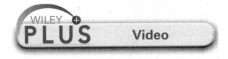

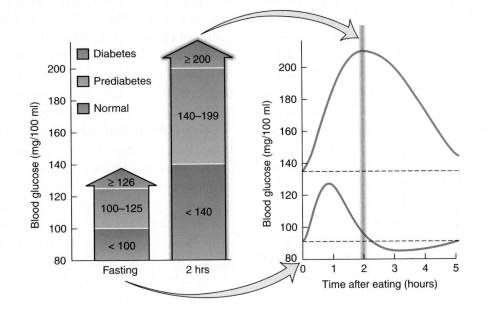

This graph compares the number of cases of type 1 and type 2 diabetes diagnosed per year in adolescents (ages 10 to 19) by race/ethnicity. Twenty years ago, type 2 diabetes was rare in this age group, but as in adults, the incidence is rising, especially in certain minority groups. Reducing type 2 diabetes in minority groups will require culturally sensitive strategies to modify diet and lifestyle.

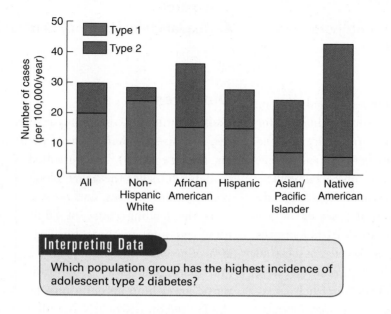

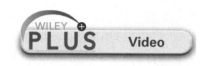

Interpreting Data

Which population group has the highest incidence of adolescent type 2 diabetes?

Types of diabetes

Type 1 diabetes is an **autoimmune disease** in which the insulin-secreting pancreatic cells are destroyed by the body's immune system. This form of diabetes accounts for only 5 to 10% of diagnosed cases and is usually diagnosed before age 30. Because no insulin is produced, people with type 1 diabetes must inject insulin in order to keep blood glucose levels in the normal range. When insulin levels are low, the lack of glucose inside cells leads to ketone formation. In uncontrolled type 1 diabetes, ketone levels can get high enough to increase the acidity of the blood. This condition, called **ketoacidosis**, can lead to coma and death.

The more common form of diabetes is **type 2 diabetes**, which accounts for 90 to 95% of all cases. It occurs when the body does not produce enough insulin to keep blood glucose in the normal range. This can occur because body cells lose their sensitivity to insulin, a condition called **insulin resistance**, or when the amount of insulin secreted is reduced. Type 2 diabetes is believed to be due to both genetic and lifestyle factors. Type 2 diabetes is more commonly diagnosed in adulthood, but we now know that people can develop this disease at any age (**Figure 4.14**). A progressive disease, it usually begins with **prediabetes**, a condition in which glucose levels are above normal but not high enough to be diagnosed as diabetes (see Figure 4.13 on previous page). In many cases, adjustments in diet and lifestyle can keep prediabetes from progressing to type 2 diabetes.

Gestational diabetes is an elevation of blood sugar that is first recognized during pregnancy.[7] The high levels of glucose in the mother's blood are passed to the fetus, frequently resulting in a baby that is large for gestational age and at increased risk of complications. Gestational diabetes usually resolves after the pregnancy, but women with gestational diabetes are at increased risk of developing type 2 diabetes later in life.

type 1 diabetes The form of diabetes caused by autoimmune destruction of insulin-producing cells in the pancreas, usually leading to absolute insulin deficiency.

autoimmune disease A disease that results from immune reactions that destroy normal body cells.

type 2 diabetes The form of diabetes characterized by insulin resistance and relative (rather than absolute) insulin deficiency.

Symptoms and complications of diabetes The symptoms and complications of all types of diabetes result from the inability to use glucose normally and from high glucose levels in the blood. Cells that require insulin in order to take up glucose are starved for glucose, and cells that can use glucose without insulin are exposed to damaging high levels.

Early symptoms of diabetes include frequent urination, excessive thirst, blurred vision, and weight loss. Frequent urination and excessive thirst occur because as blood glucose levels rise, the kidneys excrete the extra glucose and as a result must also excrete extra water, increasing the volume of urine. The additional loss of water from the body makes the individual thirsty. Blurred vision occurs when excess glucose enters the lens of the eye, drawing in water and causing the lens to swell.

Weight loss occurs because cells are unable to use glucose for energy, and so the body must break down fat to obtain the energy it needs.

The long-term complications of diabetes include damage to the heart, blood vessels, kidneys, eyes, and nerves (**Figure 4.15**). These complications are believed to be due to prolonged exposure to high glucose levels.

Managing blood glucose The goal in treating diabetes is to maintain blood glucose levels within the normal range. This requires a program of diet, exercise, and, in many cases, medication, along with frequent monitoring of blood glucose levels.[8] Carbohydrate intake must be coordinated with exercise and medication schedules so that glucose and insulin are available in the right proportions.

Diabetes complications • Figure 4.15

The long-term complications of diabetes result from damage to both the large blood vessels, which leads to an increased risk of heart attack and stroke, and changes in small blood vessels, which can cause blindness, kidney failure, and nerve dysfunction.

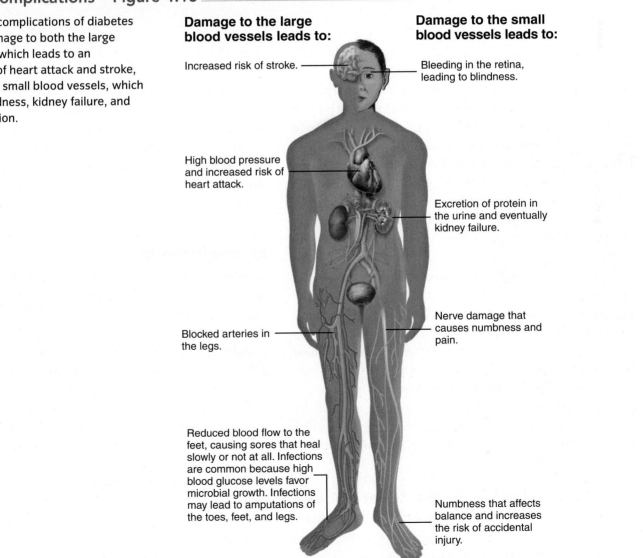

Damage to the large blood vessels leads to:

Increased risk of stroke.

High blood pressure and increased risk of heart attack.

Blocked arteries in the legs.

Reduced blood flow to the feet, causing sores that heal slowly or not at all. Infections are common because high blood glucose levels favor microbial growth. Infections may lead to amputations of the toes, feet, and legs.

Damage to the small blood vessels leads to:

Bleeding in the retina, leading to blindness.

Excretion of protein in the urine and eventually kidney failure.

Nerve damage that causes numbness and pain.

Numbness that affects balance and increases the risk of accidental injury.

Carbohydrates and calorie intake • Figure 4.16

It is the fat we add to high-carbohydrate foods that increases their calorie count. A medium-sized baked potato provides about 200 Calories. Adding a tablespoon of butter brings the total to over 300 Calories.

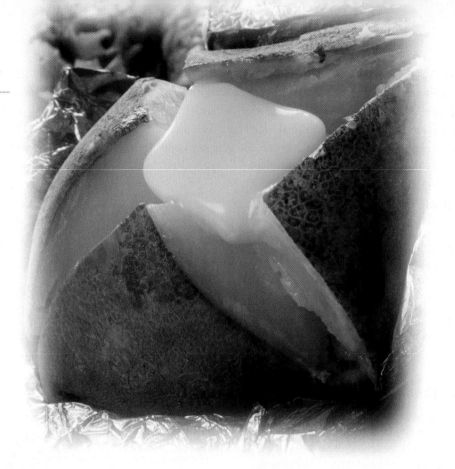

Dietary management of diabetes involves limiting the amount of carbohydrate consumed at each meal to prevent a rapid or prolonged rise in blood glucose.[8] A diet providing unrefined carbohydrates is recommended because these carbohydrate sources cause a slower rise in blood glucose than refined carbohydrates. Diets for individuals with diabetes should also be limited in saturated fat, *trans* fat, and cholesterol in order to reduce the risk for cardiovascular disease. Weight management is an important component of diabetes care because excess body fat increases the resistance of body cells to insulin. Exercise is important not only because it helps to achieve and maintain a healthy body weight but also because it increases the sensitivity of body cells to insulin.[9]

Individuals with type 1 diabetes require insulin injections because they no longer make insulin. Insulin must be given by injection because it is a protein and would therefore be digested in the gastrointestinal tract if taken orally. Individuals with type 2 and gestational diabetes are often able to manage blood glucose levels with diet and exercise but may also require oral medications and/or insulin injections.

Carbohydrate intake and the risk of diabetes

Evidence is accumulating that carbohydrate consumption may play a role in the development of type 2 diabetes in susceptible individuals.[10,11] In populations in which the diet is high in whole grains, the risk of developing type 2 diabetes is lower than in populations in which the diet is high in refined starches and added sugars.[12,13] The reason for this is not fully understood. However, it has been proposed that because insulin needs are increased when the diet is high in refined carbohydrates, the insulin-producing cells in the pancreas may wear out over time.[13]

Hypoglycemia

Another condition that involves blood glucose is **hypoglycemia**. Symptoms of hypoglycemia include low blood sugar (below 70 mg glucose/100 ml blood), irritability, sweating, shakiness, anxiety, rapid heartbeat, headache, hunger, weakness, and sometimes seizures and coma. Hypoglycemia occurs most frequently in people who have diabetes as a result of overmedication. It can also be caused by abnormalities in insulin production or by abnormalities in the way the body responds to insulin or to other hormones.

hypoglycemia Abnormally low blood glucose levels.

Fasting hypoglycemia, which occurs when an individual has not eaten, is often related to some underlying condition, such as excess alcohol consumption, hormonal deficiencies, or tumors. Treatment involves identifying and treating the underlying disease. **Reactive hypoglycemia**

occurs in response to the consumption of high-carbohydrate foods. The rise in blood glucose from the carbohydrate meal stimulates insulin release. However, too much insulin is secreted, resulting in a rapid fall in blood glucose to abnormally low levels. To prevent the rapid changes in blood glucose that occur with reactive hypoglycemia, the diet should consist of small, frequent meals that are low in carbohydrate and high in protein and fiber.

Dental Caries

Dental caries, or cavities, are the best-documented health problem associated with carbohydrate intake. Eighty-five percent of people 18 years and older have had caries. They occur when bacteria on the teeth metabolize carbohydrates, producing acids. These acids can dissolve tooth enamel and the underlying tooth structure, forming dental caries. Simple carbohydrates, especially sucrose, are easiest for the bacteria to metabolize into acids, but starchy foods also promote tooth decay. The longer teeth are exposed to carbohydrates—for example, through frequent snacking, consuming foods that stick to the teeth, sucking hard candy, and slowly sipping soda—the greater the risk of caries. Limiting intake of sweet or sticky foods and proper dental hygiene can help prevent dental caries.

Weight Management

As low-carbohydrate diets have gained popularity, carbohydrates have gotten a reputation for being fattening. In reality, carbohydrates are no more fattening than other nutrients, and there is no evidence that the proportion of total carbohydrate in the diet affects energy intake.[14] Weight gain is caused by excess intake of calories, no matter whether the excess is from carbohydrate, fat, or protein. Carbohydrates provide only 4 Calories/gram, less than half the 9 Calories/gram provided by fat (**Figure 4.16**).

Carbohydrates and weight loss

The type of carbohydrates you consume can affect how hungry you feel and whether you lose or gain weight (**Figure 4.17**). A diet high in unrefined carbohydrates is high in fiber, which increases the sense of fullness by adding bulk and slowing digestion, allowing you to feel satisfied with less food. This can help promote weight loss.[15] However, diets high in fiber may be problematic for children, who have a small stomach capacity, because they may become satiated before meeting their nutrient requirements.

Foods high in refined carbohydrates cause a rapid rise in blood glucose and therefore stimulate release of insulin. Insulin promotes fat storage. Therefore, a diet high in refined carbohydrate, which causes more insulin release, may shift

Refined versus unrefined carbohydrates • Figure 4.17

A diet high in sugar-sweetened beverages may increase caloric intake because beverages do not induce satiety to the same extent as high-carbohydrate foods. Increases in the consumption of sugar-sweetened soft drinks are associated with weight gain.[14]

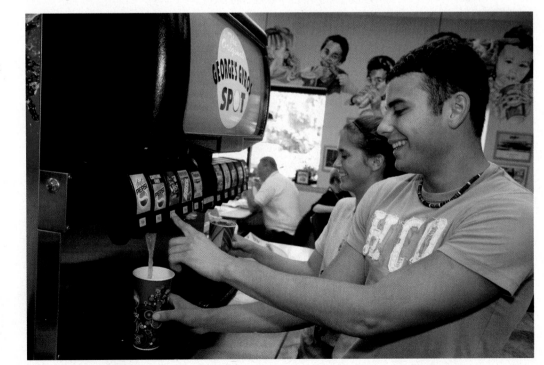

Debate   Should You Avoid High-Fructose Corn Syrup?

The Issue: High-fructose corn syrup is the most common added sweetener in the American diet. Based on the media hype, you might think it is poison. But is high-fructose corn syrup really worse than other sweeteners?

A host of processed foods are sweetened with high-fructose corn syrup (HFCS). Magazine articles and Internet blogs tell you that HFCS is unhealthy because it's not a natural sweetener. They accuse it of causing the obesity epidemic and implicate it in heart disease and diabetes. They even point out that the overuse of corn, particularly genetically modified (GM) corn, is a threat to the environment. That's a lot of blame for a simple sweetener!

To understand the pros and cons of HFCS, you have to know what it is. HFCS is made by extracting starch from corn and treating it to break the bonds between the glucose molecules. The resulting corn syrup is then treated to convert about half the glucose to fructose, hence high-fructose corn syrup. This obviously is not a natural food, but neither is sucrose, which starts as sugar beets or sugar cane and undergoes processing to extract, purify, and crystallize the sucrose. In 1970, the most common sweetener in the American diet was sucrose (see graph). Over the next four decades, HFCS use increased dramatically, and it almost completely replaced sucrose in soft drinks. Manufacturers prefer HFCS because it is cheaper and more stable during storage than other sweeteners.[17]

HFCS has been implicated as a cause of obesity because the increase in its use parallels the increase in obesity (see graph), which in turn increases the risk of diabetes and heart disease. A study of fructose metabolism provides good evidence that this sugar may promote weight gain. Fructose is converted to fat more readily than glucose. Fructose is also not as effective as glucose at stimulating the release of hormones that suppress appetite and promote

weight loss or at inhibiting the release of hormones that stimulate appetite.[18] So, when compared to glucose, fructose contributes more to fat synthesis and less to appetite suppression, leading to overeating and weight gain. This would incriminate HFCS if it provided more fructose than sucrose. In fact, both sucrose and HFCS are about half fructose and half glucose, and once digested and absorbed, the fructose from sucrose is no different than that in HFCS.[18] Eliminating HFCS will help fight obesity and other health problems only if people do not replace it with other added sweeteners.

Is concern about the environment a reason to avoid this corn sweetener? The agricultural methods used to grow corn in the United States deplete soil nutrients and introduce pesticides and fertilizers into the environment. About half of the corn grown in the United States are GM varieties that have been designed to reduce the use of pesticides. Advocates and opponents of GM crops argue about whether they are harmful for people and the environment (see Chapter 13).[19] Regardless of the answer, only about 6% of the corn crop is used to produce HFCS,[20] so eliminating it without changing agricultural practices will have a relatively minor environmental impact.

Is HFCS worse than other sweeteners? When consumed in large amounts, HFCS has the potential to increase body fat. In addition, the production of HFCS may have an impact on the environment. But will eliminating HFCS from our food supply necessarily make our diets healthier or protect the environment?

Think critically: Compare the relationship between the percentage of adults who are obese and the intake of HFCS from 1970 to 2000 and from 2000 to 2005. Do they correlate with each other over both these time periods? What do these relationships tell you about the role of HFCS in obesity?

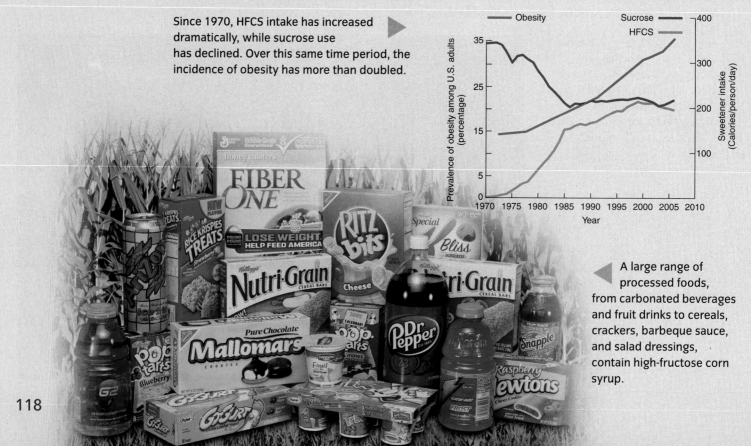

Since 1970, HFCS intake has increased dramatically, while sucrose use has declined. Over this same time period, the incidence of obesity has more than doubled.

A large range of processed foods, from carbonated beverages and fruit drinks to cereals, crackers, barbeque sauce, and salad dressings, contain high-fructose corn syrup.

118

metabolism toward fat storage (see *Debate: Should You Avoid High-Fructose Corn Syrup?*). In contrast, a low-carbohydrate diet causes less insulin release and hence does not promote fat storage. Low-carbohydrate diets lead to weight loss because they reduce insulin levels and raise blood ketone levels, both of which suppress appetite. In addition, these diets limit food choices to such an extent that the monotony of the diet causes the dieter to eat less.[16] The weight loss that is achieved with these diets is therefore caused by consuming fewer calories.

Pros and cons of nonnutritive sweetners One way to reduce the amount of refined sugar in the diet is to replace sugar with **nonnutritive sweeteners** (also called **artificial sweeteners**). The FDA has approved saccharin, aspartame, sucralose, acesulfame K, neotame, and rebiana as nonnutritive sweeteners and defined **acceptable daily intakes (ADIs)**—levels that should not be exceeded when using these products (**Table 4.1**).[21]

Nonnutritive sweeteners Table 4.1

Sweetener	Brand names	What is it?	ADI
Saccharin	Sweet'N Low, SugarTwin	The oldest of the nonnutritive sweeteners, developed in 1879. It was once considered a carcinogen but was taken off the government's list of cancer-causing substances in 2000. It is 300 times sweeter than sucrose and has a bitter aftertaste.	5 mg/kg of body weight/day; One packet contains 36 mg of saccharin. A 154-lb (70-kg) person would exceed the ADI by consuming 10 packets or about three 12-oz saccharin-sweetened beverages.
Aspartame	Equal, NutraSweet	Made of two amino acids (phenylalanine and aspartic acid; see *What a Scientist Sees: Phenylketonuria*, in Chapter 6). Because it breaks down when heated, it is typically used in cold products or added after cooking. It is 200 times sweeter than sucrose.	50 mg/kg of body weight/day; One packet contains 37 mg of aspartame. To exceed the ADI, a 154-lb (70-kg) person would have to consume 95 packets or 16 12-oz aspartame-sweetened beverages. It must be limited in the diets of people with phenylketonuria (see Chapter 6).
Acesulfame K	Sunett, Sweet One	A heat-stable sweetener that is often used in combination with other sweeteners. It is 200 times sweeter than sucrose.	15 mg/kg of body weight/ day; A 154-lb (70-kg) person could consume 2 gallons of beverages containing acesulfame K without exceeding the ADI.
Neotame	No brand name. Neotame is not sold as a tabletop sweetener.	Made from the same two amino acids as aspartame, but because the bond between them is harder to break than the bond in aspartame, it is heat stable and can be used in baking. It is used in soft drinks, dairy products, and gum but is not sold as a tabletop sweetener. It is 8000 times sweeter than sucrose.	18 mg/kg of body weight/day.
Sucralose	Splenda	Made from sucrose molecules that have been modified so that they cannot be digested or absorbed. It is heat stable so it can be used in cooking. It is 600 times sweeter than sucrose.	5 mg/kg of body weight/ day; One packet contains about 12 mg of sucralose. A 154-lb (70-kg) person could consume 29 packets without exceeding the ADI.
Rebiana	Truvia, Pure Via	A natural sweetener made from the leaf of the stevia plant.[22] It is the newest sweetener on the market and is about 300 times sweeter than sucrose.	12 mg/kilogram of body weight/day; To exceed the ADI, a 154-lb (70-kg) person would have to consume more than 30 packets of a rebiana sweetener or drink about six 12-oz cans of a rebiana-sweetened soda.

When nonnutritive sweeteners are used to replace added sugars in the diet, they can help reduce the incidence of dental caries and manage blood sugar levels. Whether use of these products promotes weight loss, however, depends on whether the calories they spare are added back from other food sources. When the effect of nonnutritive sweeteners on body weight was examined, their use was actually associated with weight gain, not weight loss. One hypothesis to explain this is that the sweet taste increases appetite, causing users to actually increase their food intake.[23]

If you think switching to nonnutritive sweeteners will make your diet healthier, think again. Foods that are high in added sugar tend to be nutrient poor. Replacing them with artificially sweetened alternatives does not necessarily increase the nutrient density of the diet or improve overall diet quality.

Heart Disease

The impact of carbohydrates on heart disease risk depends on the type of carbohydrate. There is evidence that diets high in sugar can raise blood lipid levels and thereby increase the risk of heart disease,[24] whereas diets high in fiber have been found to reduce the risk of heart disease.[15, 25]

Foods containing soluble fiber, such as legumes, oats, flaxseed, and brown rice, may reduce the risk of heart disease by lowering blood cholesterol levels. In the digestive tract, soluble fiber binds dietary cholesterol and bile acids, which are made from cholesterol, preventing them from being absorbed (**Figure 4.18**).[26] Soluble fiber may also help lower blood cholesterol because the by-products of the bacterial breakdown of the fiber may inhibit cholesterol synthesis in the liver or increase its removal from the blood.[26]

Cholesterol and soluble fiber • Figure 4.18

a. When the diet is low in soluble fiber, dietary cholesterol and bile, which contains cholesterol and bile acids made from cholesterol, are absorbed into the blood and transported to the liver, where they are reused.

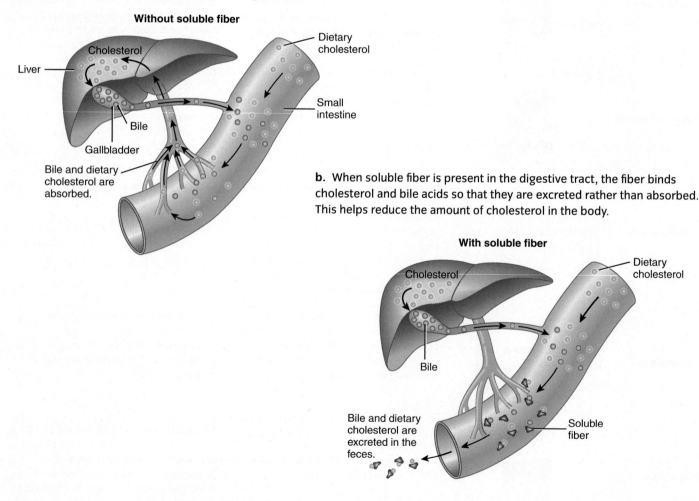

b. When soluble fiber is present in the digestive tract, the fiber binds cholesterol and bile acids so that they are excreted rather than absorbed. This helps reduce the amount of cholesterol in the body.

Diverticulosis is a condition in which outpouches form in the wall of the colon. These diverticula form at weak points due to pressure exerted when the colon contracts.

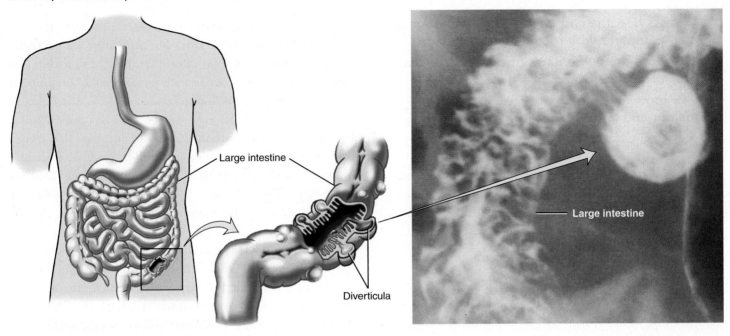

Insoluble fibers, such as wheat bran and cellulose, do not lower blood cholesterol, but a diet high in any type of fiber may help lower blood pressure, normalize blood glucose levels, prevent obesity, and affect a number of other parameters that help reduce the risk of heart disease.[27]

Bowel Health

Fiber and other indigestible carbohydrates add bulk and absorb water in the gastrointestinal tract, making the feces larger and softer and reducing the pressure needed for defecation. This helps reduce the incidence of constipation and **hemorrhoids**, the swelling of veins in the rectal or anal area. It also reduces the risk of developing outpouches in the wall of the colon called **diverticula** (the singular is *diverticulum*) (**Figure 4.19**). Fecal matter can accumulate in these pouches, causing irritation, pain, and inflammation—a condition known as **diverticulitis**. Diverticulitis may lead to infection. Treatment usually includes antibiotics to eliminate the infection and a low-fiber diet to prevent irritation of inflamed tissues. Once the inflammation is resolved, a high-fiber diet is recommended to ease stool elimination and reduce future attacks of diverticulitis.

Although fiber speeds movement of the intestinal contents, when the diet is low in fluid, fiber can contribute to constipation. The more fiber in the diet, the more water is needed to keep the stool soft. When too little fluid is consumed, the stool becomes hard and difficult to eliminate. In severe cases of excessive fiber intake and low fluid intake, intestinal blockage can occur.

A diet high in fiber, particularly from whole grains, may reduce the risk of colon cancer, although not all studies support this finding.[15,28,29] Fiber reduces contact between the cells lining the colon and potentially cancer-causing substances in the feces. Fiber in the colon also affects the intestinal microflora and their by-products. These by-products may directly affect colon cells or may change the environment of the colon in a way that can affect the development of colon cancer. Some of the protective effect may also be due to antioxidant vitamins and phytochemicals present in fiber-rich whole grains.

CONCEPT CHECK STOP

1. **What** health problems are common in people who have uncontrolled diabetes?

2. **Why** does frequent snacking on high-carbohydrate foods promote dental caries?

3. **When** does a low-carbohydrate diet promote weight loss?

4. **How** does fiber benefit colon health?

Meeting Carbohydrate Needs

LEARNING OBJECTIVES

1. **Discuss** how the carbohydrate intake of Americans compares with recommendations.
2. **Calculate** the percentage of calories from carbohydrate in a food or in a diet.
3. **Use** food labels to identify foods that are high in fiber and low in added sugar.

R ecommendations for carbohydrate intake focus on two main points: getting enough carbohydrate to meet the need for glucose and choosing the types that promote health and prevent disease.

Carbohydrate Recommendations

The RDA for carbohydrate is 130 g/day, based on the average minimum amount of glucose used by the brain.[30] In a diet that meets energy needs, this amount provides adequate glucose and prevents ketosis. Additional carbohydrate provides an important source of energy in the diet, and carbohydrate-containing foods can add vitamins,

minerals, fiber, and phytochemicals. Therefore, the Acceptable Macronutrient Distribution Range for carbohydrate is 45 to 65% of total calorie intake. A diet within this range meets energy needs without excessive amounts of protein or fat (**Figure 4.20**).

The typical U.S. diet meets the recommendation for the amount of carbohydrate, but most of this comes from refined sources, making the diet lower in fiber and higher in added sugar than recommended (see *Thinking It Through*). The Adequate Intake for fiber is 38 g/day for men and 25 g/day for women; the typical intake is only about 15 g/day.

There is no RDA or Daily Value for added sugars, but the 2010 Dietary Guidelines recommend reducing the consumption of added sugars, which add calories without contributing to the overall nutrient adequacy of the diet. Reducing added sugars reduces calorie intake without reducing essential nutrients.[31]

Because no specific toxicity is associated with high intake of any type of carbohydrate, no UL has been established for total carbohydrate intake, for fiber intake, or for added sugar intake.

How much carbohydrate do you eat? • Figure 4.20

To calculate the percentage of calories from carbohydrate in a diet, first determine the number of grams of carbohydrate and multiply this value by 4 Calories/gram. For example, the vegetarian food shown here, which represents a day's intake, provides about 300 g of carbohydrate:

300 g × 4 Calories/g = 1200 Calories from carbohydrate

Next divide the number of Calories from carbohydrate by the total number of Calories in the diet and multiply by 100 to convert it to a percentage. In this example, the diet contains 2000 total Calories, and so it provides:

(1200 Calories from carbohydrate/2000 Calories total) × 100 = 60% of Calories from carbohydrate

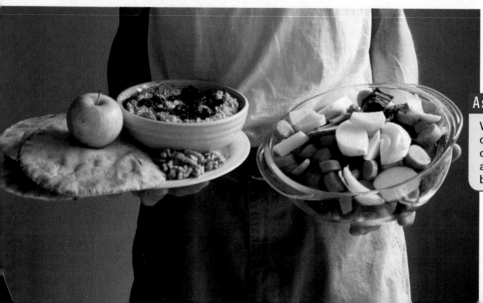

Ask Yourself

What is the percentage of calories from carbohydrate in a diet that provides 240 g of carbohydrate and 2400 Calories?
a. 10   c. 50
b. 40   d. 60

THINKING IT THROUGH

A Case Study on Healthy Carbohydrates

Trina is busy and tends to grab whatever is quick and easy to eat. She just read an article that says Americans eat the wrong kinds of carbohydrates. To see how she is doing, Trina analyzes a typical day's intake using 🌀 iProfile. For breakfast she has a bowl of presweetened cereal and a piece of fruit, lunch is chips and a soda, and dinner is a burrito. She always drinks milk with dinner. She has another soda at night while studying. Her iProfile analysis shows that she eats 2199 Calories, 70 g protein, 71 g fat, 320 g carbohydrate, and 12 g fiber per day.

How does her intake compare with the recommended amounts of carbohydrate and fiber?

▼

By calculating the percentage of calories from carbohydrate (320 g carbohydrate × 4 Calories/gram ÷ 2199 Calories × 100 = 58%), Trina is surprised to see that despite her poor choices, her carbohydrate intake is in the recommended range of 45 to 65% of calories. However, she consumes only 12 g of fiber, 13 g less than the 25 g recommended for women her age.

Compared to her MyPlate Daily Food Plan, Trina is not consuming enough fruits, vegetables, or whole grains. Boosting her intake of these will help increase her fiber intake. She decides to switch to whole-grain bread and cereal and increase her servings of high-fiber fruits and vegetables.

🌀 **Use iProfile to look up the fiber content of the fruits and vegetables listed below and choose a combination of these that will add at least 13 g of fiber to Trina's diet.**

▼

Vegetables	Fruits
Black beans, 1/2 cup	Pear, 1 medium
Green beans, 1/2 cup	Kiwi, 2 small
Iceberg lettuce, 1 cup	Apple, 1 medium
Broccoli, 1/2 cup	Banana, 1 medium
Asparagus, 1/2 cup	Watermelon, 1 cup
Raw spinach, 1 cup	Orange, 1 medium

Your answer:

Looking at her typical choices, Trina can see that much of her carbohydrate intake is from added sugars in her beverages and breakfast cereal.

If Trina replaces the two 20-oz sodas she drinks per day with water, how many calories and how much sugar will this eliminate from her diet?

▼

Your answer:

To reduce the sugar and increase the fiber in her breakfast, Trina plans to choose between these two healthy-sounding breakfast cereals.

Raisin and Bran Cereal

Nutrition Facts
Serving Size 1 Cup (59g/2.1 oz.)
Servings Per Container about 8

Amount Per Serving	Cereal	Cereal with ½ cup Vitamins A&D Fat Free Milk
Calories	190	230
Calories from Fat	10	10

	% Daily Value**	
Total Fat 1g*	2%	2%
Saturated Fat 0g	0%	0%
Trans Fat 0g		
Cholesterol 0mg	0%	0%
Sodium 250mg	10%	13%
Potassium 320mg	9%	15%
Total Carbohydrate 46g	15%	17%
Dietary Fiber 5g	20%	20%
Sugars 17g		
Other Carbohydrate 24g		
Protein 5g		

INGREDIENTS: WHOLE GRAIN WHEAT, RAISINS, WHEAT BRAN, SUGAR, HIGH FRUCTOSE CORN SYRUP, CONTAINS 2% OR LESS OF SALT, MALT FLAVORING, INVERT SUGAR…

Multigrain Cereal

Nutrition Facts
Serving Size 1 cup (29g)
Servings Per Container about 8

Amount Per Serving	MultiGrain Cheerios	with ½ cup skim milk
Calories	110	150
Calories from Fat	10	10

	% Daily Value**	
Total Fat 1g*	2%	2%
Saturated Fat 0g	0%	3%
Trans Fat 0g		
Cholesterol 0mg	0%	1%
Sodium 160mg	7%	9%
Potassium 85mg	2%	8%
Total Carbohydrate 23g	8%	10%
Dietary Fiber 4g	16%	16%
Sugars 6g		
Other Carbohydrate 13g		
Protein 2g		

INGREDIENTS: WHOLE GRAIN CORN, WHOLE GRAIN OATS, SUGAR, WHOLE GRAIN BARLEY, WHOLE GRAIN WHEAT, WHOLE GRAIN RICE, CORN STARCH, BROWN SUGAR SYRUP, CORN BRAN, SALT…

Use the ingredient list to identify the sources of whole grains and added sugars in these two products.

▼

Your answer:

Based on the amounts of sugars and fiber in each, which one would you recommend?

▼

Your answer:

(Check your answers in Appendix J.)

Healthy MyPlate carbohydrate choices • Figure 4.21

The healthiest carbohydrate choices are whole grains, legumes, and fresh fruits and vegetables, which are low in added sugar and often are good sources of fiber. Foods containing refined carbohydrates should be limited because they are typically low in fiber and contain added sugars, which add empty calories.

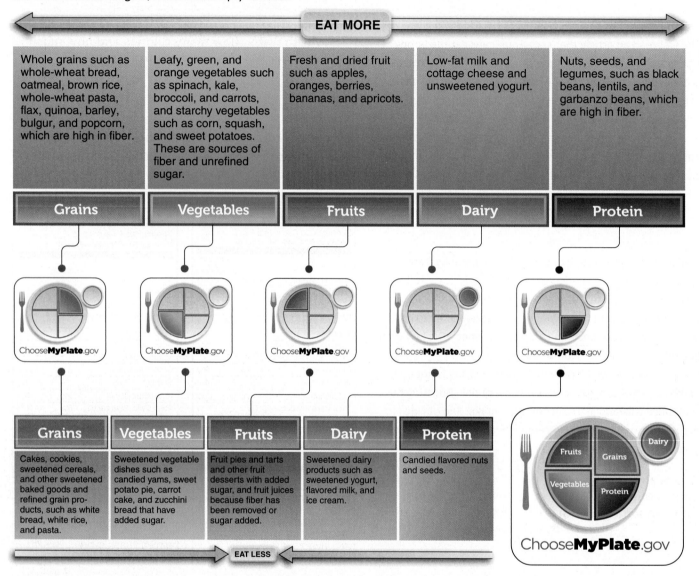

EAT MORE

Grains
Whole grains such as whole-wheat bread, oatmeal, brown rice, whole-wheat pasta, flax, quinoa, barley, bulgur, and popcorn, which are high in fiber.

Vegetables
Leafy, green, and orange vegetables such as spinach, kale, broccoli, and carrots, and starchy vegetables such as corn, squash, and sweet potatoes. These are sources of fiber and unrefined sugar.

Fruits
Fresh and dried fruit such as apples, oranges, berries, bananas, and apricots.

Dairy
Low-fat milk and cottage cheese and unsweetened yogurt.

Protein
Nuts, seeds, and legumes, such as black beans, lentils, and garbanzo beans, which are high in fiber.

ChooseMyPlate.gov

Grains
Cakes, cookies, sweetened cereals, and other sweetened baked goods and refined grain products, such as white bread, white rice, and pasta.

Vegetables
Sweetened vegetable dishes such as candied yams, sweet potato pie, carrot cake, and zucchini bread that have added sugar.

Fruits
Fruit pies and tarts and other fruit desserts with added sugar, and fruit juices because fiber has been removed or sugar added.

Dairy
Sweetened dairy products such as sweetened yogurt, flavored milk, and ice cream.

Protein
Candied flavored nuts and seeds.

EAT LESS

ChooseMyPlate.gov

Choosing Carbohydrates Wisely

To promote a healthy, balanced diet, the 2010 Dietary Guidelines and MyPlate recommend increasing consumption of whole grains, fruits and vegetables, and low-fat dairy products while limiting foods high in refined grains and added sugars, such as soft drinks and other sweetened beverages, sweet bakery products, and candy. Because the majority of the added sugars Americans consume come from beverages, the Dietary Guidelines specifically recommend reducing intake of sugar-sweetened beverages such as soda, energy drinks, sports drinks, and sugar-sweetened fruit drinks.

Using MyPlate to make healthy choices For a 2000-Calorie diet, MyPlate recommends 6 oz of grains (half of which should be whole grains), 2 cups of fruit, and 2½ cups of vegetables. As **Figure 4.21** suggests, refined carbohydrates can be replaced with unrefined ones to make the diet healthier. For example, an apple provides about 80 Calories and 3.7 g of fiber, making it a better choice than 1 cup of apple juice, which has the same amount of energy but almost no fiber (0.2 g).

Interpreting food labels Food labels can help in choosing the right mix of carbohydrates (**Figure 4.22**).

Choosing carbohydrates from the label • Figure 4.22

Whole Wheat Bread

Nutrition Facts	Amount/Serving	%DV*	Amount/Serving	%DV*
Serving Size 1 Slice (27g) Servings Per Container 17 Calories 70 Calories from Fat 10	**Total Fat** 1g	**2%**	**Total Carb.** 12g	**4%**
	Sat. Fat 0g	**0%**	Dietary Fiber 2g	**8%**
	Trans Fat 0g	**0%**	Sugars 2g	
	Cholesterol 0mg	**0%**	**Protein** 2g	
	Sodium 10mg	**0%**		
Vitamin A 0% • Vitamin C 0% • Calcium 4% • Iron 4% Thiamin 4% • Riboflavin 2% • Niacin 4%				

*Percent Daily Values (DV) are based on a 2,000-calorie diet. Your daily values may be higher or lower depending on your calorie needs:

	Calories:	2,000	2,500
Total Fat	Less than	65g	80g
Sat Fat	Less than	20g	25g
Cholesterol	Less than	300mg	300mg
Sodium	Less than	2,400mg	2,400mg
Total Carbohydrate		300g	375g
Dietary Fiber		25g	30g

NOT A SODIUM FREE FOOD

INGREDIENTS: WHOLE WHEAT FLOUR, WATER, SWEETENERS (HIGH FRUCTOSE CORN SYRUP MOLASSES), WHEAT GLUTEN, SOYBEAN CONTAINS 2% OR LESS OF THE FOLLOWING: YEAST DOUGH CONDITIONERS (MONO-DIGLYCERIDES, ETHOXYLATED MONO & GLYCERIDES, CALCIUM STEAROYL-2-LACTYLATE), YEAST NUTRIENTS (CALCIUM SULFATE, MONO- CALCIUM PHOSPHA CALCIUM PRO IONATE (A PRESERVATIVE).

The Nutrition Facts panel of a food label lists the number of grams of total carbohydrate, fiber, and sugars. The total carbohydrate and fiber values are also given as a percentage of the Daily Value.

The Daily Value for total carbohydrate is 60% of the diet's energy content, or 300 g for a 2000-Calorie diet. The Daily Value for fiber in a 2000-Calorie diet is 25 g.

To identify products made mostly from *whole* grains, look for the word "whole" before the name of the grain. If this is the first ingredient listed, the product is made from mostly whole grain. "Wheat flour" simply means it was made with wheat, not whole wheat. Note that foods labeled with the words "multigrain," "stone-ground," "100% wheat," "cracked wheat," "seven-grain," or "bran" are not necessarily 100% whole-grain products and may not contain any whole grains.

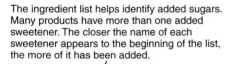

Foods labeled "high fiber" contain 20% or more of the Daily Value per serving.

Foods labeled "good source of fiber" contain between 10 and 19% of the Daily Value per serving.

Ask Yourself

Is a product that lists wheat flour as the first ingredient and whole-wheat flour as the second made mostly from whole grains? Why or why not?

Products labeled "reduced sugar" contain 25% less sugar than the regular, or reference, product.

The ingredient list helps identify added sugars. Many products have more than one added sweetener. The closer the name of each sweetener appears to the beginning of the list, the more of it has been added.

INGREDIENTS: CULTURED PASTEURIZED GRADE A REDUCED FAT MILK, SUGAR, NONFAT MILK, HIGH FRUCTOSE CORN SYRUP, STRAWBERRY PUREE, MODIFIED CORN STARCH, KOSHER GELATIN, TRI-CALCIUM PHOSPHATE, NATURAL FLAVOR, COLORED WITH CARMINE, VITAMIN A ACETATE, VITAMIN D₃

On the ingredient list, all these mean added sugar: Brown sugar, corn sweetener, corn syrup, dextrose, fructose, fruit juice, glucose, high fructose corn syrup, honey, invert sugar, lactose, maltose, malt syrup, molasses, raw sugar, sucrose, and sugar syrup concentrates.

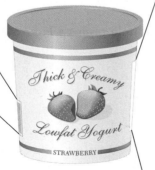

Nutrition Facts
Serving Size 1 Container

Amount Per Serving	
Calories 190	**Calories from Fat** 30

Amount/Serving	% DV*
Total Fat 3.5g	**5%**
Saturated Fat 2g	**10%**
Trans Fat 0g	
Cholesterol 15mg	**4%**
Sodium 100mg	**4%**
Potassium 310g	**9%**
Total Carbohydrate 32g	**11%**
Dietary Fiber 0g	**0%**
Sugars 28g	
Protein 7g	**14%**
Vitamin A 15% • Calcium 30%	

*Percent Daily Values (DV) are based on a 2,000 calorie diet.

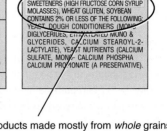

Foods labeled "sugar free" contain less than 0.5 g of sugar per serving.

The number of grams of sugars listed under Nutrition Facts tells you the total amount of mono-saccharides plus disaccharides in a food, but this number does not distinguish between added sugar and the sugar occurring naturally in the food.

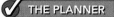

WHAT SHOULD I EAT?
Carbohydrates

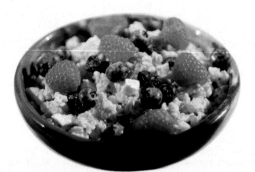

Make half your grains whole
- Have your sandwich on whole-wheat, oat bran, rye, or pumpernickel bread.
- Switch to whole-wheat pasta and brown rice.
- Fill your cereal bowl with plain oatmeal and add a few raisins for sweetness.
- Check the ingredient list for the words *whole* or *whole grain* before the grain ingredient's name.

Increase your fruits and veggies
- Don't forget beans. Kidney beans, chickpeas, black beans, and others have more fiber and resistant starch than any other vegetables.
- Add berries, bananas, and oats to cereal and desserts.
- Pile the veggies on your sandwich.
- Have more than one vegetable at dinner.

Limit added sugars
- Switch to a 12-oz can instead of a 20-oz bottle when you grab a soft drink or, better yet, have a glass of water or low-fat milk.
- Use one-quarter less sugar in your recipe next time you bake.
- Snack on a piece of fruit instead of a candy bar.
- Swap your sugary breakfast cereal for an unsweetened whole-grain variety.

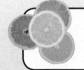

Use iProfile to look up the fiber content of some of your favorite foods.

The Nutrition Facts panel helps consumers find foods that are good sources of fiber and low in sugar. The ingredient list helps identify whole-grain products and the sources of added sugars. Nutrient content claims such as "high in fiber" or "no sugar added" and health claims such as those highlighting the relationship between fiber intake and the risk of heart disease and cancer help identify foods that meet the recommendations for fiber and added sugar intake (see *What Should I Eat?* and Appendix F).

CONCEPT CHECK STOP

1. **How** does the U.S. diet compare with recommendations for fiber and added sugar?

2. **What** is the percentage of calories from carbohydrate in your breakfast cereal?

3. **Where** on a food label can you find information about added sugars?

THE PLANNER ✓

Summary

1 Carbohydrates in Our Food 100

- Unrefined whole grains, fruits, and vegetables are good sources of fiber and micronutrients. When these foods are **refined**, nutrients and fiber are lost. Whole grains contain the entire kernel, as shown here, which includes the **endosperm**, **bran**, and **germ**; refined grains include only the endosperm. **Enrichment**, one type of **fortification**, adds back some but not all of the nutrients lost in refining.

Whole grains • Figure 4.2

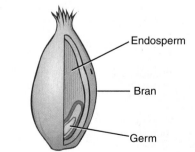

Endosperm

Bran

Germ

- Refined sugars contain calories but few nutrients; for this reason, foods high in added refined sugar are low in nutrient density.

2 Types of Carbohydrates   102

- Carbohydrates contain carbon as well as hydrogen and oxygen, in the same proportion as water. **Simple carbohydrates** include **monosaccharides** and **disaccharides** and are found in foods such as table sugar, honey, milk, and fruit. **Complex carbohydrates** are **polysaccharides**; they include **glycogen** in animals and **starches**, illustrated here, and **fiber** in plants.

Structures and sources of carbohydrates: Complex carbohydrates • Figure 4.4c

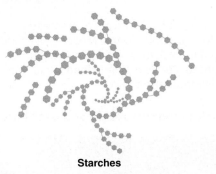

Starches

- Fiber cannot be digested in the stomach or small intestine and therefore is not absorbed into the body. **Soluble fiber** dissolves in water to form a viscous solution and is digested by bacteria in the colon; **insoluble fiber** is not digested by bacteria and adds bulk to fecal matter.

3 Carbohydrate Digestion and Absorption   105

- Disaccharides and starches must be digested to monosaccharides, as shown here, before they can be absorbed. In individuals with **lactose intolerance**, lactose passes into the colon undigested, causing cramps, gas, and diarrhea. Indigestible complex carbohydrates, including fiber, some **oligosaccharides**, and **resistant starch**, can increase intestinal gas, but they benefit health by increasing bulk in the stool, promoting growth of healthy microflora, and slowing nutrient absorption.

Carbohydrate digestion • Figure 4.7

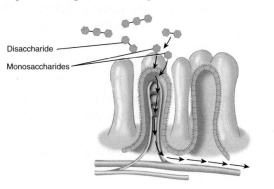

Disaccharide

Monosaccharides

- After a meal, blood **glucose** levels rise. The rate, magnitude, and duration of this rise are referred to as the **glycemic response**. Glycemic response is affected by the amount and type of carbohydrate consumed and by other nutrients ingested with the carbohydrate.

4 Carbohydrate Functions   109

- Carbohydrate, primarily as glucose, provides energy to the body. Blood glucose levels are maintained by the hormones **insulin** and **glucagon**. As depicted here, when blood glucose levels rise insulin from the pancreas allows cells to take up glucose from the blood and promotes the synthesis of glycogen, fat, and protein. When blood glucose levels fall, glucagon increases them by causing glycogen breakdown and glucose synthesis.

Blood glucose regulation Figure • 4.10

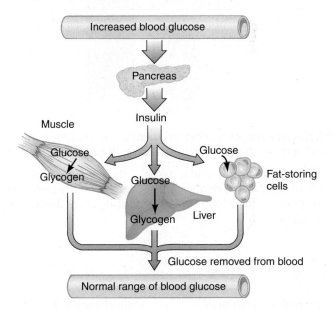

Increased blood glucose

Pancreas

Insulin

Muscle

Glucose

Glycogen

Glucose

Glycogen   Liver

Glucose

Fat-storing cells

Glucose removed from blood

Normal range of blood glucose

- Glucose is metabolized through cellular respiration. It begins with **glycolysis**, which breaks each six-carbon glucose molecule into two three-carbon pyruvate molecules, producing ATP even when oxygen is unavailable. The complete breakdown of glucose through **aerobic metabolism** requires oxygen and produces carbon dioxide, water, and more ATP than glycolysis.

- When carbohydrate intake is limited, amino acids from the breakdown of body proteins can be used to synthesize glucose. Therefore, an adequate carbohydrate intake is said to spare protein. Limited carbohydrate intake also results in the formation of **ketones (ketone bodies)** by the liver. These can be used as an energy source by other tissues. Ketones that accumulate in the blood can cause symptoms that range from headache and lack of appetite to coma and even death if levels are extremely high.

5 Carbohydrates in Health and Disease 113

- As shown in the graph, **diabetes mellitus** is characterized by high blood glucose levels, that occur either because insufficient insulin is produced or because of a decrease in the body's sensitivity to insulin. Over time, high blood glucose levels damage tissues and contribute to the development of heart disease, kidney failure, blindness, and infections that may lead to amputations. Treatment includes diet, exercise, and medication to keep glucose levels in the normal range.

Blood glucose levels in diabetes • Figure 4.13

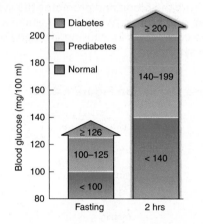

- **Hypoglycemia**, or low blood glucose, causes symptoms such as sweating, headaches, and rapid heartbeat.

- Diets high in carbohydrate, particularly refined sugars, increase the risk of dental caries. Bacteria on the teeth use carbohydrate as a food supply, producing acids that damage the teeth.

- Gram for gram, carbohydrates provide less energy than fat. High-fiber diets can prevent weight gain by making you feel full longer so that you eat less. Low-carbohydrate diets promote weight loss by causing a spontaneous reduction in food intake. **Nonnutritive sweeteners** aid weight loss if the sugar calories they replace are not added back from other food sources.

- Diets high in unrefined carbohydrates from whole grains, vegetables, fruits, and legumes may reduce the risk of heart disease, bowel disorders, and colon cancer. Soluble fiber helps prevent heart disease because it can lower blood cholesterol.

6 Meeting Carbohydrate Needs 122

- Guidelines for a healthy diet recommend 45 to 65% of energy from carbohydrates. Most of this should come from whole grains, legumes, fruits, and vegetables, such as those in this photo. Foods high in added sugar should be consumed in moderation.

How much carbohydrate do you eat? Figure 4.20

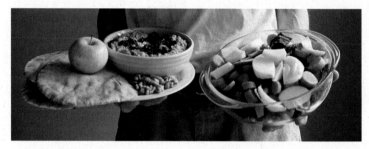

- The recommendations of MyPlate and the information on food labels can be used to select healthy amounts and sources of carbohydrate.

Key Terms

Online Resources

- For more information on diabetes, go to http://diabetes.niddk.nih.gov.

- For more information on how beverages affect our calorie intake, go to www.cdc.gov/healthyweight/healthy_eating/drinks.html.

- For more information on choosing whole grains, go to www.mayoclinic.com/health/whole-grains/NU00204.

- For more information on the 2010 Dietary Guidelines, go to www.health.gov/dietaryguidelines/.

- Visit your *WileyPLUS* site for videos, animations, podcasts, self-study, and other media that will aid you in studying and understanding this chapter.

Critical and Creative Thinking Questions

1. Record everything you eat for three days. Use iProfile to calculate your fiber intake. How does it compare with the recommendations? How could you increase your fiber intake?

2. For each high-carbohydrate food on your food record, indicate whether it is refined or unrefined. Suggest some changes that would increase your intake of unrefined carbohydrates. List some foods in your diet that are high in added sugars. Suggest some changes that would reduce your intake of these sugars.

3. Adam is 19 and plays basketball. Recently, he has been thirsty all the time, and he needs to get up several times a night to urinate. He has lost 10 pounds and is so tired that he has been missing basketball practice. What type of diabetes is most likely affecting Adam? How does it need to be managed? Why is it important to keep blood sugar levels within the normal range in both type 1 and type 2 diabetes?

4. Are carbohydrates good for you? Explain why or why not.

5. Imagine that you have gained 20 pounds over the past 5 years, and you decide to use a low-carbohydrate diet to return to a healthy weight. You are happy with your initial weight loss but begin to have headaches and bad breath. What is causing these symptoms, and why?

6. This is the label from a hot breakfast cereal. How much fiber and sugars does it provide? Is it a whole-grain product? What does this label tell you about the amount of added sugar it contains? Would you recommend this product to a friend? Why or why not?

Nutrition Facts

Serving Size 1 packet (43g)
Servings Per Container 10

Amount Per Serving	Cereal
Calories	160
Calories from Fat	15

	% Daily Value**
Total Fat 1.5g	2%
Saturated Fat 0g	0%
Trans Fat 0g	
Cholesterol 0mg	0%
Sodium 230mg	10%
Total Carbohydrate 33g	11%
Dietary Fiber 3g	12%
Soluble Fiber 1g	
Sugars 13g	
Protein 4g	

INGREDIENTS: WHOLE GRAIN ROLLED OATS (WITH OAT BRAN), SUGAR, SALT, NATURAL AND ARTIFICIAL FLAVORS, CALCIUM CARBONATE (A SOURCE OF CALCIUM), GUAR GUM, CARAMEL COLOR, VITAMIN A PALMITATE, NIACINAMIDE*, REDUCED IRON, PYRIDOXINE HYDROCHLORIDE*, RIBOFLAVIN*, THIAMIN MONONITRATE*, FOLIC ACID*. *ONE OF THE B VITAMINS.

What is happening in this picture?

These students are choosing fruit drinks, sports drinks, and iced tea because they believe these beverages are healthier choices than soda.

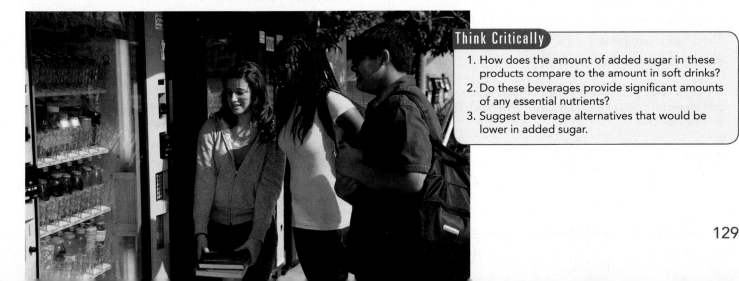

Think Critically

1. How does the amount of added sugar in these products compare to the amount in soft drinks?
2. Do these beverages provide significant amounts of any essential nutrients?
3. Suggest beverage alternatives that would be lower in added sugar.

Self-Test

(Check your answers in Appendix K.)

1. Which of the following is a source of unrefined carbohydrate?
   a. white bread
   c. corn on the cob
   b. white rice
   d. donut

2. Which of these molecules is a disaccharide?
   a. A
   c. C
   b. B
   d. D

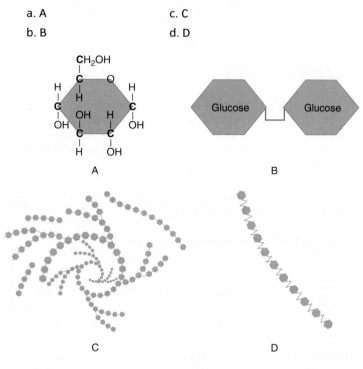

3. Which of the following is most likely to occur soon after you eat a large carbohydrate-rich meal?
   a. You break down body fat stores.
   b. Your pancreas releases insulin.
   c. Your pancreas releases glucagon.
   d. Your liver breaks down glycogen.
   e. You produce ketones.

4. Which of the following is contributing to the increase in type 2 diabetes?
   a. the increase in obesity
   b. consuming more fiber
   c. changes in our genes
   d. more sensitive immune systems

5. The Daily Value for fiber is 25 g. If a product label indicates that it provides 20% of the Daily Value, how much fiber does a serving contain?
   a. 2 g
   c. 4 g
   b. 3 g
   d. 5 g

6. Which part of this whole-wheat kernel contains most of the grain's fiber as well as many vitamins?
   a. A
   b. B
   c. C

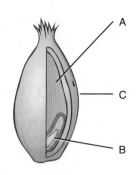

7. Foods high in added sugar provide _____.
   a. many vitamins in each calorie
   b. empty calories
   c. soluble fiber
   d. insoluble fiber

8. Which statement about simple carbohydrates is false?
   a. Fructose is found in fruit.
   b. Lactose is milk sugar.
   c. Glucose is blood sugar.
   d. Maltose is table sugar.

9. The digestive enzymes that break disaccharides into monosaccharides are located in the _____.
   a. stomach
   c. microvilli
   b. saliva
   d. colon

10. When blood glucose levels drop, all except which of the following may occur?
    a. Glucagon is released.
    b. Glycogen is broken down.
    c. Fatty acids are used to make glucose.
    d. Amino acids from protein are used to make glucose.

11. Which one of the following statements about insoluble fiber is true?
    a. It holds water in the gastrointestinal tract.
    b. It is digested by bacteria in the colon.
    c. It dissolves in water and forms a viscous solution.
    d. It adds bulk to the intestinal contents.

12. People who are lactose intolerant do not produce enough of the enzyme _____.

   a. lactase   c. galactose

   b. lactose   d. amylase

13. This graph shows an individual's glycemic response after consuming a sugar-sweetened beverage. Which of the following individuals does this graph represent?

   a. a person who has a normal glycemic response

   b. a person who has hypoglycemia

   c. a person who has prediabetes

   d. a person who has diabetes

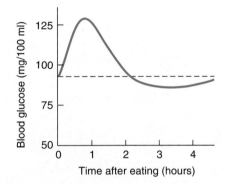

14. A high-fiber diet may help protect against which of the following?

   a. heart disease   c. large swings in blood glucose

   b. diverticulosis   d. all of the above

15. Which steps in the diagram proceed in the absence of oxygen?

   a. only step 1   c. only step 4

   b. steps 1, 2, and 3   d. steps 1 and 3

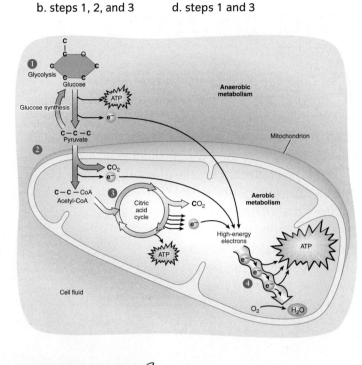

THE PLANNER ✓

Review your Chapter Planner on the chapter opener and check off your completed work.

5

Lipids: Fats, Phospholipids, and Sterols

For Colorado black bears, fall is a time of nonstop foraging; they consume about 65 pounds of apples and berries each day. Why the continuous buffet? Bears need this food to accumulate body fat that they use for energy during their long winter slumber.

Fat is an important source of energy for humans as well. Of course, our metabolism is vastly different from that of bears. If we were to eat as many calories as they do during the fall months, the equivalent of 10 double cheeseburgers everyday, sleeping through the winter would be

the least of our concerns. But the fat in our diet and in our bodies is important. Excess body fat is usually detrimental, but in some situations, having a bit more stored fat and eating more fat can be advantageous. An increase in body fat can protect against the depletion of

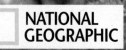

intramuscular fat during extended periods of exertion. And a diet high in fat may help prepare one for arduous, sustained exercise such as ultramarathons or survival in extreme environments.

The universality of a taste for fat among many animals indicates its importance to survival. It plays a tremendous role in the resilience of mammals—including a pair of interesting omnivores: the slumbering bear and the more wakeful humans.

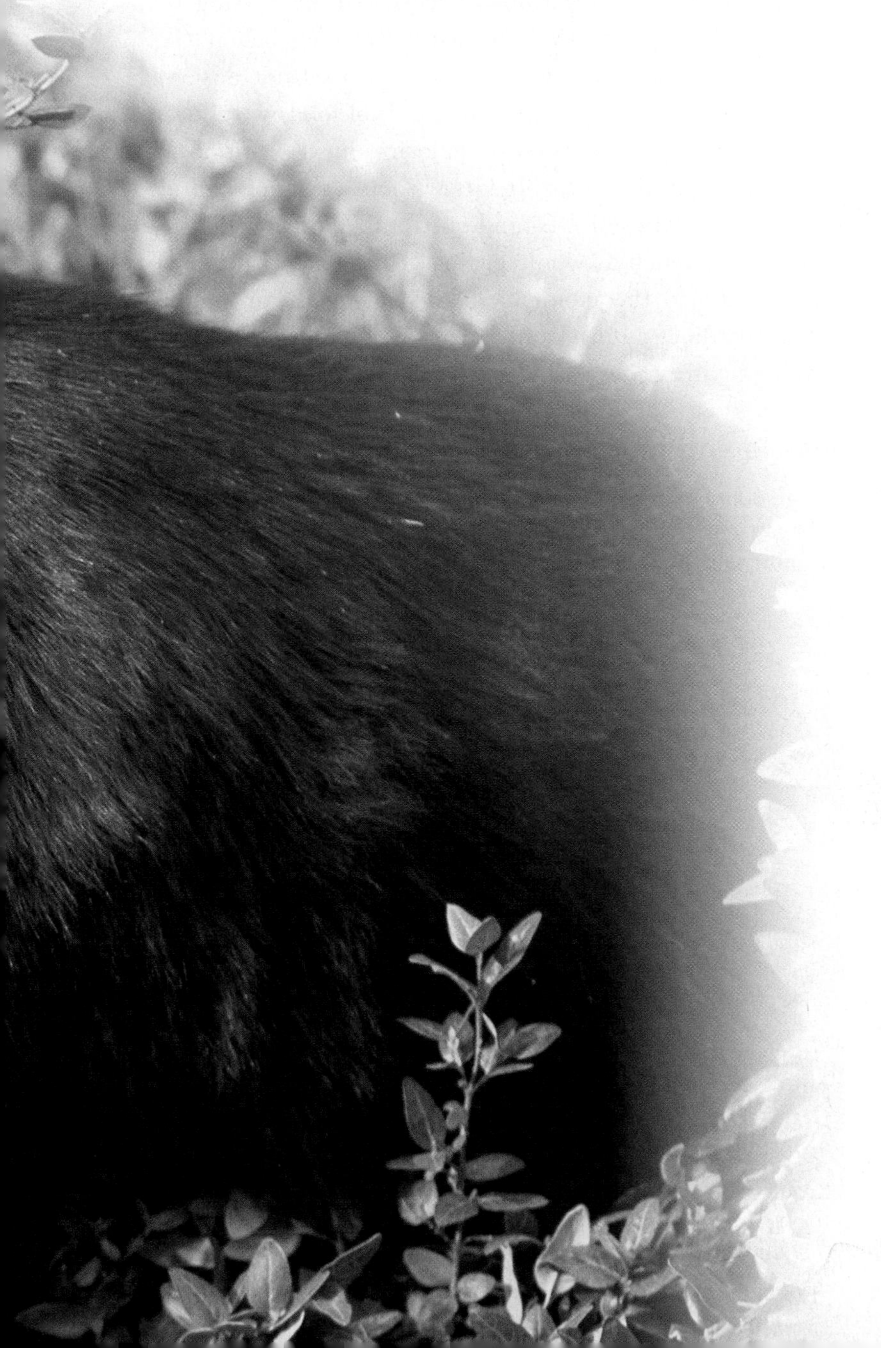

CHAPTER OUTLINE

CHAPTER PLANNER ✔

- ❏ Stimulate your interest by reading the introduction and looking at the visual.
- ❏ Scan the Learning Objectives in each section:
  p. 134 ❏   p. 135 ❏   p. 141 ❏   p. 144 ❏   p. 148 ❏   p. 154 ❏
- ❏ Read the text and study all figures and visuals. Answer any questions.

Analyze key features

- ❏ Nutrition InSight, pp. 136–137 ❏   p. 139 ❏
- ❏ Process Diagram,
  p. 141 ❏   p. 143 ❏   p. 146 ❏   pp. 148–149 ❏
- ❏ Thinking it Through, p. 155 ❏
- ❏ What a Scientist Sees, p. 156 ❏
- ❏ Stop: Answer the Concept Checks before you go on:
  p. 135 ❏   p. 140 ❏   p. 144 ❏   p. 147 ❏   p. 154 ❏   p. 160 ❏

End of chapter

- ❏ Review the Summary, Key Terms, and Online Resources.
- ❏ Answer the Critical and Creative Thinking Questions.
- ❏ Answer What is happening in this picture?
- ❏ Complete the Self-Test and check your answers.

Fats in Our Food

LEARNING OBJECTIVES

1. **Describe** the qualities that fat adds to foods.
2. **Identify** sources of hidden fat in the diet.
3. **Discuss** how fat intake in the United States has changed since the 1970s.

The fats in our foods contribute to their texture, flavor, and aroma. It is the fat that gives ice cream its smooth texture and rich taste. Olive oil imparts a unique flavor to salads and many traditional Italian and Greek dishes. Sesame oil gives egg rolls and other Chinese foods their distinctive aroma. But while the fats in our foods contribute to their appeal, they also add more calories than other nutrients (9 Calories/gram) so consuming too much can contribute to weight gain. The types of fats we eat also can affect our health; too much of the wrong types can increase the risk of heart disease and cancer.

Sources of Fat in Our Food

Sometimes the fat in our food is obvious. You can see the stripes of fat in a slice of bacon sizzling in a frying pan, for example, or the layer of fat around the outside of your steak. Other visible sources of fat in our diets are the fats we add to foods at the table—the pat of butter melting on your steaming baked potato and the dressing you pour over your salad. When you choose these items you know you are eating a high-fat food.

Not all sources of dietary fat are obvious. Cheese, ice cream, and whole milk are high in fat, and foods that we think of as sources of carbohydrate, such as crackers, doughnuts, cookies, and muffins, may also be quite high in fat (**Figure 5.1**). We also add invisible fat when we fry foods: French fries start as potatoes, which are low in fat, but when they are immersed in hot oil for frying, they soak up fat, increasing their calorie content.

America's Changing Fat Intake

Eating patterns in the United States have changed significantly over the past 40 years, even though total fat intake hasn't changed much. Beginning in the 1950s, Americans were told that too much fat made them fat, increased their risk of heart disease, and maybe even increased their risk of cancer. In response to these messages, many Americans switched from whole milk to low-fat, chose chicken in place of beef, consumed fewer eggs, and used less butter and high-fat salad dressing. But in addition to these changes, they consumed more hidden fats from foods such as pizza, pasta dishes, snack foods, and fried potatoes.[1] Thus, even though the sources of fat in the U.S. diet have changed since 1970, the types of fat and the number of grams of fat Americans consume daily have changed little.

What has changed in the past 40 years is our energy intake: It has increased. While the number of calories we eat has increased, the number of grams of fat we eat has remained constant, causing the percentage of calories from fat to drop from about 37% to 34% (**Figure 5.2**).[2,3]

Efforts to reduce chronic disease risk by cutting fat from our diets have failed not just because we haven't really cut our fat intake but because fat does not deserve its bad reputation. Changing the kinds of foods we choose without paying attention to calories hasn't promoted weight loss. Limiting visible fats without considering hidden fats, the types of fats, and our intake of other dietary components, such as whole grains, fruits, and vegetables, hasn't reduced the incidence of heart disease or cancer. A healthy diet requires eating the right kinds of fats and making healthy choices from all the food groups.

Visible and hidden fats • Figure 5.1

The amount of fat in a food is not always obvious. The two strips of bacon in this breakfast provide a total of 8 grams of fat, and the muffin provides 16 grams.

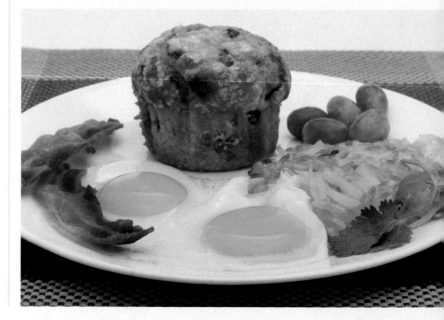

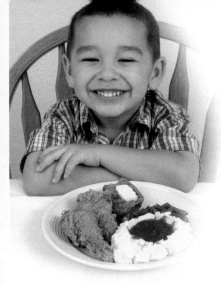

U.S. food intake in the 1970s and today • Figure 5.2

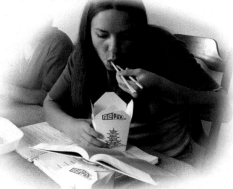

a. In the 1970s, a typical dinner included high-fat meat, bread with butter, and mashed potatoes with lots of gravy, and it was usually served with a glass of whole milk.

b. Today we drink low-fat milk and eat leaner meats, but we eat more fat from takeout Chinese and Mexican foods and fast-food pizza, French fries, hamburgers, and cheeseburgers than we did in the 1970s.[1]

c. In 1971, U.S. men consumed an average of 2450 Calories/day and women 1540 Calories/day.[2] Today, men consume over 2500 Calories/day and women over 1750 Calories/day.[3] Because of this increase in energy intake, the percentage of calories from fat has decreased, but we don't consume any less total fat today than we did in the 1970s.

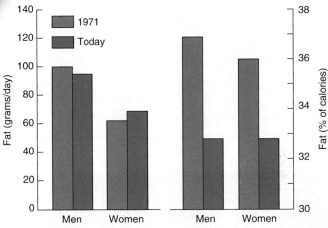

Interpreting Data

If the number of grams of fat in the U.S. diet has not changed, why has the percentage of fat in the diet gone down?

CONCEPT CHECK **STOP**

1. **How** does adding fat affect the calorie content of a food?

2. **What** are some invisible sources of fat in the diet?

3. **How** have the sources of fat in the U.S. diet changed since the 1970s?

Types of Lipids

LEARNING OBJECTIVES

1. **Explain** the relationship between triglycerides and fatty acids.

2. **Compare** the structures of saturated, monounsaturated, polyunsaturated, omega-6, omega-3, and *trans* fatty acids.

3. **Describe** how phospholipids and cholesterol are used in the body.

4. **Name** foods that are sources of saturated, monounsaturated, polyunsaturated, omega-6, omega-3, and *trans* fatty acids.

Lipids are substances that do not dissolve in water. We tend to use the term *fat* to refer to lipids, but we are usually referring to types of lipids called **triglycerides**. Triglycerides make up most of the lipids in our food and in our bodies. The structure of triglycerides includes lipid molecules called **fatty acids**. Two other types of

triglyceride The major type of lipid in food and the body, consisting of three fatty acids attached to a glycerol molecule.

fatty acid A molecule made up of a chain of carbons linked to hydrogens, with an acid group at one end of the chain.

lipids that are important in nutrition but are present in the body in smaller amounts are **phospholipids** and **sterols**.

Triglycerides and Fatty Acids

A triglyceride consists of the three-carbon molecule glycerol with three fatty acids attached to it (**Figure 5.3**). A fatty acid is a chain of carbon atoms with an acid group at one end of the chain. Fatty acids vary in the length of their carbon chains and the types and locations of carbon–carbon bonds within the chain. Fatty acids are what we are really talking about when we refer to *trans* fat or saturated fat—these terms really mean *trans* **fatty acids** and **saturated fatty acids**. Triglycerides may contain any combination of fatty

phospholipid A type of lipid whose structure includes a phosphorus atom.

sterol A type of lipid with a structure composed of multiple chemical rings.

saturated fatty acid A fatty acid in which the carbon atoms are bonded to as many hydrogen atoms as possible; it therefore contains no carbon–carbon double bonds.

Triglycerides • Figure 5.3

A triglyceride contains glycerol and three fatty acids. The carbon chains of the fatty acids vary in length from short-chain fatty acids (4 to 7 carbons) to medium-chain (8 to 12 carbons) and long-chain fatty acids (more than 12 carbons). Most fatty acids in plants and animals contain between 14 and 22 carbons.

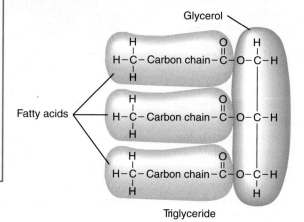
Triglyceride

Nutrition InSight Fatty acids • Figure 5.4

a. Each carbon atom in the carbon chain of a fatty acid is attached to up to four other atoms. At the omega or methyl (CH_3) end of the carbon chain, three hydrogen atoms are attached to the carbon. At the other end of the chain, an acid group (COOH) is attached to the carbon. Each of the carbon atoms in between is attached to two carbon atoms and up to two hydrogen atoms.

Saturated Fatty Acids:
Saturated fatty acids contain no carbon–carbon double bonds. Red meat, butter, cheese, and whole milk are high in saturated fatty acids, such as palmitic acid.

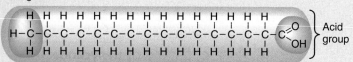
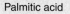
Palmitic acid

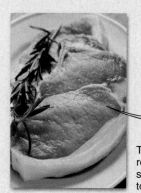

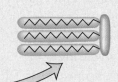

The fat on the outside of a steak is solid at room temperature because it is high in saturated fatty acids, which pack tightly together.

b. If the carbon chain of a fatty acid has adjacent carbons with only one hydrogen atom attached, a double bond forms between them. These unsaturated fatty acids may have one or more carbon–carbon double bonds.

Unsaturated Fatty Acids:
Unsaturated fatty acids include monounsaturated and polyunsaturated fatty acids.

Monounsaturated Fatty Acids:
Monounsaturated fatty acids contain one carbon–carbon double bond. Canola, olive, and peanut oils, as well as nuts and avocados, are high in monounsaturated fatty acids, such as oleic acid.

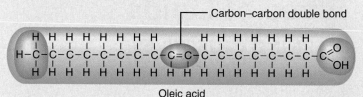
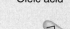
Oleic acid

Vegetable oils are a liquid at room temperature because they are high in unsaturated fatty acids. The bent chains of these fatty acids prevent tight packing, allowing the oil to flow.

acids. The fatty acids in a triglyceride determine its function in the body and the properties it gives to food.

Saturated and unsaturated fatty acids

Fatty acids are classified as saturated fatty acids or **unsaturated fatty acids**, depending on whether they contain carbon–carbon double bonds (**Figure 5.4a and b**). The number and location of these double bonds affect the characteristics that fatty acids give to food and the health effects they have in the body. Saturated fatty acids have straight carbon chains that pack tightly together. Therefore, triglycerides that are high in saturated fatty acids, such as those found in beef, butter, and lard, tend to be solid at room temperature. Diets high in saturated fatty acids have been shown to increase the risk of heart disease. Unsaturated fatty acids have bent chains. This makes triglycerides that are higher in unsaturated fatty acids, such as those found in corn, safflower, and sunflower oils, liquid at room temperature. Diets high in unsaturated fatty acids are associated with a lower risk of heart disease.

The body is capable of synthesizing most of the fatty acids it needs from glucose or other sources of carbon, hydrogen, and oxygen, but the body cannot make some of the fatty acids it needs. These must be consumed in the diet and are referred to as **essential fatty acids**.

Saturated fatty acids are more plentiful in animal foods, such as meat and dairy products, than in plant foods. Plant oils are generally low in saturated fatty acids (**Figure 5.4c**). Exceptions include

> **unsaturated fatty acid** A fatty acid that contains one or more carbon–carbon double bonds; may be either monounsaturated or polyunsaturated.

> **essential fatty acid** A fatty acid that must be consumed in the diet because it cannot be made by the body or cannot be made in sufficient quantities to meet the body's needs.

Polyunsaturated Fatty Acids:
Polyunsaturated fatty acids contain more than one carbon–carbon double bond.

Omega-6 Polyunsaturated Fatty Acids: When the first double bond occurs between the sixth and seventh carbon atoms (from the omega end), the fatty acid is called an **omega-6 fatty acid**. Corn oil, safflower oil, soybean oil, and nuts are sources of the omega-6 polyunsaturated fatty acid linoleic acid.

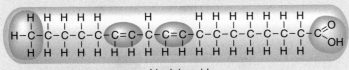

Linoleic acid

Omega-3 Polyunsaturated Fatty Acids: If the first double bond occurs between the third and fourth carbon atoms (from the omega end), the fatty acid is an **omega-3 fatty acid**. Flaxseed, canola oil, and nuts are sources of the omega-3 polyunsaturated fatty acid alpha-linolenic acid, and fish oils are high in longer-chain omega-3 fatty acids.

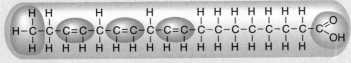

Alpha-linolenic acid

c. The fats and oils in our diets contain combinations of saturated, monounsaturated, and polyunsaturated fatty acids. The types of fatty acids in triglycerides determine their texture, taste, and physical characteristics.

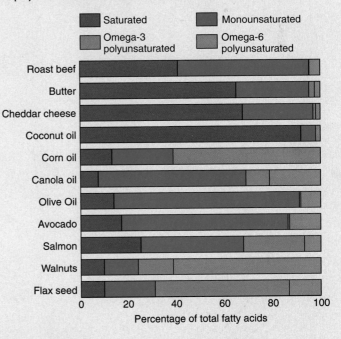

Ask Yourself

Based on the table above:
1. Which two foods are highest in omega-3 fatty acids?
2. Which two foods are highest in saturated fatty acids?

palm oil, palm kernel oil, and coconut oil, which are saturated plant oils. These are often called **tropical oils** because they are found in plants that are common in tropical climates. Saturated plant oils are useful in food processing because they are less susceptible to spoilage than are more unsaturated oils. Spoilage of fats and oils, referred to as *rancidity*, occurs when the unsaturated bonds in fatty acids are damaged by oxygen. When fats go rancid, they give food an "off" flavor.

Trans fatty acids Food manufacturers can increase the shelf life of oils by using a process called **hydrogenation**, which makes unsaturated oils more saturated. This improves the storage properties of the oils and makes them more solid at room temperature. Products such as hard margarine and shortening can be made using hydrogenation. A disadvantage of this process is that in addition to converting some double bonds into saturated bonds, it transforms some double bonds from the *cis* to the *trans* configuration (**Figure 5.5**). As discussed later, consumption of *trans* fats increases the risk of developing heart disease.

> **hydrogenation** A process whereby hydrogen atoms are added to the carbon–carbon double bonds of unsaturated fatty acids, making them more saturated.

Cis and *trans* fatty acids • Figure 5.5

a. The orientation of hydrogen atoms around the carbon–carbon double bond distinguishes *cis* fatty acids from *trans* fatty acids. Most unsaturated fatty acids found in nature have double bonds in the *cis* configuration.

b. Small amounts of *trans* fatty acids occur naturally, and larger amounts are generated by hydrogenation. Many manufacturers have reformulated their products to reduce the amounts of *trans* fatty acids.

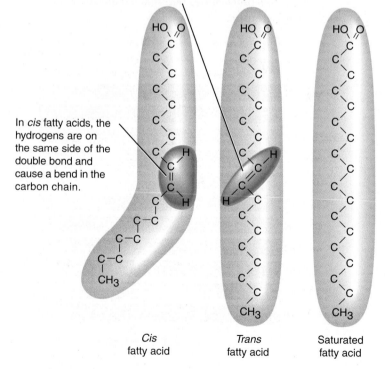

In *trans* fatty acids the hydrogens are on opposite sides of the double bond, making the carbon chain straighter, similar to the shape of a saturated fatty acid.

In *cis* fatty acids, the hydrogens are on the same side of the double bond and cause a bend in the carbon chain.

Cis fatty acid

Trans fatty acid

Saturated fatty acid

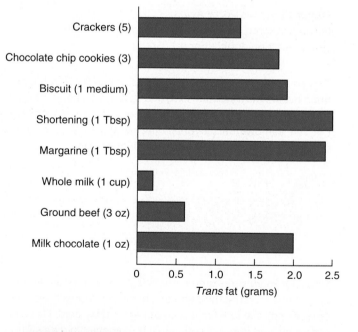

Trans fat (grams)

Ask Yourself

Which of the foods shown here contain only natural sources of *trans* fatty acids?

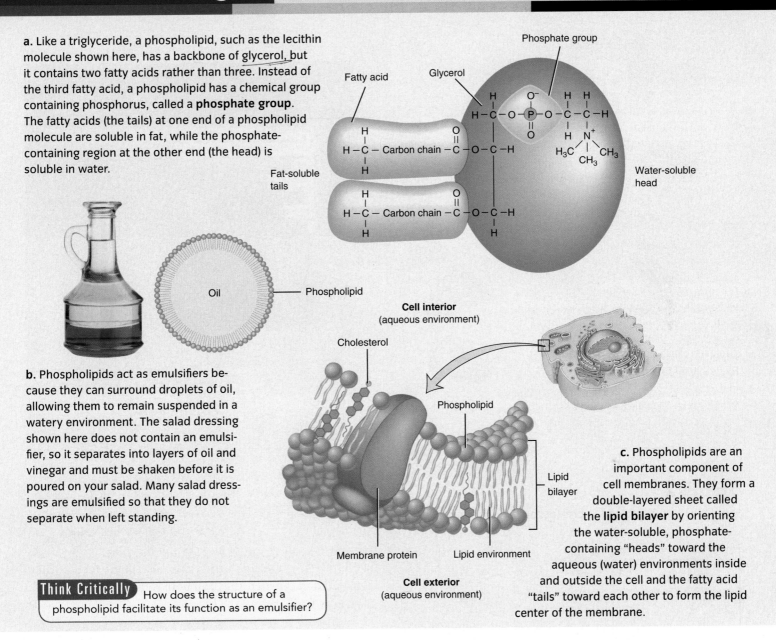

a. Like a triglyceride, a phospholipid, such as the lecithin molecule shown here, has a backbone of glycerol, but it contains two fatty acids rather than three. Instead of the third fatty acid, a phospholipid has a chemical group containing phosphorus, called a **phosphate group**. The fatty acids (the tails) at one end of a phospholipid molecule are soluble in fat, while the phosphate-containing region at the other end (the head) is soluble in water.

Fatty acid   Glycerol   Phosphate group

Fat-soluble tails

Water-soluble head

Oil   Phospholipid

b. Phospholipids act as emulsifiers because they can surround droplets of oil, allowing them to remain suspended in a watery environment. The salad dressing shown here does not contain an emulsifier, so it separates into layers of oil and vinegar and must be shaken before it is poured on your salad. Many salad dressings are emulsified so that they do not separate when left standing.

Cell interior
(aqueous environment)

Cholesterol

Phospholipid

Lipid bilayer

Membrane protein   Lipid environment

Cell exterior
(aqueous environment)

c. Phospholipids are an important component of cell membranes. They form a double-layered sheet called the **lipid bilayer** by orienting the water-soluble, phosphate-containing "heads" toward the aqueous (water) environments inside and outside the cell and the fatty acid "tails" toward each other to form the lipid center of the membrane.

Think Critically How does the structure of a phospholipid facilitate its function as an emulsifier?

Phospholipids

Phospholipids, though present in small amounts, are important in food and in the body because they allow water and fat to mix. They can do this because one side of the molecule dissolves in water, and the other side dissolves in fat (**Figure 5.6a**). In foods, substances that allow fat and water to mix are referred to as **emulsifiers**. For example, the phospholipids in egg yolks allow the oil and water in cake batter to mix; phospholipids in salad dressings prevent the oil and vinegar in the dressing from separating.

One of the best-known phospholipids is **lecithin** (shown in Figure 5.6a). Eggs and soybeans are natural sources of lecithin. The food industry uses lecithin as an emulsifier in margarine, salad dressings, chocolate, frozen desserts, and baked goods to prevent oil from separating from the other ingredients (**Figure 5.6b**). In the body, lecithin is a major constituent of cell membranes (**Figure 5.6c**). It is also used to synthesize the neurotransmitter acetylcholine, which activates muscles and plays an important role in memory.

Cholesterol • Figure 5.7

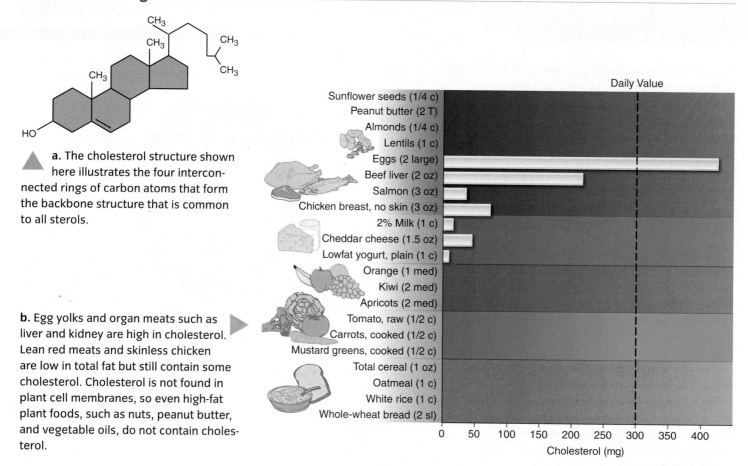

a. The cholesterol structure shown here illustrates the four interconnected rings of carbon atoms that form the backbone structure that is common to all sterols.

b. Egg yolks and organ meats such as liver and kidney are high in cholesterol. Lean red meats and skinless chicken are low in total fat but still contain some cholesterol. Cholesterol is not found in plant cell membranes, so even high-fat plant foods, such as nuts, peanut butter, and vegetable oils, do not contain cholesterol.

Sterols

The best-known sterol is **cholesterol** (**Figure 5.7**). It is needed in the body, but because the liver manufactures it, it is not essential in the diet. More than 90% of the cholesterol in the body is found in cell membranes (see Figure 5.6c). It is also part of myelin, the insulating coating on many nerve cells. Cholesterol is needed to synthesize other sterols, including vitamin D; bile acids, which are emulsifiers in bile; cortisol, which is a hormone that regulates our physiological response to stress; and testosterone and estrogen, which are hormones necessary for reproduction.

In the diet, cholesterol is found only in foods from animal sources. Plant foods do not contain cholesterol unless it has been added in the course of cooking or processing. Plants do contain other sterols, however, and these **plant sterols** have a role similar to that of cholesterol in animals: They help form plant cell membranes. Plant sterols are found in small quantities in most plant foods; when consumed in the diet, they can help reduce cholesterol levels in the body.

> **cholesterol** A sterol, produced by the liver and consumed in the diet, which is needed to build cell membranes and make hormones and other essential molecules.

CONCEPT CHECK STOP

1. **How** are triglycerides and fatty acids related?

2. **What** is the structural difference between saturated and unsaturated fatty acids?

3. **Why** are phospholipids good emulsifiers?

4. **Which** food groups contain the most saturated fat?

Absorbing and Transporting Lipids

LEARNING OBJECTIVES

1. **Discuss** the steps involved in the digestion and absorption of lipids.
2. **Describe** how lipids are transported in the blood and delivered to cells.
3. **Compare** the functions of LDLs and HDLs.

he fact that oil and water do not mix poses a problem for the digestion and absorption of lipids in the watery environment of the small intestine and their transport in the blood, which is mostly water. Therefore, the body has special mechanisms that allow it to digest, absorb, and transport lipids.

Digestion and Absorption of Lipids

In healthy adults, most fat digestion and absorption occurs in the small intestine (**Figure 5.8**). Here, bile acts as an emulsifier, breaking down large lipid droplets into small globules. The triglycerides in the globules can then be digested by enzymes from the pancreas. The resulting

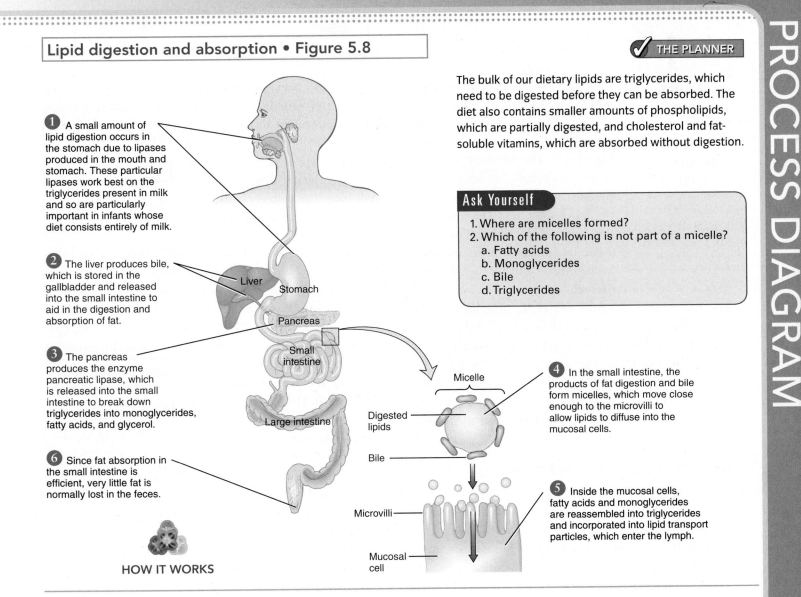

Lipid digestion and absorption • Figure 5.8

✔ THE PLANNER

PROCESS DIAGRAM

The bulk of our dietary lipids are triglycerides, which need to be digested before they can be absorbed. The diet also contains smaller amounts of phospholipids, which are partially digested, and cholesterol and fat-soluble vitamins, which are absorbed without digestion.

Ask Yourself

1. Where are micelles formed?
2. Which of the following is not part of a micelle?
   a. Fatty acids
   b. Monoglycerides
   c. Bile
   d. Triglycerides

1 A small amount of lipid digestion occurs in the stomach due to lipases produced in the mouth and stomach. These particular lipases work best on the triglycerides present in milk and so are particularly important in infants whose diet consists entirely of milk.

2 The liver produces bile, which is stored in the gallbladder and released into the small intestine to aid in the digestion and absorption of fat.

3 The pancreas produces the enzyme pancreatic lipase, which is released into the small intestine to break down triglycerides into monoglycerides, fatty acids, and glycerol.

6 Since fat absorption in the small intestine is efficient, very little fat is normally lost in the feces.

HOW IT WORKS

Liver
Stomach
Pancreas
Small intestine
Large intestine

Micelle
Digested lipids
Bile
Microvilli
Mucosal cell

4 In the small intestine, the products of fat digestion and bile form micelles, which move close enough to the microvilli to allow lipids to diffuse into the mucosal cells.

5 Inside the mucosal cells, fatty acids and monoglycerides are reassembled into triglycerides and incorporated into lipid transport particles, which enter the lymph.

Lipoprotein structure • Figure 5.9

A lipoprotein consists of a core of triglycerides and cholesterol surrounded by a shell of protein, phospholipids, and cholesterol. Phospholipids orient with their fat-soluble "tails" toward the interior and their water-soluble "heads" toward the outside. This allows the fat-soluble substances in the interior to travel through the aqueous blood.

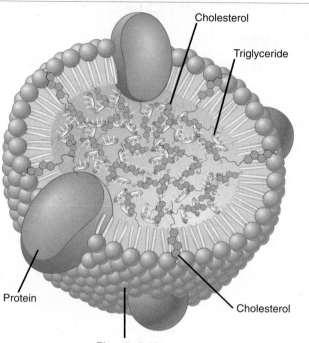

Cholesterol

Triglyceride

Protein

Cholesterol

Phospholipid

---

monoglyceride A glycerol molecule with one fatty acid attached.

micelle A particle that is formed in the small intestine when the products of fat digestion are surrounded by bile. It facilitates the absorption of lipids.

mixture of fatty acids, **monoglycerides**, cholesterol, and bile forms smaller droplets called **micelles**, which facilitate absorption (see Figure 5.8). The bile in the micelles is also absorbed and returned to the liver to be reused. Once inside the mucosal cells of the intestine, the fatty acids, cholesterol, and other fat-soluble substances must be processed further before they can be transported in the blood.

The fat-soluble vitamins (A, D, E, and K) are absorbed through the same process as other lipids. These vitamins are not digested but must be incorporated into micelles to be absorbed. The amounts absorbed can be reduced if dietary fat is very low or if disease, other dietary components, or medications such as the diet drug Alli, interfere with fat absorption (see *What a Scientist Sees* in Chapter 9).

Transporting Lipids in the Blood

Lipids that are consumed in the diet are absorbed into the intestinal mucosal cells. From here, small fatty acids, which are soluble in water, are absorbed into the blood and travel to the liver for further processing. Long-chain fatty acids, cholesterol, and fat-soluble vitamins, which are not soluble in water, are not absorbed directly into the blood

and must be packaged for transport. They are covered with a water-soluble envelope of protein, phospholipids, and cholesterol to form particles called **lipoproteins** (**Figure 5.9**). Different types of lipoproteins transport dietary lipids from the small intestine to body cells, from the liver to body cells, and from body cells back to the liver for disposal.

lipoprotein A particle that transports lipids in the blood.

Transport from the small intestine After long-chain fatty acids (from the digestion of triglycerides) have been absorbed into the mucosal cells, they are reassembled into triglycerides. These triglycerides, along with cholesterol and fat-soluble vitamins, are packaged with phospholipids, and protein to form lipoproteins called **chylomicrons**. Chylomicrons are too large to enter the capillaries in the small intestine, so they pass from the intestinal mucosa into the lymph, which then delivers them to the blood (**Figure 5.10**). They circulate in the blood, delivering triglycerides to body cells. To enter the cells, the triglycerides must first be broken down into fatty acids and glycerol, which can diffuse across the cell membrane. Once inside the cells, fatty acids can either be used to provide energy or reassembled into triglycerides for storage.

chylomicron A lipoprotein that transports lipids from the mucosal cells of the small intestine and delivers triglycerides to other body cells.

Lipid transport and delivery • Figure 5.10

THE PLANNER ✓

Chylomicrons and very-low-density lipoproteins transport triglycerides and deliver them to body cells. Low-density lipoproteins transport and deliver cholesterol, and high-density lipoproteins help return cholesterol to the liver for reuse or elimination.

VLD

HOW IT WORKS

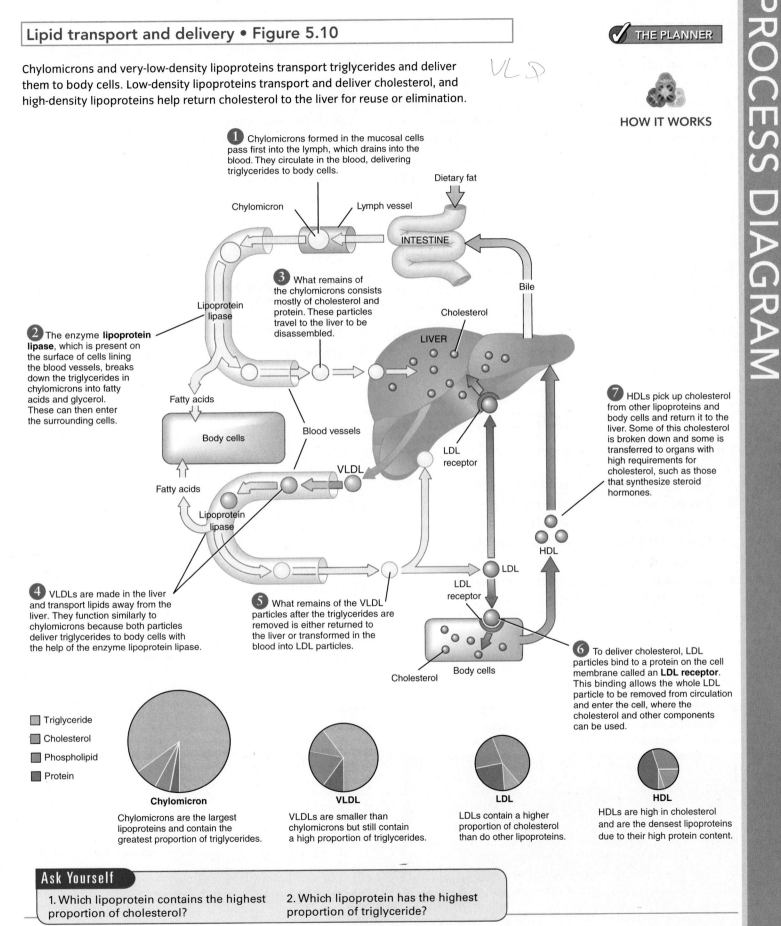

1 Chylomicrons formed in the mucosal cells pass first into the lymph, which drains into the blood. They circulate in the blood, delivering triglycerides to body cells.

Dietary fat

Chylomicron   Lymph vessel

INTESTINE

Bile

3 What remains of the chylomicrons consists mostly of cholesterol and protein. These particles travel to the liver to be disassembled.

Cholesterol

Lipoprotein lipase

LIVER

2 The enzyme **lipoprotein lipase**, which is present on the surface of cells lining the blood vessels, breaks down the triglycerides in chylomicrons into fatty acids and glycerol. These can then enter the surrounding cells.

Fatty acids

7 HDLs pick up cholesterol from other lipoproteins and body cells and return it to the liver. Some of this cholesterol is broken down and some is transferred to organs with high requirements for cholesterol, such as those that synthesize steroid hormones.

Body cells   Blood vessels

LDL receptor

VLDL

Fatty acids

HDL

Lipoprotein lipase

LDL

4 VLDLs are made in the liver and transport lipids away from the liver. They function similarly to chylomicrons because both particles deliver triglycerides to body cells with the help of the enzyme lipoprotein lipase.

LDL receptor

5 What remains of the VLDL particles after the triglycerides are removed is either returned to the liver or transformed in the blood into LDL particles.

6 To deliver cholesterol, LDL particles bind to a protein on the cell membrane called an **LDL receptor**. This binding allows the whole LDL particle to be removed from circulation and enter the cell, where the cholesterol and other components can be used.

Cholesterol   Body cells

☐ Triglyceride
☐ Cholesterol
☐ Phospholipid
■ Protein

Chylomicron

Chylomicrons are the largest lipoproteins and contain the greatest proportion of triglycerides.

VLDL

VLDLs are smaller than chylomicrons but still contain a high proportion of triglycerides.

LDL

LDLs contain a higher proportion of cholesterol than do other lipoproteins.

HDL

HDLs are high in cholesterol and are the densest lipoproteins due to their high protein content.

Ask Yourself

1. Which lipoprotein contains the highest proportion of cholesterol?

2. Which lipoprotein has the highest proportion of triglyceride?

Transport from the liver The liver can synthesize lipids. Lipids are transported from the liver in **very-low-density lipoproteins (VLDLs)**. Like chylomicrons, VLDLs are lipoproteins that circulate in the blood, delivering triglycerides to body cells. When the triglycerides have been removed from the VLDLs, a denser, smaller particle remains. About two-thirds of these particles are returned to the liver, and the rest are transformed in the blood into **low-**

> **low-density lipoprotein (LDL)** A lipoprotein that transports cholesterol to cells.

density lipoproteins (LDLs). LDLs are the primary cholesterol delivery system for cells. They contain a higher proportion of cholesterol than do chylomicrons or VLDLs (see Figure 5.10). High levels of LDLs in the blood have been associated with an increased risk for heart disease. For this reason, they are sometimes referred to as "bad cholesterol."

Eliminating cholesterol Because most body cells have no system for breaking down cholesterol, cholester-ol must be returned to the liver to be eliminated from the body. This reverse cholesterol transport is accomplished by **high-density lipoproteins (HDLs)** (see Figure 5.10). HDL cholesterol is often called "good cholesterol" because high levels of HDL in the blood are associated with a reduction in the risk of heart disease.

> **high-density lipoprotein (HDL)** A lipoprotein that picks up cholesterol from cells and transports it to the liver so that it can be eliminated from the body.

CONCEPT CHECK 🛑 STOP

1. **How** does bile help in the digestion and absorption of lipids?
2. **Why** are lipoproteins needed to transport lipids?
3. **What** is the primary function of LDLs?

Lipid Functions

LEARNING OBJECTIVES

1. **List** the functions of lipids in the body.
2. **Explain** why we need the right balance of omega-3 and omega-6 fatty acids.
3. **Summarize** how fatty acids are used to provide energy.
4. **Describe** how fat is stored and how it is retrieved from storage.

 ipids are necessary to maintain health. In our diet, fat is needed to absorb fat-soluble vitamins and is a source of essential fatty acids and energy. In our bodies, lipids form structural and regulatory molecules and are broken down to provide ATP. As discussed earlier, cholesterol plays both regulatory and structural roles: It is used to make steroid hormones, and it is an important component of cell membranes and the myelin coating that is necessary for brain and nerve function.

Most lipids in the body are triglycerides stored in **adipose tissue**, which is body fat that lies under the skin and around internal organs (**Figure 5.11**). The triglycerides

---

Adipose tissue • Figure 5.11

a. The amount and location of adipose tissue affect our body size and shape. When people have liposuction to slim their hips, the surgeon is actually vacuuming out fat cells from the adipose tissue in the region.

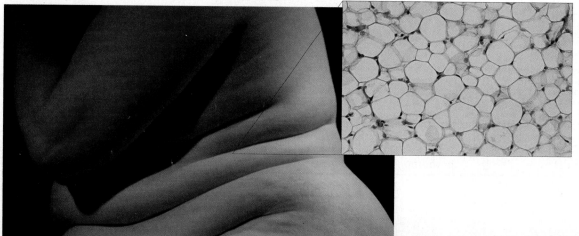

b. Adipose tissue cells contain large droplets of triglyceride that push the other cell components to the perimeter of the cell. As weight is gained, the triglyceride droplets enlarge.

a. Linoleic acid is an omega-6 fatty acid that is found in vegetable oils, such as corn and safflower oils. **Arachidonic acid** is an omega-6 fatty acid synthesized from linoleic acid; it is found in both animal and vegetable fats.

b. α-linolenic acid is an omega-3 fatty acid that is found in nuts, flaxseed, and canola oil. **Eicosapentaenoic acid (EPA)** and **docosahexaenoic acid (DHA)** are omega-3 fatty acids that are synthesized from α-linolenic acid; in our diet, they are found in fatty fish.

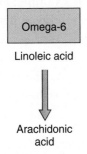

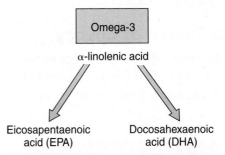

Essential Fatty Acids

in our adipose tissue provide a lightweight energy storage molecule, help cushion our internal organs, and insulate us from changes in temperature. Triglycerides are also found in oils that lubricate body surfaces, keeping the skin soft and supple.

Essential Fatty Acids

Humans are not able to synthesize fatty acids that have double bonds in the omega-6 and omega-3 positions (see Figure 5.4b). Therefore, the fatty acids **linoleic acid** (omega-6) and **alpha-linolenic acid (α-linolenic acid)** (omega-3) are considered essential fatty acids. They must be consumed in the diet because they cannot be made in the body. If the diet is low in linoleic acid and/or α-linolenic acid, other fatty acids that the body would normally synthesize from them become dietary essentials as well (**Figure 5.12**).

Omega-6 and omega-3 fatty acids are important for health. They are needed for the formation of the phospholipids that give cell membranes their structure and functional properties. Therefore, they are essential for growth, development, fertility, and maintaining the structure of red blood cells and cells in the skin and nervous system. The omega-3 fatty acid DHA is particularly important in the retina of the eye. Both DHA and the omega-6 fatty acid arachidonic acid are needed to synthesize cell membranes in the central nervous system and are therefore important for normal brain development in infants and young children.

If adequate amounts of linoleic and α-linolenic acid are not consumed, an **essential fatty acid deficiency** will result. Symptoms include scaly, dry skin, liver abnormalities, poor healing of wounds, impaired vision and hearing, and growth failure in infants. Because the requirement

for essential fatty acids is well below the typical intake in the United States, essential fatty acid deficiencies are rare in this country. However, deficiencies have occurred in infants and young children consuming low-fat diets and in individuals who are unable to absorb lipids.

Getting enough essential fatty acids in your diet will prevent deficiency, but the ratio of dietary omega-6 to omega-3 fatty acids also affects your health. This is because the omega-6 and omega-3 polyunsaturated fatty acids made from them are used to make hormone-like molecules called **eicosanoids**. Eicosanoids help regulate blood clotting, blood pressure, immune function, and other body processes. The effect of an eicosanoid on these functions depends on the fatty acid from which it is made. For example, when the omega-6 fatty acid arachidonic acid is the starting material, the eicosanoid synthesized increases blood clotting; when the omega-3 fatty acid EPA is the starting material, the eicosanoid made decreases blood clotting. The ratio of dietary omega-6 to omega-3 fatty acids affects the balance of the omega-6 and omega-3 fatty acids in the body and, therefore, the balance of the omega-6 and omega-3 eicosanoids produced.

The U.S. diet contains a higher ratio of omega-6 to omega-3 fatty acids than is optimal for health. Increasing consumption of foods that are rich in omega-3 fatty acids increases the proportion of omega-3 eicosanoids (see Figure 5.4c). This reduces the risk of heart disease

> **essential fatty acid deficiency** A condition characterized by dry, scaly skin and poor growth that results when the diet does not supply sufficient amounts of linoleic acid and α-linolenic acid.
>
> **eicosanoids** Regulatory molecules that can be synthesized from omega-3 and omega-6 fatty acids.

by decreasing inflammation, lowering blood pressure, and reducing blood clotting.[4] The American Heart Association recommends eating two or more servings per week of fish, which is a good source of EPA and DHA, along with plant sources of omega-3 fatty acids, such as walnuts, canola oil, and flaxseed.[5]

Fat as a Source of Energy

Fat is an important source of energy in the body (**Figure 5.13**). Triglycerides that are consumed in the diet can be either used immediately to fuel the body or stored in adi-

pose tissue. Depositing fat in adipose tissue is an efficient way to store energy because each gram of fat provides 9 Calories, compared with only 4 Calories per gram from carbohydrate or protein. This allows a large amount of energy to be stored in the body without a great increase in body size or weight. For example, even a lean man stores over 50,000 Calories of energy in his adipose tissue.

Throughout the day, as we eat and then go for hours without eating, triglycerides are stored and then retrieved from storage, depending on the body's immediate energy needs. For example, after we have feasted on a meal, some

---

Metabolism of fat • Figure 5.13

✔ THE PLANNER

Triglycerides are broken down to fatty acids and a small amount of glycerol. The fatty acids provide most of the energy stored in a triglyceride molecule. Fatty acids are transported into the mitochondria, where, in the presence of oxygen, they are broken down to form acetyl-CoA, which can be further metabolized to generate ATP. The glycerol molecules, which contain three carbon atoms, can also be used to generate ATP or small amounts of glucose.

HOW IT WORKS

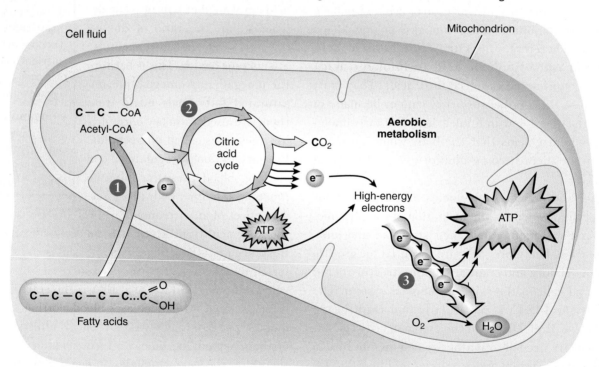

❶ Beta-oxidation splits fatty acids into two-carbon units that form acetyl-CoA and releases high-energy electrons (purple balls).

❷ If oxygen and enough carbohydrate are available, acetyl-CoA enters the citric acid cycle releasing two molecules of carbon dioxide and more high-energy electrons.

❸ In the final step of aerobic metabolism, the high-energy electrons released in beta-oxidation and the citric acid cycle combine with oxygen and hydrogen to form water and their energy is trapped and used to generate ATP.

Feasting and fasting • Figure 5.14

When we eat too much, excess energy is stored as triglycerides. When we don't eat enough, triglycerides in adipose tissue are broken down, releasing fatty acids, which can be used to provide energy.

Feasting: When excess energy is consumed, it is stored as triglycerides in adipose tissue.

Fasting: When no food has been eaten for a while, triglycerides from adipose tissue are broken down, releasing fatty acids as an energy source.

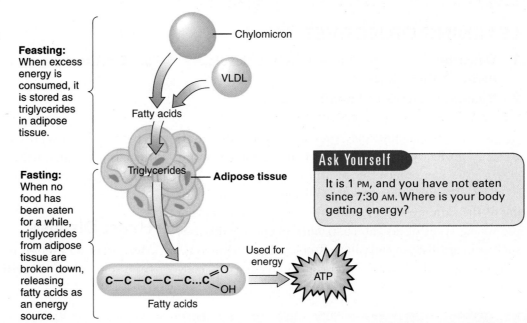

Ask Yourself

It is 1 PM, and you have not eaten since 7:30 AM. Where is your body getting energy?

---

triglycerides will be stored; then, in the small fasts between meals, some of the stored triglycerides will be broken down to provide energy. When the energy consumed in the diet equals the body's energy requirements, the net amount of body fat does not change.

Feasting When we consume more calories than we need, the excess is stored primarily as fat. Excess fat from our diet is packaged in chylomicrons and transported directly from the intestines to the adipose tissue. Because the fatty acids in our body fat come from the fatty acids we eat, what we eat affects the fatty acid composition of our adipose tissue; therefore, if you eat more saturated fat, there will be more saturated fat in your adipose tissue. Excess calories that are consumed as carbohydrate or protein must first go to the liver, where they can be used to synthesize fatty acids, which are then assembled into triglycerides, packaged in VLDLs, and transported in the blood to adipose tissue (**Figure 5.14**).

The ability of the body to store excess triglycerides is theoretically limitless. Cells in your adipose tissue can increase in weight by about 50 times, and new fat cells can be made when existing cells reach their maximum size.

Fasting When you eat fewer calories than you need, your body takes energy from its fat stores. In this situation, an enzyme inside the fat cells receives a signal to break down stored triglycerides. The fatty acids and glycerol that re-

sult are released directly into the blood and circulate throughout the body. They are taken up by cells and used to produce ATP (see Figures 5.13 and 5.14).

To be used for energy, fatty acids are broken into two-carbon units that form acetyl-CoA. When oxygen and carbohydrate are available, acetyl-CoA can be used to generate ATP. If there is not enough carbohydrate available in cells to allow the acetyl-CoA to enter the citric acid cycle, it will be used to make *ketones* (see Chapter 4). Many tissues in the body can use ketones as an energy source. During prolonged fasting, even the brain can adapt itself to use ketones to meet about half of its energy needs. For the other half, the brain continues to require glucose. Fatty acids cannot be used to make glucose, and only a small amount of glucose can be made from the glycerol released from triglyceride breakdown.

CONCEPT CHECK STOP

1. **Why** does a deficiency of essential fatty acids cause health problems?

2. **How** does eating fish regularly affect the types of eicosanoids produced?

3. **How** are fatty acids used to produce ATP?

4. **What** happens to excess dietary fat after it has been absorbed?

Lipids in Health and Disease

LEARNING OBJECTIVES

1. **Describe** the events that lead to the development of atherosclerosis.

2. **Evaluate** your risk of heart disease.

3. **Discuss** the roles of dietary fat in cancer and obesity.

The amount and types of fat you eat can affect your health. A diet that is too low in fat can reduce the absorption of fat-soluble vitamins, slow growth, and impair the functioning of the skin, eyes, liver, and other body organs. Eating the wrong types of fat can contribute to chronic diseases such as heart disease and cancer. Consuming too much fat can increase calorie intake and contribute to extra body fat storage and therefore weight gain. Excess body fat, in turn, is associated with an increased risk of diabetes, cardiovascular disease, and high blood pressure.

Heart Disease

More than 80 million people in the United States suffer from some form of **cardiovascular disease**, which is any

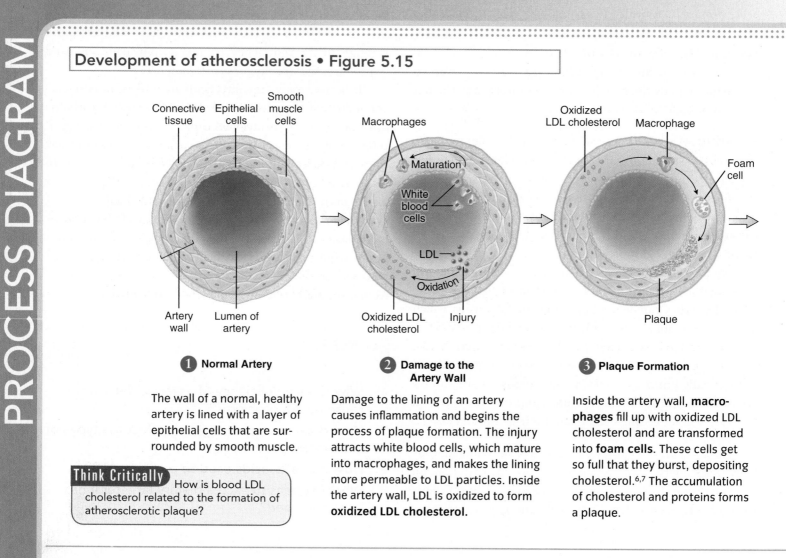

Development of atherosclerosis • Figure 5.15

① Normal Artery

The wall of a normal, healthy artery is lined with a layer of epithelial cells that are surrounded by smooth muscle.

> **Think Critically** How is blood LDL cholesterol related to the formation of atherosclerotic plaque?

② Damage to the Artery Wall

Damage to the lining of an artery causes inflammation and begins the process of plaque formation. The injury attracts white blood cells, which mature into macrophages, and makes the lining more permeable to LDL particles. Inside the artery wall, LDL is oxidized to form **oxidized LDL cholesterol.**

③ Plaque Formation

Inside the artery wall, **macrophages** fill up with oxidized LDL cholesterol and are transformed into **foam cells**. These cells get so full that they burst, depositing cholesterol.[6,7] The accumulation of cholesterol and proteins forms a plaque.

atherosclerosis A type of cardiovascular disease that involves the buildup of fatty material in the artery walls.

disease that affects the heart and blood vessels. It is the number-one cause of death for both men and women in the United States.[8] **Atherosclerosis** is a type of cardiovascular disease in which cholesterol is deposited in the artery walls, reducing their elasticity and eventually blocking the flow of blood. The development of atherosclerosis has been linked to diets that are high in cholesterol, saturated fat, and *trans* fat.[9]

How atherosclerosis develops **Inflammation**, the process whereby the body responds to injury, drives the formation of **atherosclerotic plaque**. For example, cutting yourself triggers an inflammatory response. White blood cells, which are part of the immune system,

rush to the injured area, blood clots form, and soon new tissue grows to heal the wound. Similar inflammatory responses occur when an artery is injured, but instead of resulting in healing, they lead to the development of atherosclerotic plaque (**Figure 5.15**). Therefore, the atherosclerotic process begins with an injury, and the response to this injury causes changes in the lining of the artery wall.

The exact cause of the injuries that initiate the development of atherosclerosis is not known but may be related to elevated blood levels of LDL cholesterol, glucose, or the amino acid homocysteine or to high blood pressure, smoking, diabetes, genetic alterations, or infection.[6] The specific cause may be different in different people.

atherosclerotic plaque Cholesterol-rich material that is deposited in the arteries of individuals with atherosclerosis.

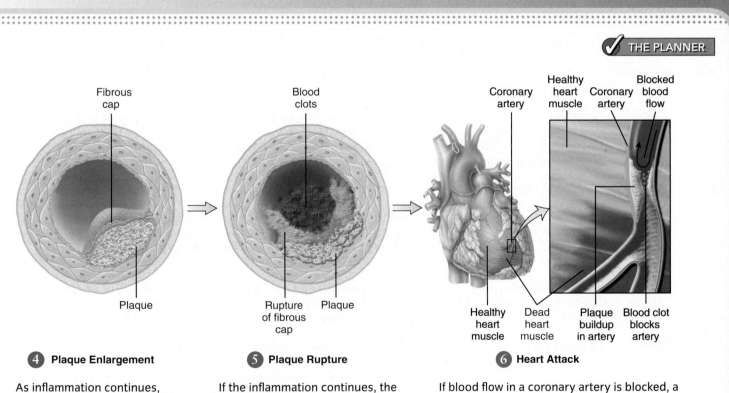

4 **Plaque Enlargement**

As inflammation continues, plaque builds up, causing the artery to narrow and lose its elasticity. A cap of smooth muscle cells and fibrous proteins forms over the plaque, walling it off from the lumen of the artery.

5 **Plaque Rupture**

If the inflammation continues, the fibrous cap covering the plaque degrades. If the cap ruptures or erodes, blood clots can rapidly form around it. The blood clots can completely block the artery at that spot or break loose and block an artery elsewhere.

6 **Heart Attack**

If blood flow in a coronary artery is blocked, a heart attack results. Heart muscle cells are cut off from their blood supply and die, causing pain and reducing the heart's ability to pump blood. If the blood flow to the brain is interrupted, a stroke results. Brain cells are cut off from their blood supply and die.

Risk factors for heart disease Diabetes, high blood pressure, obesity, and high blood cholesterol levels are considered primary risk factors for heart disease because they directly increase risk. Other factors that affect risk include age, gender, genetics, and lifestyle factors such as smoking, exercise, and diet (**Table 5.1**).

Diet and heart disease risk The risk of heart disease is affected by individual nutrients and particular whole foods. For example, diets high in sodium and saturated fat increase heart disease risk. Diets high in fiber and certain vitamins can reduce heart disease risk. Consuming fish, nuts, and whole grains may decrease risk, while diets that are high in red meat may increase risk. More important than any individual dietary factor, though, are overall dietary and lifestyle patterns. For example, diets that are plentiful in fruits, vegetables, and whole grains and low in high-fat meats and dairy products reduce the risk of heart disease.[18] The importance of dietary patterns is exemplified by the fact that the incidence of heart disease is lower in Asian and Mediterranean countries than in the United States (**Figure 5.16**). The heart-protective effect that these traditional diets seem to have has prompted nutrition experts to promote a Mediterranean dietary pattern to reduce the risk of heart disease in the United States.

What affects the risk of heart disease?   Table 5.1

Risk factor	How it affects risk
Obesity	Obesity increases blood pressure, blood cholesterol levels, and the risk of developing diabetes. It also increases the amount of work the heart must do to pump blood throughout the body.
Diabetes	High blood glucose damages blood vessel walls, initiating atherosclerosis.
High blood pressure	High blood pressure can damage blood vessel walls, initiating atherosclerosis. It forces the heart to work harder, causing it to enlarge and weaken over time.
Gender	Men and women are both at risk for heart disease, but men are generally affected a decade earlier than are women. This difference is due in part to the protective effect of the hormone estrogen in women. As women age, the effects of menopause—including a decline in estrogen level and a gain in weight—increase heart disease risk.
Age	The risk of heart disease is increased in men age 45 and older and in women age 55 and older.
Family history	Individuals with a male family member who exhibited heart disease before age 55 or a female family member who exhibited heart disease before age 65 are considered to be at increased risk. African Americans have a higher risk of heart disease than the general population, in part due to the high incidence of high blood pressure among African Americans.[16]
Lifestyle	Smoking increases risk. Regular exercise decreases risk by reducing blood pressure, increasing healthy HDL cholesterol levels, reducing the risk of diabetes, and promoting a healthy weight. Diet, including the types of lipids and the amounts of fiber, as well as other dietary components, can affect the risk of heart disease.
Blood lipid level	Blood levels of total cholesterol, LDL cholesterol, HDL cholesterol, and triglycerides all affect risk.[17]

	Low risk/optimal	Near optimal	Borderline high	High risk
Cholesterol (mg/100 ml)	< 200		200–239	≥ 240
LDL cholesterol (mg/100 ml)	< 100	100–129	130–159	≥ 160
HDL cholesterol (mg/100 ml)	≥ 60			< 40
Triglycerides (mg/100 ml)	< 150			

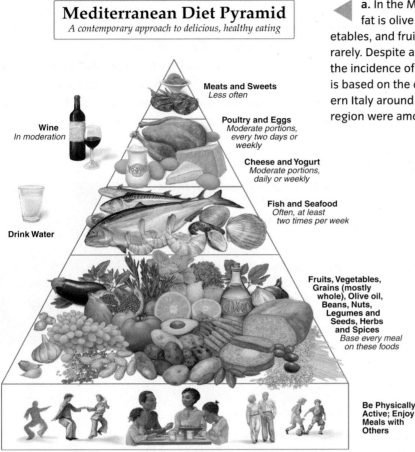

Mediterranean Diet Pyramid
A contemporary approach to delicious, healthy eating

Meats and Sweets
Less often

Wine
In moderation

Poultry and Eggs
Moderate portions, every two days or weekly

Cheese and Yogurt
Moderate portions, daily or weekly

Fish and Seafood
Often, at least two times per week

Drink Water

Fruits, Vegetables, Grains (mostly whole), Olive oil, Beans, Nuts, Legumes and Seeds, Herbs and Spices
Base every meal on these foods

Be Physically Active; Enjoy Meals with Others

Illustration by George Middleton. © 2009 Oldways Preservation & Exchange Trust. www.oldwayspt.org

a. In the Mediterranean region, the main source of dietary fat is olive oil, and the typical diet is high in nuts, vegetables, and fruits. Fish is consumed routinely and red meat rarely. Despite a fat intake that is similar to that of the U.S. diet, the incidence of heart disease is much lower. This diet pyramid is based on the dietary patterns of Crete, Greece, and southern Italy around 1960, when the rates of chronic disease in this region were among the lowest in the world.

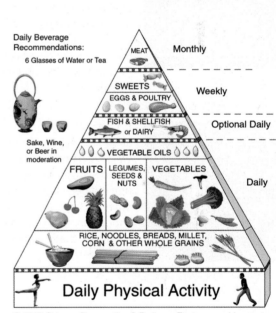

The Traditional Healthy Asian Diet Pyramid

Daily Beverage Recommendations:
6 Glasses of Water or Tea

MEAT   Monthly

SWEETS   Weekly
EGGS & POULTRY

FISH & SHELLFISH or DAIRY   Optional Daily

Sake, Wine, or Beer in moderation

VEGETABLE OILS

FRUITS   LEGUMES, SEEDS & NUTS   VEGETABLES   Daily

RICE, NOODLES, BREADS, MILLET, CORN & OTHER WHOLE GRAINS

Daily Physical Activity

© 2000 Oldways Preservation & Exchange Trust. www.oldwayspt.org

b. In Asian countries, plant foods that are rich in fiber and antioxidants form the base of the diet, and animal products are more peripheral. Traditional Asian diets include more fish and seafood than red meat. Combined with small amounts of vegetable oil, this pattern produces a balance of omega-6 to omega-3 fatty acids that helps prevent heart disease.[19] Routine consumption of green tea, which is high in antioxidants, may also contribute to the low rate of chronic disease in the region.[20] This diet pyramid was inspired by the traditional cuisines of southern and eastern Asia.

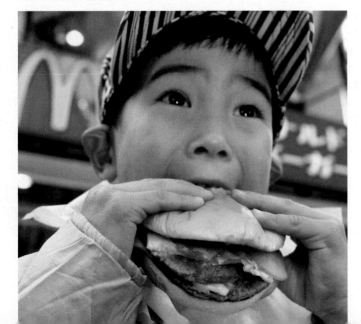

c. Traditional Asian and Mediterranean diets often protect against heart disease, but as younger generations abandon these long-established dietary patterns for more modern ones, the incidence of high blood pressure, elevated blood lipids, diabetes, and obesity is likely to rise.

Lipids in Health and Disease 151

Much of the impact that a dietary pattern has on heart disease risk depends on the abundance of nutrients and other dietary components that affect blood cholesterol levels. For example, saturated fatty acids and cholesterol from high-fat meats and dairy products can cause an increase in blood levels of total and LDL cholesterol. High intakes of *trans* fat from products that contain hydrogenated vegetable oils increase blood levels of LDL cholesterol and the risk of heart attack. Replacing foods that are high in cholesterol-raising fats with foods that provide omega-3 fatty acids, monounsaturated fat, soluble fiber, and plant sterols, which have been shown to lower total and LDL cholesterol, can reduce the risk of heart disease (**Figure 5.17**) (see *Debate: Good Egg, Bad Egg?*).[21]

Nutrients and other dietary components can also affect heart disease risk through mechanisms unrelated to blood cholesterol level. For example, adequate intakes of vitamin B$_6$, vitamin B$_{12}$, and folate help protect against heart

Eating to reduce the risk of heart disease • Figure 5.17

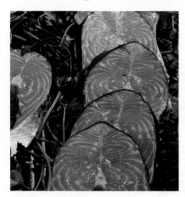

a. Fish, flaxseed, and vegetable oils are high in omega-3 fatty acids, which reduce the risk of heart disease and decrease mortality due to heart attacks. In addition to lowering LDL cholesterol and triglyceride levels, omega-3 fatty acids protect against heart disease by decreasing blood clotting, lowering blood pressure, improving the function of the cells lining blood vessels, reducing inflammation, and modulating heartbeats.[22]

b. Nuts, olives, and avocados are all good sources of monounsaturated fat, which lowers LDL cholesterol and makes it less susceptible to oxidation. Nuts are also high in omega-3 fatty acids, fiber, vegetable protein, antioxidants, and plant sterols. Diets containing nuts may lower heart disease risk by decreasing total and LDL cholesterol, increasing HDL cholesterol, and improving the functioning of cells lining the artery wall.[23]

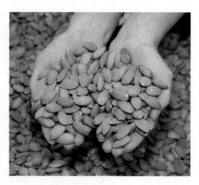

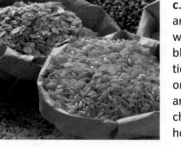

c. Oatmeal, legumes, and brown rice are good sources of soluble fiber, which has been shown to reduce blood cholesterol levels. In addition to fiber, whole grains provide omega-3 fatty acids, B vitamins, and antioxidants, as well as other phytochemicals that may protect against heart disease.

d. Moderate alcohol consumption—that is, one drink a day for women and two a day for men (one drink is equivalent to 5 ounces wine, 12 ounces beer, or 1.5 ounces distilled spirits)—reduces blood clotting and increases HDL cholesterol but also raises blood triglyceride levels. Higher alcohol intake increases the risk of heart disease and causes other health and social problems.

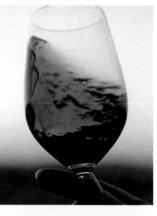

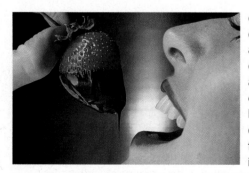

e. Modest consumption of dark chocolate is associated with reduced risk of heart disease. This is attributed to the phytochemicals in dark chocolate.[15] In addition, most of the fat in chocolate is from stearic acid, which is a saturated fatty acid that does not cause an increase in blood levels of LDL cholesterol.

f. Consuming plant sterols reduces cholesterol absorption in the small intestine, lowering total and LDL cholesterol levels.[21] Small quantities of plant sterols are found in vegetable oils, nuts, seeds, cereals, legumes, and many fruits and vegetables. Larger amounts have been added to products such as margarines, salad dressings, and orange juice.

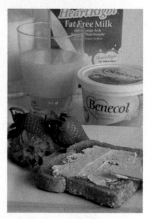

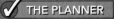
The Issue: Does eating eggs increase your risk of cardiovascular disease?

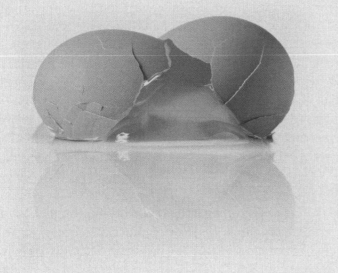

Dietary recommendations in the United States have been telling us to limit egg consumption since the 1960s. What could be bad about this high-protein, easy-to-prepare food? The problem is that one egg has over 200 mg of cholesterol. An ounce of lean meat has only about 30 mg. The Dietary Guidelines and the American Heart Association recommend limiting cholesterol to less than 300 mg per day. So, is it okay to eat eggs for breakfast?

The cholesterol in our bodies comes from what we eat as well as cholesterol synthesized by our livers. Even if you don't eat any cholesterol, your liver will make all you need. For many people, when they eat cholesterol, their liver production slows, so blood levels don't rise; others are missing this regulation. For them, an increase in dietary cholesterol results in an increase in blood cholesterol. However, the increase is typically due to increases in "good" HDL cholesterol as well as "bad" LDL cholesterol, so the risk of atherosclerosis does not change.[10] Furthermore, the LDL particles that form when dietary cholesterol increases are large. These larger LDL particles are thought to be less of a cardiovascular risk than smaller ones.[10]

Currently, the vast majority of epidemiological studies do not find a relationship between dietary cholesterol or egg consumption and cardiovascular disease.[10,11] For example, an evaluation of more than 20,000 male physicians participating in the Physicians' Health Study found that eating up to six eggs per week did not affect the risk or incidence of cardiovascular disease.[12] However, eating seven or more eggs per week caused an increased risk of death from cardiovascular disease, and eating any eggs was found to increase the risk of cardiovascular disease in people with type 2 diabetes.[12,13]

Nutrition professionals recognize that it is the overall dietary pattern, not the avoidance of particular foods, that is most important for health and wellness. Eggs are part of the Asian and Mediterranean dietary patterns, and both of these patterns are associated with good cardiovascular health. One large egg contains 6 grams of high-quality protein, and unlike many other sources of cholesterol, eggs are low in cholesterol-raising saturated fat (see table). Eggs are also a good source of zinc, B vitamins, vitamin A, and iron. The yolk is rich in lutein and zeaxanthin, two phytochemicals that help protect against age-related eye disorders. Eggs may also help you maintain your weight. A recent study found that people who eat an egg-based breakfast ate fewer overall calories during the day than people who have a bagel-based breakfast.[14]

The 2010 Dietary Guidelines has concluded that eating one egg per day is not harmful and does not result in increased risk of cardiovascular disease in healthy individuals. Despite this, they continue to recommend limiting dietary cholesterol to less than 300 mg per day, with further reductions to less than 200 mg per day for persons with or at high risk for cardiovascular disease.[15] If you eat an egg every day, is your diet likely to exceed 300 mg of cholesterol per day?

Think critically: What food or foods in this table other than eggs are high in cholesterol but low in saturated fat? How might they impact the risk of cardiovascular disease?

Cholesterol and saturated fat content of foods		
Food	Cholesterol (mg)	Saturated fat (g)
Egg, one	212	1.6
Shrimp, 3 oz, raw	129	0.3
Salmon, 3 oz, cooked	57	0.6
Hamburger patty, 3 oz, broiled	71	7.5
Chicken breast, 3 oz, roasted, no skin	72	0.9
Bacon, 3 oz, pan fried	94	11.7
Pork sausage, 3 oz, cooked	71	7.8
Butter, 2 Tbsp	61	14.6
Milk, whole, 8 fluid oz	24	4.6
Cheese, cheddar, 1 oz	30	6.0
Ice cream, vanilla, ½ cup	32	4.9

disease because they help maintain low blood levels of the amino acid homocysteine (discussed further in Chapter 7). Elevated homocysteine levels are associated with a higher incidence of heart disease.[24] Much of the heart-protective effect of omega-3 fatty acids, such as those found in fish, is due to the eicosanoids made from omega-3 fatty acids; these eicosanoids prevent the growth of atherosclerotic plaque, reduce blood clotting and blood pressure, and decrease inflammation.[22] Plant foods add soluble fiber to the diet, which can reduce blood cholesterol, but in addition they provide vitamins, minerals, and phytochemicals, some of which protect against heart disease because they perform antioxidant functions. **Antioxidants** decrease the oxidation of LDL cholesterol and, therefore, the development of plaque in artery walls (see Figure 5.15) (see *Thinking It Through*).[25]

> **antioxidant** A substance that decreases the adverse effects of reactive molecules.

Cancer

Cancer is the second-leading cause of death in the United States. As with heart disease, there is evidence that the risk of cancer can be reduced with changes in diet and activity patterns.[26] Populations consuming diets that are high in fruits and vegetables tend to have a lower risk of cancer than populations with lower intakes. These foods are rich in antioxidants such as vitamin C, vitamin E, and β-carotene. In contrast, in populations that consume diets that are high in fat, particularly animal fats, the incidence of cancer is higher.

The good news is that the same type of diet that protects you from cardiovascular disease may also reduce the risk of certain forms of cancer. For example, the Mediterranean diet, which is high in monounsaturated fat from olive oil and omega-3 fatty acids from fish, is associated with a low risk of cancers of the breast, ovary, colon, and upper digestive and respiratory tracts.[27–29] *Trans* fatty acids, on the other hand, not only raise LDL cholesterol levels but are also believed to increase the risk of breast cancer.[30]

Obesity

Excess dietary fat consumption contributes to weight gain and obesity. One reason is that fat contains 9 Calories/gram, more than twice the calorie content of carbohydrate or protein. Therefore, a high-fat meal contains more calories in the same volume than does a lower-fat meal. Because people have a tendency to eat a certain weight or volume of food, consuming meals that are high in fat leads to more calories being consumed.[31,32] Dietary fat may also contribute to weight gain because it is stored very efficiently as body fat.

Despite the fact that fat is fattening, the fat content of the U.S. diet is unlikely to be the sole reason for the high rate of obesity in the United States.[33] Weight gain occurs when energy intake exceeds energy expenditure, regardless of whether the extra energy comes from fat, carbohydrate, or protein. The increasing prevalence of overweight and obesity in the United States and worldwide is likely due to a general increase in calorie intake combined with a decrease in energy expenditure.[15]

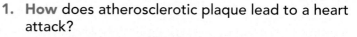

CONCEPT CHECK

1. **How** does atherosclerotic plaque lead to a heart attack?

2. **What** are three dietary factors that increase the risk of heart disease?

3. **Why** might eating a high-fat diet increase the number of calories you consume?

Meeting Lipid Needs

LEARNING OBJECTIVES

1. **Discuss** the recommendations for fat and cholesterol intake.

2. **Choose** heart-healthy foods from each section of MyPlate.

3. **Use** food labels to choose foods containing healthy fats.

The amount of fat the body requires from the diet is small, but a diet that provides only the minimum amount would be very high in carbohydrate, would not be very palatable, and would not necessarily be any healthier than diets with more fat. Therefore, the recommendations for fat intake focus on getting enough to meet the need for essential fatty acids and choosing the amounts and types of fat that will promote health and prevent disease.

THINKING IT THROUGH

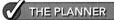

A Case Study on Improving Heart Health

Rafael is a financial advisor who spends much of his day sitting at his computer. When he is home with his family, he enjoys watching his children play soccer and basketball but rarely finds time to exercise himself. Rafael's doctor recently told him that his blood cholesterol levels are elevated. His blood lipids and other information from his medical history are given below:

Sex	Male
Age	35
Family history	Mother had heart attack at age 60
Height/weight	68 inches/160 lb
Blood pressure	145/80 (optimal is < 120/80)
Smoker	Yes
Activity level	Sedentary
Blood values:	
Total cholesterol	210 mg/100 ml
LDL cholesterol	160 mg/100 ml
HDL cholesterol	34 mg/100 ml
Triglycerides	120 mg/100 ml

Which of the factors listed here increase Rafael's risk of developing cardiovascular disease?
▼

Your answer:

Rafael meets with a dietitian. A diet recall reveals that his breakfast typically consists of a bagel with cream cheese and coffee with cream and sugar. For lunch, he goes out with his colleagues for a fast-food hamburger, fries, and a soda. Dinner at home with his family consists of beef or chicken, a green or orange vegetable, and rice or potatoes.

An analysis of his diet indicates that his total fat intake is within the recommended range of 20 to 35% of calories, but he consumes more saturated fat than is recommended. In addition, he does not consume enough omega-3 fatty acids relative to the amounts of omega-6 fatty acids, and he eats few foods that are high in heart-healthy monounsaturated fatty acids.

To reduce Rafael's intake of saturated fat, the dietitian suggests that he switch to cereal with low-fat milk for breakfast and make better fast-food choices at lunchtime.

What substitutions could Rafael make in his fast-food meal to reduce his intake of saturated fat?
▼

Your answer:

At home, to increase intake of omega-3 and monounsaturated fatty acids, the family switches to canola oil and olive oil for cooking and has fish or shellfish twice a week. Because his modified diet has fewer calories and Rafael does not need to lose weight, he starts bringing granola bars to work for a snack.

Look at the labels from these two granola bars. Based on the amounts of saturated fat, *trans* fat, fiber, and calories in each, explain which one you would recommend.
▼

Your answer:

(Check your answers in Appendix J.)

Granola Bar A

Nutrition Facts
Serving Size 1 bar (35g)
Servings Per Container 6

Amount Per Serving	
Calories	140
Calories from Fat	30

	% Daily Value*
Total Fat 3.5g	6%
Saturated Fat 2g	10%
Trans Fat 0g	
Cholesterol 0mg	0%
Sodium 130mg	5%
Total Carbohydrate 26g	9%
Dietary Fiber 1g	5%
Sugars 13g	
Protein 2g	

Granola Bar B

Nutrition Facts
Serving Size 1 bar (68g)
Servings Per Container 6

Amount/Serving	
Calories	230
Calories from Fat	30

	% Daily Value*
Total Fat 3g	5%
Saturated Fat 0.5g	3%
Trans Fat 0g	
Cholesterol 0mg	0%
Sodium 125mg	5%
Total Carbohydrate 45g	15%
Dietary Fiber 5g	20%
Sugars 21g	
Protein 10g	20%

Fat and Cholesterol Recommendations

The DRIs recommend a total fat intake of 20 to 35% of calories for adults. Of this, a small proportion needs to come from the essential fatty acids. The AI for linoleic acid is 12 grams/day for women and 17 grams/day for men. You can meet your requirement by consuming a half-cup of almonds or 2 tablespoons of corn oil. For α-linolenic acid, the AI is 1.1 grams/day for women and 1.6 grams/day for men. Your requirement can be met by eating a quarter-cup of walnuts or 1 tablespoon of ground flaxseed. Consuming these amounts provides the recommended ratio of linoleic to α-linolenic acid of between 5:1 and 10:1.[9]

WHAT A SCIENTIST SEES

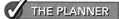

Looking for Lean Meat

Fresh meats are not required to carry Nutrition Facts labels, but they often provide information about the fat content of the meat. The terms *lean* and *extra lean* are used to describe the fat content of packaged meats, such as hot dogs and lunch meat, and fresh meats, such as pork chops, poultry, and steaks. "Lean" means that the meat contains less than 10% fat by weight, and "extra lean" means that it contains less than 5% fat by weight (see Appendix F). So a package of ground beef like this one that is 85% lean looks like a good choice.

What a scientist sees is that "lean" and "percent lean" are not the same thing. "Percent lean" refers to the weight of the meat that is lean, not the percentage of calories provided by lean meat. So when the label says it is 85% lean, it means that 15% of the weight of the meat is fat, or that there are 15 grams of fat in

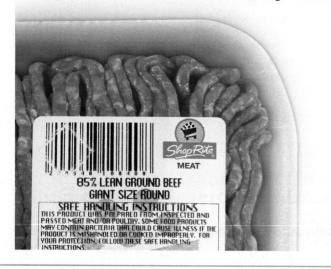

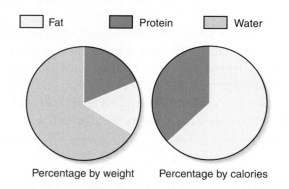

The chart on the left shows what percentage of the weight of the ground beef consists of fat, protein, and water. The chart on the right shows the percentage of calories contributed by fat and protein.

100 grams (3.5 ounces) of raw meat. This is a relatively small percentage by weight, but because fat contains 9 Calories per gram, the fat contributes 63% of the calories in the meat (see charts).

Should you pass on the ground beef and select ground turkey instead? Check the label. If the package is labeled "ground turkey," it may contain skin and leg meat and actually have more fat than the ground beef. Only poultry labeled "ground turkey (or chicken) breast" is made with just the lean breast meat.

Think Critically If you want to purchase ground beef that fits the definition of a "lean" meat, what "percent lean" should you look for on the label?

To reduce the risk of heart disease the 2010 Dietary Guidelines recommend limiting saturated fat intake to less than 10% of total calories by replacing foods high in saturated fat with sources of mono or polyunsaturated fat. Reducing saturated fat intake to 7% of calories and keeping *trans* fat intake as low as possible can lower risk even more. The guidelines recommend limiting cholesterol to less than 300 mg per day for the general population and suggest that those at high risk for heart disease reduce their cholesterol intake to less than 200 mg/day. Limiting sources of solid fats in the diet will help to reduce saturated fat, *trans* fat, and cholesterol.[15]

Children need more fat than adults to allow for growth and development so their acceptable ranges of fat intake are higher: 30% to 40% of calories for ages 1 to 3 and 25% to 35% of calories for ages 3 to 18. Like adults, adolescents and children over age 2 should consume a diet that is low in saturated fat, cholesterol, and *trans* fat.[15]

Choosing Fats Wisely

The typical U.S. diet falls within the recommended 20 to 35% of calories from fat. Our *trans* fat intake is declining because food manufacturers have reduced the *trans* fat content of fats and oils used in processing. However, our intake of cholesterol and saturated fat often exceeds recommendations, and most people don't get enough omega-3 polyunsaturated fatty acids.[3, 15]

Shifting the sources of dietary fat can improve the proportion of healthy fats in your diet. Limiting fatty cuts of meat, full-fat dairy products, and high-fat processed meats, and trimming the fat from meat and removing the skin from poultry will reduce your intake of saturated fat and cholesterol (see *What a Scientist Sees*). Avoiding foods such

Healthy MyPlate choices • Figure 5.18

MyPlate recommends limiting intake of solid fats, which includes fats that are high in saturated or *trans* fat, and choosing liquid oils, which are high in mono- and polyunsaturated fats.

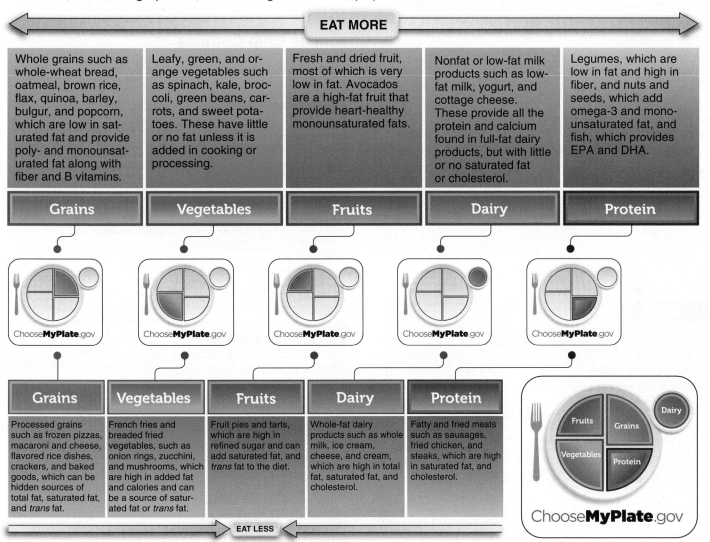

EAT MORE

Grains	Vegetables	Fruits	Dairy	Protein
Whole grains such as whole-wheat bread, oatmeal, brown rice, flax, quinoa, barley, bulgur, and popcorn, which are low in saturated fat and provide poly- and monounsaturated fat along with fiber and B vitamins.	Leafy, green, and orange vegetables such as spinach, kale, broccoli, green beans, carrots, and sweet potatoes. These have little or no fat unless it is added in cooking or processing.	Fresh and dried fruit, most of which is very low in fat. Avocados are a high-fat fruit that provide heart-healthy monounsaturated fats.	Nonfat or low-fat milk products such as low-fat milk, yogurt, and cottage cheese. These provide all the protein and calcium found in full-fat dairy products, but with little or no saturated fat or cholesterol.	Legumes, which are low in fat and high in fiber, and nuts and seeds, which add omega-3 and mono-unsaturated fat, and fish, which provides EPA and DHA.

Grains	Vegetables	Fruits	Dairy	Protein
Processed grains such as frozen pizzas, macaroni and cheese, flavored rice dishes, crackers, and baked goods, which can be hidden sources of total fat, saturated fat, and *trans* fat.	French fries and breaded fried vegetables, such as onion rings, zucchini, and mushrooms, which are high in added fat and calories and can be a source of saturated fat or *trans* fat.	Fruit pies and tarts, which are high in refined sugar and can add saturated fat, and *trans* fat to the diet.	Whole-fat dairy products such as whole milk, ice cream, cheese, and cream, which are high in total fat, saturated fat, and cholesterol.	Fatty and fried meats such as sausages, fried chicken, and steaks, which are high in saturated fat, and cholesterol.

EAT LESS

ChooseMyPlate.gov

as hard margarines and baked goods that contain hydrogenated fats will limit your intake of *trans* fat. Eating more nuts and avocados and cooking with canola and olive oils will boost your intake of monounsaturated fat, and eating more fish and flaxseed will boost your omega-3 intake.

Making wise MyPlate choices Your choices from each food group can have a significant impact on the amounts and types of fats in your diet (**Figure 5.18**). Generally, grains, fruits, and vegetables are low in total fat and saturated fat, and they contain no cholesterol. However, choices from these groups need to be made with care to avoid fats that are added in processing or preparation. Smart choices from the protein group and the dairy group can reduce your intake of unhealthy fats.

Oils, butter, margarine, fatty sauces, and salad dressings used in cooking or added at the table are the most concentrated sources of fat in the diet. Limiting these can reduce your total fat and calorie intake, and choosing liquid oils rather than solid fats can increase the proportion of unsaturated fats in your diet. Solid fats such as butter, shortening, beef fat, and lard are high in saturated or *trans* fats. These solid fats provide the same number of calories per gram as oils but few essential nutrients. Therefore MyPlate considers them to be empty calories. Consuming too many empty calories makes it difficult to meet your nutrient needs without gaining weight. If you consume a 2000-Calorie diet, you can include only about 260 empty Calories. Spreading 1 tablespoon of butter on your morning bagel uses up 100 Calories, over one-third of your empty Calorie allowance.

Lipids on food labels • Figure 5.19

a. Understanding how to use food labels can help you make more informed choices about the foods you include in your diet. By noting the grams of fat and the total number of Calories, you can determine the percentage of calories from fat in a product as follows:

1. Multiply the grams of fat by 9 Calories/gram. For example, this product provides 8 grams of fat:

   8 grams × 9 Calories/gram = 72 Calories from fat

2. Divide Calories from fat by total Calories and multiply by 100 to obtain the percentage. For example, this food contains 160 Calories/serving and 72 Calories from fat:

   72 Calories ÷ 160 Calories × 100 = 45% of Calories from fat

The Nutrition Facts panel lists Calories from fat; grams of total fat, saturated fat, and *trans* fat; and milligrams of cholesterol in a serving. The amount of monounsaturated and polyunsaturated fat is voluntarily included on the labels of some products.

The Daily Values recommend consuming less than 30% of calories as fat, no more than 300 mg of cholesterol per day, and no more than 10% of calories as saturated fat. It is recommended that *trans* fat intake be limited to the amounts present naturally in meats and dairy products (≤0.5% of calories).

The sources of fat in a product are listed in the ingredient list with the other ingredients, in order of prominence by weight.

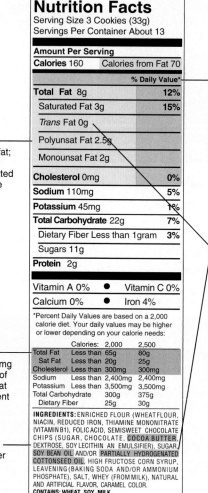

Chocolate Chip Cookies

Nutrition Facts
Serving Size 3 Cookies (33g)
Servings Per Container About 13

Amount Per Serving

Calories 160	Calories from Fat 70

	% Daily Value*
Total Fat 8g	12%
Saturated Fat 3g	15%
Trans Fat 0g	
Polyunsat Fat 2.5g	
Monounsat Fat 2g	
Cholesterol 0mg	0%
Sodium 110mg	5%
Potassium 45mg	1%
Total Carbohydrate 22g	7%
Dietary Fiber Less than 1gram	3%
Sugars 11g	
Protein 2g	

Vitamin A 0%	●	Vitamin C 0%
Calcium 0%	●	Iron 4%

*Percent Daily Values are based on a 2,000 calorie diet. Your daily values may be higher or lower depending on your calorie needs:

		Calories:	2,000	2,500
Total Fat	Less than		65g	80g
Sat Fat	Less than		20g	25g
Cholesterol	Less than		300mg	300mg
Sodium	Less than		2,400mg	2,400mg
Potassium	Less than		3,500mg	3,500mg
Total Carbohydrate			300g	375g
Dietary Fiber			25g	30g

INGREDIENTS: ENRICHED FLOUR (WHEAT FLOUR, NIACIN, REDUCED IRON, THIAMINE MONONITRATE (VITAMIN B1), FOLIC ACID, SEMISWEET CHOCOLATE CHIPS (SUGAR, CHOCOLATE, COCOA BUTTER, DEXTROSE, SOY LECITHIN AN EMULSIFIER), SUGAR, SOY BEAN OIL AND/OR PARTIALLY HYDROGENATED COTTONSEED OIL, HIGH FRUCTOSE CORN SYRUP, LEAVENING (BAKING SODA AND/OR AMMONIUM PHOSPHATE), SALT, WHEY (FROM MILK), NATURAL AND ARTIFICIAL FLAVOR, CARAMEL COLOR.
CONTAINS: WHEAT, SOY, MILK

A % Daily Value is listed for total fat, saturated fat, and cholesterol. This allows consumers to tell how a food fits the recommendations. Generally, ≤5% of the Daily Value is low, and ≥20% is high. There are no Daily Values for *trans*, polyunsaturated, and monounsaturated fats.

If the product has less than 0.5 gram of *trans* fat per serving, the nutrition facts panel will list the amount of *trans* fat as 0, even if partially hydrogenated oil is an ingredient.

Fat free: Contains < 0.5 g fat per serving

Reduced fat: Contains at least 25% less fat per serving than the regular or reference product

Low fat: Contains ≤ 3 g fat per serving

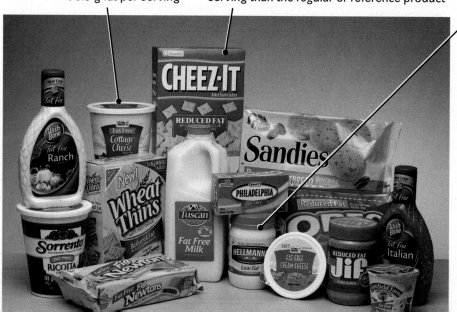

b. Food labeling regulations have developed standard definitions for descriptors such as "low fat" and "low cholesterol," and such terms can be used only in ways that will not confuse the consumer. For example, because saturated fat in the diet raises blood cholesterol, to be labeled "low cholesterol," a food must contain ≤ 20 mg cholesterol per serving and ≤ 2 g saturated fat per serving. So crackers containing coconut oil, which are low in cholesterol but are high in saturated fat, cannot be labeled "low cholesterol."

Looking at food labels Food labels are an accessible source of information about the fat content of packaged foods. The Nutrition Facts panel shows the amounts of total fat, saturated fat, cholesterol, and *trans* fat, and the ingredient list indicates the source of the fat—for example, whether a food contains corn oil, soybean oil, coconut oil, or partially hydrogenated vegetable oil. Nutrient content claims such as "low fat," "fat free," and "low cholesterol" on food labels can also be used to identify foods that help you meet the recommendations for fat intake. Health claims can help you choose foods that will meet your nutritional goals. For example, foods that are low in saturated fat and cholesterol may state that they help reduce the risk of heart disease (**Figure 5.19** and Appendix F).

The Role of Fat Replacers

People often choose low-fat and reduced-fat products in order to reduce the total amount of fat in their diets. Some of these foods, such as low-fat and nonfat milk and yogurt, are made by simply removing the fat, but in other products, the fat is replaced with ingredients that mimic the taste and texture of the fat. Some reduced-fat foods contain added sugars to improve the taste and texture. Some contain soluble fiber or modified proteins that simulate fat, and others contain fats that have been altered to reduce or prevent absorption (**Figure 5.20**).[34] A problem with nonabsorbable fats is that they reduce the absorption of the fat-soluble substances in the diet, including the fat-soluble vitamins, A, D, E, and K. To avoid depleting these vitamins, products made with the nonabsorbable fat substitute Olestra have been fortified with them. However, these products are not fortified with β-carotene and other fat-soluble substances that may be important for health. Another potential problem with Olestra is that it can cause abdominal cramping and loose stools in some individuals because it passes into the colon without being digested.

Will using low-fat and reduced-fat products improve your diet? Some low-fat foods make an important contribution to a healthy diet. Low-fat dairy products are recommended because they provide all the essential nutrients contained in the full-fat versions but have fewer calories

Fat replacers • Figure 5.20

Carbohydrates and proteins added to replace fat add calories to foods. In some cases, so much is added that the low-fat food is not much lower in calories than the original product. Some fat replacers are made from fats that have been modified to reduce how well they can be digested and absorbed. The calories they provide depend on how much is absorbed.

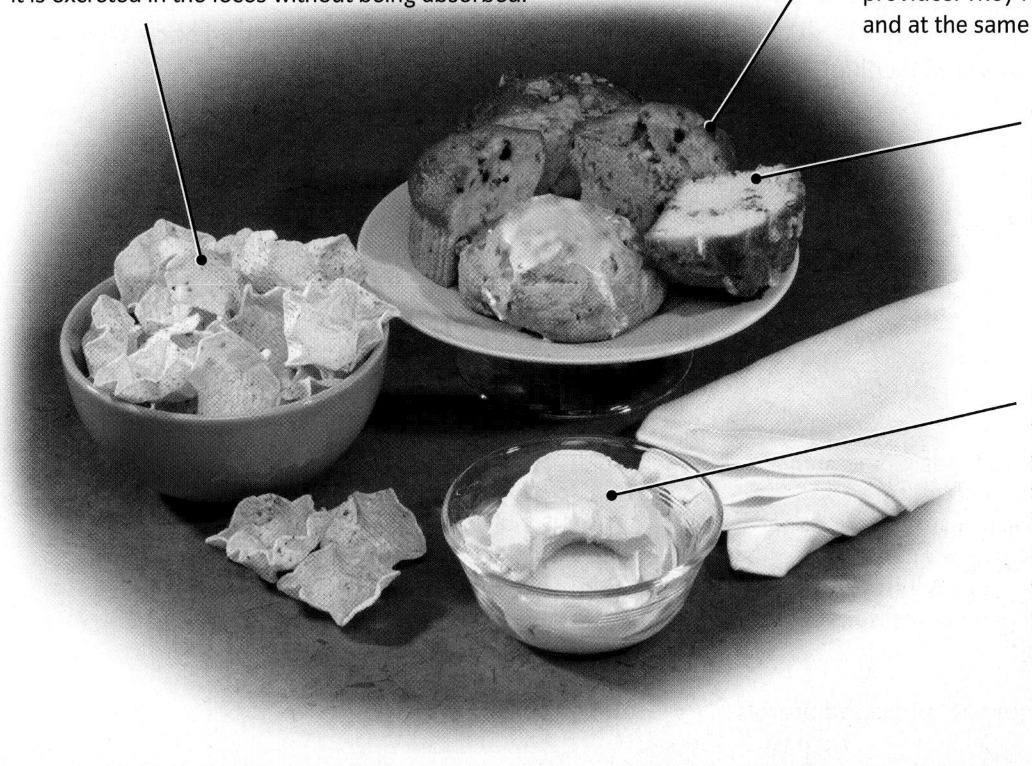

The artificial fat Olestra (sucrose polyester) is made from sucrose with fatty acids attached. Olestra cannot be digested by either human enzymes or bacterial enzymes in the gastrointestinal tract. Therefore, it is excreted in the feces without being absorbed.

Polysaccharides such as pectins and gums are often used in baked goods, as well as salad dressings, sauces, and ice cream, to mimic the texture that fat provides. They reduce the amount of fat in a product and at the same time add soluble fiber.

The sugar sucrose is usually added to low-fat and nonfat baked goods to improve flavor and add volume. Sucrose adds 4 Calories per gram.

Protein-based fat replacers are made from milk and egg proteins processed to form millions of microscopic balls that slide over each other, mimicking the creamy texture of fat.[34] They are used in frozen desserts, cheese foods, and other products but cannot be used for frying because they break down at high temperatures.

Meeting Lipid Needs **159**

WHAT SHOULD I EAT?
Fats and Cholesterol

Limit your intake of cholesterol, *trans* fat, and saturated fat
- Choose low-fat milk and yogurt.
- Trim the fat from your meat and serve chicken and fish but don't eat the skin.
- Cut in half your usual amount of butter and use soft rather than stick margarine.
- Watch your fast food choices—choose chicken over burgers and skip the special sauce.

Increase the proportion of polyunsaturated and monounsaturated fats
- Snack on nuts and seeds.
- Add olives and avocados to your salads.
- Use olive, peanut, or canola oil for cooking and salad dressing.
- Use corn, sunflower, or safflower oil for baking.

Up your omega-3 intake
- Sprinkle ground flax seeds on your cereal or yogurt.
- Have a serving of mackerel, lake trout, sardines, tuna, or salmon.
- Pick a leafy green vegetable with dinner.
- Add walnuts to your salad or cereal.

Use iProfile to find the varieties of nuts and fish that are highest in omega-3 fatty acids.

and less saturated fat and cholesterol. Using these products increases the nutrient density of the diet as a whole. However, not all reduced-fat foods are nutrient dense. Low-fat baked goods often have more sugar than the full-fat versions because extra sugar is needed to add volume and make up for the flavor that is lost when the fat is removed. Some are just lower-fat versions of nutrient-poor choices, such as baked goods and chips. If these reduced-fat desserts and snack foods replace whole grains, fruits, and vegetables, the resulting diet could be low in fat but also low in fiber, vitamins, minerals, and phytochemicals (see *What Should I Eat?*).

Using low-fat foods does not necessarily transform a poor diet into a healthy one or improve overall diet quality, but if used appropriately, fat-modified foods can be part of a healthy diet.[34] For example, if a low-fat salad dressing replaces a full-fat version, it allows you to enhance the appeal of a nutrient-rich salad without as much added fat and calories from the dressing. Low-fat products can also be used in conjunction with weight-loss diets because they are often lower in calories. But check the label. Although most are lower in calories, they are by no means calorie free and cannot be consumed liberally without adding calories to the diet and possibly contributing to weight gain.

CONCEPT CHECK STOP

1. **How** much fat is recommended in a healthy diet?
2. **Which** food groups contribute the most foods that are high in saturated fat and cholesterol?
3. **How** can labels help you identify foods that are low in saturated and *trans* fat?

Summary

1 Fats in Our Food 134

- Fat adds calories, texture, and flavor to foods. Some of the fats we eat are visible, but others are hidden.
- Over the past 40 years, Americans have changed the sources of fat in their diets, but the number of grams of fat consumed daily has changed little, as seen in this graph, and the incidence of obesity and other chronic diseases has continued to rise.

U.S. food intake in the 1970s and today • Figure 5.2c

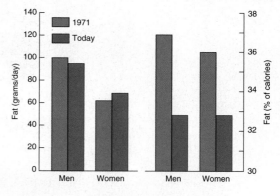

2 Types of Lipids 135

- **Lipids** are a diverse group of organic compounds, most of which do not dissolve in water. **Triglycerides**, commonly referred to as fat, are the type of lipid that is most abundant in our food and in our **adipose tissue**. As shown here, a triglyceride contains three **fatty acids** attached to a molecule of glycerol.

Triglycerides • Figure 5.3

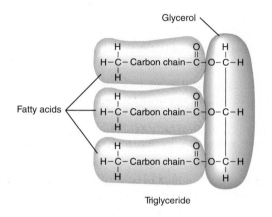

Triglyceride

- The structure of fatty acids affects their chemical properties and functions in the body. Each carbon atom in the carbon chain of a **saturated fatty acid** is attached to as many hydrogen atoms as possible, so no carbon–carbon double bonds form. Saturated fatty acids are found primarily in animal products. Exceptions include saturated plant oils often called **tropical oils**. A **monounsaturated fatty acid** contains one carbon–carbon double bond. A **polyunsaturated fatty acid** contains more than one carbon–carbon double bond. The location of the first double bond determines whether it is an **omega-3** or **omega-6 fatty acid**. The orientation of hydrogen atoms around a carbon–carbon double bond distinguishes *cis* fatty acids from *trans* **fatty acids**. **Hydrogenation** transforms some carbon–carbon double bonds to the *trans* configuration.

- A **phospholipid** contains a **phosphate group** and two fatty acids attached to a backbone of glycerol. One end of the molecule is water soluble, and one end is fat soluble. Phospholipids therefore make good **emulsifiers**. In the human body, they are an important structural component of cell membranes and **lipoproteins**.

- **Sterols**, of which **cholesterol** is the best known, are made up of multiple chemical rings. Cholesterol is made by the body and consumed in animal foods in the diet. In the body, it is a component of cell membranes and is used to synthesize vitamin D, bile acids, and some hormones.

3 Absorbing and Transporting Lipids 141

- In the small intestine, muscular churning mixes chyme with bile from the gallbladder to break fat into small globules. This allows pancreatic lipase to access triglycerides for digestion. The products of triglyceride digestion, cholesterol, phospholipids, and other fat-soluble substances combine with bile to form **micelles**, as depicted here, which facilitate the absorption of these materials.

Lipid digestion and absorption • Figure 5.8

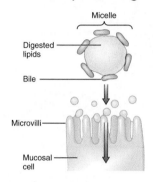

- Lipids absorbed from the intestine are packaged with protein to form **chylomicrons**. The triglycerides in chylomicrons are broken down by **lipoprotein lipase** on the surface of cells lining the blood vessels. The fatty acids released are taken up by surrounding cells, and what remains is taken up by the liver.

- **Very-low-density lipoproteins (VLDLs)** are synthesized by the liver. With the help of lipoprotein lipase, they deliver triglycerides to body cells. **Low-density lipoproteins (LDLs)** deliver cholesterol to tissues by binding to **LDL receptors** on the cell surface. **High-density lipoproteins (HDLs)** help remove cholesterol from cells and transport it to the liver for disposal.

4 Lipid Functions 144

- Dietary fat is needed for the absorption of fat-soluble vitamins and to provide essential fatty acids. In the body, triglycerides in adipose tissue provide a concentrated source of energy and insulate the body against shock and temperature changes. **Essential fatty acids** are needed for normal structure and function of cell membranes, particularly those in the retina and central nervous system. Omega-6 and omega-3 polyunsaturated fatty acids are used to synthesize **eicosanoids**, which help regulate blood clotting, blood pressure, immune function, and other body processes. The ratio of dietary omega-6 to omega-3 fatty acids affects the balance of omega-6 and omega-3 eicosanoids made and hence their overall physiological effects.

- Throughout the day triglycerides are continuously stored in adipose tissue and then broken down to release fatty acids, as shown in the illustration, depending on the immediate energy needs of the body. To generate ATP from fatty acids, the carbon chain is broken into two carbon units that form acetyl-CoA, which can then be metabolized in the presence of oxygen.

Feasting and fasting • Figure 5.14

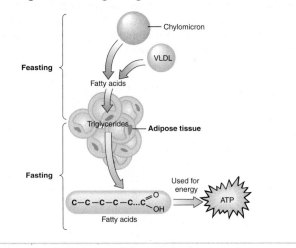

5 **Lipids in Health and Disease   148**

• **Atherosclerosis** is a disease characterized by the formation of **atherosclerotic plaque** in the artery wall. It starts with an injury to the artery wall that triggers **inflammation**, leading to plaque formation. A key event in the process is the oxidation of LDL cholesterol in the artery wall. **Oxidized LDL cholesterol** promotes inflammation and is taken up by macrophages, as depicted here, forming **foam cells**, that deposit in the artery wall. High blood levels of total and LDL cholesterol are risk factors for heart disease. High blood HDL cholesterol levels protect against heart disease. The risk of atherosclerosis is also increased by diabetes, high blood pressure, and obesity.

Development of atherosclerosis • Figure 5.15

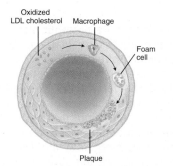

• Diets high in saturated fat, *trans* fat, and cholesterol increase the risk of heart disease. Diets high in omega-6 and omega-3 polyunsaturated fatty acids, monounsaturated fatty acids, certain B vitamins, and plant foods containing fiber, antioxidants, and phytochemicals reduce the risk of

heart disease. The total dietary and lifestyle pattern is more important than any individual dietary factor in reducing heart disease risk.

• Diets high in fat correlate with an increased incidence of certain types of cancer. In general, the same types of lipids and other dietary components that protect you from heart disease will also protect you from certain forms of cancer.

• Fat contains 9 Calories per gram. A high-fat diet may therefore increase energy intake and promote weight gain, but it is not the primary cause of obesity. Consuming more energy than expended leads to weight gain, regardless of whether the energy is from fat, carbohydrate, or protein.

6 **Meeting Lipid Needs   154**

• The DRIs recommend that adults consume a diet that provides 20 to 35% of energy from fat and is low in cholesterol, saturated fat, and *trans* fat. The Dietary Guidelines recommend limiting saturated fatty acid intake to less than 10% of total calories, limiting cholesterol to 300 mg per day, avoiding *trans* fat.

• The U.S. diet is not too high in fat, but it often does not contain the healthiest types of fats. To reduce saturated fat and cholesterol intake, limit solid fats and choose liquid oils, fish, and nuts and seeds often. Use food labels like the one shown here to avoid processed foods that are high in saturated and *trans* fat. A diet based on whole grains, fruits, vegetables, and lean meats and low-fat dairy products will meet the recommendations for fat intake.

Lipids on food labels • Figure 5.19a

Chocolate Chip Cookies

Nutrition Facts	
Serving Size 3 Cookies (33g)	
Servings Per Container About 13	

Amount Per Serving	
Calories 160 Calories from Fat 70	

	% Daily Value*
Total Fat 8g	**12%**
Saturated Fat 3g	**15%**
Trans Fat 0g	
Polyunsat Fat 2.5g	
Monounsat Fat 2g	
Cholesterol 0mg	**0%**
Sodium 110mg	**5%**
Potassium 45mg	**1%**
Total Carbohydrate 22g	**7%**
Dietary Fiber Less than 1gram	**3%**
Sugars 11g	
Protein 2g	

• Fat replacers are used to create reduced-fat products with taste and texture similar to the original. Some low-fat products are made by using mixtures of carbohydrates or proteins to simulate the properties of fat, and some use lipids that are modified to reduce their digestion and absorption. Products containing fat replacers can help reduce fat and energy intake when used in moderation as part of a balanced diet.

Key Terms

- adipose tissue 144
- alpha-linolenic acid (α-linolenic acid) 145
- antioxidant 154
- arachidonic acid 145
- atherosclerosis 149
- atherosclerotic plaque 149
- cardiovascular disease 148
- cholesterol 140
- chylomicron 142
- docosahexaenoic acid (DHA) 145
- eicosapentaenoic acid (EPA) 145
- eicosanoids 145
- emulsifier 139
- essential fatty acid 137
- essential fatty acid deficiency 145
- fatty acid 135
- foam cell 148
- high-density lipoprotein (HDL) 144
- hydrogenation 138
- inflammation 149
- LDL receptor 143
- lecithin 139
- linoleic acid 145
- lipids 135
- lipid bilayer 139
- lipoprotein 142
- lipoprotein lipase 143
- low-density lipoprotein (LDL) 144
- macrophage 148
- micelle 142
- monoglyceride 142
- monounsaturated fatty acid 136
- omega-3 fatty acid 137
- omega-6 fatty acid 137
- oxidized LDL cholesterol 148
- phosphate group 139
- phospholipid 136
- plant sterol 140
- polyunsaturated fatty acid 137
- saturated fatty acid 136
- sterol 136
- *trans* fatty acid 136
- triglyceride 135
- tropical oil 138
- unsaturated fatty acid 137
- very-low-density lipoprotein (VLDL) 144

Online Resources

- For more information on diet, lifestyle, and heart disease go to Statements and Practice Guidelines at the American Heart Association at http://www.americanheart.org/presenter.jhtml?identifier=3003999

- For more information on diet, lifestyle, and cancer go to the American Cancer Society at http://www.cancer.org/Healthy/EatHealthyGetActive/ACSGuidelinesonNutritionPhysicalActivityforCancerPrevention/nupa-guidelines-toc

- For more information on omega-3 fatty acid supplements and heart disease go to the Office of Dietary Supplements at http://ods.od.nih.gov/health_information/omega_3_fatty_acids.aspx

- For more information the Mediterranean diet go to http://www.mayoclinic.com/health/mediterranean-diet/CL00011

- For more information on high blood cholesterol levels go to the NIH at http://www.nlm.nih.gov/medlineplus/cholesterol.html

- Visit your *WileyPLUS* site for videos, animations, podcasts, self-study, and other media that will aid you in studying and understanding this chapter.

Critical and Creative Thinking Questions

1. Record everything you eat for three days. Use iProfile to determine your nutrient intake. How does your intake of total fat, saturated fat, and cholesterol compare with the recommendations?

2. Using your food record from question 1, list the dairy products in your diet and indicate whether they are full fat or reduced fat. List the grain products you typically consume. How many of them are baked goods with added fats? How many of them are eaten with an added high-fat spread or sauce? Suggest changes you could make to reduce the fats added to your carbohydrates. List the foods in your diet that are from the meat and beans food group. Use iProfile to determine the types and amounts of fats these provide. Suggest some other foods from this group that would increase your intake of monounsaturated and omega-3 fatty acids.

3. Jessica is 18, at a healthy weight, and eats a vegetarian diet. Explain how she could still have high blood cholesterol levels.

4. The table shown here illustrates the percentage of calories from fat in the diets of American men and women and the incidence of obesity among adults between 1971 and 2000. Use these values to construct a graph. Based on your graph, discuss what happened to each over time and how these two factors might be related.

Year[2,35,36]	1971–1974	1976–1980	1988–1994	1999–2000
% Calories from fat (men)	36.9	36.8	33.9	32.8
% Calories from fat (women)	36.1	36	33.4	32.8
Percentage of adults who are obese	14.5	15	23.3	30.5

5. Ka Ming is a second generation Chinese American. At his college health fair a blood cholesterol screening reveals that his total blood cholesterol is 280 mg/100 ml. He is at a healthy weight and does not smoke. He gets little exercise and consumes a diet that is a mixture of American foods and traditional Chinese foods. A medical history reveals that none of Ka Ming's relatives in China have had cardiovascular disease. Why might the lack of cardiovascular disease in his family history not be a true indication of Ka Ming's risk?

6. Relate the functions of LDL and HDL cholesterol to how levels of each in the blood affect heart disease risk.

7. What are the similarities and differences in how the body responds to a cut on the finger and to an injury to the inside of an artery wall?

8. Why might taking fish oil supplements reduce the rate at which your blood clots?

What is happening in this picture?

This individual has familial hypercholesterolemia, a rare genetic disease in which there are no LDL receptors on cells. It causes cholesterol levels so high that the cholesterol deposits in body tissues, seen here as raised lumps.

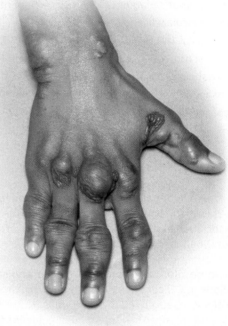

Think Critically

1. Why would this condition cause elevated blood cholesterol?
2. How would this condition affect the risk of developing heart disease?

Self-Test

(Check your answers in Appendix K.)

1. What type of fatty acid is labeled C in the illustration?

   a. saturated

   c. omega-3 polyunsaturated

   b. monounsaturated

   d. omega-6 polyunsaturated

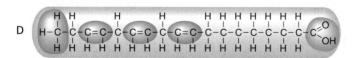

2. Which of the following is unlikely to occur after you eat a fatty meal?

   a. Fatty acids stored in adipose tissue are released into the blood and taken up by body cells as an energy source.

   b. The gallbladder releases bile into the small intestine.

   c. Micelles are formed in the small intestine.

   d. Pancreatic lipase releases fatty acids from triglycerides.

   e. The concentration of chylomicrons in the blood increases.

3. Omega-3 fatty acids have a beneficial effect on blood lipid levels but also reduce the risk of cardiovascular diseases because they _____.

   a. inhibit the absorption of cholesterol from the diet

   b. increase the formation of oxidized LDL cholesterol

   c. cause mutations in cellular DNA

   d. break down *trans* fatty acids

   e. are converted into eicosanoids

4. Which of the following statements about cholesterol is false?

   a. It is used to synthesize vitamin D.

   b. It is needed to make bile.

   c. It is an essential component of animal cell membranes.

   d. It is found in peanut butter, leafy green vegetables, and avocados.

   e. It is needed to make the hormones estrogen and testosterone.

5. Which two fatty acids are considered essential?

   a. saturated and unsaturated

   b. linoleic and α-linolenic

   c. stearic and palmitic

   d. EPA and DHA

   e. short and medium chain

Use the diagram to answer questions 6 and 7.

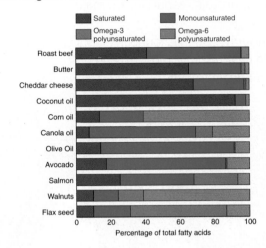

6. Which of the following statements about dietary sources of fat is true?

   a. Coconut oil is high in polyunsaturated fat.

   b. Canola oil is high in monounsaturated fat.

   c. Olive oil is high in omega-3 fatty acids.

   d. Butter is high in omega-6 fatty acids.

   e. Avocados are high in saturated fat.

7. Which of the following is highest in omega-3 fatty acids?

   a. corn oil   c. flax seed   e. salmon

   b. canola oil   d. walnuts

8. Which one of the following is associated with an increased risk of developing heart disease?

   a. a high concentration of HDL in the blood

   b. daily exercise

   c. a high-fiber, low-fat diet

   d. a diet made up mostly of plant foods

   e. a high concentration of LDL in the blood

9. Which of the following contribute to the lower heart disease risk associated with eating nuts?

   a. They are high in monounsaturated fat and omega-3 fatty acids.

   b. They are a good source of fiber and vegetable protein.

   c. They provide antioxidants.

   d. They contain plant sterols.

   e. All of the above are correct.

10. The transport of cholesterol to the liver for elimination is accomplished by _____.

    a. chylomicrons   c. HDLs

    b. VLDLs   d. LDLs

11. Which of the following statements about *trans* fatty acids is true?

    a. They have carbon–carbon double bonds, with the hydrogen atoms on the same side of the bond.

    b. They have straighter carbon chains than a corresponding *cis* fatty acid.

    c. They are formed during deep fat frying.

    d. High levels in the diet decrease the risk of heart disease.

12. Based on the label shown here, what is the approximate percentage of calories from saturated fat in this product?

    a. 3.5%   c. 13%   e. 22.5%

    b. 2%   d. 17%

Nutrition Facts		
Serving Size 1 bar (35g)		
Servings Per Container 6		
Amount Per Serving		
Calories 140		
Calories from Fat		30
		% Daily Value*
Total Fat 3.5g		6%
Saturated Fat 2g		10%
Trans Fat 0g		
Cholesterol 0mg		0%
Sodium 130mg		5%
Total Carbohydrate 26g		9%
Dietary Fiber 1g		5%
Sugars 13g		
Protein 2g		

13. Which one of the following statements about micelles is true?

    a. They help facilitate the absorption of lipids in the small intestine.

    b. They help transport lipids in the bloodstream.

    c. They are essential in the diet.

    d. They break the bonds that hold fatty acids to glycerol.

    e. They are transformed into chylomicrons in the blood.

14. Which MyPlate group contains the most foods that are high in saturated fat and cholesterol?

    a. vegetables   c. dairy

    b. grains   d. fruit

15. Identify the molecule in the animal cell membrane labeled B.

    a. cholesterol   c. starch

    b. protein   d. phospholipid

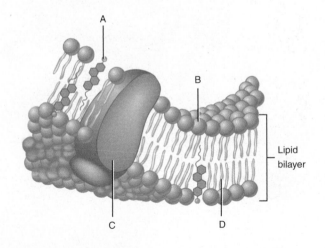

THE PLANNER ✓

Review your Chapter Planner on the chapter opener and check off your completed work.

Proteins and Amino Acids

The word *protein* comes from the Greek *proteios*, meaning "of primary importance." Proteins are essential to every cellular function. Proteins catalyze chemical reactions, are fundamental components of skeletal and muscular tissue, and are vital to immune response. The generation, development, processing, and renewal of protein resources are major human activities.

Although protein is found in plants and animals, Western cultures fulfill most of their protein needs from animal products. As affluence increases in non–Western societies, those societies adopt Western habits, including increasing the amount of beef in their diets, placing greater demands on agriculture to provide grain

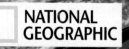

NATIONAL GEOGRAPHIC

for cattle, which will convert it to the preferred beef protein.

Today, agricultural production is facing a challenge from biofuels. In the United States, more and more grain crops are being grown not as food but as biofuel. One may argue that it is inefficient to feed grain to cattle in order to consume beef protein, but at least this process is a nutrition cycle. Corn that is converted into ethanol to fuel an automobile feeds no one. Obtaining enough protein and maintaining an adequate balance of plant and animal protein for the world's population, like protein itself, is clearly of primary importance.

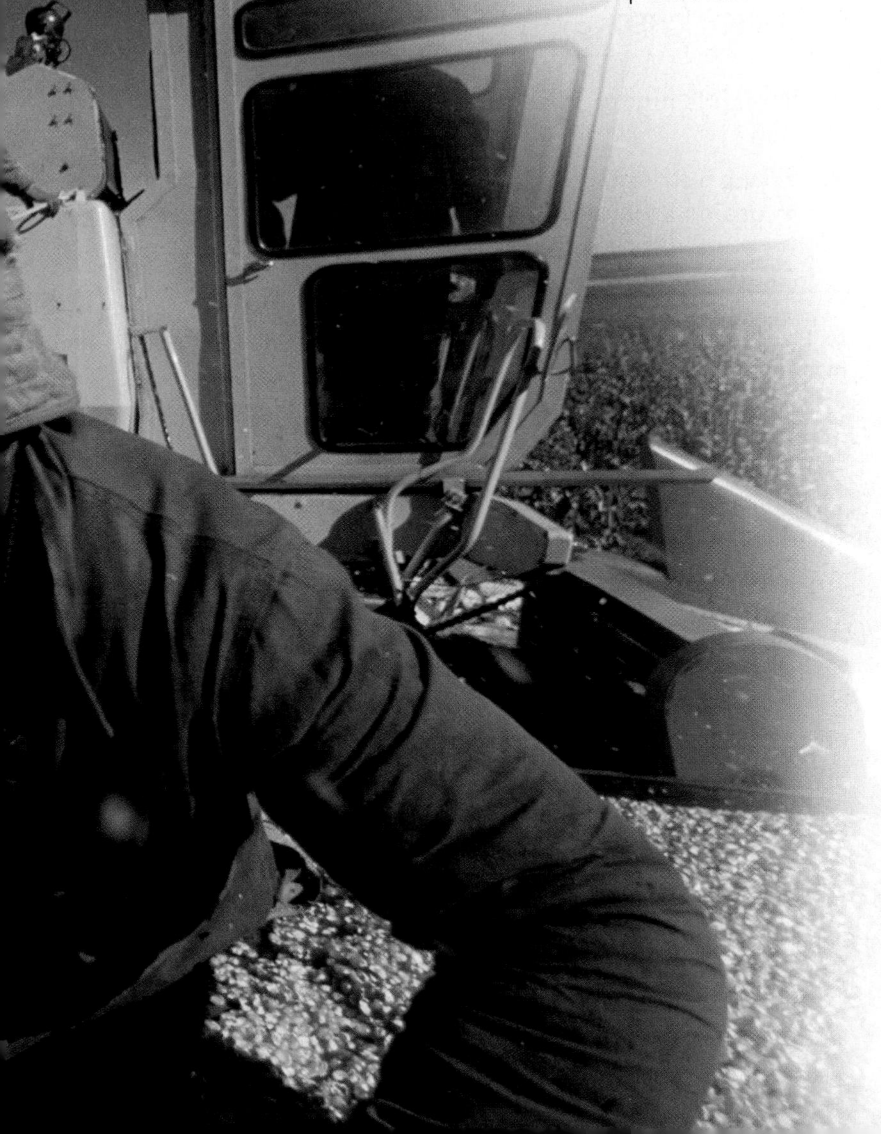

CHAPTER PLANNER ✓

- ❑ Stimulate your interest by reading the opening story and looking at the visual.
- ❑ Scan the Learning Objectives in each section:
  p. 168 ❑   p. 169 ❑   p. 173 ❑   p. 173 ❑   p. 179 ❑   p. 183 ❑
- ❑ Read the text and study all figures and visuals. Answer any questions.

Analyze key features

- ❑ Nutrition InSight, p. 170 ❑   p. 175 ❑   p. 176 ❑
- ❑ What a Scientist Sees, p. 171 ❑
- ❑ Process Diagram, p. 172 ❑   p. 178 ❑
- ❑ Thinking It Through, p. 192 ❑
- ❑ Stop: Answer the Concept Checks before you go on:
  p. 168 ❑   p. 171 ❑   p. 173 ❑   p. 179 ❑   p. 182 ❑   p. 193 ❑

End of chapter

- ❑ Review the Summary, Key Terms, and Online Resources.
- ❑ Answer the Critical and Creative Thinking Questions.
- ❑ Answer What is happening in this picture?
- ❑ Complete the Self-Test and check your answers.

Proteins in Our Food

LEARNING OBJECTIVES

1. **Describe** the types of foods that provide the most concentrated sources of protein.

2. **Compare** the nutrients in plant sources of protein with those in animal sources of protein.

legume The starchy seed of a plant that produces bean pods; includes peas, peanuts, beans, soybeans, and lentils.

amino acids The building blocks of proteins. Each amimo acid contains an amino group, an acid group, and a unique side chain.

When we think of protein, we usually think of a steak, a plate of scrambled eggs, or a glass of milk. These animal foods provide the most concentrated sources of protein in our diet, but plant foods such as grains, nuts, and **legumes** are also important sources of dietary protein. The proteins found in plants are made up of different combinations of **amino acids** than proteins found in animals. Because of this difference, most plant proteins are not used as efficiently as animal proteins to build proteins in the human body. Nevertheless, a diet that includes a variety of plant proteins can easily meet most people's protein needs.

The sources of protein in your diet have an impact not only on the amount of protein and variety of amino acids available to your body but also on what other nutrients you are consuming (**Figure 6.1**). Animal products provide B vitamins and readily absorbable sources of minerals, such as iron, zinc, and calcium. They are low in fiber, however, and are often high in saturated fat and cholesterol—a nutrient mix that increases the risk of heart disease.

Plant sources of protein provide most, but not all, B vitamins and also supply iron, zinc, and calcium, but often these are in less absorbable forms. Plant foods are generally excellent sources of fiber, phytochemicals, and unsaturated fats—dietary substances that promote health. Recommendations for a healthy diet, including the Dietary Guidelines and MyPlate, suggest that our diets be based on whole-grain products, vegetables, and fruits and include smaller amounts of meats and dairy products. Following these guidelines will provide plenty of protein from a mixture of plant and animal sources.

CONCEPT CHECK STOP

1. **Which** is higher in protein: an egg or a cup of rice?

2. **What** nutrients are plentiful in meat and milk? in grains and legumes?

Animal versus plant proteins • Figure 6.1

a. Animal products are high in protein, iron, zinc, and calcium but also add saturated fat and cholesterol to the diet.

b. Plant sources of protein are rich in fiber, phytochemicals, and monounsaturated and polyunsaturated fats.

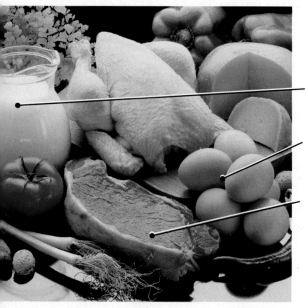

One cup milk: 8 grams protein

One egg: 7 grams protein

3 ounces meat: over 20 grams protein

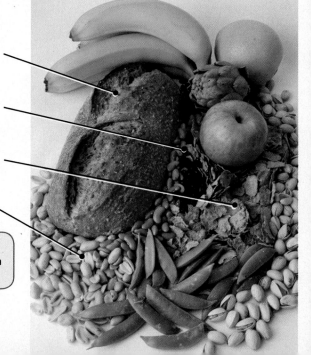

1 slice bread: about 2 grams protein

½ cup legumes: 6–10 grams protein

½ cup rice, pasta, or cereal: 2–4 grams protein

½ cup nuts or seeds: 5–10 grams protein

Ask Yourself

Why might a diet high in animal protein increase the risk of heart disease?

The Structure of Amino Acids and Proteins

LEARNING OBJECTIVES

1. **Describe** the general structure of an amino acid and of a protein.
2. **Distinguish** between essential and nonessential amino acids.
3. **Discuss** how the order of amino acids in a polypeptide chain affects protein structure.
4. **Explain** how a protein's structure is related to its function.

What do the proteins in a lamb chop, a kidney bean, and your thigh muscle have in common? They are all constructed of amino acids linked together to form one or more folded, chainlike strands. Twenty amino acids are commonly found in proteins. Each kind of protein contains a different number, combination, and sequence of amino acids. These differences give proteins their specific functions in living organisms and their unique characteristics in foods.

Amino Acid Structure

Each amino acid consists of a carbon atom that is bound to a hydrogen atom; an amino group, which contains nitrogen; an acid group; and a side chain (**Figure 6.2a** on next page). The nitrogen in amino acids distinguishes protein from carbohydrate and fat; all three contain carbon, hydrogen, and oxygen, but only protein contains nitrogen. The side chains of amino acids vary in size and structure; they give different amino acids their unique properties.

Nine of the amino acids needed by the adult human body must be consumed in the diet because they cannot be made in the body (**Figure 6.2b**). If the diet is deficient in one or more of these **essential amino acids** (also called **indispensable amino acids**), the body cannot make new proteins without breaking down existing proteins to provide the needed amino acids. The other 11 amino acids that are commonly found in protein are **nonessential**, or **dispensable**, **amino acids** because they can be made in the body.

Under certain conditions, some of the nonessential amino acids cannot be synthesized in

> **essential amino acid** (or **indispensable amino acid**) An amino acid that cannot be synthesized by the body in sufficient amounts to meet its needs and therefore must be included in the diet.

sufficient amounts to meet the body's needs. These are therefore referred to as **conditionally essential amino acids**. For example, the amino acid tyrosine can be made in the body from the essential amino acid phenylalanine. In individuals who have the inherited disease **phenylketonuria (PKU)**, phenylalanine cannot be converted into tyrosine, so tyrosine is an essential amino acid for these individuals (see *What a Scientist Sees* on page 171).

> **phenylketonuria (PKU)** A genetic disease in which the amino acid phenylalanine cannot be metabolized normally, causing it to build up in the blood. If untreated, the condition results in brain damage.

Protein Structure

To form proteins, amino acids are linked together by **peptide bonds**, which join the acid group of one amino acid to the amino group of another amino acid (**Figure 6.2c**). Many amino acids bonded together constitute a **polypeptide**. A protein is made up of one or more polypeptide chains that are folded into three-dimensional shapes. The order and chemical properties of the amino acids in a polypeptide

> **polypeptide** A chain of amino acids linked by peptide bonds that is part of the structure of a protein.

determine its final shape because the folding of the chain occurs in response to forces that attract or repel amino acids from one another or from water (**Figure 6.2d**). The folded polypeptide chain may constitute the final protein, or it may join with several other folded polypeptide chains to form the final structure of the protein (**Figure 6.2e**).

The shape of a protein is essential to its function. For example, the elongated shape of the protein collagen, found in connective tissue, helps it give strength to tendons and ligaments. The spherical shape of the protein hemoglobin

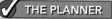
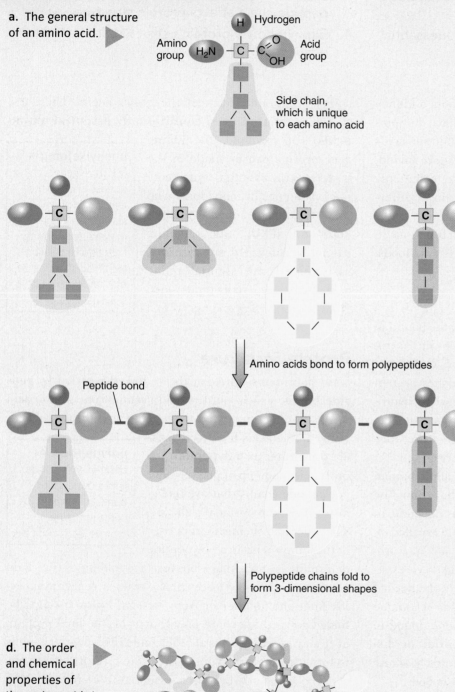

a. The general structure of an amino acid.

Hydrogen

Amino group H_2N

Acid group

Side chain, which is unique to each amino acid

Amino acids bond to form polypeptides

Peptide bond

Polypeptide chains fold to form 3-dimensional shapes

d. The order and chemical properties of the amino acids in a polypeptide chain determine how the polypeptide folds and, hence, the three-dimensional shape of the protein.

b. Twenty amino acids are commonly found in proteins. The table shown here lists them based on whether they are essential or nonessential and indicates those that are conditionally essential.

Essential Amino Acids	Nonessential Amino Acids
Histidine	Alanine
Isoleucine	Arginine*
Leucine	Asparagine
Lysine	Aspartic acid
Methionine	Cysteine*
Phenylalanine	Glutamic acid
Threonine	Glutamine*
Tryptophan	Glycine*
Valine	Proline*
	Serine
	Tyrosine*

*Considered conditionally essential by the Institute of Medicine, Food and Nutrition Board

c. Amino acids linked by peptide bonds are called **peptides**. When two amino acids are linked, they form a **dipeptide**; three form a **tripeptide**. Many amino acids bonded together constitute a polypeptide. Polypeptide chains may contain hundreds of amino acids.

e. The final structure of a protein molecule consists of one or more folded polypeptide chains.

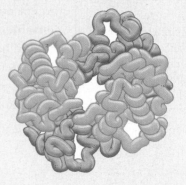

WHAT A SCIENTIST SEES

✓ THE PLANNER

Phenylketonuria

This warning on a can of diet soda probably doesn't mean much unless you have the genetic disease phenylketonuria (PKU). Individuals with PKU must limit their intake of the amino acid phenylalanine. Usually this means limiting their consumption of high-protein foods. When a scientist looks at this label, she recognizes that the artificial sweetener aspartame in this soda is the source of the phenylalanine. The breakdown of aspartame in the digestive tract releases phenylalanine, which cannot be properly metabolized by individuals with PKU. If they consume large amounts of this amino acid, compounds called phenylketones build up in their blood. In infants and young children, phenylketones interfere with brain development, and in pregnant women they cause birth defects in the baby. To prevent this, these individuals must consume a diet that provides just enough phenylalanine to meet the body's needs but not so much that phenylketones build up in their blood.

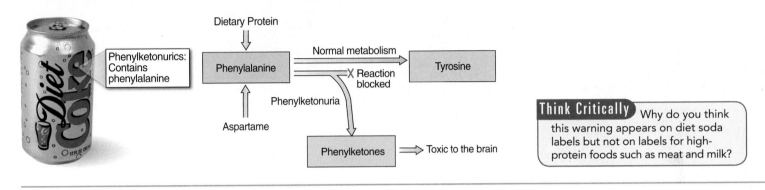

Think Critically Why do you think this warning appears on diet soda labels but not on labels for high-protein foods such as meat and milk?

---

contributes to the proper functioning of red blood cells, and the linear shape of muscle proteins allows them to overlap and shorten muscles during contraction.

Protein denaturation • Figure 6.3

When an egg is cooked, the heat denatures the protein. The protein in a raw egg white forms a clear, viscous liquid, but when cooking denatures it, the egg white becomes white and firm and cannot be restored to its original form. The denaturation of proteins in our food also creates other characteristics we desire. For example, whipped cream is made when mechanical agitation denatures the protein in cream.

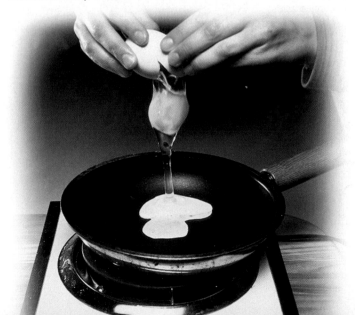

When the shape of a protein is altered, the protein no longer functions normally. For example, when the enzyme salivary amylase, which is a protein, enters the stomach, the acid causes the structure of the protein to change, and it no longer functions in the digestion of starch. This change in structure is called **denaturation**, referring to a change from the natural. Proteins in food are often denatured during processing and cooking (**Figure 6.3**).

> **denaturation** Alteration of a protein's three-dimensional structure.

CONCEPT CHECK 🛑 STOP

1. **Which** chemical elements are found in all amino acids?

2. **What** determines whether an amino acid must be consumed in the diet?

3. **What** determines the shape of a protein?

4. **How** does denaturation affect the function of proteins?

Protein digestion and absorption • Figure 6.4

Protein must be broken down into small peptides and amino acids to be absorbed into the mucosal cells.

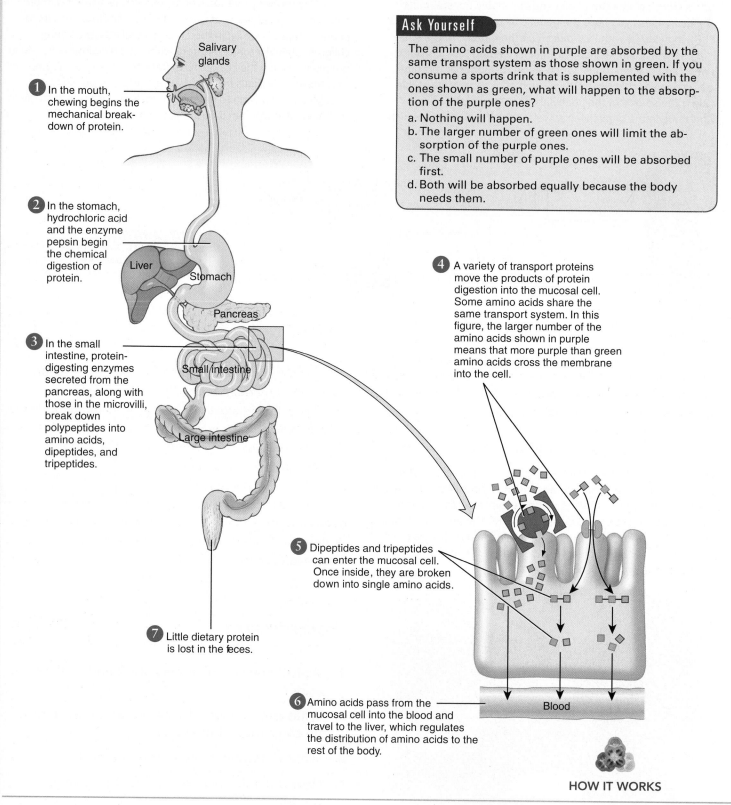

1 In the mouth, chewing begins the mechanical breakdown of protein.

2 In the stomach, hydrochloric acid and the enzyme pepsin begin the chemical digestion of protein.

3 In the small intestine, protein-digesting enzymes secreted from the pancreas, along with those in the microvilli, break down polypeptides into amino acids, dipeptides, and tripeptides.

7 Little dietary protein is lost in the feces.

Ask Yourself

The amino acids shown in purple are absorbed by the same transport system as those shown in green. If you consume a sports drink that is supplemented with the ones shown as green, what will happen to the absorption of the purple ones?

a. Nothing will happen.
b. The larger number of green ones will limit the absorption of the purple ones.
c. The small number of purple ones will be absorbed first.
d. Both will be absorbed equally because the body needs them.

4 A variety of transport proteins move the products of protein digestion into the mucosal cell. Some amino acids share the same transport system. In this figure, the larger number of the amino acids shown in purple means that more purple than green amino acids cross the membrane into the cell.

5 Dipeptides and tripeptides can enter the mucosal cell. Once inside, they are broken down into single amino acids.

6 Amino acids pass from the mucosal cell into the blood and travel to the liver, which regulates the distribution of amino acids to the rest of the body.

HOW IT WORKS

Protein Digestion and Absorption

LEARNING OBJECTIVES

1. **Describe** the process of protein digestion.
2. **Discuss** how amino acids are absorbed.

Proteins must be digested before their amino acids can be absorbed into the body (**Figure 6.4**). The chemical digestion of protein begins in the acid environment of the stomach. Here, hydrochloric acid denatures proteins, opening up their folded structure to make the polypeptide chains more accessible for breakdown by enzymes. Stomach acid also activates the protein-digesting enzyme *pepsin*, which breaks some of the peptide bonds in the polypeptide chains, leaving shorter polypeptides. Most protein digestion occurs in the small intestine, where polypeptides are broken into even smaller peptides and amino acids by protein-digesting enzymes produced in the pancreas and small intestine. Single amino acids, dipeptides, and tripeptides are absorbed into the mucosal cells of the small intestine.

Amino acids enter your body by crossing from the lumen of the small intestine into the mucosal cells and then into the blood. This process involves one of several energy-requiring amino acid transport systems. Amino acids with similar structures use the same transport system (see Figure 6.4). As a result, amino acids may compete with one another for absorption. If there is an excess of any one of the amino acids sharing a transport system, more of it will be absorbed, slowing the absorption of competing amino acids. This competition for absorption is usually not a problem because foods contain a variety of amino acids, none of which are present in excessive amounts. However, when people consume amino acid supplements, the supplemented amino acid may overwhelm the transport system, reducing the absorption of other amino acids that share the same transport system. For example, weight lifters often take supplements of the amino acid arginine. Because arginine shares a transport system with lysine, large doses of arginine can inhibit the absorption of lysine, upsetting the balance of amino acids in the body.

CONCEPT CHECK 　　　　　　　　　　　　　　 **STOP**

1. **Where** does the chemical digestion of protein begin?

2. **Why** might supplementing one amino acid reduce the absorption of other amino acids?

Protein Synthesis and Functions

LEARNING OBJECTIVES

1. **Discuss** the steps involved in synthesizing proteins.
2. **Explain** what is meant by the term limiting amino acid.
3. **Name** four functions of body proteins.
4. **Describe** the conditions under which the body uses protein to provide energy.

As discussed earlier, proteins are made from amino acids. Amino acids are also used to make other nitrogen-containing molecules, including neurotransmitters; the units that make up DNA and RNA; the skin pigment melanin; the vitamin niacin; creatine phosphate, which is used to fuel muscle contraction; and histamine, which causes blood vessels to dilate. In some situations, amino acids from proteins are also used to provide energy or synthesize glucose or fatty acids.

The amino acids available for these functions come from the proteins consumed in the diet and from the

amino acid pool All the amino acids in body tissues and fluids that are available for use by the body.

breakdown of body proteins. These amino acids are referred to collectively as the **amino acid pool** (**Figure 6.5**). There is not actually a "pool" in the body containing a collection of amino acids, but these molecules are available in body fluids and cells to provide the raw materials needed to synthesize proteins and other molecules.

Synthesizing Proteins

gene A length of DNA that contains the information needed to synthesize a polypeptide chain.

The instructions for making proteins are contained in the nucleus of the cell in stretches of DNA called **genes**. When a protein is needed, the process of protein synthesis begins, and the information contained in the gene is used to make the necessary protein (**Figure 6.6**).

Regulating protein synthesis The types of proteins made and when they are made are carefully regulated by increasing or decreasing **gene expression**. When a gene is expressed, the protein it codes for is made. Not all genes are expressed in all cells or at all times; only the proteins that are needed are made at any given time. This allows the body to save energy and resources. For example, when your diet is high in iron, expression of the gene that codes for the protein ferritin, which stores iron, is increased.

This causes more ferritin to be synthesized and allows the body to store extra iron in this protein. When the diet is low in iron, the production of ferritin is suppressed so that the body doesn't waste amino acids and energy making large amounts of a protein that it doesn't need.

Limiting amino acids During the synthesis of a protein, a shortage of one amino acid can stop the process. This is similar to an assembly line, where if one part is missing, the line stops; a different part cannot be substituted. If the missing amino acid is a nonessential amino acid, it can be made in the body, and protein synthesis can continue. Most nonessential amino acids are made through a process called **transamination**, which involves transferring the amino group from one amino acid to a carbon-containing molecule to form the needed amino acid (**Figure 6.6a**). If the missing amino acid is an essential amino acid, the body cannot make the amino acid, but it can break down its own protein to obtain it. If an amino acid cannot be supplied, protein synthesis will stop.

transamination The process by which an amino group from one amino acid is transferred to a carbon compound to form a new amino acid.

limiting amino acid The essential amino acid that is available in the lowest concentration relative to the body's need.

The essential amino acid that is present in shortest supply relative to the body's need for it is called the **limiting amino acid** because lack of this amino acid limits the ability to synthesize protein (**Figure 6.6c**). Different food sources of protein

Amino acid pool • Figure 6.5

Amino acids enter the available pool from the diet and from the breakdown of body proteins. Of the approximately 300 grams of protein synthesized by the body each day, only about 100 g are made from amino acids consumed in the diet. The other 200 g are produced by the recycling of amino acids from protein broken down in the body. Amino acids in the pool can be used to synthesize body proteins and other nitrogen-containing molecules, to provide energy, or to synthesize glucose or fatty acids.

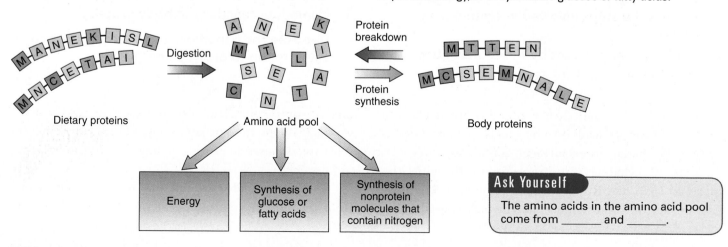

Dietary proteins → Digestion → Amino acid pool → Protein synthesis / Protein breakdown → Body proteins

Energy | Synthesis of glucose or fatty acids | Synthesis of nonprotein molecules that contain nitrogen

Ask Yourself
The amino acids in the amino acid pool come from _____ and _____.

a. Protein is synthesized from amino acids. These protein building blocks come from the diet and from the breakdown of body proteins.

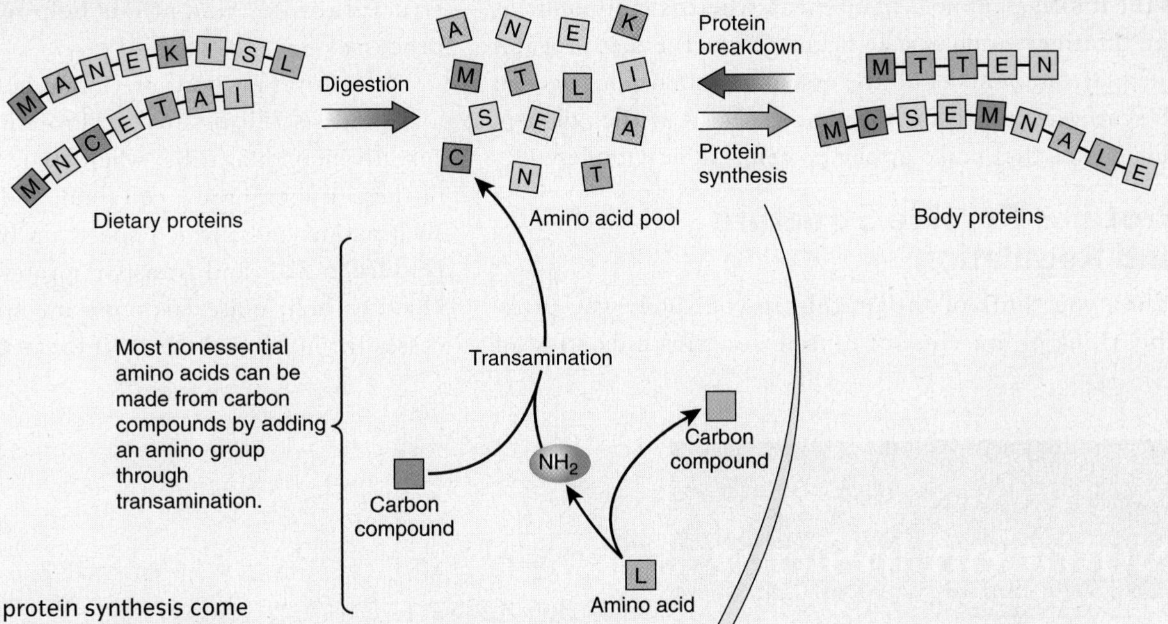

Dietary proteins

Digestion →

Amino acid pool

← Protein breakdown

→ Protein synthesis

Body proteins

Most nonessential amino acids can be made from carbon compounds by adding an amino group through transamination.

Transamination

Carbon compound

NH₂

Carbon compound

Amino acid

L

b. The instructions for protein synthesis come from genes. The process of protein synthesis involves **transcription** and **translation**.

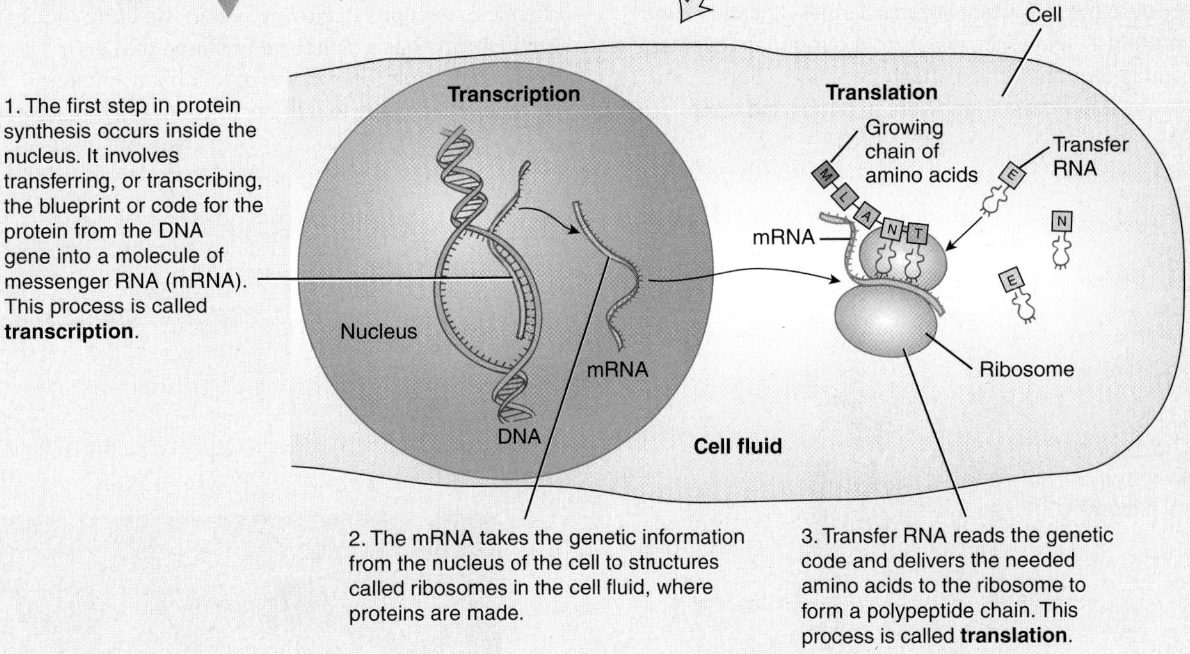

1. The first step in protein synthesis occurs inside the nucleus. It involves transferring, or transcribing, the blueprint or code for the protein from the DNA gene into a molecule of messenger RNA (mRNA). This process is called **transcription**.

Cell

Transcription

Translation

Growing chain of amino acids

Transfer RNA

mRNA

Nucleus

mRNA

DNA

Cell fluid

Ribosome

2. The mRNA takes the genetic information from the nucleus of the cell to structures called ribosomes in the cell fluid, where proteins are made.

3. Transfer RNA reads the genetic code and delivers the needed amino acids to the ribosome to form a polypeptide chain. This process is called **translation**.

c. The amino acids needed for protein synthesis come from the amino acid pool. If the protein to be made requires more of a particular amino acid than is available, that amino acid limits protein synthesis and is referred to as the *limiting amino acid*.

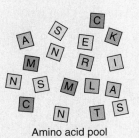

Amino acid pool

A shortage of amino acid A, represented by the orange squares, limits the ability to synthesize a protein that is high in this amino acid.

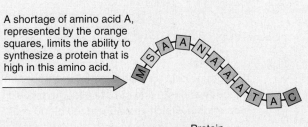

Protein

provide different combinations of amino acids. The limiting amino acid in a food is the one supplied in the lowest amount relative to the body's need. For example, lysine is the limiting amino acid in wheat, whereas methionine is the limiting amino acid in beans. When the diet provides adequate amounts of all the essential amino acids needed to synthesize a specific protein, synthesis of the polypeptide chains that make up the protein can be completed.

Proteins Provide Structure and Regulation

When you think of the protein in your body, you probably think of muscle, but muscle contains only a few of the many types of proteins found in your body. There are more than 500,000 proteins in the human body, each with a specific function. Some perform important structural roles, and others help regulate specific body processes.

Structural proteins are found in skin, hair, ligaments, and tendons (**Figure 6.7a**). Proteins also provide structure to individual cells, where they are an integral part of the cell membrane, cell fluid, and organelles. Proteins such as enzymes, which speed up biochemical reactions (**Figure 6.7b**), and transport proteins that travel in the blood or help materials cross membranes, regulate processes throughout the body (**Figure 6.7c**).

Nutrition InSight   Protein functions • Figure 6.7

a. Collagen, which is the most abundant protein in the body, plays important structural roles. It is the major protein in ligaments, which hold our bones together, and in tendons, which attach muscles to bones, and it forms the protein framework of bones and teeth.

b. Enzymes, such as this one, are protein molecules. Almost all the chemical reactions occurring within the body require the help of enzymes. Each enzyme has a structure or shape that allows it to interact with the specific molecules in the reaction it accelerates. Without enzymes, metabolic reactions would occur too slowly to support life.

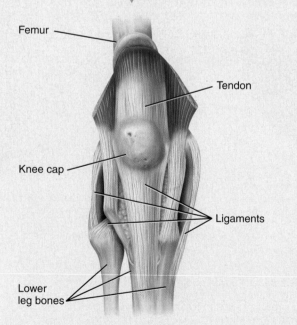

Femur

Tendon

Knee cap

Ligaments

Lower leg bones

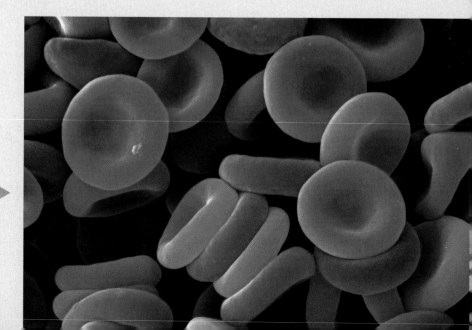

Enzyme

Enzyme

c. Proteins help transport materials throughout the body and into and out of cells. The protein hemoglobin, which gives these red blood cells their color, shuttles oxygen to body cells and carries away carbon dioxide.

Proteins are an important part of the body's defense mechanisms. Skin, which is made up primarily of protein, is the first barrier against infection and injury. Foreign particles such as dirt or bacteria that are on the skin cannot enter the body and can be washed away. If the skin is broken and blood vessels are injured, blood-clotting proteins help prevent too much blood from being lost. If a foreign material does get into the body, *antibodies*, which are immune system proteins, help destroy it (**Figure 6.7d**).

Some proteins have contractile properties, which allow muscles to move various parts of the body (**Figure 6.7e**). Others are hormones, which regulate biological processes.

The hormones insulin, growth hormone, and glucagon are made from amino acids. These protein hormones act rapidly because they affect the activity of proteins that are already present in the cell.

Proteins also help regulate fluid balance (**Figure 6.7f**) and prevent the level of acidity in body fluids from deviating from the normal range. The chemical reactions of metabolism require a specific level of acidity, or pH, to function properly. Inside the body, pH must be maintained at a relatively neutral level in order to allow metabolic reactions to proceed normally. If the pH changes, these reactions slow or stop. Proteins both within cells and in the blood help prevent large changes in pH.

THE PLANNER

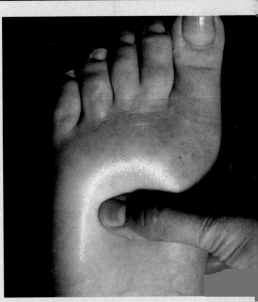

e. Proteins help us move. The proteins actin and myosin in the arm and leg muscles of this rock climber are able to slide past each other to contract the muscles. A similar process causes contraction in the heart muscle and in the muscles of the digestive tract, blood vessels, and body glands. ▼

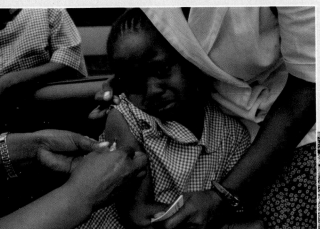

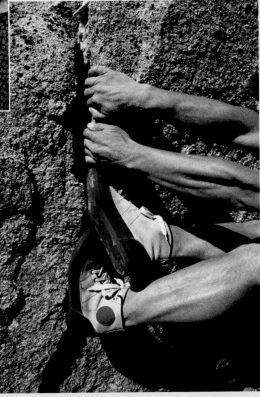

d. Proteins help protect us from disease. This child is being immunized against measles. The vaccine contains a small amount of dead or inactivated measles virus. It does not make the child sick, but it does stimulate his immune system to make proteins called *antibodies*, which help destroy the measles virus and prevent the child from contracting the disease.

f. Proteins help regulate fluid balance through their effect on *osmosis*. Blood proteins help hold fluid in the blood because they contribute to the number of dissolved particles in the blood. If protein levels in the blood fall too low, water leaks out of the blood vessels and accumulates in the tissues, causing swelling known as **edema**, shown here. Proteins also regulate fluid balance because some are membrane transporters, which pump dissolved substances from one side of a membrane to the other.

Producing ATP from amino acids • Figure 6.8

Amino acids from dietary or body protein can be used to produce ATP. First, the amino group (NH_2) must be removed through a process called **deamination**. The remaining compound, composed of carbon, hydrogen, and oxygen, can then be broken down to produce ATP or used to make glucose or fatty acids.

① The amino group is removed by deamination and converted into the waste product **urea**. Urea is removed from the blood by the kidneys and excreted in the urine.

② Deamination of some amino acids results in three-carbon molecules that can be used to synthesize glucose.

③ Deamination of some amino acids results in acetyl-CoA that enters the citric acid cycle.

④ Deamination of some amino acids forms molecules that enter the citric acid cycle directly.

⑤ The acetyl-CoA derived from the breakdown of amino acids can be used to synthesize fatty acids. This occurs when calories are consumed in excess of needs.

⑥ In the final step of aerobic metabolism, the energy from the amino acid molecules is trapped and used to produce ATP.

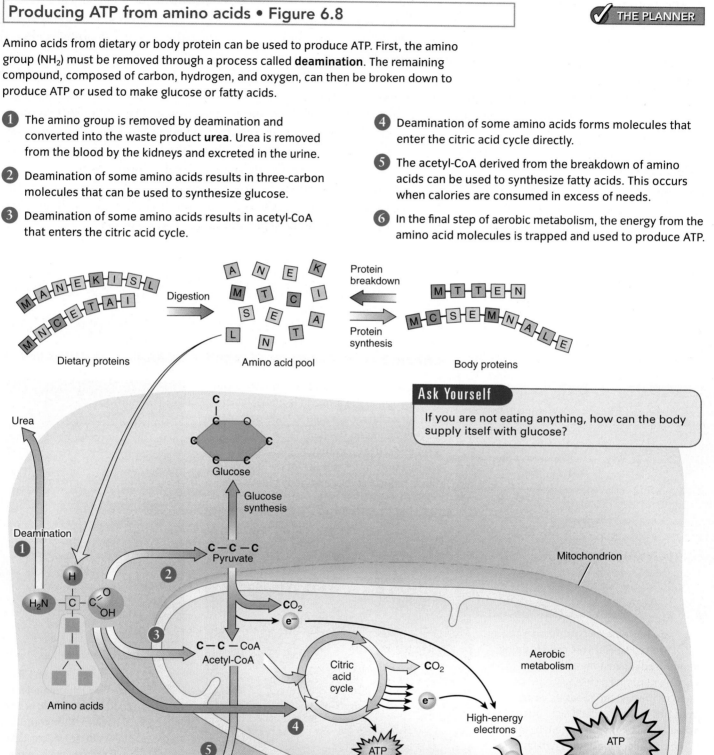

Ask Yourself

If you are not eating anything, how can the body supply itself with glucose?

Protein as a Source of Energy

In addition to all the essential functions performed by body proteins, under some circumstances, proteins can be broken down and their amino acids used to provide energy or synthesize glucose or fatty acids (**Figure 6.8**). When the diet does not provide enough energy to meet the body's needs, such as during starvation or when consuming a weight-loss diet, body protein is used to provide energy. Because our bodies do not store protein, functional body proteins, such as enzymes and muscle proteins, must be broken down to yield amino acids, which can then be used as fuel or to make glucose. This ensures that cells have a constant energy supply but also robs the body of the functions performed by these proteins.

Amino acids are also used for energy when the amount of protein consumed in the diet is greater than that needed to make body proteins and other molecules. This occurs in most Americans every day because our typical diet contains more protein than we need. The body first uses amino acids from the diet to make body proteins and other nitrogen-containing molecules. Then, because extra amino acids can't be stored, they are metabolized to provide energy. When your diet includes more calories than you need, amino acids can be converted into fatty acids, which are stored as triglycerides, thus contributing to weight gain.

CONCEPT CHECK 🛑 STOP

1. **How** does the body know in what order to assemble the amino acids when making a protein?
2. **Why** does protein synthesis stop when the supply of an amino acid is limited?
3. **What** type of protein speeds up chemical reactions?
4. **When** is protein used as an energy source?

Protein in Health and Disease

LEARNING OBJECTIVES

1. **Distinguish** kwashiorkor from marasmus.
2. **Explain** why protein-energy malnutrition is more common in children than in adults.
3. **Discuss** the potential risks associated with high-protein diets.
4. **Explain** how a dietary protein can trigger a food allergy.

We need to eat protein to stay healthy. If we don't eat enough of it, less-essential body proteins are broken down, and their amino acids are used to synthesize proteins that are critical for survival. For example, when the diet is deficient in protein, muscle protein is broken down to provide amino acids to make hormones and enzymes for which there is an immediate need. If protein deficiency continues, eventually so much body protein is lost that all life-sustaining functions cannot be supported. In some cases, too much protein or the wrong proteins can also contribute to health problems.

Protein Deficiency

Protein deficiency is a great concern in the developing world but generally not a problem in economically developed societies, where plant and animal sources of protein are abundant. Usually, protein deficiency occurs along with a general lack of food and other nutrients. The term **protein-energy malnutrition (PEM)** is used to refer to a continuum of

protein-energy malnutrition (PEM) A condition characterized by loss of muscle and fat mass and an increased susceptibility to infection that results from the long-term consumption of insufficient amounts of energy and/or protein to meet the body's needs.

conditions ranging from pure protein deficiency, called **kwashiorkor**, to an overall energy deficiency, called **marasmus** (**Figure 6.9**).

Protein deficiency occurs when the diet is very low in protein or when protein needs are high, as they are in young children. Hence, kwashiorkor is typically a disease found in children (**Figure 6.9a**). The word *kwashiorkor* comes from the Ga tribe of the African Gold

Protein-energy malnutrition • Figure 6.9

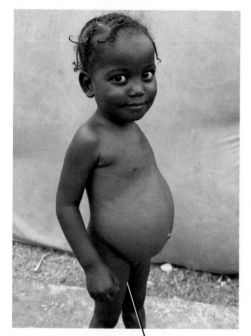

a. Kwashiorkor, seen in this child from Haiti, is characterized by a swollen belly, which results from fluid accumulating in the abdomen and fat accumulating in the liver. Growth is impaired, but because energy intake is not necessarily low, the child may not appear extremely thin. The lack of protein also causes poor immune function and an increase in infections, changes in hair color, and impaired nutrient absorption.

b. Marasmus, seen in this Somalian boy, is characterized by depletion of fat stores and wasting of muscle. It has devastating effects on infants because most brain growth takes place in the first year of life; malnutrition in the first year causes decreases in intelligence and learning ability that persist throughout the individual's life.

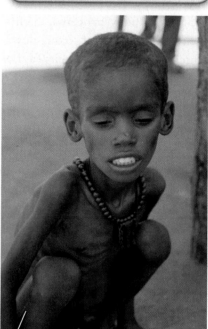

c. Protein-energy malnutrition is uncommon in the United States and other developed nations, but in developing countries, it is a serious public health problem that results in high infant and child mortality. The highest prevalence is in sub-Saharan Africa and south Asia.

% of population undernourished

- 35%
- 20–34%
- 5–19%
- 2.5–4%
- <2.5%
- No data

Coast. It means "the disease that the first child gets when a second child is born."[1] When the new baby is born, the older child is no longer breast-fed. Rather than receiving protein-rich breast milk, the young child is fed a watered-down version of the diet eaten by the rest of the family. This diet is low in protein and often high in fiber and difficult to digest. The child, even if he or she is able to obtain adequate calories from the diet, may not be able to eat a large enough quantity to get adequate protein. Because children are growing, their protein needs per unit of body weight are higher than those of adults, and a deficiency occurs more quickly.

At the other end of the continuum of protein-energy malnutrition is marasmus, meaning "to waste away" (**Figure 6.9b**). Marasmus is caused by starvation; the diet doesn't supply enough calories or nutrients to meet the body's needs. Marasmus may have some of the same symptoms as kwashiorkor, but there are differences. In kwashiorkor, some fat stores are retained because energy intake is adequate. In marasmus, individuals appear emaciated because their stores of body fat have been depleted to provide energy. Although they are most common in children, both marasmus and kwashiorkor can occur in individuals of all ages.

High-Protein Diets and Health

The recent popularity of high-protein, low-carbohydrate diets for weight loss (see Chapters 4 and 9) has raised questions about whether consuming too much protein can be harmful. As protein intake increases, so does the production of protein-breakdown products, such as urea, which must be eliminated from the body by the kidneys. To excrete more waste, more water must be lost in the urine. High-protein diets therefore increase water loss. Although not a concern for most people, this can be a problem if the kidneys are not able to concentrate urine, as is the case for infants. Feeding a newborn an infant formula that is too high in protein increases the amount of water lost in the urine and can lead to dehydration. High protein intake may also be detrimental for people with kidney disease; the increased wastes produced with a high-protein diet may speed the progression of renal failure. However, there is no evidence that a high-protein diet will precipitate kidney disease in a person with normal kidney function.[2]

It has also been suggested that the amount and source of protein in the diet affect calcium status and bone health.[3] Adequate protein is essential for healthy

bones, but too much protein has been shown to increase the amount of calcium lost in the urine. Some studies suggest that the amount of calcium lost in the urine is greater when protein comes from animal rather than vegetable sources.[3] These findings have contributed to a widely held belief that high-protein diets (especially diets that are high in animal protein) result in bone loss. However, clinical studies do not support the idea that animal protein has a detrimental effect on bone health or that vegetable-based proteins are better for bone health.[3,4] In fact, when calcium intake is adequate, high-protein diets are associated with greater bone mass and fewer fractures.[3] This is likely the case because in healthy adults, a high protein intake increases intestinal calcium absorption as well as urinary excretion, so the increase in the amount of calcium lost in the urine does not cause an overall loss of body calcium.

The increase in urinary calcium excretion associated with high-protein diets has led to speculation that a high protein intake may increase the risk of kidney stones. Kidney stones are deposits of calcium and other substances in the kidneys and urinary tract. Higher concentrations of calcium and acid in the urine increase the likelihood that the calcium will be deposited, forming these stones. Epidemiological studies suggest that diets that are rich in animal protein and low in fluid contribute to the formation of kidney stones.[5]

The best-documented concern with high-protein diets is related more to the rest of the diet than to the amount of protein consumed. Typically, high-protein diets are also high in animal products; this dietary pattern is high in saturated fat and cholesterol and low in fiber, and it therefore increases the risk of heart disease. These diets are also typically low in grains, vegetables, and fruits, a pattern associated with an increased risk of cancer.[6]

Proteins and Food Allergies and Intolerances

When a protein from the diet is absorbed without being completely digested, it can trigger a **food allergy**. The first time the protein is consumed and a piece of it is absorbed intact, it stimulates the immune system. When the same protein is consumed again, the immune system sees it as a foreign substance and mounts an attack, causing an allergic reaction (see Chapter 3). Allergic reactions cause symptoms throughout the body and can be life threatening. The proteins from milk, eggs, peanuts, tree

food allergy An adverse immune response to a specific food protein.

Food allergy labeling • Figure 6.10

Food labels provide life-saving information for individuals with food allergies. A label must indicate whether the product contains any of the eight major food allergens: milk, eggs, peanuts, tree nuts, fish, shellfish, soy, and wheat. Sometimes these are just included in the ingredient list, but often, as on this label, they are also highlighted at the end of the list in a statement such as "Contains soy ingredients." Warnings such as "manufactured in a facility that processes peanuts" are included on products that may be cross-contaminated with these allergens.

Ask Yourself

If you had an allergy to soy, would this soup be a safe choice?

The ingredient list includes sources of protein in food as well as sources of **hydrolyzed protein** or **protein hydrolysates**. These are proteins that have been treated with acid or enzymes to break them down into amino acids and small peptides. They are added as flavorings, flavor enhancers, stabilizers, and thickening agents.

INGREDIENTS: CHICKEN BROTH, CARROTS, COOKED WHITE CHICKEN MEAT (WHITE CHICKEN MEAT, WATER, SALT, SODIUM PHOSPHATE, ISOLATED SOY PROTEIN, MODIFIED CORN STARCH, CORN STARCH, CARRAGEENAN), TOMATOES, WILD RICE, RICE, CELERY. LESS THAN 2% OF: SALT, MONOSODIUM GLUTAMATE, HYDROLYZED CORN PROTEIN, CHICKEN FAT, ONION POWDER, AUTOLYZED YEAST EXTRACT, PARSLEY FLAKES, NATURAL FLAVOR. **CONTAINS SOY INGREDIENTS.**

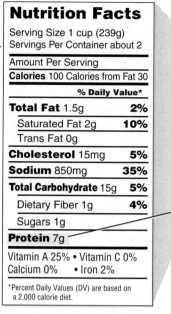

Nutrition Facts

Serving Size 1 cup (239g)
Servings Per Container about 2

Amount Per Serving	
Calories 100	Calories from Fat 30

	% Daily Value*
Total Fat 1.5g	2%
Saturated Fat 2g	10%
Trans Fat 0g	
Cholesterol 15mg	5%
Sodium 850mg	35%
Total Carbohydrate 15g	5%
Dietary Fiber 1g	4%
Sugars 1g	
Protein 7g	

Vitamin A 25% • Vitamin C 0%
Calcium 0% • Iron 2%

*Percent Daily Values (DV) are based on a 2,000 calorie diet.

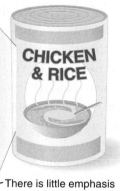

There is little emphasis on protein in the Nutrition Facts panel, where the grams of protein are given without any % Daily Value. A % Daily Value for protein is required only on products that make a claim about the product's protein content.

---

nuts, wheat, soy, fish, and shellfish are common causes of food allergies (**Figure 6.10**).

Not all adverse reactions to proteins and amino acids are due to allergies; some are due to **food intolerances**, also called **food sensitivities**. These reactions do not involve the immune system. The symptoms of a food intolerance can range from minor discomfort, such as the abdominal distress some people feel after eating raw onions, to more severe reactions. For example, some people report having a reaction after consuming **monosodium glutamate (MSG)**. MSG is a flavor enhancer made up of the amino acid glutamic acid bound to sodium. It is used in meat tenderizers and commonly added to Chinese food. Although research has been unable to confirm that MSG ingestion causes any adverse reactions, some people report experiencing a collection of symptoms such as flushed face, tingling or burning sensations, headache, rapid heartbeat, chest pain, and general weakness that are collectively referred to as **MSG symptom complex**, commonly called **Chinese restaurant syndrome**.[7] Sensitive individuals should ask for food to be prepared without added MSG and should check ingredient lists for monosodium glutamate or potassium glutamate before consuming packaged foods.

food intolerance or **food sensitivity** An adverse reaction to a food that does not involve the production of antibodies by the immune system.

Gluten intolerance, also called **celiac disease**, celiac sprue, or gluten-sensitive enteropathy, is another form of food intolerance (see Chapter 3). Individuals with celiac disease cannot tolerate gluten, a protein found in wheat, rye, and barley. Celiac disease is an autoimmune disease in which gluten causes the body to attack the villi in the small intestine, causing symptoms such as diarrhea, abdominal bloating and cramps, weight loss, and anemia. Once thought to be a rare childhood disease, it is now known to affect more than 2 million people in the United States.[8] The only treatment is to avoid gluten by eliminating from the diet all products containing wheat, rye, or barley and proteins isolated from these foods.

celiac disease A disorder that causes damage to the intestines when the protein gluten is eaten.

CONCEPT CHECK   STOP

1. **Why** do children with marasmus appear more emaciated than those with kwashiorkor?

2. **Why** is kwashiorkor more common in children than in adults?

3. **Who** should be concerned about excessive protein intake?

4. **How** can allergic reactions to food be avoided?

Meeting Protein Needs

LEARNING OBJECTIVES

1. **Describe** how protein needs are determined.
2. **Explain** what is meant by protein quality.
3. **Review** a diet and replace the animal proteins with complementary plant proteins.
4. **Discuss** the benefits and risks of vegetarian diets.

In order to stay healthy, you have to eat enough protein to replace the amount you lose every day. Most Americans get plenty of protein, and healthy diets can contain a wide range of intakes from both plant and animal sources. An individual's protein needs may be increased by growth, injury, and illness, as well as by some types of physical activity.

Balancing Protein Intake and Losses

Current protein intake recommendations are based on **nitrogen balance** studies. These studies compare the amount of nitrogen consumed with the amount excreted. Studying nitrogen balance allows researchers to evaluate protein balance because most of the nitrogen we consume comes from dietary protein. Most of the nitrogen we lose is excreted in urine.

> **nitrogen balance**
> The amount of nitrogen consumed in the diet compared with the amount excreted over a given period.

Smaller amounts are lost in feces, skin, sweat, menstrual fluids, hair, and nails. When your body is in nitrogen balance, your nitrogen intake equals your nitrogen losses; in other words, you are consuming enough protein to replace losses. You are not gaining or losing body protein; you are maintaining it at a constant level. Nitrogen balance is negative if you're losing body protein and positive if the amount of body protein is increasing (**Figure 6.11**).

Nitrogen balance • Figure 6.11

a. Nitrogen balance
Nitrogen intake = Nitrogen output. This indicates that the amount of protein being synthesized is equal to the amount being broken down, so the total amount of protein in the body is not changing. Healthy adults who consume adequate amounts of protein and are maintaining a constant body weight are in nitrogen balance.

Nitrogen intake

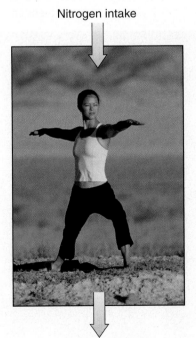

Nitrogen output

b. Negative nitrogen balance
Nitrogen intake < Nitrogen output. This indicates that more protein is being broken down than is being synthesized so body protein is decreasing. Negative nitrogen balance occurs due to injury or illness as well as when the diet is too low in protein or calories.

Nitrogen intake

Nitrogen output

c. Positive nitrogen balance
Nitrogen intake > Nitrogen output. This indicates that there is more protein synthesis than degradation so the body is gaining protein. This occurs when the body is growing, during pregnancy, and in individuals who are increasing their muscle mass by lifting weights.

Nitrogen intake

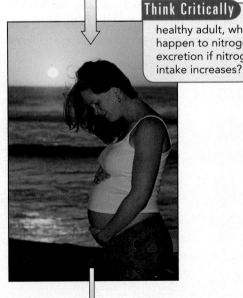

Think Critically In a healthy adult, what will happen to nitrogen excretion if nitrogen intake increases?

Nitrogen output

Protein requirements • Figure 6.12

During the first year of life, growth is rapid, so a large amount of protein is required per unit of body weight. As growth rate slows, requirements per unit of body weight decrease, but continue to be greater than adult requirements, until age 19.

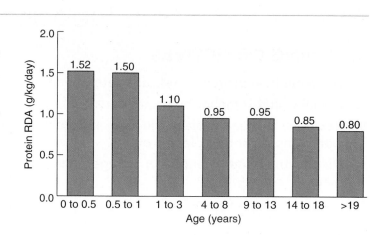

Interpreting Data

What is the RDA for a 2-year-old child who weighs 14 kg?
a. 14 g/day
b. 15.4 g/day
c. 11.2 g/day
d. 21 g/day

Recommended Protein Intake

Most of us eat more protein than we need: The typical young adult in the United States consumes about 90 g of protein/day.[9] The RDA for protein for adults is 0.8 g/kg of body weight. For a person weighing 70 kg (154 lb), the RDA is 56 g of protein/day. RDAs have also been developed for each of the essential amino acids;[2] these are not a concern in typical diet planning but are important when developing solutions for intravenous feeding.

Protein recommendations are expressed per unit of body weight because protein is needed to maintain and repair the body. The more a person weighs, the more protein he or she needs for those purposes. Because children are small, they need less total protein than adults do, but because new protein must be synthesized for growth to occur, protein requirements per unit of body weight are much greater for infants and children than for adults (**Figure 6.12**). To calculate protein needs per day, multiply weight in kilograms (which equals weight in pounds multiplied by 0.45) by the recommended amount for the individual's age.

Protein needs are also increased during pregnancy and lactation. Additional protein is needed during pregnancy to support the expansion of maternal blood volume,

Protein needs of athletes • Figure 6.13

a. Endurance athletes need extra protein because some protein is used for energy and to maintain blood glucose during endurance events, such as triathlons and long distance cross country skiing. Endurance athletes may benefit from the daily consumption of 1.2 to 1.4 g/kg of body weight.[10]

b. Strength athletes, such as weight lifters and body builders, need extra protein because it provides the raw materials needed for muscle growth; 1.2 to 1.7 g/kg/day is recommended.[10]

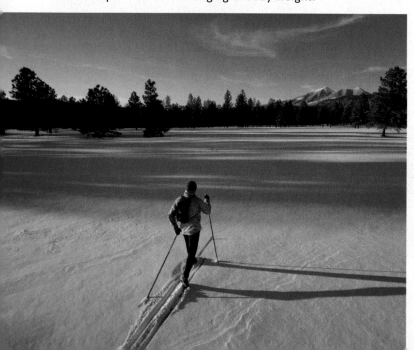

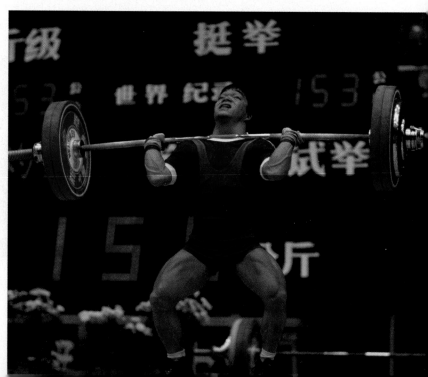

the growth of the uterus and breasts, the formation of the placenta, and the growth and development of the fetus. The RDA for pregnant women is 25 g of protein/day higher than the recommendation for nonpregnant women. An extra 25 g/day is also needed during lactation to provide protein for the production of breast milk.

Extreme stresses on the body, such as infections, fevers, burns, or surgery, increase the amount of protein that is broken down. For the body to heal and rebuild, the amount of protein lost must be replaced. The extra amount needed for healing depends on the injury. A severe infection may increase the body's protein needs by about 30%; a serious burn can increase protein requirements by 200 to 400%.

Although most athletes can meet their protein needs by consuming the RDA of 0.8 g/kg of body weight, extreme endurance athletes and strength athletes benefit from higher protein intakes (**Figure 6.13**).[10] Athletes often think they need supplements to meet their higher protein needs (**Figure 6.14**). However, supplements tend to be an expensive way to increase protein intake. Because athletes

Protein and amino acid supplements • Figure 6.14

Protein and amino acid supplements are rarely needed to meet protein needs. Nonetheless, supplements are marketed to boost total protein intake, to add individual amino acids, and to provide enzyme activity.

Protein supplements are marketed to promote proper immune function, make hair healthy, and stimulate muscle growth, but increasing protein intake above the level required for good health does not protect you from disease, make your hair shine, or give you larger biceps.

Many promises are made about amino acid supplements, from aiding sleep to enhancing athletic performance. There is weak evidence to support some of these, but consuming large amounts of one amino acid may interfere with the absorption of others. Due to insufficient research, no ULs have been set for amino acids.

Supplements of enzymes that function inside body tissues provide no benefits because the enzyme is broken down into amino acids during digestion. Supplements of enzymes that function in the gut, such as lactase for lactose intolerance, retain enzyme activity long enough to breakdown the lactose but are also eventually digested.

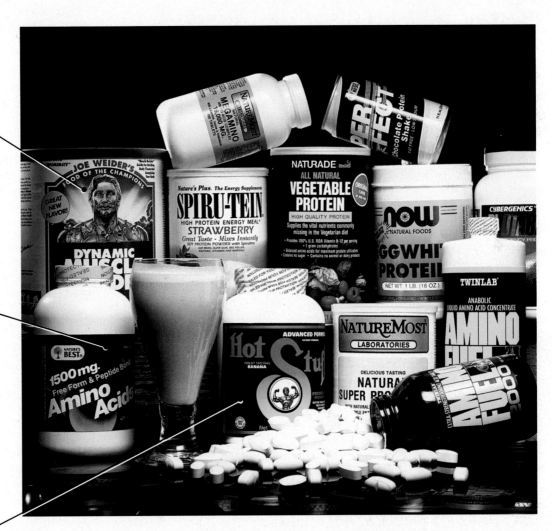

typically need to consume more calories to meet their energy needs, they also consume more dietary protein and can easily meet their protein needs through diet alone.

In addition to the RDA, the DRIs include a recommendation for protein intake as a percentage of calories: The Acceptable Macronutrient Distribution Range for protein is 10 to 35% of calories.[2] This range allows for different food preferences and eating patterns. A protein intake in this range will meet protein needs and allow sufficient intakes of other nutrients to promote health. A diet that provides 10% of calories from protein will meet the RDA but is a relatively low-protein diet compared with typical eating patterns in the United States. The upper end of this healthy range—35% of calories—is a relatively high-protein diet, about twice as much protein as the average American eats. This amount of protein is not harmful, but if the diet is this high in protein, it is probably high in animal products, which tend to be high in saturated fat and cholesterol. Therefore, unless protein sources are chosen carefully, a diet that contains 35% protein would tend to include more saturated fat and cholesterol than would a diet with the same number of calories that contains only 10% protein. For example, a 2500-Calorie diet that provides 35% of calories from protein would include the protein equivalent of a 16-oz steak and 2 quarts of milk daily.

Debate Should You Switch to Soy?

The Issue: Many people have switched from cow's milk to soy milk and chosen to snack on edamame (boiled green soybeans), soy nuts, and soy-based protein bars. Will increasing your intake of soy benefit your health or cause health problems?

Soy is found in many traditional Asian foods, such as tofu and miso, and it is used as a meat substitute in vegetarian hotdogs and chicken nuggets. A high intake of soy has been linked to a lower incidence of heart disease, type 2 diabetes, osteoporosis, and certain types of cancer.[12] This association has contributed to a dramatic rise in the number of available soy products; more than 2700 new foods with soy as an ingredient were introduced between 2000 and 2007.[13] But there has also been concern about the safety of soy for certain segments of the population. So should we be adding tofu to our soups, salads, and stir-fries; spreading soy butter on our toast; and snacking on soy protein bars?

Soy provides high-quality protein—comparable to the protein in eggs and milk. Soy products are also high in healthy polyunsaturated fat, fiber, vitamins, and minerals, and they are low in unhealthy saturated fat. Soy protein is believed to lower blood lipid levels. The FDA has even approved a food label health claim related to soy intake and a lower risk of heart disease. Soy also provides phytochemicals called *isoflavones*, which have estrogen-like effects. This has led to speculation that consuming soy isoflavones will reduce the symptoms of menopause (including hot flashes), reduce bone loss, and have preventive effects in terms of certain forms of cancer, including breast cancer.

It sounds like we should all switch to soy. However, a more careful look at the research on soy suggests that it may not be as beneficial as initially hoped, and there is now concern that it might not be safe for everyone. A review of the effect of soy on blood cholesterol concluded that it has only a small LDL cholesterol-lowering effect, and this occurs only when large amounts, about 50 g/day, are consumed.[14] But, because soy contains substances that may interfere with thyroid gland function, overconsumption has been accused of contributing to low levels of thyroid hormones in individuals with compromised thyroid function and/or whose iodine intake is marginal.[15] The health effects of those estrogen-like soy isoflavones are also confusing. Clinical trials support a role of isoflavones in the prevention of bone loss, but results are inconsistent.[16] Research has not shown soy to reduce the symptoms of menopause.[16] Isoflavones have been found to promote the growth of breast tumors in animals, and therefore women who have breast cancer are typically advised to avoid soy.[17] In women who do not have breast cancer, soy appears to be protective if it is consumed in moderate amounts throughout life, but switching to soy milk after menopause may have no effect.[17]

So, is soy good for you? Choosing soy products, such as those shown in the photo, will provide plant protein equivalent in quality to animal proteins, and can help you meet your protein needs without much saturated fat. High intakes of soy may help reduce the risk of heart disease. But it is not clear what effect these amounts will have on breast cancer risk or thyroid function. Studies in Asian populations that typically consume soy support its benefits, but there is little evidence that switching to soy will have the same effect as a moderate soy intake throughout life.

Choosing Protein Wisely

To evaluate protein intake, it is important to consider both the amount and the quality of protein in the diet. **Protein quality** is a measure of how good the protein in a food is at providing the essential amino acids the body needs to synthesize proteins. Because animal amino acid patterns are similar to those of humans, the animal proteins in our diet generally provide a mixture of amino acids that better matches our needs than the amino acid mixtures provided by plant proteins. Animal proteins also tend to be digested more easily than plant proteins; only protein that is digested can contribute amino acids to meet the body's requirements.[11] Because they are easily digested and supply essential amino acids in the proper proportions for human use, foods of animal origin are generally sources of **high-quality protein**, or **complete dietary protein**. When your diet contains high-quality protein, you don't have to eat as much total protein to meet your needs.

Compared to animal proteins, plant proteins are usually more difficult to digest and are lower in one or more of the essential amino acids. They are therefore generally referred to as **incomplete dietary protein**. Exceptions include quinoa and soy protein, which are both high-quality plant proteins (see *Debate: Should You Switch to Soy?*).

Think critically: An intake of about 50 g of soy protein per day has been shown to lower blood cholesterol in some people. Based on the protein content of foods in the table, is this a reasonable way for Americans to lower cholesterol? Why or why not?

Good sources of soy		
Food	**Serving**	**Protein (g)**
Soy milk, regular	1 cup	7
Tofu, regular	1 oz	2.5
Miso	1 Tbsp	2
Tempeh	1 Tbsp	2
Roasted soybeans	1/4 cup	15
Soybean sprouts	1 cup	9
Texturized soy protein (TSP)	1 oz	14
Veggie hotdog	1	13
Soy veggie burger	3 oz	12
Tofutti frozen dessert, regular	1/2 cup	2
Soy flour, regular	1 Tbsp	2
Soy butter	2 Tbsp	7

Soy milk is a substitute for cow's milk.

Soy flour can be incorporated into baked goods.

Soy butter is similar to peanut butter and can be spread on crackers and sandwiches.

Tofu, also known as bean curd, is added to soups, salads, and stir-fries.

Texturized soy protein (TSP), also known as texturized vegetable protein (TVP), is formed into chunks, woven or spun into fibers, or otherwise shaped and flavored to produce vegetarian versions of burgers, hotdogs, meatballs, and chicken.

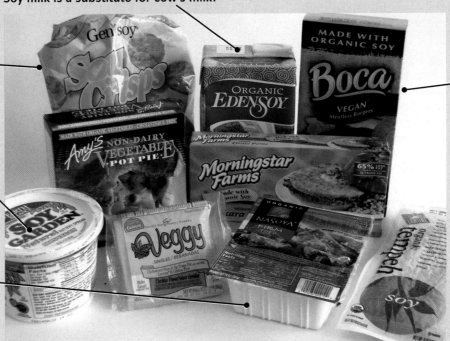

Complementary proteins If you get your protein from a single source and that source is an incomplete protein, it will be difficult to meet your body's protein needs. However, combining proteins that are limited in different amino acids can supply a complete mixture of essential amino acids. For example, legumes are limited in methionine but high in lysine. When legumes are consumed with grains, which are high in methionine and low in lysine, the combination provides all the needed amino acids (**Figure 6.15**). Vegetarian diets rely on this technique, called **protein complementation**, to meet protein needs. By eating plant proteins that have complementary amino acid patterns, a person can meet his or her essential amino acid requirements without consuming any animal proteins.

> **protein complementation** The process of combining proteins from different sources so that they collectively provide the proportions of amino acids required to meet the body's needs.

Protein complementation • Figure 6.15

a. The amino acids that are most often limited in plant proteins are lysine (lys), methionine (met), and cysteine (cys). As a general rule, legumes are deficient in methionine and cysteine but high in lysine. Grains, nuts, and seeds are deficient in lysine but high in methionine and cysteine.

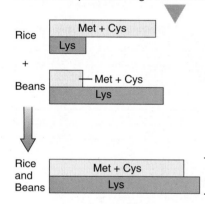

Rice
Met + Cys
Lys

+

Beans
Met + Cys
Lys

Rice and Beans
Met + Cys
Lys

When rice, which is limited in lys but high in met and cys, is eaten with beans, which are high in lys but limited in met and cys, the combination provides all the amino acids needed by the body.

Grains, nuts, or seeds + Legumes = Complete protein

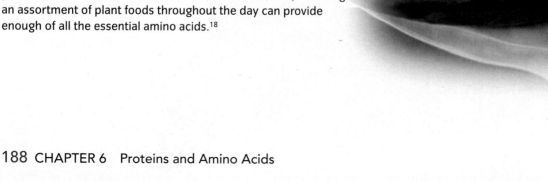

b. Many of the food combinations consumed in traditional diets take advantage of complementary plant proteins, such as lentils and rice or chickpeas and rice in India, rice and beans in Mexico and South America, hummus (chickpeas and sesame seeds) in the Middle East, and bread and peanut butter (peanuts are a legume) in the United States. Complementary proteins do not have to be consumed in the same meal, so eating an assortment of plant foods throughout the day can provide enough of all the essential amino acids.[18]

Choosing healthy protein sources • Figure 6.16

The protein group and the dairy group provide the most concentrated sources of protein. Nuts, dry beans, and peas are the most concentrated sources of plant protein. When you eat dry beans or peas, you can count them in either the vegetables group or the protein group. There is very little protein in fruits.

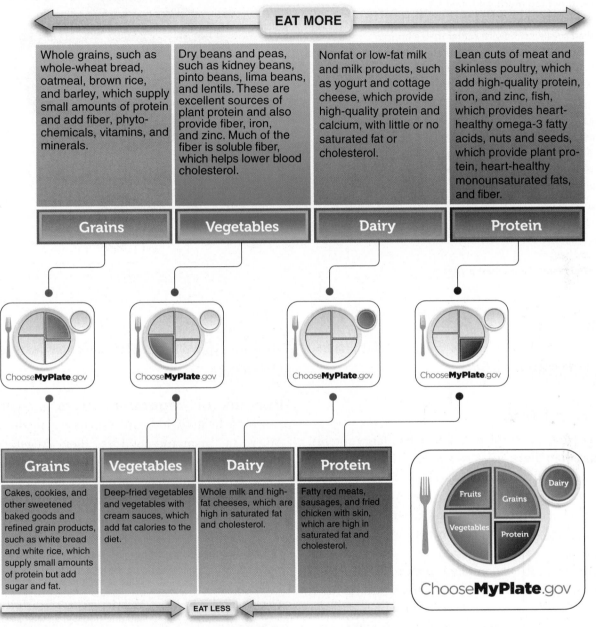

EAT MORE

Grains	Vegetables	Dairy	Protein
Whole grains, such as whole-wheat bread, oatmeal, brown rice, and barley, which supply small amounts of protein and add fiber, phytochemicals, vitamins, and minerals.	Dry beans and peas, such as kidney beans, pinto beans, lima beans, and lentils. These are excellent sources of plant protein and also provide fiber, iron, and zinc. Much of the fiber is soluble fiber, which helps lower blood cholesterol.	Nonfat or low-fat milk and milk products, such as yogurt and cottage cheese, which provide high-quality protein and calcium, with little or no saturated fat or cholesterol.	Lean cuts of meat and skinless poultry, which add high-quality protein, iron, and zinc, fish, which provides heart-healthy omega-3 fatty acids, nuts and seeds, which provide plant protein, heart-healthy monounsaturated fats, and fiber.

Grains	Vegetables	Dairy	Protein
Cakes, cookies, and other sweetened baked goods and refined grain products, such as white bread and white rice, which supply small amounts of protein but add sugar and fat.	Deep-fried vegetables and vegetables with cream sauces, which add fat calories to the diet.	Whole milk and high-fat cheeses, which are high in saturated fat and cholesterol.	Fatty red meats, sausages, and fried chicken with skin, which are high in saturated fat and cholesterol.

EAT LESS

ChooseMyPlate.gov

MyPlate and Dietary Guidelines recommendations MyPlate and the Dietary Guidelines include recommendations regarding both animal and plant sources of protein to meet your need for protein and essential amino acids (**Figure 6.16**). The MyPlate food groups that provide the most protein per serving are the dairy and protein groups; 1 cup of milk provides about 8 g of protein, 1 ounce of meat about 7 g, 1/2 cup of beans 7 to 10 g. Each serving from the grains group and the vegetables group provides 2 to 4 g, so choosing the recommended number of servings from these groups will provide a significant proportion of your protein needs. To assure an overall healthy diet, the 2010 Dietary Guidelines recommend that we choose a variety of protein foods, including seafood, lean meat and poultry, eggs, beans, soy products, and unsalted nuts and seeds. They recommend increasing consumption of seafood and low-fat or fat-free dairy products and replacing protein foods that are high

WHAT SHOULD I EAT?
Protein Sources

✓ THE PLANNER

Get protein without too much saturated fat
- Eat more fish.
- Have a grilled chicken sandwich rather than a burger.
- Choose lean cuts of red meat, such as round steaks and loin chops.
- Grill, roast, or broil so the fat will end up in the pan or the fire.
- Choose low-fat milk, yogurt, and cheese.

Eat both animal and plant proteins
- Have your beef or chicken in a stir-fry with lots of vegetables.
- Serve a small portion of meat over noodles.
- Add nuts and seeds to snacks and salads.
- Have a meatless meal at least once a week.
- Try a veggie burger.

Go with beans
- Have some hummus.
- Order beans in your burrito.
- Snack on soy beans.
- Choose baked beans rather than potatoes.

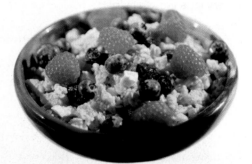

Use iProfile to look up the protein content of your favorite vegetarian entrée.

---

in solid fats with those that are lower in solid fats and calories (see *What Should I Eat?*).

Vegetarian Diets

In many parts of the world, diets based on plant proteins, called **vegetarian diets**, have evolved mostly out of necessity because animal sources of protein are limited, either physically or economically, in those areas. Animals require more land and resources to raise and are more expensive to purchase than are plants. The developing world relies primarily on plant foods to meet protein needs. For example, in rural Mexico, most of the protein in the diet comes from beans, rice, and tortillas (corn), and in India, protein comes from lentils and rice. As a population's economic prosperity rises, the proportion of animal foods in its diet typically increases, but in developed countries, people eat vegetarian diets for a variety of reasons other than economics, such as health, religion, personal ethics, or environmental awareness. **Vegan diets** eliminate all animal products, but there

> **vegetarian diet** A diet that includes plant-based foods and eliminates some or all foods of animal origin.
>
> **vegan diet** A plant-based diet that eliminates all animal products.

are other types of vegetarian diets that are less restrictive (**Table 6.1**).

Benefits of vegetarian diets A vegetarian diet can be a healthy, low-cost alternative to the traditional American meat-and-potatoes diet. Vegetarians have been shown to have lower body weight relative to height and a reduced incidence of obesity and of other chronic diseases, such as diabetes, cardiovascular disease, high

Types of vegetarian diets   Table 6.1

Diet	What it excludes and includes
Semivegetarian	Excludes red meat but may include fish and poultry, as well as dairy products and eggs
Pescetarian	Excludes all animal flesh except fish
Lacto-ovo vegetarian	Excludes all animal flesh but does include eggs and dairy products such as milk and cheese
Lacto vegetarian	Excludes animal flesh and eggs but does include dairy products
Vegan	Excludes all food of animal origin

blood pressure, and some types of cancer.[18] The lower body weight of vegetarians is a result of lower energy intake, primarily due to higher intake of fiber, which makes the diet more filling. The reductions in the risk of other chronic diseases may be due to lower body weight and to the fact that these diets are lower in saturated fat and cholesterol, which increase disease risk. Or it could be that vegetarian diets are higher in whole grains, legumes, nuts, vegetables, and fruits, which add fiber, vitamins, minerals, antioxidants, and phytochemicals—substances that have been shown to lower disease risk. It is likely that the total dietary pattern, rather than a single factor, is responsible for the health-promoting effects of vegetarian diets.

In addition to reducing disease risks, diets that rely more heavily on plant protein than on animal protein are more economical. For example, a vegetarian stir-fry over rice costs about half as much as a meal of steak and potatoes. Yet both meals provide a significant portion of the day's protein requirement. A small steak, a baked potato with sour cream, and a tossed salad provides about 50 g of protein, whereas a dish of rice with tofu and vegetables provides about 30 g.

Risks of vegetarian diets Despite the health and economic benefits of vegetarian diets, a poorly planned vegetarian diet can cause nutrient deficiencies. Protein deficiency is a risk when vegan diets that contain little high-quality protein are consumed by small children or by adults with increased protein needs, such as pregnant women and those recovering from illness or injury. Most people can easily meet their protein needs with lacto and lacto-ovo vegetarian diets. These diets contain high-quality animal proteins from eggs or milk, which complement the limiting amino acids in the plant proteins.

Vitamin and mineral deficiencies are a greater concern for vegetarians than is protein deficiency.[18] Of primary concern to vegans is vitamin B_{12}. Because this B vitamin is found almost exclusively in animal products, vegans must take vitamin B_{12} supplements or consume foods fortified with vitamin B_{12} to meet their needs for this nutrient. Another nutrient of concern is calcium. Dairy products are the major source of calcium in the North American diet, so diets that eliminate these foods must rely on plant sources of calcium. Likewise, because much of the dietary vitamin D comes from fortified milk, this vitamin must be made in the body from exposure to sunlight or consumed in other sources. Iron and zinc may be deficient in vegetarian diets because they exclude red meat, which is an excellent source of these minerals, and iron and zinc are poorly absorbed from plant sources. Because dairy products are low in iron and zinc, lacto-ovo and lacto vegetarians as well as vegans are at risk for deficiencies of these minerals. Vegan diets may also be low in iodine and the omega-3 fatty acids EPA and DHA (see Chapter 5).[18] **Table 6.2** provides suggestions for how vegans can meet the need for the nutrients just discussed.

Meeting nutrient needs with a vegan diet[18] Table 6.2	
Nutrient at risk	**Sources in vegan diets**
Protein	Soy-based products, legumes, seeds, nuts, grains, and vegetables
Vitamin B_{12}	Products fortified with vitamin B_{12}, such as soy beverages, rice milk, and breakfast cereals; fortified nutritional yeast; dietary supplements
Calcium	Tofu processed with calcium; broccoli, kale, bok choy, and legumes; products fortified with calcium, such as soy beverages, rice milk, grain products, and orange juice
Vitamin D	Sunshine; products fortified with vitamin D, such as soy beverages, rice milk, breakfast cereals, and margarine
Iron	Legumes, tofu, dark green leafy vegetables, dried fruit, whole grains, iron-fortified grain products (absorption is improved when iron-containing foods are consumed with vitamin C found in citrus fruit, tomatoes, strawberries, and dark green vegetables)
Zinc	Whole grains, wheat germ, legumes, nuts, tofu, and fortified breakfast cereals
Iodine	Iodized salt, sea vegetables (seaweed), and foods grown near the sea
Omega-3 fatty acids	Canola oil, flaxseed and flaxseed oil, soybean oil, walnuts, and sea vegetables (seaweed), which provide fatty acids that can be used to synthesize EPA and DHA; DHA-rich microalgae

THINKING IT THROUGH ✓ THE PLANNER
A Case Study on Healthy Vegetarian Diets

Simon is 26 years old and weighs 154 pounds. A year ago, he decided to stop eating meat because he thought it would make his diet healthier. Now that he is studying nutrition, he has become concerned that his vegetarian diet may not be as healthy as he thought. First, he wants to see if he meets his protein needs.

What is the RDA for protein for someone of Simon's age and weight?
▼

Your answer:

Simon records his food intake for one day and then uses ⬤ iProfile to assess his nutrient intake. He is pleased to discover that his diet provides 66 g of protein, which exceeds his RDA, but he is shocked to discover that his diet is high in saturated fat.

This is a photo of Simon's typical lunch. Why is it high in saturated fat?
▼

Your answer:

Simon typically has cereal with milk for breakfast, and he has cheese pizza or cheese lasagna for dinner. He snacks on chips and ice cream.

Vegetarian diets are often deficient in calcium, vitamin D, zinc, and iron. Which of these are likely low in Simon's diet?
▼

Your answer:

What could Simon have for dinner that would provide less saturated fat and more of the nutrients that are lacking in his diet?
▼

Your answer:

To reduce his saturated fat intake, Simon wants to try a vegan lunch. Suggest a vegan sandwich Simon could have that makes use of complementary plant proteins.
▼

Your answer:

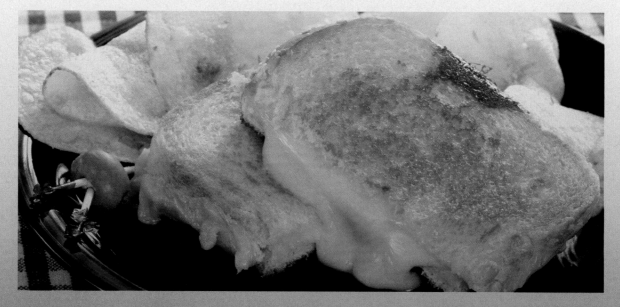

(Check your answers in Appendix J.)

Planning vegetarian diets Well-planned vegetarian diets, including vegan diets, can meet nutrient needs at all stages of the life cycle, from infancy, childhood, and adolescence to early, middle, and late adulthood, and during pregnancy and lactation (See *Thinking It Through*).[18] One way to plan a healthy vegetarian diet is to modify the selections from MyPlate. The food choices and recommended amounts from the grains, vegetables, and fruits groups should stay the same for vegetarians. Including 1 cup of dark green and colorful vegetables daily will help meet iron and calcium needs. The dairy group and the protein group include foods of animal origin. Vegetarians who consume eggs and milk can still choose these foods. Those who avoid all animal foods can choose dry beans, nuts and seeds, and soy products from the protein group. Fortified soy milk and protein-enriched rice milk can be substituted for dairy foods. To obtain adequate vitamin B_{12}, vegans must take supplements or use products fortified with vitamin B_{12}. Obtaining plenty of omega-3 fatty acids from foods such as canola oil, nuts, and flaxseed ensures adequate synthesis of the long-chain omega-3 fatty acids DHA and EPA.

CONCEPT CHECK 🛑 STOP

1. **What** circumstances result in a positive nitrogen balance?

2. **Why** is the quality of animal protein generally considered to be higher than that of plant protein?

3. **What** could you serve with rice to increase the overall protein quality of the meal?

4. **Why** are vegans at risk for vitamin B_{12} deficiency?

THE PLANNER ✓

Summary

1 Proteins in Our Food 168

- Dietary protein comes from both animal and plant sources. Animal sources of protein are generally good sources of iron, zinc, and calcium but are high in saturated fat and cholesterol. Plant sources of protein, such as the nuts, peas, and beans shown in the photo, are higher in unsaturated fat, fiber, and phytochemicals.

Plant proteins • Figure 6.1b

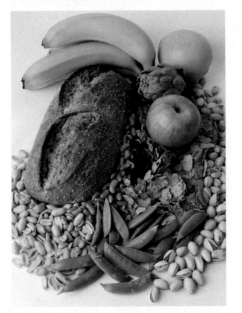

2 The Structure of Amino Acids and Proteins 169

- **Amino acids** are the building blocks from which proteins are made. Each amino acid contains an amino group, an acid group, and a unique side chain. The amino acids that the body is unable to make in sufficient amounts are called **essential amino acids** and must be consumed in the diet.

- Proteins are made by linking amino acids by **peptide bonds**, as shown here, to form **polypeptides**. Polypeptide chains fold to create unique three-dimensional protein structures. The shape of a protein determines its function.

Amino acid and protein structure • Figure 6.2c

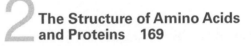

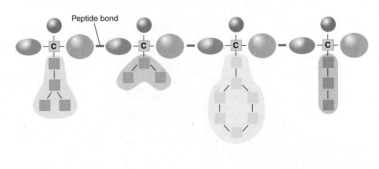

3 Protein Digestion and Absorption 173

- Digestion breaks dietary protein into small **peptides** and amino acids that can be absorbed. Because amino acids that share the same transport system, such as those pictured here in green and purple, compete for absorption, an excess of one can inhibit the absorption of another.

Protein digestion and absorption • Figure 6.4

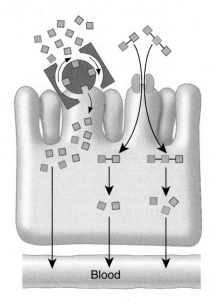

Blood

4 Protein Synthesis and Functions 173

- Amino acids are used to synthesize proteins and other nitrogen-containing molecules. **Genes** located in the nucleus of the cell code for the order of amino acids in the **polypeptide** chains that make up proteins. Regulatory mechanisms ensure that proteins are made only when they are needed. For a protein to be synthesized, all the amino acids it contains must be available. The essential amino acid present in shortest supply relative to need, depicted here as amino acid A (orange), is called the **limiting amino acid**.

- In the body, protein molecules form structures, regulate body functions, transport molecules through the blood and in and out of cells, function in the immune system, and aid in muscle contraction, fluid balance, and acid balance.

- When the diet is deficient in energy or when the diet contains more protein than needed, amino acids are used as an energy source and to synthesize glucose or fatty acids. Before amino acids can be used for these purposes, the amino group must be removed via **deamination**.

Protein synthesis • Figure 6.6c

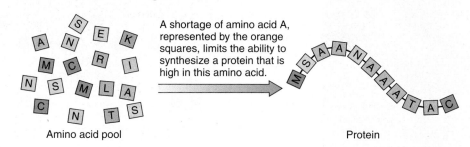

A shortage of amino acid A, represented by the orange squares, limits the ability to synthesize a protein that is high in this amino acid.

Amino acid pool

Protein

5 Protein in Health and Disease 179

- **Protein-energy malnutrition (PEM)** is a health concern primarily in developing countries. **Kwashiorkor**, shown here, occurs when the protein content of the diet is deficient but energy is adequate. It is most common in children. **Marasmus** occurs when total energy intake is deficient.

Protein-energy malnutrition • Figure 6.9a

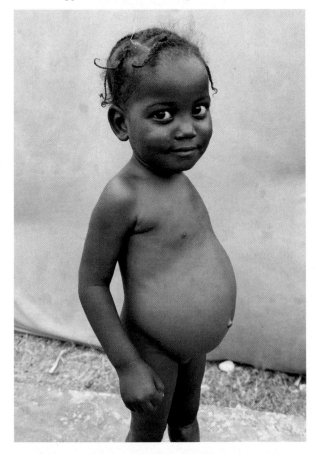

- High-protein diets increase the production of urea and other waste products that must be excreted in the urine and therefore can increase water losses. High protein intakes increase urinary calcium losses, but when calcium intake is adequate, high-protein diets are associated with greater bone mass and fewer fractures. Diets high in animal proteins and low in fluid are associated with an increased risk of kidney stones. High-protein diets can be high in saturated fat and cholesterol.

- If proteins are absorbed without being completely digested, they can trigger an immune system reaction, resulting in a **food allergy**. Some amino acids and proteins can also cause **food intolerances**.

6 Meeting Protein Needs 183

- Protein requirements are determined by looking at **nitrogen balance**, the amount of nitrogen consumed as dietary protein compared with the amount excreted as protein waste products.

- For healthy adults, the RDA for protein is 0.8 g/kg of body weight. Growth, pregnancy, lactation, illness, injury, and certain types of physical exercise increase requirements. Recommendations for a healthy diet are to ingest 10 to 35% of calories from protein.

- Animal proteins are considered **high-quality proteins** because their amino acid composition matches that needed to synthesize body proteins. Most plant proteins are limited in one or more of the essential amino acids needed to make body protein; therefore, they are considered **incomplete proteins**. The **protein quality** of plant sources can be increased through **protein complementation**. As illustrated here, it combines proteins with different limiting amino acids to supply enough of all the essential amino acids.

Protein complementation • Figure 6.15b

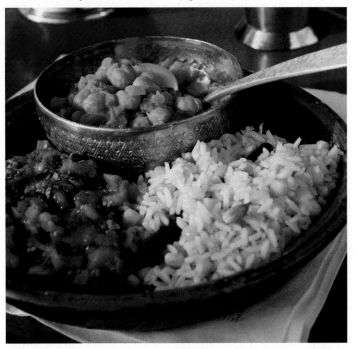

- Compared with meat-based diets, **vegetarian diets** are lower in saturated fat and cholesterol and higher in fiber, certain vitamins and minerals, antioxidants, and phytochemicals. People consuming **vegan diets** must plan their diets carefully to meet their needs for vitamin B_{12}, calcium, vitamin D, iron, zinc, and omega-3 fatty acids.

Key Terms

- amino acid pool 174
- amino acid 168
- celiac disease 182
- conditionally essential amino acid 169
- deamination 178
- denaturation 171
- dipeptide 170
- edema 177
- essential, or indispensable, amino acid 169
- food allergy 181
- food intolerance or food sensitivity 182
- gene 174
- gene expression 174
- high-quality protein or complete dietary protein 187
- hydrolyzed protein or protein hydrolysate 182
- incomplete dietary protein 187
- kwashiorkor 180
- legume 168
- limiting amino acid 174
- marasmus 180
- monosodium glutamate (MSG) 182
- MSG symptom complex or Chinese restaurant syndrome 182
- nitrogen balance 183
- nonessential, or dispensable, amino acid 169
- peptide bond 169
- peptide 170
- phenylketonuria (PKU) 169
- polypeptide 169
- protein complementation 188
- protein quality 187
- protein-energy malnutrition (PEM) 179
- transamination 174
- transcription 175
- translation 175
- tripeptide 170
- urea 178
- vegan diet 190
- vegetarian diet 190

Online Resources

- For more information on choosing a healthy vegetarian diet, go to www.choosemyplate.gov/tipsresources/vegetarian_diets.html.

- For more information on vegetarian diets for children, go to www.pcrm.org/health/veginfo/vegetarian_kids.html.

- For more information on the health effects of high-protein diets, go to www.americanheart.org/presenter.jhtml?identifier=11234.

- For more information on food allergies, go to www.webmd.com/allergies/foods-allergy-intolerance.

- For more information on protein needs of athletes, go to www.aces.edu/pubs/docs/H/HE-0748/.

- Visit your *WileyPLUS* site for videos, animations, podcasts, self-study, and other media that will aid you in studying and understanding this chapter.

Critical and Creative Thinking Questions

1. Syed is a body builder. He is concerned about his protein intake. If Syed weighs 200 pounds and consumes about 3600 Calories/day, 15% of which comes from protein, will his diet supply enough protein to meet the recommendation for strength athletes of 1.2 to 1.7 g of protein/kilogram of body weight per day? What if he consumed only 2500 Calories/day?

2. Make a vegetarian meal plan for yourself for one day. Use 🌐 iProfile to make sure it meets your calorie and protein needs. Then plan a day that includes meat. Go to the grocery store and calculate how much each day's meals will cost. Use this information to explain the economic benefits or pitfalls of these two eating plans.

3. For each food in column A, select one or more in column B that could be combined with it to provide a meal of high-quality protein.

A	B
Rice	Tofu
Wheat bread	Peanut butter
Corn tortilla	Cheese
Pasta	Kidney beans
Tofu	Cashews
Peanut butter	Corn tortilla
Corn bread	Wheat bread
Soybeans	Chickpeas
Black-eyed peas	Chicken

4. Children with the genetic disease phenylketonuria must consume a low-phenylalanine diet to prevent the accumulation of damaging phenylketones. Why not just eliminate the essential amino acid phenylalanine from the diet altogether?

5. Jack consumes about 120 g of protein/day. Of this, about 30 g is broken down and used to make ATP, and 30 g is used to synthesize body fat. What does this tell you about Jack's protein and energy intake?

6. Fluid accumulates in the bellies of children with kwashiorkor. Use your understanding of how protein helps regulate fluid balance to explain why this occurs.

7. The graph shows the amount of animal protein and saturated fat in four different diets. Based on the data here, what is the relationship between the two? How might the animal protein choices in a diet affect this relationship—for example, if a skinless chicken breast replaced a cheeseburger?

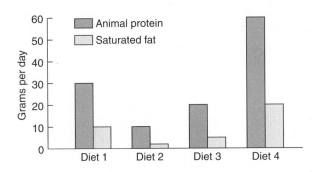

What is happening in this picture?

Sickle cell anemia is an inherited disease caused by an abnormality in the gene for the protein hemoglobin. It causes red blood cells to take on a sickle shape.

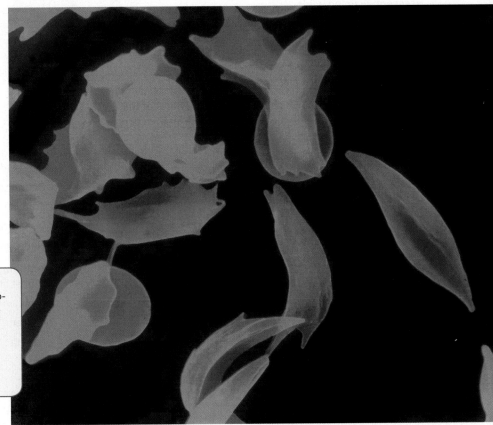

Think Critically

1. Sickle cell hemoglobin differs from normal hemoglobin by one amino acid. Why might this difference change the shape of the hemoglobin?

2. Do you think sickle-shaped red blood cells can travel easily through narrow capillaries?

3. How might this disorder affect the ability to get oxygen to the body's cells?

Self-Test

(Check your answers in Appendix K.)

1. Which part of this amino acid will differ, depending on the particular amino acid?

    a. A   b. B   c. C   d. D

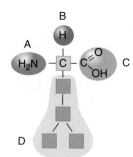

2. Amino acids that cannot be made by the adult human body in sufficient amounts are called _____.

    a. essential amino acids

    b. complete proteins

    c. incomplete amino acids

    d. hydrolyzed proteins

    e. nonessential amino acids

3. Based on the diagram, which letters label the parts of the digestive tract where chemical digestion of protein occurs?

    a. A and B   d. B and C

    b. A and C   e. B and D

    c. C and D

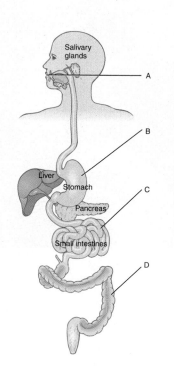

4. Which one of the following is made from amino acids?

    a. triglycerides

    b. glycogen

    c. lecithin

    d. cholesterol

    e. enzymes

5. Which of the following letters best labels transcription?

    a. A

    b. B

    c. C

    d. D

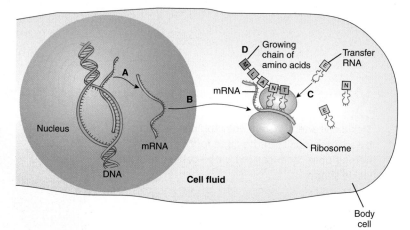

6. _____ is the process of transferring an amino group from an amino acid to another molecule to form a second amino acid.

    a. Deamination

    b. Transamination

    c. Denaturation

    d. Hydrogenation

7. The amino acid colored _____ would be considered the most limiting for the synthesis of this specific protein?

    a. yellow

    b. green

    c. orange

    d. red

    e. blue

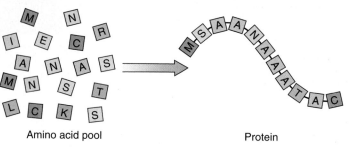

Amino acid pool   Protein

8. Which of the following groups requires the least protein per kilogram of body weight?

a. adult men

b. pregnant women

c. infants

d. young children

9. What element is found in amino acids but not in glucose and triglycerides?

a. carbon

b. nitrogen

c. phosphorous

d. oxygen

e. hydrogen

10. Which of the following is least likely to be low in a vegan diet?

a. calcium

b. vitamin D

c. iron

d. fiber

e. vitamin B_{12}

11. Which of the following values for nitrogen intake and output are most likely to belong to a healthy 9-year-old boy?

a. nitrogen in = 14 g, nitrogen out = 16 g

b. nitrogen in = 15 g, nitrogen out = 15 g

c. nitrogen in = 14 g, nitrogen out = 10 g

d. nitrogen in = 20 g, nitrogen out = 22 g

12. When extra protein is consumed, it is stored in the muscle for later use.

a. true

b. false

13. When amino acids are broken down to generate energy or synthesize glucose, the amino group must be removed. What waste product is generated from it?

a. ketones

b. urea

c. free fatty acids

d. carbon dioxide

e. oxygen

14. Which of the following is *not* a good example of protein complementation?

a. sunflower seeds and peanuts

b. rice and beans

c. chickpeas and sesame seeds

d. corn and rice

e. lentils and rice

15. Which one of the following statements about children with kwashiorkor is false?

a. Their fat stores are completely depleted.

b. They are more susceptible to infections than healthy children.

c. They have swollen bellies.

d. They have hair color changes.

e. They do not grow well.

THE PLANNER ✓

Review your Chapter Planner on the chapter opener and check off your completed work.

7 Vitamins

Britons have long been referred to as "Limeys." If you eat a lot of carrots, your night vision will improve. Mom says to go outside and get some sunshine.

These statements are related to an alphabet soup of essential compounds known as *vitamins*. In times past, British sailors on long voyages developed scurvy due to a lack of vitamin C. Adding citrus fruits—such as limes—to their diet prevented this condition, and a nickname was born. Carrots provide vitamin A, needed for the perception of light. Sun exposure allows our bodies to synthesize vitamin D, which we need to absorb calcium.

Populations enduring sunless Arctic winters have traditionally acquired vitamin D from a diet of fish, eggs, seal, walrus, and whale blubber. But as consumption of these traditional foods has declined, vitamin D deficiency has increased. If we who live in more temperate regions do not get enough sunlight, we must also obtain vitamin D from our diet.

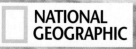

As the British Royal Navy discovered—and diverse cultures have appreciated for thousands of years—certain foods can counteract certain ailments. Only relatively recently have the agents in these foods been isolated and recognized for their specific roles in preventing illness and ensuring good health.

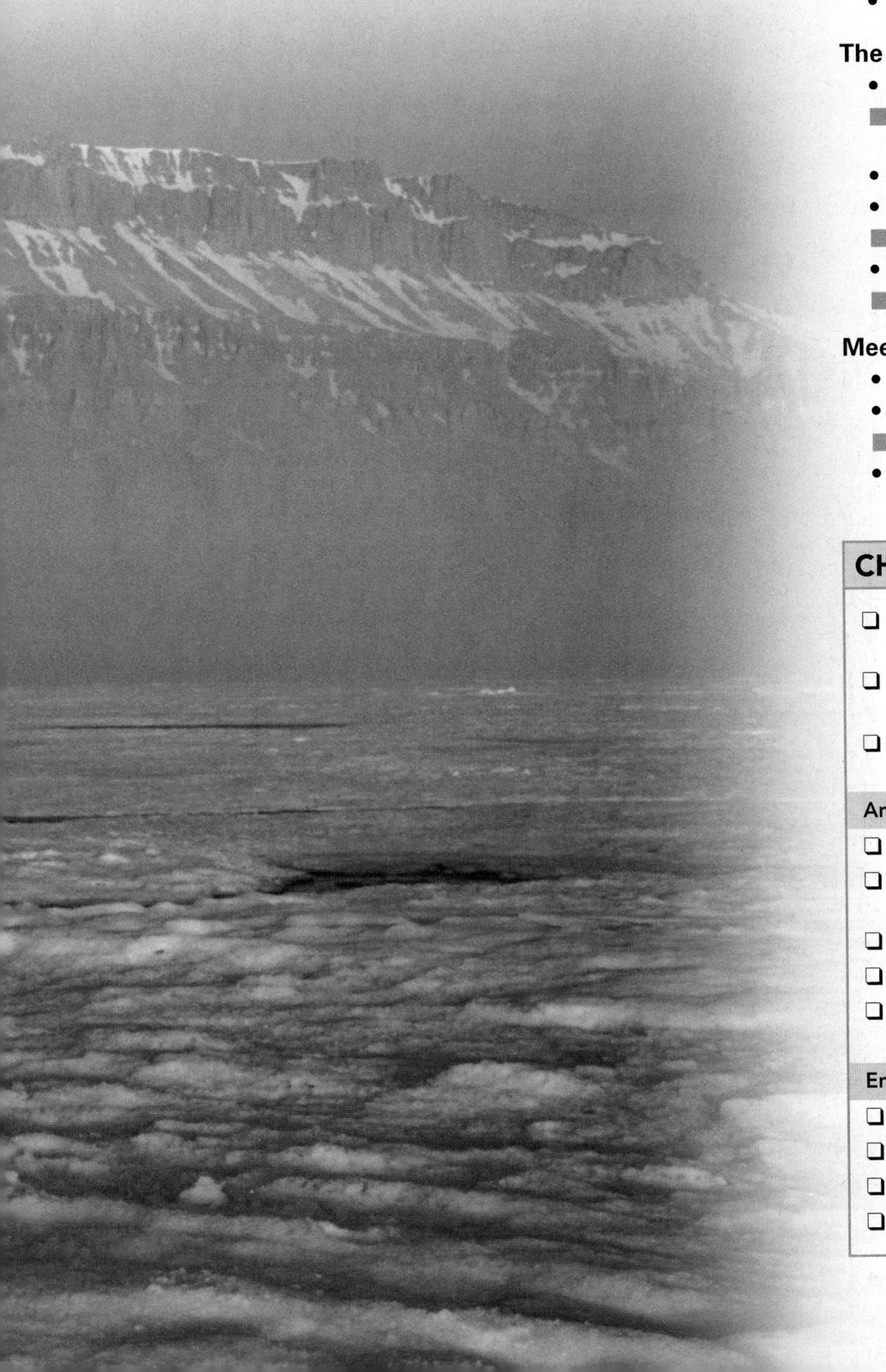

CHAPTER PLANNER ✓

- ❏ Stimulate your interest by reading the opening story and looking at the visual.
- ❏ Scan the Learning Objectives in each section:
  p. 202 ❏   p. 209 ❏   p. 228 ❏   p. 244 ❏
- ❏ Read the text and study all figures and visuals. Answer any questions.

Analyze key features

- ❏ What a Scientist Sees, p. 203 ❏   p. 241 ❏
- ❏ Process Diagram, p. 205 ❏   p. 207 ❏   p. 222 ❏ p. 230 ❏   p. 234 ❏
- ❏ Nutrition InSight, p. 206 ❏   p. 216 ❏   p. 232 ❏   p. 236 ❏
- ❏ Thinking It Through, p. 231 ❏
- ❏ Stop: Answer the Concept Checks before you go on:
  p. 209 ❏   p. 227 ❏   p. 243 ❏   p. 249 ❏

End of chapter

- ❏ Review the Summary, Key Terms, and Online Resources.
- ❏ Answer the Critical and CreativeThinking Questions.
- ❏ Answer What is happening in this picture?
- ❏ Complete the Self-Test and check your answers.

A Vitamin Primer

LEARNING OBJECTIVES

1. **Discuss** the dietary sources of vitamins.
2. **Describe** how bioavailability affects vitamin requirements.
3. **Explain** the function of coenzymes.
4. **Describe** the function of antioxidants.

Vitamins are organic compounds that are essential in the diet in small amounts to promote and regulate body processes necessary for growth, reproduction, and the maintenance of health. When a vitamin is lacking in the diet, deficiency symptoms occur. When the vitamin is restored to the diet, the symptoms resolve.

Vitamins have traditionally been assigned to two groups, based on their solubility in water or fat. This chemical characteristic allows generalizations to be made about how the vitamins are absorbed, transported, excreted, and stored in the body. The **water-soluble vitamins** include the B vitamins and vitamin C. The **fat-soluble vitamins** include vitamins A, D, E, and K (**Table 7.1**). The vitamins were initially named alphabetically, in approximately the order in which they were identified. The B vitamins were first

The vitamins Table 7.1	
Water-soluble vitamins	**Fat-soluble vitamins**
B vitamins	Vitamin A
• Thiamin (B$_1$)	Vitamin D
• Riboflavin (B$_2$)	Vitamin E
• Niacin (B$_3$)	Vitamin K
• Biotin	
• Pantothenic acid	
• Vitamin B$_6$ (pyridoxine)	
• Folate (folic acid)	
• Vitamin B$_{12}$ (cobalamin)	
Vitamin C (ascorbic acid)	

thought to be a single chemical substance but were later found to be many different vitamins so they were distinguished by numbers. Vitamins B$_6$ and B$_{12}$ are the only ones that are still routinely referred to by their numbers.

Vitamins in Our Food

Almost all foods contain some vitamins, and all the food groups contain foods that are good sources of a variety of vitamins (**Figure 7.1**). The amount of a vitamin in a food

Vitamins in MyPlate
• Figure 7.1

Vitamins are found in foods from all the food groups, as well as in oils, but some groups are lacking in specific vitamins. For example, grains, fruits, and vegetables lack vitamin B$_{12}$, and grains and protein foods are low in vitamin C.

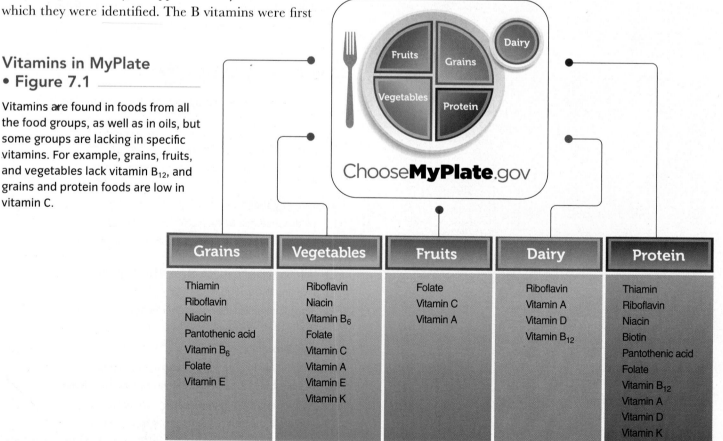

Grains	Vegetables	Fruits	Dairy	Protein
Thiamin	Riboflavin	Folate	Riboflavin	Thiamin
Riboflavin	Niacin	Vitamin C	Vitamin A	Riboflavin
Niacin	Vitamin B$_6$	Vitamin A	Vitamin D	Niacin
Pantothenic acid	Folate		Vitamin B$_{12}$	Biotin
Vitamin B$_6$	Vitamin C			Pantothenic acid
Folate	Vitamin A			Folate
Vitamin E	Vitamin E			Vitamin B$_{12}$
	Vitamin K			Vitamin A
				Vitamin D
				Vitamin K

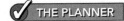

Fortified Breakfast Cereal

Nutrition Facts

| Serving Size | 1 Cup (50g/1.8 oz.) |
| Servings per Container | About 10 |

Amount Per Serving	Cereal	Cereal with 1/2 Cup Vitamins A&D Fat-Free Milk
Calories	180	220
Calories from Fat	5	5

	% Daily Value**	
Total Fat 0.5g*	1%	1%
Saturated Fat 0g	0%	0%
Trans Fat 0g		
Cholesterol 0mg	0%	0%
Sodium 280mg	12%	14%
Potassium 100mg	3%	9%
Total Carbohydrate 35g	12%	14%
Dietary Fiber 2g	9%	9%
Sugars 7g		
Other Carbohydrate 26g		
Protein 3g		
Vitamin A	15%	20%
Vitamin C	25%	25%
Calcium	0%	15%
Iron	100%	100%
Vitamin D	10%	25%
Vitamin E	100%	100%
Thiamin	100%	100%
Riboflavin	100%	110%
Niacin	100%	100%
Vitamin B$_6$	100%	100%
Folic Acid	100%	100%
Vitamin B$_{12}$	100%	110%
Pantothenate	100%	100%
Phosphorus	10%	20%
Magnesium	8%	10%
Zinc	100%	100%
Copper	4%	6%

Fortification: Benefits and Risks

The Nutrition Facts panel on a box of breakfast cereal shows an abundance of vitamins and minerals, many of which have been added through fortification. A consumer sees an easy way to meet nutrient needs. A scientist sees both the health benefits and the risks of fortification.

Fortification began as a way to address nutrient deficiencies. In the early 1900s, the niacin deficiency disease *pellagra* caused more than 3,000 deaths annually in the southern United States. In 1938, bakers voluntarily began enriching flour with B vitamins, a move that led to a decline in mortality from pellagra (see graph).[1] By 1943, enrichment of flour was becoming mandatory. Other government-supported fortification programs in the United States have helped to prevent vitamin A and D deficiencies.

Not all fortification is mandated by the government. Scientists recognize that indiscriminate fortification of foods, such as breakfast cereals, can increase the risk of nutrient toxicities. A recent analysis of nutrient intakes in toddlers and preschoolers showed that a significant percentage had intakes of preformed vitamin A, folate, and zinc that exceeded the ULs. Much of the excess zinc is likely to be from fortified breakfast cereals.[2]

Think Critically Should the government regulate all fortification of food?

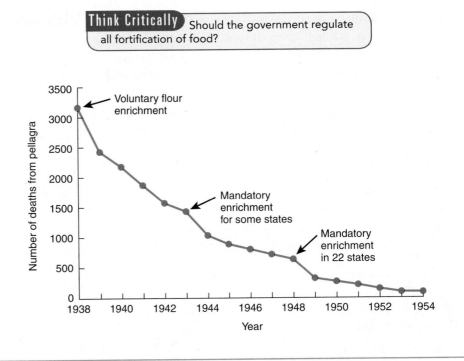

depends on the amount that is naturally present in the food, what is added to it, and how the food is processed, prepared, and stored.

Fortification adds nutrients to foods. Sometimes nutrients are added to foods to comply with government fortification programs that mandate such additions in order to prevent vitamin or mineral deficiencies and promote health in the population (see *What a Scientist Sees*). For example, grains are enriched with B vitamins and iron to prevent deficiencies, and milk is fortified with vitamin D to promote bone health. In other cases, manufacturers add nutrients with the goal of increasing product sales.

Which choice is highest in vitamins? • Figure 7.2

Because heat, light, air, and the passage of time all cause foods to lose nutrients, most of us try to purchase fresh produce, but is fresh always best?

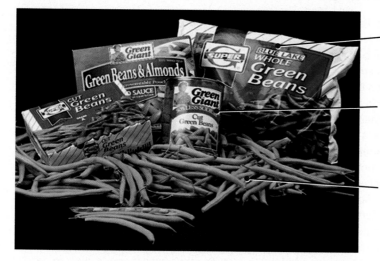

Frozen foods are often frozen in the field in order to minimize nutrient losses. Thus, frozen fruits and vegetables may supply more vitamins than "fresh" ones.

The high temperatures used in canning reduce nutrient content. However, because canned foods keep for a long time, do not require refrigeration, and are often less expensive than fresh or frozen foods, they provide an available, affordable source of nutrients that may be the best choice in some situations.

Sometimes "fresh" produce is lower in nutrients than you would expect because it has spent a week in a truck, traveling to your store, several days on a shelf, and maybe another week in your refrigerator.

The vitamins in foods can be damaged by exposure to light or oxygen, washed away during preparation, or destroyed by cooking. Thus, processing steps used by food producers can cause nutrient losses, as can cooking and storage methods used at home (**Figure 7.2**). Vitamin losses can be minimized through food preparation methods that reduce exposure to heat and light, which destroy some vitamins, and to water, which washes away water-soluble vitamins (**Table 7.2**).

Tips for preserving the vitamins in your food   Table 7.2

- Store food away from heat and light and eat it soon after purchasing it.

- Cut fruits and vegetables as close as possible to the time when they will be cooked or served.

- Don't soak vegetables.

- Cook vegetables with as little water as possible by microwaving, pressure-cooking, roasting, grilling, stir-frying, or baking rather than boiling them.

- If foods are cooked in water, use the cooking water to make soups and sauces so that you can retrieve some of the nutrients.

- Don't rinse rice before cooking, in order to avoid washing away water-soluble vitamins.

Vitamin Bioavailability

About 40 to 90% of the vitamins in food are absorbed, primarily from the small intestine (**Figure 7.3**). The composition of the diet and conditions in the digestive tract and the rest of the body influence vitamin **bioavailability**. For example, fat-soluble vitamins are absorbed along with dietary fat. If the diet is very low in fat, absorption of these vitamins is impaired.

> **bioavailability** The extent to which the body can absorb and use a nutrient.

Once they have been absorbed into the blood, vitamins must be transported to the cells. Most of the water-soluble vitamins are bound to blood proteins for transport. Fat-soluble vitamins are incorporated into chylomicrons for transport from the intestine. The bioavailability of a vitamin depends on the availability of these transport systems.

Some vitamins are absorbed in an inactive form called either a **provitamin** or a **vitamin precursor**. To perform vitamin functions, provitamins must be converted into active vitamin forms once they are inside the body. How much of each provitamin can be converted into the active vitamin and the rate at which this process occurs affect the amount of a vitamin available to function inside the body.

> **provitamin** or **vitamin precursor** A compound that can be converted into the active form of a vitamin in the body.

Vitamin absorption • Figure 7.3

THE PLANNER

Most vitamin absorption takes place in the small intestine. The mechanism by which vitamins are absorbed and transported affects their bioavailability.

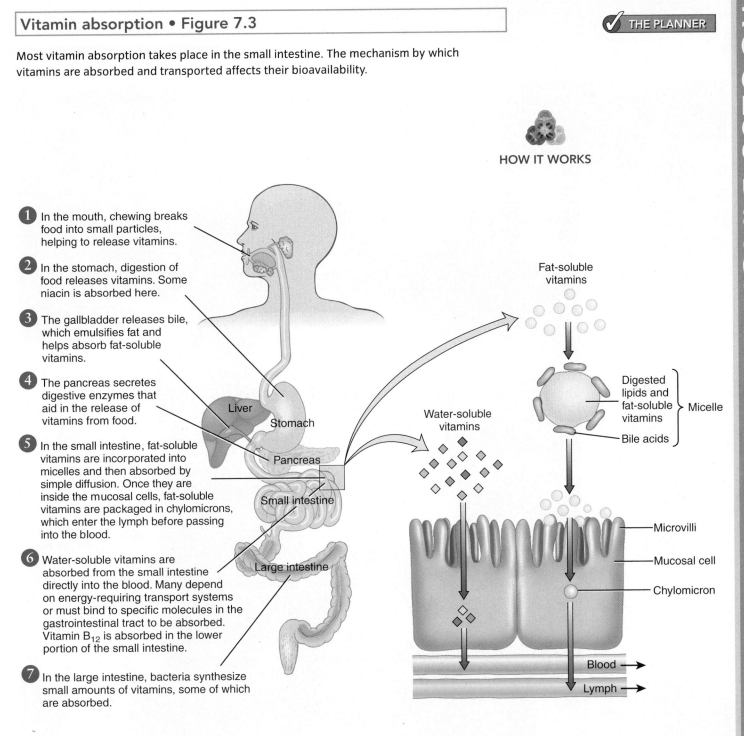

HOW IT WORKS

1. In the mouth, chewing breaks food into small particles, helping to release vitamins.

2. In the stomach, digestion of food releases vitamins. Some niacin is absorbed here.

3. The gallbladder releases bile, which emulsifies fat and helps absorb fat-soluble vitamins.

4. The pancreas secretes digestive enzymes that aid in the release of vitamins from food.

5. In the small intestine, fat-soluble vitamins are incorporated into micelles and then absorbed by simple diffusion. Once they are inside the mucosal cells, fat-soluble vitamins are packaged in chylomicrons, which enter the lymph before passing into the blood.

6. Water-soluble vitamins are absorbed from the small intestine directly into the blood. Many depend on energy-requiring transport systems or must bind to specific molecules in the gastrointestinal tract to be absorbed. Vitamin B_{12} is absorbed in the lower portion of the small intestine.

7. In the large intestine, bacteria synthesize small amounts of vitamins, some of which are absorbed.

Liver
Stomach
Pancreas
Small intestine
Large intestine

Fat-soluble vitamins

Water-soluble vitamins

Digested lipids and fat-soluble vitamins } Micelle

Bile acids

Microvilli
Mucosal cell
Chylomicron
Blood →
Lymph →

Ask Yourself

Why would a very low-fat diet decrease the absorption of fat-soluble vitamins?

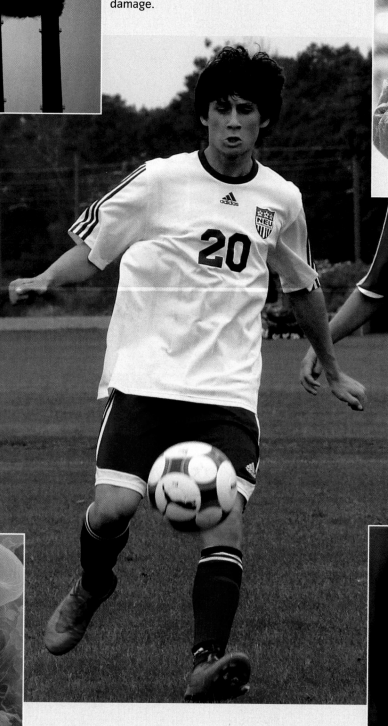

Vitamin C, vitamin E, and provitamin A are antioxidants that can help protect us from molecules that cause oxidative damage.

Vitamins A, B₆, C, and D, as well as folate, are needed for healthy immune function, and thus help protect us from infection.

Vitamin A and vitamin D are needed for normal growth and development.

The B vitamins thiamin, riboflavin, niacin, biotin, pantothenic acid, and vitamin B₆ are needed to produce ATP from carbohydrate, fat, and protein.

Folate, vitamin B₆, and vitamin B₁₂ are important for protein and amino acid metabolism.

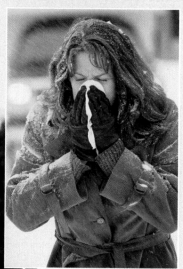

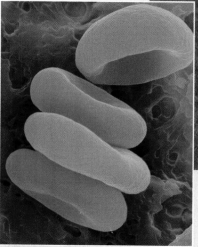

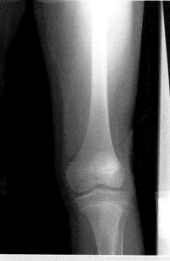

Folate, vitamin B₆, vitamin B₁₂, and vitamin K are needed to keep blood healthy.

Vitamins A, D, K, and C are needed for bone health.

Vitamin Functions

Vitamins promote and regulate the body's activities. Each vitamin has one or more important functions (**Figure 7.4**). For example, vitamin A is needed for vision as well as normal growth and development. Vitamin K is needed for blood clotting and bone health. Often more than one vitamin is needed to ensure the health of a particular organ or system. Some vitamins act in a similar manner to do their jobs. For example, all the B vitamins act as **coenzymes** (**Figure 7.5**).

coenzyme An organic nonprotein substance that binds to an enzyme to promote its activity.

A few vitamins function as **antioxidants**, substances that protect against **oxidative damage**. Oxidative damage is caused when reactive oxygen molecules steal electrons from other compounds, causing changes in their structure and function. Reactive oxygen molecules such as **free radicals** can be generated by normal oxygen-requiring reactions inside the body, such as cellular respiration, or can come from

antioxidant A substance that decreases the adverse effects of reactive molecules on normal physiological function.

free radical A type of highly reactive atom or molecule that causes oxidative damage.

Coenzymes • Figure 7.5

THE PLANNER

Coenzymes bind to enzymes to promote their activity. They act as carriers of electrons, atoms, or chemical groups that participate in the reaction. All the B vitamins are coenzymes, but there are also coenzymes that are not dietary essentials and therefore are not vitamins. Coenzymes are essential for the proper functioning of numerous enzymes involved in metabolism.

HOW IT WORKS

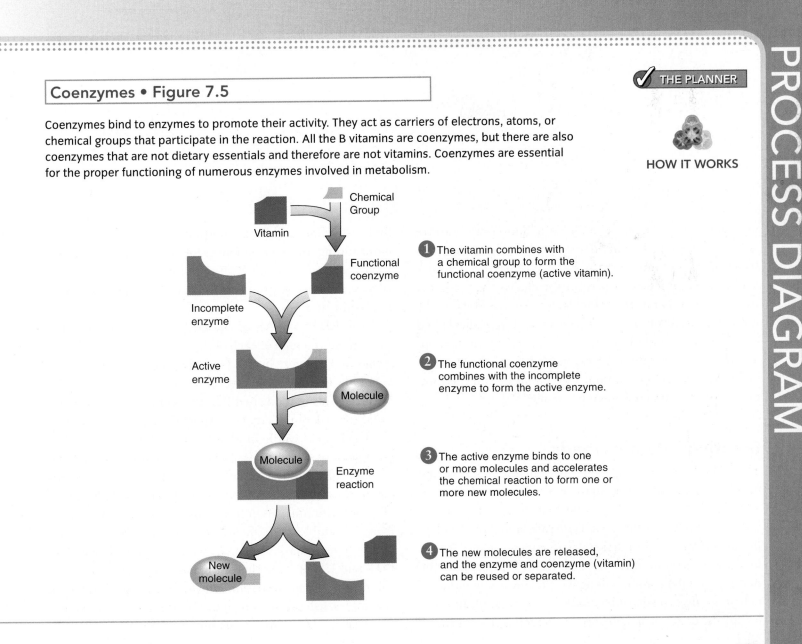

1 The vitamin combines with a chemical group to form the functional coenzyme (active vitamin).

2 The functional coenzyme combines with the incomplete enzyme to form the active enzyme.

3 The active enzyme binds to one or more molecules and accelerates the chemical reaction to form one or more new molecules.

4 The new molecules are released, and the enzyme and coenzyme (vitamin) can be reused or separated.

Many antioxidants, including vitamin C, function by donating electrons to free radicals. A donated electron stabilizes the free radical so that it is no longer reactive and cannot steal electrons from important molecules in and around cells.

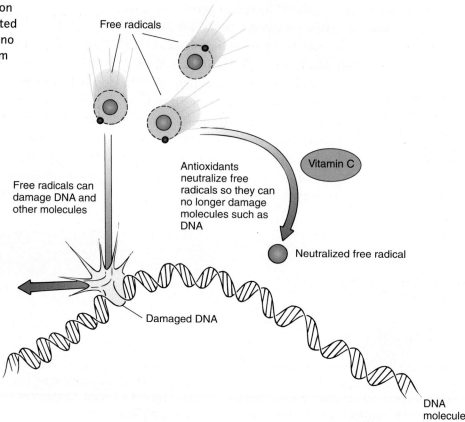

Free radicals

Antioxidants neutralize free radicals so they can no longer damage molecules such as DNA

Vitamin C

Free radicals can damage DNA and other molecules

Neutralized free radical

Damaged DNA

DNA molecule

environmental sources such as air pollution or cigarette smoke. Free radicals cause damage by snatching electrons from DNA, proteins, carbohydrates, or unsaturated fatty acids. This loss of electrons results in changes in the structure and function of these molecules. Antioxidants act by reducing the formation of or destroying free radicals and other reactive oxygen molecules before they can do damage (**Figure 7.6**). Some antioxidants are produced in the body; others, such as vitamin C, vitamin E, and the mineral selenium, are consumed in the diet.[3]

Meeting Vitamin Needs

The right amounts and combinations of vitamins and other nutrients are essential to health. Despite our knowledge of what vitamins do and how much of each we need, not everyone consumes the right amounts. In developing countries, vitamin deficiencies remain a major public health problem. In industrialized countries, thanks to the more varied food supply, along with fortification, vitamin-deficiency diseases have been almost eliminated. In these countries, concern now focuses on meeting the needs of

high-risk groups, such as children and pregnant women; determining the consequences of marginal deficiencies, such as the effect of low B vitamin intake on heart disease risk; and evaluating the risk of consuming large amounts of certain vitamins.

The RDAs and AIs of the DRIs recommend amounts that provide enough of each of the vitamins to prevent deficiency and promote health (see Chapter 2). Because more is not always better when it comes to nutrient intake, the DRIs have also established ULs as a guide to amounts that avoid the risk of toxicity (see Appendix A).

Food labels can help identify packaged foods that are good sources of vitamins. Labels are required to list the amounts of vitamin A and vitamin C in foods as a percentage of the Daily Values (**Figure 7.7**). The % Daily Values of other vitamins are often provided voluntarily. Fresh fruits, vegetables, fish, meat, and poultry, which are excellent sources of many vitamins, do not carry food labels. The FDA and USDA have therefore asked that grocery stores voluntarily provide nutrition information for the raw fruits, vegetables, fish, meat, and poultry that are most frequently purchased, and about 75% of stores comply.[4]

Vitamins on food labels • Figure 7.7

As a general guideline, if the % Daily Value is 20% or more, the food is an excellent source of that nutrient; if it is 10 to 19%, the food is a good source; and if it is 5% or less, the food is a poor source of that nutrient.

To determine the exact amount of a vitamin in a food, look up the Daily Value (see Appendix F) and multiply it by the % Daily Value on the label.

Orange Juice

Nutrition Facts
Serving Size 8 fl oz (250 mL)
Servings Per Container 8

Amount Per Serving

Calories 110   Calories from Fat 0

	%Daily Value**
Total Fat 0g	**2%**
Sodium 0mg	**0%**
Potassium 450mg	**13%**
Total Carbohydrate 26g	**9%**
Sugars 7g	
Protein 2g	

Vitamin C 120%	•	Calcium	2%
Thiamin 10%	•	Riboflavin	4%
Niacin 4%	•	Vitamin B₆	6%
Folate 15%	•	Magnesium	6%

Not a significant source of saturated fat, cholesterol, dietary fiber, vitamin A and iron.

*Percent Daily Values are based on a 2,000 calorie diet.

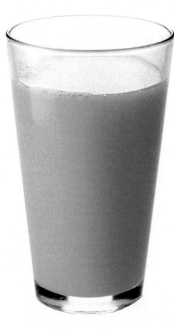

Interpreting Data

The Daily Value for vitamin C is 60 mg. Based on the information on this label, how many milligrams of vitamin C are in 4 fluid ounces of orange juice?

a. 36   b. 60   c. 72   d. 120

CONCEPT CHECK STOP

1. **What** food groups contain the greatest variety of vitamins?

2. **Why** might a low-fat diet affect the bioavailability of fat-soluble vitamins?

3. **What** is the principal function of coenzymes?

4. **How** do antioxidants protect our cells?

The Water-Soluble Vitamins

LEARNING OBJECTIVES

1. **Discuss** the role of thiamin, riboflavin, and niacin in producing ATP.

2. **Explain** why vitamin B₆ is so important for protein metabolism.

3. **Compare** the functions of folate and vitamin B₁₂.

4. **Relate** the role of vitamin C in the body to the symptoms of scurvy.

he water-soluble vitamins include the B vitamins and vitamin C. The B vitamins are directly involved in converting the energy in carbohydrate, fat, and protein into ATP, the form of energy that is used to run the body. Vitamin C is needed to synthesize connective tissue and to protect us from damage by oxidation.

Because water-soluble vitamins are not stored to any great extent, supplies of most of these vitamins are rapidly depleted. For this reason, water-soluble vitamins must be consumed regularly. Nevertheless, it takes more than a few days to develop deficiency symptoms, even when one of these vitamins is completely eliminated from the diet. For years, we thought that because most water-soluble vitamins are not stored in the body and are excreted in the urine, high doses were not harmful. However, we now recognize that high doses of some of these vitamins are toxic.

Thiamin

Thiamin, the first of the B vitamins to be discovered, is sometimes called vitamin B_1. **Beriberi**, the disease that results from a deficiency of this vitamin, came to the attention of Western medicine in colonial Asia in the 19th century. It became such a problem that the Dutch East India Company sent a team of scientists to determine its cause. A young physician named Christian Eijkman worked on this problem for over 10 years. His success came as a result of a twist of fate. He ran out of food for his experimental chickens and, instead of the usual brown rice, fed them white rice. Shortly thereafter, the chickens displayed beriberi-like symptoms. When he fed them brown rice again, their health was restored. These events provided evidence that the cause of beriberi was not a poison or a microorganism, as had previously been thought, but rather something that was missing from the diet.

Knowledge gained from Eijkman's studies made it possible to prevent and cure beriberi by feeding people a diet adequate in thiamin; however, the vitamin itself was

> **beriberi** A thiamin deficiency disease that causes weakness, nerve degeneration, and, in some cases, heart changes.

not isolated until 1926. We now know that polishing the bran layer off rice kernels to make white rice removes the thiamin-rich portion of the grain. Therefore, in populations where white rice was the staple of the diet, beriberi became a common health problem. The incidence of beriberi in eastern Asia increased dramatically in the late 1800s due to the rising popularity of polished rice.

Thiamin is a coenzyme that is needed for the breakdown of glucose to provide energy. It is particularly important for nerve function because glucose is the energy source for nerve cells. In addition to its role in energy metabolism, thiamin is needed for the synthesis of **neurotransmitters**, the metabolism of other sugars and certain amino acids, and the synthesis of ribose and deoxyribose, sugars that are part of the structure of RNA (ribonucleic acid) and DNA, respectively.

In addition to being found in the bran layer of brown rice and other whole grains, thiamin is added to enriched grains and is particularly abundant in pork, legumes, and seeds (**Figure 7.8**). When inadequate amounts of thiamin are consumed, the deficiency affects

> **neurotransmitter** A chemical substance produced by a nerve cell that can stimulate or inhibit another cell.

Meeting thiamin needs • Figure 7.8

A large proportion of the thiamin consumed in the United States comes from enriched grain products that we consume in abundance, such as pasta, rice dishes, baked goods, and breakfast cereals. The dashed lines indicate the RDAs for adult men and women, which are 1.2 mg/day and 1.1 mg/day, respectively.

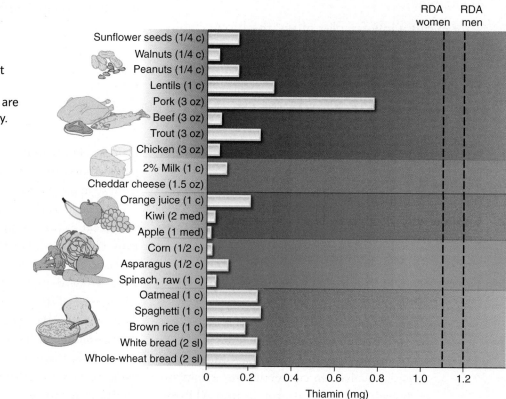

How thiamin functions • Figure 7.9

a. The active thiamin coenzyme is needed to convert pyruvate into acetyl-CoA. Acetyl-CoA can continue through cellular respiration to produce ATP. Acetyl-CoA is also needed to synthesize the neurotransmitter acetylcholine. Without thiamin, the body cannot synthesize acetylcholine or properly use glucose, which is the primary fuel for the brain and nerve cells.

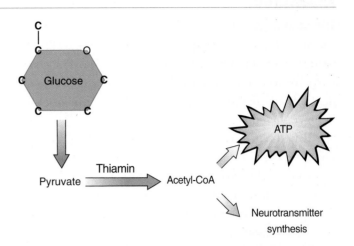

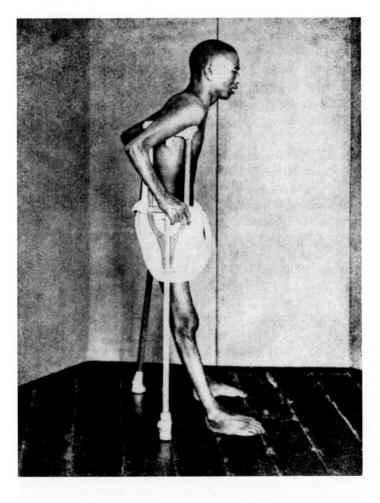

Ask Yourself

How would a deficiency of thiamin affect the amounts of ATP and neurotransmitters available?

b. For over 1000 years, beriberi flourished in East Asian countries. In Sri Lanka, the word *beriberi* means "I cannot," referring to the extreme weakness and depression that are the earliest symptoms of the disease. These symptoms may result from the inability of nerve cells to produce ATP from glucose. Other neurological symptoms, such as poor coordination, tingling sensations, and paralysis, may be related to the body's inability to synthesize certain neurotransmitters when thiamin is deficient.

the nervous and cardiovascular systems. The neurological symptoms of beriberi can be related to the functions of thiamin (**Figure 7.9**), but it is not clear why thiamin deficiency causes cardiovascular symptoms such as rapid heartbeat and enlargement of the heart.[5]

Beriberi is rare in North America today, but a form of thiamin deficiency called **Wernicke-Korsakoff syndrome** occurs in alcoholics. People with this condition experience mental confusion, psychosis, memory disturbances, and eventually coma. Alcoholics are particularly vulnerable because thiamin absorption is decreased due to the effect of alcohol on the gastrointestinal tract. In addition, their thiamin intake is low because alcoholic beverages contribute calories to the diet but add almost no nutrients.

Although thiamin is needed to provide energy, unless the diet is deficient in thiamin, increasing thiamin intake does not increase the ability to produce ATP. There is no UL for thiamin because no toxicity has been reported when an excess of this vitamin is consumed from either food or supplements.[5]

Riboflavin

Riboflavin is a B vitamin that provides a visible indicator of excessive consumption; the excess is excreted in the urine, turning it a bright fluorescent yellow. The color may surprise you, but it is harmless. No adverse effects of high doses of riboflavin from either foods or supplements have been reported.

Riboflavin forms two active coenzymes that serve as electron carriers. They function in the reactions needed to produce ATP from carbohydrate, fat, and protein. Riboflavin is also involved directly or indirectly in converting a number of other vitamins, including folate, niacin, vitamin B_6, and vitamin K, into their active forms.

One of the best sources of riboflavin in the diet is milk (**Figure 7.10**). When riboflavin is deficient, injuries heal poorly because new cells cannot grow to replace the damaged ones. The tissues that grow most rapidly, such as the skin and the linings of the eyes, mouth, and tongue, are the first to be affected. Deficiency causes symptoms such as cracking of the lips and at the corners of the mouth; increased sensitivity to light; burning, tearing, and itching of the eyes; and flaking of the skin around the nose, eyebrows, and earlobes.

A deficiency of riboflavin usually occurs in conjunction with deficiencies of other B vitamins because the same foods are also sources of those vitamins and because riboflavin is needed to convert other vitamins into their active forms. Some of the symptoms seen in cases of riboflavin deficiency therefore reflect deficiencies of these other nutrients as well.

Meeting riboflavin needs • Figure 7.10

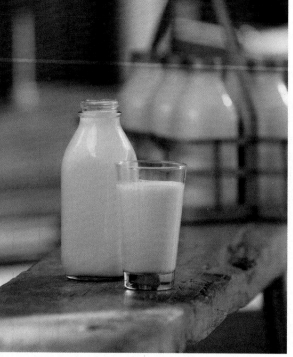

a. Ever wonder why milk doesn't come in glass bottles anymore? The reason is that riboflavin is destroyed by light. Cloudy plastic containers block some of the light, but opaque ones, such as cardboard containers, are the most effective. Exposure to light can also cause an "off" flavor and losses of vitamins A and D.[6]

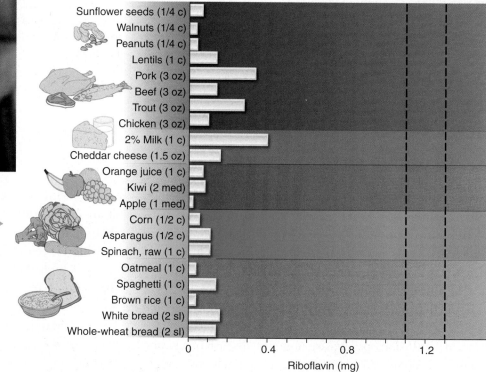

b. Major dietary sources of riboflavin include dairy products, liver, red meat, poultry, fish, whole grains, and enriched breads and cereals. Vegetable sources include asparagus, broccoli, mushrooms, and leafy green vegetables such as spinach. The dashed lines indicate the RDAs for adult men and women, which are 1.3 mg/day and 1.1 mg/day, respectively.[5]

Niacin

In the early 1900s, psychiatric hospitals in the southeastern United States were filled with patients with the niacin-deficiency disease **pellagra** (**Figure 7.11**). **Niacin** is a B vitamin that forms coenzymes essential for glucose metabolism and the synthesis of fatty acids and cholesterol. The need for niacin is so widespread

pellagra A disease resulting from niacin deficiency, which causes dermatitis, diarrhea, dementia, and, if not treated, death.

in metabolism that a deficiency causes major changes throughout the body. The early symptoms of pellagra include fatigue, decreased appetite, and indigestion. These are followed by symptoms that can be remembered as the three Ds: dermatitis, diarrhea, and dementia. If left untreated, niacin deficiency results in a fourth D—death.

Tracking down the cause of pellagra • Figure 7.11

In 1914, Dr. Joseph Goldberger was appointed by the U.S. Public Health Service to investigate the pellagra epidemic in the South. He unraveled the mystery of its cause by using the scientific method.

Observation

Goldberger observed that individuals in institutions such as hospitals, orphanages, and prisons suffered from pellagra, but the staff did not. If pellagra were an infectious disease, both populations would be equally affected.

Hypothesis

Goldberger hypothesized that pellagra was due to a deficiency in the diet.

Experiments

Experimental design: Goldberger and coworkers added nutritious foods, including meat, milk, and vegetables, to the diets of children in two orphanages.
Results: Those consuming the healthier diets recovered from pellagra. Those without the disease who ate the new diet did not contract pellagra, supporting the hypothesis that it was caused by a dietary deficiency.
Experimental design: Goldberger and colleagues fed eleven volunteers a diet believed to be lacking in the dietary substance that prevents pellagra.
Results: Six of the eleven developed symptoms of pellagra after 5 months of consuming the experimental diet, supporting the hypothesis that it was caused by a dietary deficiency.
Continued experiments: Human and animal studies by a number of scientists lead to the identification of nicotinic acid, better known as the water-soluable B vitamin niacin, in 1937, as the dietary component that cures and prevents pellagra.

Theory

Pellagra is caused by a deficiency of the B vitamin niacin.

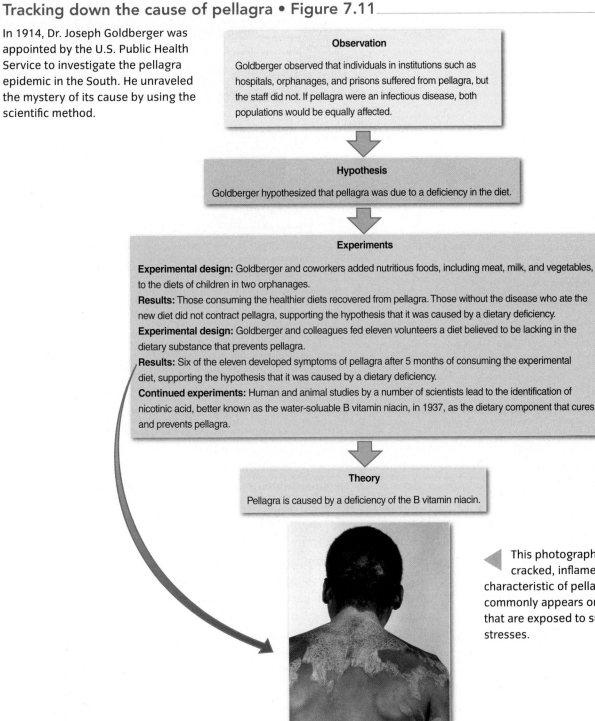

This photograph illustrates the cracked, inflamed skin that is characteristic of pellagra. The rash most commonly appears on areas of the skin that are exposed to sunlight or other stresses.

Meat, fish, peanuts, and whole and enriched grains are the best sources of niacin. Other sources include legumes and wheat bran. Food composition tables and databases do not include the amount of niacin that could be made from the tryptophan in a food. The dashed lines indicate the RDAs for adult men and women, which are 16 mg NE/day and 14 mg NE/day, respectively.

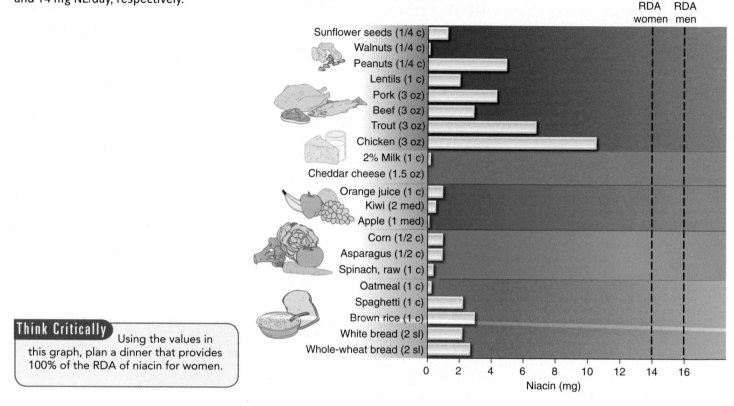

Think Critically Using the values in this graph, plan a dinner that provides 100% of the RDA of niacin for women.

Meats and grains are good sources of niacin (**Figure 7.12**). Niacin can also be synthesized in the body from the essential amino acid tryptophan. Tryptophan, however, is used to make niacin only if enough of it is available to first meet the needs of protein synthesis. When the diet is low in tryptophan, it is not used to synthesize niacin. Because some of the requirement for niacin can be met through the synthesis of niacin from tryptophan, the RDA is expressed as **niacin equivalents (NEs)**. One NE is equal to 1 mg of niacin or 60 mg of tryptophan, the amount needed to make 1 mg of niacin.[5]

The reason niacin deficiency was so prevalent in the South in the early 1900s is that the local diet among the poor was based on corn. Corn is low in tryptophan, and the niacin found naturally in corn is bound to other molecules and therefore not well absorbed. Today, as a result of the enrichment of grains with an available form of niacin, pellagra is rare in the United States, but it remains a problem in areas of Africa where the diet is based on corn.[7] Despite the corn-based diet in Mexico and Central American countries, pellagra is uncommon in those countries, in part because the treatment of corn with limewater, as is done during the making of tortillas, enhances the bioavailability of niacin. The diet in these regions also includes legumes, which provide both niacin and a source of tryptophan for the synthesis of niacin.

There is no evidence of any adverse effects due to the consumption of niacin that occurs naturally in foods, but niacin supplements can be toxic. Excess niacin supplementation can cause flushing of the skin, a tingling sensation in the hands and feet, a red skin rash, nausea, vomiting, diarrhea, high blood sugar levels, abnormalities in liver function, and blurred vision. The UL for adults is 35 mg. Doses of 50 mg or greater of one form of niacin are used as a drug to treat elevated blood cholesterol; this amount should be consumed only when prescribed by a physician.

Biotin

The B vitamin **biotin** is a coenzyme that functions in energy metabolism and glucose synthesis. It is also important in the metabolism of fatty acids and amino acids. Good sources of biotin in the diet include cooked eggs, liver, yogurt, and nuts. Fruit and meat are poor sources. Bacteria in the gastrointestinal tract synthesize biotin, and some of this is absorbed into the body and helps meet our biotin needs. An AI of 30 μg/day has been established for adults.[5]

Although biotin deficiency is uncommon, it has been observed in people with malabsorption and those taking certain medications for long periods.[5] Eating raw eggs can also cause biotin deficiency (**Figure 7.13**). Biotin deficiency in humans causes nausea, thinning hair, loss of hair color, a red skin rash, depression, lethargy, hallucinations, and tingling of the extremities. High doses of biotin have not resulted in toxicity symptoms; there is no UL for biotin.

Pantothenic Acid

Pantothenic acid, which gets its name from the Greek word *pantothen* (meaning "from everywhere"), is a B vitamin that is widely distributed in foods. It is particularly abundant in meat, eggs, whole grains, and legumes, and it is found in lesser amounts in milk, vegetables, and fruits.

In addition to being "from everywhere" in the diet, pantothenic acid seems to be needed everywhere in the body. It is part of coenzyme A (CoA), which is needed for the breakdown of carbohydrates, fatty acids, and amino acids, as well as for the modification of proteins and the synthesis of neurotransmitters, steroid hormones, and hemoglobin. Pantothenic acid is also needed to form a molecule that is essential for the synthesis of cholesterol and fatty acids.

The wide distribution of pantothenic acid in foods makes deficiency rare in humans. The AI is 5 mg/day for adults. Pantothenic acid is relatively nontoxic, and there are insufficient data to establish a UL.[5]

Raw eggs and biotin bioavailability • Figure 7.13

Raw egg whites contain a protein called avidin that tightly binds biotin and prevents its absorption. Even if you were not concerned with biotin deficiency, raw eggs should never be eaten because they can contain harmful bacteria. Thoroughly cooking eggs kills bacteria and denatures avidin so that it cannot bind biotin.

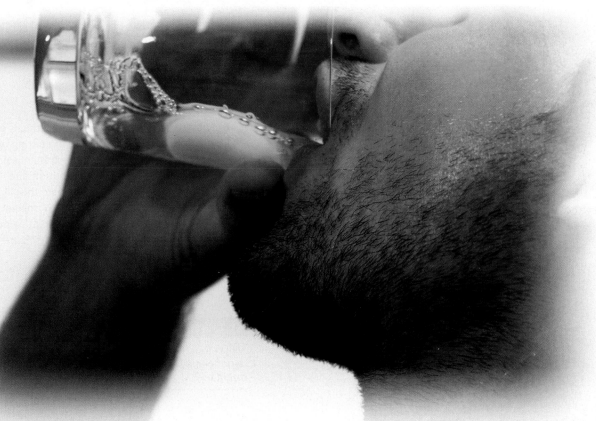

Vitamin B₆

Vitamin B₆ is a B vitamin that is particularly important for amino acid and protein metabolism. It is needed to synthesize nonessential amino acids, make neurotransmitters, synthesize hemoglobin, convert tryptophan into niacin, and break down glycogen to release glucose into the blood. There are three forms of vitamin B₆: pyridoxal, pyridoxine, and pyridoxamine. These can be converted into the active coenzyme **pyridoxal phosphate**, which is needed for the activity of more than 100 enzymes involved in the metabolism of protein, carbohydrate, and fat.

Nutrition InSight | Vitamin B₆ functions and deficiency symptoms • Figure 7.14

a. Vitamin B₆ is needed for *transamination* reactions, which synthesize nonessential amino acids by transferring an amino group to a carbon compound, and for *deamination* reactions, which remove the amino group from amino acids so that the remaining carbon compound can be used to provide energy or synthesize glucose. Vitamin B₆ is also needed to remove the acid group from amino acids so that the remaining molecule can be used to synthesize neurotransmitters.

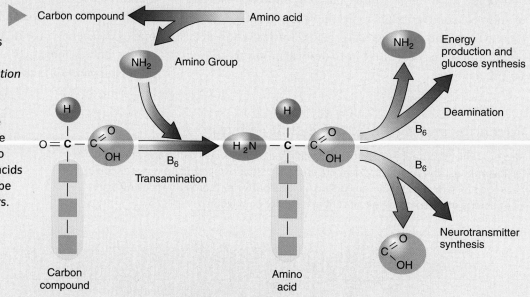

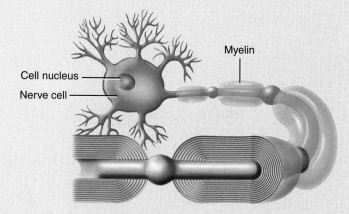

b. Vitamin B₆ is needed for the synthesis of lipids that are part of the **myelin** coating on nerves. Myelin is essential for nerve transmission. The role of vitamin B₆ in myelin formation and neurotransmitter synthesis may explain the neurological symptoms that occur with deficiency, such as numbness and tingling in the hands and feet, depression, headaches, confusion, and seizures.

Ask Yourself

What functions of vitamin B₆ might explain why a deficiency of this vitamin interferes with nerve function?

Vitamin B$_6$ deficiency leads to poor growth, skin lesions, decreased immune function, anemia, and neurological symptoms. Because vitamin B$_6$ is needed for amino acid metabolism, the onset of a deficiency can be hastened by a diet that is low in vitamin B$_6$ but high in protein. Many of the symptoms can be linked to the chemical reactions that depend on this vitamin coenzyme (**Figure 7.14**). For example, poor growth, skin lesions, and decreased antibody formation may occur with a diet that is low in vitamin B$_6$ because of the central role of vitamin B$_6$ in protein and energy metabolism.

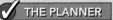
THE PLANNER

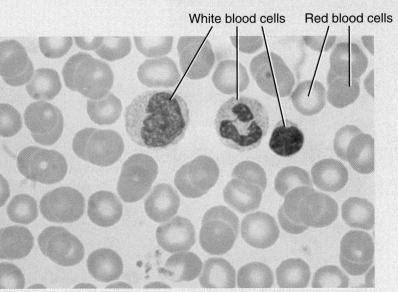
White blood cells   Red blood cells

c. Vitamin B$_6$ is needed to synthesize hemoglobin, the oxygen-carrying protein in red blood cells. When vitamin B$_6$ is deficient, hemoglobin cannot be made; the result is a type of anemia characterized by small, pale red blood cells. Vitamin B$_6$ is also needed to form white blood cells, which are part of the immune system, so deficiency reduces immune function.

d. If vitamin B$_6$ status is low, homocysteine, which is formed from the amino acid methionine, cannot be converted to cysteine, so levels rise. Even a mild elevation in blood homocysteine levels has been shown to increase the risk of heart disease.[8]

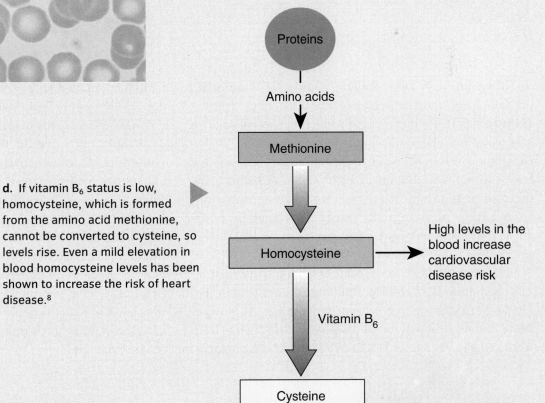

Proteins

Amino acids

Methionine

Homocysteine → High levels in the blood increase cardiovascular disease risk

Vitamin B$_6$

Cysteine

The Water-Soluble Vitamins **217**

Meeting vitamin B₆ needs • Figure 7.15

Animal sources of vitamin B₆ include chicken, fish, pork, and organ meats. Good plant sources include whole-wheat products, brown rice, soybeans, sunflower seeds, and some fruits and vegetables, such as bananas, broccoli, and spinach. The dashed line indicates the RDA for adult men and women ages 19 to 50, which is 1.3 mg/day. [5]

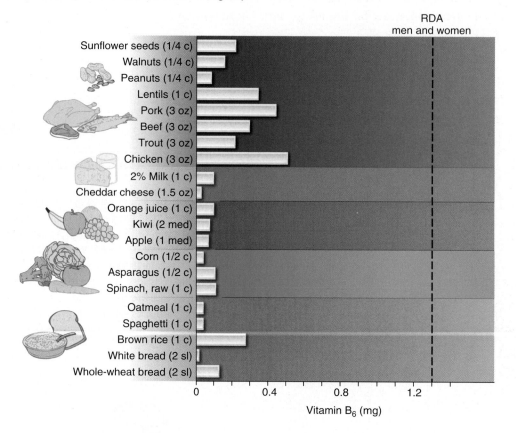

Meat and fish are excellent sources of vitamin B₆, and whole grains and legumes are good plant sources (**Figure 7.15**). Refined grain products such as white rice and white bread are not good sources of vitamin B₆ because the vitamin is lost during refining but is not added back through enrichment. It is, however, added to many fortified breakfast cereals, so these make an important contribution to vitamin B₆ intake.[9] Vitamin B₆ is destroyed by heat and light, so it can easily be lost during processing.

No adverse effects have been associated with high intake of vitamin B₆ from foods, but large doses found in supplements can cause severe nerve impairment. To prevent nerve damage, the UL for adults is set at 100 mg/day from food and supplements.[5] Despite the potential for toxicity, high-dose supplements of vitamin B₆ containing 100 mg/dose (5000% of the Daily Value) are available over the counter, making it easy to obtain a dose that exceeds the UL.

People take vitamin B₆ supplements to reduce the symptoms of premenstrual syndrome (PMS), treat carpal tunnel syndrome, and strengthen immune function. There is little evidence that supplements consistently relieve the symptoms of carpal tunnel syndrome or provide significant benefit for women with PMS.[10,11] Vitamin B₆ supplements have been found to improve immune function in older adults.[5] However, because elderly people frequently have low intakes of vitamin B₆, it is unclear whether the beneficial effects of supplements are due to an improvement in vitamin B₆ status or to stimulation of the immune system.

Folate (Folic Acid)

Folate is a B vitamin that is important during pregnancy for the development of the embryo. Low folate intake increases the risk of birth defects called **neural tube defects** (**Figure 7.16**). The formation of the neural tube, which later develops into the brain and spinal cord, occurs very early during pregnancy. Therefore, to reduce the risk of neural tube defects, a woman's folate status must be adequate before she becomes pregnant and during the critical early days of pregnancy. To help ensure adequate folate intake in women of childbearing age, in 1998 the FDA mandated that the **folic acid** form of the vitamin be added to all enriched grains and cereal products. Since then, the incidence of neural tube defects in the United States has decreased by almost 50%, and a similar reduction has been observed in other countries where folic acid fortification has been introduced (see Chapter 11: *What a Scientist Sees: Folate Fortification and Neural Tube Defects*).[12,13]

Folate and *folacin* are general terms for compounds whose chemical structures and nutritional properties are similar to those of folic acid. The folic acid form, which is added to enriched grains and other fortified products and used in dietary supplements, is more easily absorbed, so its bioavailability is about twice that of folate found naturally in foods. The RDA for folate is expressed in **dietary folate equivalents (DFEs)**. DFEs correct for differences in the bioavailability of different forms of folate. One DFE is equal to 1 microgram (µg) of food folate, 0.6 µg of

> **neural tube defect** An abnormality in the brain or spinal cord that results from errors that occur during pre-natal development.
>
> **folic acid** An easily absorbed form of the vitamin folate that is used in dietary supplements and forti-fied foods.

Neural tube defects • Figure 7.16

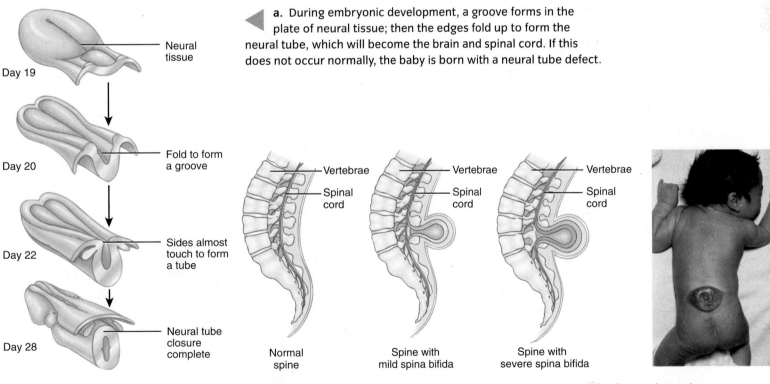

a. During embryonic development, a groove forms in the plate of neural tissue; then the edges fold up to form the neural tube, which will become the brain and spinal cord. If this does not occur normally, the baby is born with a neural tube defect.

Day 19 — Neural tissue

Day 20 — Fold to form a groove

Day 22 — Sides almost touch to form a tube

Day 28 — Neural tube closure complete

Normal spine — Vertebrae, Spinal cord

Spine with mild spina bifida — Vertebrae, Spinal cord

Spine with severe spina bifida — Vertebrae, Spinal cord

b. If a lower portion of the neural tube does not close normally, the result is **spina bifida** (shown here), a condition in which the spinal cord forms abnormally. Many babies with spina bifida have learning disabilities and nerve damage that causes varying degrees of paralysis of the lower limbs. If the head end of the neural tube does not close properly, the brain doesn't form completely; the result is anencephaly (partial or total absence of the brain). Babies with anencephaly are usually blind, deaf, and unconscious, and they die soon after birth.

Folate deficiency and anemia • Figure 7.17

Folate is needed for DNA replication. Without folate, developing red blood cells, cannot divide. Instead, they just grow bigger. The abnormally large immature red blood cells, called megaloblasts, then mature into abnormally large red blood cells called macrocytes. Because fewer mature red cells are produced when folate is deficient, the blood's oxygen-carrying capacity is reduced.

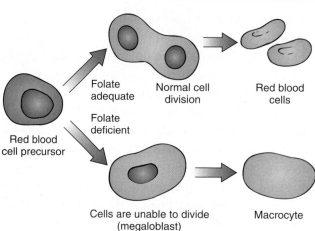

Red blood cell precursor

Folate adequate → Normal cell division → Red blood cells

Folate deficient → Cells are unable to divide (megaloblast) → Macrocyte

synthetic folic acid from fortified food or supplements consumed with food, or 0.5 μg of synthetic folic acid consumed on an empty stomach.[5]

Folate coenzymes are needed for the synthesis of DNA and the metabolism of some amino acids. Cells must synthesize DNA in order to replicate, so folate is particularly important in tissues in which cells are dividing rapidly, such as the intestines, skin, embryonic and fetal tissues, and bone marrow, where red blood cells are made. When folate is deficient, cells cannot divide

normally. This leads to one of the most notable symptoms of folate deficiency a type of anemia called **macrocytic anemia**, or **megalo-blastic anemia (Figure 7.17)**. Other symptoms of folate deficiency include poor growth, problems with nerve development and function, diarrhea, and inflammation of the tongue.

> **macrocytic anemia** or **megalo-blastic anemia** A reduction in the blood's capacity to carry oxygen that is characterized by abnormally large immature and mature red blood cells.

The relationship between folate and vitamin B$_{12}$ • Figure 7.18

Vitamin B$_{12}$ deficiency prevents folate from being converted into one of its active forms, so vitamin B$_{12}$ deficiency causes folate to also be deficient. This interrelationship has raised concerns that our folate-fortified food supply will prevent folate-deficiency symptoms from occurring and allow B$_{12}$ deficiencies to go unnoticed. The UL for adults, set at 1000 μg/day of folic acid from supplements and/or fortified foods, is based on an amount that will not mask the macrocytic anemia caused by vitamin B$_{12}$ deficiency.

Supplemental folic acid can prevent macrocytic anemia, thus "hiding" vitamin B$_{12}$ deficiency. Untreated vitamin B$_{12}$ deficiency can cause irreversible nerve damage.

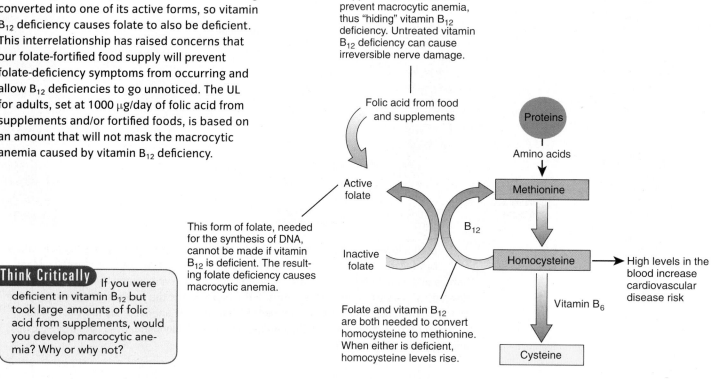

Folic acid from food and supplements

Proteins

Amino acids

Active folate

Methionine

B$_{12}$

This form of folate, needed for the synthesis of DNA, cannot be made if vitamin B$_{12}$ is deficient. The resulting folate deficiency causes macrocytic anemia.

Inactive folate

Homocysteine → High levels in the blood increase cardiovascular disease risk

Vitamin B$_6$

Folate and vitamin B$_{12}$ are both needed to convert homocysteine to methionine. When either is deficient, homocysteine levels rise.

Cysteine

Think Critically If you were deficient in vitamin B$_{12}$ but took large amounts of folic acid from supplements, would you develop marcocytic anemia? Why or why not?

Meeting folate needs • Figure 7.19

Folate is named after the Latin word for *foliage*, because leafy greens, such as spinach, are good sources of this vitamin. Legumes, nuts, enriched grains, and orange juice are also good sources. Whole grains and many vegetables are fair sources, and only small amounts of folate are found in meats, cheese, milk, and most fruits. The dashed line indicates the RDA for adult men and women, which is 400 μg/day.

Ask Yourself

Which three of the foods shown here provide the most folate? Are any of these foods fortified?

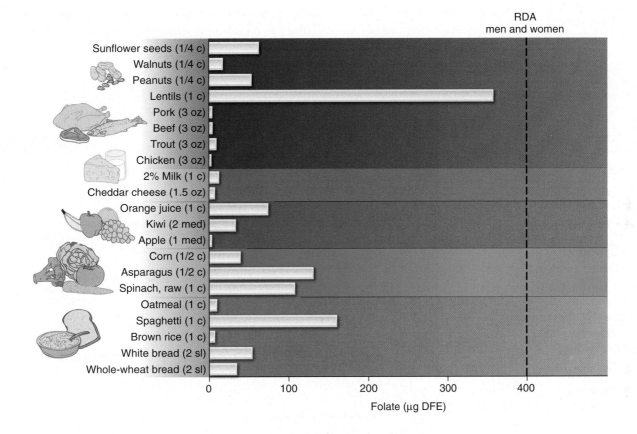

Low folate status may also increase the risk of developing heart disease and cancers of the ovary, pancreas, breast, and colon.[14–16] Folate's connection with heart disease has to do with the metabolism of homocysteine. Elevated levels of homocysteine have been associated with increased risk of heart disease. Folate and vitamins B_{12} and B_6 are all needed to prevent homocysteine levels from rising (**Figure 7.18**). Despite this, supplementation with these vitamins has failed to exert significant effects on cardiovascular risk.[8]

Population groups most at risk of folate deficiency include pregnant women and premature infants (because of their rapid rates of cell division and growth), the elderly (because of their limited intake of foods high in folate), alcoholics (because alcohol inhibits the absorption of folate),

and tobacco smokers (because smoke inactivates folate in the cells lining the lungs).[5]

Asparagus, oranges, legumes, liver, and yeast are excellent food sources of folate (**Figure 7.19**). Whole grains are a fair source, and, as discussed earlier, folic acid is added to enriched grain products, including enriched breads, flours, corn meal, pasta, grits, and rice. Because supplementing folic acid early in pregnancy has been shown to reduce neural tube defects in the fetus, it is recommended that women who are capable of becoming pregnant consume 400 μg of synthetic folic acid from fortified foods and/or supplements in addition to the food folate consumed in a varied diet.[5] To get 400 μg of folic acid, women of childbearing age would need to eat four to six servings of fortified grain products each day or take a supplement containing folic acid.

Vitamin B$_{12}$

In the early 1900s, **pernicious anemia** amounted to a death sentence. There was no cure. In the 1920s, researchers George Minot and William Murphy pursued their belief that pernicious anemia could be cured by something in the diet. They discovered that they could restore patients' health by feeding them about 4 to 8 ounces of slightly cooked liver at every meal. Today we know that eating liver cured pernicious anemia because liver is a concentrated source of **vitamin B$_{12}$**. Individuals with pernicious anemia lack a protein produced in the stomach, called **intrinsic factor**, that enhances vitamin B$_{12}$ absorption (**Figure 7.20**). Today, pernicious anemia is treated with injections or megadoses of vitamin B$_{12}$ rather than with plates full of liver.

> **pernicious anemia** A macrocytic anemia resulting from vitamin B$_{12}$ deficiency that occurs when dietary vitamin B$_{12}$ cannot be absorbed due to a lack of intrinsic factor.

> **intrinsic factor** A protein produced in the stomach that is needed for the absorption of adequate amounts of vitamin B$_{12}$.

Vitamin B$_{12}$ digestion and absorption • Figure 7.20

✓ THE PLANNER

The body stores and reuses vitamin B$_{12}$ more efficiently than it does most other water-soluble vitamins, so deficiency is typically caused by poor absorption rather than by low intake alone. Absorption of adequate amounts of vitamin B$_{12}$ depends on the presence of stomach acid, protein-digesting enzymes, and intrinsic factor.

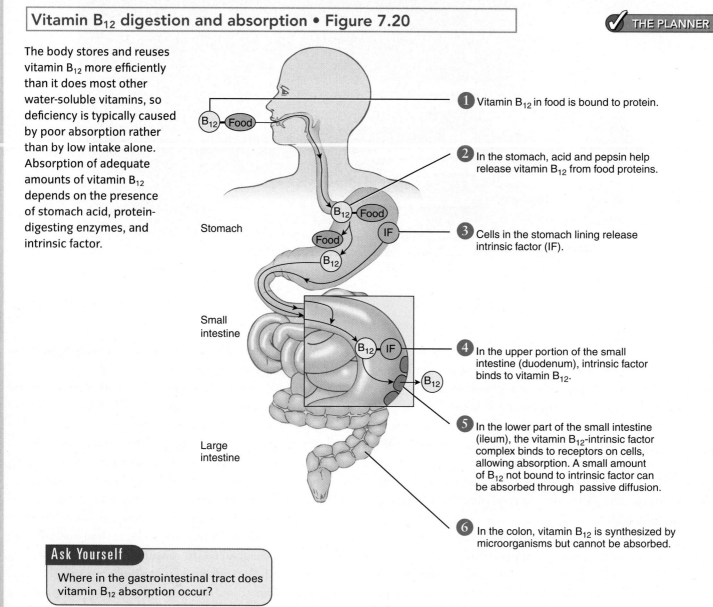

1 Vitamin B$_{12}$ in food is bound to protein.

2 In the stomach, acid and pepsin help release vitamin B$_{12}$ from food proteins.

3 Cells in the stomach lining release intrinsic factor (IF).

4 In the upper portion of the small intestine (duodenum), intrinsic factor binds to vitamin B$_{12}$.

5 In the lower part of the small intestine (ileum), the vitamin B$_{12}$-intrinsic factor complex binds to receptors on cells, allowing absorption. A small amount of B$_{12}$ not bound to intrinsic factor can be absorbed through passive diffusion.

6 In the colon, vitamin B$_{12}$ is synthesized by microorganisms but cannot be absorbed.

Ask Yourself

Where in the gastrointestinal tract does vitamin B$_{12}$ absorption occur?

Meeting vitamin B₁₂ needs • Figure 7.21

Animal foods provide vitamin B$_{12}$, but plant foods do not unless they have been fortified with it or contaminated by bacteria, soil, insects, or other sources of B$_{12}$. The dashed line indicates the RDA for adult men and women of all ages, which is 2.4 μg/day. No toxic effects have been reported for vitamin B$_{12}$ intakes of up to 100 μg/day from food or supplements. Insufficient data are available to establish a UL for vitamin B$_{12}$.[5]

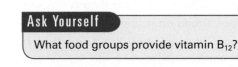

Ask Yourself

What food groups provide vitamin B$_{12}$?

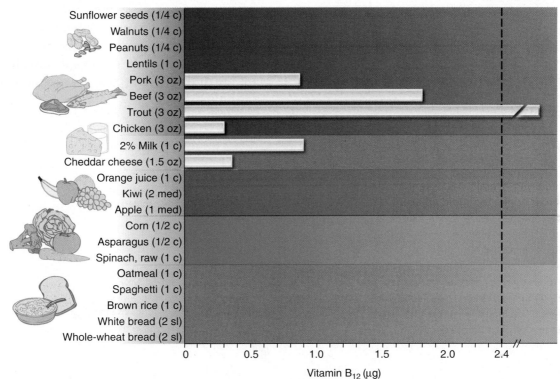

Vitamin B$_{12}$, also known as **cobalamin**, is necessary for the production of ATP from certain fatty acids, to convert homocysteine to methionine (see Figure 7.18), and to maintain the myelin coating on nerves (see Figure 7.14b). When vitamin B$_{12}$ is deficient, homocysteine levels rise, and folate cannot be converted into its active form. The lack of folate causes macrocytic anemia. Lack of vitamin B$_{12}$ also leads to degeneration of the myelin that coats the nerves in the spinal cord and brain, resulting in symptoms such as numbness and tingling, abnormalities in gait, memory loss, and disorientation. If not treated, vitamin B$_{12}$ deficiency eventually causes paralysis and death.

Vitamin B$_{12}$ is found naturally only in animal products (**Figure 7.21**). Therefore, meeting vitamin B$_{12}$ needs is a concern among vegans—those who consume no animal products. Vegans must consume supplements or foods fortified with vitamin B$_{12}$ in order to meet their needs for this vitamin.[17] Vitamin B$_{12}$ deficiency is also a concern in older

adults because of a condition called **atrophic gastritis**, which reduces the secretion of stomach acid. Without sufficient stomach acid, the enzymes that release the vitamin B$_{12}$ bound to proteins in food cannot function properly, so vitamin B$_{12}$ remains bound to the food proteins and cannot be absorbed (see Figure 7.20). In addition, lack of stomach acid allows large numbers of microbes to grow in the gut and compete for available vitamin B$_{12}$, reducing absorption. Atrophic gastritis affects 10 to 30% of adults over age 50. To ensure adequate B$_{12}$ absorption, it is recommended that individuals over age 50 meet their RDA by consuming foods fortified with vitamin B$_{12}$ or taking vitamin B$_{12}$ supplements.[5] The vitamin B$_{12}$ in these products is not bound to proteins, so it is absorbed even when stomach acid levels are low.

atrophic gastritis An inflammation of the stomach lining that results in reduced secretion of stomach acid, microbial overgrowth, and, in severe cases, a reduction in the production of intrinsic factor.

Vitamin C

Vitamin C, also called **ascorbic acid**, is best known for its role in the synthesis and maintenance of **collagen** (**Figure 7.22**). Collagen, the most abundant protein in the body, can be thought of as the glue that holds the body together. It forms the base of all connective tissue. It is the framework for bones and teeth; it is the main component of ligaments, tendons, and the scars that bind a wound together; and it gives structure to the walls of blood vessels. When vitamin C is lacking, collagen cannot be formed and maintained, and the symptoms of **scurvy** appear. In the 17th and 18th centuries, sailors were far more likely to die of scurvy than to be killed in shipwrecks or battles.

> **scurvy** A vitamin C deficiency disease characterized by bleeding gums, tooth loss, joint pain, bleeding into the skin and mucous membranes, and fatigue.

In addition to its role in the synthesis and maintenance of collagen, vitamin C functions in reactions that synthesize neurotransmitters, hormones, bile acids, and carnitine, which is needed for the breakdown of fatty acids. It is also an antioxidant that acts in the blood and other body fluids. Because its antioxidant properties help maintain the immune system, the ability to fight infection is decreased when this vitamin is deficient. Vitamin C's antioxidant action also regenerates the active antioxidant form of vitamin E and enhances iron absorption in the small intestine by keeping iron in its more readily absorbed form.

Vitamin C function and deficiency • Figure 7.22

a. A reaction requiring vitamin C is essential for the formation of bonds that hold adjacent collagen strands together and give the protein strength. Like all other body proteins, collagen is continuously being broken down and reformed. Without vitamin C, the bonds holding adjacent collagen molecules together cannot be formed, so the collagen that is broken down is replaced with abnormal collagen. The inability to form healthy collagen causes the symptoms of scurvy.

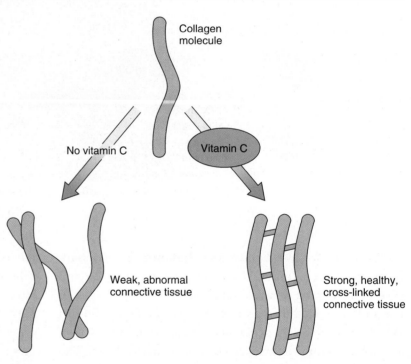

Collagen molecule

No vitamin C

Vitamin C

Weak, abnormal connective tissue

Strong, healthy, cross-linked connective tissue

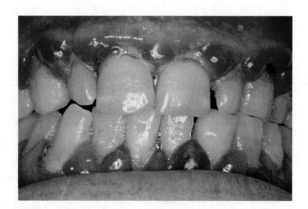

b. When vitamin C intake is below 10 mg/day, the symptoms of scurvy begin to appear. The gums become inflamed, swell, and bleed. The teeth loosen and eventually fall out. The capillary walls weaken and rupture, causing bleeding under the skin and into the joints. This causes raised red spots on the skin, joint pain and weakness, and easy bruising. Wounds do not heal, old wounds may reopen, and bones fracture. People with scurvy become tired and depressed, and they suffer from hysteria.

Meeting vitamin C needs • Figure 7.23

Fruits that are high in vitamin C include citrus fruits, strawberries, kiwis, and cantaloupe. Vegetables in the cabbage family, such as broccoli, cauliflower, bok choy, and Brussels sprouts, as well as dark-green vegetables, green and red peppers, okra, tomatoes, and potatoes, are also good sources of vitamin C. Meat, fish, poultry, eggs, dairy products, and grains are poor sources.

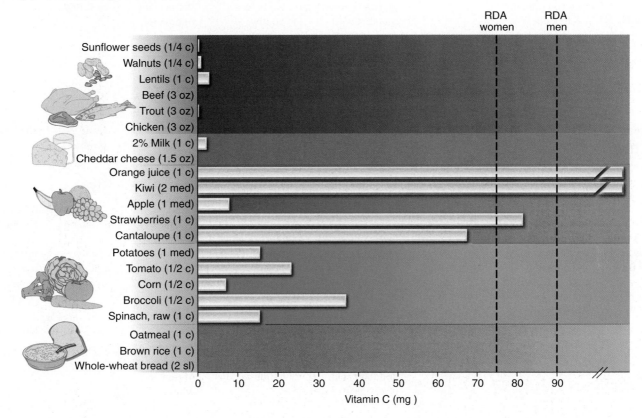

Citrus fruits are an excellent source of vitamin C. A large orange contains enough vitamin C to meet the RDA of 90 mg/day for men and 75 mg/day for women.[3] Other fruits and vegetables are also good sources of this vitamin (**Figure 7.23**).

Vitamin C is destroyed by oxygen, light, and heat, so it is readily lost in cooking. This loss is accelerated in low-acid foods and by the use of copper or iron cooking utensils. Although most Americans consume enough vitamin C to prevent severe deficiency, marginal vitamin C deficiency is a concern for individuals who consume few fruits and vegetables. Cigarette smoking increases the requirement for vitamin C because the vitamin is used to break down compounds in cigarette smoke. It is recommended that cigarette smokers consume an extra 35 mg of vitamin C daily—an amount that can easily be supplied by a half-cup of broccoli.[3]

One-third of the population of the United States takes vitamin C supplements—usually in the hope that they will prevent the common cold. Although vitamin C does not prevent colds or reduce their severity, regular vitamin C supplementation may help reduce the duration of cold symptoms.[18] It has also been suggested that vitamin C supplements reduce the risk of cardiovascular disease and cancer, but there is insufficient evidence to support this claim.[3]

Taking high doses of supplemental vitamin C can cause diarrhea, nausea, and abdominal cramps, and it may increase the risk of kidney stone formation. In individuals who are unable to regulate iron absorption, taking vitamin C supplements, which increase iron absorption, increases the risk that toxic amounts of iron will be stored. For those with sickle cell anemia, excess vitamin C can worsen symptoms. In those taking medication to reduce blood clotting, taking more than 3000 mg/day of vitamin C can interfere with the effectiveness of the medication. In large doses, chewable vitamin C supplements can dissolve tooth enamel. The UL for vitamin C has been set at 2000 mg/day from food and supplements.[3]

A summary of the water-soluble vitamins and choline Table 7.3

Vitamin	Sources	Recommended intake for adults	Major functions	Deficiency diseases and symptoms	Groups at risk of deficiency	Toxicity	UL
Thiamin (vitamin B$_1$, thiamin mononitrate)	Pork, whole and enriched grains, seeds, nuts, legumes	1.1–1.2 mg/day	Coenzyme in glucose and energy metabolism; needed for neurotransmitter synthesis and normal nerve function	Beriberi: weakness, apathy, irritability, nerve tingling, poor coordination, paralysis, heart changes	Alcoholics, those living in poverty	None reported	ND
Riboflavin (vitamin B$_2$)	Dairy products, whole and enriched grains, dark green vegetables, meats	1.1–1.3 mg/day	Coenzyme in energy and lipid metabolism	Inflammation of the mouth and tongue, cracks at corners of the mouth	None	None reported	ND
Niacin (nicotinamide, nicotinic acid, vitamin B$_3$)	Beef, chicken, fish, peanuts, legumes, whole and enriched grains; can be made from tryptophan	14–16 mg NE/day	Coenzyme in energy metabolism and lipid synthesis and breakdown	Pellagra: diarrhea, dermatitis on areas exposed to sun, dementia	Those consuming a limited diet based on corn; alcoholics	Flushing nausea, rash, tingling extremities	35 mg/day from fortified foods and supplements
Biotin	Liver, egg yolks; synthesized in the gut	30 μg/day	Coenzyme in glucose synthesis and energy and fatty acid metabolism	Dermatitis, nausea, depression, hallucinations	Those consuming large amounts of raw egg whites; alcoholics	None reported	ND
Pantothenic acid (calcium pantothenate)	Meat, legumes, whole grains; widespread in foods	5 mg/day	Coenzyme in energy metabolism and lipid synthesis and breakdown	Fatigue, rash	Alcoholics	None reported	ND

Choline

Choline is a water-soluble substance that you may see included in supplements called "vitamin B complex." It is needed for the synthesis of the neurotransmitter acetylcholine, the structure and function of cell membranes, lipid transport, and homocysteine metabolism. It can be synthesized to a limited extent by humans. Although it is not currently classified as a vitamin, it is recognized as an essential nutrient. Deficiency during pregnancy can interfere with brain development in the fetus and deficiency in adults causes fatty liver and muscle damage.[19] The DRIs have set AIs for this compound: 550 mg/day for men and 425 mg/day for women.[5]

Choline is found in many foods, with large amounts in egg yolks, liver, meat and fish, wheat germ, and nuts.[20] Because the average daily choline intake in the United States exceeds the recommended intake, a deficiency is unlikely in healthy humans in this country.[5]

Excess choline intake can cause a fishy body odor, sweating, reduced growth rate, low blood pressure, and liver damage. The amounts needed to cause these symptoms are much higher than can be obtained from foods. The UL for choline for adults is 3.5 g/day.[5]

A summary of the water-soluble vitamins and choline is provided in **Table 7.3**.

Vitamin	Sources	Recommended intake for adults	Major functions	Deficiency diseases and symptoms	Groups at risk of deficiency	Toxicity	UL
Vitamin B₆ (pyridoxine, pyridoxal phosphate, pyridoxamine)	Meat, fish, poultry, legumes, whole grains, nuts and seeds	1.3–1.7 mg/day	Coenzyme in protein and amino acid metabolism, neurotransmitter and hemoglobin synthesis, many other reactions	Headache, convulsions, other neurological symptoms, nausea, poor growth, anemia	Alcoholics	Numbness, nerve damage	100 mg/day
Folate (folic acid, folacin, pteroyglutamic acid)	Leafy green vegetables, legumes, seeds, enriched grains, orange juice	400 μg DFE/ day	Coenzyme in DNA synthesis and amino acid metabolism	Macrocytic anemia, inflammation of tongue, diarrhea, poor growth, neural tube defects	Pregnant women, alcoholics	Masks B₁₂ deficiency	1000 μg/day from fortified food and supplements
Vitamin B₁₂ (cobalamin, cyanocobalamin)	Animal products	2.4 μg/day	Coenzyme in folate and homocysteine metabolism; nerve function	Pernicious anemia, macrocytic anemia, nerve damage	Vegans, elderly, people with stomach or intestinal disease	None reported	ND
Vitamin C (ascorbic acid, ascorbate)	Citrus fruit, broccoli, strawberries, greens, peppers	75–90 mg/day	Coenzyme in collagen (connective tissue) synthesis; hormone and neurotransmitter synthesis; antioxidant	Scurvy: poor wound healing, bleeding gums, loose teeth, bone fragility, joint pain, pinpoint hemorrhages	Alcoholics, elderly people	GI distress, diarrhea	2000 mg/day
Choline*	Egg yolks, organ meats, wheat germ, meat, fish, nuts, synthesis in the body	425–550 mg/ day	Synthesis of cell membranes and neurotransmitters	Fatty liver, muscle damage, abnormal prenatal development	None	Sweating, low blood pressure, liver damage	3500 mg/day

*Choline is technically not a vitamin, but recommendations have been made for its intake.

Note: UL, Tolerable Upper Intake Level; NE, niacin equivalent; DFE, dietary folate equivalent; ND, not determined due to insufficient data.

CONCEPT CHECK

1. **Why** do people think B vitamin supplements give them energy?

2. **What** is the role of vitamin B₆ in amino acid metabolism?

3. **How** can folate and vitamin B₁₂ deficiency both cause macrocytic anemia?

4. **What** is the role of vitamin C in collagen formation?

The Fat-Soluble Vitamins

LEARNING OBJECTIVES

1. **Explain** the roles of vitamin A in keeping eyes healthy.

2. **Relate** the functions of vitamin D to the symptoms that occur when it is deficient in the body.

3. **Describe** the function of vitamin E.

4. **Discuss** how vitamin K is involved in blood clotting.

The fat-soluble vitamins—A, D, E, and K—are found along with fats in foods. They require special handling for absorption into and transport through the body. Because excesses of these vitamins can be stored in the liver and fatty tissues, intakes can vary without a risk of deficiency as long as average intake over a period of weeks or months meets the body's needs. Their solubility in fat, however, limits their routes of excretion and therefore increases the risk of toxicity.

Vitamin A

Did you ever hear that eating carrots would help you see in the dark? It turns out to be true. Carrots are a good source of **beta-carotene (β-carotene)**, a provitamin that can be converted into vitamin A in your body. **Vitamin A** is needed for vision and healthy eyes.

Vitamin A in the diet Vitamin A is found both preformed and in provitamin form in our diet. Preformed vitamin A compounds are known as **retinoids**. Three retinoids are active in the body: retinal, retinol, and retinoic acid. **Carotenoids** are yellow-orange pigments found in plants, some of which are vitamin A precursors; once inside the body, they can be converted into retinoids (**Figure 7.24a**). Beta-carotene is the most potent

> **retinoids** Chemical forms of preformed vitamin A: includes retinol, retinal, and retinoic acid.
>
> **carotenoids** Yellow, orange, and red pigments synthesized by plants and many microorganisms. Some can be converted to vitamin A.

Meeting vitamin A needs • Figure 7.24

a. Provitamin A is found in fruits and vegetables. Beta-carotene is plentiful in carrots, squash, apricots, and other orange and yellow vegetables and fruits. It is also found in dark green vegetables such as broccoli and spinach, in which the yellow-orange pigment is masked by green chlorophyll. Other carotenoids that provide some provitamin A activity include α-carotene, found in dark green vegetables, carrots, and squash, and β-cryptoxanthin, found in papaya, sweet red peppers, and winter squash.

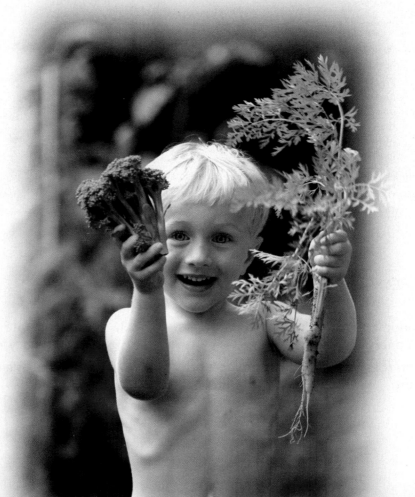

vitamin A precursor. **Alpha-carotene** (α-**carotene**) and **beta-cryptoxanthin** (β-**cryptoxanthin**) are also provitamin A carotenoids, but they are not converted into retinoids as efficiently as β-carotene. Carotenoids that are not converted into retinoids may function as antioxidants and thus may play a role in protecting against cancer and heart disease.

You can meet your needs for vitamin A by eating animal products, such as eggs and dairy products, that are sources of retinoids, and by eating fruits and vegetables that are sources of provitamin A carotenoids (**Figure 7.24b**). Because carotenoids are not absorbed as well as retinoids and are not completely converted into vitamin A in the body, you get less functional vitamin A from this form. To account for this difference, **retinol activity equivalents (RAEs)** are used to express the amount of usable vitamin A in foods; 1 RAE is the amount of retinol, β-carotene, α-carotene, or β-cryptoxanthin that provides vitamin A activity equal to 1 μg of retinol (see Appendix I).[21]

Both carotenoids and retinoids are bound to proteins in food. To be absorbed they must be released from protein by pepsin and other protein-digesting enzymes. In the small intestine, they combine with bile acids and other dietary fats in order to be absorbed. The fat content of the diet can affect the amount of vitamin A absorbed. When dietary fat intake is very low (less than 10 g/day), vitamin A absorption is impaired. This is rarely a problem in the United States and other industrialized countries, where typical fat intake is greater than 50 g/day. However, in developing countries, vitamin A deficiency may occur not only because the diet is low in vitamin A but also because the diet is too low in fat for the vitamin to be absorbed efficiently. Diseases that cause fat malabsorption can also interfere with vitamin A absorption and cause deficiency.

Protein and zinc status are also important for healthy vitamin A status. To move from liver stores to other body tissues, vitamin A must be bound to a protein called **retinol-binding protein**. When protein is deficient, the amount of retinol-binding protein made is inadequate, so vitamin A cannot be transported to the tissues where it is needed. Likewise, when zinc is deficient, a vitamin A deficiency may occur because zinc is needed to make proteins involved in vitamin A transport and metabolism.

Vitamin A functions and deficiency
Vitamin A is needed for vision and eye health because it is involved in

b. Grains and meats are generally poor sources of vitamin A. The dashed lines indicate the RDA for adult men and women, which are 900 μg/day and 700 μg/day, respectively. No specific recommendations have been made for intakes of carotenoids; their intake is considered only with regard to the amount of retinol they provide.

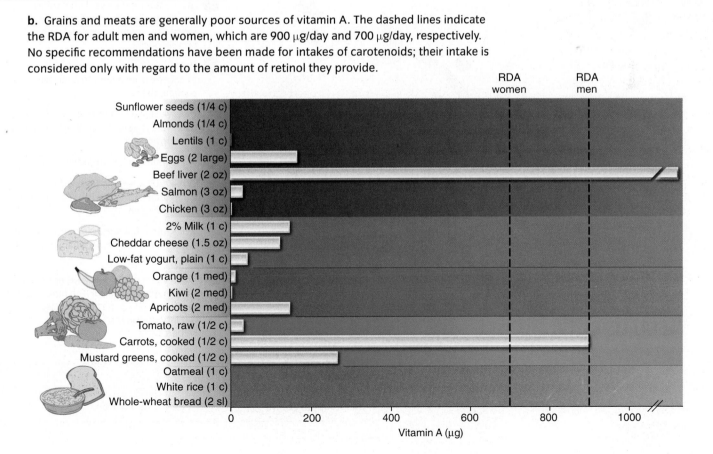

the perception of light and because it is needed for normal **cell differentiation**, the process whereby immature cells change in structure and function to become specialized.

Vitamin A helps us see because retinal is part of **rhodopsin**, a visual pigment in the eye. When light strikes rhodopsin, it initiates a series of events that result in a nerve signal being sent to the brain, which allows us to see (**Figure 7.25**). After the light stimulus has passed, rhodopsin is re-formed. Because some retinal is lost in these reactions, it must be replaced by vitamin A from the blood. If blood levels of vitamin A are low, as they are in someone who is vitamin A deficient, there is a delay in the regeneration of rhodopsin. This delay causes difficulty seeing in dim light, a condition called **night blindness**. Night blindness is one of the first and most easily reversible symptoms of vitamin A deficiency. If the deficiency progresses, more serious and less reversible symptoms can occur.

Vitamin A deficiency is uncommon in developed countries, but many Americans may have marginal deficiencies.[21] Intakes below the RDA can be caused by poor food choices even when the food supply is plentiful. In the United States, intake of fruits and vegetables, many of which are excellent sources of provitamin A, does not meet recommendations. A typical fast-food meal of a hamburger

The visual cycle • Figure 7.25

THE PLANNER ✓

Looking into the bright headlights of an approaching car at night is temporarily blinding for all of us, but for someone with vitamin A deficiency, the blindness lasts a lot longer. This occurs because of the role of vitamin A in the visual cycle.

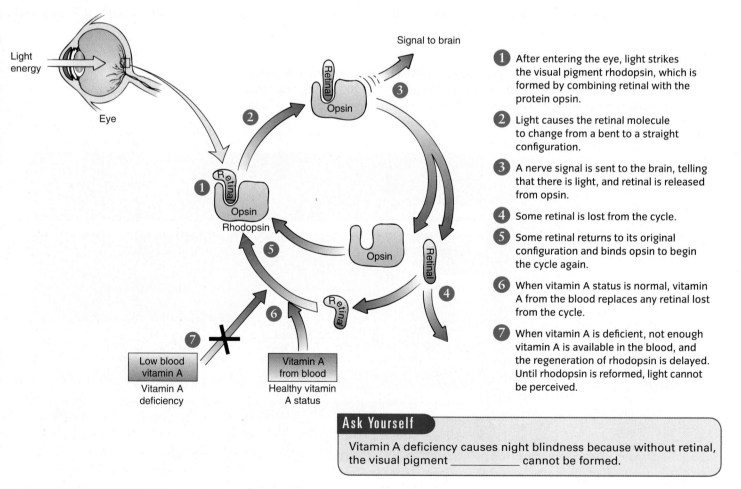

1. After entering the eye, light strikes the visual pigment rhodopsin, which is formed by combining retinal with the protein opsin.

2. Light causes the retinal molecule to change from a bent to a straight configuration.

3. A nerve signal is sent to the brain, telling that there is light, and retinal is released from opsin.

4. Some retinal is lost from the cycle.

5. Some retinal returns to its original configuration and binds opsin to begin the cycle again.

6. When vitamin A status is normal, vitamin A from the blood replaces any retinal lost from the cycle.

7. When vitamin A is deficient, not enough vitamin A is available in the blood, and the regeneration of rhodopsin is delayed. Until rhodopsin is reformed, light cannot be perceived.

Ask Yourself

Vitamin A deficiency causes night blindness because without retinal, the visual pigment _____ cannot be formed.

THINKING IT THROUGH

A Case Study on Vitamin A and Fast Food

John lives on his own, goes to school, and works part time. He eats breakfast at home and usually takes a sandwich for lunch; dinner is always fast food. He recently heard that fast food is low in some vitamins, particularly vitamin A. To check on his vitamin A intake, John uses 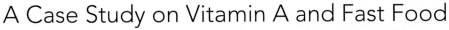 iProfile to look up the nutrient content of his favorite fast-food meals.

Which of the meals shown here is higher in vitamin A? Which ingredients are sources of the vitamin?
▼

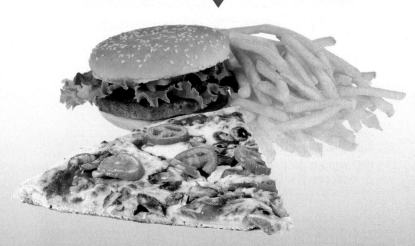

Your answer:

John doesn't want to give up his fast food, so he looks at his other meals to make sure they provide plenty of vitamin A. For breakfast, he has Cheerios with milk, toast with jelly, and coffee,

and for lunch, he packs a ham-and-cheese sandwich on whole-wheat bread, potato chips, an apple, and a soda.

Which foods in John's breakfast and lunch are good sources of vitamin A?
▼

The cereal is fortified with vitamin A, and the milk and cheese also contain vitamin A. The bread, meat, and chips contain little or none. Together, these foods provide only about 20% of the vitamin A John should consume on an average day.

What could John add to his breakfast and lunch to provide some good sources of vitamin A?
▼

Your answer:

John also discovers that his diet is low in vitamin C. Suggest one fruit and one vegetable that he could add to his breakfast and/or lunch to increase his intake of vitamin C.
▼

Your answer:

(Check your answers in Appendix J.)

---

and French fries provides almost no vitamin A (see *Thinking It Through*).

> **gene expression**
> The events of protein synthesis in which the information coded in a gene is used to synthesize a protein.

Vitamin A affects cell differentiation through its role in **gene expression**: It can increase or decrease the expression of certain genes. When a specific gene is expressed, it instructs the cell to make a particular protein. Proteins have structural and regulatory functions within cells and throughout the body. Altering the expression of specific

genes increases (or decreases) the production of certain proteins and thereby affects various cellular and body functions. By affecting gene expression, vitamin A can determine what type of cell an immature cell will become.

Vitamin A is necessary for the maintenance of epithelial tissue, which makes up the skin, and the linings of the eyes, intestines, lungs, vagina, and bladder. When vitamin A is deficient, epithelial cells do not differentiate normally because vitamin A is not there to regulate the production of particular proteins. All epithelial tissues are affected by vitamin A deficiency, but the eye is

The lining of the eye normally contains cells that secrete mucus, which lubricates the eye. When these cells die, immature cells differentiate to become new mucus-secreting cells that replace the dead ones. Without vitamin A, the immature cells can't differentiate normally, and instead of mucus-secreting cells, they become cells that produce a hard protein called keratin.

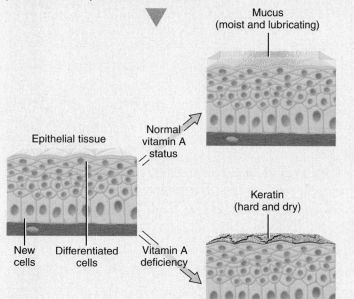

Epithelial tissue

Normal vitamin A status

Mucus (moist and lubricating)

New cells   Differentiated cells   Vitamin A deficiency

Keratin (hard and dry)

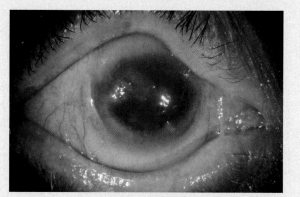

When mucus-secreting cells are replaced by keratin-producing cells, the surface of the eye becomes dry and cloudy. As xerophthalmia progresses, the drying of the cornea results in ulceration and infection. If left untreated, the damage is irreversible and causes permanent blindness.

Ask Yourself

On which continents is clinical vitamin A deficiency most prevalent?

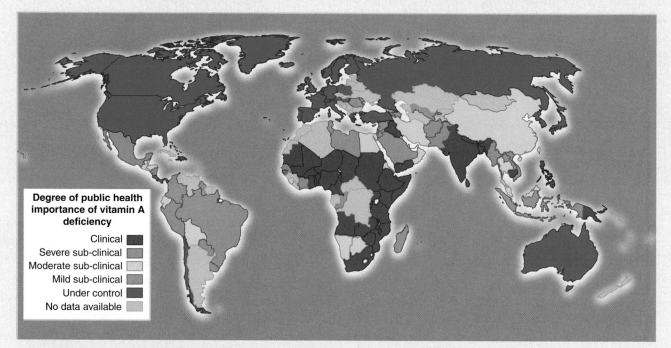

Degree of public health importance of vitamin A deficiency

- Clinical
- Severe sub-clinical
- Moderate sub-clinical
- Mild sub-clinical
- Under control
- No data available

Vitamin A deficiency is a threat to the health, sight, and lives of millions of children in the developing world. It is estimated that more than 250 million preschool children worldwide are vitamin A deficient and that 250,000 to 500,000 children go blind annually due to vitamin A deficiency. Children with clinical vitamin A deficiency have poor appetites, are anemic, are more susceptible to infections, and are more likely to die in childhood.[22]

Vitamin A and carotenoid toxicity • Figure 7.27

a. Foods generally do not naturally contain large enough amounts of nutrients to be toxic. Polar bear liver is an exception. It contains about 100,000 μg of vitamin A in just 1 ounce and has caused vitamin A toxicity in Arctic explorers who consumed it. Polar bear liver is not a common dish at most dinner tables, but supplements of preformed vitamin A also have the potential to deliver a toxic dose.

b. β-carotene supplements or regular consumption of large amounts of carrot juice can cause hypercarotenemia. The hand on the right, illustrates this harmless buildup of carotenoids in the adipose tissue, which makes the skin look yellow-orange, particularly on the palms of the hands and the soles of the feet.

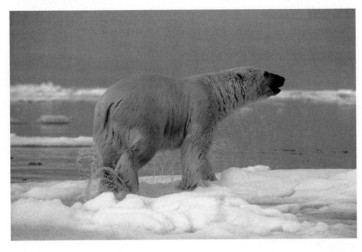

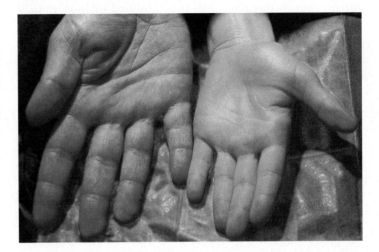

particularly susceptible (**Figure 7.26**). The eye disorders associated with vitamin A deficiency are collectively

> **xerophthalmia** A spectrum of eye conditions resulting from vitamin A deficiency that may lead to blindness.

known as **xerophthalmia**. Night blindness is an early stage of xeropthalmia and can be treated by increasing vitamin A intake. If left untreated, xerophthalmia affects the epithelial lining of the eye and can result in permanent blindness.

The ability of vitamin A to regulate the growth and differentiation of cells makes it essential throughout life for normal reproduction, growth, and immune function. In reproduction, vitamin A is needed to direct cells to differentiate and to form the shapes and patterns needed for the development of a complete organism. In growing children, vitamin A affects the activity of cells that form and break down bone; a deficiency early in life can cause abnormal jawbone growth, resulting in crooked teeth and poor dental health. In the immune system, vitamin A is needed for the differentiation that produces the different types of immune cells. When vitamin A is deficient, the activity of specific immune cells cannot be stimulated; the result is increased susceptibility to infections.

Vitamin A toxicity Preformed vitamin A is toxic in large doses, causing symptoms such as nausea, vomiting,

headache, dizziness, blurred vision, and lack of muscle coordination. Excess vitamin A is a particular concern for pregnant women because it may contribute to birth defects. Derivatives of vitamin A that are used to treat acne (Retin-A and Accutane) should never be used by pregnant women because they cause birth defects. High intakes of vitamin A have also been found to cause liver damage and increase the incidence of bone fractures.[23,24] The UL is set at 2800 mg/day of preformed vitamin A for 14- to 18-year-olds and 3000 mg/day for adults (**Figure 7.27a**).[21]

Because preformed vitamin A can be toxic, dietary supplements typically contain β-carotene. Carotenoids are not toxic because when they are consumed in high doses, their absorption from the diet decreases, and their conversion to active vitamin A is limited. However, large daily intakes of carotenoids from supplements or the diet can lead to a harmless condition known as **hypercarotenemia** (**Figure 7.27b**). β-carotene supplements have also been associated with an increase in lung cancer in cigarette smokers.[25] Therefore, smokers are advised to avoid

> **hypercarotenemia** A condition caused by the accumulation of carotenoids in the adipose tissue, causing the skin to appear yellow-orange.

β-carotene supplements. There is no UL for carotenoids, and the small amounts found in standard-strength multivitamin supplements are not likely to be harmful for any group.

Vitamin D

Vitamin D is known as the sunshine vitamin because it can be made in the skin with exposure to ultraviolet (UV) light. Because vitamin D can be made in the body, it is essential in the diet only when exposure to sunlight is limited or the body's ability to synthesize it is reduced.

Vitamin D, whether from the diet or from synthesis in the skin, is inactive until it is modified by biochemical reactions in both the liver and the kidney (**Figure 7.28**). Active vitamin D is needed to maintain normal levels of the minerals calcium and phosphorus in the blood. Calcium is important for bone health, but it is also needed for proper functioning of nerves, muscles, glands, and other tissues. Blood levels of calcium are regulated so that a steady supply of the mineral is available when and where it is needed.

PROCESS DIAGRAM

Vitamin D activation and function • Figure 7.28

THE PLANNER

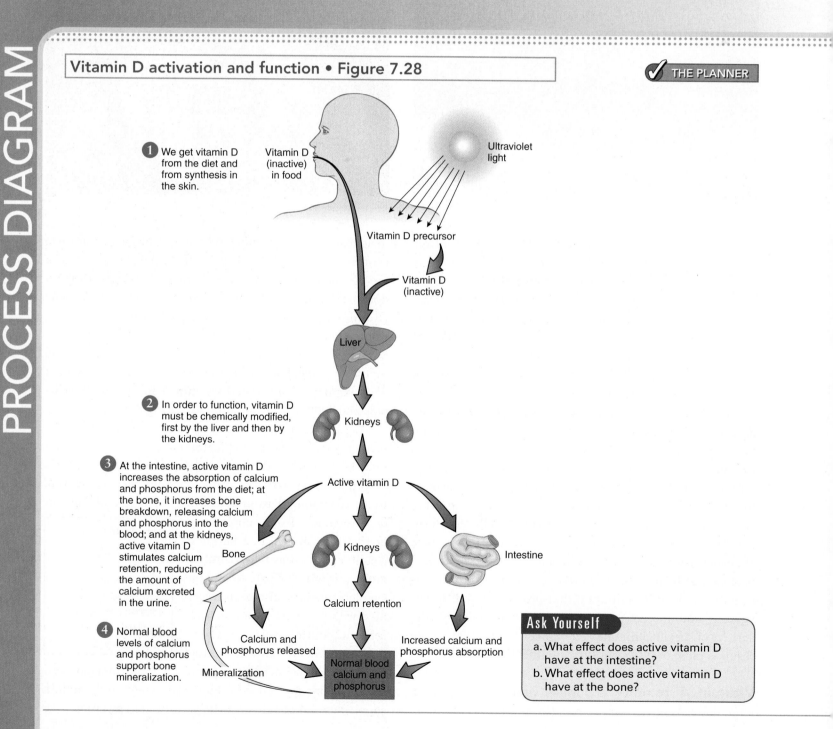

① We get vitamin D from the diet and from synthesis in the skin.

Vitamin D (inactive) in food

Ultraviolet light

Vitamin D precursor

Vitamin D (inactive)

Liver

② In order to function, vitamin D must be chemically modified, first by the liver and then by the kidneys.

Kidneys

③ At the intestine, active vitamin D increases the absorption of calcium and phosphorus from the diet; at the bone, it increases bone breakdown, releasing calcium and phosphorus into the blood; and at the kidneys, active vitamin D stimulates calcium retention, reducing the amount of calcium excreted in the urine.

Active vitamin D

Bone

Kidneys

Intestine

Calcium retention

④ Normal blood levels of calcium and phosphorus support bone mineralization.

Calcium and phosphorus released

Mineralization

Normal blood calcium and phosphorus

Increased calcium and phosphorus absorption

Ask Yourself

a. What effect does active vitamin D have at the intestine?

b. What effect does active vitamin D have at the bone?

When calcium levels in the blood drop too low, the body responds immediately to correct the problem. The

parathyroid hormone (PTH) A hormone released by the parathyroid gland that acts to increase blood calcium levels.

response starts with the release of **parathyroid hormone (PTH)**, which stimulates the activation of vitamin D by the kidneys. Active vitamin D enters the blood and travels to its major target tissues—intestine, bone, and kidneys—where it acts to increase calcium and phosphorus levels in the blood (see Figure 7.28). The functions of vitamin D, like vitamin A, are due to its role in gene expression. In the intestine, it increases the production of proteins needed for the absorption of calcium. In the bone, it increases the production of proteins that are needed for the differentiation of cells that break down bone.

Vitamin D deficiency When vitamin D is deficient, only about 10 to 15% of the calcium in the diet can be absorbed.

rickets A vitamin D deficiency disease in children, characterized by poor bone development due to inadequate calcium absorption.

osteomalacia A vitamin D deficiency disease in adults, characterized by loss of minerals from bone, bone pain, muscle aches, and an increase in bone fractures.

Without adequate calcium, bone structure becomes abnormal. In children, vitamin D deficiency causes **rickets**; it is characterized by narrow rib cages known as pigeon breasts and by bowed legs (**Figure 7.29**). In adults, vitamin D deficiency causes a condition called **osteomalacia**. Bone deformities do not occur with osteomalacia because adults are no longer growing, but the bones are weakened because not enough calcium is available to form the mineral deposits needed to maintain healthy bone. Insufficient bone mineralization leads to fractures of the weight-bearing bones, such as those in the hips and spine. This lack of calcium in bones can precipitate or exacerbate **osteoporosis**, which is a loss of total bone mass, not just minerals (discussed further in Chapter 8). Osteomalacia is common in adults with kidney failure because the conversion of vitamin D to the active form is reduced in these patients.

Over the past decade, it has been recognized that vitamin D may have functions that affect tissues other than bone. Vitamin D deficiency has been suggested to contribute to the development of cancer, cardiovascular disease, type 2 diabetes, and autoimmune disorders.[26] However,

Rickets • Figure 7.29

The vitamin D deficiency disease rickets causes short stature and bone deformities. The characteristic bowed legs occur because the bones are too weak to support the body. It is seen in children with poor diets and little exposure to sunlight, in those with disorders that affect fat absorption, and in some vegan children who do not receive adequate exposure to sunlight.

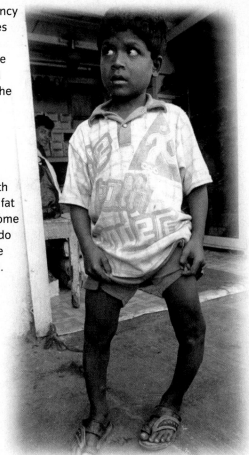

the current evidence that vitamin D provides health benefits beyond bone health is mixed and inconclusive.[27]

Meeting vitamin D needs Vitamin D is not very widespread in the diet. It is found naturally in liver, egg yolks, and oily fish such as salmon (**Figure 7.30a** on next page). Foods fortified with vitamin D include milk, margarine, and some yogurts, cheeses, and breakfast cereals. National surveys indicate that average vitamin D intake is below recommendations, but average blood levels of vitamin D are above the level needed for good bone health. This dichotomy suggests that vitamin D synthesis from sun exposure contributes enough vitamin D to allow the majority of the population to meet vitamin D needs even when intake is below recommendations.[27] Anything that interferes with the transmission of UV radiation to Earth's surface or its penetration into the skin will affect the synthesis of vitamin D. Therefore, living at higher latitudes, staying indoors, and keeping the skin covered when outdoors increase the risk of vitamin D deficiency (**Figure 7.30b–d**).

a. Only a few foods are natural sources of vitamin D. Without adequate sun exposure, supplements, or fortified foods, it is difficult to meet the body's needs for this vitamin, particularly for vegans. The dashed line indicates the RDA for ages 1 to 70, which is 600 IU (15 μg)/day. It would take about 5 cups of vitamin D–fortified milk to provide this much vitamin D.

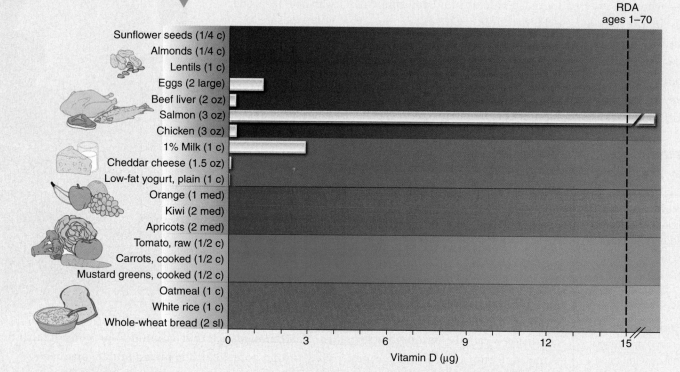

b. The angle at which the sun strikes the earth affects the body's ability to synthesize vitamin D in the skin. During the winter at latitudes greater than about 40 degrees north or south, there is not enough UV radiation to synthesize adequate amounts. However, during the spring, summer, and fall at 42 degrees latitude, as little as 5 to 10 minutes of midday sun exposure three times weekly can provide a light-skinned individual with adequate vitamin D.[28]

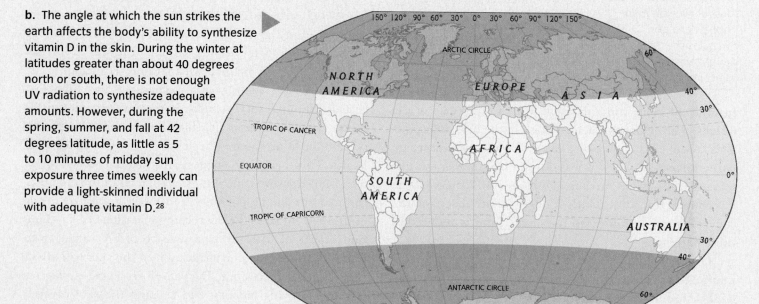

c. Sunscreen with an SPF of 15 decreases vitamin D synthesis by 99%.[29] Sunscreen is important for reducing the risk of skin cancer, but some time in the sun without sunscreen may be needed to meet vitamin D needs. In the summer, children and active adults usually spend enough time outdoors without sunscreen to meet their vitamin D requirements.

d. Dark skin pigmentation prevents UV light rays from penetrating into the layers of the skin where vitamin D is formed and reduces the body's ability to make vitamin D in the skin by as much as 99%. Dark-skinned individuals living in temperate climates have a higher rate of vitamin D deficiency than do those living near the equator.

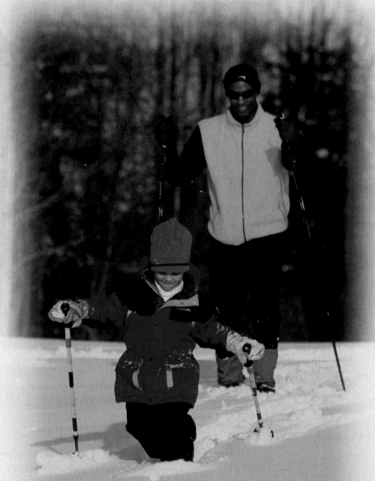

e. Concealing clothing worn by certain cultural and religious groups prevents sunlight from striking the skin. This explains why vitamin D deficiency occurs in women and children in some of the sunniest regions of the world. The elderly also typically cover their skin with clothing when they are outdoors. Risk of vitamin D deficiency in elderly people is further compounded because they consume a diet that is low in vitamin D, and the ability to synthesize vitamin D in the skin declines with age.

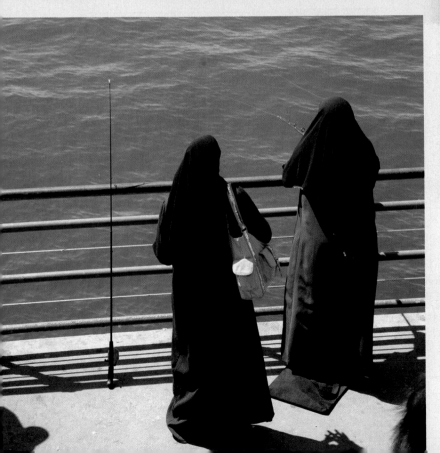

The Fat-Soluble Vitamins **237**

The RDA for vitamin D is expressed both in International Units (IUs) and in μg. The amount of vitamin D listed on dietary supplement labels is given in IUs. One IU is equal to 0.025 μg of vitamin D (40 IU = 1 μg of vitamin D; see Appendix I). The RDA for vitamin D for children and adults 70 and under is set at 600 IU (15 μg)/day—an amount that ensures that vitamin D levels in the blood are high enough to support bone health even when sun exposure is minimal.[27] Due to physiological changes that occur with aging, such as a reduction in vitamin D activation at the kidney and less efficient vitamin D synthesis in the skin, the amount of vitamin D needed to reduce the risk of fractures is higher in older adults. The RDA for adults older than 70 is 800 IU (20 μg)/day.

Too much vitamin D in the body can cause high calcium concentrations in the blood and urine, deposition of calcium in soft tissues such as the blood vessels and kidneys, and cardiovascular damage. Synthesis of vitamin D from exposure to sunlight does not produce toxic amounts because the body regulates vitamin D formation. The UL for ages 9 and older for vitamin D is 4000 IU (100 μg)/day.[27]

Vitamin E

Vitamin E is an antioxidant that protects lipids throughout the body by neutralizing reactive oxygen compounds before they can cause damage (**Figure 7.31**). Vitamin E protects membranes in red blood cells, white blood cells, nerve cells, and lung cells, where it is particularly important because oxygen concentrations in the lung are high.[30] Vitamin E can also defend cells against damage caused by heavy metals, such as lead and mercury, and toxins, such as carbon tetrachloride, benzene, and a variety of drugs.

Vitamin E deficiency
Because vitamin E is needed to protect cell membranes, a deficiency causes those membranes to break down. Red blood cells and nerve tissue are particularly susceptible. With a vitamin E deficiency, red blood cell membranes may rupture, causing a type of anemia called **hemolytic anemia**. This is most common in premature infants. All newborn infants have low blood vitamin E levels because there is little transfer of this vitamin from mother to fetus until the last weeks

The antioxidant role of vitamin E • Figure 7.31

By neutralizing free radicals, vitamin E guards not only cell membranes, as shown here, but also body proteins, DNA, and cholesterol.

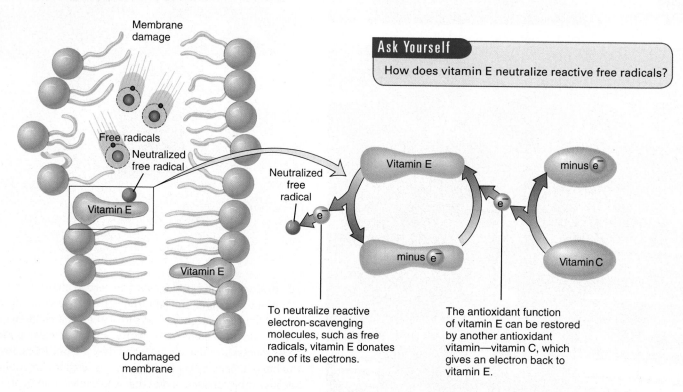

Ask Yourself

How does vitamin E neutralize reactive free radicals?

To neutralize reactive electron-scavenging molecules, such as free radicals, vitamin E donates one of its electrons.

The antioxidant function of vitamin E can be restored by another antioxidant vitamin—vitamin C, which gives an electron back to vitamin E.

WHAT SHOULD I EAT?

Vitamins

Focus on foliage for folate, vitamin A, and vitamin K

- Snack on an orange—you'll get your folate as well as vitamin C.
- Add beans—such as lentils and kidneys—to soups and tacos.
- Munch on a hidden source of β-carotene by eating something dark green.
- Have a salad with a heaping helping of leafy greens to add folate, vitamin K, and β-carotene.

B (vitamin) sure

- Don't forget the whole grains—you'll get vitamin B_6 as well as fiber.
- Enrich your diet with some enriched grains.
- Have a bowl of fortified breakfast cereal for B_{12} insurance.
- Enjoy lean meats, poultry, and fish to get a B_6 and B_{12} boost.

Get your antioxidants

- Snack on nuts and seeds and cook with canola oil to increase your vitamin E.
- Try for five different colors of fruits and veggies each day.
- Add carrot sticks to your lunch or snack to increase your vitamin A intake.
- Savor some strawberries and kiwis for dessert—they are loaded with vitamin C.

Soak up some D

- Get outside to stay fit and make some vitamin D.
- Have three servings of dairy per day to boost your intake of vitamin D.

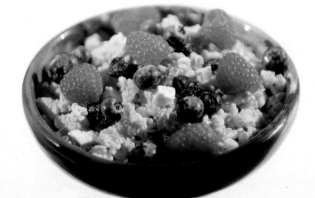

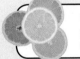

Use iProfile to calculate your vitamin C intake for a day.

of pregnancy. The levels are lower in premature infants because they are born before much vitamin E has been transferred from the mother. To prevent vitamin E deficiency in premature infants, special formulas for these infants contain higher amounts of vitamin E.

Vitamin E deficiency is rare in adults, occurring only when other health problems interfere with fat absorption, which reduces vitamin E absorption. In such cases, the vitamin E deficiency is usually characterized by symptoms associated with nerve degeneration, such as poor muscle coordination, weakness, and impaired vision.

The antioxidant role of vitamin E suggests that it may help reduce the risk of heart disease, cancer, Alzheimer's disease, macular degeneration, and a variety of other chronic diseases associated with oxidative damage. Particular attention has been paid to its possible benefits in guarding against heart disease. In addition to the potential for vitamin E to protect against cardiovascular disease through its antioxidant function, there is evidence that it may also have anti-inflammatory functions and be involved in modulating the immune response, regulating genes that affect cell growth and cell death, and detoxifying harmful substances.[31] Studies examining the relationship between blood levels of vitamin E or vitamin E intake and the incidence of cardiovascular disease have been mixed, and studies investigating the effect of vitamin E supplements on the incidence of cardiovascular disease and other chronic diseases have failed to provide evidence of any benefits.[31,32] The best approach is to get plenty of dietary vitamin E; however, most Americans do not consume enough vitamin E to meet the RDA (see *What Should I Eat?*).[33]

Dietary sources of vitamin E include sunflower seeds, nuts, peanuts, and refined plant oils such as canola, safflower, and sunflower oils. Vitamin E is also found in leafy green vegetables, such as spinach and mustard greens, and in wheat germ and fortified breakfast cereals. The dashed line represents the RDA for adults of 15 mg α-tocopherol/day.

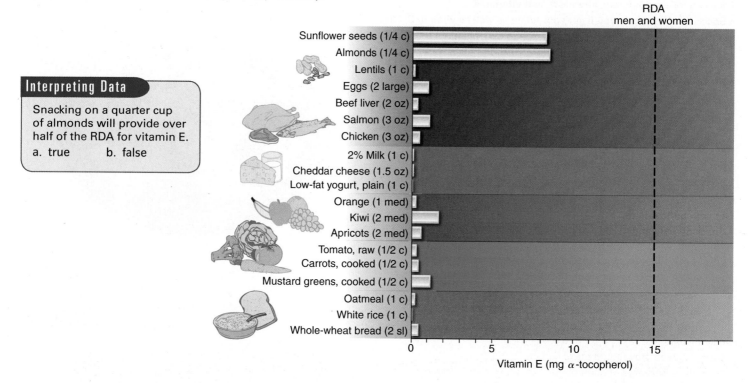

Interpreting Data

Snacking on a quarter cup of almonds will provide over half of the RDA for vitamin E.
a. true   b. false

Meeting vitamin E needs Nuts, seeds, and plant oils are the best sources of vitamin E; fortified products such as breakfast cereals also make a significant contribution to our vitamin E intake (**Figure 7.32**). The need for vitamin E increases as polyunsaturated fat intake increases because polyunsaturated fats are particularly susceptible to oxidative damage; fortunately, polyunsaturated oils are one of the best sources of dietary vitamin E. However, because vitamin E is sensitive to destruction by oxygen, metals, light, and heat, when vegetable oils are repeatedly used for deep-fat frying, most of the vitamin E in them is destroyed.

Vitamin K and blood clotting • Figure 7.33

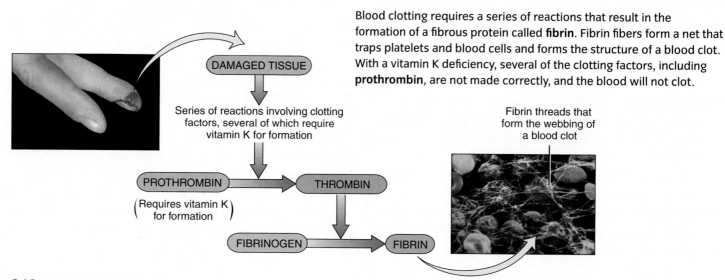

Blood clotting requires a series of reactions that result in the formation of a fibrous protein called **fibrin**. Fibrin fibers form a net that traps platelets and blood cells and forms the structure of a blood clot. With a vitamin K deficiency, several of the clotting factors, including **prothrombin**, are not made correctly, and the blood will not clot.

The chemical name for vitamin E is **tocopherol**. Several forms of vitamin E occur naturally in food, but the body can use only the **alpha-tocopherol (α-tocopherol)** form to meet vitamin E requirements. Therefore, the RDA is expressed as mg α-tocopherol. Synthetic α-tocopherol used in supplements and fortified foods provides only half as much vitamin E activity as the natural form. Supplement labels often express vitamin E content in IUs. Appendix J contains information for converting IUs into mg α-tocopherol.

There is no evidence of adverse effects from consuming large amounts of vitamin E naturally present in foods. The amounts typically contained in supplements are also safe for most people; however, large doses can interfere with blood clotting, so individuals taking blood-thinning medications should not take vitamin E supplements. The UL is 1000 mg/day from supplemental sources.[3]

Vitamin K

Blood is a fluid that flows easily through your blood vessels, but when you cut yourself, blood must solidify or clot to stop your bleeding. **Vitamin K** is needed in the production of several blood proteins, called clotting factors, that cause blood to clot (**Figure 7.33**). The *K* in vitamin K comes from the Danish word for coagulation, *koagulation*, which means "blood clotting." Abnormal blood coagulation is the major symptom of vitamin K deficiency. Without vitamin K, even a bruise or small scratch could cause you to bleed to death (see *What a Scientist Sees*).

Vitamin K is also needed for the synthesis of several proteins involved in bone formation and breakdown. With a vitamin K deficiency, bone mineral density is reduced, and the risk of fractures increases.[34] Therefore, adequate

WHAT A SCIENTIST SEES ✓ THE PLANNER

Anticoagulants Take Lives and Save Them

Consumers see using warfarin as way to eliminate some unwanted houseguests. A scientist sees that this rat poison can also be used to save lives. Warfarin is an anticoagulant, which means it prevents blood from clotting. It acts by blocking the activation of vitamin K. When rats eat warfarin, minor bumps and scrapes cause them to bleed to death. Dicoumarol, a derivative of warfarin, was first isolated from moldy clover hay in 1940. At that time, cows across the Midwest were bleeding to death because they were being fed this moldy hay during the winter months.

Blood clot formation is essential to survival, but blood clots in the arteries cause heart attacks and strokes and are responsible for killing about half a million Americans annually. Scientists have taken advantage of what they learned about dicoumarol and vitamin K and used it to save human lives. Dicoumarol was the first anticoagulant used to treat humans that could be taken orally rather than by injection. In the 1950s, the more potent anticoagulant warfarin, also known by the brand name Coumadin, was developed. It was used to treat President Eisenhower when he had a heart attack in 1955, and this "rat poison" is still used to treat heart attack patients today.

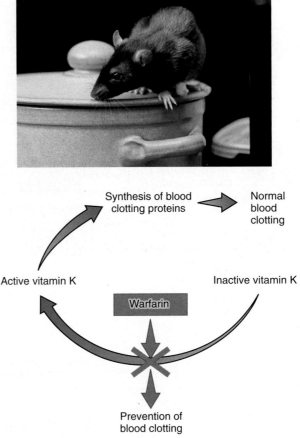

Think Critically Why might patients taking warfarin need to avoid vitamin K supplements?

vitamin K may be important for the prevention or treatment of osteoporosis.[35]

Vitamin K is used more rapidly than other fat-soluble vitamins, so a constant supply is necessary. Although only a small number of foods provide a significant amount of vitamin K, typical intakes in North America meet recommendations, and deficiency is very rare among healthy adults (**Figure 7.34**).[21] Another source of vitamin K is synthesis by bacteria in the large intestine. Deficiency can be precipitated by long-term antibiotic use, which kills the bacteria in the gastrointestinal tract that synthesize the vitamin. Newborns are at risk of deficiency because when a baby is born, no bacteria are present in the GI tract to synthesize vitamin K. In addition, newborns are at risk because little vitamin K is transferred to the baby from the mother before birth, and breast milk is a poor source of this vitamin. To ensure normal blood clotting, infants are typically given a vitamin K injection within six hours of birth.

A summary of the fat-soluble vitamins is provided in **Table 7.4**.

Meeting vitamin K needs • Figure 7.34

Leafy green vegetables, such as spinach, broccoli, Brussels sprouts, kale, and turnip greens, and some vegetable oils are good sources of vitamin K. The dashed lines indicate the AIs for adult men and women, which are 120 µg/day and 90 µg/day, respectively.

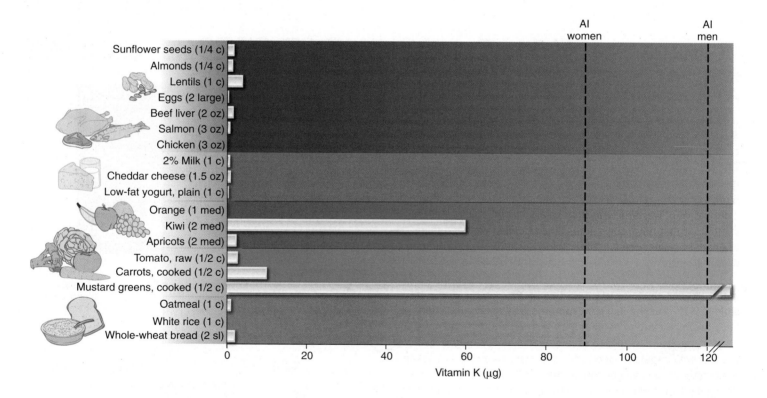

A summary of the fat-soluble vitamins   Table 7.4

Vitamin	Sources	Recommended intake for adults	Major functions	Deficiency diseases and symptoms	Groups at risk of deficiency	Toxicity	UL
Vitamin A (retinol, retinal, retinoic acid, vitamin A acetate, vitamin A palmitate, retinyl palmitate, provitamin A, carotene, β-carotene, carotenoids)	Retinol: liver, fish, fortified milk and margarine, butter, eggs; carotenoids: carrots, leafy greens, sweet potatoes, broccoli, apricots, cantaloupe	700–900 μg/day	Vision, health of cornea and other epithelial tissue, cell differentiation, reproduction, immune function	Xerophthalmia: night blindness, dry cornea, eye infections; poor growth, dry skin, impaired immune function	People living in poverty (particularly children and pregnant women), people who consume very low-fat or low-protein diets	Headache, vomiting, hair loss, liver damage, skin changes, bone pain, fractures, birth defects	3000 μg/day of preformed vitamin A
Vitamin D (calciferol, chole-calciferol, calcitriol, ergo-calciferol, dihydroxy vitamin D)	Egg yolk, liver, fish oils, tuna, salmon, fortified milk, synthesis from sunlight	600–800 IU/day (15–20 μg/day)	Absorption of calcium and phosphorus, maintenance of bone	Rickets in children: abnormal growth, misshapen bones, bowed legs, soft bones; osteomalacia in adults: weak bones and bone and muscle pain	Some breast-fed infants; children and elderly people (especially those with dark skin and little exposure to sunlight); people with kidney disease	Calcium deposits in soft tissues, growth retardation, kidney damage	4000 IU/day (100 μg/day)
Vitamin E (tocopherol, alpha-tocopherol)	Vegetable oils, leafy greens, seeds, nuts, peanuts	15 mg/day	Antioxidant, protects cell membranes	Broken red blood cells, nerve damage	People with poor fat absorption, premature infants	Inhibition of vitamin K activity	1000 mg/day from supplemental sources
Vitamin K (phylloquin-ones, mena-quinone)	Vegetable oils, leafy greens, synthesis by intestinal bacteria	90–120 μg/day	Synthesis of blood-clotting proteins and proteins in bone	Hemorrhage	Newborns (especially premature), people on long-term antibiotics	Anemia, brain damage	ND

Note: UL, Tolerable Upper Intake Level; ND, not determined due to insufficient evidence.

CONCEPT CHECK

1. **How** does vitamin A help us see in the dark?

2. **Why** do the leg bones bow when children are vitamin D deficient?

3. **How** does vitamin E protect membranes?

4. **What** is the role of vitamin K in blood clotting?

Meeting Needs with Dietary Supplements

LEARNING OBJECTIVES

1. **List** some population groups that may benefit from taking vitamin and mineral supplements.
2. **Explain** how the safety of dietary supplements is monitored.
3. **Evaluate** the safety of a dietary supplement using a Supplement Facts panel.

Currently 66% all adult Americans consider themselves supplement users.[36] We take them for a variety of reasons—to energize ourselves, to protect ourselves from disease, to cure illnesses, to lose weight, to enhance what we obtain from the foods we eat, and simply to ensure against deficiencies. These products may be beneficial and even necessary under some circumstances for some people, but they also have the potential to cause harm.

Some dietary supplements contain vitamins and minerals, some contain herbs and other plant-derived substances, and some contain compounds that are found in the body but are not essential in the diet. While supplements can help us obtain adequate amounts of specific nutrients, they do not provide all the benefits of foods. A pill that meets a person's vitamin needs does not provide the energy, protein, minerals, fiber, or phytochemicals supplied by food sources of these vitamins.

Who Needs Vitamin/Mineral Supplements?

Eating a variety of foods is the best way to meet nutrient needs, and most healthy adults who consume a reasonably good diet do not need supplements. In fact, an argument against the use of supplements is that supplement use gives people a false sense of security, causing them to pay less attention to the nutrient content of the foods they choose. For some people, however, taking supplements may be the only way to meet certain nutrient needs because of low intakes, increased needs, or excess losses (**Table 7.5**).

Groups for whom dietary supplements are recommended[37] Table 7.5	
Group	**Recommendation**
Dieters	People who consume fewer than 1600 Calories/day should take a multivitamin/multimineral supplement.
Vegans and those who eliminate all dairy foods	To obtain adequate vitamin B_{12}, people who do not eat animal products need to take supplements or consume vitamin B_{12}–fortified foods. Because dairy products are an important source of calcium and vitamin D, those who do not consume dairy products may benefit from taking supplements that provide calcium and vitamin D.
Infants and children	Supplemental fluoride, vitamin D, and iron are recommended under certain circumstances.
Young women and pregnant women	Women of childbearing age should consume 400 µg of folic acid daily from either fortified foods or supplements. Supplements of iron and folic acid are recommended for pregnant women, and multivitamin/multimineral supplements are usually prescribed during pregnancy.
Older adults	Because of the high incidence of atrophic gastritis in adults over age 50, vitamin B_{12} supplements or fortified foods are recommended. It may also be difficult for older adults to meet the RDAs for vitamin D and calcium, so supplements of these nutrients are often recommended.
Individuals with dark skin pigmentation	People with dark skin may be unable to synthesize enough vitamin D to meet their needs for this vitamin and may therefore require supplements.
Individuals with restricted diets	Individuals with health conditions that affect what foods they eat or how nutrients are used may require vitamin and mineral supplements.
People taking medications	Medications may interfere with the body's use of certain nutrients.
Cigarette smokers and alcohol users	People who smoke heavily require more vitamin C and possibly vitamin E than do nonsmokers.[3,38] Alcohol consumption inhibits the absorption of B vitamins and may interfere with B vitamin metabolism.

Herbal Supplements

Technically, an herb is a nonwoody, seed-producing plant that dies at the end of the growing season. However, the term *herb* is generally used to refer to any botanical or plant-derived substance. Throughout history, folk medicine has used herbs to prevent and treat disease. Today, herbs and herbal supplements are still popular (**Figure 7.35**). They are readily available and relatively inexpensive, and

Popular herbal supplements • Figure 7.35

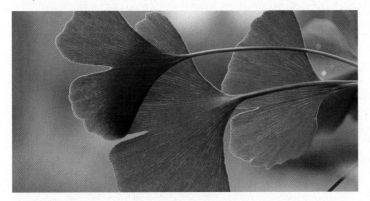

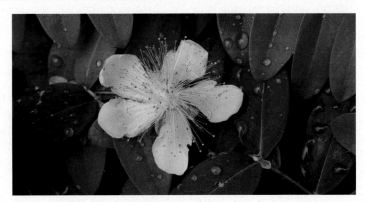

▲ *Ginkgo biloba*, also called "maidenhair," is one of the top-selling herbal medicinal supplements in the United States.[40] It is marketed to enhance memory and to treat a variety of circulatory ailments. Supplements have not been found to reduce the incidence of dementia or protect against cognitive decline in the elderly,[41] but there is evidence that it may benefit mood and attention in healthy adults.[42] Taking *Ginkgo biloba* may cause side effects that include headaches and gastrointestinal symptoms.[43] *Ginkgo biloba* also interacts with a number of medications. It can cause bleeding when combined with warfarin or aspirin, elevated blood pressure when combined with a thiazide diuretic, and coma when combined with the antidepressant trazodone.[44]

▲ St. John's wort, taken to promote mental well-being, contains low doses of the chemical found in the antidepressant drug fluoxetine (Prozac). The results of clinical trials suggest that it is effective for the treatment of depression.[45] Side effects include nausea and sensitivity to sunlight. St John's wort should not be used in conjunction with prescription antidepressant drugs, and it has been found to interact with anticoagulants, heart medications, birth control pills, immunosupressants, antibiotics, medications used to treat HIV infection, and others.[44,45]

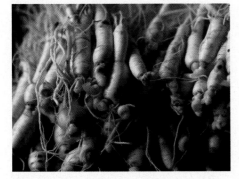

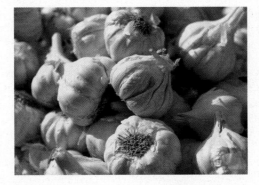

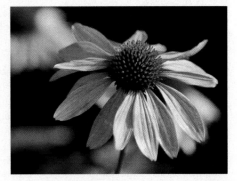

▲ Ginseng has been used in Asia for centuries for its energizing, stress-reducing, and aphrodisiac properties. Today it is popular for its effects on cardiovascular, central nervous system, endocrine, and sexual function. Although ginseng contains substances that have antioxidant, anti-inflammatory, immunostimulating, and central nervous system effects, controlled trials investigating its health benefits have been equivocal.[46] It can cause diarrhea, headache, and insomnia.[44]

▲ Hippocrates recommended garlic for treating pneumonia and other infections, as well as cancer and digestive disorders. Although it is no longer recommended for those purposes, recent research has shown that garlic may cause a modest reduction in blood cholesterol and triglyceride levels.[47] Even though we often spice our food with garlic, garlic supplements are not safe for everyone. They could be harmful for people undergoing treatment for HIV infection and could lead to bleeding in those taking the anticoagulant drug warfarin.[44]

▲ Native Americans used petals of the Echinacea plant as a treatment for colds, flu, and infections. Today, the plant's root is typically used, and it is a popular herbal cold remedy. Echinacea is believed to act as an immune system stimulant, but there is little evidence that it is beneficial in either preventing or treating the common cold.[48] Although side effects have not been reported, allergies are possible.

Potential benefits and side effects of common herbal ingredients   Table 7.6

Product	Suggested benefit and uses	Side effects
Astragalus (bei qi, huang qi, ogi, hwang ki, milk vetch)	Enhances the immune system	Can interact with drugs that suppress the immune system and affect blood sugar levels and blood pressure
Bitter orange (Seville orange, sour orange, Zhi shi)	Relieves heartburn and nasal congestion, stimulates appetite, promotes weight loss	Increased heart rate and blood pressure, fainting, heart attack, stroke
Cat's Claw (uña de gato)	Relieves arthritis and stimulates the immune system	Headache, dizziness, vomiting; Should not be taken by individuals who are pregnant
Chamomile	Aids gastrointestinal upset, promotes relaxation and sleep	Allergic reactions
Dandelion (lion's tooth, blowball)	Relieves minor digestive problems, increases urine production, supports liver and kidney health	Upset stomach and diarrhea, allergic reactions
Echinacea (purple coneflower, coneflower)	Stimulates the immune system, prevents and treats colds and other upper respiratory infections.	Allergic reactions
Ephedra (Ma Huang, Chinese ephedra)	Treats colds and nasal congestion, aids in weight loss, increases energy, and enhances athletic performance	High blood pressure, irregular heartbeat, heart attack, stroke, death; banned by the FDA, but the ban does not apply to traditional Chinese herbal remedies or to products like herbal teas regulated as conventional foods
Ginger	Relieves motion sickness and nausea	Gas, bloating, heartburn, nausea
Ginkgo (Ginkgo biloba, maidenhair tree, fossil tree)	Improves memory and mental function, improves circulation	Gastrointestinal distress, headache, dizziness, allergic skin reactions
Ginseng (Asian ginseng, Chinese ginseng)	Increases sense of well-being and stamina, improves mental and physical performance, enhances immune function, improves sexual function, lowers blood glucose, controls blood pressure	Headache, insomnia, gastrointestinal upset with prolonged use
Hawthorn	Strengthens heart muscle	Possible drug interactions
Hoodia (Kalahari cactus, Xhoba)	Suppresses appetite	Safety unknown; potential risks, side effects, and interactions with medicines and other supplements have not been studied
Kava (kava kava, awa, kava pepper)	Relieves anxiety, stress, insomnia, menopausal symptoms	Liver damage, including hepatitis and liver failure (which can cause death); FDA has issued a warning that using kava supplements has been linked to a risk of severe liver damage
Milk thistle (Mary thistle, holy thistle)	Protects against liver disease, improves liver function	Gastrointestinal upset, allergic reactions, low blood sugar
Red clover (cow clover, meadow clover, wild clover)	Relieves menopausal symptoms, breast pain associated with menstrual cycles, and symptoms of prostate enlargement; lowers blood cholesterol	Headache, nausea, rash
Saw palmetto (American dwarf palm tree, cabbage palm)	Improves urinary flow with enlarged prostate	Mild stomach discomfort
St. John's wort (hypericum, Klamath weed, goatweed)	Promotes mental well-being; treats depression, anxiety, and/or sleep disorders	Increased sensitivity to sunlight, anxiety, dry mouth, dizziness, gastrointestinal symptoms, fatigue, headache, sexual dysfunction; interacts with many medications, including antidepressants, birth control pills, digoxin, warfarin, and seizure-control drugs
Valerian (all-heal, garden heliotrope)	Mild sedative, relieves sleep disorders and anxiety	Gastrointestinal upset, headache, and tiredness possible with prolonged use
Yohimbe (yohimbe bark)	Acts as aphrodisiac; treats sexual dysfunction, including erectile dysfunction in men	High blood pressure, increased heart rate, headache, anxiety, dizziness, nausea, vomiting, tremors, and sleeplessness

Sources: National Center for Complementary and Alternative Medicine, *Herbs at a Glance*, http://nccam.nih.gov/health/herbsataglance.htm; Office of Dietary Supplements, *Dietary Supplement Fact Sheets*, http://ods.od.nih.gov/factsheets/list-all; and Office of Dietary Supplements, *Botanical Supplement Fact Sheets*, http://ods.od.nih.gov/factsheets/list-Botanicals/.

they can be purchased without a trip to the doctor or a prescription. Although these features are appealing to consumers who want to manage their own health, some herbs may be toxic, either alone or in combination with other herbs and drugs (**Table 7.6**). They should not be taken to replace prescribed medication without the knowledge of your physician (see *Debate: Are Herbal Supplements Helpful or Harmful?*).[39]

Debate   Are Herbal Supplements Helpful or Harmful?

✓ THE PLANNER

The Issue: Herbal supplements are popular as "natural" remedies. Are these products a helpful addition to traditional health care, or are they a health risk?

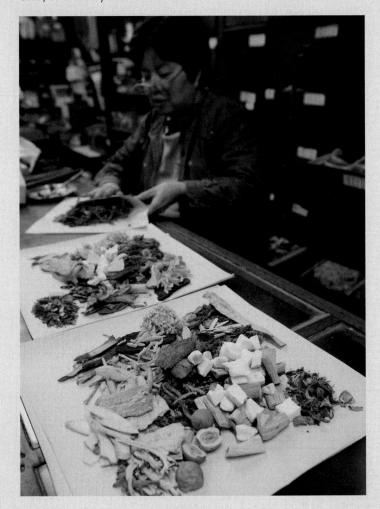

Many cultures, including the ancient Greeks and Native Americans have used herbal products to treat everything from coughs, constipation, and poison ivy to arthritis and heart ailments. Today, about one in six Americans uses herbs to treat maladies or boost health.[49] These products are affordable and widely available, and they do not require prescriptions. Advocates of herbal supplements feel that this availability allows people more control of their own health care. Opponents fear that self-dosing with herbs may lead to toxic reactions and prevent people from seeking traditional medical care and proven treatments. How effective and safe are herbal supplements?

Herbs have demonstrated physiological effects. In fact, some of the prescription drugs used today were derived from plants. Aspirin comes from willow bark; digitalis, a drug prescribed for certain heart conditions, comes from foxglove flowers. Herbs are made from all or part of the plant, so the amounts of active ingredients are affected by growing conditions, harvesting, and processing, and they vary with the brand and batch.[50] In contrast, drugs are purified compounds and are tested to ensure consistent amounts in each pill. Advocates believe that having a mixture of compounds is an advantage because some ingredients can enhance the effects of others. Opponents argue that these interactions may be negative, diminishing the effect of one of the active ingredients.[50]

Proponents of herbal supplements argue that most herbal medicines are well tolerated and have fewer unintended consequences than prescription drugs. Prescription drugs are certainly not without side effects, but because of the levels of regulation, we are assured that a prescribed drug is an effective treatment, and any side effects are documented. Herbal products, like other dietary supplements, do not require FDA approval before they are marketed. Opponents believe that this lack of regulation allows dangerous products to enter the marketplace. Many botanical compounds are toxic. The FDA has issued warnings about ingredients such as comfrey, kava, and aristolochic acid; it took ephedra off the market.[51] Because herbal products are made from unpurified plant material, there is also a risk of contamination with pesticides, microbes, metals, and other toxins.[52]

Another concern when people self-dose with herbs is that the herbs may interact with drugs and cause unwanted side effects.[50] For example, gingko biloba and garlic can interfere with blood clotting so should not be used with blood-thinning medication or before surgery. St. John's wort may interact with anesthetics and antidepressants, and Echinacea can limit the effect of some steroids.[53] Prescription drugs come with instructions and warnings about potential side effects; in addition, a physician or pharmacist considers the other medications and conditions that may alter the safety and effectiveness of the drug, and a prescribing physician monitors patient health. This is not the case with dietary supplements.

Herbs are medicines, and like taking other medications, taking herbs has some advantages and risks. Whether herbal supplements are helpful or harmful depends on the supplement, the dose, and the consumer.

Think critically: Would you purchase a remedy from the selection of herbs at the shop shown in the photo? Why or why not?

Choose Supplements with Care

Using dietary supplements can be part of an effective strategy to promote good health, but supplements are not a substitute for a healthy diet, and they are not without risks. The Dietary Supplement Health and Education Act (DSHEA) of 1994 defined the term *dietary supplement* and created standards for labeling these products (see Chapter 2). However, it left most of the responsibility for manufacturing practices and safety in the hands of manufacturers.

To help ensure that dietary supplements contain the right ingredients and the right amount per dose, the FDA established dietary supplement "current Good Manufacturing Practice" regulations. These regulations require manufacturers to test their products to ensure identity, purity, strength, and composition.[54] Supplement manufacturers are responsible for ensuring that their products are safe and effective, so the FDA does not approve most of these products before they are marketed. The only dietary supplements that do require pre-market review by the FDA are those containing an ingredient that was not sold in the United States before October 15, 1994. Ingredients sold prior to this date are presumed to be safe, based on their history of safe use by humans. Prior to marketing a supplement containing a new ingredient, the manufacturer must notify the FDA of its intention to market the product and provide safety data. If a problem arises with a specific product, the FDA must prove that the supplement represents a risk before it can require the manufacturer to remove the supplement from the market.

Because supplements are not regulated as strictly as drugs, consumers need to use care and caution if they choose to use them. A safe option is a multivitamin/multimineral supplement that does not exceed 100% of the Daily Values. Although there is little evidence that the average person benefits from such a supplement, there is also little evidence of harm. Here are a number of suggestions that will help you when choosing or using dietary supplements:

- **Consider why you want it.** If you are taking it to ensure good health, does it provide both vitamins and minerals? If you want to supplement specific nutrients, are they contained in the product?

- **Compare product costs.** Just as more isn't always better, more expensive is not always better either.

- **Read the label.** Does the supplement contain potentially toxic levels of any nutrient? Are you taking the amount recommended on the label? For any nutrients that exceed 100% of the Daily Value, check to see if they exceed the UL (see Appendix A). Does it contain any nonvitamin/nonmineral ingredients? If so, have any of them been shown to be toxic to someone like you (**Figure 7.36**)?

Check the Supplement Facts • Figure 7.36

This Supplement Facts panel is from a supplement marketed to reduce appetite and therefore promote weight loss. Would you recommend it? Why or why not?

Supplement Facts		
Serving Size: 2 Capsules		
Servings Per Container: 60		
	Amount Per Serving	**DV%**
Vitamin C (as ascorbic acid)	60mg	100%
Pantothenic Acid (as calcium, pantothenate)	20mg	200%
Vitamin B-6 (as pyridoxine HCL)	8mg	400%
Niacin	5mg	25%
Folate (as folic acid)	100mcg	25%
Zinc (as zinc gluconate)	5mg	33%
Copper (as copper gluconate)	500mcg	25%
NADH (Nicotinamide Adenine Dinucleotide)	1000mcg	*
Hoodia Gordonii Extract (20:1 Extract- Equal to 2000 mg of whole plant)	100mg	*
5-Hydroxytryptophan (Griffonia Simplicifolia)	25mg	*
N, N Dimethylglycine	50mg	*
Trimethylglycine	75mg	*
L-Phenylalanine	600mg	*
Decaffinated Green Tea Extract (Total Catechins 130mg, Epigaliocatechin Galiate (EGCG) 70mg)	175mg	*
Salvia Scalarea Extract	50mg	*
Choline (as bitartrate)	75mg	*

*Daily Value (DV, not established)

This supplement contains more than 100% of the Daily Value for vitamin B$_6$. Does this amount exceed the UL?

This supplement contains many ingredients that are not vitamins or minerals and therefore have no Daily Value or UL. The ones shown in blue are herbs. Are they safe when taken in these amounts?

Recommended Use: As a dietary supplement take two capsules before breakfast on a empty stomach (or before exercise) and two capsules at mid-afternoon preferably with 8 oz of water.

- **Check the expiration date.** Some nutrients degrade over time, so expired products will have a lower nutrient content than is shown on the label. This is particularly true if the product has not been stored properly.

- **Consider your medical history.** Do you have a medical condition that recommends against certain nutrients or other ingredients? Are you taking prescription medication that an ingredient in the supplement may interact with? Check with a physician, dietitian, or pharmacist to help identify these interactions.

- **Approach herbal supplements with caution.** If you are pregnant, ill, or taking medications, consult your physician before taking herbs. Do not give them to children. Do not take combinations of herbs. Do not use herbs for long periods. Stop taking any product that causes side effects.

- **Report harmful effects.** If you suffer a harmful effect or an illness that you think is related to the use of a supplement, seek medical attention and go to the FDA Reporting Web site, at www.fda.gov/safety/medwatch/howtoreport/ucm053074.htm, for information about how to proceed.

CONCEPT CHECK STOP

1. **Why** is it recommended that vegans and older adults take vitamin B_{12} supplements?
2. **Who** regulates the safety of dietary supplements?
3. **How** can the UL be used when evaluating a dietary supplement?

THE PLANNER ✓

Summary

1 A Vitamin Primer 202

- **Vitamins** are essential organic nutrients that do not provide energy and are required in small quantities in the diet to maintain health. Vitamins are classified by their solubility in either water or fat. Vitamins are present naturally in foods and are also added through fortification and enrichment.

- Vitamin **bioavailability** is affected by the composition of the diet, conditions in the digestive tract, and the ability to transport and activate the vitamin once it has been absorbed.

- Vitamins promote and regulate body activities. The B vitamins act as **coenzymes,** as illustrated here. Some vitamins are **antioxidants**, which protect the body from **oxidative damage** by **free radicals**.

- In developing countries, vitamin deficiencies remain a major public health problem. They are less common in industrialized countries due to fortification and a more varied food supply.

Coenzymes • Figure 7.5

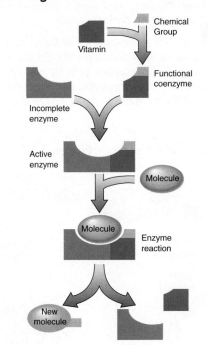

2 The Water-Soluble Vitamins 209

- **Thiamin** is a coenzyme that is particularly important for glucose metabolism and **neurotransmitter** synthesis; a deficiency of thiamin, called **beriberi**, causes nervous system abnormalities. Thiamin is found in whole and enriched grains.

- **Riboflavin** coenzymes are needed for ATP production and for the utilization of several other vitamins. Milk is one of the best food sources of riboflavin.

- **Niacin** coenzymes are needed for the breakdown of carbohydrate, fat, and protein and for the synthesis of fatty acids and cholesterol. A deficiency results in **pellagra**, which is characterized by dermatitis, diarrhea, and dementia. The amino acid tryptophan can be converted into niacin. High doses lower blood cholesterol but can cause toxicity symptoms.

- **Biotin** is needed for the synthesis of glucose and for energy, fatty acid, and amino acid metabolism. Some of our biotin need is met by bacterial synthesis in the gastrointestinal tract.

- **Pantothenic acid** is part of coenzyme A. It is required for the production of ATP from carbohydrate, fat, and protein and for the synthesis of cholesterol and fat. It is widespread in the food supply.

- **Vitamin B$_6$** is particularly important for amino acid and protein metabolism. Deficiency causes numbness and tingling and may increase the risk of heart disease because it is needed to keep levels of homocysteine low. Food sources include meats and whole grains. Large doses of vitamin B$_6$ can cause nervous system abnormalities.

- **Folate** is necessary for the synthesis of DNA, so it is especially important for rapidly dividing cells. Folate deficiency prevents red blood cell precursor cells from dividing, as shown here, resulting in **macrocytic anemia**. Low levels of folate before and during early pregnancy are associated with an increased incidence of **neural tube defects**. Food sources include liver, legumes, oranges, leafy green vegetables, and fortified grains. A high intake of folate can mask some of the symptoms of vitamin B$_{12}$ deficiency.

- Absorption of **vitamin B$_{12}$** requires stomach acid and **intrinsic factor**. Without intrinsic factor, only tiny amounts of vitamin B$_{12}$ are absorbed, and **pernicious anemia** occurs. Vitamin B$_{12}$ is needed for the metabolism of folate and fatty acids and to maintain **myelin**. Deficiency results in macrocytic anemia and nerve damage. Vitamin B$_{12}$ is found almost exclusively in animal products. Deficiency is a concern in vegans and in older individuals with **atrophic gastritis**.

- **Vitamin C** is necessary for the synthesis of **collagen**, hormones, and neurotransmitters. Vitamin C deficiency, called **scurvy**, is characterized by poor wound healing, bleeding, and other symptoms related to the improper formation and maintenance of collagen. Vitamin C is also a water-soluble antioxidant. The best food sources are citrus fruits.

3 The Fat-Soluble Vitamins 228

- **Vitamin A** is a fat-soluble vitamin needed in the visual cycle and for growth and **cell differentiation**. Its role in **gene expression** makes it essential for maintenance of epithelial tissue, reproduction, and immune function. Vitamin A deficiency causes blindness and death. Preformed vitamin A **retinoids** are found in liver, eggs, fish, and fortified dairy products. High intakes are toxic and have been linked to birth defects and bone loss. Provitamin A **carotenoids**, such as β-**carotene**, are found in yellow-orange fruits and vegetables such as mangoes, carrots, and apricots, as well as leafy greens. Some carotenoids are antioxidants. Carotenoids are not toxic, but a high intake can give the skin a yellow-orange appearance.

- **Vitamin D** can be made in the skin by exposure to sunlight, as depicted to the right, so dietary needs vary depending on the amount synthesized. Vitamin D is found in fish oils and fortified milk. It is essential for maintaining proper levels of calcium and phosphorus in the body. A deficiency in children results in **rickets**; in adults, vitamin D deficiency causes **osteomalacia**. Adequate vitamin D is associated with reduced incidence of certain cancers.

Folate deficiency and anemia • Figure 7.17

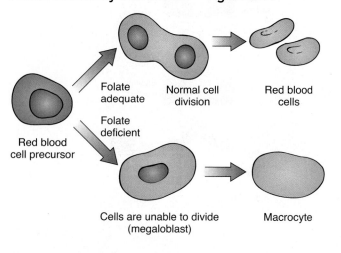

Red blood cell precursor

Folate adequate → Normal cell division → Red blood cells

Folate deficient → Cells are unable to divide (megaloblast) → Macrocyte

Vitamin D activation and function • Figure 7.28

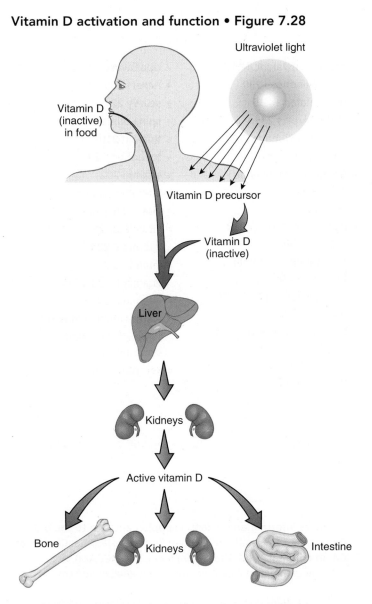

- **Vitamin E** functions primarily as a fat-soluble antioxidant. It is necessary for reproduction and protects cell membranes from oxidative damage. It is found in nuts, plant oils, green vegetables, and fortified cereals.

- **Vitamin K** is essential for blood clotting. Because vitamin K deficiency is a problem in newborns, they are routinely given vitamin K injections at birth. Warfarin, a substance that inhibits vitamin K activity, is used medically as an anti-coagulant. Vitamin K is found in plants and is synthesized by bacteria in the gastrointestinal tract.

4 Meeting Needs with Dietary Supplements 244

- About half the adult population in the United States takes some type of dietary supplement. Vitamin and mineral supplements are recommended for dieters, vegetarians, pregnant women and women of childbearing age, older adults, and other nutritionally vulnerable groups.

- Herbal supplements are currently popular. These products, which are made from plants (such as the St. John's wort shown here) may have beneficial physiological actions, but their dosage is not regulated, and they can be toxic either on their own or in combination with other herbs, medications, or medical conditions.

Popular herbal supplements: St. John's wort • Figure 7.35

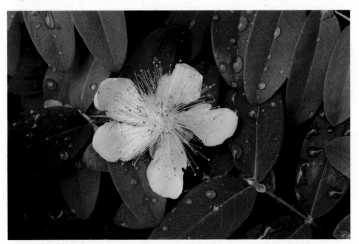

- Manufacturers are responsible for the consistency and safety of supplements before they are marketed. The FDA regulates dietary supplement labeling and can monitor their safety once they are being sold. When choosing a dietary supplement, it is important to carefully consider both the potential risks and benefits of the product.

Key Terms

- alpha-carotene (α-carotene) 229
- alpha-tocopherol (α-tocopherol) 241
- antioxidant 207
- ascorbic acid 224
- atrophic gastritis 223
- beriberi 210
- beta-carotene (β-carotene) 228
- beta-cryptoxanthin (β-cryptoxanthin) 229
- bioavailability 204
- biotin 215
- carotenoids 228
- cell differentiation 230
- choline 226
- cobalamin 223
- coenzyme 207

- collagen 224
- dietary folate equivalent (DFE) 219
- fat-soluble vitamin 202
- fibrin 240
- folate 219
- folic acid 219
- free radical 207
- gene expression 231
- hemolytic anemia 238
- hypercarotenemia 233
- intrinsic factor 222
- macrocytic anemia or megaloblastic anemia 220
- myelin 216
- neural tube defect 219
- neurotransmitter 210
- niacin 213

- niacin equivalent (NE) 214
- night blindness 230
- osteomalacia 235
- osteoporosis 235
- oxidative damage 207
- pantothenic acid 215
- parathyroid hormone (PTH) 235
- pellagra 213
- pernicious anemia 222
- prothrombin 240
- provitamin or vitamin precursor 204
- pyridoxal phosphate 216
- retinoids 228
- retinol activity equivalent (RAE) 229
- retinol-binding protein 229
- rhodopsin 230

- riboflavin 212
- rickets 235
- scurvy 224
- spina bifida 219
- thiamin 210
- tocopherol 241
- vitamin 202
- vitamin A 228
- vitamin B_{12} 222
- vitamin B_6 216
- vitamin C 224
- vitamin D 234
- vitamin E 238
- vitamin K 241
- water-soluble vitamin 202
- Wernicke-Korsakoff syndrome 211
- xerophthalmia 233

Online Resources

- For more information on vitamins and their food sources, go to the National Library of Medicine, at www.nlm.nih.gov/medlineplus/ency/article/002399.htm.

- For more information on vitamin A deficiency as a world health issue, go to the World Health Organization, at www.who.int/nutrition/topics/vad/en/.

- For more information on vitamin and mineral supplements, go to the Office of Dietary Supplements, at http://ods.od.nih.gov/factsheets/list-VitaminsMinerals.

- For more information on herbal supplements, go to the U.S. Department of Health and Human Service's National Center for Complementary and Alternative Medicine (NCCAM), at http://nccam.nih.gov/health/supplements/wiseuse.htm.

- Visit your *WileyPLUS* site for videos, animations, podcasts, self-study, and other media that will aid you in studying and understanding this chapter.

Critical and Creative Thinking Questions

1. The dietary supplement products listed in the table below are on sale at a local nutrition store:

Supplement	Ingredients/tablet	Dose (tablets/day)
Vitamin B$_6$	100 mg pyridoxine	1
Stress tabs	35 mg pyridoxine 1 mg thiamin 1.1 mg riboflavin 30 mg niacin 500 mg choline	2
Folic acid	800 μg folic acid	1
Cold relief	1000 mg vitamin C	3

Do any of these supplements pose a risk for toxicity at the dose listed above? Which ones and why? Would the risk of toxicity change if a consumer took all four of these supplements together? Would you recommend them for everyone? Would you recommend them for a specific group? Why or why not?

2. Sam is a fast-food fanatic. For breakfast, he stops for coffee and donuts. For lunch he has iced tea, a roast beef sub with lettuce and mayonnaise, and a cookie. For dinner he has a soft drink, burger, and fries. Name two vitamins likely to be lacking in Sam's diet if he eats like this every day. Why is he likely to be deficient in these vitamins?

3. Anna is 28 years old. She and her husband plan to start a family soon. Because Anna is overweight and knows she will put on more weight during her pregnancy, she begins a low-carbohydrate diet to slim down before she gets pregnant. She eliminates breads, grains, legumes, starchy vegetables, and fruit from her diet. What nutrient that is important early in pregnancy would be lacking in this diet? What could Anna add to her diet to increase her intake of this nutrient? Will taking a prenatal vitamin supplement once she knows she is pregnant be enough to reduce the risk of neural tube defects?

4. Why might someone with kidney failure develop a vitamin D deficiency?

5. Explain why a dark-skinned Nigerian exchange student living in Buffalo, New York, is at risk for vitamin D deficiency.

6. Explain why a deficiency either of vitamin B$_{12}$ or of folate causes red blood cells to be larger than normal.

7. Explain why infections are more common and immunization programs are less successful in regions where vitamin A deficiency is prevalent.

What is happening in this picture?

These children, who live in Russia, are being exposed to UV radiation to prevent vitamin D deficiency.

Think Critically

1. Why does this treatment help them meet their need for vitamin D?
2. Why are children in Russia at risk for vitamin D deficiency?
3. What else could be done to ensure that they get adequate amounts of vitamin D?

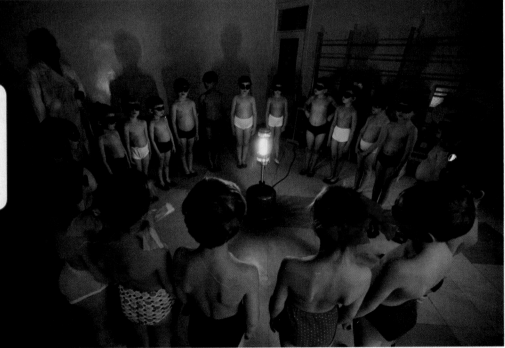

Self-Test

(Check Your Answers In Appendix K.)

1. Which of the following vitamins is *not* added to grains during enrichment?
   a. thiamin
   b. riboflavin
   c. niacin
   d. vitamin B$_6$

2. Which vitamin is needed for the reaction labeled with the letter A?
   a. thiamin
   b. vitamin C
   c. vitamin B$_6$
   d. vitamin A
   e. vitamin K

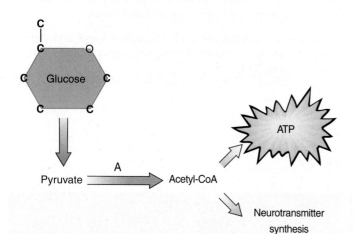

3. Which of the following descriptions of the water-soluble vitamins is false?
   a. niacin—a deficiency causes pellagra
   b. thiamin—can be synthesized from tryptophan
   c. pantothenic acid—found in most foods
   d. vitamin C—needed for the cross-linking of collagen
   e. vitamin B$_6$—needed for amino acid metabolism

4. Which of the following statements is true of all the B vitamins?
   a. They are all electron carriers.
   b. They are all needed for DNA synthesis.
   c. They are all coenzymes.
   d. They all contain energy that is used to fuel body activities.
   e. They are all fat soluble.

5. Which of the following nutrients is not essential in the diet when sun exposure is adequate?
   a. riboflavin
   b. vitamin E
   c. vitamin K
   d. vitamin D

6. Which of the following statements about folate is false?
   a. Adequate amounts decrease the incidence of neural tube defect–affected pregnancies.
   b. It is needed for DNA synthesis.
   c. A deficiency causes macrocytic anemia.
   d. It can be made in the body from methionine.
   e. It is added to enriched grain products.

7. The disease scurvy is due to a deficiency of _____.
   a. vitamin K
   b. vitamin D
   c. vitamin C
   d. vitamin A
   e. thiamin

8. A deficiency of vitamin K leads to _____.
   a. rickets
   b. blindness
   c. scurvy
   d. pellagra
   e. decreased blood clotting

9. Which of the following is a poor source of β-carotene?
   a. milk
   b. carrots
   c. sweet potatoes
   d. spinach
   e. apricots

10. The food sources of _____ are illustrated by this graph.

    a. vitamin C

    b. folate

    c. vitamin B₁₂

    d. thiamin

    e. vitamin B₆

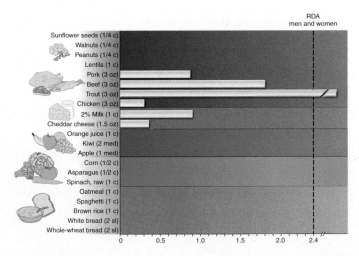

11. The actions of _____ are illustrated in this diagram.

    a. vitamin C

    b. vitamin D

    c. vitamin B₆

    d. vitamin K

    e. vitamin E

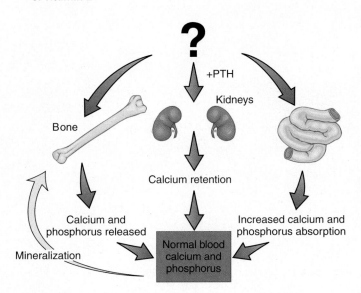

12. It is recommended that older adults get their vitamin B₁₂ from fortified foods and supplements because _____.

    a. they eat a poor diet

    b. their requirement for B₁₂ is higher than that of younger people

    c. many have atrophic gastritis and are not able to absorb the vitamin B₁₂ found in foods

    d. they have higher vitamin B₁₂ losses than other groups

13. Vitamin A deficiency causes the eye condition illustrated here because _____.

    a. the visual pigment rhodopsin cannot be synthesized

    b. collagen is not made correctly

    c. there is insufficient antioxidant protection

    d. bone development is abnormal

    e. mucus-secreting cells do not differentiate normally

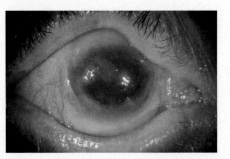

14. Which of the following statements is true of vitamin E?

    a. It is needed in energy metabolism.

    b. It protects cell membranes from oxidative damage.

    c. Severe deficiency is a common problem in North America.

    d. Supplements increase fertility even in people with adequate vitamin E status.

    e. It is needed for night vision.

15. Elevated blood homocysteine has been associated with an increased risk of cardiovascular disease. Deficiencies of _____ may increase levels of homocysteine in the blood.

    a. pantothenic acid, riboflavin, and vitamin C

    b. biotin, thiamin, and vitamin B₆

    c. vitamin B₆, folate, and vitamin B₁₂

    d. thiamin, riboflavin, and niacin

THE PLANNER ✓

Review your Chapter Planner on the chapter opener and check off your completed work.

Water and Minerals

8

It is in the water of Earth's first seas that scientists propose life itself originally appeared. These primitive seas were not plain water but rather a complex mixture of minerals, organic compounds, and water. Over time, as simple organisms developed greater complexity, many left this mineral-rich external marine environment behind. To survive, they needed to bring with them a similar internal environment. Within our bodies today, minerals and water make up an "internal sea" that allows the chemistry of life to function.

Getting the right amounts of minerals and water remains essential to survival. Inadequate and excessive

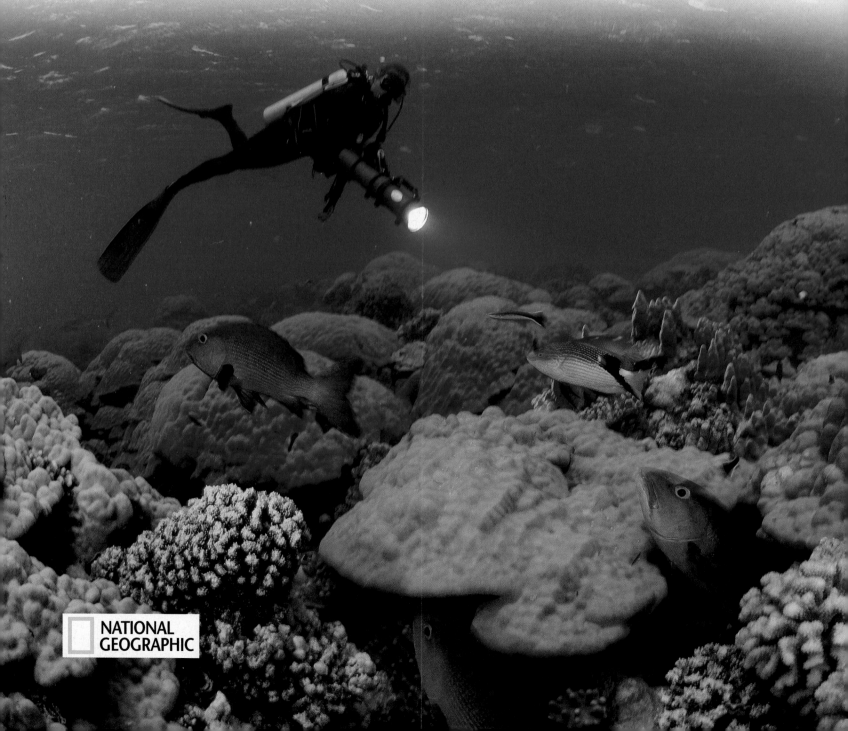

intakes of certain minerals are world health problems contributing to such conditions as high blood pressure, bone fractures, anemia, and increased risk of infection. Getting enough clean, fresh water may prove to be an even greater challenge to human survival than meeting mineral needs. Pollution and population growth are making fresh water an increasingly rare commodity: Approximately one in eight people around the world lack access to a safe water supply.[1] In the United States clean water is accessible to most, but the huge aquifers beneath the surface are diminishing. The water crisis may make shrinking oil supplies seem like a minor inconvenience for the simple reason that without water, we die.

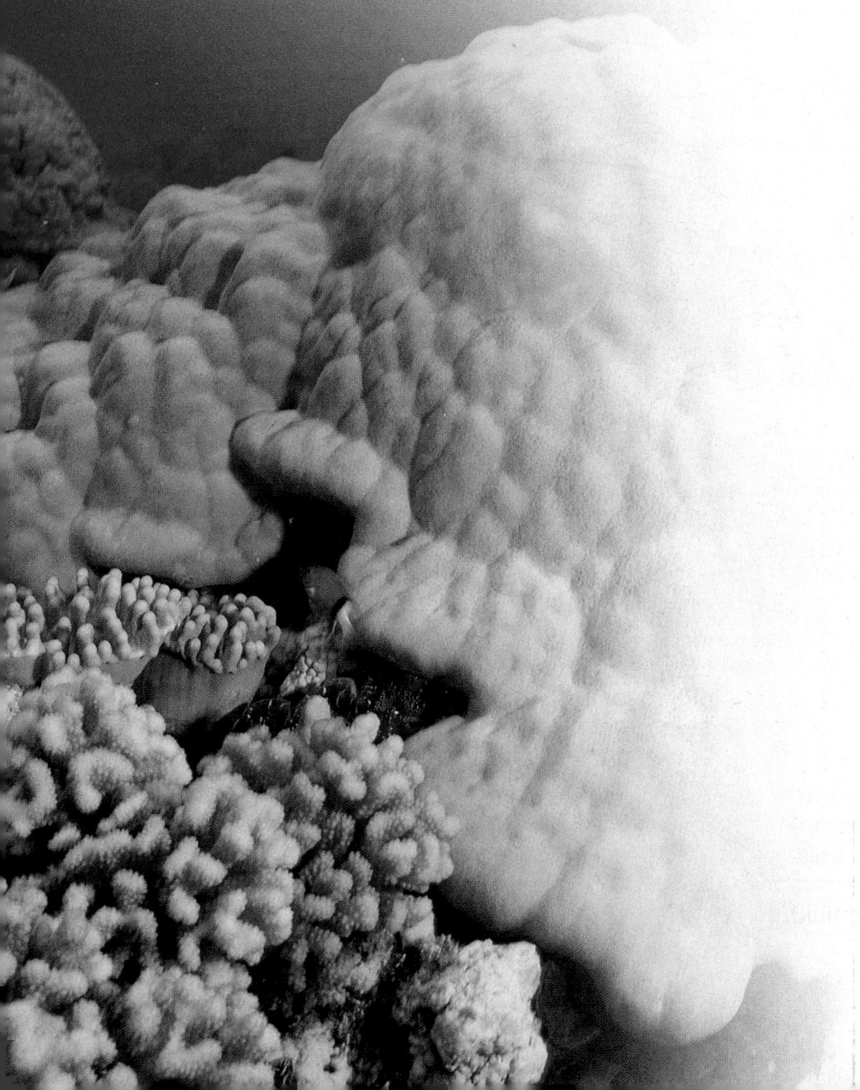

CHAPTER OUTLINE

CHAPTER PLANNER ✓

- ❏ Stimulate your interest by reading the introduction and looking at the visual.
- ❏ Scan the Learning Objectives in each section:
  p. 258 ❏   p. 265 ❏   p. 269 ❏   p. 277 ❏   p. 287 ❏
- ❏ Read the text and study all figures and visuals. Answer any questions.

Analyze key features

- ❏ Process Diagram, p. 260 ❏   p. 261 ❏   p. 269 ❏   p. 271 ❏
- ❏ InSight, p. 268 ❏   p. 272 ❏   p. 278 ❏   p. 290 ❏   p. 296 ❏
- ❏ What a Scientist Sees, p. 280 ❏
- ❏ Thinking It Through, p. 291 ❏
- ❏ Stop: Answer the Concept Checks before you go on:
  p. 265 ❏   p. 269 ❏   p. 277 ❏   p. 287 ❏   p. 301 ❏

End of chapter

- ❏ Review the Summary, Key Terms, and Online Resources.
- ❏ Answer the Critical and Creative Thinking Questions.
- ❏ Answer What is happening in this picture?
- ❏ Complete the Self-Test and check your answers.

Water

LEARNING OBJECTIVES

1. **Describe** how osmosis affects water distribution.
2. **Explain** the role of the kidneys in regulating the amount of water in the body.
3. **List** five functions of water in the body.
4. **Discuss** factors that increase water needs.

ater is an overlooked but essential nutrient. Lack of sufficient water in the body causes deficiency symptoms more rapidly than does a deficiency of any other nutrient. These symptoms can be alleviated almost as rapidly as they appeared by drinking enough water to restore the body's water balance.

Water in the Body

In adults, water accounts for about 60% of body weight. Water is found in different proportions in different tissues. For example, about 75% of muscle weight is water, whereas only about 25% of the weight of bone is due to water. Water is found both inside cells (intracellular) and outside cells (extracellular) in the blood, the lymph, and the spaces between cells (**Figure 8.1**). The cell membranes that separate the intracellular and extracellular spaces are not watertight; water can pass right through them.

Water distribution • Figure 8.1

About two-thirds of the water in the body is intracellular (located inside the cells). The other one-third is extracellular (located outside the cells). The extracellular portion includes the water in the blood and lymph, the water between cells, and the water in the digestive tract, eyes, joints, and spinal cord. The amount of water in the blood, between cells, and inside cells is affected by blood pressure and the force generated by osmosis.

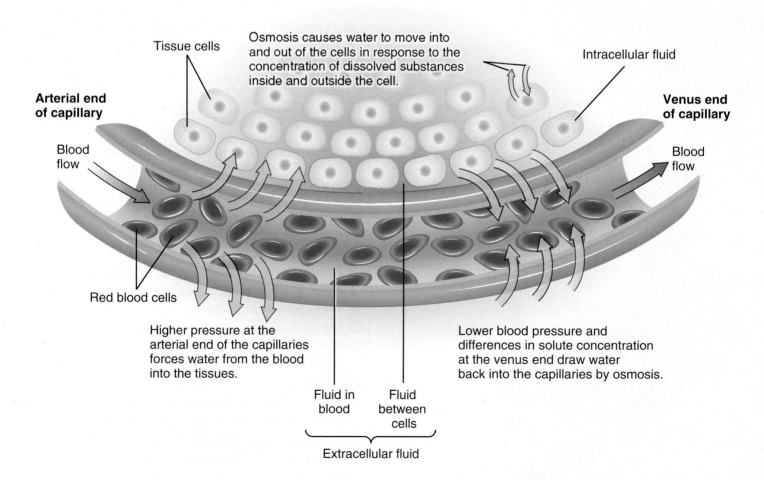

Tissue cells

Osmosis causes water to move into and out of the cells in response to the concentration of dissolved substances inside and outside the cell.

Intracellular fluid

Arterial end of capillary

Venus end of capillary

Blood flow

Blood flow

Red blood cells

Higher pressure at the arterial end of the capillaries forces water from the blood into the tissues.

Lower blood pressure and differences in solute concentration at the venus end draw water back into the capillaries by osmosis.

Fluid in blood

Fluid between cells

Extracellular fluid

Water balance • Figure 8.2

To maintain water balance, intake from food and drink and water produced by metabolism must equal water output from evaporation, sweat, urine, and feces. This figure illustrates approximate amounts of water that enter and leave the body daily in a typical woman who is in water balance. Increases in temperature or activity increase evaporative losses; increasing water consumption proportionately increases urinary excretion.

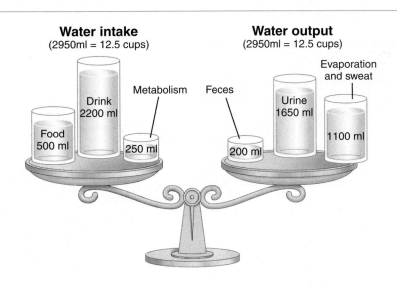

The distribution of water between various intra- and extracellular spaces depends on differences in the concentrations of dissolved substances, or **solutes**, such as proteins, sodium, potassium, and other small molecules. The concentration differences of these substances drive *osmosis*, the diffusion of water in a direction that equalizes the concentration of dissolved substances on either side of a membrane (see Chapter 3). Water is also moved by **blood pressure**, which forces water from the capillary blood vessels into the spaces between the cells of the surrounding tissues (see Figure 8.1). The body regulates the amount of water in cells and in different extracellular spaces by adjusting the concentration of dissolved particles and relying on osmosis to move the water.

blood pressure
The amount of force exerted by the blood against the walls of arteries.

Water Balance

The amount of water in the body remains relatively constant over time. Because water cannot be stored in the body, water intake and output must be balanced to maintain the right amount. Most of the water we consume comes from water and other liquids that we drink. Solid foods also provide water; most fruits and vegetables are over 80% water, and even roast beef is about 50% water. A small amount of water is also produced in the body as a by-product of metabolic reactions. We lose water from our bodies in urine and feces, through evaporation from the lungs and skin, and in sweat (**Figure 8.2**).

The amount of water lost in the urine varies with water intake and the amount of waste that needs to be excreted in the urine. In a healthy person, the amount of water lost in the feces is small—usually less than a cup per day. This is remarkable because every day about 9 L (38 cups) of fluid enters the gastrointestinal tract, but more than 95% of this is absorbed before the feces are eliminated. However, in cases of severe diarrhea, large amounts of water can be lost via this route, which can compromise health.

We are continuously losing water from our skin and respiratory tract due to evaporation. The amount of water lost through evaporation varies greatly, depending on activity, temperature, humidity, and body size. In a temperate climate, an inactive person loses about 1 L (4 cups) per day; the amount increases with increases in activity, environmental temperature, and body size, as well as when humidity is low.

In addition to being lost through evaporation, water is lost through sweat when you exercise or when the environment is hot. More sweat is produced as exercise intensity increases and as the environment becomes hotter and more humid. An individual doing light work at a temperature of 84°F will lose about 2 to 3 L of sweat per day. Strenuous exercise in a hot environment can increase this to 2 to 4 L in an hour.[2] Clothing that permits the evaporation of sweat helps keep the body cool and therefore decreases the amount of sweat produced.

Stimulating water intake • Figure 8.3

The sensation of thirst motivates fluid intake in order to restore water balance.

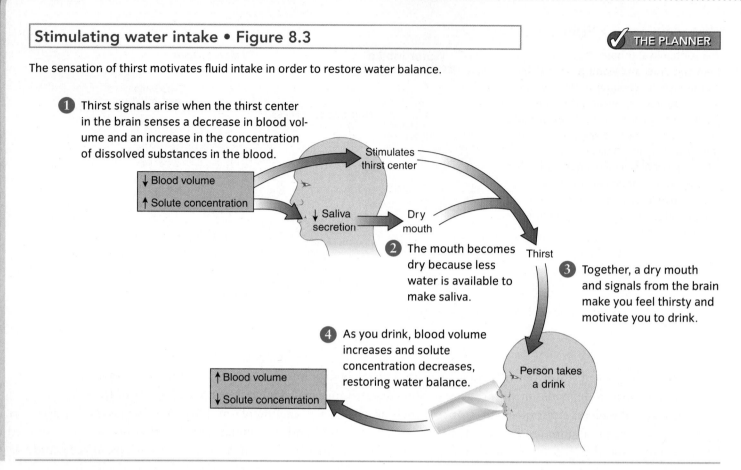

1 Thirst signals arise when the thirst center in the brain senses a decrease in blood volume and an increase in the concentration of dissolved substances in the blood.

↓ Blood volume

↑ Solute concentration

Stimulates thirst center

↓ Saliva secretion

Dry mouth

Thirst

2 The mouth becomes dry because less water is available to make saliva.

3 Together, a dry mouth and signals from the brain make you feel thirsty and motivate you to drink.

4 As you drink, blood volume increases and solute concentration decreases, restoring water balance.

↑ Blood volume

↓ Solute concentration

Person takes a drink

Regulating water intake When water losses increase, intake must increase to keep body water at a healthy level. The need to consume water is signaled by the sensation of **thirst**. Thirst is caused by dryness in the mouth as well as by signals from the brain (**Figure 8.3**). It is a powerful urge but often lags behind the need for water, and we don't or can't always drink when we are thirsty. Therefore, thirst alone cannot be relied on to maintain water balance.

Regulating water loss: The kidneys To maintain water balance, the kidneys regulate water loss in urine. The kidneys typically produce about 1 to 2 L (4 to 8 cups) of urine per day, but urine production varies, depending on the amount of water consumed and the amount of waste that needs to be excreted. Wastes that must be eliminated in the urine include urea and other nitrogen-containing molecules (produced by protein breakdown), ketones (from incomplete fat breakdown), sodium, and other minerals.

The kidneys function like a filter. As blood flows through them, water molecules and other small molecules move through the filter and out of the blood, while blood cells and large molecules are retained in the blood.

Some of the water and other molecules that are filtered out are reabsorbed into the blood, and the rest are excreted in the urine.

The amount of water that is reabsorbed into the blood rather than excreted in the urine depends on conditions in the body. When the solute concentration in the blood is high, as it would be in someone who has exercised strenuously and not consumed enough water, a hormone called **antidiuretic hormone (ADH)** signals the kidneys to reabsorb water, reducing the amount lost in the urine (**Figure 8.4**). This reabsorbed water is returned to the blood, preventing the concentration of dissolved particles from increasing further. When the solute concentration in the blood is low, as it might be after someone has guzzled several glasses of water, ADH levels decrease. Now the kidneys reabsorb less water, and more water is excreted in the urine, allowing the solute concentration in the blood to increase to its normal level.

The amount of water lost from the kidneys can also be affected by regulating the amount of sodium and other substances dissolved in the blood (as discussed later in the chapter).

Even though the kidneys work to control how much water is lost, their ability to concentrate urine is limited because there is a minimum amount of water that must be lost as dissolved wastes are excreted. If there are a lot of wastes to be excreted, more water must be lost.

The Functions of Water

Water doesn't provide energy, but it is essential to life. Water in the body serves as a medium for and participant in metabolic reactions, helps regulate acid–base balance, transports nutrients and wastes, provides protection, and helps regulate body temperature.

Water in metabolism and transport Water is an excellent **solvent**; glucose, amino acids, minerals, proteins, and many other molecules dissolve in water. The chemical reactions of metabolism that support life take place in water. Water also participates in a number of reactions that join small molecules together or break apart large ones. Some of the reactions in which water participates help maintain the proper level of acidity in the body. Water is the primary constituent of blood, which flows through our bodies, delivering oxygen and nutrients to cells and delivering waste products to the lungs and kidneys for excretion.

Water as protection Water bathes the cells of the body and lubricates and cleanses internal and external body surfaces. Water in tears lubricates the eyes and washes away dirt; water in synovial fluid lubricates the joints; and water in saliva lubricates the mouth, helping us chew and swallow food. Because water resists compression, it cushions the joints and other parts of the body against shock. The cushioning effect of water in the amniotic sac protects a fetus as it grows inside the uterus.

Regulating urinary water losses • Figure 8.4

✓ THE PLANNER

The kidneys help regulate water balance by adjusting the amount of water lost in the urine in response to the release of ADH.

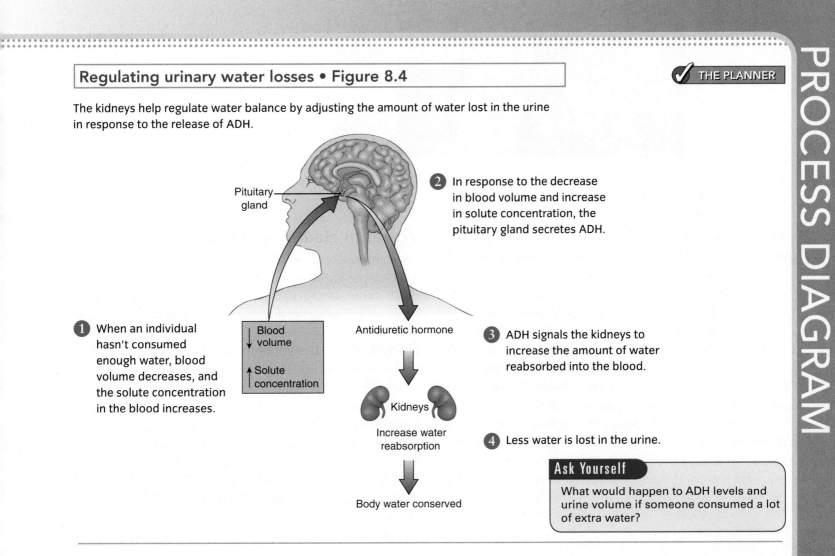

Pituitary gland

2 In response to the decrease in blood volume and increase in solute concentration, the pituitary gland secretes ADH.

1 When an individual hasn't consumed enough water, blood volume decreases, and the solute concentration in the blood increases.

↓ Blood volume

↑ Solute concentration

Antidiuretic hormone

3 ADH signals the kidneys to increase the amount of water reabsorbed into the blood.

Kidneys

Increase water reabsorption

4 Less water is lost in the urine.

Body water conserved

Ask Yourself

What would happen to ADH levels and urine volume if someone consumed a lot of extra water?

Water helps cool the body • Figure 8.5

Increased blood flow at the surface of the body causes the skin to become red in hot weather and during strenuous activity. Shunting blood to the skin allows heat to be transferred from the blood to the surroundings. Evaporation of sweat cools the skin and the blood near the surface of the skin.

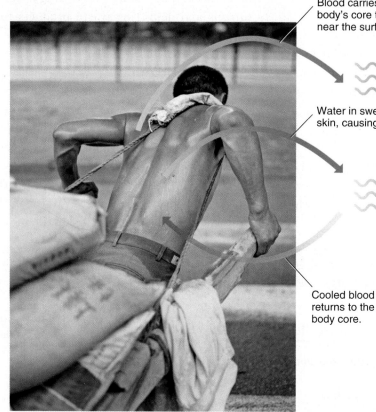

Blood carries heat from the body's core to the capillaries near the surface of the skin.

Heat is released from the skin to the environment.

Water in sweat evaporates from the skin, causing heat to be lost.

Evaporation cools the skin and the blood at the skin's surface.

Cooled blood returns to the body core.

Water and body temperature The fact that water holds heat and changes temperature slowly helps keep body temperature constant, but water is also actively involved in temperature regulation (**Figure 8.5**). The water in blood helps regulate body temperature by increasing or decreasing the amount of heat lost at the surface of the body. When body temperature starts to rise, the blood vessels in the skin dilate, causing more blood to flow close to the surface, where it can release some of the heat to the surrounding air. Cooling is aided by the production of sweat. When body temperature increases, the brain triggers the sweat glands in the skin to produce sweat, which is mostly water. As sweat evaporates from the skin, additional heat is lost, cooling the body.

Water in Health and Disease

Without food, you could probably survive for about eight weeks, but without water, you would last only a few days. Too much water can also be a problem if it changes the osmotic balance, disrupting the distribution of water within the body.

Dehydration Dehydration occurs when water loss exceeds water intake. It causes a reduction in blood volume, which impairs the ability to deliver oxygen and nutrients to cells and remove waste products. Early symptoms of dehydration include thirst, headache, fatigue, loss of appetite, dry eyes and mouth, and dark-colored urine (**Figure 8.6**). Dehydration affects

dehydration A state that occurs when not enough water is present to meet the body's needs.

Are you at risk for dehydration? • Figure 8.6

Urine color is an indication of whether you are drinking enough. Pale yellow urine indicates you are well hydrated. The darker the urine, the greater the level of dehydration.

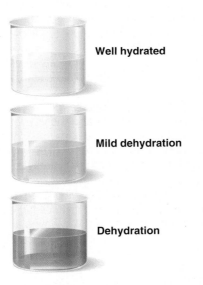

Well hydrated

Mild dehydration

Dehydration

physical and cognitive performance. As dehydration worsens, it causes nausea, difficulty concentrating, confusion, and disorientation. The milder symptoms of dehydration disappear quickly after water or some other beverage is consumed, but if left untreated, dehydration can become severe enough to require medical attention (**Figure 8.7**). A water loss amounting to about 10 to 20% of body weight can be fatal. Athletes are at risk for dehydration because they may lose large amounts of water in sweat. Older adults are at risk because the thirst mechanism becomes less sensitive with age. Infants are at risk because their body surface area relative to their weight is much greater than that of adults, so they lose proportionately more water through evaporation; also, their kidneys cannot concentrate urine efficiently, so they lose more water in urine. In addition, they cannot tell us they are thirsty.

Water intoxication It is difficult to consume too much water under normal circumstances. However, overhydration, or **water intoxication**, can occur under some conditions (see Chapter 10). When there is too much water relative to the amount of sodium in the body, the concentration of sodium in the blood drops—a condition called **hyponatremia**. When this occurs, water moves out of the blood vessels and into the tissues by osmosis, causing them to swell. Swelling in the brain can cause disorientation, convulsions, coma, and death. The early symptoms of water intoxication may be similar to those of dehydration: nausea, muscle cramps, disorientation, slurred speech, and confusion. It is important to determine whether the symptoms are due to dehydration or water intoxication because while drinking water will alleviate dehydration, it will worsen the symptoms of water intoxication.

> **water intoxication** A condition that occurs when a person drinks enough water to significantly lower the concentration of sodium in the blood.

Rehydration saves lives • Figure 8.7

Dehydration due to diarrhea is a major cause of child death in the developing world. Replacing fluids and electrolytes in the right combinations can save lives. In some cases, oral rehydration therapy is sufficient. Drinking mixtures made by simply dissolving a large pinch of salt (1/2 tsp) and a fistful of sugar (2 Tbsp) in 1 L of clean water can restore the body's water balance by promoting the absorption of water and sodium. In severe cases of diarrhea, administration of intravenous fluids, as seen in this hospital in Bangladesh, is needed to restore hydration.

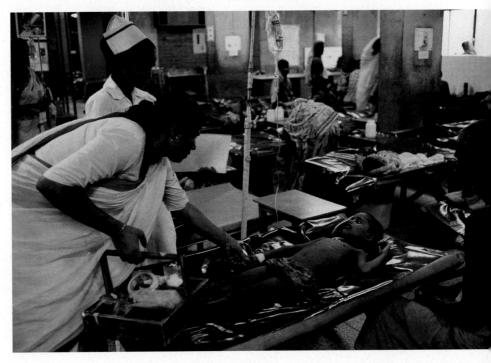

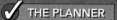

The Issue: Americans consume almost 28 gallons of bottled water per person per year.[4] We choose it because it is convenient and because we think it tastes better and is safer than tap water. But the cost to our pocketbooks and our environment is high. Should we be drinking from the tap instead?

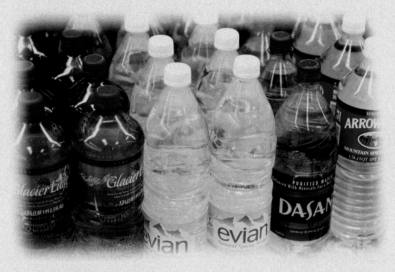

It is easy to grab a bottle of water, and most bottled water has no chlorine or other unpleasant aftertaste. Words like *pure, crisp,* and *fresh tasting* on the label lead consumers to buy bottled water because they think it is better than water that comes from the tap. But about 25% of the bottled water sold in the United States is tap water, and some is tap water that has been filtered, disinfected, or otherwise treated. By definition, bottled water can be any water, as long as it has no added ingredients (except antimicrobial agents or fluoride). Labels may help you distinguish: Distilled water and purified water are treated tap water; artesian water, spring water, well water, and mineral water come from underground sources.

Is bottled water safer than tap water? Municipal (tap) water is regulated by the Environmental Protection Agency (EPA), and bottled water sold in interstate commerce is regulated by the Food and Drug Administration (FDA). The FDA uses most of the EPA's tap water standards, so it would make sense that tap water and bottled water would be equally safe. However, tap water advocates argue that tap water may actually be safer. A certified outside laboratory tests municipal water supplies every year, while bottled water companies are permitted to do their own tests for purity.[5] Tap water must also be filtered and disinfected; there are no federal filtration or disinfection requirements for bottled water.

Contamination is a safety concern for both bottled water and tap water. A study of contaminants in bottled water found that 10 popular brands contained a total of 38 chemical pollutants—everything from caffeine and Tylenol to bacteria, radioactive

isotopes, and fertilizer residue.[6] Sounds scary, but bottled water advocates argue that public drinking water may also fall short of pollutant standards. Since 2004, testing by water utilities has found 315 pollutants in tap water. Some of these are substances that are regulated but were found at levels above guidelines, but more than half of the chemicals detected are not subject to health or safety regulations and can legally be present in any amount.[7]

One of the strongest arguments against bottled water is the cost, both to the consumer and the environment. Bottled water typically costs about $3.79 per gallon—1900 times the cost of public tap water. Bottled water drinkers may feel that the added cost is worth it because of the advantages in terms of taste and convenience. Opponents argue that even if you can afford it, the planet can't. Globally, bottled water generates 1.5 million tons of plastic waste per year and consumes oil, which is used to produce the bottles as well as the gasoline and jet fuel needed to transport it.[8] About three-quarters of the water bottles produced in the United States are not recycled.[5] Bottled water proponents argue that despite the large amount of plastic waste, discarded water bottles still represent less than 1% of total municipal waste. And even though bottled water production is more energy-intensive than the production of tap water, it comprises only a small share of total U.S. energy demand.[5]

So which is better? In the United States, bottled water and tap water are both generally safe. If you recycle your bottle, does it matter which you choose?

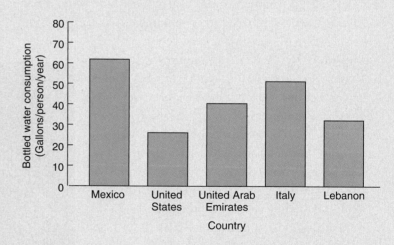

Think critically: Based on this graph, which country has the highest per capita bottled water consumption? What factors might increase a country's consumption of bottled water?

Meeting Water Needs

The AI for water is 3.7 L/day for men and 2.7 L/day for women. As discussed above, however, the amount of water you need each day varies, depending on your activity level, the environmental temperature, and the humidity. Diet can also affect water needs. A high-protein diet increases water needs because the urea produced from protein breakdown is excreted in the urine. A low-calorie diet increases water needs because as body fat and protein are broken down to fuel the body, ketones and urea are produced and must be excreted in the urine. A high-salt diet increases water losses because the excess must be excreted in the urine. A high-fiber diet increases water needs because more water is held in the intestines and lost in the feces.

In the United States beverages provide about 80% of the body's requirement for water—about 3 L (13 cups) for men and 2.2 L (9 cups) for women.[3] The rest comes from the water consumed in food. Most beverages, whether water, milk, juice, or soda, help meet the overall need for water (see *Debate: Is Bottled Water Better?*). Beverages containing caffeine, such as coffee, tea, and cola, increase water losses in the short term because caffeine is a **diuretic**. However, the increase in water loss is small, so the net amount of water that caffeinated beverages add to the body is similar to the amount contributed by noncaffeinated beverages. Alcohol is also a diuretic; the overall effect it has on water balance depends on the relative amounts of water and alcohol in the beverages being consumed.[3]

> **diuretic** A substance that increases the amount of urine passed from the body.

CONCEPT CHECK   STOP

1. **How** does osmosis affect the distribution of water in the body?
2. **What** is the role of ADH?
3. **How** does water help cool the body?
4. **Why** do water needs increase when you exercise more?

An Overview of Minerals

LEARNING OBJECTIVES

1. **Define** minerals in terms of nutrition.
2. **Describe** factors that affect mineral bioavailability.
3. **Discuss** the functions of minerals in the body

 inerals are found in the ground on which we walk, the jewels we wear on our fingers, and even some of the makeup we wear on our faces. But perhaps the most significant impact of minerals on our lives comes from their importance in our nutritional health. You need to consume more than 20 **minerals** in your food to stay healthy. Some of these make up a significant portion of your body weight; others are found in minute quantities. If more than 100 milligrams of a mineral is required in the diet each day, an amount equivalent in weight to about two drops of water, the mineral is considered a **major mineral**; these include sodium, potassium, chloride, calcium, phosphorus, magnesium, and sulfur. Minerals that are needed in smaller amounts are referred to as **trace minerals**; these include iron, copper, zinc, selenium, iodine, chromium, fluoride, manganese, molybdenum, and others. Just because you need more of the major minerals than of the trace minerals doesn't mean that one group is more important than the other. A deficiency of a trace mineral is just as damaging to your health as a deficiency of a major mineral.

> **mineral** In nutrition, an element needed by the body to maintain structure and regulate chemical reactions and body processes.

> **major mineral** A mineral required in the diet in an amount greater than 100 mg/day or present in the body in an amount greater than 0.01% of body weight.

> **trace mineral** A mineral required in the diet in an amount of 100 mg or less per day or present in the body in an amount of 0.01% of body weight or less.

Minerals On MyPlate • Figure 8.8

Minerals are found in all the MyPlate food groups, but some groups are particularly good sources of specific minerals. Eating a variety of foods, including fresh fruits, vegetables, nuts, legumes, whole grains and cereals, milk, seafood, and lean meats can maximize your diet's mineral content.

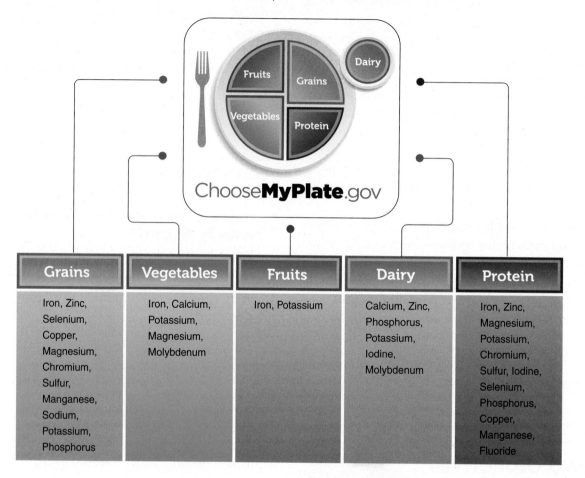

Grains	Vegetables	Fruits	Dairy	Protein
Iron, Zinc, Selenium, Copper, Magnesium, Chromium, Sulfur, Manganese, Sodium, Potassium, Phosphorus	Iron, Calcium, Potassium, Magnesium, Molybdenum	Iron, Potassium	Calcium, Zinc, Phosphorus, Potassium, Iodine, Molybdenum	Iron, Zinc, Magnesium, Potassium, Chromium, Sulfur, Iodine, Selenium, Phosphorus, Copper, Manganese, Fluoride

Ask Yourself

Which MyPlate food groups provide the greatest variety of minerals?

Minerals in Our Food

Minerals in the diet come from both plant and animal sources (**Figure 8.8**). Some minerals are present as functioning components of the plant or animal and are therefore present in consistent amounts. For instance, the iron content of beef is predictable because iron is part of the muscle protein that gives beef its red color. In other foods, some minerals are present as contaminants from the soil or from processing. For example, plants grown in an area where the soil is high in selenium are higher in selenium than plants grown in other areas, and milk from dairies that use sterilizing solu-

tions that contain iodine is a source of iodine. Minerals are also added to food intentionally during processing. Sodium is added to soups and crackers as a flavor enhancer; iron is added to enriched grain products; and calcium, iron, and other minerals are typically added to fortified breakfast cereals.

Processing can also remove minerals from foods. For example, when vegetables are cooked, the cells are broken down, and potassium is lost in the cooking water. When the skins of fruits and vegetables or the bran and germ of grains are detached, magnesium, iron, selenium, zinc, and copper are lost.

Mineral Bioavailability

The *bioavailability* of the minerals that we consume in foods varies. For some minerals, such as sodium, we absorb almost all that is present in our food, but for others, we absorb only a small percentage. For instance, we typically absorb only about 25% of the calcium in our diet, and iron absorption may be as low as 5%. How much of a particular mineral is absorbed may vary from food to food, meal to meal, and person to person.

In general, the minerals in animal products are better absorbed than those in plant foods. The difference in absorption is due in part to the fact that plants contain substances such as phytates (also called phytic acid), tannins, oxalates, and fiber that bind minerals in the gastrointestinal tract and can reduce absorption (**Figure 8.9**). The North American diet generally does not contain enough of any of these components to cause a mineral deficiency, but diets in developing countries may. For example, in some populations, the phytate content of the diet is high enough to cause a zinc deficiency.

> **ion** An atom or a group of atoms that carries an electrical charge.

The presence of one mineral can also interfere with the absorption of another. For example, mineral **ions** that carry the same charge compete for absorption in the gastrointestinal tract. Calcium, magnesium, zinc, copper, and iron all carry a 2+ charge, so a high intake of one may reduce the absorption of another. Although this is generally not a problem when whole foods are consumed, a large dose of one mineral from a dietary supplement may interfere with the absorption of other minerals.

The body's need for a mineral may also affect how much of that mineral is absorbed. For instance, if plenty of iron is stored in your body, you will absorb less of the iron you consume. Life stage can also affect absorption; for example, calcium absorption doubles during pregnancy, when the body's needs are high.

Mineral Functions

Minerals contribute to the body's structure and help regulate body processes. Many serve more than one function. For example, we need calcium to keep our bones strong as well as to maintain normal blood pressure, allow muscles to contract, and transmit nerve signals from cell to cell. Some minerals help regulate water balance, others help regulate energy metabolism, and some affect growth and development through their role in the

---

Compounds that interfere with mineral absorption • Figure 8.9

Plant foods such as these contain substances that can reduce mineral absorption when consumed in large amounts.

Oxalates, found in spinach, rhubarb, beet greens, and chocolate, have been found to interfere with the absorption of calcium and iron.

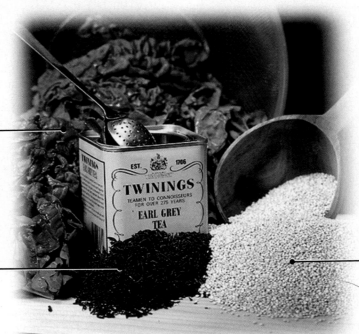

Tannins, found in tea and some grains, can interfere with the absorption of iron.

Phytates, found in whole grains, bran, and soy products, bind calcium, zinc, iron, and magnesium, limiting the absorption of these minerals. Phytates can be broken down by yeast, so the bioavailability of minerals is higher in yeast-leavened foods such as breads.

Selenium, sulfur, zinc, copper, and manganese are needed for the functioning of antioxidant enzymes and molecules that can defend the body against damaging chemicals.

Sodium, potassium, and chloride help regulate fluid balance.

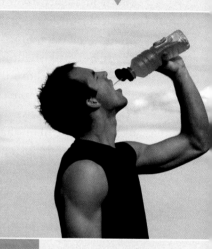

Zinc, iodine, and calcium are needed for normal growth and development.

Iron, magnesium, zinc, chromium, selenium, iodine, phosphorus, and calcium are needed to provide energy for physical activity and to regulate metabolism.

Calcium, sodium, potassium, and chloride are needed for the transmission of nerve impulses and for muscle contraction.

Iron, copper, calcium, zinc, selenium, and magnesium are needed to keep blood healthy and immune function strong.

Calcium, phosphorus, magnesium, and fluoride are needed to maintain the health of bones and teeth.

Cofactors • Figure 8.11

The binding of a cofactor to an enzyme activates the enzyme. For example, zinc is essential for the activity of an enzyme needed for DNA synthesis. Coenzymes, discussed in Chapter 7, are a type of cofactor.

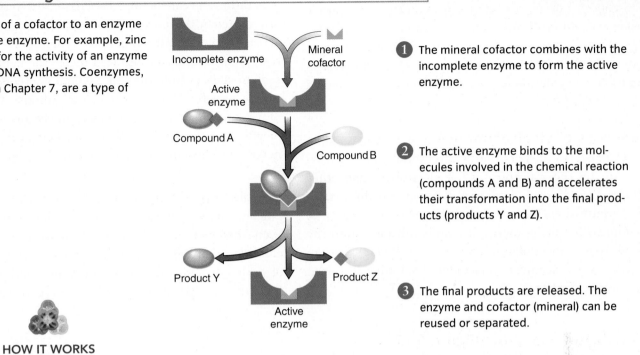

1 The mineral cofactor combines with the incomplete enzyme to form the active enzyme.

2 The active enzyme binds to the molecules involved in the chemical reaction (compounds A and B) and accelerates their transformation into the final products (products Y and Z).

3 The final products are released. The enzyme and cofactor (mineral) can be reused or separated.

HOW IT WORKS

---

expression of certain genes (**Figure 8.10**). Many minerals act as **cofactors** needed for enzyme activity (**Figure 8.11**). None of the minerals we require acts in isolation. Instead, they interact with each other as well as with other nutrients and other components of the diet.

cofactor An inorganic ion or coenzyme that is required for enzyme activity.

CONCEPT CHECK STOP

1. **How** do minerals differ from vitamins?
2. **How** do phytates, oxalates, and tannins decrease mineral bioavailability?
3. **What** is the function of a cofactor?

Electrolytes: Sodium, Potassium, and Chloride

LEARNING OBJECTIVES

1. **Explain** how electrolytes function in the body.
2. **Define** hypertension and describe its symptoms and consequences.
3. **Discuss** how diet affects blood pressure.
4. **Contrast** the dietary sources of sodium and potassium.

the body are electrolytes, in nutrition and in sports drinks, the term *electrolyte* refers to the three principal electrolytes in body fluids: sodium, potassium, and chloride. Sodium and potassium carry a positive charge, and chloride carries a negative charge. In the diet, sodium is most commonly found combined with chloride as **sodium chloride**, what we call either "salt" or "table salt." In our bodies, these electrolytes are important in maintaining fluid balance and allowing nerve impulses to travel throughout our bodies, signaling the activities that are essential for life.

electrolyte A positively or negatively charged ion that conducts an electrical current in solution. Commonly refers to sodium, potassium, and chloride.

We think of **electrolytes** as the things we get by guzzling a sports drink. But what exactly are they, and why do we need them? Electrolytes are ions. Although many substances in

Electrolytes in the Body

The concentrations of sodium, potassium, and chloride inside cells differ dramatically from those outside. Potassium is the principal positively charged intracellular ion, sodium is the most abundant positively charged extracellular ion, and chloride is the principal negatively charged extracellular ion.

Functions of electrolytes

Electrolytes help regulate fluid balance; the distribution of water throughout the body depends on the concentration of electrolytes and other solutes. Water moves by osmosis in response to differences in concentration. So, for example, if the concentration of sodium in the blood increases, water will move into the blood from intracellular and other extracellular spaces to equalize the concentration of sodium and other dissolved substances (**Figure 8.12a**).

Sodium, potassium, and chloride are also essential for generating and conducting nerve impulses. Nerve impulses are created by the movement of sodium and potassium ions across the nerve cell membrane. When a nerve cell is at rest, potassium is concentrated inside the nerve cell, and sodium stays outside the cell. Sodium and potassium ions cannot pass freely across the cell membrane. But when a nerve is stimulated, the cell membrane becomes more permeable to sodium, allowing sodium ions to rush into the nerve cell, which initiates a nerve impulse (**Figure 8.12b**).

Regulating electrolyte balance

Our bodies are efficient at regulating the concentration of electrolytes, even when dietary intake varies dramatically. Sodium and chloride balance is regulated to some extent by the intake of both salt and water. When sodium chloride intake is high, thirst is stimulated in order to increase water intake.

Electrolyte functions • Figure 8.12

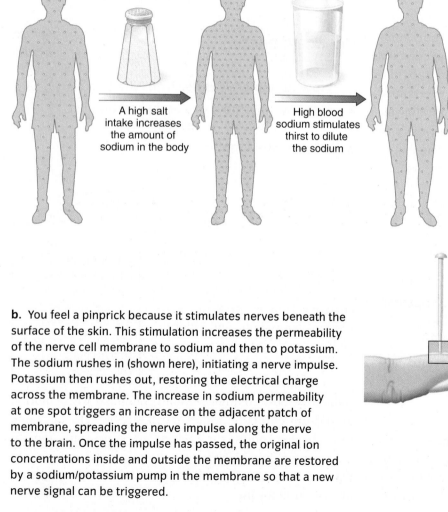

A high salt intake increases the amount of sodium in the body

High blood sodium stimulates thirst to dilute the sodium

a. Have you ever noticed that your weight is a few pounds higher the morning after you eat a salty dinner? The sodium you consume in such a meal increases your blood sodium concentration and stimulates you to drink enough to dilute it. The extra pounds you see on the scale reflect the extra water you have temporarily stowed away.

b. You feel a pinprick because it stimulates nerves beneath the surface of the skin. This stimulation increases the permeability of the nerve cell membrane to sodium and then to potassium. The sodium rushes in (shown here), initiating a nerve impulse. Potassium then rushes out, restoring the electrical charge across the membrane. The increase in sodium permeability at one spot triggers an increase on the adjacent patch of membrane, spreading the nerve impulse along the nerve to the brain. Once the impulse has passed, the original ion concentrations inside and outside the membrane are restored by a sodium/potassium pump in the membrane so that a new nerve signal can be triggered.

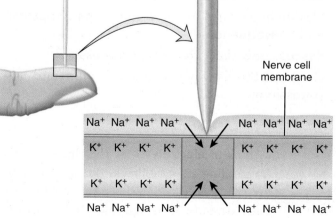

Nerve cell membrane

Na^+ Na^+ Na^+ Na^+ Na^+ Na^+ Na^+ Na^+

K^+ K^+ K^+ K^+ K^+ K^+ K^+ K^+

K^+ K^+ K^+ K^+ K^+ K^+ K^+ K^+

Na^+ Na^+ Na^+ Na^+ Na^+ Na^+ Na^+ Na^+

Regulation of blood pressure • Figure 8.13

A drop in blood pressure triggers events that cause blood vessels to constrict and the kidneys to retain water. An increase in blood pressure inhibits these events so that blood pressure does not continue to rise.

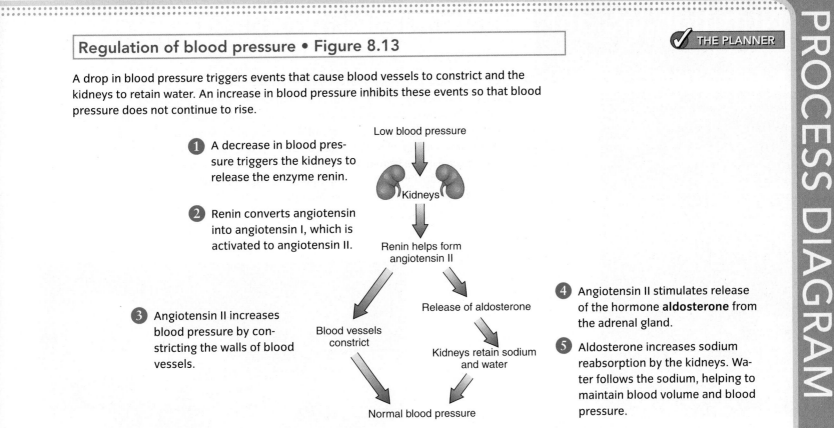

1 A decrease in blood pressure triggers the kidneys to release the enzyme renin.

2 Renin converts angiotensin into angiotensin I, which is activated to angiotensin II.

3 Angiotensin II increases blood pressure by constricting the walls of blood vessels.

4 Angiotensin II stimulates release of the hormone **aldosterone** from the adrenal gland.

5 Aldosterone increases sodium reabsorption by the kidneys. Water follows the sodium, helping to maintain blood volume and blood pressure.

Low blood pressure

Kidneys

Renin helps form angiotensin II

Release of aldosterone

Blood vessels constrict

Kidneys retain sodium and water

Normal blood pressure

Very low salt intake stimulates a "salt appetite" that causes you to crave salt. The craving that triggers your desire to plunge into a bag of salty chips, however, is not due to this salt appetite. It is a learned preference, not a physiological drive. If you cut back on your salt intake, you will find that your taste buds become more sensitive to the presence of salt, and foods taste saltier.

Thirst and salt appetite help ensure that appropriate proportions of sodium chloride and water are taken in, but the kidneys are the primary regulator of sodium, potassium, and chloride concentrations in the body. Excretion of these electrolytes in the urine is decreased when intake is low and increased when intake is high.

Because water follows sodium by osmosis, the ability of the kidneys to conserve sodium provides a mechanism for conserving water in the body. This mechanism also helps regulate blood pressure. When the concentration of sodium in the blood increases, water follows, causing an increase in blood volume. Changes in blood volume can change blood pressure. Changes in blood pressure, in turn, trigger the production and release of proteins and hormones that affect the amount of sodium, and hence water, retained by the kidneys (**Figure 8.13**).

Regulation of blood potassium levels is also important. Even a small increase can be dangerous. If blood potassium levels begin to rise, body cells are stimulated to take up potassium. This short-term regulation prevents the amount of potassium in the extracellular fluid from getting lethally high. Long-term regulation of potassium balance depends on the release of proteins that cause the kidney to excrete potassium and retain sodium.

Electrolytes in Health and Disease

Electrolyte deficiencies are uncommon in healthy people. Sodium, potassium, and chloride are plentiful in most diets, and the kidneys of healthy individuals are efficient at regulating the amounts of these electrolytes in the body. Acute deficiencies and excesses can occur due to illness or extreme conditions. The health problem most commonly associated with electrolyte imbalance is **hypertension**, or high blood pressure. Hypertension is a serious public health concern in the United States; about one-third of adult Americans ages 20 and older have hypertension. Only about 44% of those with hypertension have their blood pressure under control.[9]

> **hypertension** Blood pressure that is consistently elevated to 140/90 millimeters (mm) mercury or greater.

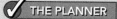
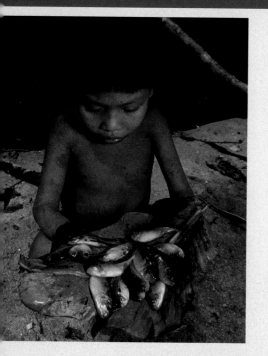

This Yanomami Indian boy lives in the rain forest of Brazil. The Yanomami diet consists of locally grown crops, nuts, insects, fish, and game. It contains less than 1 gram of sodium chloride a day, the lowest salt intake recorded for any population. The Yanomami have very low average blood pressure and no hypertension. Studying the salt intake and blood pressure of the Yanomami and 51 other populations around the world helped to establish a relationship between salt intake and hypertension; diets that are high in salt are associated with an increased incidence of hypertension.[17]

A diet that is high in fruits and vegetables, which are good sources of potassium, magnesium, and fiber, reduces blood pressure compared to a similar diet containing fewer fruits and vegetables. The amounts in the measuring cups shown here, about 2 cups of fruit and 2 1/2 cups of vegetables, represent the amount recommended for a 2000-Calorie diet.[18]

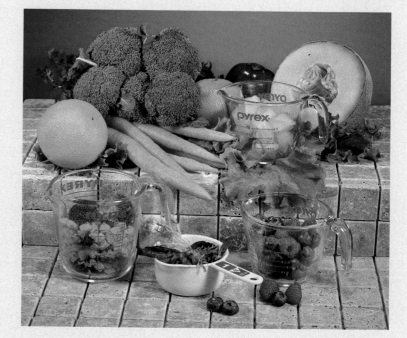

Electrolyte deficiency Deficiencies of any of the electrolytes can lead to electrolyte imbalance, which can cause disturbances in acid–base balance, poor appetite, muscle cramps, confusion, apathy, constipation, and, eventually, irregular heartbeat. For example, the sudden death that can occur as a result of fasting, anorexia nervosa, or starvation may be due to heart failure caused by potassium deficiency. Sodium, chloride, and potassium depletion can occur when losses of these electrolytes are increased by heavy and persistent sweating, chronic diarrhea or vomiting, or kidney disorders that lead to excessive excretion. Medications can also interfere with electrolyte balance. For example, certain diuretic medications that are used to treat high blood pressure cause potassium loss.

Electrolyte toxicity It is not possible for healthy people to consume too much potassium from foods. If,

however, supplements are consumed in excess or kidney function is compromised, blood levels of potassium can increase and potentially cause death due to an irregular heartbeat. A high oral dose of potassium generally causes vomiting, but if too much potassium enters the blood, it can cause the heart to stop.

It is difficult to consume more sodium than the body can handle because we usually drink more water when we consume more sodium. Though rare, elevation of blood sodium can result from massive ingestion of salt, such as may occur from drinking seawater or consuming salt tablets. The most common cause of high blood sodium is dehydration, and the symptoms of high blood sodium are similar to those of dehydration.

Hypertension Hypertension, or high blood pressure, has been called "the silent killer" because it has no

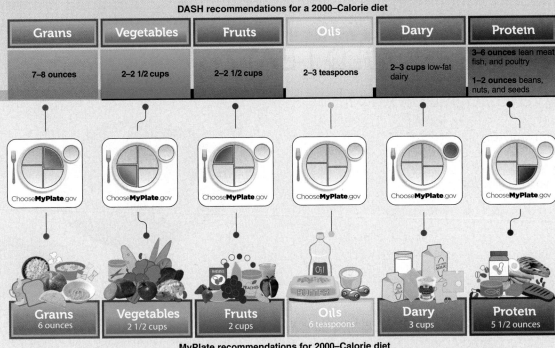

DASH recommendations for a 2000–Calorie diet

Grains	Vegetables	Fruits	Oils	Dairy	Protein
7–8 ounces	2–2 1/2 cups	2–2 1/2 cups	2–3 teaspoons	2–3 cups low-fat dairy	3–6 ounces lean meat, fish, and poultry; 1–2 ounces beans, nuts, and seeds

The recommendations of the DASH Eating Plan (DASH stands for Dietary Approaches to Stop Hypertension) are shown in the upper portion of the figure. This diet is abundant in fruits and vegetables; includes low-fat dairy products, whole grains, legumes, nuts, and seafood; and incorporates moderate amounts of lean meat. The amounts recommended are similar to those of MyPlate, which are shown at the bottom of the figure. MyPlate also recommends eating plenty of fruits and vegetables; choosing whole grains; having beans, nuts, seeds, and fish more often; and choosing lean meats and low-fat dairy products.

Grains	Vegetables	Fruits	Oils	Dairy	Protein
6 ounces	2 1/2 cups	2 cups	6 teaspoons	3 cups	5 1/2 ounces

ChooseMyPlate.gov

MyPlate recommendations for 2000–Calorie diet

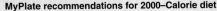

A blood pressure measurement is two numbers: systolic over diastolic **120/80**

Systolic is the maximum pressure in the arteries

Diastolic is the minimum pressure in the arteries

Reductions in blood pressure are seen with the DASH diet pattern compared with a typical American eating pattern. When the sodium content of either diet is lowered, there is a reduction in blood pressure.[16]

(Bar graph: Systolic blood pressure (mm mercury) 120–135 left axis; Diastolic blood pressure (mm mercury) 75–85 right axis. Legend: Typical American diet, DASH diet. X-axis Dietary sodium level (mg/day): 2400, 1500, 2400, 1500.)

outward symptoms but can lead to atherosclerosis, heart attack, stroke, kidney disease, and early death. It is caused by an increase in blood volume or a narrowing of the blood vessels. Hypertension is a complex disorder resulting from disturbances in one or more of the mechanisms that control body fluid and electrolyte balance.

Elevated blood pressure is treated with diet, exercise, and medication. To allow early treatment and avoid the potentially lethal side effects of elevated blood pressure, people should have their blood pressure monitored regularly. A healthy blood pressure is 120/80 mm of mercury or less. Blood pressure between 120/80 and 140/90 is referred to as **prehypertension**, and blood pressure that is consistently 140/90 mm of mercury or greater indicates hypertension (see Appendix C).[10]

Some of the risk of developing hypertension is genetic; your risk is increased if you have a family history of the dis-

ease. It is more common in African Americans than in Mexican Americans or non-Hispanic whites.[11] Whether you are genetically predisposed to hypertension or not, your risk of developing high blood pressure increases as you grow older and is higher if you are overweight, particularly if the excess fat is in your abdominal region. Lack of physical activity, heavy alcohol consumption, and stress can also increase blood pressure.[12] Regular exercise can prevent or delay the onset of hypertension, and weight loss can help reduce blood pressure in obese individuals. Your risk of developing high blood pressure can also be increased or decreased by your dietary choices (**Figure 8.14**).

Diet and blood pressure

Dietary intake of sodium, chloride, potassium, calcium, and magnesium can affect your blood pressure and your risk of hypertension. In general, as the sodium content of the diet increases, so

WHAT SHOULD I EAT?
Water and Electrolytes

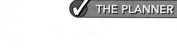

Stay hydrated
- Drink before, during, and after exercise.
- Guzzle two extra glasses of water when you are outside on a hot day.
- Bring a bottle of water with you in your car.

Boost your potassium intake
- Double your vegetable serving at dinner.
- Take two pieces of fruit for lunch.
- Drink orange juice instead of soda or punch.

Reduce your sodium intake
- Choose more unprocessed foods.
- Do not add salt to the water when cooking rice, pasta, and cereals.
- Flavor foods with lemon juice, onions, garlic, pepper, curry, basil, oregano, or thyme rather than with salt.
- Limit salty snacks such as salted potato chips, nuts, popcorn, and crackers.
- Limit condiments such as soy sauce, barbecue sauce, ketchup, and mustard; they are high in sodium.

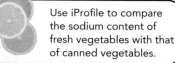

Use iProfile to compare the sodium content of fresh vegetables with that of canned vegetables.

does blood pressure.[13] In contrast, diets that are high in potassium, calcium, and magnesium are associated with a lower average blood pressure.[14] Other components of the diet, such as the amount of fiber and the type and amount of fat, may also affect your risk of developing hypertension. A dietary pattern, such as the **DASH**

Processing adds sodium • Figure 8.15

a. About 77% of the salt we eat comes from processed foods. Only about 12% comes from salt found naturally in food, while 11% comes from salt added in cooking and at the table.[19]

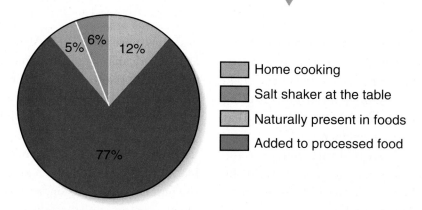

- Home cooking
- Salt shaker at the table
- Naturally present in foods
- Added to processed food

5% 6% 12%

77%

Ask Yourself

For a typical American, which of the following will result in the greatest reduction in sodium intake?

a. Taking away the salt shaker during meals
b. Reducing the amount of salt added during meal preparation
c. Consuming fewer processed foods

(Dietary Approaches to Stop Hypertension) **Eating Plan**, that incorporates the recommended amounts of each of these can cause a significant reduction in blood pressure and is a dietary pattern recommended by the 2010 Dietary Guidelines. This pattern provides plenty of fiber, potassium, magnesium, and calcium; is low in total fat, saturated fat, and cholesterol; and is lower in sodium than the typical American diet (see Appendix D). Consuming a diet that follows the DASH pattern lowers blood pressure in individuals with elevated blood pressure even when sodium levels are not severely restricted. Reductions in blood pressure are greater when sodium intake is lower (see Figure 8.14).[15,16]

Meeting Electrolyte Needs

Most people in the United States need to reduce their salt intake and increase their potassium intake to meet recommendations for a healthy diet (see *What Should I Eat?*). The 2010 Dietary Guidelines recommend a daily sodium intake of less than 2300 mg. This value is the same as the UL for sodium, which is set to avoid the increase in blood pressure seen with higher sodium intakes. For people who are 51 years or older and those of any age who are African American or have hypertension, diabetes, or kidney disease, sodium intake should be reduced to 1500 mg/day. The typical daily intake of sodium in the United States is about 3400 mg.[13] Because salt is 40% sodium and 60% chloride by weight, this represents 8.5 grams (8500 mg) of salt per day.

The DRIs recommend a potassium intake of 4700 mg/day; the Daily Value is at least 3500 mg/day for adults. This amount is significantly higher than the typical 2000 to 3000 mg consumed by most Americans. No UL has been set for potassium.

One of the reasons our diet is high in salt (sodium chloride) and low in potassium is that we eat a lot of processed foods, which are high in sodium and chloride, and too few fresh unprocessed foods, such as fruits, vegetables, whole grains, and fresh meats, which are high in potassium. Over three-quarters of the salt we eat is from foods that have had salt added during processing and manufacturing (**Figure 8.15**).

You can lower the amount of sodium in your diet by limiting your intake of processed foods and cutting down on the amount of salt added in cooking and at the table.

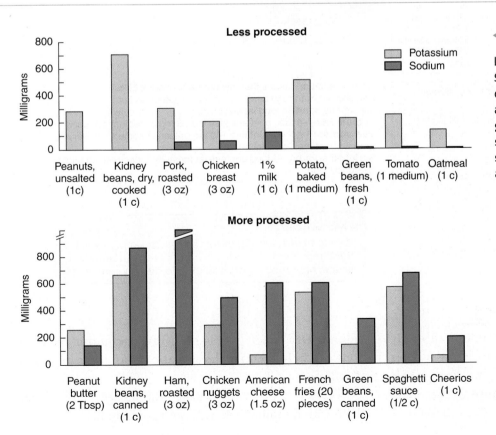

b. Processed foods are generally higher in sodium and may also be lower in potassium than unprocessed foods. Some of the sodium in processed foods comes from salt added for flavoring; some is added as a preservative to inhibit microbial growth. In addition to sodium chloride, sodium bicarbonate, sodium citrate, and sodium glutamate are added to preserve and flavor foods.

Sodium on food labels • Figure 8.16

Food labels are an important source of information about the sodium content of packaged foods. In addition to the information illustrated here, a food that meets the definition for *low sodium* and provides 20% or less of the Daily Value for fat, saturated fat, and cholesterol per serving can include on the label the health claim that diets that are low in sodium may reduce the risk of high blood pressure.

Nutrition Facts

Serving Size 1/2 cup (125g)
Servings Per Container about 3½

Amount Per Serving

Calories 50	Calories from Fat 10

	%Daily Value**
Total Fat 1g	**2%**
Saturated Fat 0g	**0%**
Trans Fat 0g	
Cholesterol 0mg	**0%**
Sodium 250mg	**10%**
Potassium 530mg	**15%**
Total Carbohydrate 9g	**3%**
Dietary Fiber 1g	**4%**
Sugars 7g	
Protein 2g	

Vitamin A 10%	•	Vitamin C 25%
Calcium 2%	•	Iron 10%

*Percent Daily Values are based on a 2,000 calorie diet. Your daily values may be higher or lower depending on your calorie needs.

	Calories:	2,000	2,500
Total Fat	Less than	65g	80g
Sat Fat	Less than	20g	25g
Cholesterol	Less than	300mg	300mg
Sodium	Less than	2,400mg	2,400mg
Potassium		3,500mg	3,500mg
Total Carbohydrate		300g	375g
Dietary Fiber		25g	30g

The Nutrition Facts section lists the total amount of sodium per serving and the % Daily Value this amount represents.

The Daily Value for sodium for a 2000-Calorie diet is given at the bottom of the label.

Light Spaghetti Sauce, 250 milligrams (mg) per serving
Regular Spaghetti Sauce, 500 mg per serving

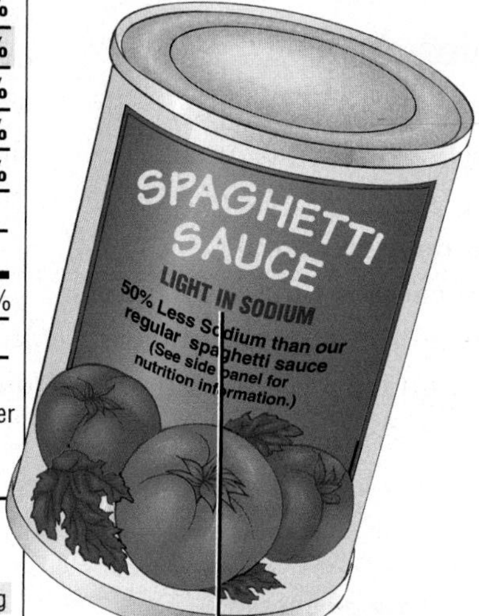

SPAGHETTI SAUCE
LIGHT IN SODIUM
50% Less Sodium than our regular spaghetti sauce (See side panel for nutrition information.)

"Light in sodium" means that this product contains 50% less sodium than regular spaghetti sauce. Other sodium descriptors seen on food labels include:
Sodium free—a food contains less than 5 mg of sodium per serving
Low sodium—a food contains 140 mg or less of sodium per serving (about 5% of the Daily Value)
Reduced sodium—a food contains at least 25% less sodium than a reference food.

Ask Yourself

If instead of a serving of this spaghetti sauce, which is light in sodium, you ate a serving of regular spaghetti sauce, how much more sodium would you consume?

A diet that is high in fruits and vegetables will easily meet potassium intake recommendations; daily intakes of 8000 to 11,000 mg are not uncommon.[3] Food labels can help identify low-sodium foods (**Figure 8.16**). Some medications can also contribute a significant amount of sodium. Drug facts labels on over-the-counter medications can help identify those that contain large amounts of sodium.

Table 8.1, on the next page, summarizes information about water, sodium, chloride, and potassium.

A summary of water and the electrolytes   Table 8.1

Nutrient	Sources	Recommended intake for adults	Major functions	Deficiency diseases and symptoms	Groups at risk of deficiency	Toxicity	UL
Water	Drinking water, other beverages, and food	2.7–3.7 L/day	Solvent, reactant, protector, transporter, regulator of temperature and pH	Thirst, dark-colored urine, weakness, poor endurance, confusion, disorientation	Infants, people with fever and diarrhea, elderly individuals, athletes	Confusion, coma, convulsions	ND
Sodium	Table salt, processed foods	<2300 mg; ideally 1500 mg/day	Major positive extracellular ion, nerve transmission, muscle contraction, fluid balance	Muscle cramps	People consuming a severely sodium-restricted diet, those who sweat excessively	High blood pressure in sensitive people	2300 mg/day
Potassium	Fresh fruits and vegetables, legumes, whole grains, milk, meat	4700 mg/day or more	Major positive intracellular ion, nerve transmission, muscle contraction, fluid balance	Irregular heartbeat, fatigue, muscle cramps	People consuming poor diets high in processed foods, those taking thiazide diuretics	Abnormal heartbeat	ND
Chloride	Table salt, processed foods	<3600 mg/day; ideally 2300 mg/day	Major negative extracellular ion, fluid balance	Unlikely	None	None likely	3600 mg/day

Note: UL, Tolerable Upper Intake Level; ND, not determined.

CONCEPT CHECK

1. **Why** does eating a salty meal cause your weight to increase temporarily?
2. **Why** is hypertension called "the silent killer"?
3. **What** is the DASH Eating Plan?
4. **Which** types of foods contribute the most sodium to the American diet?

Major Minerals and Bone Health

LEARNING OBJECTIVES

1. **Describe** factors that affect peak bone mass and the rate of bone loss.
2. **Explain** how blood calcium levels are regulated.
3. **List** foods that are good sources of calcium.
4. **Describe** functions of calcium, phosphorus, and magnesium that are unrelated to their role in bone.

B ones are the hardest, strongest structures in the human body. They support our weight, whether we are stepping off a curb or jumping rope. Age, however, heralds a loss of bone strength. For many people, the loss is so great that the force of stepping off a curb is enough to cause their bones to fracture.

Bone is strong because it is composed of a protein framework, or matrix, that is hardened by deposits of minerals.

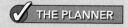
THE PLANNER

a. Changes in the balance between bone formation and bone breakdown cause bone mass to increase in children and adolescents and decrease in adults as they grow older. ▼

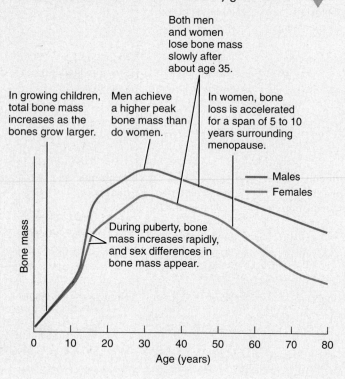

Both men and women lose bone mass slowly after about age 35.

In growing children, total bone mass increases as the bones grow larger.

Men achieve a higher peak bone mass than do women.

In women, bone loss is accelerated for a span of 5 to 10 years surrounding menopause.

— Males
— Females

During puberty, bone mass increases rapidly, and sex differences in bone mass appear.

Bone mass

Age (years)

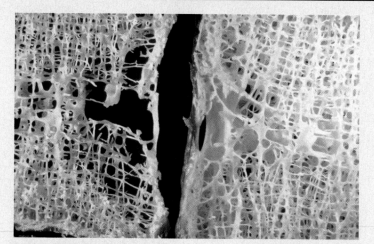

Bone weakened by osteoporosis   Normal bone

▲ **b.** Osteoporosis, shown here compared to normal bone, is a major public health problem in the United States and elsewhere around the world. In the United States, more than 5 million people over age 50 have osteoporosis, and another 34.5 million are at risk due to low bone mass, called **osteopenia**.[21]

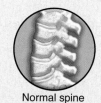

Normal spine   Osteoporotic spine

When weakened by osteoporosis, the front edge of the vertebrae collapses more than the back edge, so the spine bends forward.

c. Osteoporosis leads to 1.5 million fractures annually, which account for $18 billion per year in direct medical costs.[22] Spinal compression fractures, shown here, are common and may result in loss of height and a stooped posture (called a "dowager's hump").

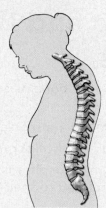

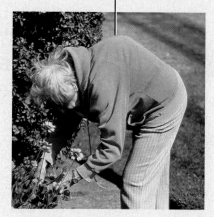

Interpreting Data

Based on the information in this graph, why would women over 50 be at greater risk of osteoporosis than men over 50?

This matrix consists primarily of the protein collagen. The mineral portion of bone is composed mainly of calcium associated with phosphorus, but it also contains magnesium, sodium, fluoride, and a number of other minerals. Healthy bone requires adequate dietary protein and vitamin C to maintain the collagen and a sufficient supply of calcium and other minerals to ensure solidity. Adequate vitamin D (discussed in Chapter 7) is needed to maintain appropriate levels of calcium and phosphorus. There is also growing evidence of the importance of vitamin K for bone health.[20]

Bone in Health and Disease

Like other tissues in the body, bone is alive, and it is constantly being broken down and reformed through a process called **bone remodeling**. Most bone is formed early in life. During childhood, bones grow larger; even after growth stops, bone mass continues to increase into young adulthood (**Figure 8.17a**). The maximum amount of bone that you have in your lifetime, called **peak bone mass**, is achieved somewhere between ages 16 and 30. Up to this point, bone formation occurs more rapidly than breakdown, so the total amount of bone increases.

> **bone remodeling** A continuous process in which small amounts of bone are removed and replaced by new bone.
>
> **peak bone mass** The maximum bone density attained at any time in life, usually occurring in young adulthood.

After about age 35 to 45, the amount of bone that is broken down begins to exceed the amount that is formed, so total bone mass decreases. Over time, if enough bone is lost, the skeleton is weakened and fractures occur more easily, a condition referred to as **osteoporosis** (**Figure 8.17b** and **c**).

Factors affecting the risk of osteoporosis

The risk of developing osteoporosis depends on the level of peak bone mass and the rate at which bone is lost. These variables are affected by genetics, gender, age, hormone levels, and lifestyle factors such as smoking, alcohol consumption, exercise, and diet (**Table 8.2**).

Women have a higher risk of osteoporosis because they have less bone than men and lose it faster as they age. **Age-related bone loss** occurs in both men and women, but women lose additional bone for period of about 5 to 10 years surrounding **menopause**. This **postmenopausal bone loss** is related to the decline in estrogen level, which increases calcium release from bone and decreases the amount of

> **osteoporosis** A bone disorder characterized by reduced bone mass, increased bone fragility, and increased risk of fractures.
>
> **age-related bone loss** Bone loss that occurs in both men and women as they advance in age.
>
> **menopause** The time in a woman's life when the menstrual cycle ends.
>
> **postmenopausal bone loss** Accelerated bone loss that occurs in women for about 5 to 10 years surrounding menopause.

Factors affecting the risk of osteoporosis	Table 8.2
Risk factor	**How it affects risk**
Gender	Fractures due to osteoporosis are about twice as common in women as in men. Men are larger and heavier than women and therefore have a greater peak bone mass. Women lose more bone than men due to postmenopausal bone loss.
Age	Bone loss is a normal part of aging, and risk increases with age.
Race	African Americans have denser bones than do Caucasians and Southeast Asians, so their risk of osteoporosis is lower.[21]
Family history	Having a family member with osteoporosis increases risk.
Body size	Individuals who are thin and light have an increased risk because they have less bone mass.
Smoking	Tobacco use weakens bones.
Exercise	Weight-bearing exercise, such as walking and jogging, throughout life strengthens bone, and increasing weight-bearing exercise at any age can increase your bone density.
Alcohol abuse	Long-term alcohol abuse reduces bone formation and interferes with the body's ability to absorb calcium.
Diet	A diet that is lacking in calcium and vitamin D plays a major role in the development of osteoporosis. Low calcium intake during the years of bone formation results in a lower peak bone mass, and low calcium intake in adulthood can accelerate bone loss.

WHAT A SCIENTIST SEES

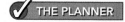 THE PLANNER

Soda versus Milk

Carbonated beverages have become a part of U.S. culture. The average woman in her 20s drinks two 12-ounce sodas a day; teenage boys drink about two and a half.[24] When you grab a can of soda from a vending machine, convenience store, fast-food restaurant, or grocery store, you see a cold, delicious beverage. What a scientist sees is the beverage's nutritional impact. A 12-ounce can of soda contains about 10 teaspoons of sugar and few other nutrients. Replacing a glass of milk with a soda increases the amount of added sugar in the diet by about 40 grams and reduces protein, calcium, vitamin A, vitamin D, and riboflavin intake.

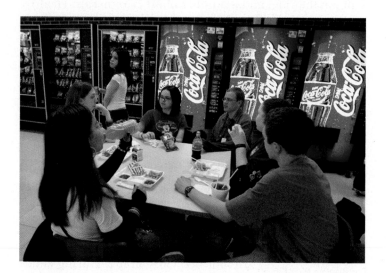

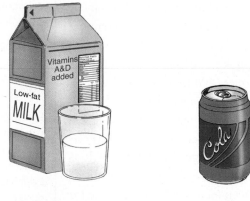

	Low–fat milk	Cola soft drink
Serving size (oz)	12	12
Energy (Cal)	153	150
Protein (g)	12	0
Calcium (mg)	450	0
Phosphorus (mg)	588	45
Riboflavin (mg)	0.6	0
Vitamin A (µg)	216	0
Vitamin D (µg)	3.8	0
Caffeine (mg)	0	40

Teenage boys and girls today drink twice as much soda as milk, whereas 20 years ago, boys drank more than twice as much milk as soda, and girls drank 50% more milk than soda.[24] Milk is the major source of calcium in the U.S. diet. The reduction in calcium intake that occurs when milk is replaced by soda is of great concern. Teenage girls consume only 60% of the recommended amount of calcium, with soda drinkers consuming almost one-fifth less calcium than those who don't drink soda.[24] Osteoporosis is a major problem among older adults today, and when these adults were children, they drank twice as much milk as kids do today.

Think Critically How do you think the current trend away from milk consumption will affect the incidence of osteoporosis 30 years from now?

calcium absorbed in the intestines. A low calcium intake is the most significant dietary factor contributing to osteoporosis (see *What a Scientist Sees*). The effect of diet on bone mass is discussed in more depth later in the chapter.

A factor that is associated with a reduced risk of osteoporosis is excess body weight.[23] Having greater body weight, whether that weight is due to an increase in muscle mass or to excess body fat, increases bone mass because it increases the amount of weight the bones must support. In other words, stressing the bones makes them grow stronger. A similar effect is seen in people of all body weights who engage in weight-bearing exercise. In postmenopausal women, excess body fat may also reduce risk because adipose tissue is an important source of estrogen, which helps maintain bone mass and enhances calcium absorption.

Preventing and treating osteoporosis You can't feel your bones weakening, so people with osteoporosis may not know that their bone mass is dangerously low until they are in their 50s or 60s and experience a bone fracture. Once osteoporosis has developed, it is difficult to restore lost bone. Therefore, the best treatment for osteoporosis is to prevent it by achieving a high peak bone mass and slowing the rate of bone loss. During childhood, adolescence, and young adulthood, diet and exercise can help prevent osteoporosis by ensuring maximum peak bone density. A diet that contains adequate amounts of calcium and vitamin D produces greater peak bone mass during the early years and slows bone loss as adults age. Adequate intakes of zinc, magnesium, potassium, fiber, vitamin K, and vitamin C—nutrients that are plentiful in fruits and vegetables—are also important for bone health. Weight-bearing exercise before about age 35 helps to increases peak bone mass, and maintaining an active lifestyle that includes weight-bearing exercise throughout life helps maintain bone density. Limiting smoking and alcohol consumption can also help to increase and maintain bone density.

Some dietary factors can have a negative impact on calcium status and may affect the risk of osteoporosis. High intakes of phytates, oxalates, and tannins can reduce calcium absorption. High intakes of dietary sodium and protein have been found to increase calcium loss in the urine. However, when intakes of calcium and vitamin D are adequate, neither high protein nor high sodium are believed to adversely affect bone health and the risk of osteoporosis.[25-27]

Osteoporosis is commonly treated with estrogen to reduce bone breakdown and increase calcium absorption, along with supplements of calcium and vitamin D and regular weight-bearing exercise. Treatments also include other hormones and drugs, called bisphosphonates, that inhibit the activity of cells that break down bone. Bisphosphonates have been shown to prevent postmenopausal bone loss, increase bone mineral density, and reduce the risk of fractures.[28]

Calcium

In an average person, about 1.5% of body weight is due to calcium, and 99% of this is found in the bones and teeth. The remaining calcium is located in body cells and fluids, where it is needed for muscle contraction, release of neurotransmitters, blood pressure regulation, cell communication, blood clotting, and other essential functions. Neurotransmitter release is critical to nerve function because neurotransmitters relay nerve impulses from one nerve to another and from nerves to other cells. Calcium in muscle cells is essential for muscle contraction because it allows the muscle proteins actin and myosin to interact. Calcium may help regulate blood pressure by controlling the contraction of muscles in the blood vessel walls and signaling the secretion of substances that regulate blood pressure.

Calcium in health and disease The various roles of calcium are so vital to survival that powerful regulatory mechanisms maintain calcium concentrations both inside and outside cells. Slight changes in blood calcium levels trigger the release of hormones that work to keep calcium levels constant. When calcium levels drop, parathyroid hormone (PTH) is released (see Chapter 7). PTH acts in a number of tissues to increase blood calcium levels (**Figure 8.18**). If blood calcium levels become too

Raising blood calcium levels • Figure 8.18

Low blood calcium triggers the secretion of PTH from the parathyroid gland. PTH stimulates the release of calcium from bone and causes the kidneys to reduce calcium loss in the urine and to activate vitamin D. Activated vitamin D increases the absorption of calcium from the gastrointestinal tract and acts with PTH to stimulate calcium release from the bone. The overall effect of PTH is to rapidly restore blood calcium levels to normal.

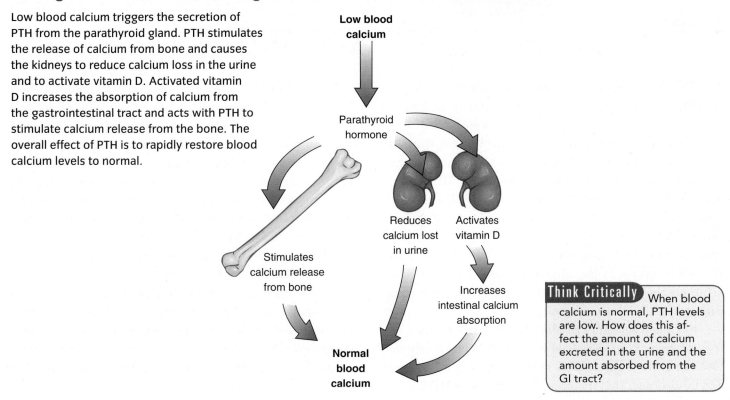

Low blood calcium

Parathyroid hormone

Stimulates calcium release from bone

Reduces calcium lost in urine

Activates vitamin D

Increases intestinal calcium absorption

Normal blood calcium

Think Critically When blood calcium is normal, PTH levels are low. How does this affect the amount of calcium excreted in the urine and the amount absorbed from the GI tract?

Food sources of calcium • Figure 8.19

Dairy products are an important source of calcium. Fish, such as sardines, that are consumed with the bones are also a good source, as are legumes, almonds, and some dark green vegetables, such as kale and broccoli. Grains are a moderate source, but because we consume them in large quantities, they make a significant contribution to our calcium intake.

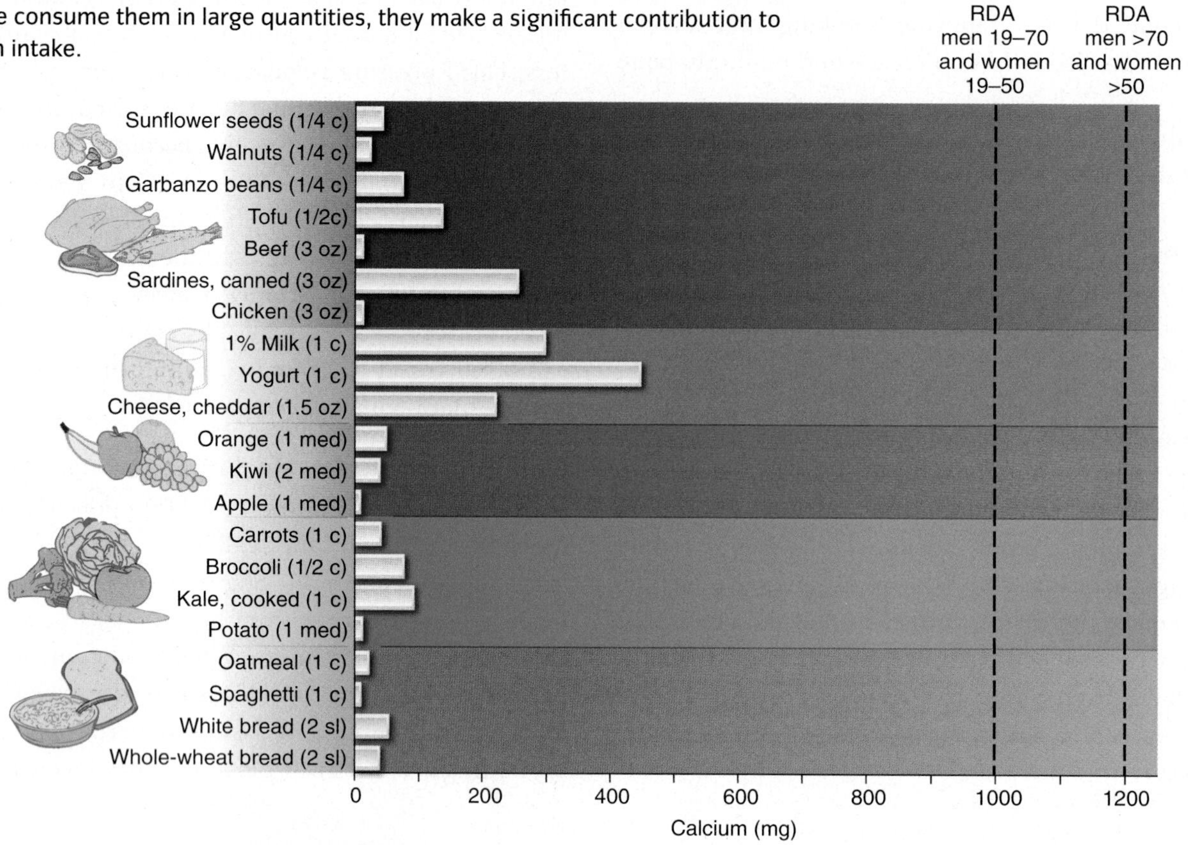

| | RDA men 19–70 and women 19–50 | RDA men >70 and women >50 |

Sunflower seeds (1/4 c)
Walnuts (1/4 c)
Garbanzo beans (1/4 c)
Tofu (1/2c)
Beef (3 oz)
Sardines, canned (3 oz)
Chicken (3 oz)
1% Milk (1 c)
Yogurt (1 c)
Cheese, cheddar (1.5 oz)
Orange (1 med)
Kiwi (2 med)
Apple (1 med)
Carrots (1 c)
Broccoli (1/2 c)
Kale, cooked (1 c)
Potato (1 med)
Oatmeal (1 c)
Spaghetti (1 c)
White bread (2 sl)
Whole-wheat bread (2 sl)

0   200   400   600   800   1000   1200
Calcium (mg)

Ask Yourself

If bioavailability were the same, how much cooked kale would you need to eat to get as much calcium as you do from a cup of milk?

high, PTH secretion stops, and **calcitonin** is released. Calcitonin is a hormone that acts primarily on bone to inhibit the release of calcium into the blood.

When too little calcium is consumed, the body maintains normal blood levels by breaking down bone to release calcium, a process called **bone resorption**. This process provides a steady supply of calcium and causes no short-term symptoms. Over time, however, a calcium deficiency can reduce bone mass. Low calcium intake during the years of bone formation results in lower peak bone mass. If calcium intake is low after peak bone mass has been achieved, the rate of bone loss may be increased and, along with it, the risk of osteoporosis.

Too much calcium can also affect health. Because the level of calcium in the blood is finely regulated, elevated blood calcium is rare and is most often caused by cancer and by disorders that increase the secretion of PTH. It can also result from increases in intestinal calcium absorption due to excessive vitamin D intake or high intakes of calcium. Consuming too much calcium from foods is unlikely, but high intakes of calcium from supplements can interfere with the availability of iron, zinc, magnesium, and phosphorus; cause constipation; and contribute to elevated blood and urinary calcium levels. Elevated blood calcium levels can cause symptoms such as loss of appetite, abnormal heartbeat, weight loss, fatigue, frequent urination, and soft tissue calcification. High urinary calcium can damage the kidneys and increase the risk of kidney stones.[29]

The UL for calcium in young adults ages 19 to 50 is 2500 mg/day. In older adults the UL is lower, only 2000 mg/day, based on the occurrence of kidney stones in older age groups.[29] Some postmenopausal women taking supplements may be getting too much calcium and increasing their risk of kidney stones.

Meeting calcium needs For adults ages 19 to 50, 1000 mg/day of calcium is recommended to maintain bone health. Since bone loss is accelerated in women due to menopause, the RDA for women 51 to 70 is set at 1200 mg/day to slow bone loss. For men in this age group it remains at 1000 mg/day. Bone loss and resulting osteoporotic fractures is a concern for both men and women 70 and older, so the RDA for both genders in this age group is 1200 mg/day.[29]

The main source of calcium in the North American diet is dairy products (**Figure 8.19**). Those who do not consume dairy products can meet their calcium needs by consuming dark green vegetables, fish consumed with bones, foods processed with calcium, and foods fortified with calcium, such as juices and breakfast cereals.

Individuals who do not meet their calcium needs through their diet alone can benefit from calcium supplements (**Figure 8.20**). In young individuals, supplemental calcium can increase peak bone mass. In postmenopausal women, calcium supplements are not effective at increasing bone mass, but they can help reduce the rate of bone loss.[30]

Whether your calcium comes from foods or from supplements, bioavailability must be considered. Vitamin D is the nutrient that has the most significant impact on calcium absorption. When calcium intake is high, calcium is absorbed by diffusion, but when intake is low to moderate, as it typically is, absorption depends on the active form of vitamin D. When vitamin D is deficient, less than 10% of dietary calcium may be absorbed, compared to the typical 25% when it is present. Other dietary components that affect calcium absorption include acidic foods, lactose, and fat, which increase calcium absorption, and oxalates, phytates, tannins, and fiber, which inhibit calcium absorption. For example, spinach is a high-calcium vegetable, but only about 5% of its calcium is absorbed; the rest is bound by oxalates and excreted in the feces.[31] Vegetables such as kale, collard greens, turnip greens, mustard greens, and Chinese cabbage are low in oxalates, so their calcium is more readily absorbed. Chocolate also contains oxalates, but chocolate milk is still a good source of calcium because the amount of oxalates from the chocolate added to a glass of milk is small.

Calcium supplements • Figure 8.20

If you are not getting enough calcium from foods, a supplement that contains a calcium compound alone or calcium with vitamin D can help you meet your calcium needs. A multivitamin/multimineral supplement will provide only a small amount of the calcium you need. Use the Supplement Facts label to choose an appropriate supplement.

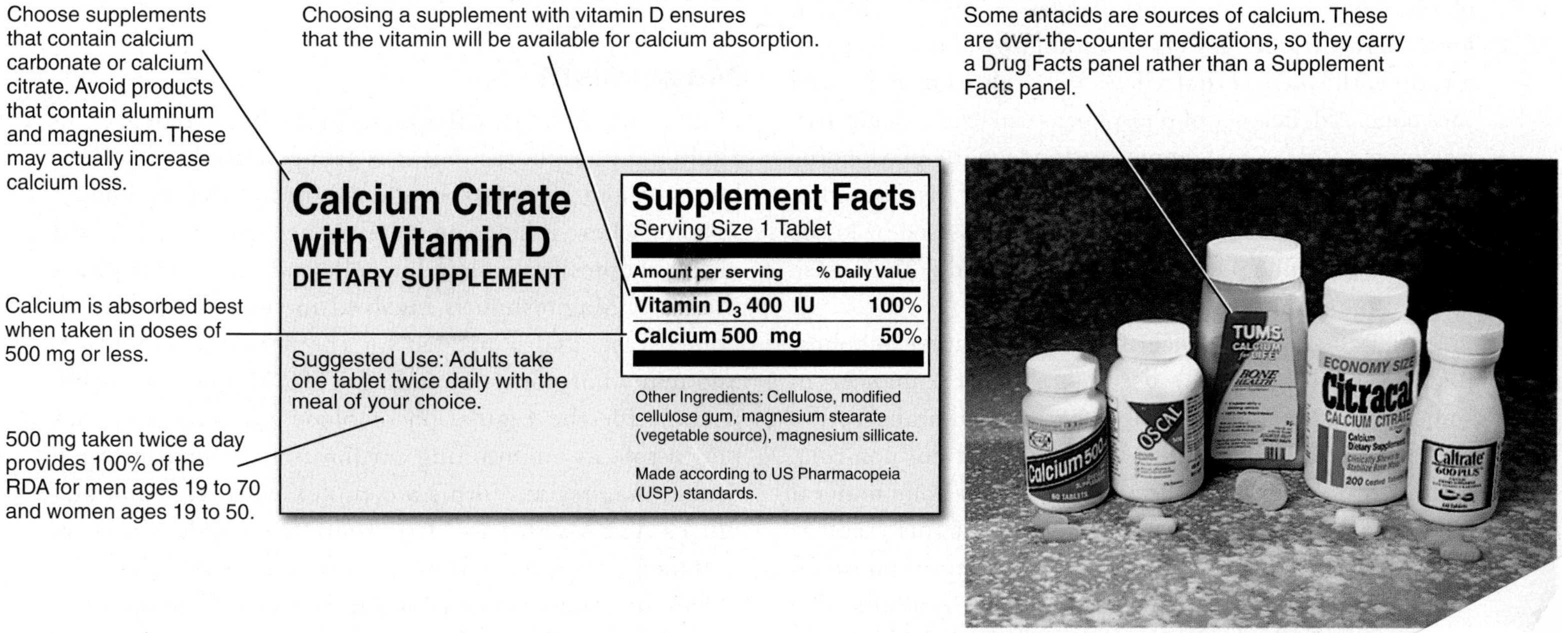

Choose supplements that contain calcium carbonate or calcium citrate. Avoid products that contain aluminum and magnesium. These may actually increase calcium loss.

Choosing a supplement with vitamin D ensures that the vitamin will be available for calcium absorption.

Some antacids are sources of calcium. These are over-the-counter medications, so they carry a Drug Facts panel rather than a Supplement Facts panel.

Calcium is absorbed best when taken in doses of 500 mg or less.

500 mg taken twice a day provides 100% of the RDA for men ages 19 to 70 and women ages 19 to 50.

Calcium Citrate with Vitamin D
DIETARY SUPPLEMENT

Suggested Use: Adults take one tablet twice daily with the meal of your choice.

Supplement Facts
Serving Size 1 Tablet

Amount per serving	% Daily Value
Vitamin D$_3$ 400 IU	100%
Calcium 500 mg	50%

Other Ingredients: Cellulose, modified cellulose gum, magnesium stearate (vegetable source), magnesium sillicate.

Made according to US Pharmacopeia (USP) standards.

Major Minerals and Bone Hea

Nonskeletal functions of phosphorus • Figure 8.21

Most of the phosphorus in the body helps form the structure of bones and teeth. Phosphorus also plays an important role in a host of cellular activities.

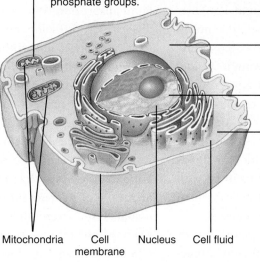

Phosphorus is important in energy metabolism because the high-energy bonds of ATP are formed between phosphate groups.

Phosphorus is a component of phospholipids, which form the structure of cell membranes.

Phosphorus is involved in regulating enzyme activity; the addition of a phosphorus-containing group to certain enzymes can activate or inactivate them.

Phosphorus is a major constituent of DNA and RNA, which orchestrate the synthesis of proteins.

Phosphorus is part of a compound that can prevent changes in acidity so that chemical reactions inside the cell can proceed normally.

Mitochondria   Cell membrane   Nucleus   Cell fluid

Phosphorus

Most of the phosphorus in your body is associated with calcium as part of the hard mineral crystals in bones and teeth. The smaller amount of phosphorus in soft tissues performs an essential role as a structural component of phospholipids, DNA and RNA, and ATP. It is also important in regulating the activity of enzymes and maintaining the proper level of acidity in cells (**Figure 8.21**).

Phosphorus in health and disease Blood levels of phosphorus are not controlled as strictly as calcium levels, but the kidneys help maintain phosphorus levels in a ratio with calcium that allows minerals to be deposited into bone. A deficiency of phosphorus can lead to bone loss, weakness, and loss of appetite. Inadequate phosphorus intake is rare because phosphorus is widely distributed in food. Marginal phosphorus status may be caused by losses due to chronic diarrhea or poor absorption due to overuse of aluminum-containing antacids.

There has been concern that high intake of phosphoric acid (phosphate) used as a flavor enhancer in some soft drinks may interfere with calcium absorption and contribute to bone loss. Cola-type, but not non-cola, soft drinks have been associated with lower bone mineral density, but there is no good evidence that this result is due to phosphate consumption.[32] High dietary phosphorus does not appear to be harmful for healthy adults. The UL for phosphorus is 4000 mg/day for adults, based on an amount associated with the upper limits of normal blood phosphorus levels.[33]

Meeting phosphorus needs The RDA for phosphorus is 700 mg/day for adults; most diets provide this amount.[33] Dairy products such as milk, yogurt, and cheese, as well as meat, cereals, bran, eggs, nuts, and fish, are good sources of phosphorus. Food additives used in baked goods, cheese, processed meats, and soft drinks also provide phosphorus.

Magnesium

Magnesium is far less abundant in the body than are calcium and phosphorus, but it is still essential for healthy bones. About 50 to 60% of the magnesium in the body is in bone, where it helps maintain bone structure. The rest of the magnesium is found in cells and fluids throughout the body. Magnesium is involved in regulating calcium homeostasis and is needed for the action of vitamin D and many hormones, including PTH. Magnesium is important for the regulation of blood pressure and may play a role in maintaining cardiovascular health. In addition, magnesium forms a complex with ATP that stabilizes ATP's structure. It is therefore needed in every metabolic reaction that generates or uses ATP. This includes reactions needed for the release of energy from carbohydrate, fat, and protein; the functioning of the nerves and muscles; and the synthesis of DNA, RNA, and protein, making it particularly important for dividing, growing cells.

Magnesium in health and disease

Although overt magnesium deficiency is rare, the typical intake of magnesium in the United States is below the RDA. Low intakes of magnesium have been associated with a number of chronic diseases, including osteoporosis.[34] Magnesium deficiency can cause nausea, muscle weakness and cramping, irritability, mental derangement, and changes in blood pressure and heartbeat. As discussed earlier, dietary patterns that are high in magnesium are associated with lower blood pressure, and the risk of other types of cardiovascular disease is lower for people with adequate magnesium intake than for those with less magnesium in their diet.[35] Low blood magnesium levels affect levels of blood calcium and potassium; therefore, some of the symptoms of magnesium deficiency may be due to alterations in the levels of these other minerals.

No adverse effects have been observed from magnesium consumed in foods, but toxicity may occur from drugs containing magnesium, such as milk of magnesia and supplements that include magnesium. Magnesium toxicity causes nausea, vomiting, low blood pressure, and other cardiovascular changes. The UL for adults and adolescents over age 9 is 350 mg of magnesium from nonfood sources such as supplements and medications.[33]

Meeting magnesium needs

Magnesium is found in many foods but in small amounts, so you can't get all you need from a single food (**Figure 8.22**). Enriched grain products are poor sources because magnesium is lost in processing, and it is not added back by enrichment. For example, removing the bran and germ from wheat kernels reduces the magnesium content of 1 cup of white flour to only 28 mg, compared with the 166 mg in 1 cup of whole-wheat flour. Magnesium absorption is enhanced by the active form of vitamin D and decreased by the presence of phytates and calcium.

Sources of magnesium • Figure 8.22

Magnesium is a component of the green pigment chlorophyll, so leafy greens such as spinach and kale are good sources of this mineral. Nuts, seeds, legumes, bananas, and the germ and bran of whole grains are also good sources of magnesium. The dashed lines represent the RDAs of 420 and 320 mg/day for adult men and women over age 30, respectively.[33]

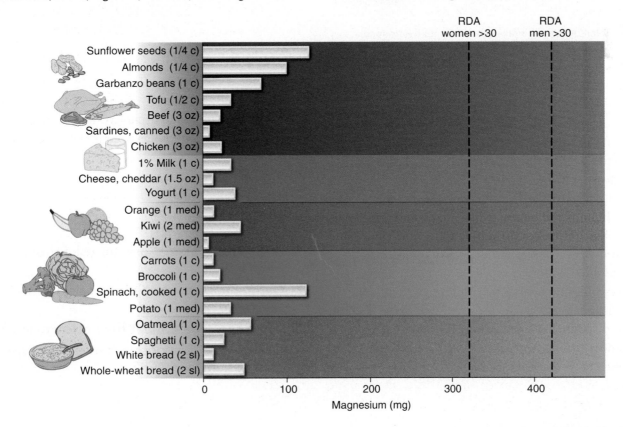

A summary of calcium, phosphorus, magnesium, and sulfur Table 8.3

Mineral	Sources	Recommended intake for adults	Major functions	Deficiency diseases and symptoms	Groups at risk of deficiency	Toxicity	UL
Calcium	Dairy products, fish consumed with bones, leafy green vegetables, fortified foods	1000–1200 mg/day	Bone and tooth structure, nerve transmission, muscle contraction, blood clotting, blood pressure regulation, hormone secretion	Increased risk of osteoporosis	Postmenopausal women; elderly people; those who consume a vegan diet, are lactose intolerant, or have kidney disease	Elevated blood calcium, kidney stones, and other problems in susceptible individuals	2000–2500 mg/day from food and supplements
Phosphorus	Meat, dairy, cereals, baked goods	700 mg/day	Structure of bones and teeth, membranes, ATP, and DNA; acid–base balance	Bone loss, weakness, lack of appetite	Premature infants, alcoholics, elderly people	None likely	4000 mg/day
Magnesium	Greens, whole grains, legumes, nuts, seeds	310–420 mg/day	Bone structure, ATP stabilization, enzyme activity, nerve and muscle function	Nausea, vomiting, weakness, muscle pain, heart changes	Alcoholics, individuals with kidney and gastrointestinal disease	Nausea, vomiting, low blood pressure	350 mg/day from nonfood sources
Sulfur	Protein foods, preservatives	None specified	Part of some amino acids and vitamins, acid–base balance	None when protein needs are met	None	None likely	ND

Note: UL, Tolerable Upper Intake Level; ND, not determined.

Sulfur

Sulfur is part of the proteins in the body because the amino acids methionine and cysteine, needed for protein synthesis, contain sulfur. Cysteine is also part of glutathione, a molecule that plays an important role in detoxifying drugs and protecting cells from oxidative damage. The vitamins thiamin and biotin, which are essential for energy metabolism, also contain sulfur, and sulfur-containing ions are important in regulating acidity in the body.

We consume sulfur as a part of dietary proteins and the sulfur-containing vitamins. Sulfur is also found in some food preservatives, such as sulfur dioxide, sodium sulfite, and sodium and potassium bisulfite. There is no recommended intake for sulfur, and no deficiencies are known when protein needs are met.

Table 8.3 provides a summary of the sources and functions of calcium, phosphorus, magnesium, and sulfur and *What Should I Eat?* helps you meet your needs for these minerals.

CONCEPT CHECK STOP

1. **Why** are women at greater risk for osteoporosis than men?

2. **What** happens when blood calcium levels decrease?

3. **How** can vegans meet their calcium needs?

4. **What** is the relationship between phosphorus, magnesium, and ATP?

WHAT SHOULD I EAT?
Calcium, Phosphorus, and Magnesium

✓ THE PLANNER

Get calcium into your body and your bones
- Have three servings of dairy a day: milk, yogurt, cheese.
- Bone up on calcium by eating sardines or canned salmon, which are eaten with the bones.
- Choose leafy greens—they are a source of calcium.
- Walk, jog, or jump up and down; weight-bearing exercises build up bone.

Don't fret about phosphorus—it's in almost everything you eat.

Maximize your magnesium
- Choose whole grains.
- Sprinkle nuts and seeds on your salad, cereal, and stir-fry.
- Go for the green: Whenever you eat green, you are eating magnesium; most greens contain calcium, too.

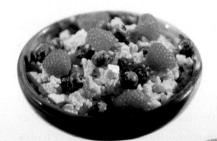

Use iProfile to find a nondairy source of calcium.

Trace Minerals

LEARNING OBJECTIVES

1. **Relate** the primary function of iron to the effects of iron deficiency.
2. **Compare** the antioxidant functions of selenium and vitamin E.
3. **Explain** why iodine deficiency causes the thyroid gland to enlarge.
4. **Describe** the functions of copper, zinc, chromium, and fluoride.

Just as a pinch of this or a dash of that can enhance the flavor of a special dish, the presence of minute quantities of certain minerals can boost the nutritional impact of a person's diet. The trace minerals, so called because they are needed in extremely small amounts, are essential to health. For some trace minerals, the amount in food is affected by where the food is grown and/or how it is handled. When modern transportation systems make available foods produced in many locations, these variations balance each other and are unlikely to affect an individual's mineral status. In countries where the diet consists predominantly of locally grown foods, trace mineral deficiencies and excesses are more likely to occur.

Iron

In the 1800s, iron tablets were used to treat young women whose blood lacked "coloring matter." Today we know that the "coloring matter" is the iron-containing protein **hemoglobin**. The hemoglobin in red blood cells transports oxygen to body cells and carries carbon dioxide away from them for elimination by the lungs. Most of the iron in the body is part of hemoglobin, but iron is also needed for the production of other iron-containing proteins. It is part of **myoglobin**, a protein found in muscle that enhances the amount of oxygen available for use in muscle contraction. Iron is essential for ATP production because it is a part of several proteins needed in aerobic metabolism. Iron-containing proteins are also involved in drug metabolism and immune function.

Iron absorption and transport The amount of iron absorbed from the intestine depends on the form of the iron and on the dietary components consumed along with it. Much of the iron in meats is **heme iron**—iron that is part of a chemical complex found in proteins such as hemoglobin and myoglobin. Heme iron is absorbed

heme iron A readily absorbable form of iron found in meat, fish, and poultry that is chemically associated with certain proteins.

more than twice as efficiently as the nonheme iron found in plant sources such as leafy green vegetables, legumes, and grains. The amount of nonheme iron absorbed can be enhanced or reduced by the foods and nutrients consumed in the same meal.

Once iron is absorbed, the amount that is delivered to the cells of the body depends to some extent on the body's needs. When the body's iron status is high, less iron is delivered to body cells and more is trapped in the mucosal cells of the small intestine and lost when the cells die and are sloughed into the intestinal lumen. When iron status is low, more iron is transported out of the mucosal cells for use by the body (**Figure 8.23**). This regulation is important because once iron has entered the blood and other tissues, it is not easily eliminated. Even when red blood cells die, the iron in their hemoglobin is not lost from the body; instead, it is recycled and can be incorporated into new red blood cells. Even in healthy individuals, most iron loss occurs through blood loss, including blood lost during menstruation and the small amounts lost from the gastrointestinal tract. Some iron is also lost through the shedding of cells from the intestines, skin, and urinary tract.

Meeting iron needs Iron in the diet comes from both plant and animal sources (**Figure 8.24**). Animal products provide both heme and nonheme iron, but only the less readily absorbed nonheme iron is found in plants. Nonheme iron absorption can be enhanced as much as

Iron absorption, uses, and loss • Figure 8.23

The amount of iron available to the body depends on both the amount absorbed into the mucosal cells of the small intestine and the amount transported to the rest of the body. The iron that is transported may be used to synthesize iron-containing proteins, such as hemoglobin needed for red blood cell formation, or increase iron stores in the liver or spleen.

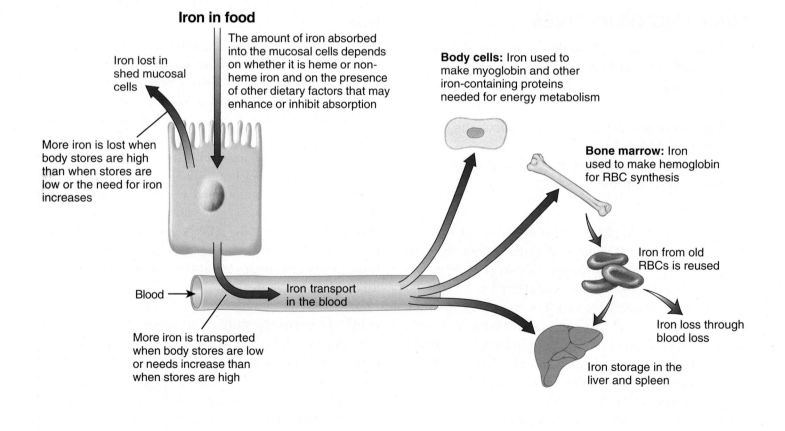

Iron in food

The amount of iron absorbed into the mucosal cells depends on whether it is heme or non-heme iron and on the presence of other dietary factors that may enhance or inhibit absorption

Iron lost in shed mucosal cells

More iron is lost when body stores are high than when stores are low or the need for iron increases

Blood

Iron transport in the blood

More iron is transported when body stores are low or needs increase than when stores are high

Body cells: Iron used to make myoglobin and other iron-containing proteins needed for energy metabolism

Bone marrow: Iron used to make hemoglobin for RBC synthesis

Iron from old RBCs is reused

Iron loss through blood loss

Iron storage in the liver and spleen

Sources of iron • Figure 8.24

The best sources of highly absorbable heme iron are red meats and organ meats such as liver and kidney. Legumes, leafy greens, and whole grains are good sources of nonheme iron; enriched grains are also good sources of nonheme iron because it is added during enrichment. The RDA for adult men and postmenopausal women is 8 mg/day of iron. Due to menstrual losses, the RDA for women of childbearing age is set much higher, 15 mg/day for young women 14 to 18 years and 18 mg/day for women 19 to 50.

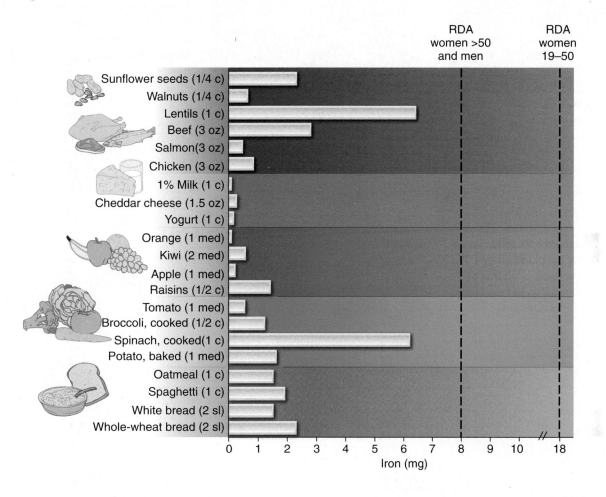

sixfold if it is consumed along with foods that are rich in vitamin C. Consuming beef, fish, or poultry in the same meal as nonheme iron also increases absorption. For example, a small amount of hamburger in a pot of chili will enhance the body's absorption of iron from the beans. If the pot is made of iron, it increases iron intake because the iron leaches into food. Iron absorption is decreased by fiber, phytates, tannins, and oxalates, which bind iron in the gastrointestinal tract. The presence of other minerals with the same charge, such as calcium, may also decrease iron absorption.

The RDA for iron assumes that the diet contains both plant and animal sources of iron.[36] A separate RDA category has been created for vegetarians. These recommendations are higher, to take into account lower iron absorption from plant sources. People who have difficulty consuming enough iron can increase their iron intake by choosing foods fortified with iron.

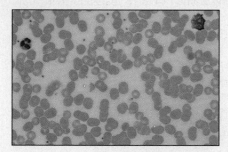

Normal red blood cells

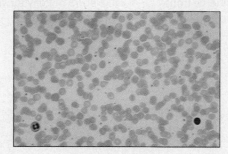

Iron deficiency anemia

Iron deficiency anemia occurs when there is too little iron to synthesize adequate amounts of hemoglobin. It results in red blood cells that are small and pale and unable to transport as much oxygen as red blood cells containing normal amounts of hemoglobin.

Iron deficiency anemia is the final stage of iron deficiency. Inadequate iron intake first causes a decrease in the amount of stored iron, followed by low iron levels in the blood plasma. It is only after plasma levels drop that there is no longer enough iron to maintain hemoglobin in red blood cells.

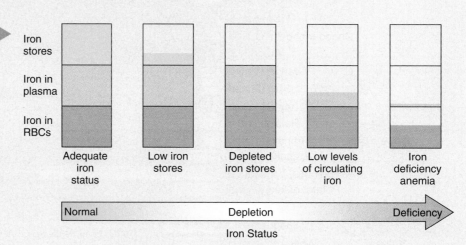

Iron stores
Iron in plasma
Iron in RBCs

Adequate iron status | Low iron stores | Depleted iron stores | Low levels of circulating iron | Iron deficiency anemia

Normal — Depletion — Deficiency

Iron Status

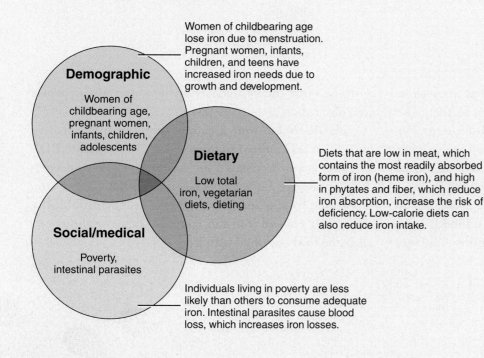

Women of childbearing age lose iron due to menstruation. Pregnant women, infants, children, and teens have increased iron needs due to growth and development.

Demographic

Women of childbearing age, pregnant women, infants, children, adolescents

Dietary

Low total iron, vegetarian diets, dieting

Social/medical

Poverty, intestinal parasites

Diets that are low in meat, which contains the most readily absorbed form of iron (heme iron), and high in phytates and fiber, which reduce iron absorption, increase the risk of deficiency. Low-calorie diets can also reduce iron intake.

Individuals living in poverty are less likely than others to consume adequate iron. Intestinal parasites cause blood loss, which increases iron losses.

The risk of iron deficiency is highest among individuals with greater iron losses, those with greater needs due to growth and development, and those who are unable to obtain adequate dietary iron. In the United States, it affects 3% of adolescent girls and women of childbearing age and 2% of children between the ages of 1 and 2 years.[39] The incidence is greatest among low-income and minority women and children.

Iron in health and disease When there is too little iron in the body, hemoglobin cannot be produced. When sufficient hemoglobin is not available, the red blood cells that are formed are small and pale, and they are unable to deliver adequate oxygen to the tissues. This condition is known as **iron deficiency anemia** (**Figure 8.25**). Symptoms of iron deficiency anemia include fatigue, weakness, headache, decreased work capacity, inability to maintain body temperature in a cold environment, changes in behavior, decreased resistance to infection, impaired development in infants, and increased risk of lead poisoning in young children. Anemia is the last stage of iron deficiency. Earlier stages have no symptoms because they do not affect the amount of iron in red blood cells, but levels of iron in the blood plasma and in body stores are low (see *Thinking It Through*). Iron deficiency anemia is the most common nutritional deficiency; more than 2 billion people, or over 30% of the world's population, suffer from anemia, many due to iron deficiency.[37,38]

> **iron deficiency anemia** An iron deficiency disease that occurs when the oxygen-carrying capacity of the blood is decreased because there is insufficient iron to make hemoglobin.

THINKING IT THROUGH
A Case Study on Iron Deficiency

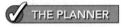

Hanna is a 23-year-old graduate student from South Carolina. She has been working long hours and is always tired. She tries to eat a healthy diet; she has been a lacto-ovo vegetarian for the past six months.

What factors increase Hanna's risk for iron deficiency anemia?
▼

Your answer:

Hanna goes to the health center to see if there is a medical reason for her exhaustion. A nurse draws her blood to check her for anemia. The results of Hanna's blood work are summarized in the figure below.

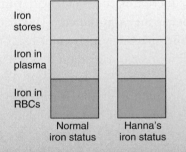

What does the blood test reveal about Hanna's iron status? Is she tired due to iron deficiency anemia? Why or why not?
▼

Your answer:

Hanna meets with a dietitian. A diet analysis reveals that because she consumes no meat, most of her protein comes from dairy products. She consumes about eight servings of whole grains, three fresh fruits, and about a cup of cooked vegetables daily. She drinks four glasses of iced tea daily. Her average iron intake is about 12 mg/day.

Name three dietary factors that put Hanna at risk for iron deficiency.
▼

Your answer:

How could Hanna increase her iron intake?
▼

Your answer:

What could Hanna do to increase the absorption of the nonheme iron in her diet?
▼

Your answer:

(Check your answers in Appendix J.)

Trace Minerals 291

To protect children, the labels of iron-containing drugs and supplements are required to display this warning. Iron-containing products should be stored out of the reach of children or other individuals who might consume them in excess.[40]

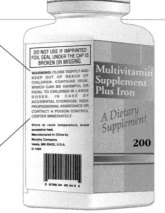

WARNING: CLOSE TIGHTLY AND KEEP OUT OF REACH OF CHILDREN. CONTAINS IRON, WHICH CAN BE HARMFUL OR FATAL TO CHILDREN IN LARGE DOSES. IN CASE OF ACCIDENTAL OVERDOSE, SEEK PROFESSIONAL ASSISTANCE OR CONTACT A POISON CONTROL CENTER IMMEDIATELY.

Iron also causes health problems if too much is consumed. Acute iron toxicity caused by excessive consumption of iron-containing supplements is one of the most common forms of poisoning among children under age 6. Iron poisoning may cause damage to the lining of the intestine, abnormalities in body acidity, shock, and liver failure. Even a single large dose can be fatal (**Figure 8.26**). A UL has been set at 45 mg/day from all sources.[36]

Accumulation of iron in the body over time, referred to as **iron overload**, is most commonly due to an inherited condition called **hemochromatosis**, which permits increased iron absorption.[41] More than 1 million people in the United States have the gene mutation that can lead to hemochromatosis. The gene mutation is most common in people of European descent.[42] It has no symptoms early in life, but in middle age, nonspecific symptoms such as weight loss, fatigue, weakness, and abdominal pain develop. If allowed to progress, the accumulation of excess iron can damage the heart and liver and increase the individual's risks for diabetes and cancer. The treatment for hemochromatosis is simple: regular blood withdrawal. Iron loss through blood withdrawal will prevent the complications of iron overload, but to be effective, the treatment must be initiated before organs have been damaged. Therefore, genetic screening is essential to identify and treat individuals before any damage occurs.

hemochromatosis An inherited disorder that results in increased iron absorption.

Copper

It is logical that consuming too little iron will cause iron deficiency anemia, but consuming too little copper can also cause this problem. Iron status and copper status are interrelated because a copper-containing protein is needed for iron to be transported from the intestinal cells. Even if iron intake is adequate, iron can't get to tissues if copper is not present. Thus copper deficiency results in iron deficiency that may lead to anemia. Copper also functions as a component of a number of important proteins and enzymes that are involved in connective tissue synthesis, lipid metabolism, maintenance of heart muscle, and function of the immune and central nervous systems.[36]

We consume copper in seafood, nuts and seeds, whole-grain breads and cereals, and chocolate; the richest dietary sources of copper are organ meats such as liver and kidney. As with many other trace minerals, soil content affects the amount of copper in plant foods. The RDA for copper for adults is 900 micrograms (μg)/day.[36]

When there is too little copper in the body, the protein collagen does not form normally, resulting in skeletal changes similar to those seen in vitamin C deficiency. Copper deficiency also causes elevated blood cholesterol, reflecting copper's role in cholesterol metabolism. Copper deficiency has been associated with impaired growth, degeneration of the heart muscle and the nervous system, and changes in hair color and structure. Because copper is needed to maintain the immune system, a diet that is low in copper increases the incidence of infections. Also, because copper is an essential component of one form of the antioxidant enzyme superoxide dismutase, a copper deficiency will weaken antioxidant defenses.

Severe copper deficiency is relatively rare, although it may occur in premature infants. It can also occur if zinc intake is high because high dietary zinc interferes with the absorption of copper. Copper toxicity from dietary sources is also rare but has occurred as a result of drinking from contaminated water supplies or consuming acidic foods or beverages that have been stored in copper containers. Toxicity is more likely to occur from supplements containing copper. Excessive copper intake causes abdominal pain, vomiting, and diarrhea. The UL has been set at 10 mg/day of copper.[36]

Zinc and gene expression • Figure 8.27

One of zinc's most important roles is in gene expression. Zinc-containing DNA-binding proteins allow vitamin A, vitamin D, and a number of hormones to interact with DNA. The zinc forms "fingers" in the protein structure. When the vitamins or hormones bind to the protein, the zinc fingers bind to regulatory regions of DNA, increasing or decreasing the expression of specific genes and thus the synthesis of the proteins for which they code. Without zinc, these vitamins and hormones cannot function properly.

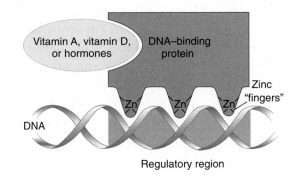

Ask Yourself

How could a zinc deficiency lead to a secondary vitamin A deficiency?

Zinc

Zinc, the most abundant intracellular trace mineral, is involved in the functioning of approximately 100 different enzymes, including a form of superoxide dismutase that is vital for protecting cells from free-radical damage. Zinc is needed to maintain adequate levels of metal-binding proteins, which also scavenge free radicals. Zinc is needed by enzymes that function in the synthesis of DNA and RNA, in carbohydrate metabolism, in acid–base balance, and in a reaction that is necessary for the absorption of folate from food. Zinc plays a role in the storage and release of insulin, the mobilization of vitamin A from the liver, and the stabilization of cell membranes. It influences hormonal regulation of cell division and is therefore needed for the growth and repair of tissues, the activity of the immune system, and the development of sex organs and bone. Some of the functions of zinc can be traced to its role in gene expression (**Figure 8.27**).[43]

Zinc transport from the mucosal cells of the intestine into the blood is regulated. When zinc intake is high, more zinc is held in the mucosal cells and lost in the feces when these cells die. When zinc intake is low, more dietary zinc passes into the blood for delivery to tissues.

Meeting zinc needs We consume zinc in red meat, liver, eggs, dairy products, vegetables, and seafood (**Figure 8.28**). Because many plant foods are high in substances that bind zinc, zinc is absorbed better from animal sources than from plant sources.

Food sources of zinc • Figure 8.28

Meat, seafood, dairy products, legumes, and seeds are good sources of zinc. Refined grains are not because zinc is lost in milling and not added back. Yeast-leavened grain products are better sources of zinc than are unleavened products because yeast leavening reduces phytate content. The dashed lines represent the RDAs for adult men and women, which are 11 and 8 mg/day, respectively.

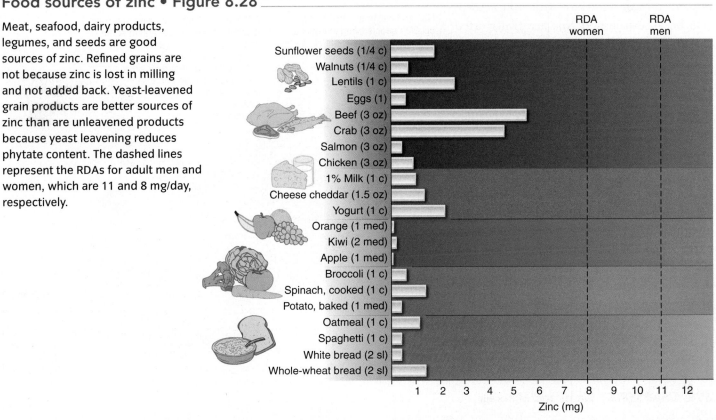

Zinc in health and disease Symptomatic zinc deficiency is relatively uncommon in North America, but in developing countries, it has important health and developmental consequences. Zinc deficiency interferes with growth and development, impairs immune function, and causes skin rashes and diarrhea. Diminished immune function is a concern even when zinc deficiency is mild.[44] Because zinc is needed for the proper functioning of vitamins A and D and the activity of numerous enzymes, deficiency symptoms can resemble those of other essential nutrient deficiencies.

The risk of zinc deficiency is greater in areas where the diet is high in phytate, fiber, tannins, and oxalates, which limit zinc absorption. In the 1960s, a syndrome of growth depression and delayed sexual development was observed in Iranian and Egyptian men consuming a diet based on plant protein. The diet was not low in zinc, but it was high in grains containing phytates, which interfered with zinc absorption, thus causing the deficiency.

It is difficult to consume a toxic amount of zinc from food. However, high doses from supplements can cause toxicity symptoms. A single dose of 1 to 2 g can cause gastrointestinal irritation, vomiting, loss of appetite, diarrhea, abdominal cramps, and headaches. High intakes have been shown to decrease immune function, reduce concentrations of HDL cholesterol in the blood, and interfere with the absorption of copper. High doses of zinc can also interfere with iron absorption because iron and zinc are transported through the blood by the same protein. The converse is also true: Too much iron can limit the transport of zinc. Zinc and iron are often found together in foods, but food sources do not contain large enough amounts of either to cause imbalances.

Zinc supplements are marketed to improve immune function, enhance fertility and sexual performance, and cure the common cold. For individuals consuming adequate zinc, there is no evidence that extra zinc enhances immune function, fertility, or sexual performance. However, in individuals with a mild zinc deficiency, supplementation can have beneficial immune, antioxidant, and anti-inflammatory effects that can help in the treatment of a variety of diseases, including diarrhea, pneumonia,

and tuberculosis. In older adults improving zinc status with supplements can decrease the incidence of infections and prevent a type of age-associated blindness; in children, it can reduce the incidence of respiratory infections and improve growth.[45,46] Zinc supplements are most often taken to cure colds. When administered within 24 hours of the onset of cold symptoms, zinc supplements have been found to reduce the duration and severity of the common cold in healthy people; the mechanism by which they work is unclear.[47] A UL has been set at 40 mg/day from all sources.[36]

Selenium

The amount of selenium in food varies greatly, depending on the concentration of selenium in the soil where the food is produced. In regions of China with low soil selenium levels, a form of heart disease called **Keshan disease** occurs in children and young women. This disease can be prevented and cured with selenium supplements. In contrast, people living in regions of China with very high selenium in the soil may develop symptoms of selenium toxicity (**Figure 8.29**).

Soil selenium and health • Figure 8.29

The amount of selenium in the soil varies widely from one region of China to another. When the diet consists primarily of locally grown food, these differences affect selenium intake and, therefore, health. When the diet includes foods from many different locations, the low selenium content of foods grown in one geographic region is offset by the high selenium content of foods from other regions.

Hair and nail brittleness and loss occur in people living in regions of China with high levels of selenium in the soil. Other toxicity symptoms include nausea, diarrhea, abdominal pain, nervous system abnormalities, fatigue, and irritability.

Selenium deficiency causes muscular discomfort, weakness, and in some cases Keshan disease. However, Keshan disease is not caused entirely by selenium deficiency. It is believed to be due to a combination of selenium deficiency and a viral infection.[48]

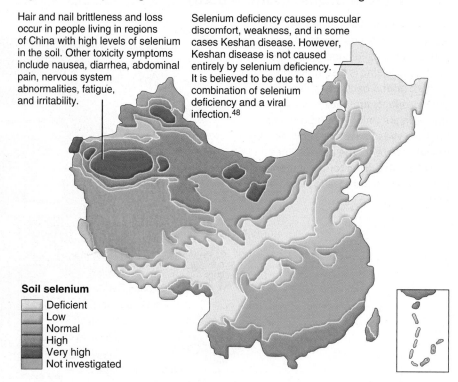

Soil selenium
- Deficient
- Low
- Normal
- High
- Very high
- Not investigated

Selenium is incorporated into the structure of certain proteins. One of these proteins is the antioxidant enzyme **glutathione peroxidase**. Glutathione peroxidase neutralizes peroxides before they can form free radicals, which cause oxidative damage (**Figure 8.30**). In addition to its antioxidant role in glutathione peroxidase, selenium is part of a protein needed for the synthesis of the **thyroid hormones**, which regulate metabolic rate.

> **glutathione per-oxidase** A selenium-containing enzyme that protects cells from oxidative damage by neutralizing peroxides.

Meeting selenium needs Selenium deficiencies and excesses are not a concern in the United States because the foods we consume come from many different locations around the country and around the world. The RDA for selenium for adults is 55 µg/day.[49] The average intake in the United States meets, or nearly meets, this recommendation for all age groups. Seafood, kidney, liver, and eggs are excellent sources of selenium. Grains, nuts, and seeds can be good sources, depending on the selenium content of the soil in which they were grown. Fruits, vegetables, and drinking water are generally poor sources. The UL for adults is 400 µg/day from food and supplements.[49]

Selenium and cancer An increased incidence of cancer has been observed in regions where selenium intake is low, suggesting that selenium plays a role in preventing cancer. In 1996, a study investigating the effect of selenium supplements on people with a history of skin cancer found that the supplement had no effect on the recurrence of skin cancer but that the incidence of lung, prostate, and colon cancer decreased in the selenium-supplemented group.[50] This result caused speculation that selenium supplements could reduce the risk of cancer. Continued study, however, has led to the conclusion that the reduction in the incidence of cancer seen in the 1996 study occurred primarily in people who began the study with low levels of selenium. It appears that an adequate level of selenium is necessary to prevent cancer, but the role of supplemental selenium in preventing cancer is still under investigation.[51]

Glutathione peroxidase • Figure 8.30

Glutathione peroxidase is a selenium-containing enzyme that neutralizes peroxides before they can form free radicals. Selenium therefore can reduce the body's need for vitamin E, which neutralizes free radicals.

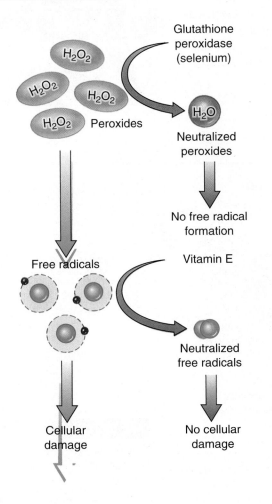

Iodine

About three-fourths of the iodine in the body is found in a small gland in the neck called the **thyroid gland**. The reason iodine is concentrated in this gland is that it is an essential component of the thyroid hormones, which are produced here. Thyroid hormones regulate metabolic rate, growth, and development, and they promote protein synthesis.

Iodine in health and disease Thyroid hormone levels are carefully regulated. If blood levels drop, **thyroid-stimulating hormone** is released. This hormone signals the thyroid gland to take up iodine and synthesize more thyroid hormones. When the supply of iodine is adequate, thyroid hormones can be produced, and the return of thyroid hormones to normal levels turns off the synthesis of thyroid-stimulating hormone. If iodine is

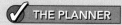

WILEY PLUS   Video

When thyroid hormone levels drop too low, thyroid-stimulating hormone stimulates the thyroid gland to take up iodine and synthesize more hormones. If iodine is not available, thyroid hormones cannot be made, and the stimulation continues, causing the thyroid gland to enlarge.

Low thyroid hormones levels

Anterior pituitary

Inhibits TSH release

Thyroid-stimulating hormone (TSH)

TSH release continues

Thyroid gland

Thyroid hormones made

No thyroid hormones made

Thyroid gland enlarges

Iodine available

Iodine deficient

Cretinism is characterized by symptoms that include impaired mental development, deaf mutism, and growth failure. Unlike with a mild goiter, the damage is permanent.

A goiter, which is an enlarged thyroid gland, can be seen as a swelling in the neck. In milder cases of goiter, treatment with iodine causes the thyroid gland to return to its normal size, but it may remain enlarged in more severe cases.

Although iodine deficiency remains a global health issue, its incidence has declined dramatically since universal salt iodization was adopted in 1993. UNICEF estimates that 70% of all households now have access to iodized salt.[52] Excessive iodine intake can occur if the level of iodine added to salt is too high.

No data
Severe iodine deficiency
Moderate iodine deficiency
Mild iodine deficiency
Optimal iodine status
Risk of iodine-induced hyperthyroidism
Risk of adverse health consequences

Ask Yourself

Why does the thyroid gland enlarge when iodine is deficient?

Source: de Benoist B et al., eds. Iodine status worldwide. WHO Global Database on Iodine Deficiency. Geneva, World Health Organization, 2004.
Data was produced by WHO using the best available evidence and do not necessarily correspond to the official statistics of Member States.

deficient, thyroid hormones cannot be synthesized (**Figure 8.31**). Without sufficient thyroid hormones, metabolic rate slows, causing fatigue and weight gain.

The most obvious outward sign of iodine deficiency is an enlarged thyroid gland, called a **goiter**, but because of the importance of the thyroid hormones for growth and development, other iodine deficiency disorders are also prevalent (see Figure 8.31). If iodine is deficient during pregnancy, the risk of stillbirth and spontaneous abortion increases; insufficient iodine during pregnancy can cause a condition called **cretinism** in the child. Iodine deficiency impairs mental function and reduces intellectual capacity in children and adolescents. Though easily prevented, it is the world's most prevalent cause of brain damage.[52]

goiter An enlargement of the thyroid gland caused by a deficiency of iodine.

cretinism A condition resulting from poor maternal iodine intake during pregnancy that impairs mental development and growth in the offspring.

Iodine deficiency is most common in regions where the soil is low in iodine and there is little access to fish and seafood. The risk of iodine deficiency is also increased by the consumption of foods that contain **goitrogens**, substances that interfere with iodine utilization or with thyroid function. Goitrogens are found in turnips, rutabaga, cabbage, millet, and cassava. When these foods are boiled, the goitrogen content is reduced because some of these compounds leach into the cooking water. Goitrogens are primarily a problem in African countries where cassava is a dietary staple. Goitrogens are not a problem in the United States because the typical diet does not include large amounts of foods containing them.

Chronically high intakes or a sudden increase in iodine intake can also cause an enlargement of the thyroid gland. For example, in a person with a marginal intake, a large dose from supplements could cause thyroid enlargement, even at levels that would not be toxic in a healthy person. The UL for adults is 1100 mg/day of iodine from all sources.[36]

Meeting iodine needs The iodine content of food varies, depending on the soil in which plants are grown or where animals graze. When the Earth was formed, all soils were high in iodine, but today mountainous areas and river valleys have little iodine left in the soil because it has been washed out by glaciers, snow, rain, and floodwaters. The iodine washed from the soil has accumulated in the oceans. Therefore, foods from the sea, such as fish, shellfish, and seaweed, are the best sources of iodine.

Today most of the iodine in the North American diet comes from **iodized salt** (**Figure 8.32**). Iodine deficiency is rare in North America, and typical iodine intake meets or exceeds the RDA of 150 μg/day for adult men and women.[36]

We also obtain iodine from contaminants and other additives in foods. Iodine-containing additives used in cattle feed and disinfectants used on milking machines and milk storage tanks increase the iodine content of dairy products. Iodine-containing sterilizing agents are also used in restaurants, and iodine is used in dough conditioners and some food colorings. Despite our intake of iodine from iodized salt and contaminants, toxicity is rare in the United States.

iodized salt Table salt to which a small amount of sodium iodide or potassium iodide has been added in order to supplement the iodine content of the diet.

Iodized salt • Figure 8.32

Iodized salt was first introduced in Switzerland in the 1920s as a way to combat iodine deficiency. Salt was chosen because it is readily available, inexpensive, and consumed in regular amounts throughout the year. It takes only about half a teaspoon of iodized salt to provide the recommended amount of iodine. Iodized salt should not be confused with sea salt, which is a poor source of iodine because its iodine is lost in the drying process.

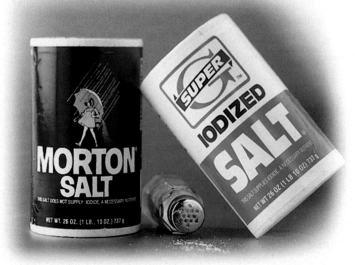

WHAT SHOULD I EAT?
Trace Minerals

Use iProfile to find the iron and zinc content of 1 cup of pinto beans.

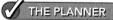
THE PLANNER

Add more iron
- Have some meat—red meat, poultry, and fish are all good sources of heme iron.
- Add raisins to your oatmeal.
- Fortify your breakfast by eating iron-fortified cereal.
- Cook in an iron skillet to add iron to food.
- Have some beans; they are a good source of iron.

Increase iron absorption
- Have orange juice with your iron-fortified cereal.
- Don't take your calcium supplement with your iron sources.

Think zinc
- Scramble some eggs.
- Beef up your zinc by having a few ounces of meat.
- Eat whole grains but make sure they are yeast leavened.

Trace down your minerals
- Check to see if your water is fluoridated.
- See if your salt is iodized.
- Replace refined grains with whole grains to increase your chromium intake.
- Have some seafood to add selenium to your diet.

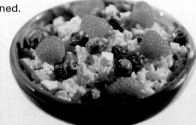

Chromium

Chromium is required to maintain normal blood glucose levels. It is believed to act by enhancing the effects of insulin.[36] Insulin facilitates the entry of glucose into cells and stimulates the synthesis of proteins, lipids, and glycogen. When chromium is deficient, more insulin is required to produce the same effect. A deficiency of chromium therefore affects the body's ability to regulate blood glucose, causing diabetes-like symptoms such as elevated blood glucose levels and increased insulin levels.[36]

Dietary sources of chromium include liver, brewer's yeast, nuts, and whole grains. Milk, vegetables, and fruits are poor sources. Refined carbohydrates such as white breads, pasta, and white rice are also poor sources because chromium is lost in milling and is not added back in the enrichment process. Chromium intake can be increased by cooking in stainless-steel cookware because chromium leaches from the steel into the food. The recommended intake for chromium is 35 µg/day for men age 19 to 50 and 25 µg/day for women age 19 to 50.[36]

Overt chromium deficiency is not a problem in the United States; nevertheless, chromium, in the form of chromium picolinate, is a common dietary supplement. Because chromium is needed for insulin action and insulin promotes protein synthesis, chromium picolinate is popular with athletes and dieters who take it to reduce body fat and increase muscle mass. However, studies of chromium picolinate and other chromium supplements in healthy human subjects have not found them to have beneficial effects on muscle strength, body composition, or weight loss.[53] Toxicity is always a concern with nutrient supplements, but in the case of chromium, there is little evidence of dietary toxicity in humans. The DRI committee concluded that there was insufficient data to establish a UL for chromium.[36]

Fluoride

Fluoride helps prevent **dental caries** (cavities) in both children and adults. During tooth formation, fluoride is incorporated into the crystals that make up tooth enamel. These fluoride-containing crystals are more resistant to acid than are crystals formed when fluoride is not present. Fluoride therefore helps protect the teeth from the cavity-causing acids produced by bacteria in the mouth. Adequate fluoride has its greatest effect during the period of maximum tooth development (up to age 13), but it continues to have benefits throughout life. In addition to making tooth enamel more acid resistant, fluoride in saliva prevents cavities by reducing the amount of acid produced by bacteria, inhibiting the dissolution of tooth enamel by acid, and increasing enamel re-mineralization after acid exposure.

Fluoride is also incorporated into the mineral crystals in bone. There is evidence that fluoride stimulates bone formation and therefore might strengthen bones in adults who have osteoporosis. Fluoride supplementation has been shown to increase bone mass and reduce the risk of fractures.[54]

Meeting fluoride needs Fluoride is present in small amounts in almost all soil, water, plants, and animals. The richest dietary sources of fluoride are toothpaste, tea, marine fish consumed with their bones, and fluoridated water (see *What Should I Eat?*). Because food readily absorbs the fluoride in cooking water, the fluoride content of food can be significantly increased when it is handled and prepared using water that contains fluoride. Cooking utensils also affect the fluoride content of foods. Foods cooked with Teflon utensils can pick up fluoride from the Teflon, whereas aluminum cookware can decrease the fluoride content of foods. Bottled water usually does not contain fluoride, so people who habitually drink bottled water need to obtain fluoride from other sources.

The recommended intake for fluoride for people 6 months of age and older is 0.05 mg/kg/day. This is equivalent to about 3.8 mg/day for a 76-kg man and 3.1 mg/day for a 61-kg woman. Fluoridated water provides about 0.7 to 1.2 mg/L of fluoride. The American Academy of Pediatrics suggests a fluoride supplement of 0.25 mg/day for children 6 months to 3 years of age, 0.5 mg/day for children ages 3 to 6 years, and 1.0 mg/day for those ages 6 to 16 years who are receiving less than 0.3 mg/liter of fluoride in the water supply. These supplements are available by prescription for children living in areas with low fluoride concentrations in the water supply.

Fluoridation of water

To promote dental health, fluoride is added to public water supplies in many communities. Currently about 70% of people served by public water systems receive fluoridated water.[55] When fluoride intake is low, tooth decay is more frequent (**Figure 8.33**). Water fluoridation is a safe, inexpensive way to prevent dental caries, but some people still believe that the added fluoride increases the risk of cancer and other diseases. These beliefs are not supported by scientific facts; the small amounts of fluoride consumed in drinking water promote dental health and do not pose a risk for health problems such as cancer, kidney failure, or bone disease.[56]

Although the levels of fluoride included in public water supplies are safe, too much fluoride can be toxic. In children, too much fluoride causes **fluorosis** (see Figure 8.33). Recently, there has been an increase in fluorosis in the United States due to chronic ingestion of fluoride-containing toothpaste.[57] The fluoride in toothpaste is good for your teeth, but swallowing it can increase fluoride intake to dangerous levels. Swallowed toothpaste is estimated to contribute about 0.6 mg/day of fluoride in young children. Due to concern over excess fluoride intake, the following warning is now required on all fluoride-containing toothpastes: "If you accidentally swallow more than used for brushing, seek professional help or contact a poison control center immediately."

fluorosis A condition caused by chronic overconsumption of fluoride, characterized by black and brown stains and cracking and pitting of the teeth.

In adults, doses of 20 to 80 mg/day of fluoride can result in changes in bone health that may be crippling, as well as changes in kidney function and possibly nerve and muscle function. Death has been reported in cases involving

---

Just the right amount of fluoride • Figure 8.33

This graph illustrates that the incidence of dental caries in children increases when the concentration of fluoride in the water supply is lower. If the fluoride concentration of the water is too high, it increases the risk of fluorosis.

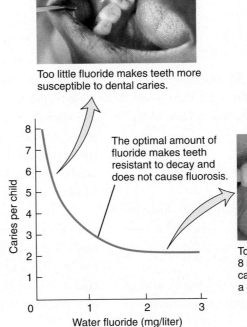

Too little fluoride makes teeth more susceptible to dental caries.

The optimal amount of fluoride makes teeth resistant to decay and does not cause fluorosis.

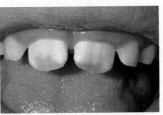

Too much fluoride (intakes of 2 to 8 mg/day or greater in children) causes teeth to appear mottled, a condition called fluorosis.

Interpreting Data

Based on this graph, what concentration of water fluoride will protect against dental caries but not cause fluorosis?

a. 2.5 mg/liter   b. 2 mg/liter
c. 1 mg/liter   d. 0.5 mg/liter

A summary of the trace minerals   Table 8.4

Mineral	Sources	Recommended intake for adults	Major functions	Deficiency diseases and symptoms	Groups at risk of deficiency	Toxicity	UL
Iron	Red meats, leafy greens, dried fruit, legumes, whole and enriched grains	8–18 mg/day	Part of hemoglobin (which delivers oxygen to cells), myoglobin (which holds oxygen in muscle), and proteins needed for ATP production; needed for immune function	Iron deficiency anemia: fatigue; weakness; small, pale red blood cells; low hemoglobin levels; inability to maintain normal body temperature	Infants and preschool children, adolescents, women of childbearing age, pregnant women, athletes, vegetarians	Acute: Gastro-intestinal upset, liver damage Chronic: fatigue, heart and liver damage, increased risk of diabetes and cancer	45 mg/day
Copper	Organ meats, nuts, seeds, whole grains, seafood, cocoa	900 μg/day	A component of proteins needed for iron transport, lipid metabolism, collagen synthesis, nerve and immune function, protection against oxidative damage	Anemia, poor growth, skeletal abnormalities	People who consume excessive amounts of zinc in supplements	Vomiting, abdominal pain, diarrhea, liver damage	10 mg/day
Zinc	Meat, seafood, whole grains, dairy products, legumes, nuts	8–11 mg/day	Regulates protein synthesis; functions in growth, development, wound healing, immunity, and antioxidant enzymes	Poor growth and development, skin rashes, decreased immune function	Vegetarians, low-income children, elderly people	Decreased copper absorption, depressed immune function	40 mg/day
Selenium	Meats, seafood, eggs, whole grains, nuts, seeds	55 μg/day	Antioxidant as part of glutathione peroxidase, synthesis of thyroid hormones, spares vitamin E	Muscle pain, weakness, Keshan disease	Populations in areas where the soil is low in selenium	Nausea, diarrhea, vomiting, fatigue, changes in hair and nails	400 μg/day

an intake of 5 to 10 g/day. The UL for fluoride is set at 0.1 mg/kg/day for infants and children younger than 9 years of age and at 10 mg/day for those 9 years and older.[33]

Manganese, Molybdenum, and Other Trace Minerals

In addition to the seven we have just examined, there are many other trace minerals in the human body. DRI recommendations have been set for two of them: manganese and molybdenum.[36]

Manganese is a constituent of some enzymes and an activator of others. Enzymes that require manganese are involved in carbohydrate and cholesterol metabolism, bone formation, synthesis of urea, and prevention of oxidative damage because manganese is a component of a form of superoxide dismutase. The recommended intake for manganese is 2.3 mg/day for adult men and 1.8 mg/day for adult women. The best dietary sources of manganese are whole grains, nuts, legumes, and leafy green vegetables.

Molybdenum is also needed to activate enzymes. It functions in the metabolism of sulfur-containing amino acids and nitrogen-containing compounds that are present in DNA and RNA, in the production of a waste product called uric acid, and in the oxidation and detoxification of various other compounds. The recommended intake

(Continued) Table 8.4

Mineral	Sources	Recommended intake for adults	Major functions	Deficiency diseases and symptoms	Groups at risk of deficiency	Toxicity	UL
Iodine	Iodized salt, seafood, seaweed, dairy products	150 µg/day	Needed for synthesis of thyroid hormones	Goiter, cretinism, impaired brain function, growth and developmental abnormalities	Populations in areas where the soil is low in iodine and iodized salt is not used	Enlarged thyroid	1110 µg/day
Chromium	Brewer's yeast, nuts, whole grains, meat, mushrooms	25–35 µg/day	Enhances insulin action	High blood glucose	Malnourished children	None reported	ND
Fluoride	Fluoridated water, tea, fish, toothpaste	3–4 mg/day	Strengthens tooth enamel, enhances re-mineralization of tooth enamel, reduces acid production by bacteria in the mouth	Increased risk of dental caries	Populations in areas with unfluoridated water, those who drink mostly bottled water	Fluorosis: mottled teeth, kidney damage, bone abnormalities	10 mg/day
Manganese	Nuts, legumes, whole grains, tea, leafy vegetables	1.8–2.3 mg/day	Functions in carbohydrate and cholesterol metabolism and antioxidant enzymes	Growth retardation	None	Nerve damage	11 mg/day
Molybdenum	Milk, organ meats, grains, legumes	45 µg/day	Cofactor for a number of enzymes	Unknown in humans	None	Arthritis, joint inflammation	2 mg/day

Note: UL, Tolerable Upper Intake Level; ND, not determined.

for molybdenum is 45 µg/day for adult men and women. The molybdenum content of food varies with the molybdenum content of the soil in the regions where the food is produced. The most reliable sources include milk and milk products, organ meats, breads, cereals, and legumes. Molybdenum is readily absorbed from foods; the amount in the body is regulated by excretion in the urine and bile.

There is evidence that arsenic, boron, nickel, silicon, and vanadium play a role in human health. The DRI committee reviewed the need for and functions of these minerals, but there was insufficient data to establish a recommended intake for any of them. Other trace minerals that are believed to play a physiological role in human health include aluminum, bromine, cadmium, germanium, lead, lithium, rubidium, and tin. Their specific functions have not been defined, and the DRI committee has not evaluated them. All the minerals, both those that are known to be essential and those that are still being assessed for their role in human health, can be obtained by choosing a variety of foods from each of the MyPlate food groups.

Table 8.4 provides a summary of the trace minerals.

CONCEPT CHECK STOP

1. **Why** does iron deficiency cause fatigue?
2. **How** does selenium reduce the body's need for vitamin E?
3. **What** is the function of iodine?
4. **How** does fluoride protect the teeth?

Summary

1 Water 258

- Water, which is found intracellularly and extracellularly, accounts for about 60% of adult body weight. The amount of water in the blood is a balance between the forces of **blood pressure** and osmosis.

- Because water isn't stored in the body, intake from fluids and foods, as shown in the illustration, must replace losses in urine, feces, sweat, and evaporation. Water intake is stimulated by the sensation of **thirst**. The kidneys regulate urinary water losses.

Water balance • Figure 8.2

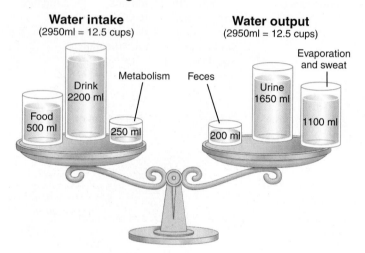

- In the body, water is a **solvent** where chemical reactions occur; it also transports nutrients and wastes, provides protection, helps regulate temperature, and participates in chemical reactions and acid–base balance.

- **Dehydration** occurs when there is too little water in the body. **Water intoxication** causes **hyponatremia**, which can result in abnormal fluid accumulation in body tissues.

- The recommended intake of water is 2.7 L/day for women and 3.7 L/day for men; needs vary depending on environmental conditions and activity level.

2 An Overview of Minerals 265

- **Major minerals** and **trace minerals** are distinguished by the amounts needed in the diet and found in the body. Both plant and animal foods are good sources of minerals.

- Mineral bioavailability is affected by the food source of the mineral, the body's need, and interactions with other minerals, vitamins, and dietary components such as fiber, phytates, oxalates, and tannins, which are plentiful in the foods shown here.

Compounds that interfere with mineral absorption • Figure 8.9

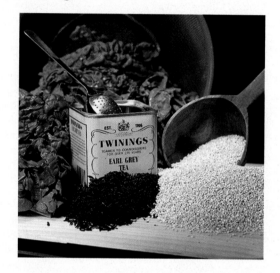

- Minerals are needed to provide structure and to regulate biochemical reactions, often as **cofactors**.

3 Electrolytes: Sodium, Potassium, and Chloride 269

- The minerals sodium, potassium, and chloride are **electrolytes** that are important in the maintenance of fluid balance and the functioning of nerves and muscles. The kidneys are the primary regulator of electrolyte and fluid balance.

- Sodium, potassium, and chloride depletion can occur when losses are increased by heavy and persistent sweating, chronic diarrhea, or vomiting. Diets high in sodium and low in potassium are associated with an increased risk of **hypertension**. The **DASH Eating Plan**—a dietary pattern moderate in sodium; high in potassium, magnesium, calcium, and fiber; and low in fat, saturated fat, and cholesterol—lowers blood pressure.

- As shown in the graph, processed foods add sodium to the diet. Potassium is highest in unprocessed foods such as fresh fruits and vegetables. Recommendations for health suggest that we increase our intake of potassium and consume less sodium.

Processing adds sodium • Figure 8.15b

Less processed

Potassium / Sodium

(Bar graph, y-axis "Milligrams" from 0 to 800)
- Peanuts, unsalted (1c)
- Kidney beans, dry, cooked (1 c)
- Pork, roasted (3 oz)
- Chicken breast (3 oz)
- 1% milk (1 c)

More processed

(Bar graph, y-axis "Milligrams" from 0 to 800)
- Peanut butter (2 Tbsp)
- Kidney beans, canned (1 c)
- Ham, roasted (3 oz)
- Chicken nuggets (3 oz)
- American cheese (1.5 oz)

4 Major Minerals and Bone Health   277

- Bone is a living tissue that is constantly remodeled. **Peak bone mass** occurs in young adulthood. **Age-related bone loss** occurs in adults when more bone is broken down than is made. Bone loss is accelerated in women after **menopause**. **Osteoporosis**, occurs when bone mass is so low that it increases the risk of bone fractures.

- Most of the calcium in the body is found in bone, but calcium is also needed for essential functions such as nerve transmission, muscle contraction, blood clotting, and blood pressure regulation. Good sources of calcium in the U.S. diet include dairy products, fish consumed with bones, and leafy green vegetables. As shown in the illustration, low blood calcium causes the release of **parathyroid hormone (PTH)**, which affects the amount of calcium excreted in the urine, absorbed from the diet, and released from bone. When blood calcium is high, **calcitonin** blocks calcium release from bone.

Raising blood calcium levels • Figure 8.18

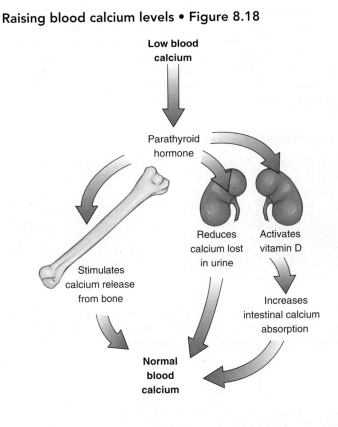

Low blood calcium → Parathyroid hormone →
- Stimulates calcium release from bone
- Reduces calcium lost in urine
- Activates vitamin D → Increases intestinal calcium absorption

→ **Normal blood calcium**

- Phosphorus is widely distributed in foods. It plays an important structural role in bones and teeth. Phosphorus helps prevent changes in acidity and is an essential component of phospholipids, ATP, DNA, and RNA.

- Magnesium is important for bone health and blood pressure regulation, and it is needed as a cofactor and to stabilize ATP. The best dietary sources are whole grains and green vegetables.

- Sulfur is found in protein and is part of the structure of certain vitamins and of glutathione, which protects cells from oxidative damage.

- Iron functions as part of **hemoglobin**, **myoglobin**, and proteins involved in energy metabolism. The amount of iron absorbed depends on the form of iron and other dietary components. **Heme iron**, found in meats, is more absorbable than nonheme iron, which is the only form found in plant foods. **Iron deficiency anemia** is characterized by small, pale red blood cells such as those in the right-hand photo. It causes fatigue and decreased work capacity. The amount of iron transported from the intestinal cells to body cells depends on the amount needed. If too much iron is absorbed, as in **hemochromatosis**, the heart and liver can be damaged, and diabetes and cancer are more likely. A single large dose of iron is toxic and can be fatal.

Iron deficiency • Figure 8.25

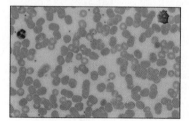 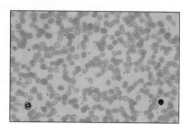

Normal red blood cells   Iron deficiency anemia

- Copper functions in proteins that affect iron and lipid metabolism, synthesis of connective tissue, antioxidant capacity, and iron transport. High levels of zinc can cause copper deficiency. A copper deficiency can result in anemia and skeletal abnormalities. Seafood, nuts, seeds, and whole-grain breads and cereals are good sources of copper.

- Zinc is needed for the activity of many enzymes, and zinc-containing proteins are needed for gene expression. Good sources of zinc include red meats, eggs, dairy products, and whole grains. The amount of zinc in the body is regulated primarily by the amount absorbed and lost through the small intestine. Zinc deficiency depresses immunity. Too much zinc depresses immune function and contributes to copper and iron deficiency.

- Selenium is part of the antioxidant enzyme **glutathione peroxidase** and is needed for the synthesis of **thyroid hormones**. Dietary sources include seafood, eggs, organ meats, and plant foods grown in selenium-rich soils. Selenium deficiency causes muscle discomfort and weakness and is associated with **Keshan disease**. Low selenium intake has been linked to increased cancer risk.

- Iodine is an essential component of thyroid hormones. The best sources of iodine are seafood, foods grown near the sea, and **iodized salt**. When iodine is deficient, the **thyroid gland** enlarges, forming a **goiter**. Iodine deficiency also affects growth and development. The use of iodized salt has reduced the incidence of iodine deficiency worldwide.

- Chromium is needed for normal insulin action and glucose utilization. It is found in liver, brewer's yeast, nuts, and whole grains.

- Fluoride is necessary for the maintenance of bones and teeth and the prevention of **dental caries**. Dietary sources of fluoride include fluoridated drinking water, toothpaste, tea, and marine fish consumed with bones. Too much fluoride causes **fluorosis** in children.

Key Terms

- age-related bone loss 279
- aldosterone 271
- antidiuretic hormone (ADH) 260
- blood pressure 259
- bone remodeling 279
- bone resorption 282
- calcitonin 282
- cofactor 269
- cretinism 297
- DASH (Dietary Approaches to Stop Hypertension) eating plan 274
- dehydration 262
- dental cary 298
- diuretic 265
- electrolyte 269
- fluorosis 299

- glutathione peroxidase 295
- goiter 297
- goitrogen 297
- heme iron 287
- hemochromatosis 292
- hemoglobin 287
- hypertension 271
- hyponatremia 263
- iodized salt 297
- ion 267
- iron deficiency anemia 291
- iron overload 292
- Keshan disease 294
- major mineral 265
- menopause 279
- mineral 265

- myoglobin 287
- osteopenia 278
- osteoporosis 279
- peak bone mass 279
- postmenopausal bone loss 279
- prehypertension 273
- sodium chloride 269
- solute 259
- solvent 261
- thirst 260
- thyroid gland 295
- thyroid hormone 295
- thyroid-stimulating hormone 295
- trace mineral 265
- water intoxication 263

Online Resources

- For more information on the incidence, causes, and treatment of high blood pressure, go to the National Heart Lung and Blood Institute site, at www.nhlbi.nih.gov.

- For information about milk, calcium intake, and bone health, go to the Milk Matters site of the National Institutes of Child Health and Human Development, at www.nichd.nih.gov/milk/kids/kidsteens.cfm.

- For more information on osteoporosis, go to the National Institutes of Health Osteoporosis and Related Bone Disease National Resource Center, at www.niams.nih.gov/Health_Info/Bone/.

- For more information on iron and iodine deficiency, go to the World Health Organization site, at www.who.int/nutrition/topics/en/, and click on Iron Deficiency Anemia or Iodine Deficiency Disorders.

- Visit your *WileyPLUS* site for videos, animations, podcasts, self-study, and other media that will aid you in studying and understanding this chapter.

Critical and Creative Thinking Questions

1. Mary Beth has just been diagnosed with anemia that is believed to be due to a deficiency in her diet. The total amount of hemoglobin in her blood is low, as is her hematocrit (the percentage of her blood that is made up of red blood cells). What other information can help determine what nutrient deficiency is the cause of Mary Beth's anemia?

2. Evaluate your risk of developing osteoporosis, based on your age, ethnicity, gender, diet, and lifestyle.

3. Why might a thirsty sailor who drank sea water die of dehydration?

4. Virginia works at a desk. The only exercise she gets is when she takes care of her nieces and nephews one weekend a month. Her typical diet includes a breakfast of cereal, tomato juice, and coffee. She has a snack of donuts and coffee at work, and for lunch she joins coworkers for a fast-food cheeseburger, fries, and a milkshake. When she gets home, she snacks on a soda and peanuts or chips. Dinner is usually a frozen meal with milk. A recent physical exam indicated that her blood pressure is elevated. What dietary and lifestyle changes would you recommend to help Virginia lower her blood pressure?

5. Use food labels to identify three processed foods you commonly eat that contain more than 10% of the Daily Value for sodium per serving. What less-processed choices might you substitute for these? If you typically consumed a serving of each of these processed foods per day, by how much would these substitutions lower your sodium intake?

6. Many people in the United States must limit their milk consumption due to lactose intolerance. What foods can they include in their diets to help meet their calcium needs?

7. This table shows the incidence of hip fractures in different groups within a population of older adults. Use your knowledge of bone physiology to explain the differences observed among Caucasian women, Caucasian men, African American women, and African American men.

Population group	Annual incidence of hip fracture per 1000
Caucasian women	30
Caucasian men	13
African American women	11
African American men	7

8. A researcher asked his new technician to prepare a diet for his laboratory animals. The technician is interrupted several times while mixing the diet and is unfamiliar with the scale he is using to weigh the diet ingredients. After the diet is fed to the animals for several months, they begin to show signs of anemia. An error in diet preparation is suspected. Errors in the amounts (deficiencies or excesses) of which of the diet ingredients listed below (vitamins, minerals, or others) could lead to anemia? For each, explain why.

Diet ingredients
Starch, Sucrose, Casein (protein), Corn oil, Mixed plant fibers, Vitamin A, Vitamin D, Vitamin E, Vitamin K, B vitamin mix, Calcium, Sodium, Potassium, Magnesium, Chloride, Zinc, Iron, Iodine, Selenium, Copper, Manganese, Chromium, Molybdenum

What is happening in this picture?

This photo shows astronaut Pete Conrad riding a stationary bike during his 28-day stay aboard Skylab in 1973. Weight-bearing exercise and adequate nutrient intake are important for the maintenance of bone.

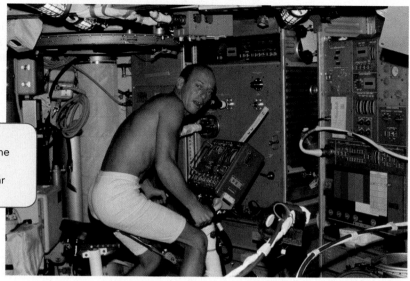

Think Critically

1. Why is scheduled exercise even more important for bone health in space than it is on Earth?
2. What nutrients other than calcium might be of particular concern for the bone health in an astronaut? Why?

Self-Test

(Check your answers in Appendix K.)

1. In a sedentary individual at room temperature, most water is lost via _____.
   a. evaporation from the skin and lungs
   b. sweat
   c. saliva
   d. urine
   e. feces

2. _____ will increase water needs.
   a. A high-salt diet
   b. A high-protein diet
   c. A high-fiber diet
   d. A very low-calorie diet
   e. All of the above

3. If the concentration of solutes in your blood increases (that is, the blood is more concentrated), which one of the following is most likely to occur?
   a. You will lose more water in the urine.
   b. Antidiuretic hormone will be released.
   c. You will begin to sweat.
   d. Your body temperature will go up.
   e. You will feel hungry.

4. The risk of high blood pressure is increased by _____.
   a. obesity
   b. family history
   c. high salt diet
   d. sedentary lifestyle
   e. all of the above

5. Which of the following statements about iron is true?
   a. When iron levels are high, more iron is eliminated from the body in the urine.
   b. Heme iron is better absorbed than nonheme iron.
   c. Vitamin C inhibits iron absorption.
   d. Iron and calcium supplements should be taken together.
   e. Tomatoes are good source of heme iron.

6. Which one of the following is occurring at the point labeled with the arrow?
   a. Bone formation is occurring more rapidly than bone breakdown.
   b. Peak bone mass has been reached.
   c. Bone breakdown exceeds bone formation due to normal aging.
   d. Bone loss is accelerated around menopause.

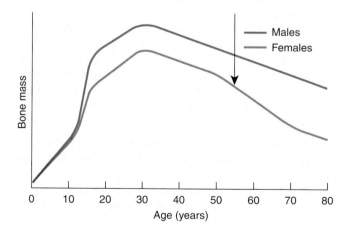

7. Hemochromatosis is treated with iron supplements.
   a. True
   b. False

8. Which of the following occurs when blood calcium levels get too high?
   a. More calcium is excreted in the urine.
   b. Bone is broken down, releasing calcium into the blood.
   c. Vitamin D is activated by the kidney.
   d. Parathyroid hormone is released.
   e. Intestinal absorption of calcium increases.

9. Which of the following is a function of iodine?
   a. It is an antioxidant.
   b. It is needed for insulin action.
   c. It is a component of the thyroid hormones.
   d. It is a component of superoxide dismutase.
   e. It is needed to cross-link collagen.

10. Women of childbearing age need more iron than men of the same age because they _____.
    a. are more active
    b. are growing
    c. lose more iron in the digestive tract
    d. have more muscle mass
    e. lose iron through menstruation

11. Selenium is said to spare vitamin E. Indicate at which step in the diagram the selenium-dependent enzyme glutathione peroxidase acts and at what step vitamin E would be needed to protect cells.

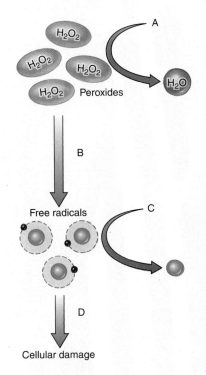

a. glutathione peroxidase—step A, vitamin E—step B
b. glutathione peroxidase—step A, vitamin E—step C
c. glutathione peroxidase—step B, vitamin E—step C
d. glutathione peroxidase—step C, vitamin E—step D

12. Which of the following statements about zinc is false?
    a. The amount of zinc that moves from the intestinal cells into the blood is regulated.
    b. Phytates present in grain products enhance zinc absorption.
    c. Zinc is involved in regulating protein synthesis.
    d. Zinc is part of the protein that allows vitamin A to affect gene expression.
    e. Zinc is absorbed better from meat than from plant foods.

13. The woman shown here has a deficiency of which of the following minerals?

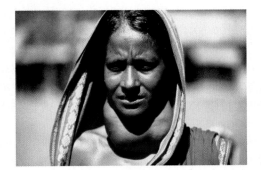

a. calcium   d. chromium
b. iodine   e. magnesium
c. iron

14. Chromium increases the effectiveness of _____.
    a. insulin   d. antidiuretic hormone
    b. thyroid hormone   e. parathyroid hormone
    c. thyroid-stimulating hormone

15. Which of the following is most likely to have caused the condition shown here?

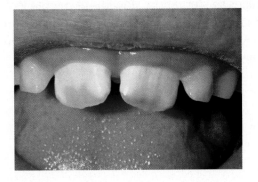

a. living in a community that does not have fluoridated water
b. taking calcium supplements
c. swallowing toothpaste
d. absorbing too much iron

THE PLANNER ✓

Review your Chapter Planner on the chapter opener and check off you completed work.

Energy Balance and Weight Management

Cultural and societal perceptions of attractiveness and good health present challenges to responsible weight management. One person may be perfectly healthy yet somewhat plump and be judged harshly by peers or the media. Another person may be frightfully unhealthy but willowy thin, and because of an arbitrary standard of body type and appearance, that person might be hailed as a paragon of health and beauty. The impact of this dynamic to personal esteem alone is staggering.

Managing body weight involves choosing the right amount of food and exercise to keep weight in the healthy range. But food producers and sellers urge us to buy, eat, and supersize, while the weight-loss and diet industry "experts" urge us to try the latest device, diet plan, or superfood. Is there a middle ground?

As developing nations strive for Western patterns of consumption—as well as Western perceptions of health and beauty—weight problems manifest themselves in their populations as well. Sadly, vast numbers of humans still lack access to food that provides adequate nutrients and are subject to afflictions ranging from vitamin deficiencies to starvation. How these people look may be the least of their concerns; for them, weight management may mean simply having enough food to meet the body's energy demands.

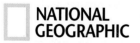

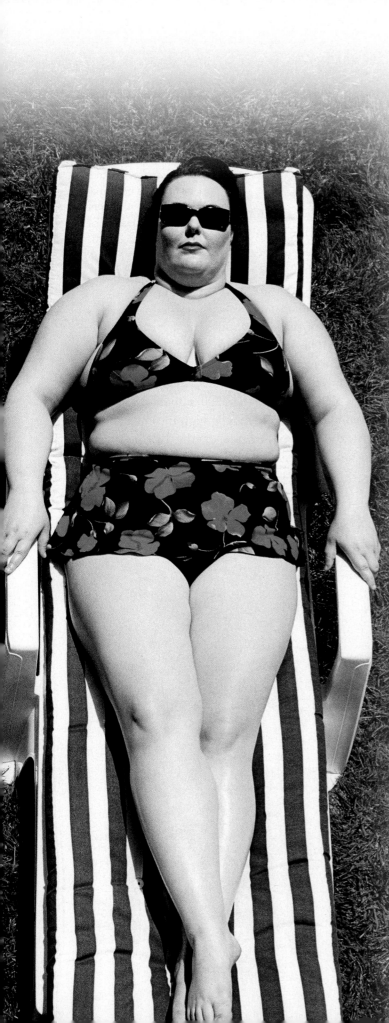

CHAPTER OUTLINE

CHAPTER PLANNER ✓

❑ Stimulate your interest by reading the introduction and looking at the visual.

❑ Scan the Learning Objectives in each section:
   p. 310 ❑   p. 315 ❑   p. 322 ❑   p. 327 ❑   p. 337 ❑

❑ Read the text and study all figures and visuals. Answer any questions.

Analyze key features

❑ Nutrition InSight, p. 314 ❑   p. 318 ❑   p. 340 ❑

❑ What a Scientist Sees, p. 326 ❑   p. 334 ❑

❑ Process Diagram, p. 328 ❑   p. 331 ❑

❑ Thinking It Through, p. 323 ❑

❑ Stop: Answer the Concept Checks before you go on:
   p. 315 ❑   p. 321 ❑   p. 327 ❑   p. 336 ❑   p. 345 ❑

End of chapter

❑ Review the Summary, Key Terms, and Online Resources.

❑ Answer the Critical and Creative Thinking Questions.

❑ Answer What is happening in this picture?

❑ Complete the Self-Test and check your answers.

Body Weight and Health

LEARNING OBJECTIVES

1. **Discuss** the obesity epidemic.
2. **Describe** the health consequences of excess body fat.
3. **Calculate** your BMI and determine whether it indicates increased health risks.
4. **Discuss** how the amount and location of body fat affect the health risks associated with being overweight.

n the United States today, a staggering 68% of adults are either **overweight** or **obese**. The numbers have increased dramatically over the past 5 decades (**Figure 9.1**). In 1960, only 13.4% of American adults were obese. By 1990, about 23% were obese, and today, only two decades later, almost 34% are obese. Obesity affects both men and women and all racial and ethnic groups. Obesity rates for minorities often exceed those in the general population: Among African Americans, more than 49% of women and 37% of men are obese, and among Hispanic Americans, more than 34% of men and about 43% of women are obese.[1]

Obesity is a growing concern worldwide. It is such an important trend that the term *globesity* has been coined to reflect the escalation of global obesity and overweight. Around the world, approximately 1.5 billion adults are overweight, and of these, 500 million are obese. The World Health Organization projects that by 2015, approximately 2.3 billion adults will be overweight and more than 700 million will be obese.[2] Once considered a problem only in high-income countries, overweight and obesity are now on the rise in low- and middle-income countries, particularly in urban settings.

> **overweight** Being too heavy for one's height, usually due to an excess of body fat. Overweight is defined as having a body mass index (ratio of weight to height squared) of 25 to 29.9 kilograms/meter² (kg/m²).
>
> **obese** Having excess body fat. Obesity is defined as having a body mass index (ratio of weight to height squared) of 30 kg/m² or greater.

Obesity on the rise • Figure 9.1

These maps show the percentage of the adult population classified as obese in each state in 1990 and 2009. The dramatic rise in overweight and obesity in the United States over the past few decades has led medical and public health officials to label the situation an epidemic.

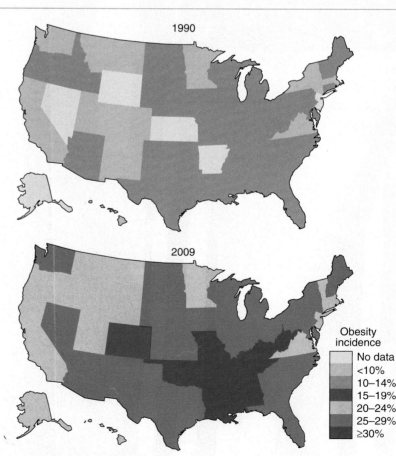

1990

2009

Obesity incidence
- No data
- <10%
- 10–14%
- 15–19%
- 20–24%
- 25–29%
- ≥30%

Interpreting Data

In 2009, how many states still had an obesity rate of less than 15% of their population?

Health consequences of excess body fat • Figure 9.2

Obesity-related health complications such as those highlighted here have reached epidemic proportions in the United States and around the world.

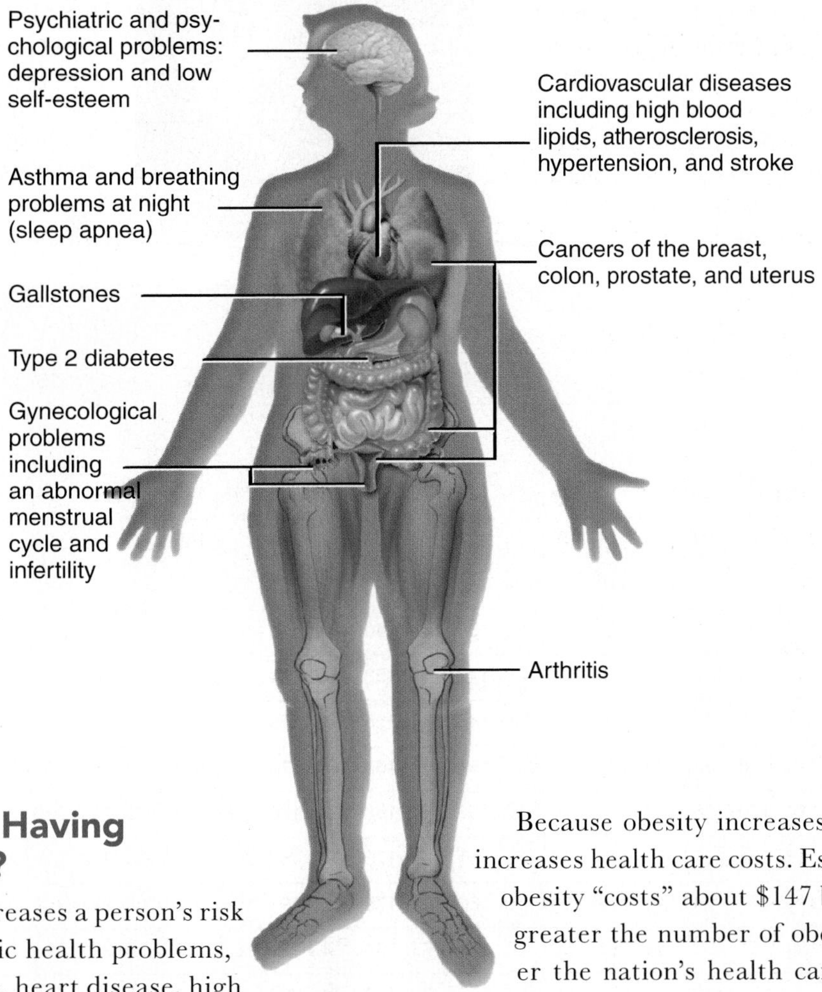

Psychiatric and psychological problems: depression and low self-esteem

Cardiovascular diseases including high blood lipids, atherosclerosis, hypertension, and stroke

Asthma and breathing problems at night (sleep apnea)

Cancers of the breast, colon, prostate, and uterus

Gallstones

Type 2 diabetes

Gynecological problems including an abnormal menstrual cycle and infertility

Arthritis

What's Wrong With Having Too Much Body Fat?

Having too much body fat increases a person's risk of developing a host of chronic health problems, including high blood pressure, heart disease, high blood cholesterol, diabetes, gallbladder disease, arthritis, sleep disorders, respiratory problems, menstrual irregularities, and cancers of the breast, uterus, prostate, and colon (**Figure 9.2**). Obesity also increases the incidence and severity of infectious disease and has been linked to poor wound healing and surgical complications. The more excess body fat you have, the greater your health risks. The longer you carry excess fat, the greater the risks; individuals who gain excess weight at a young age and remain overweight throughout life face the greatest health risks.

Being overweight also has psychological and social consequences. Overweight and obese individuals of any age are at increased risk of experiencing depression, negative self-image, and feelings of inadequacy.[3] They may also be discriminated against in college admissions, in the workplace, and even on public transportation. The physical health consequences of excess body fat may not manifest themselves as disease for years, but the psychological and social problems are experienced every day.

Because obesity increases health problems, it increases health care costs. Estimates suggest that obesity "costs" about $147 billion per year.[4] The greater the number of obese people, the higher the nation's health care expenses and the higher the cost to society as a whole in terms of lost wages and productivity.

What Is a Healthy Weight?

A healthy weight is a weight that minimizes health risks. Your body weight is the sum of the weight of your fat and your **lean body mass**. Some body fat is essential for health, but too much increases your risk for a number of chronic health problems. How much weight and fat is too much depends on your age, gender, and lifestyle and where your fat is located.

lean body mass Body mass attributed to nonfat body components such as bone, muscle, and internal organs; also called *fat-free mass*.

body mass index (BMI) A measure of body weight relative to height that is used to compare body size with a standard.

Body mass index (BMI) The current standard for assessing the healthfulness of body weight is **body mass index (BMI)**, which is determined by dividing body weight (in kilograms) by height (in meters)

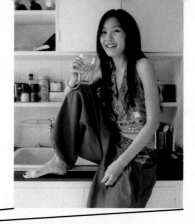

What's your BMI? • Figure 9.3

To find your BMI, locate your height in the leftmost column and read across to your weight. Follow the column containing your weight up to the top line to find your BMI. A BMI < 18.5 kg/m² is classified as **underweight**, a BMI ≥ 25 and < 30 kg/m² is classified as overweight, and a BMI of ≥ 30 kg/m² is classified as obese. A BMI ≥ 40 kg/m² is considered **extreme obesity** or **morbid obesity**.[5]

Being underweight is associated with increased risk of early death, but this does not mean that all thin people are at risk.[6] People who are naturally lean have a lower incidence of certain chronic diseases and do not face increased health risks due to their low body weight. However, low body fat due to starvation, eating disorders, or a disease process decreases energy reserves and the ability of the immune system to fight disease.

	UNDER-WEIGHT		NORMAL						OVERWEIGHT					OBESE										EXTREME OBESITY		
BMI	17	18	19	20	21	22	23	24	25	26	27	28	29	30	31	32	33	34	35	36	37	38	39	40	41	42
Height (feet/inches)	**Body Weight** (pounds)																									
4'10"	81	86	91	96	100	105	110	115	119	124	129	134	138	143	148	153	158	162	167	172	177	181	186	191	196	201
4'11"	84	89	94	99	104	109	114	119	124	128	133	138	143	148	153	158	163	168	173	178	183	188	193	198	203	208
5'0"	87	92	97	102	107	112	118	123	128	133	138	143	148	153	158	163	168	174	179	184	189	194	199	204	209	215
5'1"	90	95	100	106	111	116	122	127	132	137	143	148	153	158	164	169	174	180	185	190	195	201	206	211	217	222
5'2"	93	98	104	109	115	120	126	131	136	142	147	153	158	164	169	175	180	186	191	196	202	207	213	218	224	229
5'3"	96	102	107	113	118	124	130	135	141	146	152	158	163	169	175	180	186	191	197	203	208	214	220	225	231	237
5'4"	99	105	110	116	122	128	134	140	145	151	157	163	169	174	180	186	192	197	204	209	215	221	227	232	238	244
5'5"	102	108	114	120	126	132	138	144	150	156	162	168	174	180	186	192	198	204	210	216	222	228	234	240	246	252
5'6"	105	112	118	124	130	136	142	148	155	161	167	173	179	186	192	198	204	210	216	223	229	235	241	247	253	260
5'7"	108	115	121	127	134	140	146	153	159	166	172	178	185	191	198	204	211	217	223	230	236	242	249	255	261	268
5'8"	112	119	125	131	138	144	151	158	164	171	177	184	190	197	203	210	216	223	230	236	243	249	256	262	269	276
5'9"	115	122	128	135	142	149	155	162	169	176	182	189	196	203	209	216	223	230	236	243	250	257	263	270	277	284
5'10"	119	126	132	139	146	153	160	167	174	181	188	195	202	209	216	222	229	236	243	250	257	264	271	278	285	292
5'11"	122	129	136	143	150	157	165	172	179	186	193	200	208	215	222	229	236	243	250	257	265	272	279	286	293	301
6'0"	125	133	140	147	154	162	169	177	184	191	199	206	213	221	228	235	242	250	258	265	272	279	287	294	302	309
6'1"	129	137	144	151	159	166	174	182	189	197	204	212	219	227	235	242	250	257	265	272	280	288	295	302	310	318
6'2"	132	140	148	155	163	171	179	186	194	202	210	218	225	233	241	249	256	264	272	280	287	295	303	311	319	326
6'3"	136	144	152	160	168	176	184	192	200	208	216	224	232	240	248	256	264	272	279	287	295	303	311	319	327	335
6'4"	140	148	156	164	172	180	189	197	205	213	221	230	238	246	254	263	271	279	287	295	304	312	320	328	336	344

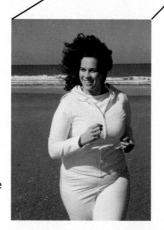

Although BMI can be a useful tool, other information is also needed to determine health risks. For example, someone who is overweight based on BMI but consumes a healthy diet and exercises regularly may be more fit and at lower risk for chronic diseases than someone with a BMI in the healthy range who is sedentary and eats a poor diet.

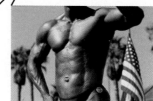
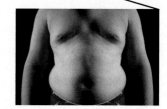

A high BMI may be caused by either too much body fat or a large amount of muscle. Therefore, in muscular athletes, BMI does not provide an accurate estimate of health risk. Both of these individuals have a BMI of 33, but only the man on the right has excess body fat. The high body weight of the man on the left is due to his large muscle mass. His body fat, and hence disease risk, is low.

squared. A healthy BMI for adults is between 18.5 and 24.9 kg/m². People with a BMI in this range have the lowest health risks. Although BMI is not actually a measure of body fat, it is recommended as a way to assess body fatness that is better than measuring weight alone.[5] You can use **Figure 9.3** to determine your BMI or calculate it according to either of these equations:

$$BMI = Weight\ in\ kilograms/(Height\ in\ meters)^2$$

or

$$BMI = [Weight\ in\ pounds/(Height\ in\ inches)^2] \times 703$$

Body composition **Body composition**, which refers to the relative proportions of fat and lean tissue that make up the body, affects the risks associated with excess body weight. Having more than the recommended percentage of body fat increases health risks, whereas having more lean body mass does not. In general, women store more body fat than men do, so the level that is healthy for women is somewhat higher than the level that is healthy for men. A healthy level of body fat for a young adult female is between 21 and 32% of total weight; for young adult males, it is between 8 and 19%.[7] With aging, lean body mass decreases and body fat increases, even if body weight remains the same. Some of this change may be prevented through exercise. Body composition can be measured using a variety of techniques (**Figure 9.4**).

Techniques for measuring body composition • Figure 9.4

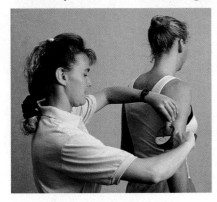

Skinfold thickness. Skinfold thickness uses calipers to measure the thickness of the fat layer under the skin at several locations. This technique assumes that the amount of fat under the skin is representative of total body fat. It is fast, easy, and inexpensive but can be inaccurate if not performed by a trained professional.

Underwater weighing. Underwater weighing relies on the fact that lean tissue is denser than fat tissue. The difference between a person's weight on land and his or her weight underwater is used to calculate body density; the higher a person's body density, the less fat he or she has. Underwater weighing is accurate but can't be used for small children or for ill or frail adults.

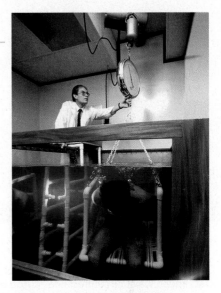

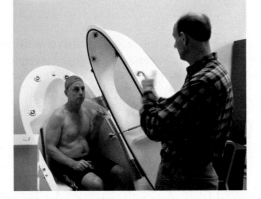

Air displacement. The BOD POD measures the amount of air displaced by the body in a closed chamber and uses this along with body weight to determine body density, which is related to body fat mass. This method is accurate and easy for the subject but expensive and not readily available.

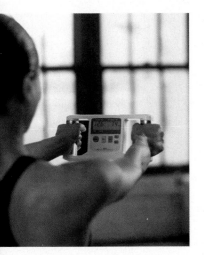

Bioelectric impedance. Bioelectric impedance analysis measures an electric current traveling through the body. It is based on the fact that current moves easily through lean tissue, which is high in water, but is slowed by fat, which resists current flow. Bioelectric impedance measurements are fast, easy, and painless but can be inaccurate if the amount of body water is higher or lower than typical. For example, in someone who has been sweating heavily, the estimate of percentage body fat obtained using bioelectric impedance will be artificially high.

Dual-energy X-ray absorptiometry (DXA). DXA distinguishes among various body tissues by measuring differences in levels of X-ray absorption. A single investigation can accurately determine total body mass, bone mineral mass, and body fat percentage, but the apparatus is expensive and not readily available.

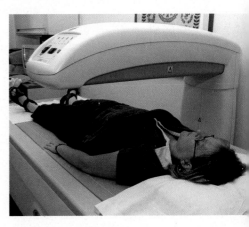

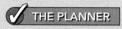

a. People who carry their excess fat around and above the waist have more visceral fat. Those who carry their extra fat below the waist, in the hips and thighs, have more subcutaneous fat. In the popular literature, these body types have been dubbed "apples" and "pears," respectively.

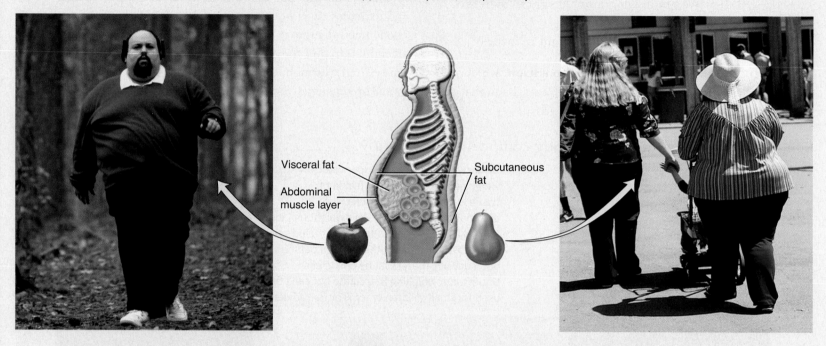

Visceral fat

Abdominal muscle layer

Subcutaneous fat

b. Waist circumference is indicative of the amount of visceral fat, the type of fat that is associated with increased health risk. Waist measurements along with BMI are used to estimate the health risk associated with excess body fat. These waist circumference "cutpoints" are not useful in patients with a BMI of 35 kg/m² or greater.

In men a BMI of 25 to 34.9 kg/m² and a waist circumference >40 inches indicates visceral fat storage.

In women a BMI of 25 to 34.9 kg/m² and a waist circumference >35 inches indicates visceral fat storage.

Location of body fat The location of body fat stores affects the risks associated with having too much fat (**Figure 9.5**). Excess **subcutaneous fat**, which is adipose tissue located under the skin, does not increase health risk as much as does excess **visceral fat**, which is adipose tissue located around the organs in the abdomen. Generally, fat in the hips and lower body is subcutaneous, whereas fat in the abdominal region is primarily visceral. Visceral fat is more metabolically active than subcutaneous fat, releasing dozens of biologically active substances that can contribute to disease.[8] An increase in visceral fat is associated with a higher incidence of heart disease, high blood cholesterol, high blood pressure, stroke, diabetes, and breast cancer.

Where your extra fat is deposited is determined primarily by your genes. Visceral fat storage is more common in men than in women, but after menopause, the amount of visceral fat in women increases. Age and environment also influence where fat is stored.[9] Visceral fat storage increases with age. Stress, tobacco use, and alcohol consumption predispose people to visceral fat deposition, and weight loss and exercise reduce the amount of visceral fat.

CONCEPT CHECK 🛑 STOP

1. **How** has the incidence of overweight and obesity changed in the United States over the past few decades?

2. **What** are two chronic disorders that are more common in obese individuals than in lean individuals?

3. **When** is a high BMI not associated with an increased health risk?

4. **What** type of body fat increases health risks?

Energy Balance

LEARNING OBJECTIVES

1. **Identify** lifestyle factors that have led to weight gain among Americans.

2. **Explain** the principle of energy balance.

3. **Describe** the components of energy expenditure.

4. **Calculate** your EER at various levels of activity.

The rising rates of overweight and obesity in virtually every population group in the United States demonstrate that many Americans are in energy imbalance.[10] According to the principle of **energy balance**, if you consume the same amount of energy—or calories—as you expend, your body weight will remain the same. If you consume more energy than you expend, you will gain weight, and if you expend more energy than you consume, you will lose weight. In the United States today, our energy intake is exceeding our energy expenditure.[10] Bringing it back into balance requires an understanding of how many calories we need and how we use energy.

energy balance The amount of energy consumed in the diet compared with the amount expended by the body over a given period.

America's Energy Imbalance

Over the past 40 years, changes in our food supply and lifestyle have affected what we eat, how much we eat, and how much exercise we get. Simply put, more Americans are overweight than ever before because we are eating more and burning fewer calories than we did 40 years ago.[10] Food is plentiful and continuously available, and little activity is required in our daily lives.

Eating more In America today, supermarkets, fast-food restaurants, and convenience marts make palatable, affordable food readily available to the majority of the population 24 hours a day. We are constantly bombarded with cues to eat: Advertisements entice us with tasty, inexpensive foods, and convenience stores, food courts, and vending machines tempt us with the sights and smells of fatty, sweet, high-calorie snacks. As a result, since 1970 the amount of energy available to us has increased by about 600 Calories per day, with the greatest increases in added fats, grains, dairy products, and sweeteners.[10] The accessibility of tempting treats stimulates **appetite**. Because appetite is triggered by external cues such as the sight or smell of food, it is usually

appetite A desire to consume specific foods that is independent of hunger.

Portion distortion • Figure 9.6

The burger and French fry portions served in fast-food restaurants today are two to five times larger than they were when fast food first appeared about 40 years ago. Soft-drink portion sizes have also escalated. A large fast-food soft drink today contains 32 ounces, providing about 300 Calories, and 20-oz bottles have replaced 12-oz cans in many vending machines.

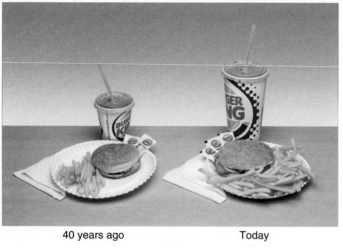

40 years ago   Today

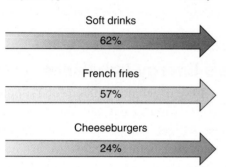

Soft drinks
62%

French fries
57%

Cheeseburgers
24%

Percentage increase in portion size

appetite, and not **hunger**, that makes us stop for an ice cream cone on a summer afternoon or give in to the smell

> **hunger** A desire to consume food that is triggered by internal physiological signals.

of freshly baked chocolate chip cookies while strolling through the mall. Studies examining the relationship between the food environment and BMI have found that people in communities with more fast-food or quick-service restaurants tend to have higher BMIs.[10]

In addition to having more enticing choices available to us, we consume more calories today because portion sizes have increased (**Figure 9.6**). The more food that is put in front of people, the more they eat.[10] Portion size is associated with body weight; being served and consuming larger portions is associated with weight gain, whereas small portions are associated with weight loss.[10]

Social changes over the past few decades have also contributed to the increase in the number of calories Americans consume. Busy schedules and an increase in the number of single-parent households and households with two working parents mean that families are often too rushed to cook meals at home. As a result, prepackaged, convenience, and fast-food meals have become mainstays. These foods are typically higher in fat and energy than foods prepared at home.

Moving less Along with America's rising energy intake, there has been a decline in the amount of energy Americans expend, both at work and at play. Fewer American adults today work in jobs that require physical labor. People drive to work rather than walk or bike, take elevators instead of stairs, use dryers rather than hang clothes outside, and cut the lawn with riding mowers rather than with push mowers. All these modern conveniences reduce the amount of energy expended daily (**Figure 9.7**). Americans are also less active during their leisure time because busy schedules and long days at work and commuting leave little time for active recreation. Instead, at the end of the day, people tend to sit in front of television sets, video games, and computers.

Inactivity is also contributing to excess body weight among children. In the 1960s, schools provided daily physical education classes, and children spent their after-school hours playing outdoors; today, they are more likely to spend their afternoons indoors with televisions, video

Activity reduces the risk of obesity • Figure 9.7

A typical office worker today walks only about 3000 to 5000 steps per day (2000 steps = approximately 1 mile). In contrast, in the Amish community—where automobiles and other modern conveniences are not allowed—a typical adult takes 14,000 to 18,000 steps a day. The overall incidence of obesity among the Amish is only 4%.[11]

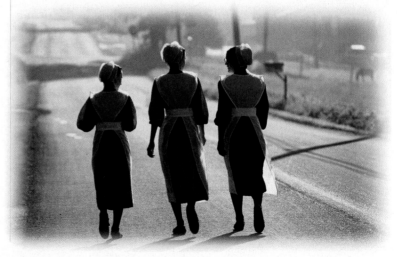

games, and computers. As a result, they burn fewer calories, snack more, and consequently gain weight. In the United States, 17% of children and adolescents ages 2 through 19 are obese.[12]

Balancing Energy Intake and Expenditure

The energy needed to fuel your body comes from the food you eat and the energy stored in your body. You use this energy to stay alive, process your food, move, and grow.

Energy intake The amount of energy you consume depends on what and how much you eat and drink. The carbohydrate, fat, protein, and alcohol consumed in food and drink all contribute energy: 4, 9, 4, and 7 Calories/gram, respectively (**Figure 9.8a**). Vitamins, minerals, and water, though essential nutrients, do not provide energy. You can determine your calorie intake by using food labels or looking up values in a food composition table or database (**Figure 9.8b**).

Energy expenditure The total amount of energy used by the body each day is called **total energy expenditure**. It includes the energy needed to maintain basic body functions as well as that needed to fuel physical activity and process food. In individuals who are growing or pregnant, total energy expenditure also includes the energy used to deposit new tissues. In women who are lactating, it includes the energy used to produce milk. A small amount of energy is also used to maintain body temperature in a cold environment.

For most people, about 60 to 75% of total energy expenditure is used for **basal metabolism**. Basal metabolism

> **basal metabolism** The energy expended to maintain an awake, resting body that is not digesting food.
>
> **basal metabolic rate (BMR)** The rate of energy expenditure under resting conditions. It is measured after 12 hours without food or exercise.

includes all the essential metabolic reactions and life-sustaining functions needed to keep you alive, such as breathing, circulating blood, regulating body temperature, synthesizing tissues, removing waste products, and sending nerve signals. The rate at which energy is used for these basic functions is the **basal metabolic rate (BMR)**. The energy expended for basal metabolism does *not* include the energy needed for physical activity or for the digestion and absorption of food.

BMR increases with increasing body weight and is affected by body composition because it takes more energy to maintain lean tissue than to maintain body fat (**Figure 9.8c**). BMR is generally higher in men than in women because men have a greater amount of lean body mass. BMR decreases with age, partly because of the decrease in lean body mass that occurs as we get older. BMR is also lower when calorie intake is consistently below the body's needs.[13] This drop in BMR reduces the amount of energy needed to maintain body weight. It is a beneficial adaptation in someone who is starving, but in someone who is trying to lose weight, it is frustrating because it makes weight loss more difficult.

Physical activity is the second major component of total energy expenditure. In most people, physical activity accounts for a smaller proportion of total energy expenditure than basal metabolism does—about 15 to 30% of energy requirements (**Figure 9.8d**). The energy we expend in physical activity includes both planned exercise and daily activities such as walking to work, typing, performing yard work, work-related activities, and even fidgeting. This **non-exercise activity thermogenesis (NEAT)** includes the energy expended for everything that is not sleeping, eating, or sports-like exercise. It accounts for the majority of the energy expended for activity and varies enormously, depending on an individual's occupation and daily movements.

The amount of energy used for activity depends on the size of the person, how strenuous the activity is, and the length of time it is performed. Because it takes more energy to move a heavier object, the amount of energy expended for many activities increases as body weight increases. More strenuous activities, such as jogging, use more energy than do less strenuous activities, such as walking, but if you walk for an hour, you will probably burn as many calories as you would by jogging for 30 minutes (Appendix I).

We also use energy to digest food and to absorb, metabolize, and store the nutrients from this food. The energy used for these processes is called either the **thermic effect of food (TEF)** or **diet-induced thermogenesis**. This energy expenditure causes body temperature to rise slightly for several hours after a person has eaten. The energy required

> **thermic effect of food (TEF)** or **diet-induced thermogenesis** The energy required for the digestion of food and absorption, metabolism, and storage of nutrients.

for TEF is estimated to be about 10% of energy intake but can vary, depending on the amounts and types of nutrients consumed (**Figure 9.8e**).

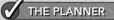
What you weigh is determined by the balance between how much energy you take in and how much energy you expend.

a. The number of calories in a food depends on how much carbohydrate, fat, and protein it contains. Each of these tacos contains 9 g of protein, 16 g of carbohydrate, and 13 g of fat. The energy content of each is:

(9 g × 4 Cal/g protein)
+ (16 g × 4 Cal/g carbohydrate)
+ (13 g × 9 Cal/g fat)
= 217 Cal.

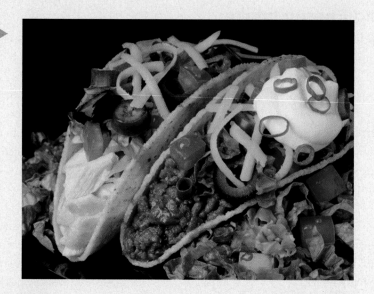

Nutrition Facts

Serving Size 8 fl oz (240mL)
Servings Per Container 2

Amount Per Serving

Calories 100

	%Daily Value*
Total Fat 0g	**0%**
Sodium 10 mg	**0%**
Total Carb 26g	**9%**
Sugars 25g	
Protein 0g	

Percent daily values are based on a 2,000 calorie diet.

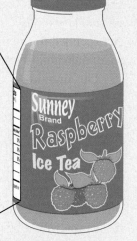

b. The Nutrition Facts panel shows the Calories per serving, but to know how many Calories your portion contains, you need to check the serving size. Often the portions of foods and beverages that people consume are larger than the servings listed on the label. As a result, they consume more calories than they think they do.

Ask Yourself

If you drank this entire bottle of iced tea, how many Calories would you be consuming?

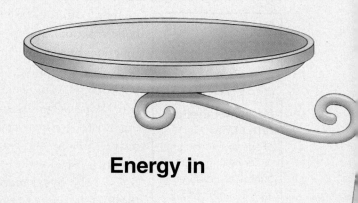

Energy in

c. The hood in the photo below collects expired air. Because aerobic metabolism uses oxygen and produces carbon dioxide, the amounts of these gases in expired air can be used to estimate the amount of energy that is being used. BMR can be measured in the morning, in a warm room, before rising, and at least 12 hours after food intake or activity. For convenience, measurements are often made after only 5 to 6 hours without food or exercise. This measurement, called the **resting metabolic rate (RMR)**, yields values about 10 to 20% higher than BMR values.[14]

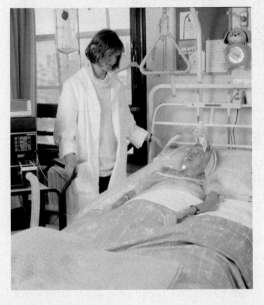

Factors that affect basal metabolism	
Factor	Effect
Higher lean body mass	↑
Greater height and weight	↑
Pregnancy	↑
Lactation	↑
Growth	↑
Low-calorie diet	↓
Starvation	↓
Fever	↑
Low thyroid hormone levels	↓
Stimulant drugs such as caffeine and tobacco	↑
Exercise	↑

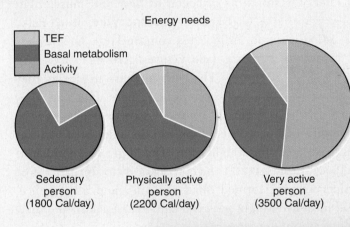

Energy needs

TEF
Basal metabolism
Activity

Sedentary person (1800 Cal/day) Physically active person (2200 Cal/day) Very active person (3500 Cal/day)

d. Sedentary people must plan their intake carefully so it does not exceed energy expenditure. More active people burn more calories for activity so they can eat more and still maintain their weight. Very active people, such as professional athletes, can actually burn more calories for activity than they do for basal metabolism.

Energy out

e. The amount of energy used to process the food we eat varies with the size and composition of the meal. A bigger meal produces a greater thermic effect of food (TEF). A high-fat meal yields a lower TEF than one high in carbohydrate or protein because dietary fat can be used and stored more efficiently.[15]

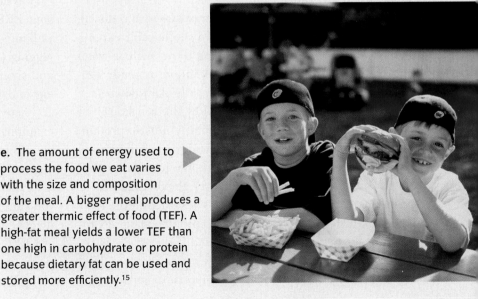

Energy balance: Storing and retrieving energy • Figure 9.9

When calories are consumed in excess of needs, they are stored, mostly as fat. If the excess calories are consumed as fat, they are easily stored as body fat. If the excess calories are consumed as carbohydrate, they are stored as glycogen or converted into fat. If excess calories are consumed as protein, they are converted into body fat. When calorie intake is less than needs, energy can be retrieved from stores. Glycogen and a small amount of body protein can be broken down to supply glucose, and triglycerides in adipose tissue can be broken down to supply fatty acids.

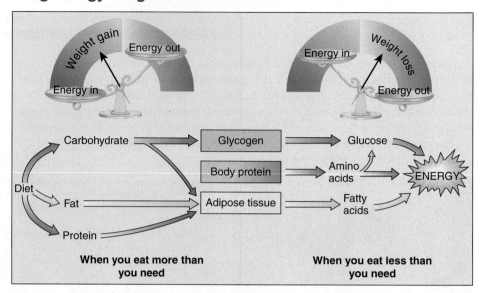

The basics of weight gain and weight loss

If you consume more energy than you expend, the excess energy is stored for later use (**Figure 9.9**). A small amount of energy is stored as glycogen in liver and muscle, but most is stored as triglycerides in **adipocytes**, which make up adipose tissue. Adipocytes contain large fat droplets

adipocyte A cell that stores fat.

(see Figure 5.11b in Chapter 5). The cells increase in size as they accumulate more fat, and they shrink as fat is removed. If intake exceeds needs over the long term, adipocytes enlarge, and the amount of body fat increases, causing weight gain. The larger the number of adipocytes, the greater the body's ability to store fat. Most adipocytes are formed during infancy and adolescence, but excessive weight gain can cause the formation of new adipocytes at any time of life.

Stored energy is used when energy intake is reduced, both in the short term, such as when you haven't eaten a meal for a few hours, and in the long term, such as when you are trying to lose weight. To maintain a steady supply of blood glucose, liver glycogen is broken down (see Figure 9.9). Glucose is also supplied by the breakdown of small amounts of body protein, primarily muscle protein, to yield amino acids. These amino acids can then be used to make glucose or produce ATP. Energy for tissues that don't require glucose is provided by the breakdown of stored fat (triglycerides). Nutrients consumed in the next meal replenish these stores, but with prolonged energy restriction, fat and protein are lost, and body weight is reduced. It is estimated that an energy deficit of about 3500 Calories results in the loss of a pound of adipose tissue.

Estimated Energy Requirements

The current recommendations for energy intake in the United States are the *Estimated Energy Requirements* (*EER*; see Chapter 2), the number of calories needed for a healthy individual to maintain his or her weight.[16] They are calculated using equations that take into account gender, age, height, weight, activity level, and life stage, all of which affect calorie needs.

To calculate your EER, you must first determine your physical activity level.[17] You can do this by keeping a daily log of your activities and recording the amount of time spent at each. Use **Figure 9.10** to help translate the amount of time you spend engaged in moderate-intensity or vigorous activity into an activity level (sedentary, low active, active, or very active). Each activity level corresponds to a numerical physical activity (PA) value that can be used to calculate your EER. For example, if you spend about an hour a day walking (a moderate-intensity activity) or about 30 minutes jogging (a vigorous activity), you are in the active category and should use the active PA value corresponding to your age and gender when calculating your EER.

Activity level has a significant effect on calorie needs. For example, a 22-year-old man who is 6 feet tall and weighs 185 pounds needs about 2770 Calories/day if he is sedentary but almost 600 more if he is at the active physical activity level.

Once you have determined your physical activity level, you can calculate your EER by entering your age, weight, height, and PA value (see Figure 9.10) into the appropriate EER prediction equation. **Table 9.1** provides equations for normal-weight adults and children age 9 and older. Equations for other groups are in Appendix A.

Physical activity level and PA value • Figure 9.10

Physical activity level, which is used to calculate EER, is categorized as sedentary, low active, active, or very active. A sedentary person spends about 2.5 hours per day engaged in the activities of daily living, such as housework, homework, and yard work. Adding activity moves the person into the low-active, active, or very-active category. Activity can be moderate or vigorous or a combination of the two; compared to moderate-intensity activity, vigorous activity will burn the same number of calories in less time.

An adult in the very-active category spends at least 2.5 hours per day in moderate-intensity activity or at least 1.25 hours in vigorous activity.

An active adult spends at least 60 minutes per day engaged in moderate-intensity activity or at least 30 minutes in vigorous activity.

An adult in the low-active category spends at least 30 minutes per day engaged in moderate-intensity activity or at least 15 minutes in vigorous activity.

An adult in the sedentary category engages only in activities of daily living and not in moderate-intensity or vigorous activities.

Ask Yourself

What are your activity level and corresponding PA value?

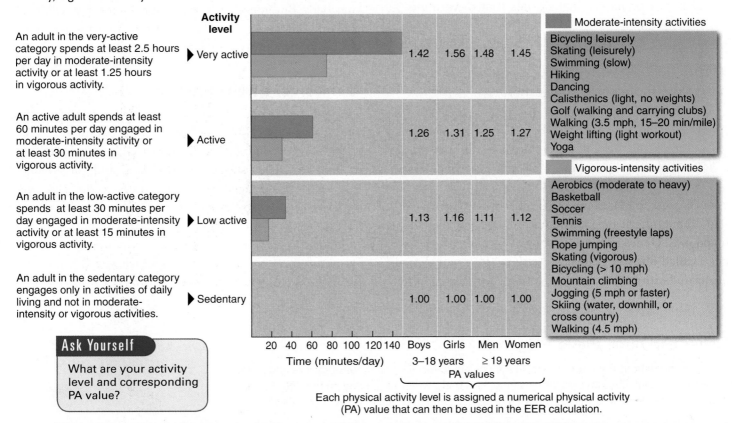

Each physical activity level is assigned a numerical physical activity (PA) value that can then be used in the EER calculation.

EER prediction equations   Table 9.1

Life stage	EER prediction equation*
Boys 9–18 years	EER = 88.5 − (61.9 × Age in yrs) + PA [(26.7 × Weight in kg) + (903 × Height in m)] + 25
Girls 9–18 years	EER = 135.3 − (30.8 × Age in yrs) + PA [(10.0 × Weight in kg) + (934 × Height in m)] + 25
Men ≥ 19 years	EER = 662 − (9.53 × Age in yrs) + PA [(15.91 × Weight in kg) + (539.6 × Height in m)]
Women ≥ 19 years	EER = 354 − (6.91 × Age in yrs) + PA [(9.36 × Weight in kg) + (726 × Height in m)]

For example, if you are an active 19-year-old male who weighs 72.7 kg and is 1.75 m tall, EER = 662 − (9.53 × 19 yrs) + 1.25[(15.91 × 72.7 kg) + (539.6 × 1.75 m)] = 3107 Cal/day

* These equations are appropriate for determining EER in normal-weight individuals. Equations that predict the amount of energy needed for weight maintenance in overweight and obese individuals are also available (see Appendix A).

CONCEPT CHECK

1. Why are more Americans obese today compared to 40 years ago?

2. What happens to energy stores when energy intake exceeds expenditure?

3. Which component of energy expenditure is easiest to modify?

4. What is your EER?

What Determines Body Size and Shape?

LEARNING OBJECTIVES

1. **Discuss** genetic and environmental factors that affect body weight.

2. **List** four physiological signals that determine whether you feel hungry or full.

3. **Describe** how hormones regulate body fat levels.

4. **Discuss** factors that cause some people to gain weight more easily than others.

 ou are probably shaped like your mother or your father. This is because the information that determines body size and shape is contained in the genes you inherit from your parents (**Figure 9.11**). Some of us inherit long, lean bodies, and others inherit huskier builds and the tendency to put on pounds. Genes involved in regulating body weight have been called **obesity genes**. More than 100 genes that are associated with body weight regulation have been identified;

it is estimated that 20 to 30 of these may contribute to obesity in humans.[17] Obesity genes are responsible for the production of proteins that affect how much food you eat, how much energy you expend, and the way fat is stored in your body. But genes are not the only factor; regardless of your genetic background, the lifestyle choices you make play an important role in determining what you weigh.

Genes vs. Environment

The genes you inherit play a major role in determining your body weight. If one or both of your parents is obese, your risk of becoming obese is increased by a factor of 2 or 3, and the risk increases with the magnitude of the obesity. By studying identical twins, who have the same genetic makeup, researchers have been able to determine that about 75% of the variation in BMI can be attributed to genes.[18,19] This means that the remaining 25% is determined by the environment in which you live and the lifestyle choices you make (see *Thinking It Through*).

Genes and body shape • Figure 9.11

The genes we inherit from our parents are important determinants of our body size and shape. The boy on the left inherited his father's long, lean body, whereas the boy on the right has his father's huskier build and will likely have a tendency to be overweight throughout his life.

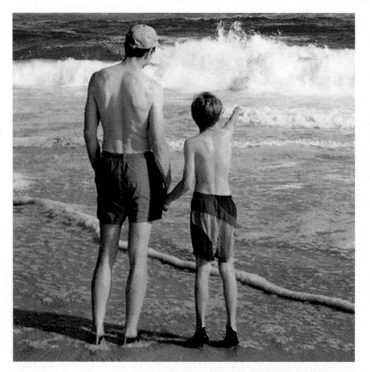 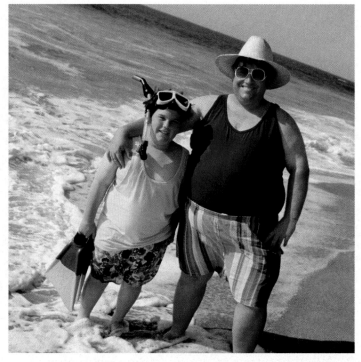

THINKING IT THROUGH

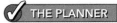
THE PLANNER

A Case Study on Genetics, Lifestyle, and Body Weight

Aysha was a chubby baby. Into her teens, she continued to be slightly overweight. Because her parents are both obese, no one was surprised by Aysha's size. During her freshman year at college, she gained 15 pounds and became resigned to the inevitability that she would be fat like her parents. Then she noticed that the choices many of her thin friends made—both in the foods they ate and how they spent their free time—were different from the choices she made. She decided to make some changes.

Aysha, now 23 years old, is 5 feet 4 inches tall and weighs 155 lb.

What is her BMI? Is it in the healthy range?
▼

Your answer:

By recording and analyzing her food intake for three days, Aysha determines that she consumes about 2450 Calories/day. By keeping an activity log, she estimates that a typical day includes 30 minutes of walking rapidly around campus—a moderate-intensity activity.

What is her EER?
▼

Your answer:

How does Aysha's EER compare with her intake? Is she in energy balance?
▼

Your answer:

Aysha decides to start exercising more and to cut down on her portions at meals and make healthier choices. Meal A, shown below, used to be her typical lunch, and Meal B is her new lunch.

How can Meal B have fewer calories even though it looks like more food?
▼

Your answer:

Why might Meal B satisfy hunger just as well as or better than Meal A?
▼

Your answer:

If Aysha adds an additional 30 minutes of moderate-intensity exercise every day, by how much will her EER increase?
▼

Your answer:

Do you think Aysha is destined to be overweight? Explain your answer.
▼

Your answer:

(Check your answers in Appendix J.)

Meal A

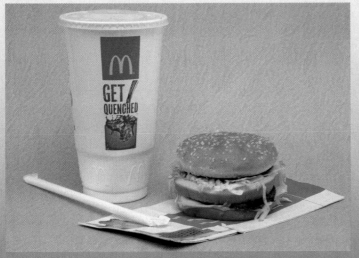

Meal B

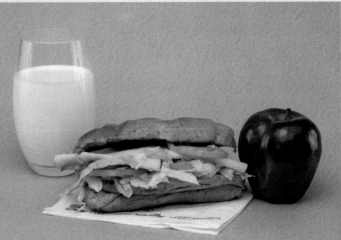

When individuals who are genetically susceptible to weight gain find themselves in an environment where food is appealing and plentiful and physical activity is easily avoided, obesity is a likely outcome but not the only possible one. If you inherit genes that predispose you to being overweight but carefully monitor your diet and exercise regularly, you can maintain a healthy weight. It is also possible for individuals with no genetic tendency toward obesity to end up overweight if they consume a high-calorie diet and get little exercise. The interplay between genetics and lifestyle is illustrated by the higher incidence of obesity in Pima Indians living in Arizona than in a genetically similar group of Pima Indians living in Mexico (**Figure 9.12**).[20]

Regulation of Food Intake and Body Weight

What we eat and how much we exercise vary from day to day, but body weight tends to stay relatively constant for long periods. The body compensates for variations in diet and exercise by adjusting energy intake and expenditure to keep weight at a particular level, or **set point**. This set point, which is believed to be determined in part by genes, explains why your weight remains fairly constant, despite the added activity of a weekend hiking trip, or why most people gain back the weight they lose when they follow a weight-loss diet.[23]

To regulate weight and fatness at a constant level, the body must be able to respond both to short-term changes in food intake and to long-term changes in the amount of stored body fat. Signals related to food intake affect hunger and **satiety** over a short period—from meal to meal—whereas signals from adipose tissue trigger the brain to adjust both food intake and energy expenditure for long-term weight regulation.

> **satiety** The feeling of fullness and satisfaction caused by food consumption that eliminates the desire to eat.

Genes vs. lifestyle • Figure 9.12

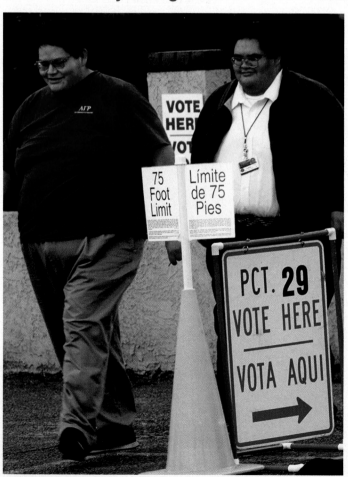

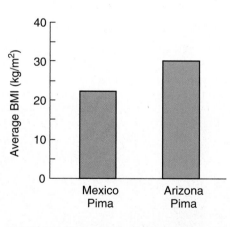

a. Genetic analysis of the Pima Indian population living in Arizona has identified a number of genes that may be responsible for this group's tendency to store excess body fat.[21] When this genetic susceptibility is combined with an environment that fosters a sedentary lifestyle and consumption of high-calorie, high-fat processed foods, the outcome is the strikingly high incidence of obesity seen in this population.

b. The Pima Indians of Mexico have the same genetic susceptibility to obesity as the Arizona Pimas but are farmers who work in the fields and consume the food they grow.[22] They still have higher rates of obesity than would be predicted from their diet and exercise patterns, suggesting that they possess genes that favor fat storage, but they are significantly less obese than the Arizona Pimas.[20]

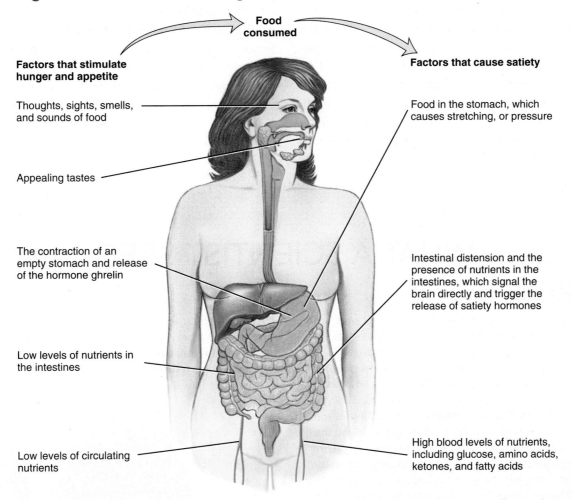

Food consumed

Factors that stimulate hunger and appetite

Thoughts, sights, smells, and sounds of food

Appealing tastes

The contraction of an empty stomach and release of the hormone ghrelin

Low levels of nutrients in the intestines

Low levels of circulating nutrients

Factors that cause satiety

Food in the stomach, which causes stretching, or pressure

Intestinal distension and the presence of nutrients in the intestines, which signal the brain directly and trigger the release of satiety hormones

High blood levels of nutrients, including glucose, amino acids, ketones, and fatty acids

Regulating how much we eat at each meal How do you know how much to eat for breakfast or when it is time to eat lunch? The physical sensations of hunger or satiety that determine how much you eat at each meal are triggered by signals from the gastrointestinal tract, levels of nutrients and hormones circulating in the blood, and messages from the brain.[24] Some signals are sent before you eat to tell you that you are hungry, some are sent while food is in the gastrointestinal tract, and some occur when nutrients are circulating in the bloodstream (Figure 9.13).

The hormone **ghrelin** may cause you to feel hungry around lunchtime, regardless of when and how much you ate for breakfast. Ghrelin, which is produced by the stomach, is believed to stimulate the desire to eat at usual mealtimes. Blood levels of ghrelin rise an hour or two before a meal and drop very low after a meal. Another hormone, peptide YY, causes a reduction in appetite. It is released from the gastrointestinal tract after a meal, and the amount released is proportional to the number of calories in the meal.[25]

Psychological factors can also affect hunger and satiety. Some people eat for comfort and to relieve stress. Others lose their appetite when they experience these emotions. Psychological distress can alter the mechanisms that regulate food intake.

Regulating how much we weigh over the long term Sometimes we don't pay attention to how full we are after a meal, and we make room for dessert anyway. If this happens often enough, it can cause an increase in body weight and fatness. To return fatness to a set level, the body must be able to monitor how much fat is present. Some of this information comes from hormones.

Leptin is a good example of a hormone that can affect body weight. Leptin is produced by the adipocytes. The amount produced is proportional to the size of the adipocytes, and the effect of leptin on energy intake and expenditure depends on the amount released (see *What a Scientist Sees*). Unfortunately, leptin regulation, like other regulatory mechanisms, is much better at preventing weight loss than at preventing weight gain. Obese individuals generally have high levels of leptin, but these levels are not effective at reducing calorie intake and increasing energy expenditure.[26]

Despite regulatory mechanisms that act to keep our weight stable, changes in physiological, psychological, and environmental circumstances cause the level at which body weight is maintained to change, usually increasing it over time. This supports the hypothesis that the mechanisms that defend against weight loss are stronger than those that prevent weight gain.[27]

WHAT A SCIENTIST SEES ✓ THE PLANNER

Leptin and Body Fat

The average person looking at the photo on the right sees a normal mouse and a very fat mouse. A scientist sees an explanation for obesity. Leptin acts in a part of the brain called the hypothalamus to help maintain body fat at a normal level. As shown in the diagram, the effect of leptin depends on how much of it is present. If the mouse loses weight, fat is lost from adipocytes, and less leptin is released, causing an increase in food intake and a decrease in energy expenditure. If the mouse gains weight, the adipocytes accumulate fat, and more leptin is released, triggering events that decrease food intake and increase energy expenditure.

The mouse on the left inherited a defective leptin gene, so it produces no leptin. Even when the adipocytes enlarge, leptin levels do not increase. The lack of leptin continues to signal the mouse to eat more and expend less energy. The mouse on the right also inherited a defective leptin gene, but treatment with leptin injections returned its weight to normal.

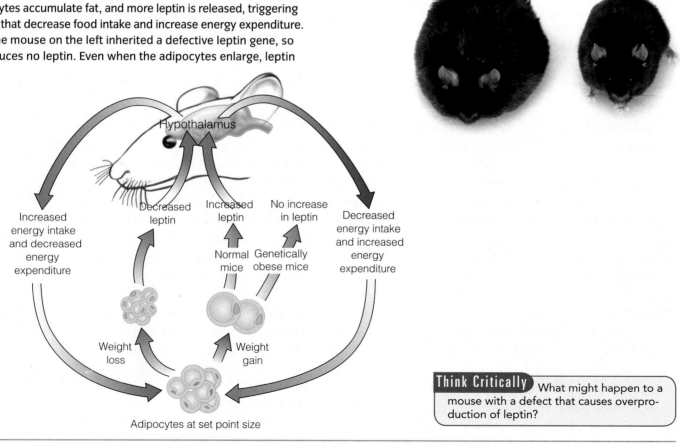

Adipocytes at set point size

> **Think Critically** What might happen to a mouse with a defect that causes overproduction of leptin?

Obese individuals use fewer calories for NEAT than their lean counterparts. When obese and lean individuals who do not engage in any planned exercise were compared, the lean people walked more and sat less, by about 2 hours per day, than the obese study subjects. If obese individuals could adopt the same patterns as the lean subjects, they would expend an extra 350 Calories per day.[28]

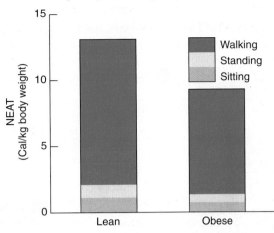

Why Do Some People Gain Weight More Easily?

A few cases of human obesity have been linked directly to defects in specific genes,[21] but mutations in single genes are not responsible for most human obesity. Rather, variations in many genes interact with one another and affect metabolic rate, food intake, fat storage, and activity level. These in turn affect body weight, determining why some of us stay lean and others put on pounds.

Some people, such as the Pima Indians discussed earlier, may gain weight more easily because they inherited genes that make them more efficient at using energy and storing fat. Throughout human history, starvation has threatened survival. Over time, the human body has evolved ways to conserve body fat stores and prevent weight loss. Individuals with the "thriftiest" metabolism would have been more likely to survive. In the United States today, however, food is abundant, so people who inherited these "thrifty genes" are more likely to be obese.

Some people may gain weight more easily because they inherit a tendency to expend less energy on activity. Even if they spend the same amount of time engaged in planned exercise as a lean person, their total energy expenditure may be lower because they expend less energy for NEAT activities, such as housework, walking between classes, fidgeting, and moving to maintain posture (**Figure 9.14**).

CONCEPT CHECK

1. **What** is the role of genes in regulating body weight?
2. **Why** do we feel hungry at about the same times every day?
3. **What** happens to leptin levels when you lose weight?
4. **Why** are some of us fat and some of us lean?

Managing Body Weight

LEARNING OBJECTIVES

1. **Evaluate** an individual's weight and medical history to determine whether weight loss is recommended.
2. **Discuss** the recommendations for the rate and amount of weight loss.
3. **Distinguish** between a good weight management program and a fad diet.
4. **Explain** how medications and surgery can promote weight loss.

Managing your body weight to keep it in the healthy range requires maintaining a balance between energy intake and energy expenditure. For some people, weight management may mean avoiding weight gain as they age by making healthy food choices, controlling portion size, and maintaining an active lifestyle. For others, it may mean making major lifestyle changes in order to reduce their weight into the healthy range and keep it there.

Weight-loss decisions • Figure 9.15

THE PLANNER ✓

To determine whether someone would benefit from weight loss, the first steps are to evaluate the person's current weight and weight history and review her or his medical history.[5]

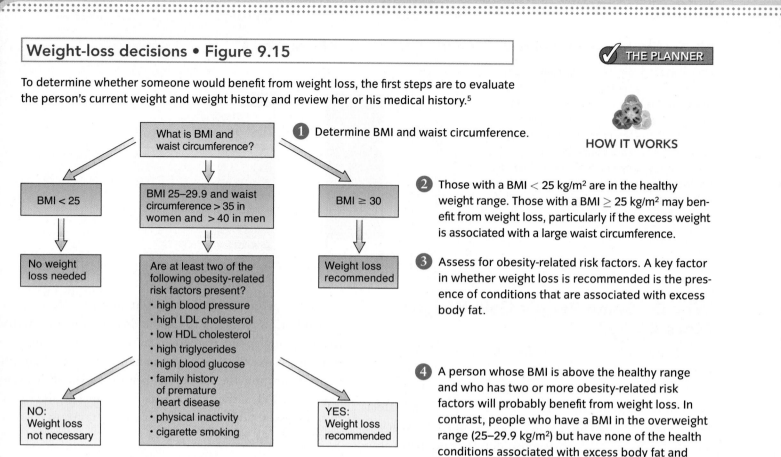

1 Determine BMI and waist circumference.

HOW IT WORKS

2 Those with a BMI < 25 kg/m² are in the healthy weight range. Those with a BMI ≥ 25 kg/m² may benefit from weight loss, particularly if the excess weight is associated with a large waist circumference.

3 Assess for obesity-related risk factors. A key factor in whether weight loss is recommended is the presence of conditions that are associated with excess body fat.

4 A person whose BMI is above the healthy range and who has two or more obesity-related risk factors will probably benefit from weight loss. In contrast, people who have a BMI in the overweight range (25–29.9 kg/m²) but have none of the health conditions associated with excess body fat and have a healthy lifestyle may not improve their health by losing weight.

Who Should Lose Weight?

These days, just about everybody wants to lose a few pounds or more, but not everyone who is concerned about their weight needs to lose weight in order to be healthy. The risks associated with carrying excess weight are related to the degree of the excess, the location of the excess fat, and the presence of other diseases or risk factors that often accompany excess body fat (**Figure 9.15**).

Weight-Loss Goals and Guidelines

Losing weight requires tipping the energy balance scale by eating less, exercising more, or some combination of the two. A pound of adipose tissue provides about 3500 Calories. Therefore, to lose a pound of fat, you need to decrease your intake and/or increase your expenditure by this amount. To lose a pound in a week, you would need to tip your energy balance by about 500 Calories/day.

The medical goal for weight loss in an overweight person is to reduce the health risks associated with being overweight. For most people, a loss of 5 to 15% of body weight will significantly reduce disease risk.[5] Losing weight slowly, at a rate of 1/2 to 2 lb/week, helps ensure that most of what is lost is fat and not lean tissue. The more severe energy restriction needed for rapid weight loss leads to greater losses of water and protein and causes a more significant drop in BMR. People who lose weight rapidly are more likely to regain the weight, leading to repeated cycles of weight loss and gain (**Figure 9.16**). Successful long-term weight management involves a combination of decreasing intake, increasing activity, and changing the behavior patterns that led to weight gain in the first place.

Decreasing energy intake For healthy weight loss, intake must be low in energy but high in nutrients in order to provide for all the body's nutrient needs (see *What Should I Eat?*). Even when choosing nutrient-dense foods, it is difficult to meet nutrient needs with an intake of fewer than 1200 Calories/day; therefore, dieters consuming less than this amount should take a multivitamin/multimineral supplement. Medical supervision is recommended if intake is below 800 Calories/day.

Yo-yo dieting • Figure 9.16

Repeated cycles of weight loss and gain, referred to as *weight cycling*, or *yo-yo dieting*, decrease the likelihood that future attempts at weight loss will be successful.[29]

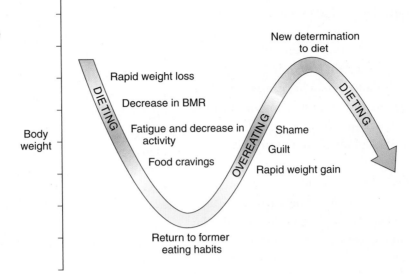

Body weight

DIETING
Rapid weight loss
Decrease in BMR
Fatigue and decrease in activity
Food cravings

OVEREATING

Return to former eating habits

New determination to diet

DIETING

Shame
Guilt
Rapid weight gain

Increasing physical activity Exercise increases energy expenditure and therefore makes weight loss easier. If food intake stays the same, adding enough exercise to expend 200 Calories five days a week will result in the loss of a pound in about three and a half weeks. Exercise also promotes muscle development, and because muscle is metabolically active tissue, increased muscle mass increases energy expenditure. In addition, physical activity improves overall fitness and relieves boredom and stress. Weight loss is maintained better when physical activity is included. The benefits of exercise are discussed more fully in Chapter 10.

WHAT SHOULD I EAT?
Weight Management

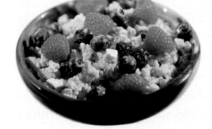

Balance your intake and output
- Know your calorie needs and monitor what you eat.
- Weigh yourself once a week; if the number goes up, cut down your calories.
- When you add dessert, add extra exercise.
- Watch your alcohol consumption and count the calories in alcoholic beverages.
- Don't snack while watching TV.

Cut down on calories
- Replace your sugar-sweetened soft drink with a glass of water with lemon.
- Have a plain burger, not one with a special sauce or an extra-large patty.
- Pour chips or crackers into a one-serving bowl rather than eating right from the bag or box.
- Bring your own lunch rather than eating out.

- Don't supersize—choose a small drink and a small order of fries.
- When you eat out, share an entrée with a friend or take some home for lunch the next day.

Increase activity
- Go for a bike ride.
- Try bowling or miniature golf instead of watching TV on Friday nights.
- Take a walk during your lunch break or after dinner.
- Play tennis; you don't have to be good to get plenty of exercise.
- Get off the bus one stop early.

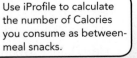

Use iProfile to calculate the number of Calories you consume as between-meal snacks.

To achieve and maintain a healthy body weight, the 2010 Dietary Guidelines for Americans recommend that adults engage in the equivalent of 150 minutes of moderate-intensity aerobic activity per week.[10] Those who are overweight may need to gradually increase their weekly minutes of aerobic physical activity over time and decrease calorie intake to achieve calorie balance and a healthy weight. The amount of activity needed to achieve and maintain a healthy body weight varies; some may need more than the equivalent of 300 minutes per week of moderate-intensity activity.

Modifying behavior After people lose weight, they typically go off their "diet." When eating patterns return to what they were previously, these dieters then regain the weight they lost. To manage your weight at a healthy level, you need to establish a pattern of food intake and exercise that allows you to enjoy foods and activities you like and that you can maintain throughout your life without gaining weight. Changing food consumption and exercise patterns requires identifying behaviors that led to weight gain and replacing them with new ones that promote and maintain weight loss. This can be accomplished through behavior modification (Figure 9.17).

> **behavior modification** A process that is used to gradually and permanently change habitual behaviors.

Managing America's weight To become a thinner nation, we need strategies that can help all Americans improve their food choices, reduce serving sizes, and increase their physical activity.[30] Although successful weight management ultimately depends on an individual's choices, food manufacturers and restaurants can help us cut calories by offering healthier foods and packaging or serving foods in smaller portions. Communities can help increase activity by providing parks, bike paths, and other recreational facilities for people of all ages. Businesses and schools can contribute by offering more opportunities for physical activity at the workplace and during the school day.

Even small changes, if they are consistent, can arrest the increase in obesity in the population. It has been estimated that a population-wide shift in energy balance of only 100 Calories/day, the equivalent of walking a mile or cutting out a scoop of ice cream, would prevent further weight gain in 90% of the population.[31]

Suggestions for Weight Gain

As difficult as weight loss is for some people, weight gain can be equally elusive for underweight individuals. The first step toward weight gain is a medical evaluation to rule out medical reasons for low body weight. This is particularly important when weight loss occurs unexpectedly. If low body weight is due to low energy intake or high energy expenditure, gradually increasing consumption of energy-dense foods is suggested. Energy intake can be increased by eating meals more frequently; adding healthy high-calorie snacks, such as nuts, peanut butter, or milkshakes, between meals; and replacing low-calorie drinks such as water and diet beverages with 100% fruit juices and milk.

To encourage a gain in muscle rather than fat, muscle-strengthening exercise should be a component of any weight gain program. This approach requires extra calories to fuel the activity needed to build muscles. These weight-gain recommendations apply to individuals who are naturally thin and have trouble gaining weight on the recommended energy intake. However, this dietary approach may not promote weight gain for those who limit intake because of an eating disorder.

Diets and Fad Diets

Want to lose 10 lb in just 5 days? What dieter wouldn't? People who are desperate to lose weight are prey to all sorts of diets that promise quick fixes. They willingly eat a single food for days at a time, select foods on the basis of special fat-burning qualities, and consume odd combinations at specific times of the day. Most diets, no matter how outlandish, will promote weight loss because they reduce energy intake. Even diets that focus on modifying fat or carbohydrate intake or promise to allow unlimited amounts of certain foods work because intake is reduced. The true test of the effectiveness of a weight-loss plan is whether it promotes weight loss that can be maintained over the long term.

People often don't recognize that if you lose weight, you need to eat less to stay at the lower weight. For example, an inactive 30-year-old, 5'4" woman who weighs 170 lb needs to consume about 2100 Calories/day to maintain her weight. If she loses 40 lb but does not change her activity level, she will need to consume only

ABCs of behavior modification • Figure 9.17

Behavior modification is based on the theory that behaviors involve three factors: antecedents or cues that lead to a behavior, the behavior itself, and the consequences of the behavior. These are referred to as the ABCs of behavior modification. The steps shown here can be used to identify and change undesirable behaviors.

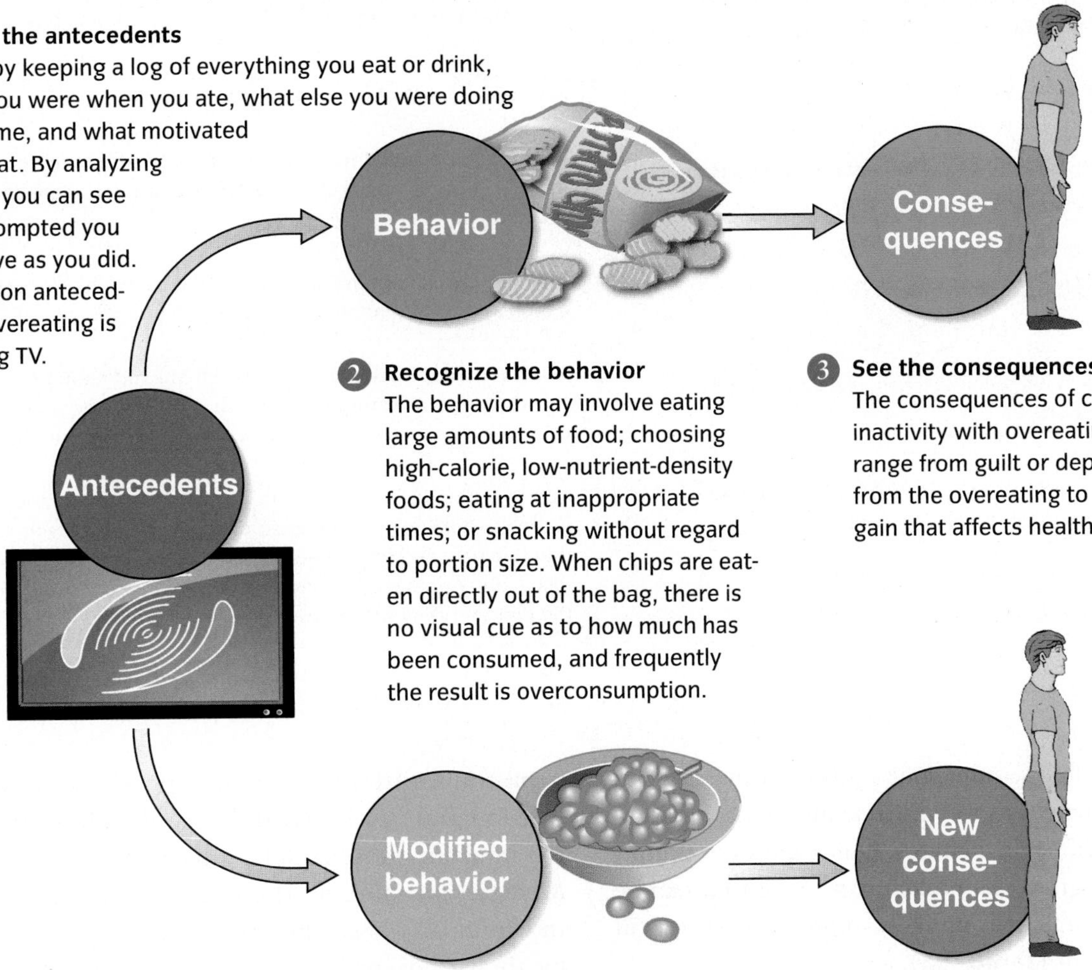

❶ **Identify the antecedents**
Do this by keeping a log of everything you eat or drink, where you were when you ate, what else you were doing at the time, and what motivated you to eat. By analyzing this log, you can see what prompted you to behave as you did. A common antecedent to overeating is watching TV.

Antecedents

Behavior

Conse-quences

❷ **Recognize the behavior**
The behavior may involve eating large amounts of food; choosing high-calorie, low-nutrient-density foods; eating at inappropriate times; or snacking without regard to portion size. When chips are eaten directly out of the bag, there is no visual cue as to how much has been consumed, and frequently the result is overconsumption.

❸ **See the consequences**
The consequences of combining inactivity with overeating may range from guilt or depression from the overeating to weight gain that affects health.

Modified behavior

New conse-quences

❹ **Modify the behavior**
The behavior can be modified by choosing smaller portions and lower-calorie snacks, such as fruit, while watching TV.

❺ **Enjoy the new consequences**
The new consequence may be a healthier weight and a sense of accomplishment.

about 1880 Calories to maintain her healthier reduced weight. If, once the weight is lost, she resumes her pre-weight-loss dietary pattern, eating 2100 Calories/day, she will regain all the lost weight.

Effective weight-management programs promote healthy weight-loss diets and encourage changes in the lifestyle patterns that led to weight gain. When selecting a program, look for one that is based on sound nutrition

Distinguishing between healthy diets and fad diets Table 9.2

A healthy diet . . .	A fad diet . . .
Promotes a healthy dietary pattern that meets nutrient needs, includes a variety of foods, suits food preferences, and can be maintained throughout life.	Limits food selections to a few food groups or promotes rituals such as eating only specific food combinations. As a result, it may be limited in certain nutrients and in variety.
Promotes a reasonable weight loss of 0.5 to 2 lb per week and does not restrict Calories to under 1200/day.	Promotes rapid weight loss of much more than 2 lb/week.
Promotes or includes physical activity.	Advertises weight loss without the need to exercise.
Is flexible enough to be followed when eating out and includes foods that are easily obtained.	May require a rigid menu or avoidance of certain foods or may include "magic" foods that promise to burn fat or speed up metabolism.
Does not require costly supplements.	May require the purchase of special foods, weight-loss patches, expensive supplements, creams, or other products.
Promotes a change in behavior. Teaches new eating habits. Provides social support.	Does not recommend changes in activity and eating habits, recommends an eating pattern that is difficult to follow for life, or provides no support other than a book that must be purchased.
Is based on sound scientific principles and may include monitoring by qualified health professionals.	Makes outlandish and unscientific claims, does not support claims that it is clinically tested or scientifically proven, claims that it is new and improved or based on some new scientific discovery, or relies on testimonials from celebrities or connects the diet to trendy places such as Beverly Hills.

and exercise principles, suits your individual preferences in terms of food choices as well as time and costs, and promotes long-term lifestyle changes. Quick fixes are tempting, but if the program's approach is not one that can be followed for a lifetime, it is unlikely to promote successful weight management (**Table 9.2**).

Some of the most common methods for reducing calorie intake include using exchange lists for diet planning, eating pre-portioned meals or liquid meals, and reducing the fat or carbohydrate content of the diet (**Figure 9.18**). All these methods cause weight loss by limiting, in one way or another, the number of calories consumed.

Weight-Loss Drugs and Supplements

Prescription drugs for the treatment of obesity include those that reduce appetite by affecting the activity of brain neurotransmitters (for example, phentermine, trade name Adipex) and those that decrease the absorption of fat in the intestine (for example, orlistat, brand name Xenical). Medications such as these are recommended only for individuals whose health is seriously compromised by their body weight: obese individuals (BMI greater than 30 kg/m^2) and overweight individuals with a BMI greater than or equal to 27 kg/m^2 who have two or more obesity-related risk factors or diseases.[5] One of the major disadvantages of drug treatment is that even if the drug promotes weight loss, the weight is usually regained when the drug is discontinued.

Like prescription drugs, over-the-counter weight-loss medications are regulated by the FDA and must adhere to strict guidelines regarding the dose per pill and the effectiveness of the ingredients. The FDA has approved only a limited number of substances for sale as nonprescription weight-loss medications. One of these is

Common dieting methods • Figure 9.18

a. Exchanges

Foods that are in the same exchange list, such as rice, bread, and potatoes, are similar in their energy and macronutrient content, so they can be exchanged for one another in a calorie-controlled diet (see Appendix E). Diets based on exchanges include a variety of foods and are likely to meet nutrient needs. They teach meal-planning skills that are easy to apply away from home and can be used over the long term.

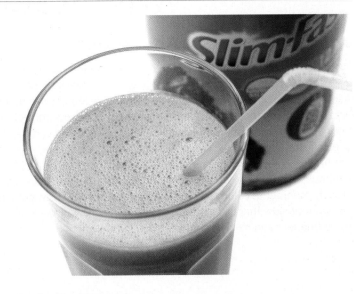

 = =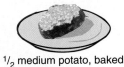

$^1/_3$ cup rice	1 slice bread	$^1/_2$ medium potato, baked
80 Calories	80 Calories	80 Calories
15 g carbohydrate	15 g carbohydrate	15 g carbohydrate
3 g protein	3 g protein	3 g protein
0–1 g fat	0–1 g fat	0–1 g fat

b. Liquid formulas

Liquid formulas and pre-portioned meals make it easier to eat less, but they are not practical when traveling or eating out, and they do not teach the food-selection skills needed to make a long-term lifestyle change. Programs that rely exclusively on liquid formulas are not recommended without medical supervision.

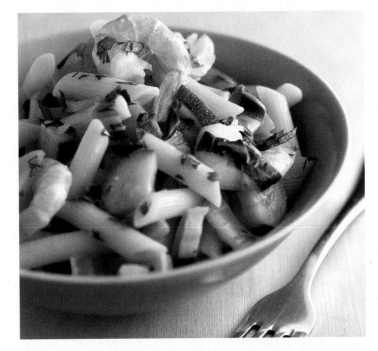

c. Low-fat diets

Low-fat diets typically reduce calorie intake because fat is high in calories. Low-fat diets can include large quantities of fresh fruits and vegetables, which are low in fat and calories and high in nutrients. But just because a food is low in fat does not mean it is low in calories. In the 1990s, low-fat cookies, crackers, and cakes flooded the market. These foods were low in fat but not in calories. When eaten in excess, they contributed to weight gain.

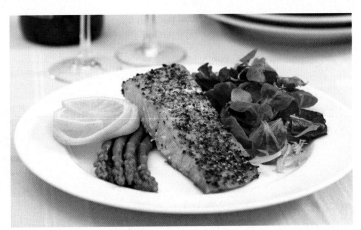

d. Low-carbohydrate diets

Where are the rice and potatoes? Low-carbohydrate diets limit grain products, fruits, some vegetables, and milk and allow unlimited quantities of meats and fats. Weight loss occurs on these diets because people eat less. This may be due to metabolic changes that suppress appetite, but intake is also reduced because of the monotony of the food choices.[32]

Think Critically Which of these diet plans will promote weight loss? Which are best for long-term weight management?

WHAT A SCIENTIST SEES

Alli: Blocking Fat Absorption

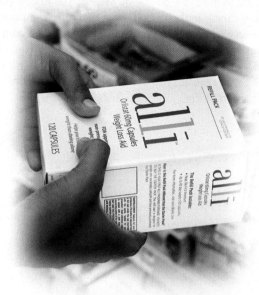

Alli is an over-the-counter version of a prescription weight-loss drug. Consumers see using it as a way to lose weight without needing to watch food intake quite so carefully. Scientists see that it acts by disabling the enzyme lipase. Lipase breaks triglycerides into fatty acids and monoglycerides, which are absorbed and can then be used or stored for energy. When Alli is present, the triglycerides are not broken down, so they cannot be absorbed. The undigested fat continues through the intestines and is eliminated in the feces. This cuts the number of calories from fat that get into your body, but it is not without side effects. Fat in the colon may cause gas, diarrhea, and more frequent and hard-to-control bowel movements.

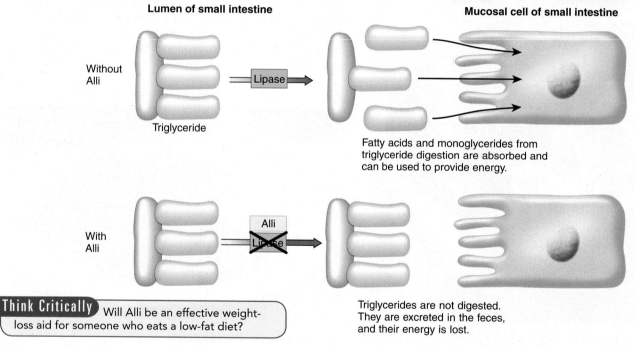

Lumen of small intestine — **Mucosal cell of small intestine**

Without Alli / Lipase / Triglyceride

Fatty acids and monoglycerides from triglyceride digestion are absorbed and can be used to provide energy.

With Alli / Alli / Lipase

Triglycerides are not digested. They are excreted in the feces, and their energy is lost.

Think Critically Will Alli be an effective weight-loss aid for someone who eats a low-fat diet?

---

a nonprescription version of orlistat (see *What a Scientist Sees*). As with prescription medications, any weight loss that occurs with over-the-counter weight-loss medications is usually regained when the product is no longer consumed.

In addition to weight-loss drugs, hundreds of dietary supplements claim to promote weight loss. As with other dietary supplements, weight-loss supplements are not strictly regulated by the FDA, so their safety and effectiveness may not have been carefully tested.

Some products claiming to be weight-loss supplements have been found to contain hidden prescription drugs or compounds that have not been adequately studied in humans.[33] It cannot be assumed that a product is safe simply because it is labeled a dietary supplement or as "herbal" or "all natural."

Weight-loss supplements that contain soluble fiber promise to reduce the amount you eat by filling up your stomach. Although they are safe, there is little evidence that they promote weight loss.[34] Hydroxycitric acid, conjugated linoleic acid, and chromium picolinate are weight-loss supplements that promise to enhance fat loss by altering metabolism so as to prevent the synthesis and deposition of fat. None of these has been shown to be effective for promoting weight loss in humans.[35–37] Supplements that boost energy expenditure, often called "fat burners," can be effective but have serious and potentially life-threatening side effects. One of the most popular and controversial herbal fat burners is ephedra, a stimulant that increases blood pressure and heart rate and constricts blood vessels. Due to safety concerns, the FDA banned it in 2004. After the ban was instituted, supplement manufacturers began substituting other herbal products, such as bitter orange, that contain similar stimulants and therefore may have similar side effects.[38] Fat burners also typically contain guarana, an herbal source of caffeine. Green tea extract is another popular supplement used to boost metabolism and aid weight loss. It appears to be safe if used in appropriate amounts, but studies have not shown it to enhance weight loss.[39]

Taking some dietary supplements results in weight loss through water loss—either because these supplements are diuretics or because they cause diarrhea. Water loss decreases body weight but does not cause a decrease in body fat. Herbal laxatives found in weight-loss teas and supplements include senna, aloe, buckthorn, rhubarb root, cascara, and castor oil. Overuse of these substances can have serious side effects, including diarrhea, electrolyte imbalances, and liver and kidney toxicity.[40]

Weight-Loss Surgery

A number of surgical procedures decrease body weight by altering the gastrointestinal tract so as to reduce food intake and absorption. At present, the most popular surgical approaches to treating obesity are **adjustable gastric banding**, which limits the amount of food that can be consumed, and **gastric bypass**, which reduces the amount of food that can be consumed and the amount that can be absorbed (**Figure 9.19**). These surgical approaches are

Gastric banding and bypass • Figure 9.19

a. Gastric banding involves surgically placing an adjustable band around the upper part of the stomach, creating a small pouch. The narrow opening between the stomach pouch and the rest of the stomach slows the rate at which food leaves the pouch. This promotes weight loss by reducing the amount of food that can be consumed at one time and slowing digestion. Gastric banding entails less surgical risk and is more easily reversible than other types of weight-loss surgery. ▼

b. Gastric bypass involves bypassing part of the stomach and small intestine by connecting the intestine to the upper portion of the stomach. Food intake is reduced because the stomach is smaller, and absorption is reduced because the small intestine is shortened. Gastric bypass entails short-term surgical risks and a long-term risk of nutrient deficiencies, particularly of vitamin B_{12}, folate, calcium, and iron, because absorption of these nutrients is reduced. ▼

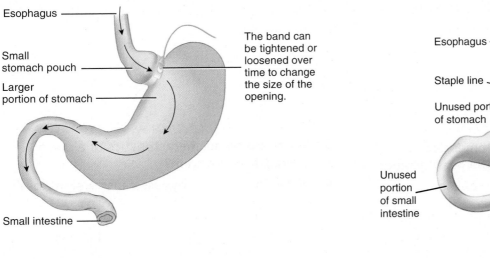

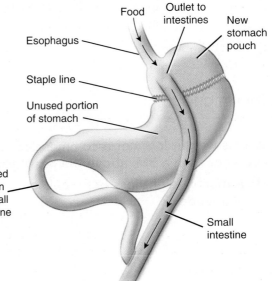

The Issue: The medical, social, and financial costs of obesity are well known. So is the fact that eating less and moving more will promote weight loss. However, these conventional methods do not always work. When they fail, is surgery a good weight-loss option?

Obesity surgery, known as bariatric surgery, is becoming increasingly common; over the past decade, there has been a 15-fold increase in the frequency of these procedures.[41] They are effective, and for some they can be lifesaving. When compared with conventional treatment, weight loss was greater at 2 years and at 10 years in those who had bariatric surgery. The incidence and control of type 2 diabetes, hypertension, high blood cholesterol, gastrointestinal reflux disease, and sleep apnea all improved with weight-loss surgery. In addition, quality of life improved in those who had surgery, and medication costs and overall mortality decreased.[41–43]

About 1 in 20 Americans is severely obese and meets the criteria for treatment with bariatric surgery, but only 0.6% of eligible patients have the surgery each year. This is because bariatric surgery is not without costs and complications.[44] Gastric bypass surgery costs about $18,000 to $22,000, and adjustable gastric banding costs about $17,000 to $30,000.[45] Complications are common; although fewer than 1% of patients die during or immediately after surgery, 20% experience adverse events.[46] The major complications, some of which require follow-up surgery, include ulcers, blockage of the opening from the stomach, leakage at the connection between the stomach and intestine, and pneumonia and blood clots. The incidence of gallstones and subsequent gallbladder removal is high because of the rapid weight loss that occurs following surgery. The reasons for the high complication rate include both the fact that anesthesia and surgery are risky in obese individuals and that there are a limited number of surgeons and surgical centers that have experience with these procedures.

In addition to surgical complications, there are long-term issues that affect digestion and lifestyle. Procedures that reduce the length of the small intestine reduce nutrient absorption and can lead to malnutrition if dietary supplements are not consumed for life. Some people feel very sleepy after eating and many experience chronic diarrhea, gas, foul-smelling stools, and other changes in bowel habits. Everyone who has this surgery must be willing to commit to changes in the types and amounts of food they consume. Eating too much or eating the wrong foods may induce vomiting or cause food to dump rapidly into the small intestine, leading to symptoms such as nausea, rapid pulse, and diarrhea. There are also emotional consequences to the changes in body size and eating habits that contribute to a post-bariatric surgery divorce rate that is higher than the national average.[47]

So is bariatric surgery a good option? It is expensive and risky, but results are impressive in the first decade after the procedures. For those who have high blood pressure, diabetes, high blood cholesterol, and arthritis, all of which are helped by weight loss,

recommended only in cases in which the health risks of obesity are greater than the health risks of the surgery (see *Debate: Is Surgery a Good Solution to Obesity?*).[5]

Another popular surgical procedure for reducing body fat is **liposuction**. This procedure involves inserting a large hollow needle under the skin into a fat deposit and literally vacuuming out the fat. Liposuction is considered a cosmetic procedure. It can reduce the amount of fat in a specific location, but it does not significantly reduce overall body weight.

CONCEPT CHECK

1. **Why** is weight loss not recommended for everyone with a BMI above the healthy range?
2. **How** much weight loss per week is recommended?
3. **What** are some characteristics of a good weight-loss program?
4. **How** does gastric bypass cause weight loss?

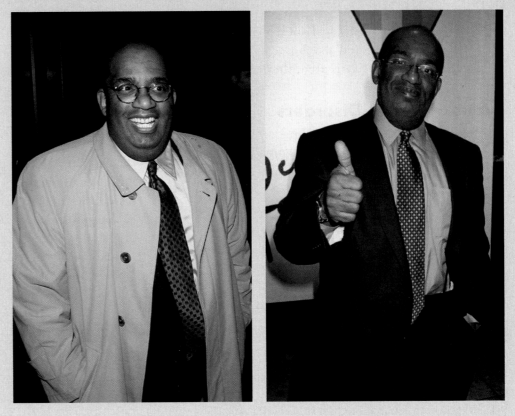

the surgery can enhance quality of life and even be lifesaving. But we still do not understand what the consequences of rearranging the GI anatomy will be in 20 or 30 years.

Think critically: In patients who have undergone bariatric surgery, some weight gain is common after 2 to 5 years. Why might this weight gain occur?

Significant weight loss is usually achieved 18 to 24 months after weight-loss surgery. NBC's *Today Show* weather anchor Al Roker lost 100 lb after undergoing gastric bypass surgery.

Eating Disorders

LEARNING OBJECTIVES

1. **Distinguish** among anorexia, bulimia, and binge-eating disorder.

2. **Describe** demographic and psychological factors associated with increased risk of developing an eating disorder.

3. **Discuss** how body ideal and the media affect the incidence of eating disorders.

4. **Explain** what is meant by the binge/purge cycle.

hat and how much people eat vary, depending on social occasions, emotions, time limitations, hunger, and the availability of food, but generally people eat when they are hungry, choose foods that they enjoy, and stop eating when they are satisfied. Abnormal or disordered eating occurs when a person is overly concerned with food, eating, and body size and shape. When the emotional

eating disorder A psychological illness characterized by specific abnormal eating behaviors, often intended to control weight.

aspects of food and eating overpower the role of food as nourishment, an **eating disorder** may develop. Eating disorders affect physical and nutritional health and psychosocial functioning. If untreated, they can be fatal.

sociocultural factors contribute to their development (**Figure 9.20**). Eating disorders can be triggered by traumatic events such as sexual abuse or by day-to-day occurrences such as teasing or judgmental comments by a friend or a coach. Eating disorders occur in people of all ages, races, and socioeconomic backgrounds, but some groups are at greater risk than others. Women are more likely than men to develop eating disorders. In the United States, eating disorders affect about 3% of girls and women between ages 18 and 30.[48] Professional dancers, models, and others who are concerned about maintaining a low body weight are most likely to develop eating disorders. Eating disorders commonly begin in adolescence, when physical, psychological, and social development is occurring rapidly.

bulimia nervosa An eating disorder characterized by the consumption of a large amount of food at one time (binge eating) followed by purging behaviors such as self-induced vomiting to prevent weight gain.

binge-eating disorder An eating disorder characterized by recurrent episodes of binge eating in the absence of purging behavior.

Types of Eating Disorders

Mental health guidelines define three categories of eating disorders: **anorexia nervosa**, **bulimia nervosa**, and **eating disorders not otherwise specified (ED-NOS)**, which includes **binge-eating disorder** and other abnormal eating behaviors that don't qualify as anorexia or bulimia (**Table 9.3**).

anorexia nervosa An eating disorder characterized by self-starvation, a distorted body image, and abnormally low body weight.

What Causes Eating Disorders?

We do not completely understand what causes eating disorders, but we do know that genetic, psychological, and

Distinguishing among eating disorders Table 9.3

Characteristic	Eating disorder		
	Anorexia nervosa	Bulimia nervosa	Binge-eating disorder
Body weight	Below normal (<85% of recommended)	Usually normal	Above normal
Binge eating	Possibly	Yes, at least twice a week for three months	Yes, at least twice a week for six months
Purging	Possibly	Yes, at least twice a week for three months	No
Restricts food intake	Yes	Yes	Yes
Body image	Dissatisfaction with body and distorted image of body size	Dissatisfaction with body and distorted image of body size	Dissatisfaction with body
Fear of being fat	Yes	Yes	Not excessive
Self-esteem	Low	Low	Low
Menstrual abnormalities	Absence of at least three consecutive periods	No	No
Typical age of onset	Preadolescence/adolescence	Adolescence/young adults	Adults of all ages

Factors contributing to eating disorders • Figure 9.20

Eating disorders are caused by a combination of genetic, psychological, and sociocultural factors. Although these disorders are not necessarily passed from parent to child, the genes that a person inherits contribute to psychological and biological characteristics that can predispose him or her to developing an eating disorder. When placed in the right sociocultural environment, an individual who carries such genes will be more likely than others to develop an eating disorder.

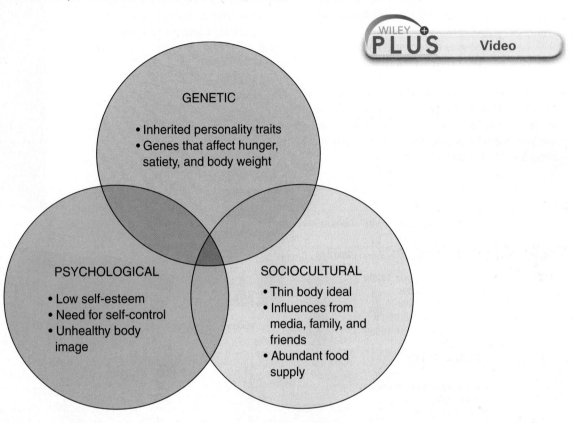

WILEY PLUS Video

GENETIC
- Inherited personality traits
- Genes that affect hunger, satiety, and body weight

PSYCHOLOGICAL
- Low self-esteem
- Need for self-control
- Unhealthy body image

SOCIOCULTURAL
- Thin body ideal
- Influences from media, family, and friends
- Abundant food supply

Psychological issues People with eating disorders often have low self-esteem. *Self-esteem* refers to the judgments people make and maintain about themselves—a general attitude of approval or disapproval about worth and capability. A poor **body image** contributes to low self-esteem. Eating disorders are characterized not only by dissatisfaction with one's body but also with distorted body image. Someone with a distorted body image is unable to judge the size of his or her own body. Thus, even if a young woman achieves a body weight comparable to that of a fashion model, she may continue to see herself as fat and strive to lose more weight.

> **body image** The way a person perceives and imagines his or her body.

People with eating disorders are often perfectionists who set very high standards for themselves and strive to be in control of their bodies and their lives. Despite their many achievements, they feel inadequate, defective, and worthless. They may use their relationship with food to gain control over their lives and boost their self-esteem. They believe that controlling their food intake and weight demonstrates their ability to control other aspects of their lives and solves other problems. Even if they feel insecure, helpless, or dissatisfied in other aspects of their lives, if they are in control of their food intake, weight, and body size, they can associate this control with success.

Nutrition InSight
Body ideal and body weight • Figure 9.21

a. A fuller figure is still desirable in many cultures. Young women in these cultures, such as the Zulu of South Africa, may struggle to gain weight in order to achieve what is viewed as the ideal female body. As television images of very thin Western women become more accessible, the Zulu cultural view of plumpness as desirable may be changing.[50]

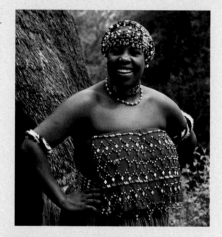

b. Thinness has not always been the beauty standard in the United States. This time line shows how the female body ideal has changed over the years. As female models, actresses, and other cultural icons have become thinner over the past several decades, the incidence of eating disorders has increased. ▼

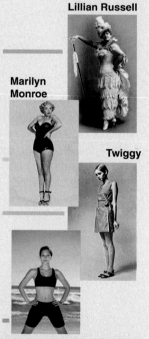

Lillian Russell

Actress Lillian Russell **1900** is considered a beauty at about 200 pounds

Marilyn Monroe

The thinner flapper **1920s** look becomes popular

The curvy figure of **1950s** Marilyn Monroe becomes the beauty standard

Twiggy

Twiggy, who weighs **1960s** less than 100 pounds, is the leading model

Jane Fonda's workout **1980s** book is a best seller

The fashion ideal today is thin but well muscled **Today**

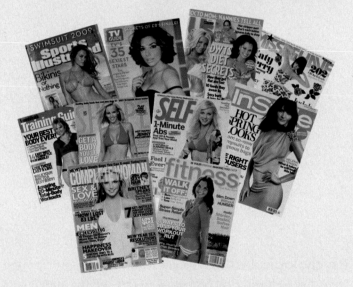

c. Magazine covers and advertisements emphasize thinness as a standard for female beauty. These "ideal" bodies are frequently atypical of normal, healthy women. Fashion models today weigh 23% less than the average female. Although many women strive for this thin ideal, only 1% of young women have a chance of being as thin as a supermodel.[51]

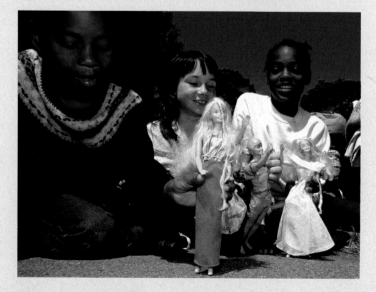

d. The toys that children play with set a cultural standard for body ideal. Little girls playing with Barbie dolls want to be like Barbie when they grow up, and boys playing with Superman, Batman, or GI Joe action figures want to be like them. This includes looking like them. Unfortunately, Barbie's measurements would be virtually unachievable if Barbie were life-sized. The same is true of the big chest, muscular arms and legs, and flat stomach with "six-pack" abs seen on male action figures.

Sociocultural issues What is viewed as an "ideal" body differs across cultures and has changed throughout history (**Figure 9.21**). Cultural ideals about body size are linked to body image and the incidence of eating disorders.[49] Eating disorders occur in societies where food is abundant and the body ideal is thin. They do not occur in societies where food is scarce and people must worry about where their next meal is coming from.

U.S. culture today is a culture of thinness. Messages about what society views as a perfect body—the ideal that we should strive for—are constantly delivered by television, movies, magazines, advertisements, and even toys. Tall, lean fashion models adorn billboards and magazine covers. Thinness is associated with beauty, success, intelligence, and vitality. A young woman facing a future in which she must be independent, have a prestigious job, maintain a successful love relationship, bear and nurture children, manage a household, and keep up with fashion trends can become overwhelmed. Unable to master all these roles, she may look for some aspect of her life that she can control. Food intake and body weight are natural choices because thinness is associated with success. These messages about how we should look are hard to ignore and can create pressure to achieve this ideal body. But it is a standard that is very difficult to meet—a standard that is contributing to disturbances in body image and eating behavior.

Although men currently represent a small percentage of people with eating disorders, the numbers are increasing.[52] This is likely due to increasing pressure to achieve an ideal male body. Advertisements directed at men are showing more and more exposed skin, with a focus on well-defined abdominal and chest muscles.

Anorexia Nervosa

Anorexia means lack of appetite, but in the case of the eating disorder anorexia nervosa, it is a desire to be thin, rather than a lack of appetite, that causes individuals to decrease their food intake. Anorexia nervosa is characterized by severe weight loss, **amenorrhea**, constipation, and restlessness. It affects about 1% of female adolescents in the United States. The average age of onset is 17 years. There is a 5% death rate in the first two years, and the death rate can reach 20% in untreated individuals.[48]

The psychological component of anorexia nervosa revolves around an overwhelming fear of gaining weight, even in individuals who are already underweight. It is not uncommon for individuals with anorexia to feel that they would rather be dead than fat. Anorexia is also characterized by disturbances in body image or perception of body size that prevent those with this disorder from seeing themselves as underweight even when they are dangerously thin. People with this disorder may use body weight and shape as a means of self-evaluation: "If I weren't so fat, everyone would like and respect me, and I wouldn't have other problems." However, no matter how much weight they lose, they do not gain self-respect, inner assurance, or the happiness they seek. Therefore, they continue to restrict their intake and use other behaviors to lose weight.

The most obvious behaviors associated with anorexia are those that contribute to the maintenance of a body weight that is 15% or more below normal. These behaviors include restriction of food intake, binge-eating and purging episodes in some patients, strange eating rituals, and excessive activity (**Figure 9.22**). For some individuals

amenorrhea
Delayed onset of menstruation or the absence of three or more consecutive menstrual cycles.

A day in the life of a person with anorexia • Figure 9.22

For individuals with anorexia, food and eating become an obsession. In addition to restricting the total amount of food they consume, people with anorexia develop personal diet rituals, limiting certain foods and eating them in specific ways. Although they do not consume very much food, they are preoccupied with food and spend an enormous amount of time thinking about it, talking about it, and preparing meals for others. Instead of eating, they move the food around the plate and cut it into tiny pieces.

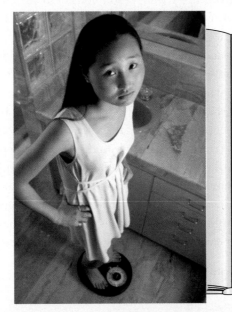

Dear Diary,
For breakfast today I had a cup of tea. For lunch I ate some lettuce and a slice of tomato, but no dressing. I cooked dinner for my family. I love to cook, but it is hard not to taste. I tried a new chicken recipe and served it with rice and asparagus. I even made a chocolate cake for dessert but I didn't even lick the bowl from the frosting. When it came time to eat, I only took a little. I told my mom I nibbled while cooking. I pushed the food around on my plate so no one would notice that I only ate a few bites. I was good today – I kept my food intake under control. The scale says I have lost 20 pounds, but I still look fat.

A day in the life of a person with bulimia • Figure 9.23

The amount of food consumed during a binge varies but is typically on the order of 3400 Calories, while a normal young woman may consume only about 2000 Calories in an entire day. Self-induced vomiting is the most common purging behavior. At first a physical maneuver such as sticking a finger down the throat is needed to induce vomiting, but patients eventually learn to vomit at will. Bingeing and purging are followed by intense feelings of guilt and shame.

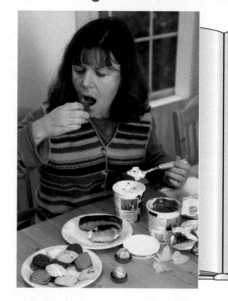

Dear Diary,

Today started well. I stuck to my diet through breakfast, lunch, and dinner, but by 8 PM I was feeling depressed and bored. I thought food would make me feel better. Before I knew it I was at the convenience store buying two pints of ice cream, a large bag of chips, a one pound package of cookies, half dozen candy bars, and a quart of milk. I told the clerk I was having a party. But it was a party of one. Alone in my dorm room I started by eating the chips, then polished off the cookies and the candy bars, washing them down with milk and finishing with the ice cream. Luckily no one was around so I was able to vomit without anyone hearing. I feel weak and guilty but also relieved that I got rid of all those calories. Tomorrow, I will start a new diet.

---

with anorexia, the increase in activity is surreptitious, such as going up and down stairs repeatedly or getting off the bus a few stops too early. For others, the activity takes the form of strenuous physical exercise. They may become fanatical athletes and feel guilty if they cannot exercise. They link exercise and eating, so a certain amount of exercise earns them the right to eat, and if they eat too much, they must pay the price by adding extra exercise. They do not stop when they are tired; instead, they train compulsively beyond reasonable endurance.

The first obvious physical manifestation of anorexia is weight loss. As weight loss becomes severe, symptoms of starvation begin to appear. Starvation affects mental function, causing the person to become apathetic, dull, exhausted, and depressed. Fat stores are depleted. Other symptoms that appear include muscle wasting, inflammation and swelling of the lips, flaking and peeling of the skin, growth of fine hair (called lanugo) on the body, and dry, thin, brittle hair on the head. In females, estrogen levels drop, and menstruation becomes irregular or stops. In males, testosterone levels decrease. In the final stages of starvation, the person experiences abnormalities in electrolyte and fluid balance and cardiac irregularities. Suppression of immune function leads to infection, which further increases nutritional needs.

The goal of treatment for anorexia nervosa is to help resolve the underlying psychological and behavioral problems while providing for physical and nutritional rehabilitation. Treatment requires an interdisciplinary team of nutritional, psychological, and medical specialists and

typically requires years of therapy. The goal of nutrition intervention is to promote weight gain by increasing energy intake and expanding dietary choices.[48] In more severe cases of anorexia hospitalization is required so food intake and exercise behaviors can be controlled. Intravenous nutrition may be necessary to keep a patient with anorexia alive. Some people with anorexia make full recoveries, but about half have poor long-term outcomes—remaining irrationally concerned about weight gain and never achieving normal body weight. Some patients with anorexia also transition to bulimia nervosa.[53]

Bulimia Nervosa

Bulimia comes from the Greek *bous* ("ox") and *limos* ("hunger"), denoting hunger of such intensity that a person could eat an entire ox. The term *bulimia nervosa* was coined in 1979 by a British psychiatrist who suggested that bulimia consists of powerful urges to overeat in combination with a morbid fear of becoming fat and avoidance of the fattening effects of food by inducing vomiting and/or abusing purgatives.[54]

Like anorexia, bulimia is characterized by an intense fear of becoming fat and a negative body image, accompanied by a distorted perception of body size. Because self-esteem is highly tied to impressions of body shape and weight, people with bulimia may blame all their problems on their appearance. They are preoccupied with the fear that once they start eating, they will not be able to stop. They may engage in continuous dieting, which leads to a preoccupation with food. They are often socially isolated and may avoid situations that will expose them to food, such as going to parties or out to dinner; thus they become further isolated.

Bulimia typically begins with food restriction motivated by the desire to be thin. Overwhelming hunger may finally cause the dieting to be interrupted by a period of overeating. Eventually a pattern develops that consists of semi-starvation interrupted by periods of gorging. During a binge-eating episode, a person with bulimia experiences a sense of lack of control. Binges usually last less than two hours and occur in secrecy. Eating stops when the food runs out or when pain, fatigue, or an interruption intervenes. The amount of food consumed in a binge may not always be enormous, but the individual perceives it as a binge episode (**Figure 9.23**).

After binge episodes, individuals with bulimia use various behaviors to eliminate the extra calories and prevent weight gain. Some use behaviors such as fasting or excessive exercise, but most use purging behaviors such as vomiting or taking laxatives, diuretics, or other medications. Self-induced vomiting does eliminate some of the food before the nutrients have been absorbed, preventing weight gain, but laxatives and diuretics cause only water loss. Nutrient absorption is almost complete before food enters the colon, where laxatives have their effect. The weight loss associated with laxative abuse is due to dehydration. Diuretics also cause water loss, but via the kidney rather than the GI tract. They do not cause fat loss.

It is the purging portion of the binge/purge cycle that is most hazardous to health. Vomiting brings stomach acid into the mouth. Frequent vomiting can cause tooth decay, sores in the mouth and on the lips, swelling of the jaw and salivary glands, irritation of the throat and esophagus, and changes in stomach capacity and the rate of stomach emptying.[48] It also causes broken blood vessels in the face due to the force of vomiting, as well as electrolyte imbalance, dehydration, muscle weakness, and menstrual irregularities. Laxative and diuretic abuse can also lead to dehydration and electrolyte imbalance.

The overall goal of therapy for people with bulimia nervosa is to reduce or eliminate bingeing and purging behavior by separating the patients' eating behavior from their emotions and their perceptions of success and promoting eating in response to hunger and satiety. Psychological issues related to body image and a sense of lack of control over eating must be resolved. Nutritional therapy must address physiological imbalances caused by purging episodes as well as provide education on nutrient needs and how to meet them. Treatment has been found to speed recovery, especially if it is provided soon after symptoms begin, but for some women, this disorder may remain a chronic problem throughout life.[55]

Binge-Eating Disorder

Binge-eating disorder is the most common eating disorder. Unlike anorexia and bulimia, binge-eating disorder is not uncommon in men, who account for about 40% of cases. It is most common in overweight individuals (**Figure 9.24**). Individuals with binge-eating disorder engage in recurrent

A day in the life of a person with binge-eating disorder • Figure 9.24

People with binge-eating disorder often seek help for their weight rather than for their disordered eating pattern. It is estimated that 10 to 15% of people enrolled in commercial weight-loss programs suffer from this disorder.[56]

Dear Diary,
I got on the scale today. What a mistake! My weight is up to 250 pounds. I hate myself for being so fat. Just seeing that I gained more weight made me feel ashamed – all I wanted to do was bury my feelings in a box of cookies or a carton of ice cream. Why do I always think the food will help? Once I started eating I couldn't stop. When I finally did I felt even more disgusted, depressed, and guilty. I am always on a diet but it is never long before I lose control and pig out. I know my eating and my weight are not healthy but I just can't seem to stop.

Other eating disorders Table 9.4

Eating disorder	Who is affected	Characteristics and consequences
Anorexia athletica	Athletes in weight-dependent sports such as dance, figure skating, gymnastics, track and field, cycling, wrestling, and horse racing	Engaging in compulsive exercise to lose weight or maintain a very low body weight. Can lead to more serious eating disorders and serious health problems, including kidney failure, heart attack, and death.
Female athlete triad	Female athletes in weight-dependent sports	A triad of disordered eating, amenorrhea, and osteoporosis. The energy restriction, along with high levels of exercise, causes amenorrhea. Low estrogen levels then interfere with calcium balance, eventually causing reductions in bone mass and an increased risk of bone fractures (discussed further in Chapter 10).
Bigorexia (muscle dysmorphia or reverse anorexia)	Bodybuilders and avid gym-goers; more common in men than in women	An obsession with being small and underdeveloped. Those affected believe that their muscles are inadequate, even when they have good muscle mass. They become avid weight lifters and may experiment with steroids or other muscle-enhancing drugs.
Avoidance emotional disorder	Children	Similar to anorexia nervosa in that the child avoids eating and experiences weight loss and the other physical symptoms of anorexia. However, there is no distorted body image or fear of weight gain.
Selective eating disorder	Children	Children with this disorder will eat only a few foods, mostly those high in carbohydrate. If the disorder continues for long periods, it increases the risk of malnutrition.
Night-eating syndrome	Obese adults and those experiencing stress	A disorder that involves consuming most of the day's calories late in the day or at night. People with this disorder—which contributes to weight gain—are tense, anxious, upset, or guilty while eating. A similar disorder, in which a person may eat while asleep and have no memory of the events, is called nocturnal sleep-related eating disorder (NS-RED) and is considered a sleep disorder, not an eating disorder.
Pica	Pregnant women, children, people with psychiatric disturbances and developmental disabilities, people whose family or ethnic customs include eating certain nonfood substances, people who are hungry and try to ease hunger and cravings with nonfood substances	Craving and eating nonfood items such as dirt, clay, paint chips, plaster, chalk, laundry starch, coffee grounds, and ashes. Depending on the items consumed, pica can cause perforated intestines and contribute to mineral deficiencies or intestinal infections (discussed further in Chapter 11).
Diabulimia (insulin misuse)	People with type 1 diabetes	Type 1 diabetes is a disease that forces patients to focus on food portions and body weight. This may cause some to become preoccupied with their weight and to control it by withholding insulin. Without insulin, glucose cannot enter cells to provide fuel, blood levels rise, and weight drops. Uncontrolled blood sugar can lead to blindness, kidney disease, heart disease, nerve damage, and amputations.

episodes of binge eating but do not regularly engage in purging behaviors.

The major complications of binge-eating disorder are the health problems associated with obesity, which include diabetes, high blood pressure, high blood cholesterol levels, gallbladder disease, heart disease, and certain types of cancer. Treatment of binge-eating disorder involves counseling to improve body image and self-acceptance; a healthy, nutritious diet; increased exercise to promote weight loss; and behavior therapy to reduce bingeing.

Eating Disorders in Special Groups

Although anorexia and bulimia are most common in women in their teens and 20s, eating disorders occur in both genders and all age groups. Both male and female athletes are at high risk for eating disorders, with an incidence of 10 to 20%.[57] Eating disorders occur during pregnancy and are becoming more frequent among younger children due to social values about food and body weight. They also occur in individuals with diabetes. A number of less common eating disorders appear in special groups in the general population (Table 9.4).

Preventing and Getting Treatment for Eating Disorders

Because eating disorders are often triggered by weight-related criticism, elimination of this type of behavior can help prevent them. Another important target for reducing the incidence of eating disorders is the media. If the unrealistically thin body ideal presented by the media could be altered, the incidence of eating disorders would likely decrease. Even with these interventions, however, eating disorders are unlikely to go away entirely. Education through schools and communities about the symptoms and complications of eating disorders can help people identify friends and family members who are at risk and persuade those with early symptoms to seek help.

The first step in preventing individuals from developing eating disorders is to recognize those who are at risk. Early intervention can help prevent at-risk individuals from developing serious eating disorders. Excessive concerns about body weight, having friends who are preoccupied with weight, being teased by peers about weight, and family problems all predispose a person to developing an eating disorder.

Once an eating disorder has developed, the person usually does not get better on his or her own. The actions of family members and friends can help people suffering from eating disorders get help before their health is impaired. But it is not always easy to persuade a friend or relative with an eating disorder to agree to seek help. People with eating disorders are good at hiding their behaviors and denying the problem, and often they do not want help. When confronted, one person might be relieved that you are concerned and willing to help, whereas another might be angry and defensive. When approaching someone about an eating disorder, it is important to make it clear that you are not forcing the person to do anything he or she doesn't want to do. Continued encouragement can help some people agree to seek professional help.

CONCEPT CHECK   STOP

1. **Which** eating disorder is characterized by extreme weight loss? Which is characterized by excess weight?

2. **What** factors contribute to the higher incidence of eating disorders among women than among men?

3. **What** is meant by body image?

4. **How** does a food binge differ from "normal" overeating?

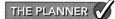

Summary

1 Body Weight and Health 310

- More Americans today are **overweight** and **obese** than ever before, as seen in this obesity map. Excess body fat increases the risk of chronic diseases such as diabetes, heart disease, high blood pressure, and certain types of cancer.

Obesity on the rise • Figure 9.1

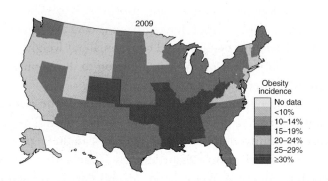

- **Body mass index (BMI)** can be used to evaluate the health risks of a particular body weight and height. Measures of **body composition** can be used to determine the proportion of a person's weight that is due to fat. Excess **visceral fat** is a greater health risk than excess **subcutaneous fat**.

2 Energy Balance 315

- Americans are getting fatter because they are consuming more calories due to poor food choices and larger portion sizes, as illustrated in the photo, and moving less due to modern lifestyles in which computers, cars, and other conveniences reduce the amount of energy expended in work and play.

Portion distortion • Figure 9.6

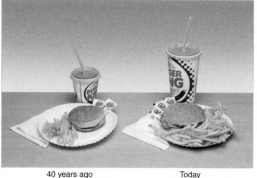

- The principle of **energy balance** states that if energy intake equals energy expenditure, body weight will remain constant. Energy is provided to the body by the carbohydrate, fat, and protein in the food we eat. This energy is used to maintain **basal metabolic rate (BMR)**, to support activity, and for the **thermic effect of food (TEF)**. When excess energy is consumed, it is stored, primarily as fat in **adipocytes**, causing weight gain. When energy in the diet does not meet needs, energy stores in the body are used, and weight is lost.

- The energy needs of healthy people can be predicted by calculating their Estimated Energy Requirements (EER). A person's EER depends on gender, age, life stage, height, weight, and level of physical activity.

3 What Determines Body Size and Shape? 322

- The genes people inherit affect their body size and shape, as illustrated by the father and son shown here, but environmental factors and personal choices concerning the amount and type of food consumed and the amount and intensity of exercise performed also affect body weight.

Genes and body shape • Figure 9.11

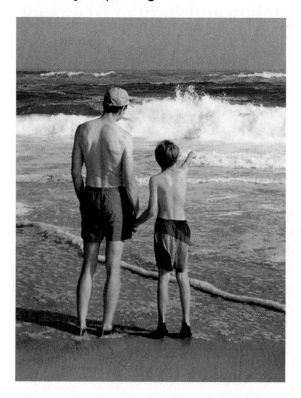

- **Hunger** and **satiety** from meal to meal are regulated by signals from the gastrointestinal tract, hormones, and levels of circulating nutrients. Signals from fat cells, such as the release of **leptin**, regulate long-term energy intake and expenditure.

- Inheriting an efficient metabolism or expending less energy through **nonexercise activity thermogenesis (NEAT)** may contribute to obesity.

4 Managing Body Weight   327

- Weight loss is recommended for those with a BMI above the healthy range who have excess body fat and a large waist circumference or who have health conditions associated with obesity.

- Weight management involves adjusting energy intake and expenditure to lose or maintain weight and **behavior modification** to keep weight in a healthy range over the long term. To lose a pound of adipose tissue, energy expenditure must be increased or intake decreased by approximately 3500 Calories. Slow, steady weight loss of 1/2 to 2 lb/week is more likely to be maintained than rapid weight loss.

- If being **underweight** is not due to a medical condition, weight gain can be accomplished by increasing energy intake and lifting weights to increase muscle mass.

- A good weight-loss program is one that promotes physical activity and a wide variety of nutrient-dense food choices, does not require the purchase and consumption of special foods or combinations of foods, and can be followed for life.

- Drug therapy and surgery are recommended only for those whose health is seriously compromised by their body weight. Currently, the most popular surgical approaches to treating obesity are **gastric bypass**, shown here, and **adjustable gastric banding**.

Gastric bypass • Figure 9.19b

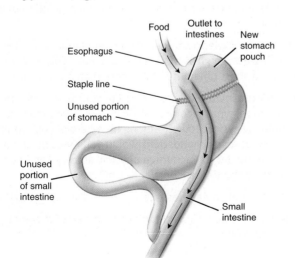

5 Eating Disorders   337

- **Eating disorders** are psychological disorders that involve dissatisfaction with body weight. **Anorexia nervosa** involves self-starvation, resulting in an abnormally low body weight as shown here. **Bulimia nervosa** is characterized by repeated cycles of binge eating followed by purging and other behaviors to prevent weight gain. **Binge-eating disorder** is characterized by bingeing without purging. People with this disorder are typically overweight.

A day in the life of a person with anorexia • Figure 9.22

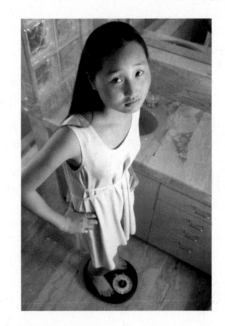

- Eating disorders are caused by a combination of genetic, psychological, and sociocultural factors. The lean body ideal in the United States is believed to contribute to disturbances in **body image** that lead to eating disorders. Treatment involves medical, psychological, and nutritional intervention to stabilize health, change attitudes about body size, and improve eating habits while supplying an adequate diet.

Key Terms

- adipocyte 320
- adjustable gastric banding 335
- amenorrhea 341
- anorexia nervosa 338
- appetite 315
- basal metabolic rate (BMR) 317
- basal metabolism 317
- behavior modification 330
- binge-eating disorder 338
- body composition 313

- body image 339
- body mass index (BMI) 311
- bulimia nervosa 338
- eating disorder 338
- eating disorders not otherwise specified (EDNOS) 338
- energy balance 315
- extreme obesity or morbid obesity 312

- gastric bypass 335
- ghrelin 325
- hunger 316
- lean body mass 311
- leptin 326
- liposuction 336
- nonexercise activity thermogenesis (NEAT) 317
- obese 310
- obesity genes 322

- overweight 310
- resting metabolic rate (RMR) 319
- satiety 324
- set point 324
- subcutaneous fat 315
- thermic effect of food (TEF) or diet-induced thermogenesis 317
- total energy expenditure 317
- underweight 312
- visceral fat 315

Online Resources

- For more information on controlling the global obesity crisis, go to www.who.int/nutrition/topics/obesity/en/index.html.

- For more information on preventing obesity in children, go to the 2010 Dietary Guidelines, at www.health.gov/dietaryguidelines/.

- For more information on balancing energy intake with expenditure, go to the 2010 Dietary Guidelines, at www.health.gov/dietaryguidelines/.

- For more information on healthy weight control, go to http://win.niddk.nih.gov.

- For more information on nutrition and eating disorders, go to www.nutrition.gov/ and click on Nutrition and Health Issues.

- Visit your *WileyPLUS* site for videos, animations, podcasts, self-study, and other media that will aid you in studying and understanding this chapter.

Critical and Creative Thinking Questions

1. Stephanie wants to lose 10 lb. She finds an app for her cell phone that allows her to track her calories in and calories out. The program says she can lose a pound a week by limiting her Calories to 1500/day and adding enough exercise to burn 300 Calories/day. Her intake and exercise Calories for three days are shown here. Is she meeting her goals? Is her current energy balance realistic and healthy for the long term?

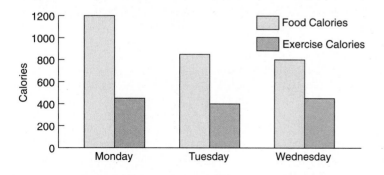

2. Beth is 22 years old and has a BMI in the healthy range. Discuss the steps she can take to prevent weight gain as she gets older.

3. If a race of humans evolved on an island where food was always abundant, how might this have affected the frequency of different types of genes that affect the regulation of body weight?

4. Use your knowledge of food intake regulation to explain why drinking a large glass of water would make you feel less hungry for a short time but not for more than an hour or so.

5. If you were invited to offer advice to your town's planning committee, what recommendations would you make to help promote physical activity among members of your community? What recommendations would you make for the middle school in order to encourage physical activity and healthy eating among the students and staff?

6. Why is leptin sometimes referred to as a *lipid thermostat*?

7. Discuss how bulimia might affect each side of the energy balance equation.

8. A late-night TV advertisement promotes a diet pill that is supposed to cause a weight loss of 10 lb in the first week. Assuming that you did not change your activity, how many Calories would you have to eliminate from your diet *each day* to lose 10 lb of adipose tissue in a week? Based on your calculation, do you think it is possible to lose 10 lb of fat in one week? Why or why not?

9. Design a weight-loss plan for someone who is 20 years old, eats in the dorm cafeteria, and is 40 lb overweight.

What is happening in this picture?

Sumo wrestlers train for many hours each day and eat huge amounts of food. The result is a high BMI and a large waist but surprisingly little visceral fat.

Think Critically

1. Why do these individuals have a low level of visceral fat?
2. Do you think they are at risk for diabetes and heart disease?
3. What type of fat is hanging over the belt of this wrestler?
4. What may happen if this wrestler retires and stops exercising but keeps eating large amounts of food?

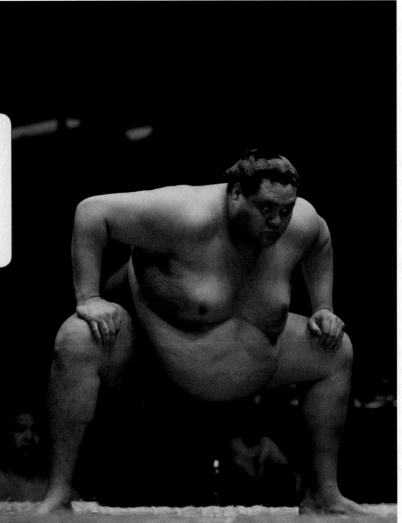

Self-Test

(Check Your Answers In Appendix K.)

1. Basal metabolic rate (BMR) _____.
   a. is a small component of energy expenditure.
   b. includes the energy needed for kidney function and heartbeat.
   c. includes the energy needed for exercise.
   d. is measured after 2 hours without food or exercise.
   e. is the energy needed to maintain body weight.

2. Excess body fat increases the risk of _____.
   a. diabetes
   b. high blood cholesterol
   c. certain cancers
   d. high blood pressure
   e. all of the above

3. In order to calculate a person's BMI, you need to know the person's _____.
   a. height and weight
   b. age and activity level
   c. lean body mass and waist circumference
   d. gender and weight
   e. gender and body composition

4. Which of the following has not contributed to the rising incidence of overweight and obesity in the United States?
   a. Americans use less energy in the activities of their daily lives than they used to.
   b. Portion sizes of our food have increased.
   c. We have ready access to food 24 hours a day.
   d. Our genetics have changed.
   e. The number of people who work at jobs requiring strenuous physical labor has decreased.

5. Which group is least likely to develop an eating disorder?
   a. ballet dancers   d. actresses
   b. fashion models   e. middle-aged men
   c. female gymnasts

6. Which eating disorder is characteristic of people who are overweight?
   a. anorexia   c. bulimia
   b. bigorexia   d. binge-eating disorder

7. The method of determining body composition shown here relies on what principle to determine the amount of body fat?
   a. Fat is less dense than water.
   b. Fat does not conduct electricity.
   c. The amount of subcutaneous fat is representative of total body fat.
   d. The extent to which X-rays penetrate fat is different from the extent to which they penetrate other tissues.

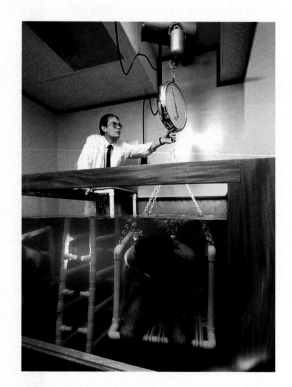

8. EER _____.
   a. is the amount of energy needed to reduce body weight to a healthy level
   b. is the amount of energy you expend daily
   c. increases if you lose weight
   d. increases in adults as they get older
   e. decreases if you exercise more

9. Which statement about leptin is true?

   a. Someone with a defective leptin gene will most likely be obese.

   b. More leptin is released as adipocytes shrink.

   c. High leptin levels stimulate food intake and reduce energy expenditure.

   d. Most human obesity is due to abnormalities in the leptin gene.

   e. Leptin is better at defending against weight gain than against weight loss.

10. Long-term healthy weight loss is based on all of the following principles except _____.

    a. increasing physical activity

    b. adopting lifelong changes in eating habits

    c. eating specific combinations of foods that increase the number of calories burned

    d. keeping portion sizes moderate

    e. making nutrient-dense choices

11. Which statement about the type of body fat labeled by the letter A is false?

    a. This type of fat storage increases the risk of heart disease, diabetes, and high blood pressure.

    b. This type of fat storage can be reduced by eating grapefruit.

    c. This type of fat storage increases after menopause.

    d. This type of fat storage is more common in men than women.

    e. This type of fat storage can be reduced through exercise.

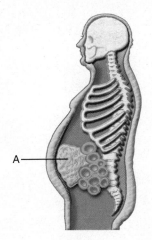

12. This chart most likely shows the distribution of energy expenditure in which of the following people?

    a. a cyclist who trains for 6 hours a day

    b. an office worker who gets no exercise other than gardening

    c. a young adult who works out for 90 minutes a day

    d. an elderly man who is bedridden

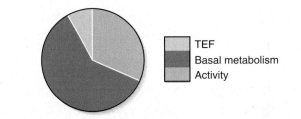

TEF
Basal metabolism
Activity

13. True or false: It is possible for someone who is 50 lb overweight to be in energy balance.

    a. True   b. False

14. True or false: Everyone with a BMI in the overweight or obese range is at risk for weight-related health problems.

    a. True   b. False

15. Which of the following is not a characteristic of anorexia nervosa?

    a. a fear of gaining weight

    b. a normal body weight

    c. a preoccupation with food

    d. an abnormal menstrual cycle

    e. a distorted body image

THE PLANNER ✓

Review your Chapter Planner on the chapter opener and check off you completed work.

Nutrition, Fitness, and Physical Activity

Introduced in 2001, the Segway revolutionized personal transport. Through a complex interaction of gyroscopes, electronics, and human control, the unusual upright contraption remains an eye-catcher a decade later. It allows vigilant security guards to zip about shopping malls or college campuses and tour groups to dash through parks and urban landscapes with barely any exertion.

Technology is a means of simplifying tasks. Even animals use "tools" of one sort or another to minimize the expenditure of energy: Chimpanzees poke sticks into anthills to gather a meal rather than exhaustively dig into the hill; sea otters break open shellfish with rocks. As human technology has produced more and more labor-saving devices, physical exertion has decreased for larger and larger segments of the population. Concurrently—

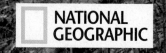

particularly in the developed world—the amount of food consumed per capita has increased.

As the Segway and other technological innovations continue to ease the daily physical challenges and exertions we face, we have to pay a lot more attention to what we eat and to how much activity we need to remain healthy. If we do not, and simply let machines do the work, we may no longer be able to move without them.

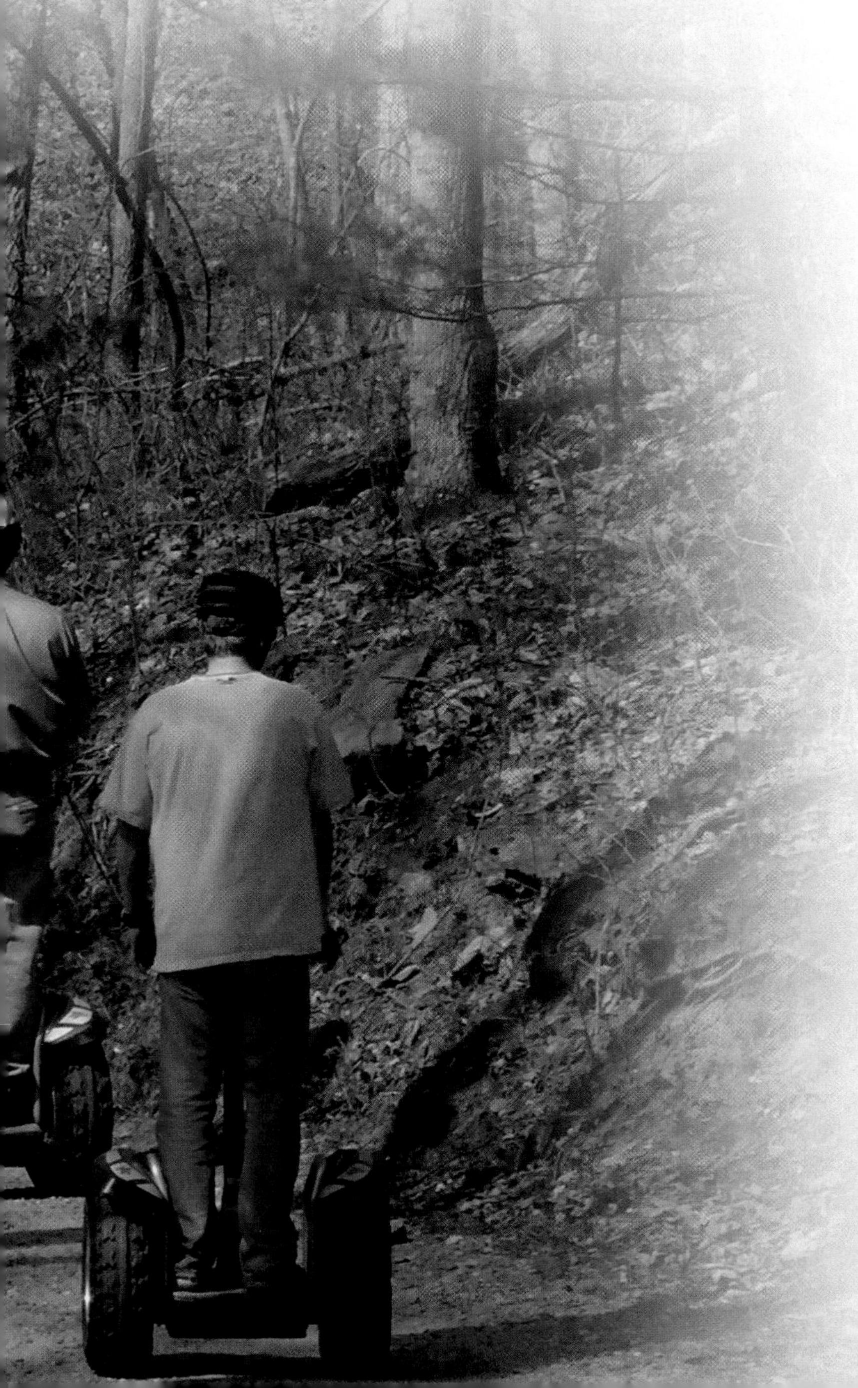

CHAPTER OUTLINE

CHAPTER PLANNER ✓

- ❑ Stimulate your interest by reading the introduction and looking at the visual.
- ❑ Scan the Learning Objectives in each section:
  p. 354 ❑   p. 357 ❑   p. 361 ❑   p. 367 ❑   p. 376 ❑
- ❑ Read the text and study all figures and visuals. Answer any questions.

Analyze key features

- ❑ Nutrition InSight, p. 354 ❑   p. 366 ❑
- ❑ Process Diagram, p. 362 ❑
- ❑ What a Scientist Sees, p. 364 ❑   p. 378 ❑
- ❑ Thinking it Through p. 375 ❑
- ❑ Stop: Answer the Concept Checks before you go on:
  p. 357 ❑   p. 360 ❑   p. 366 ❑   p. 376 ❑   p. 381 ❑

End of chapter

- ❑ Review the Summary, Online Resources, and Key Terms.
- ❑ Answer the Critical and Creative Thinking Questions.
- ❑ Answer What is happening in this picture?
- ❑ Complete the Self-Test and check your answers.

Physical Activity, Fitness, and Health

LEARNING OBJECTIVES

1. **Describe** the characteristics of a fit individual.
2. **Explain** what is meant by the overload principle.
3. **Evaluate** the impact of exercise on health.
4. **Discuss** the role of exercise in weight management.

 xercise improves your **fitness** and overall health. This is true whether your fitness goal is to be able to walk around the block easily or to perform optimally in athletic competitions. Exercise, along with an adequate diet, is important in maintaining health and reducing the risk of chronic diseases such as cardiovascular disease and obesity.

When you exercise, changes occur in your body: You breathe harder, your heart beats faster, and your muscles stretch and strain. If you exercise regularly, you adapt to the exercise you perform and as a result can continue for a few minutes longer, lift a heavier weight, or stretch a millimeter farther.

> **fitness** A set of attributes related to the ability to perform routine physical activities without undue fatigue.

This is known as the **overload principle**: The more you do, the more you are capable of doing. For example, if you run a given distance three times a week, in a few weeks you can run farther; if you lift heavy books for a few days, by the next week you have more muscle and can lift more books more easily. These adaptations improve your overall fitness.

> **overload principle** The concept that the body adapts to the stresses placed on it.

The Four Components of Fitness

A person's fitness is defined by his or her endurance, strength, flexibility, and body composition (**Figure 10.1**). A fit person can continue an activity for a longer period than an unfit person can before fatigue forces him or her to stop, but fitness is more than just stamina. Being fit also reduces the risk of chronic disease and makes weight management easier.

Cardiorespiratory endurance How long you can jog or ride your bike depends on the ability of your cardiovascular

Nutrition InSight   The components of fitness • Figure 10.1

a. The cardiovascular and respiratory systems are strengthened by aerobic exercise, such as jogging, bicycling, and swimming. To be considered aerobic, an activity must be performed at an intensity that is low enough for you to carry on a conversation but high enough that you cannot sing while exercising.

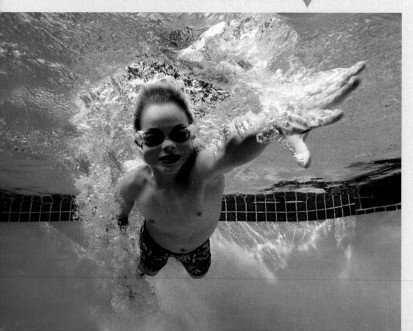

b. Weight lifting stresses the muscles, causing them to adapt by increasing in size and strength—a process called **hypertrophy**. The larger, stronger muscles can lift the same weight more easily. Muscles that are not used due to a lapse in weight training, injury, or illness become smaller and weaker. This process is called **atrophy**. Thus, there is truth to the saying "Use it or lose it."

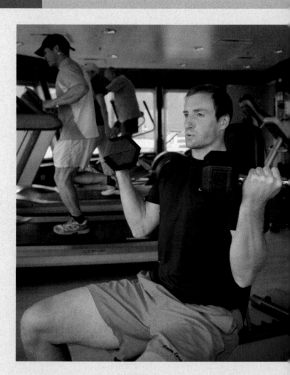

cardiorespiratory endurance The efficiency with which the body delivers to cells the oxygen and nutrients needed for muscular activity and transports waste products from cells.

aerobic exercise Endurance exercise that increases heart rate and uses oxygen to provide energy as ATP.

aerobic capacity The maximum amount of oxygen that can be consumed by the tissues during exercise. Also called maximal oxygen consumption, or VO_2 max.

and respiratory systems, referred to jointly as the cardiorespiratory system, to deliver oxygen and nutrients to your tissues and remove wastes. **Cardiorespiratory endurance** is enhanced by regular **aerobic exercise (Figure 10.1a)**.

Regular aerobic exercise strengthens the heart muscle and increases the amount of blood pumped with each heartbeat. This in turn decreases **resting heart rate**, the rate at which the heart beats when the body is at rest to supply blood to the tissues. The more fit you are, the lower your resting heart rate and the more blood your heart can pump to your muscles during exercise. In addition to increasing the amount of oxygen-rich blood that is pumped to your muscles, regular aerobic exercise increases the ability of your muscles to use oxygen to produce ATP. Your body's maximum ability to generate ATP using aerobic metabolism is called your **aerobic capacity**,

or VO_2 max. Aerobic capacity is a function of the ability of the cardiorespiratory system to deliver oxygen to the cells and the ability of the cells to use oxygen to produce ATP. The greater your aerobic capacity, the more intense activity you can perform before lack of oxygen affects your performance.

Muscle strength and endurance Greater **muscle strength** enhances the ability to perform tasks such as pushing or lifting. In daily life, this could mean lifting a gallon of milk off the top shelf of the refrigerator with one hand, carrying a full trash can out to the curb, or moving a couch into your new apartment. Greater **muscle endurance** enhances your ability to continue repetitive muscle activity, such as shoveling snow or raking leaves. Muscle strength and endurance are increased by repeatedly using muscles in activities that require moving against a resisting force. This type of exercise is called **muscle-strengthening exercise**, strength-training exercise, or resistance-training exercise and includes activities such as weight lifting and calisthenics **(Figure 10.1b)**.

muscle-strengthening exercise Activities that are specifically designed to increase muscle strength, endurance, and size; also called strength-training exercise or resistance-training exercise.

c. Flexibility makes everyday tasks easier and can improve athletic performance. Too-tight muscles, tendons, and ligaments restrict motion at the joints, decreasing stride or stroke length and increasing the amount of energy needed to move the joints. Regularly moving limbs, the neck, and the torso through their full range of motion helps increase and maintain flexibility. ▼

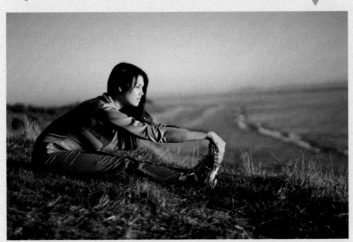

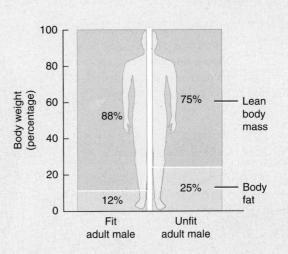

d. A fit person has more muscle mass than an unfit person of the same height and weight. Engaging in aerobic exercise and muscle-strengthening exercise has a positive impact on body composition, reducing body fat, and increasing the proportion of lean tissue.

Physical Activity, Fitness, and Health **355**

Flexibility When you think of fitness, you may picture someone with bulging muscles, but fitness also involves flexibility. Flexibility determines your range of motion—how far you can bend and stretch muscles and ligaments. If your flexibility is poor, you cannot easily bend to tie your shoes or stretch to remove packages from the car. Improving flexibility improves performance in certain activities and may reduce your risk of injuries such as pulled muscles and strained tendons (**Figure 10.1c**).

Body composition Individuals who are physically fit have a greater proportion of muscle and a smaller proportion of fat than do unfit individuals of the same weight (**Figure 10.1d**). The amount of body fat a person has is also affected by gender and age. In general, women have more stored body fat than men. For young adult women, the desirable amount of body fat is 21 to 32% of total weight; in adult men, the desirable amount is 8 to 19%.[1]

Exercise and the Risk of Chronic Disease

Regular exercise not only makes everyday tasks easier but can also prevent or delay the onset of

chronic conditions such as cardiovascular disease, hypertension, type 2 diabetes, breast and colon cancer, and bone and joint disorders (**Figure 10.2**).[2] The health benefits of exercise are so great that they can even overcome some of the health risks of carrying excess body fat. Exercise reduces overall mortality, regardless of whether the person is lean, normal weight, or obese.[2] So even if you can't take off the pounds, you'll still benefit from continuing to exercise.

In addition to decreasing the risk of disease, exercise improves mood and self-esteem and increases vigor and overall well-being. Exercise has also been shown to reduce depression and anxiety, as well as to improve the quality of life.[3] The mechanisms involved are not clear, but one hypothesis has to do with the production of **endorphins**. Exercise stimulates the release of these chemicals, which are thought to be natural mood enhancers that play a role in triggering what athletes describe as an "exercise high." In addition to causing this state of exercise euphoria, endorphins are thought to aid in relaxation, pain tolerance, and appetite control.

> **endorphins**
> Compounds that cause a natural euphoria and reduce the perception of pain under certain stressful conditions.

Health benefits of physical activity • Figure 10.2

Exercise improves strength and endurance, reduces the risk of chronic disease, aids weight management, reduces sleeplessness, improves self-image, and helps relieve stress, anxiety, and depression.

Exercise improves flexibility and balance.

Exercise increases the sensitivity of tissues to insulin and decreases the risk of developing type 2 diabetes.

Exercise reduces the risk of cardiovascular disease because it strengthens the heart muscle, lowers blood pressure, and increases HDL (good) cholesterol levels in the blood.

Regular exercise reduces the risk of colon cancer and breast cancer.

Exercise increases muscle mass, strength, and endurance.

Weight-bearing exercise stimulates bones to become denser and stronger and therefore reduces the risk of osteoporosis. The strength and flexibility promoted by exercise can help improve joint function.

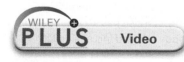

Exercise and Weight Management

Exercise makes weight management easier because it increases both energy needs and lean body mass. During exercise, energy expenditure can rise well above the resting rate, and some of this increase persists for many hours after activity slows.[4] Over time, regular exercise increases lean body mass. Even at rest, lean tissue uses more energy than fat tissue; therefore, the increase in lean body mass increases basal metabolism. The combination of increased energy output during exercise, the rise in energy expenditure that persists for a period after exercise, and the increase in basal needs over the long term can have a major impact on total energy expenditure (**Figure 10.3**). The more energy you expend, the more food you can consume while maintaining a healthy weight. As discussed in Chapter 9, exercise is an essential component of any weight-reduction program: It increases energy needs, promotes loss of body fat, and slows the loss of lean tissue that occurs with energy restriction.

CONCEPT CHECK **STOP**

1. **What** distinguishes a fit person from an unfit one?

2. **Why** do your muscles get bigger when you lift weights?

3. **How** does exercise affect heart health?

4. **How** does exercise help with weight management?

Exercise increases energy expenditure
• Figure 10.3

The total amount of energy we expend each day is the sum of the energy used for basal metabolism, physical activity, and the thermic effect of food (TEF). Adding 30 minutes of moderate activity can increase energy expenditure by as much as 300 Calories. Regular exercise increases muscle mass, which increases basal metabolism, further increasing total energy expenditure.

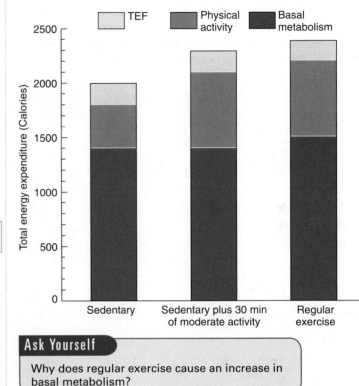

Ask Yourself

Why does regular exercise cause an increase in basal metabolism?

Exercise Recommendations

LEARNING OBJECTIVES

1. **Describe** the amounts and types of exercise recommended to improve health.

2. **Classify** activities as aerobic or anaerobic.

3. **Plan** a fitness program that can be integrated into your daily routine.

4. **Explain** overtraining syndrome.

Most Americans do not exercise regularly, and 32% of American adults get no physical activity at all during their leisure time.[5] To reduce the risk of chronic disease, public health guidelines, including the 2010 Dietary Guidelines, advise at least 150 minutes of moderate-intensity or 75 minutes of vigorous-intensity aerobic physical activity each week or an equivalent combination of both.[6,7] Greater health benefits can be obtained by exercising more vigorously or for a longer duration. Moderate-intensity exercise is the equivalent of walking 3 miles in about an hour or bicycling 8 miles in about an hour. Vigorous-intensity exercise is equivalent to jogging at a rate of 5 miles per hour or faster or bicycling at 10 miles per hour or faster.[7] Adults should also include muscle-strengthening activities on two or more days per week, but time spent in muscle-strengthening activities does not count toward meeting the aerobic activity guidelines.

If you can't find the time or motivation to exercise for an hour a day, do not give up. Even a small amount of exercise is better than none.[7]

What to Look for in a Fitness Program

A complete fitness program includes aerobic exercise for cardiovascular conditioning, stretching exercises for flexibility, and muscle-strengthening exercises to increase muscle strength and endurance and maintain or increase muscle mass.[7,8] The program should be integrated into an active lifestyle that includes a variety of everyday activities, enjoyable recreational activities, and a minimum amount of time spent in sedentary activities (**Figure 10.4**).

Exercise recommendations • Figure 10.4

A healthy lifestyle minimizes sedentary activities and includes a variety of everyday activities as well as exercise that improves muscle strength and at least 150 minutes of aerobic exercise, which increases heart rate. Achieving the recommended amounts of aerobic activity, muscle-strengthening exercise, and stretching recommended will help improve and maintain fitness and health.[7,8] In general, more exercise is better than less.

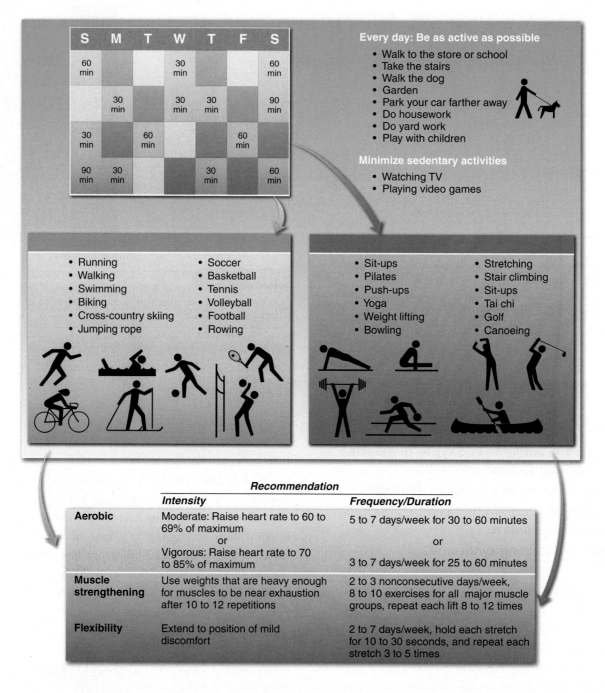

	Recommendation	
	Intensity	*Frequency/Duration*
Aerobic	Moderate: Raise heart rate to 60 to 69% of maximum or Vigorous: Raise heart rate to 70 to 85% of maximum	5 to 7 days/week for 30 to 60 minutes or 3 to 7 days/week for 25 to 60 minutes
Muscle strengthening	Use weights that are heavy enough for muscles to be near exhaustion after 10 to 12 repetitions	2 to 3 nonconsecutive days/week, 8 to 10 exercises for all major muscle groups, repeat each lift 8 to 12 times
Flexibility	Extend to position of mild discomfort	2 to 7 days/week, hold each stretch for 10 to 30 seconds, and repeat each stretch 3 to 5 times

Moderate or vigorous aerobic exercise should be performed most days of the week. An activity is aerobic if it raises your heart rate to 60 to 85% of your **maximum heart rate**; when you are exercising at an intensity in this range, you are said to be in your **aerobic zone (Figure 10.5)**. For a sedentary individual who is beginning an exercise program, mild exercise such as walking can raise the heart rate into the aerobic zone. As fitness improves, an exerciser must perform more intense activity to raise the heart rate to this level.

> **maximum heart rate** The maximum number of beats per minute that the heart can attain.

Aerobic activities of different intensities can be combined to meet recommendations and achieve health benefits. The total amount of energy expended in physical activity depends on the intensity, duration, and frequency of the activity. Vigorous physical activity, such as jogging, that raises heart rate to the high end of the aerobic zone (70 to 85%) improves fitness more and burns more calories per unit of time than does moderate-intensity activity, such as walking, that raises heart rate only to the low end of the zone (60 to 69%).

Individuals should structure their fitness program based on their needs, goals, and abilities. For example, some people might prefer a short, intense workout such as a 30 minute run, while others would rather work out for a longer time, at a lower intensity, such as a 1-hour walk. Some may choose to complete all their exercise during the same session, while others may spread their exercise throughout the day, in shorter bouts. Three short bouts of 10-minute duration can be as effective as a continuous bout of 30 minutes for reducing the risk of chronic disease.[8] It is preferable to spread your aerobic activity throughout the week rather than cram it all into the weekend. Exercising at least 3 days produces health benefits and reduces the risk of injury and fatigue. A combination of intensities, such as a brisk 30-minute walk twice during the week in addition to a 20-minute jog on 2 other days, can meet recommendations.

Muscle strengthening and stretching can be performed less often than aerobic exercise. Muscle strengthening is needed only 2 to 3 days a week at the start of an exercise program and 2 days a week after the desired strength has been achieved. Muscle strengthening should not be done on consecutive days. The rest between sessions gives the muscles time to respond to the stress by getting stronger. Increasing the amount of weight lifted increases muscle strength, whereas increasing the number of repetitions improves muscle endurance. Flexibility exercises can be performed 2 to 7 days per week. Time spent stretching does not count toward meeting aerobic or strength-training guidelines.

Finding your aerobic zone • Figure 10.5

a. You can calculate your aerobic zone by multiplying your maximum heart rate by 0.6 and 0.85. Maximum heart rate depends on age; it can be estimated by subtracting your age from 220. For example, if you are 20 years old, you have a maximum heart rate of 200 (220 − 20) beats per minute. If you exercise at a pace that keeps your heart rate between 120 (0.6 × 200) and 170 (0.85 × 200) beats per minute, you are in your aerobic zone.

b. You can check your heart rate by feeling the pulse at the side of your neck, just below the jawbone. A pulse is caused by the heart beating and forcing blood through the arteries. The number of pulses per minute equals heart rate.

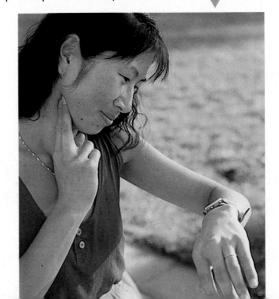

Interpreting Data

What is the aerobic zone for someone who is 30? What happens to this range when the person turns 40?

Creating an Active Lifestyle

Incorporating exercise into your day-to-day life may require a change in lifestyle, which is not always easy. Many people avoid exercise because they do not enjoy it, think it requires them to join an expensive health club, have little motivation to do it alone, or find it inconvenient or uncomfortable. Finding an exercise you enjoy, setting aside a time that is realistic and convenient, and finding a place that is appropriate and safe are important steps in starting and maintaining an exercise program (**Table 10.1**). Riding your bike to class or work rather than driving, taking a walk during your lunch break, and enjoying a game of catch or tag with your friends or family are all effective ways to increase your everyday activity level. The goal is to gradually make lifestyle changes that increase physical activity.

Before beginning an exercise program, check with your physician to be sure that your plans are appropriate for you, considering your medical history (**Figure 10.6**). If you choose to exercise outdoors rather than in a gym, reduce or curtail exercise in hot, humid weather in order

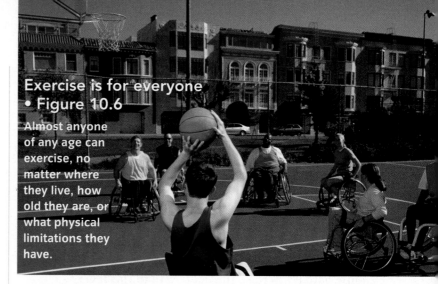

Exercise is for everyone • Figure 10.6

Almost anyone of any age can exercise, no matter where they live, how old they are, or what physical limitations they have.

to avoid heat-related illness. In cold weather, wear clothing that allows for evaporation of sweat while providing protection from the cold. Start each exercise session with a warm-up, such as mild stretching or easy jogging, to increase blood flow to the muscles. End with a cool-down period, such as walking or stretching, to prevent muscle cramps and slowly reduce heart rate.

Don't overdo it. If you don't rest enough between exercise sessions, fitness and performance will not improve. During rest, the body replenishes energy stores, repairs damaged tissues, and builds and strengthens muscles. In athletes, excessive training without sufficient rest to allow for recovery can lead to **overtraining syndrome**. The most common symptom of this condition is fatigue that limits workouts and is felt even at rest. Some athletes experience decreased appetite, weight loss, muscle soreness, increased frequency of viral illnesses, and increased incidence of injuries. They may become moody, easily irritated, or depressed; experience altered sleep patterns; or lose their competitive desire and enthusiasm. Overtraining syndrome occurs only in serious athletes who are training extensively, but rest is essential for anyone who is working to increase fitness.

> **overtraining syndrome** A collection of emotional, behavioral, and physical symptoms that occurs when the amount and intensity of exercise exceeds an athlete's capacity to recover.

Suggestions for starting and maintaining an exercise program   Table 10.1

Start slowly. Set specific, attainable goals. Once you have met them, add more

- Walk around the block after dinner.
- Get off the bus or subway one stop early.
- Use half of your lunch break to exercise.
- Do a few biceps curls each time you take the milk out of the refrigerator.

Make your exercise fun and convenient

- Opt for activities you enjoy: Bowling and dancing may be more fun for you than using a treadmill at the gym.
- Find a partner to exercise with you.
- Choose times that fit your schedule.

Stay motivated

- Vary your routine: Swim one day and mountain bike the next.
- Challenge your strength or endurance once or twice a week and do moderate workouts on other days.
- Track your progress by recording your activity.
- Reward your success with a new book, movie, or workout clothes.

Keep your exercise safe

- Warm up before you start.
- Cool down when you are done.
- Don't overdo it: Alternate hard days with easy days and take a day off when you need it.
- Listen to your body and stop before an injury occurs.

CONCEPT CHECK

1. **How** much aerobic exercise is recommended to reduce the risk of chronic disease?
2. **What** is your aerobic zone?
3. **What** types of exercise should be part of a fitness program?
4. **Who** is at risk for overtraining syndrome?

Fueling Exercise

LEARNING OBJECTIVES

1. **Compare** the fuels used to generate ATP by anaerobic and aerobic metabolism.

2. **Discuss** the effect of exercise duration and intensity on the type of fuel used.

3. **Describe** the physiological changes that occur in response to exercise.

The body runs on energy from the carbohydrate, fat, and protein in food and body stores. These fuels are needed whether you are writing a term paper, riding your bike to class, or running a marathon. Before they can be used to fuel activity, their energy must be converted into the high-energy compound ATP, the immediate source of energy for body functions. ATP can be generated both in the absence of oxygen, by **anaerobic metabolism**, and in the presence of oxygen, by **aerobic metabolism** (**Figure 10.7**). The type of metabolism that predominates during an activity determines how much carbohydrate, fat, and protein are used to fuel the activity.

Anaerobic versus aerobic metabolism • Figure 10.7

ATP is produced in the cells by anaerobic metabolism when no oxygen is available. Anaerobic metabolism produces ATP very rapidly but uses only glucose as a fuel. The **lactic acid** that is produced can be used as a fuel for aerobic metabolism. The majority of ATP is produced by aerobic metabolism. Aerobic metabolism requires oxygen, takes place in the mitochondria, and can use carbohydrate, fat, or protein to produce ATP. It is slower but more efficient at generating ATP than anaerobic metabolism.

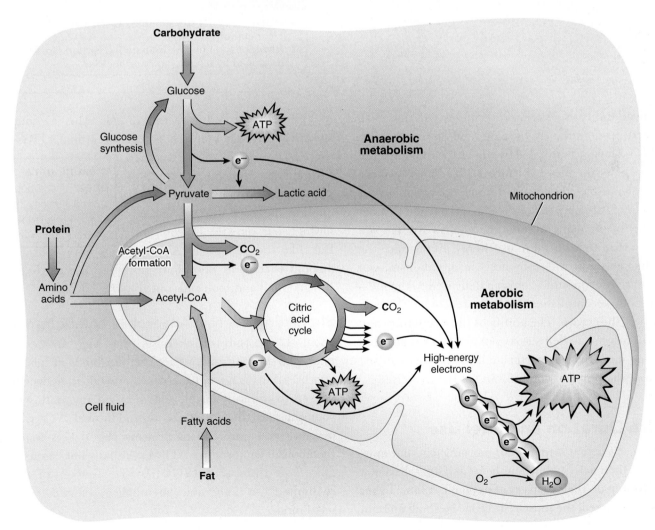

Getting oxygen to muscle cells • Figure 10.8

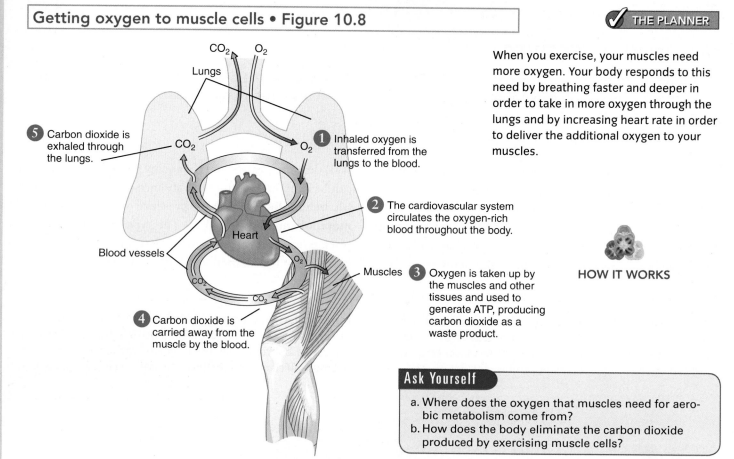

5 Carbon dioxide is exhaled through the lungs.

Lungs

CO_2 O_2

1 Inhaled oxygen is transferred from the lungs to the blood.

2 The cardiovascular system circulates the oxygen-rich blood throughout the body.

Heart

Blood vessels

Muscles

3 Oxygen is taken up by the muscles and other tissues and used to generate ATP, producing carbon dioxide as a waste product.

4 Carbon dioxide is carried away from the muscle by the blood.

When you exercise, your muscles need more oxygen. Your body responds to this need by breathing faster and deeper in order to take in more oxygen through the lungs and by increasing heart rate in order to deliver the additional oxygen to your muscles.

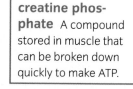

HOW IT WORKS

Ask Yourself

a. Where does the oxygen that muscles need for aerobic metabolism come from?

b. How does the body eliminate the carbon dioxide produced by exercising muscle cells?

The availability of oxygen determines whether ATP is produced predominantly by anaerobic versus aerobic metabolism. Oxygen is inhaled by the lungs and delivered to the muscle by the blood (**Figure 10.8**). When you are at rest, your muscles do not need much energy, and your heart and lungs are able to deliver enough oxygen to meet your energy needs using aerobic metabolism. When you exercise, your muscles need more energy. To increase the amount of energy provided by aerobic metabolism, you must increase the amount of oxygen delivered to the muscles. Your body accomplishes this by increasing both heart rate and breathing rate. The ability of the circulatory and respiratory systems to deliver oxygen to tissues is affected by how long an activity is performed, the intensity of the activity, and the physical conditioning of the exerciser.

Exercise Duration and Fuel Use

When you take the first steps of your morning jog, your muscles increase their activity, but your heart and lungs have not had time to step up their delivery of oxygen to them. To get the energy they need, the muscles rely on the small amount of ATP that is stored in resting muscle. This is enough to sustain activity for a few seconds. As the stored ATP is used up, enzymes break down another high-energy compound, **creatine phosphate**, to convert ADP (adenosine diphosphate) to ATP, allowing your activity to continue. But, like the amount of ATP, the amount of creatine phosphate stored in the muscle at any time is small and soon runs out (**Figure 10.9**).

creatine phosphate A compound stored in muscle that can be broken down quickly to make ATP.

Short-term energy: Anaerobic metabolism

After about 15 seconds of exercise, the ATP and creatine phosphate in your muscles are used up, but your heart rate and breathing have not increased enough to deliver more oxygen to the muscles. To get more energy at this point, your muscles must produce the additional ATP without oxygen (see Figure 10.7 on previous page). This anaerobic metabolism can produce ATP very rapidly but can use only glucose as a fuel (**Figure 10.10**). The amount of glucose is limited, so anaerobic metabolism cannot continue indefinitely.

Changes in the source of ATP over time • Figure 10.9

The source of the ATP that fuels muscle contraction changes over the first few minutes of exercise.

Instant energy
During the first few seconds of exercise, the muscles get energy from stored ATP. Then, for the next 10 seconds or so, creatine phosphate stored in the muscles is broken down to form more ATP.

Short-term energy
Anaerobic metabolism of glucose, obtained either from the blood or from muscle glycogen, becomes the predominant source of ATP when creatine phosphate stores have been depleted. Thirty seconds into the activity, anaerobic pathways are operating at full capacity.

Long-term energy
After about two to three minutes, oxygen delivery to the muscles has increased enough to support aerobic metabolism, which uses fatty acids and glucose to produce ATP.

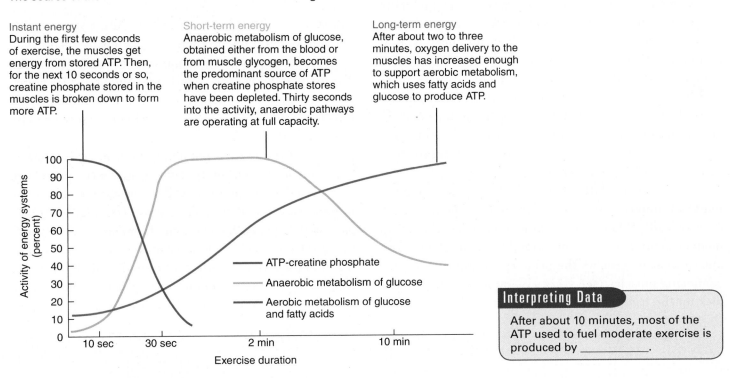

ATP-creatine phosphate

Anaerobic metabolism of glucose

Aerobic metabolism of glucose and fatty acids

Interpreting Data

After about 10 minutes, most of the ATP used to fuel moderate exercise is produced by _____.

Fuels for anaerobic and aerobic metabolism • Figure 10.10

Muscle contraction is fueled by glucose from muscle glycogen breakdown or blood glucose. Blood glucose is supplied by the breakdown of liver glycogen, glucose synthesis by the liver, and carbohydrate consumed during exercise. Some of the fatty acids used as fuel come from triglycerides stored in the muscle, but most come from adipose tissue. The amino acids available to the body come from the digestion of dietary proteins and from the breakdown of body proteins.

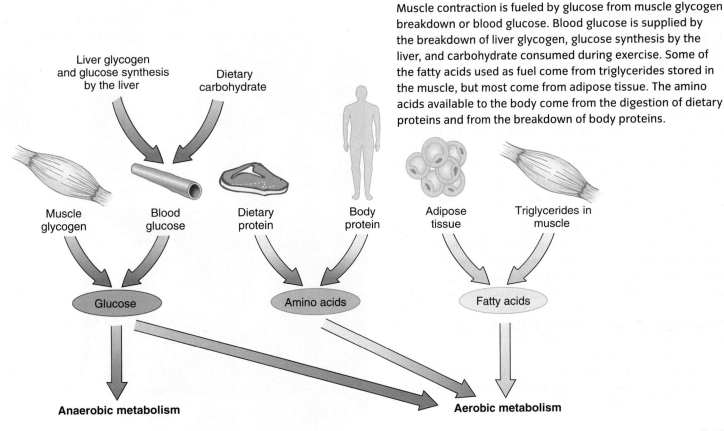

Long-term energy: Aerobic metabolism After you have been exercising for two to three minutes, your breathing and heart rate have increased to supply more oxygen to your muscles. This allows aerobic metabolism to predominate. Aerobic metabolism produces ATP at a slower rate than does anaerobic metabolism, but it is much more efficient, producing about 18 times more ATP for each molecule of glucose. As a result, glucose is used more slowly than in anaerobic metabolism. In addition, aerobic metabolism can use fatty acids, and sometimes amino acids from protein, to generate ATP (see Figure 10.10 on previous page).

In a typical adult, about 90% of stored energy is found in adipose tissue; this provides an ample supply of fatty acids. When you continue to exercise at a low to moderate intensity, aerobic metabolism predominates, and fatty acids become the primary fuel source for your exercising muscles (see *What a Scientist Sees*). When you pick up the pace, the relative amount of ATP generated by anaerobic versus aerobic metabolism and the fuels you burn will change.

Protein as a fuel for exercise Although protein is not considered a major energy source for the body, even at rest, small amounts of amino acids are used for energy. The amount increases if your diet does not provide enough total energy to meet needs, if you consume more protein than you need, or if you are involved in endurance exercise (see Chapter 6).

When the nitrogen-containing amino group is removed from an amino acid, the remaining carbon compound can be broken down to produce ATP by aerobic metabolism or, in some cases, used to make glucose (see Figure 10.7 on page 361). Exercise that continues for many hours increases the use of amino acids both as an energy source and as a raw material for glucose synthesis. Strength training does not increase the use of protein for energy, but it does increase the demand for amino acids for muscle building and repair.

WHAT A SCIENTIST SEES ✓ THE PLANNER

The Fat-Burning Zone

Have you ever jumped onto a treadmill and chosen the workout that puts you in the "fat-burning zone" rather than the one that puts you in the "cardio zone" because your goal was to lose weight? The fat-burning zone is a lower-intensity aerobic workout that keeps your heart rate between about 60 and 69% of maximum. The cardio zone is a higher-intensity aerobic workout that keeps heart rate between about 70 and 85% of maximum.

However, do you really burn more fat during a slow 30-minute jog in the fat-burning zone than during a vigorous 30-minute run in the cardio zone? A scientist sees that you do burn a higher percentage of calories from fat during a lower-intensity aerobic workout, but that's not the whole story. When you pick up the pace and exercise in what the treadmill calls the cardio zone, you continue to burn fat. The graph shows that 50% of the calories burned come from fat during the lower-intensity workout (that is, in the fat-burning zone) and only 40% come from fat during the higher-intensity workout. Looking at the actual numbers of calories burned, however, the scientist sees that at the higher intensity, you burn just as much fat (about 150 Calories/hour) but a much greater number of calories overall.

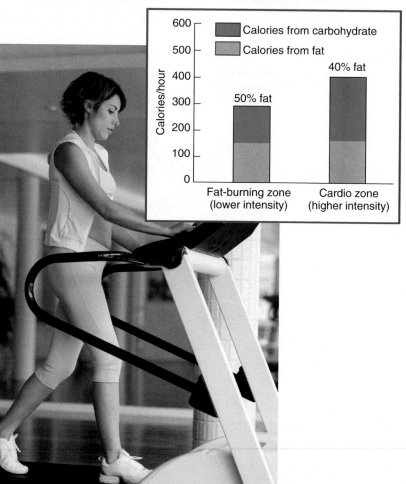

Think Critically Which workout will help you lose the most weight: 30 minutes in the cardio zone or 30 minutes in the fat-burning zone? Why?

The effect of exercise intensity on fuel use • Figure 10.11

Exercise intensity determines the contributions of carbohydrate, fat, and protein as fuels for ATP production. At rest and during low- to moderate-intensity exercise, aerobic metabolism predominates, so fatty acids are an important fuel source. As exercise intensity increases, the proportion of energy supplied by anaerobic metabolism increases, so glucose becomes the predominant fuel. Keep in mind, however, that during exercise, the total amount of energy expended is greater than the amount expended at rest.

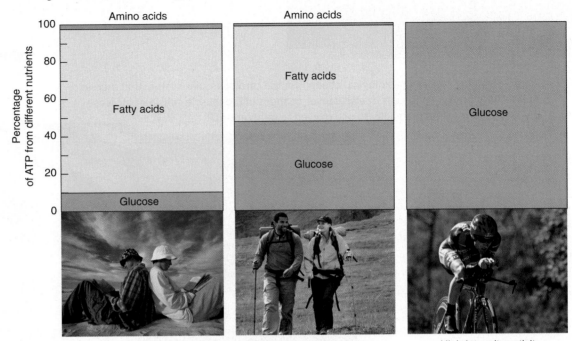

Rest   Moderate-intensity activity   High-intensity activity

Exercise Intensity and Fuel Use

The energy contributions made by anaerobic and aerobic metabolism combine to ensure that your muscles get enough ATP to meet the demands you place on them. The relative contribution of each type of metabolism depends on the intensity of your activity. With low-intensity activity, sufficient ATP can be produced by aerobic metabolism. With intense exercise, more ATP is needed, but oxygen delivery to and use by the muscles becomes limited, so the muscles must get the additional ATP they need by using anaerobic metabolism (**Figure 10.11**).

Lower-intensity exercise relies on aerobic metabolism, which is more efficient than anaerobic metabolism and uses both glucose and fatty acids to produce ATP. The body's fat reserves are almost unlimited, so if fat is the fuel, exercise can theoretically continue for a very long time. For example, it is estimated that a 130-pound woman has enough energy stored as body fat to run 1000 miles. However, even aerobic activity uses some glucose, which means that if exercise continues long enough, glycogen stores are eventually depleted, causing **fatigue**.

> **fatigue** Inability to continue an activity at an optimal level.

Fatigue occurs much more quickly with high-intensity exercise than with lower-intensity exercise because more intense exercise relies more on anaerobic metabolism, which can use only glucose for fuel. Glycogen stores thus are rapidly depleted (**Figure 10.12**). Anaerobic metabolism

Fatigue: "Hitting the wall" • Figure 10.12

Glycogen depletion is a concern for athletes because the amount of stored glycogen available to produce glucose during exercise is limited. When athletes run out of glycogen, they experience a feeling of overwhelming fatigue that is sometimes referred to as "hitting the wall" or "bonking."

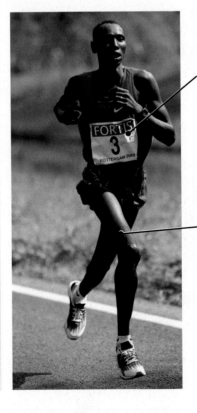

Between 60 and 120 grams of glycogen are stored in the liver; glycogen stores are highest just after a meal. Liver glycogen is used to maintain blood glucose between meals and during the night. Eating a high-carbohydrate breakfast will replenish the liver glycogen used during sleep.

There are about 200 to 500 g of glycogen in the muscles of a 70-kg (154-lb) person. The glycogen in a muscle is used to fuel that muscle's activity.

Aerobic training causes physiological changes in the cardiovascular system that increase the delivery of oxygen to cells. It also causes changes in the muscle cells that increase glycogen storage and the ability to use oxygen to generate ATP.

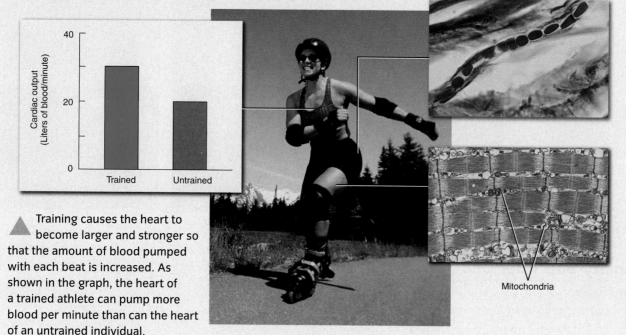

▲ Training causes the heart to become larger and stronger so that the amount of blood pumped with each beat is increased. As shown in the graph, the heart of a trained athlete can pump more blood per minute than can the heart of an untrained individual.

◀ Training causes blood volume and the number of red blood cells to expand, increasing the amount of hemoglobin so that more oxygen can be transported. It also causes the number of capillary blood vessels in the muscles to increase so that blood is delivered to muscles more efficiently.

◀ In the muscles, training enhances the ability to store glycogen and increases the number and size of muscle-cell mitochondria. Because aerobic metabolism occurs in the mitochondria, the greater size and number of mitochondria increases the capacity of cells to burn fatty acids to produce ATP.

Mitochondria

---

also produces lactic acid. With low-intensity exercise, the small amounts of lactic acid produced are carried away from the muscles and used by other tissues as an energy source or converted back into glucose by the liver. During high-intensity exercise, the amount of lactic acid produced exceeds the amount that can be used by other tissues, and the lactic acid builds up in the muscle and subsequently in the blood. Until recently, it was assumed that lactic acid buildup was the cause of muscle fatigue, but we now know that although lactic acid buildup occurs with high-intensity exercise, it is not a major factor in muscle fatigue.[9] Fatigue most likely has many causes, including glycogen depletion and changes in the muscle cells and the concentrations of molecules involved in muscle metabolism.

Fitness Training and Fuel Use

When you exercise regularly to improve your fitness, the training causes physiological changes in your body. The changes caused by repeated bouts of aerobic exercise increase the amount of oxygen that can be delivered to the muscles and the ability of the muscles to use oxygen to generate ATP by aerobic metabolism (**Figure 10.13**). This increased aerobic capacity allows fatty acids to be used for fuel so that glycogen is spared and the onset of fatigue is delayed. Training aerobically also increases the amount of glycogen stored in the muscles. Because trained athletes store more glycogen and use it more slowly, they can sustain aerobic exercise for longer periods at higher intensities than can untrained individuals.

CONCEPT CHECK

1. **What** fuels are used in anaerobic metabolism?

2. **What** type of metabolism does a marathon runner rely on?

3. **Why** is a trained athlete able to perform at a higher intensity for a longer time than an untrained person?

Energy and Nutrient Needs for Physical Activity

LEARNING OBJECTIVES

1. **Compare** the energy and nutrient needs of athletes and nonathletes.

2. **Explain** why athletes are at risk for dehydration and hyponatremia.

3. **Discuss** the recommendations for food and drink during extended exercise.

4. **Plan** pre- and post-competition meals for a marathon runner.

Good nutrition is essential to performance, whether you are a marathon runner or a mall walker. Your diet must provide enough energy to fuel activity, enough protein to maintain muscle mass, sufficient micronutrients to metabolize the energy-yielding nutrients, and enough water to transport nutrients and cool your body. The major difference between the nutritional needs of a serious athlete and those of a casual exerciser is the amount of energy and water required.

Energy Needs

The amount of energy expended for any activity depends on the intensity, duration, and frequency of the activity and the weight of the exerciser (**Figure 10.14**). Whereas casual exercise may burn only 100 additional Calories a day, the training required for an endurance athlete, such as a marathon runner, may increase energy expenditure by 2000 to 3000 Calories/day. Some athletes require 6000 Calories a day to maintain their body weight. In general, the more intense the activity, the more energy it requires, and the more time spent exercising, the more energy is expended (see Appendix H). Running for 60 minutes, for instance, involves more work than walking for the same amount of time and therefore requires more energy.

Gaining or losing weight Body weight and composition can affect exercise performance. In sports such as football and weight lifting, having a large amount of muscle is advantageous, and athletes may try to build muscle and increase body weight. Healthy weight gain can be achieved through a combination of increased energy intake, adequate protein intake, and muscle-strengthening exercise to promote an increase in lean tissue rather than fat.

In sports such as ballet, gymnastics, and certain running events, small, light bodies offer an advantage, so athletes may restrict energy intake in order to maintain a low body weight. While a slightly leaner physique may be beneficial in these sports, dieting to maintain an unrealistically low weight may threaten health and performance. An athlete who needs to lose weight should do so in advance of the competitive season to prevent the calorie restriction from affecting performance. The general guidelines for healthy weight loss should be followed: Reduce energy intake by 200 to 500 Calories/day, increase activity, and change the behaviors that led to weight gain (see Chapter 9).

Unhealthy weight-loss practices Athletes who participate in sports that require weight restriction to optimize performance are vulnerable to eating disorders. The motivation and self-discipline characteristic of successful athletes contributes to their increased risk of anorexia and bulimia (see Chapter 9). In athletes who develop anorexia, the restricted food intake can affect growth and maturation and impair exercise performance. In athletes who develop bulimia, purging can cause dehydration and electrolyte imbalance, which affect performance and endanger overall health. In addition to using restricted food intake or purging to keep body weight low, athletes are more likely than nonathletes to engage in compulsive exercise behaviors in order to increase energy expenditure.

Factors affecting energy expenditure • Figure 10.14

This graph illustrates the impact of running pace and body weight on energy expenditure per hour. The longer an individual continues to run, the greater the amount of energy expended. Body weight affects energy needs because moving a heavier body requires more energy than moving a lighter one. Therefore, if the pace is the same, a 170-lb woman requires more energy to run for an hour than does a 125-lb woman.

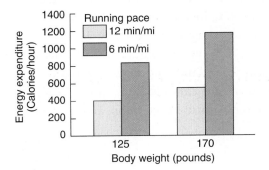

Female athlete triad • Figure 10.15

Women with female athlete triad typically have low body fat, do not menstruate regularly, and may experience multiple or recurrent stress fractures.[10] Neither adequate dietary calcium nor the increase in bone mass caused by weight-bearing exercise can compensate for the bone loss caused by low estrogen levels. Treatment involves increasing energy intake and reducing activity so that menstrual cycles resume.

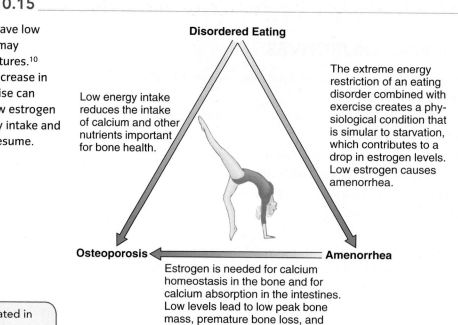

Disordered Eating

Low energy intake reduces the intake of calcium and other nutrients important for bone health.

The extreme energy restriction of an eating disorder combined with exercise creates a physiological condition that is simular to starvation, which contributes to a drop in estrogen levels. Low estrogen causes amenorrhea.

Osteoporosis ← **Amenorrhea**

Estrogen is needed for calcium homeostasis in the bone and for calcium absorption in the intestines. Low levels lead to low peak bone mass, premature bone loss, and increased risk of stress fractures.

Think Critically Why is bone loss accelerated in young girls who are not menstruating?

In female athletes, the pressure to reduce body weight and fat in order to improve performance, achieve an ideal body image, and meet goals set by coaches, trainers, or parents may lead to a combination of symptoms referred to as the **female athlete triad**. This syndrome includes energy restriction, changes in hormone levels that affect the menstrual cycle, and disturbances in bone formation and breakdown that can lead to osteoporosis (**Figure 10.15**).[10]

Athletes involved in sports that have weight classes, such as wrestling and boxing, are at particular risk for unhealthy weight-loss practices because they are under pressure to lose weight before a competition so that they can compete in a lower weight class. Competing at the high end of a weight class is thought to offer an advantage over smaller opponents. To lose weight rapidly, these athletes may use sporadic diets that severely restrict energy intake or dehydrate themselves through such practices as vigorous exercise, fluid restriction, wearing of vapor-impermeable suits, or use of hot environments, such as saunas and steam rooms, to increase sweat loss. They may also resort to even more extreme measures, such as vomiting and the use of diuretics and laxatives. These practices can be dangerous and even fatal (**Figure 10.16**). They may impair performance and can adversely affect heart and kidney function, temperature regulation, and electrolyte balance.

Making weight • Figure 10.16

After three young wrestlers died while exercising in plastic suits in order to sweat off water, wrestling guidelines were changed to improve safety.[11] Weight classes were altered to eliminate the lightest class, plastic sweat suits were banned, weigh-ins were moved to one hour before competition, and mandatory weight-loss rules were instituted. The percentage of body fat can be no less than 5% for college wrestlers and 7% for high school wrestlers.

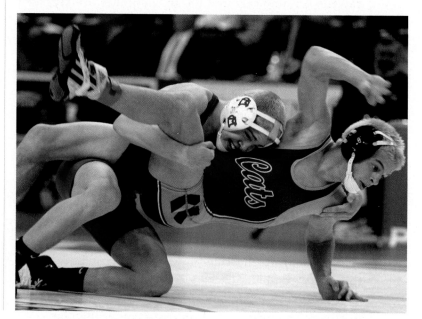

Carbohydrate, Fat, and Protein Needs

The source of energy in an athlete's diet can be as important as the amount. To maximize glycogen stores and optimize performance, a diet providing about 6 to 10 g of carbohydrate/kg of body weight per day is recommended for athletes in training (**Figure 10.17**).[12] The recommended amount of fat is the same as that for the general population—between 20 and 35% of energy. To allow for enough carbohydrate, fat intakes at the lower end of this range may be needed for some athletes. Diets that are very low in fat (less than 20% of calories) do not benefit performance. Protein is not a significant energy source, accounting for only about 5% of energy expended, but dietary protein is needed to maintain and repair lean tissues, including muscle. A diet in which 15 to 20% of calories come from protein will meet the needs of most athletes.

As discussed in Chapter 6, competitive athletes participating in endurance or strength sports may require extra protein. In endurance events, such as marathons, protein is used for energy and to maintain blood glucose. Athletes participating in these events may benefit from 1.2 to 1.4 g of protein/kilogram of body weight per day. Athletes participating in strength events require amino acids to synthesize new muscle proteins and may benefit from 1.2 to 1.7 g/kg per day.[12] While this amount is greater than the RDA (0.8 g/kg per day), it is not greater than the amount of protein habitually consumed by athletes.[13] For example, an 85-kg man consuming 3000 Calories, of which 15 to 20% is from protein, would be consuming 1.6 g of protein/kilogram body weight.

Vitamin and Mineral Needs

An adequate intake of vitamins and minerals is essential for optimal performance. These micronutrients are needed for energy production, oxygen delivery, protection against oxidative damage, and repair and maintenance of body structures.

Exercise increases the amounts of many vitamins and minerals used both in metabolism during exercise and in repairing tissues after exercise. In addition, exercise may increase losses of some micronutrients. Nevertheless, most athletes can meet their needs by consuming the amounts of vitamins and minerals recommended for the general population. Because athletes must eat more food to satisfy their higher energy needs, they consume extra vitamins and minerals with these foods, particularly if they choose nutrient-dense foods. Athletes who restrict their intake in order to maintain a low body weight may be at risk for vitamin and mineral deficiencies.

Antioxidants and oxidative damage Exercise increases the amount of oxygen used by the muscles and the rate of ATP-producing metabolic reactions. This increased oxygen use increases the production of free radicals, which can lead to oxidative damage and contribute to muscle fatigue.[14] To protect the body from oxidative damage, muscle cells contain antioxidant defenses, some of which may interact with dietary antioxidants such as vitamin C, vitamin E, β-carotene, and selenium. Despite the importance of antioxidants for health and performance, there is little evidence that supplementation with antioxidants improves human performance.[15]

Proportions of energy-yielding nutrients in an athlete's diet • Figure 10.17

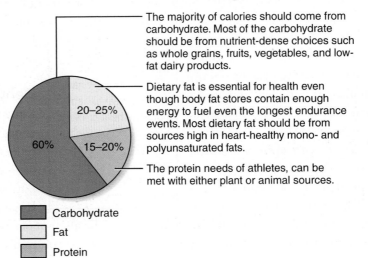

The proportions of carbohydrate, fat, and protein recommended in the diets of athletes, shown in the pie chart to the right, are within the ranges recommended for the general public: 45 to 65% of total energy from carbohydrate, 20 to 35% of energy from fat, and 10 to 35% of energy from protein.

The majority of calories should come from carbohydrate. Most of the carbohydrate should be from nutrient-dense choices such as whole grains, fruits, vegetables, and low-fat dairy products.

Dietary fat is essential for health even though body fat stores contain enough energy to fuel even the longest endurance events. Most dietary fat should be from sources high in heart-healthy mono- and polyunsaturated fats.

The protein needs of athletes, can be met with either plant or animal sources.

60%   20–25%   15–20%

- Carbohydrate
- Fat
- Protein

Sports anemia • Figure 10.18

Training causes blood volume to expand in order to increase oxygen delivery, but the synthesis of red blood cells lags behind the increase in blood volume. The result is a decrease in the percentage of blood volume that is red blood cells. However, the total number of red blood cells stays the same or increases slightly, so the transport of oxygen is not impaired. As training progresses, the number of red blood cells increases to catch up with the increase in total blood volume.

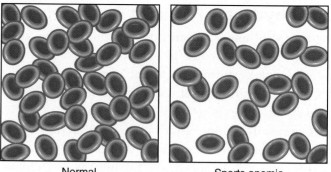

Normal   Sports anemia

Iron and anemia The body requires iron to form hemoglobin, myoglobin, and a number of iron-containing proteins that are essential for the production of ATP by aerobic metabolism. Exercise increases the need for a number of these proteins and may thereby increase iron needs. For example, exercise stimulates the production of red blood cells, so more iron is needed for hemoglobin synthesis. Prolonged training may also contribute to iron deficiency because iron losses in feces, urine, and sweat increase.[12]

Another cause of iron loss is foot strike hemolysis. This is the breaking of red blood cells due to the contraction of large muscles or impact in events such as running. Foot-strike hemolysis rarely causes anemia because most of the iron from these cells is recycled, and the breaking of red blood cells stimulates the production of new ones.

Reduced iron stores are not uncommon in athletes.[12] Female athletes are at particular risk; their needs are higher than those of male athletes because they need to replace the iron lost in menstrual blood.[16] In athletes of both sexes, inadequate iron intake often contributes to low iron stores. Iron intake may be low in athletes who are attempting to keep their body weight down and in those who do not eat meat, which is an excellent source of readily absorbable heme iron. If iron deficiency progresses to anemia, the body's ability both to transport oxygen and to provide energy by aerobic metabolism is reduced, impairing exercise performance as well as overall health.

Iron deficiency anemia (see Chapter 8) should not be confused with **sports anemia**, which is an adaptation to training that does not seem to impair the delivery of oxygen to tissues (**Figure 10.18**).[12] Although a specific iron RDA has not been set for athletes, the DRIs acknowledge that the requirement may be 30 to 70% higher for athletes than for the general population.[17]

---

heat-related illnesses Conditions, including heat cramps, heat exhaustion, and heat stroke, that can occur due to an unfavorable combination of exercise, hydration status, and climatic conditions.

Water Needs

Exercise increases water needs because it increases losses in sweat and from evaporation through the respiratory system. During exercise, most people drink only enough to assuage their thirst, but this amount typically is not enough to replace water losses. Therefore, they end their exercise session in a state of dehydration and must restore fluid balance during the remainder of the day.

The risk of dehydration is greater in hot than cold environments. However, dehydration may also occur when exercising in the cold because cold air tends to be dry, so evaporative losses from the lungs are greater. In addition, insulated clothing worn in cold weather may increase sweat loss, and fluid intake may be reduced because a chilled athlete may be reluctant to drink a cold beverage. Female athletes training in cold weather may also limit fluid intake in order to avoid the inconvenience of removing clothing in order to urinate.[12]

Even when fluids are consumed at regular intervals throughout exercise, it may not be possible to drink enough to compensate for losses. During exercise, water is needed to cool the body and to transport both oxygen and nutrients to the muscles and remove waste products from them. Not consuming enough water to replace losses can be hazardous to the performance and health of even the most casual exerciser (**Figure 10.19**).

Dehydration and heat-related illnesses

Dehydration occurs when water loss is great enough for blood volume to decrease, thereby reducing the ability of the circulatory system to deliver oxygen and nutrients to exercising muscles (see Chapter 8). A decrease in blood volume also reduces blood flow to the skin and the amount of sweat produced, thus limiting the body's ability to cool itself. As a result, core body temperature can increase, and with it the risk of various **heat-related illnesses**.

Heat cramps are involuntary muscle spasms that occur during or after intense exercise, usually in the muscles involved in the exercise. They are a form of heat-related illness caused by an imbalance of electrolytes at the muscle cell membranes. They can occur when water and salt are lost during extended exercise.

Heat exhaustion occurs when water loss causes blood volume to decrease so much that it is not possible both to cool the body and to deliver oxygen to active muscles. It is a form of heat-related illness characterized by a rapid but weak pulse, low blood pressure, disorientation, profuse sweating, and fainting. A person who is experiencing symptoms of heat exhaustion should stop exercising and move to a cooler environment.

Heat exhaustion can progress to **heat stroke**, the most serious form of heat-related illness. It occurs when core body temperature rises above 105°F, causing the brain's temperature-regulatory center to fail. When this occurs, the individual does not sweat even though body temperature is rising. Heat stroke is characterized by elevated body temperature; hot, dry skin; extreme confusion; and unconsciousness. It requires immediate medical attention.

Exercising in hot, humid weather increases the risk of heat-related illnesses. As environmental temperature rises, the body has more difficulty dissipating heat, and as humidity rises, the body's ability to cool through evaporation decreases (**Figure 10.20**).

Dehydration and performance • Figure 10.19

As the severity of dehydration increases, exercise performance declines. Even mild dehydration—a water loss of 1 to 2% of body weight—can impair exercise performance. A 3% reduction in body weight can significantly reduce the amount of blood pumped with each heartbeat because the blood volume is decreased. This, in turn, reduces the circulatory system's ability to deliver oxygen and nutrients to cells and remove waste products.

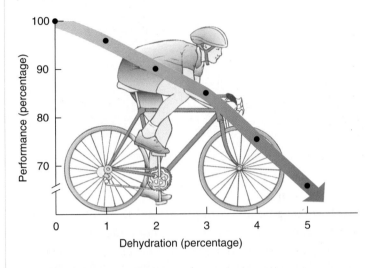

Interpreting Data

If a person loses 4% of his body weight as water during a competition, by what percentage will his performance be decreased by the end of the event?
a. 10%   b. 20%   c. 25%   d. 30%

Heat index[18] • Figure 10.20

Exercise in extreme conditions increases the risk of heat-related illness. *Heat index*, or *apparent temperature*, is a measure of how hot it feels when the relative humidity is added to the air temperature. To find the heat index, find the intersection of the temperature on the left side of the table and the relative humidity across the top. The colored zones correspond to heat index levels that contribute to increasingly severe heat illnesses with continued exposure and/or physical activity.

Relative humidity (%)

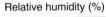

°F	40	45	50	55	60	65	70	75	80	85	90	95	100
110	136												
108	130	137											
106	124	130	137										
104	119	124	131	137									
102	114	119	124	130	137								
100	109	114	118	124	129	136							
98	105	109	113	117	123	128	134						
96	101	104	108	112	116	121	126	132					
94	97	100	102	106	110	114	119	124	129	135			
92	94	96	99	101	105	108	112	116	121	126	131		
90	91	93	95	97	100	103	106	109	113	117	122	127	132
88	88	89	91	93	95	98	100	103	106	110	113	117	121
86	85	87	88	89	91	93	95	97	100	102	105	108	112
84	83	84	85	86	88	89	90	92	94	96	98	100	103
82	81	82	83	84	84	85	86	88	89	90	91	93	95
80	80	80	81	81	82	82	83	84	84	85	86	86	87

Air temperature

Heat index (apparent temperature)

With prolonged exposure and/or physical activity

Extreme danger
Heat stroke highly likely

Danger
Heat stroke, heat cramps, and/or heat exhaustion likely

Extreme caution
Heat stroke, heat cramps, and/or heat exhaustion possible

Caution
Fatigue possible

Diluting blood sodium • Figure 10.21

Water and sodium are lost in sweat. Drinking plain water after excessive sweating can therefore dilute the sodium remaining in the blood. Hyponatremia occurs in about 6% of male ultra-endurance athletes.[19]

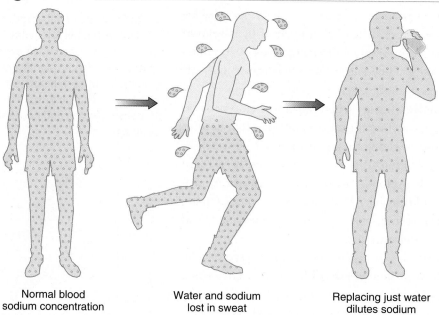

Normal blood
sodium concentration

Water and sodium
lost in sweat

Replacing just water
dilutes sodium
(hyponatremia)

Hyponatremia Sweating helps us stay cool. But if the water and sodium lost in sweat are not replaced in the right proportions, low blood sodium, or hyponatremia, may result (see Chapter 8). For most activities, sweat losses can be replaced with plain water, and lost electrolytes can be replaced during the meals following exercise. However, during endurance events such as triathalons, when sweating continues for many hours, both water and sodium need to be replenished. If an athlete replaces the lost fluid with plain water, the sodium that remains in the blood is diluted, causing hyponatremia. As sodium concentrations in the blood decrease, fluid moves into body tissues by osmosis, causing swelling. Fluid accumulation in the lungs interferes with gas exchange, and fluid accumulation in the brain causes disorientation, seizure, coma, and death (**Figure 10.21**).

The risk of hyponatremia can be reduced by consuming a sodium-containing sports drink during long-distance events, increasing sodium intake several days prior to a competition, and avoiding acetaminophen, aspirin, ibuprofen, and other nonsteroidal anti-inflammatory drugs, which may contribute to the development of hyponatremia by interfering with kidney function. The early symptoms of hyponatremia may be similar to those of dehydration: nausea, muscle cramps, disorientation, slurred speech, and confusion. A proper diagnosis is important because drinking water alone will make the problem worse. Mild symptoms of hyponatremia can be treated by eating salty foods or drinking a sodium-containing beverage, such as a sports drink. More severe symptoms require medical attention.

Fluid recommendations for exercise Anyone who is exercising should consume extra fluids. Because thirst is not a reliable short-term indicator of the body's water needs, it is important to schedule regular fluid breaks. To ensure hydration, adequate amounts of fluid should be consumed before, during, and after exercise.

Exercisers should drink generous amounts of fluid in the 24 hours before an exercise session and about 2 cups of fluid 4 hours before exercise. During exercise, whether casual or competitive, exercisers should try to drink enough fluid to prevent weight loss.[12] Drinking 6 to 12 ounces of fluid every 15 to 20 minutes for the duration of the exercise should maintain adequate hydration. To restore lost water after exercise, each pound of weight lost should be replaced with 16 to 24 oz (2 to 3 cups) of fluid.[12]

The best type of beverage to consume during exercise depends on the duration of the exercise. For exercise lasting an hour or less, water is the only fluid needed, particularly if one of your exercise goals is weight management. A typical 16-ounce sports drink provides about 100 Calories, so it will replace about half of the calories expended during a 40-minute ride on a stationary bicycle.

For exercise lasting more than 60 minutes, sports drinks or other beverages containing a small amount of carbohydrate (about 10 to 20 g of carbohydrate/cup) and electrolytes (around 150 milligrams of sodium/cup) are recommended.[12] The carbohydrate is a source of glucose for the muscle and thus delays fatigue. Commercial sports drinks contain rapidly absorbed sources of carbohydrate, such as glucose, sucrose, or glucose polymers (chains of glucose molecules). The right proportion of carbohydrate to water is important. If the concentration of carbohydrate is too low, it will not help performance; if it is too high, it will delay stomach emptying. Water and carbohydrate trapped in the stomach do not benefit the athlete and may cause stomach cramps. Because fruit juices and soft drinks contain twice as much sugar as sports drinks, they are not recommended unless they are diluted with an equal volume of water. The sodium in sports drinks helps prevent hyponatremia and also enhances intestinal absorption of water and glucose and stimulates thirst. Flavored beverages also tempt athletes to drink more, helping to ensure adequate hydration.

Food and Drink to Optimize Performance

For most of us, a trip to the gym requires no special nutritional planning, but for competitive athletes, when and what they eat before, during, and after competition are as important as a balanced overall diet. The type and amount of food eaten at these times may give or take away the extra seconds that can mean victory or defeat

Maximizing glycogen stores Glycogen stores are a source of glucose, and larger glycogen stores allow exercise to continue for longer periods. Glycogen stores and hence endurance are increased by increasing carbohydrate intake (**Figure 10.22**).

Serious endurance athletes who want to substantially increase their muscle glycogen stores before a competition may choose to follow a dietary regimen referred to as **glycogen supercompensation** or **carbohydrate loading**. Such a regimen involves resting for one to three days before competition while consuming a very high-carbohydrate diet.[21,22] The diet should provide 10 to 12 g of carbohydrate/kg of body weight per day. For a 150-lb person, this is equivalent to about 700 g of carbohydrate per day. Having a stack of pancakes with syrup and a glass of milk or a plate of pasta with garlic bread and a glass of juice provides more than 200 g of carbohydrate. A number of commercial high-carbohydrate beverages (50 to 60 g of carbohydrate in 8 fluid oz) are available to help athletes consume the amount of carbohydrate recommended to maximize glycogen stores. (These should not be confused with sports drinks designed to be consumed during competition, which contain only about 10 to 20 g of carbohydrate in 8 fluid oz.) Trained athletes who follow a carbohydrate-loading regimen can double their muscle glycogen content.[22]

Although glycogen supercompensation is beneficial to endurance athletes, it provides no benefit, and even has some disadvantages, for those exercising for less than 90 minutes. For every gram of glycogen in the muscle, about 3 g of water is also deposited. This water will cause weight gain and may cause some muscle stiffness. As glycogen is used, the water is released. This can be an advantage when exercising in hot weather, but the extra weight is a disadvantage for individuals competing in short-duration events.

What to eat before exercise Meals eaten before exercise should maximize glycogen stores and provide adequate hydration while minimizing digestion, hunger, and gastric distress. A pre-exercise meal should provide enough fluid to maintain hydration and should be high in carbohydrate (60 to 70% of calories). The carbohydrate will help maintain blood glucose and maximize glycogen stores. Muscle glycogen is depleted by activity, but liver glycogen is used to supply blood glucose and is depleted even during rest if no food is ingested.

> **glycogen supercompensation** or **carbohydrate loading** A regimen designed to increase muscle glycogen stores beyond their usual level.

Dietary carbohydrate and endurance • Figure 10.22

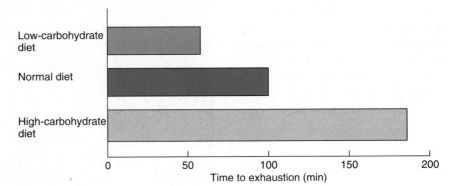

The amount of carbohydrate consumed in the diet affects the level of muscle glycogen and hence an athlete's endurance. This graph shows endurance capacity during cycling exercise after three days of a low-carbohydrate diet (less than 5% of energy from carbohydrate), a normal diet (about 55% of energy from carbohydrate), and a high-carbohydrate diet (82% of energy from carbohydrate).[20]

A pre-exercise meal should contain about 300 Calories and be moderate in protein (10 to 20%) and low in fat (10 to 25%) and fiber in order to minimize gastrointestinal distress and bloating during competition (**Figure 10.23**). Spicy foods, which can cause heartburn, and large amounts of simple sugars, which can cause diarrhea, should also be avoided unless the athlete is accustomed to eating these foods.

What to eat during exercise Most people don't need to eat while they exercise. If the activity lasts longer than an hour, however, it is important to consume carbohydrate during exercise in order to maintain glucose supplies. Carbohydrate consumption is particularly important for athletes who exercise in the morning, when liver glycogen levels are low.

For exercise that lasts longer than an hour, carbohydrate intake should begin shortly after exercise begins, and regular amounts should be consumed every 15 to 20 minutes during exercise. The carbohydrate should provide a combination of glucose and fructose. (Fructose alone is not as effective as the combination and may cause diarrhea.) This carbohydrate can be obtained from a sports drink, but consuming a solid-food snack or a carbohydrate gel with water is also appropriate. About 30 to 60 g of carbohydrate (the amount in a banana or an energy bar) each hour is recommended (see *Thinking It Through*).[12]

Snacks and sports drinks also provide sodium. Although the amount of sodium lost in sweat during exercise lasting less than three to four hours is usually not enough to affect health or performance, a snack or beverage containing sodium is recommended for exercise lasting more than an hour. This will reduce the risk of hyponatremia, improve glucose and water absorption, and stimulate thirst.

What to eat after exercise When you stop exercising, your body must shift from the task of breaking down glycogen, triglycerides, and muscle proteins for fuel to the job of restoring muscle and liver glycogen, depositing lipids, and synthesizing muscle proteins. Meals eaten after exercise should replenish lost fluid, electrolytes, and glycogen and provide protein for building and repairing muscle tissue.

After exercise, the first priority for all exercisers is to replace fluid losses. For serious athletes competing on consecutive days, glycogen replacement is also a priority. To maximize glycogen replacement, a high-carbohydrate meal or drink should be consumed within 30 minutes after the competition and again every two hours for about six hours.[12] Ideally, the meals or drinks should provide about 1.0 to 1.5 g of easily absorbed carbohydrate per kilogram of body weight, which is about 50 to 100 g of carbohydrate for a 70-kg (154-lb) person—the equivalent of 2 cups of pasta or 2 cups of chocolate milk.[23] Consuming foods such as these that contain both carbohydrate and protein enhances glycogen synthesis even more than does consuming carbohydrate alone.[24,25] Including protein with carbohydrate in postexercise meals also stimulates muscle protein

The precompetition meal • Figure 10.23

When we don't eat overnight, liver glycogen stores are reduced, so replenishing glycogen by eating is particularly important first thing on the morning of a competition. A high-carbohydrate meal—such as cereal, milk, and juice—two to four hours before competition can restore liver glycogen. The effects of different foods should be tested during training, not during competition. In addition to providing nutritional clout, a meal that includes "lucky" foods may provide an added psychological advantage.

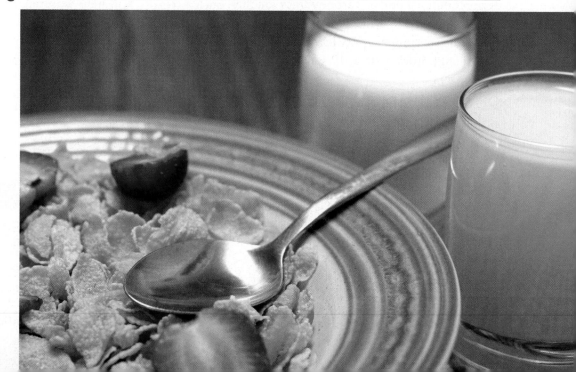

THINKING IT THROUGH

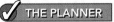

A Case Study on Snacks for Exercise

Mark enjoys long-distance cycling. On weekends, he often goes on a 40- or 50-mile ride, which takes him three to four hours. Despite the sports drink in his bike bottle, after about two hours, he gets hungry and fatigued, so he is looking for a snack that's easy to carry.

What type of snack will give Mark the energy he needs to continue his ride? Why?
▼

Carbohydrate is the fuel that is depleted during prolonged exercise. So if Mark wants to have the energy to keep pedaling, he should choose something high in carbohydrate.

The bike shop sells a variety of energy or endurance bars *that claim to prevent hunger and maintain blood glucose during extended activity. Mark should use the Nutrition Facts panel to select a bar that provides about 45 g of carbohydrate and no more than about 8 g of fat and 16 g of protein. Sports bars that are higher in fat or protein or lower in carbohydrate will not give him the blood glucose boost he needs to continue riding.*

What are the advantages and disadvantages of energy bars?
▼

Your answer:

With flavors such as chocolate coconut, tropical crisp, and sesame raisin crunch, many energy bars don't sound too different from candy bars. For about half the cost, Mark can buy a candy bar to put in his bike bag.

Based on the labels shown here, how do energy bars differ from candy bars?
▼

Your answer:

Suggest a snack for Mark that provides about the same amounts of carbohydrate and calories as an energy bar but is less expensive.
▼

Your answer:

(Check your answers in Appendix J.)

Nutrition Facts	Amount/Serving	% DV*	Amount/Serving	% DV*
Serving Size 1 bar (65g)	**Total Fat** 2g	**3%**	**Total Carb** 45g	**15%**
Calories 230	Saturated Fat 0.5g	**3%**	Dietary Fiber 3g	**12%**
Calories from Fat 20	Trans Fat 0g		Sugars 14g	
Calories from Sat Fat 5	**Cholesterol** 0mg	**0%**	Other Carb 28g	
*Percent Daily Values (DV) are based on a 2,000 calorie diet.	**Sodium** 90mg	**4%**		
	Potassium 145mg	**4%**	**Protein** 10g	

Vitamin A 0% • Vitamin C 100% • Calcium 30% • Iron 35% • Vitamin E 100% • Thiamin 100% • Riboflavin 100% • Niacin 100% • Vitamin B₆ 100% • Folate 100% • Vitamin B₁₂ 100% • Biotin 100% • Pantothenic Acid 100% • Phosphorus 35% • Magnesium 35% • Zinc 35% • Copper 35% • Chromium 20%

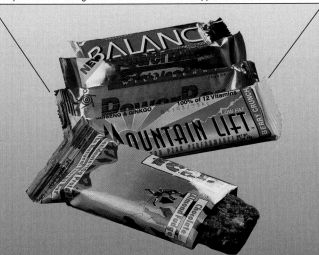

Nutrition Facts
Serving Size 1 bar (2 oz.) (57g)

Amount Per Serving

Calories 271	Calories from Fat 122
	% Daily Value*
Total Fat 14g	**21%**
Saturated Fat 5g	**26%**
Trans Fat 0g	
Cholesterol 5mg	**2%**
Sodium 140mg	**6%**
Total Carbohydrates 35g	**12%**
Dietery Fiber 1g	**5%**
Sugars 30g	
Protein 4g	

Vitamin A 2%	•	Vitamin C 0%
Calcium 5%	•	Iron 2%

*Based on a 2,000 calorie diet

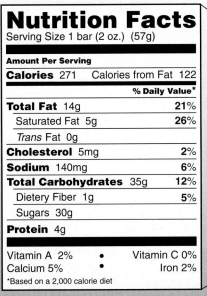

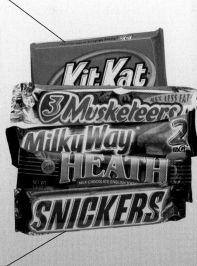

WHAT SHOULD I EAT?
Before, During, and After Exercise

Before you exercise
- Fill a water bottle four hours before exercise and finish it before you start.
- Plan to have pasta but pass on the cream sauce.
- Have a pancake breakfast.
- Fix a bowl of cereal with low-fat milk.

During your short workouts (≤ 60 min)
- Fill your water bottle with water.
- Take a swallow of water every 15 min.

During your long workouts (> 60 min)
- Fill your water bottle with a sports drink.
- Take a sip of fluid at every sign or intersection to make sure you consume at least 6 oz every 15 min.
- Carry an apple and a bagel to snack on.
- Bring a bar that's high in carbohydrates.

When you are finished
- Drink 16 to 24 oz for each pound of weight lost.
- Refuel with a sandwich or a plate of pasta and a glass of chocolate milk.

Use iProfile to plan a precompetition meal that provides at least 50 g of carbohydrate.

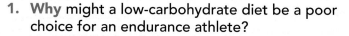

synthesis and provides the amino acids needed for muscle protein synthesis and repair (see *What Should I Eat?*).[26]

The glycogen-restoring regimen just described can replenish muscle and liver glycogen within 24 hours of an athletic event and is critical for optimizing performance on the following day. Athletes who aren't competing again the next day can replenish their glycogen stores more slowly by consuming high-carbohydrate foods for the next day or so. A diet providing about 65% of calories from carbohydrate, or about 400 g of carbohydrate in a 2500 Calorie diet, should provide sufficient carbohydrate during the recovery period.[12] More than one-third of this amount could be provided by a 6-inch sub, 12 oz of low-fat chocolate milk, a banana, and some pretzels.

Most of us are not competitive athletes, so we don't need a special glycogen replacement strategy to ensure that our glycogen stores are replenished before our next visit to the gym. If your routine includes 30 to 60 minutes at the gym, a typical diet that provides about 55% of calories from carbohydrate will replace the glycogen used so that you will be ready for a workout again the next day.

CONCEPT CHECK STOP

1. **Why** might a low-carbohydrate diet be a poor choice for an endurance athlete?

2. **Why** is dehydration more likely when it is hot and humid?

3. **How** much of what fluid should you drink during a two-hour bike ride?

4. **What** should an athlete eat as a precompetition meal and why?

Ergogenic Aids
LEARNING OBJECTIVES

1. **Assess** the health risks associated with using anabolic steroids.

2. **Explain** why creatine supplements affect sprint performance.

3. **Describe** one way in which a supplement might improve endurance.

Citius, altius, fortius—faster, higher, stronger—is the motto of the Olympic Games. For as long as there have been competitions, athletes have yearned for anything that would give them a competitive edge. Everything from bee pollen and high-dose vitamins to ancient herbs and hormones has been used as an **ergogenic aid**.

> **ergogenic aid** A substance, an appliance, or a procedure that improves athletic performance.

The impact of diet and supplements on performance • Figure 10.24

This figure illustrates the relative importance of various nutrition strategies for exercise performance. Along with talent and hard work, eating a healthy overall diet provides the most significant benefit. Sports foods and beverages can supply energy and ensure hydration during an athletic event; most ergogenic supplements provide little or no performance boost.

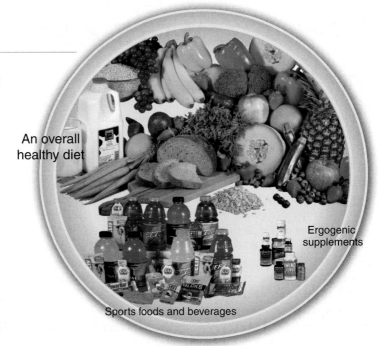

An overall healthy diet

Ergogenic supplements

Sports foods and beverages

Athletes are willing to go to great lengths to improve performance and are therefore susceptible to the lures of ergogenic supplements. Many of the vitamins, minerals, and other substances in these supplements are involved in providing energy for exercise or promoting recovery from exercise. Most supplements do not improve athletic performance, and the few that do have a small effect compared to the benefits of an overall healthy diet (**Figure 10.24**). When considering whether to use an ergogenic supplement or any other type of supplement, wise consumers weigh the health risks against the potential benefits (see Figure 7.35).

Vitamin and Mineral Supplements

Many of the promises made to athletes about the benefits of vitamin and mineral supplements are extrapolated from the biochemical functions of these micronutrients. For example, B vitamin are promoted to enhance ATP production because of their roles in muscle energy metabolism. Vitamin B_6, vitamin B_{12}, and folic acid are promoted for aerobic exercise because they are involved in the transport of oxygen to exercising muscles. These vitamins are indeed needed for energy metabolism, and a deficiency of one or more of them will interfere with ATP production and impair athletic performance. But providing more than the recommended amount does not deliver more oxygen to the muscles, cause more ATP to be produced, or enhance athletic performance.

Supplements of vitamin E, vitamin C, and selenium are promoted to athletes because of their antioxidant functions. As discussed earlier, exercise increases oxidative processes and therefore increases the production of free radicals, which cause cellular damage and have been associated with fatigue. However, antioxidant supplements have not been found to improve performance.[15]

Supplements of chromium (chromium picolinate) and vanadium (vanadyl sulfate) are marketed to increase lean body mass and decrease body fat. Chromium is needed for insulin action, and insulin promotes protein synthesis. However, studies have not consistently demonstrated that supplemental chromium has any effect on muscle strength, body composition, or other aspects of health (see Chapter 8).[27] Vanadium is also believed to assist the action of insulin, but there is no evidence that supplemental vanadium increases lean body mass.[28]

Supplements to Build Muscle

Protein supplements are often marketed to athletes with the promise of enhancing muscle growth or improving performance. Adequate protein is necessary for muscle growth, but consuming extra protein, either as food or as supplements, does not increase muscle growth or strength. Muscles enlarge in response to exercise stress. The protein provided by expensive supplements will not meet an athlete's needs any better than the protein found in a balanced diet. If an athlete's diet provides enough energy, it usually provides enough protein, without a supplement.

WHAT A SCIENTIST SEES

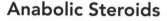 THE PLANNER

Anabolic Steroids

Athletes looking at this photograph see the bulging muscles and enhanced performance that can be achieved with anabolic steroid use. A scientist sees that these are not the only effects that anabolic steroids have. These drugs make the body think natural testosterone is being produced, and therefore, as shown in the diagram, the body shuts down its own testosterone production. Natural testosterone stimulates and maintains the male sexual organs and promotes the development of bones and muscles and the growth of skin and hair. The synthetic testosterone in anabolic steroids has a greater effect on muscle, bone, skin, and hair than it does on sexual organs. Without natural testosterone, the sexual organs are not maintained; this leads to shrinkage of the testicles and a decrease in sperm production.[33]

In adolescents, the use of anabolic steroids causes cessation of bone growth and stunted height. Anabolic steroid use may also cause oily skin and acne, water retention in the tissues, yellowing of the eyes and skin, coronary artery disease, liver disease, and sometimes death. Users may experience psychological and behavioral side effects such as violent outbursts and depression, possibly leading to suicide.[33]

When testosterone levels are low, the hypothalamus releases a hormone that stimulates the anterior pituitary to secrete a hormone that increases the production of testosterone by the testes. High levels of either natural or synthetic testosterone inhibit the release of the stimulatory hormone from the hypothalamus, shutting down the synthesis of natural testosterone.

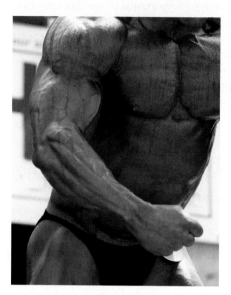

Despite the risks, between 1 million and 3 million athletes in the United States have used anabolic steroids.[34] Anabolic steroids are controlled substances and are banned by the International Olympic Committee, the National Collegiate Athletic Association (NCAA), and most other sporting organizations.[35]

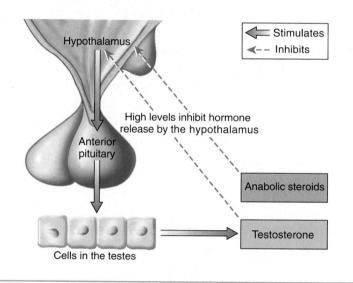

Think Critically
Why does anabolic steroid use promote muscle development while causing the testes to shrink?

Growth hormone is another hormone used as an ergogenic aid. It is appealing to athletes because it increases muscle protein synthesis. Despite this physiological effect, however, it has not been shown to enhance muscle strength, power, or aerobic exercise capacity, but there is evidence that it improves anaerobic exercise capacity.[29] Prolonged use of growth hormone can cause heart dysfunction, high blood pressure, and excessive growth of some body parts, such as hands, feet, and facial features. Growth hormone is on the World Anti-Doping Agency's list of banned substances.

Supplements of the amino acids ornithine, arginine, and lysine are marketed with the promise that they will stimulate the release of growth hormone and, in turn, enhance the growth of muscles. Large doses of these amino acids have been shown to stimulate the release of growth hormone. However, growth hormone levels in the blood of athletes taking these amino acids are no greater than levels typically resulting from exercise alone. Also, supplements of these amino acids have not been found to cause greater increases in muscle mass and strength than those achieved through strength-training exercise alone.[30, 31]

Anabolic steroids accelerate protein synthesis. When taken in conjunction with exercise and an adequate diet, they cause increases in muscle size and strength. However, they have extremely dangerous side effects (see *What a Scientist Sees*). Anabolic steroids are regulated as controlled substances. **Steroid precursors**, which are compounds that can be converted into steroid hormones in the body, are also classified as controlled substances. The best known of these is androstenedione, often referred to as "andro." It was launched to public prominence when professional baseball player Mark McGwire announced his use of it during the 1998 major league baseball season, when he hit 70 home runs, breaking the league's single-season home-run record. Contrary to marketing claims, the use of andro or other steroid precursors has not been found to increase testosterone levels or produce any ergogenic effects, and they may cause some of the same side effects as anabolic steroids.[32]

Supplements to Enhance Performance in Short, Intense Activities

A number of supplements are marketed to athletes who seek to improve performance in sports that depend on quick bursts of intense activity. Supplements of β-hydroxy-β-methylbutyrate, known as HMB, claim to increase strength and muscle growth and improve muscle recovery; however, the outcome of research studies has been variable. Overall, studies have found a small increase in strength in previously untrained men, but the effects in trained weight lifters are trivial, as is the effect of HMB on body composition.[36]

Bicarbonate is a supplement that may enhance performance in high-intensity activities. Because bicarbonate acts as a buffer in the body, supplementing it is thought to neutralize acid and thus delay fatigue and allow improved performance. Taking sodium bicarbonate, which is just baking soda from the kitchen cupboard, before exercise has been found to improve performance and delay exhaustion in sports, such as sprint cycling and sprint swimming, which entail intense exercise lasting only one to seven minutes. It has also been found to enhance endurance in longer continuous and intermittent exercise, such as running and cycling.[37] However, just because baking soda is an ingredient in your cookies does not mean that it is risk free. Many people experience abdominal cramps and diarrhea after taking sodium bicarbonate, and other possible side effects have not been carefully researched.

One of the most popular ergogenic supplements is **creatine**. This nitrogen-containing compound is found primarily in muscle, where it is used to make creatine phosphate (**Figure 10.25**). Higher levels of creatine and creatine phosphate provide more quick energy for short-term muscular activity. Creatine supplementation has been shown to improve performance in high-intensity exercise lasting 30 seconds or less. It is therefore beneficial for exercise that requires explosive bursts of energy, such as sprinting and weight lifting, but not for long-term endurance activities, such as marathons.[38]

Athletes also take creatine supplements to increase muscle mass and strength. Some of the increase in lean body mass is believed to be due to water retention related

Creatine boosts creatine phosphate • Figure 10.25

Creatine can be synthesized in the liver and kidneys and also comes from meat and milk in the diet. The more creatine consumed, the greater the amount of creatine stored in the muscles. Increasing creatine intake with supplement use has been shown to increase levels of muscle creatine and creatine phosphate, which is made from it.[38] During short bursts of intense activity, the creatine phosphate can be converted back into creatine, transforming ADP to ATP for muscle contraction.

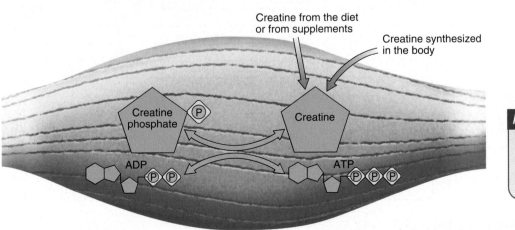

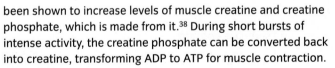

Ask Yourself

When creatine phosphate is converted into creatine, what happens to the phosphate group? What other molecule is made?

Debate   Energy Drinks for Athletic Performance?

The Issue: Energy drinks are sold alongside sports drinks, and manufacturers of these beverages often sponsor athletes and athletic events. Should they be used as ergogenic aids? Is drinking them a safe way to improve your game?

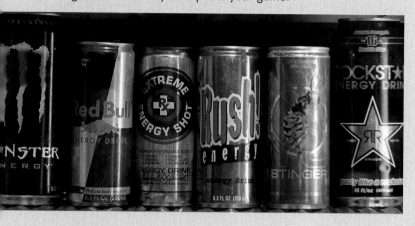

The popularity of energy drinks with names like Red Bull, Monster, and Full Throttle has soared over the past decade. They promise to keep you alert to study, work, drive, party all night, and perhaps excel at your next athletic competition. The main ingredients in these drinks are sugar and caffeine. Glucose is an important fuel for exercise, and caffeine is known to enhance endurance, so these drinks may seem like an ideal ergogenic aid.

A traditional sports drink, like Gatorade, contains about 28 g of sugar in 16 ounces; a typical energy drink provides twice this much (55 to 60 g, or about 14 teaspoons). Since carbohydrate fuels activity, it may seem that the additional sugar would provide energy for prolonged exercise. But more is not always better during activity. The double load of sugar cannot be absorbed quickly, and unabsorbed sugar in the stomach can cause GI distress and also slow fluid absorption.

The caffeine content of energy drinks ranges from 50 to about 500 mg per can or bottle. Caffeine is an effective ergogenic aid that enhances endurance when consumed before or during exercise.[44] But too much caffeine, referred to as *caffeine intoxication*, causes nervousness, anxiety, restlessness, insomnia, gastrointestinal upset, tremors, increased blood pressure, and rapid heartbeat. A number of cases of caffeine-associated death, seizure, and cardiac arrest have occurred after consumption of energy drinks.[45–47] Even if the caffeine in an energy drink increases endurance, depending on when it is consumed, it can affect timing and coordination and hurt overall performance. Caffeine is also a diuretic; at the levels contained in these drinks, it may contribute to dehydration, particularly in first-time users.[48] The FDA limits the amount of caffeine in soft drinks to 0.02% (about 71 mg in 12 oz), but energy drinks are considered dietary supplements, so the caffeine content is not regulated.

Energy drinks often also contain other ingredients that promise to improve performance, such as B vitamins, taurine, guarana, and ginseng. B vitamins are needed to produce ATP, so they are marketed to enhance energy production from sugar. But unless you are deficient in these vitamins, drinking them in an energy drink will not enhance your ATP production. Taurine is an amino acid that may reduce the amount of muscle damage and improve exercise performance and capacity, but not all research supports these claims.[47] Guarana is an herbal ingredient that contains caffeine as well as small amounts of the stimulants theobromine and theophylline. The extra caffeine from guarana (not included in the caffeine listed for these beverages) may contribute to caffeine toxicity. Ginseng is also claimed to have performance-enhancing effects, but these effects have not been demonstrated scientifically.[46,49] In general, the amounts of these ingredients are too small to have much effect, and the safety of consuming them in combination with caffeine prior to or during exercise has yet to be established.[46]

So should you down an energy drink before your next competition? They do provide a caffeine boost, but is it so much caffeine that you risk dehydration, high blood pressure, and heart problems? Energy drinks provide sugar to fuel activity, but will they upset your stomach? What about the herbal ingredients—do they offer a benefit you are looking for?

Think critically: Use the table below to assess the advantages and disadvantages of consuming an 8-oz can of Red Bull versus a 12-oz can of Coca-Cola Classic before your 30-minute run.

Caffeine content				
Beverage	Serving (fluid ounces)	Caffeine (mg)	Sugar (g)	Energy (calories)
Coffee	8	100–200	0	0
Espresso with sugar	1.5	100	15–30	60–120
Coca-Cola Classic	12	35	39	140
Mountain Dew	12	54	46	170
Monster	16	160	54	200
Jolt Cola	8	80	30	120
Arizona Caution Extreme Energy Shot	8	100	33	130
Red Bull	8	80	28	110
Rockstar	16	160	62	280
Monster	8	80	27	100
Full Throttle	16	160	57	220

to creatine uptake in the muscle. In addition, an increase in muscle mass and strength may occur when supplementation is combined with muscle-strengthening exercises because the increase in muscle creatine permits a higher level of training intensity, which leads to greater muscle hypertrophy.[39]

Creatine supplementation at intakes of up to 5 g per day appears to be safe for up to a year, but the safety of higher doses over the long term has not been established.[40] Ingestion of creatine immediately before or during exercise is not recommended, and the FDA has advised consumers to consult a physician before using creatine.

Supplements to Enhance Endurance

Sprinters and weight lifters can benefit from increases in creatine phosphate levels, but endurance athletes are more concerned about running out of glycogen. Glycogen is spared when fat is used as an energy source, allowing exercise to continue for a longer time before glycogen is depleted and fatigue sets in. Supplements that increase the amount of fat or oxygen available to the muscle cell are used to increase endurance.

Carnitine supplements are marketed as fat burners—substances that increase the utilization of fat during exercise. Carnitine is needed to transport fatty acids into the mitochondria, where they are used to produce ATP by aerobic metabolism. However, enough carnitine is made in the body to ensure efficient use of fatty acids. Carnitine supplements have not been shown to increase endurance.[41]

Medium-chain triglycerides (MCT) are composed of fatty acids with medium-length carbon chains (8 to 10 carbons). These fatty acids can be absorbed directly into the blood without first being incorporated into chylomicrons. They are therefore absorbed quickly, causing blood fatty acids levels to rise and thereby increasing the availability of fat as a fuel for exercise. Nevertheless, research has not found that supplementation with MCT increases endurance, spares glycogen, or enhances performance.[42]

Caffeine is a stimulant found in coffee, tea, soft drinks, and energy drinks (see *Debate: Energy Drinks for Athletic Performance?*).[43] Consuming 3 to 6 mg of caffeine per kilogram of body weight, an amount equivalent to about 2.5 cups of percolated coffee, up to an hour before exercising as well as consuming smaller doses of caffeine during exercise (1 to 2 mg/kg) have been shown to improve endurance.[38] Caffeine enhances the release of fatty acids. When fatty acids are used as a fuel source, less glycogen is used, and the onset of fatigue is delayed. Athletes who are unaccustomed to caffeine respond better to it than do those who consume caffeine routinely. Caffeine also improves concentration and enhances alertness, but in some athletes, it may impair performance by causing gastrointestinal upset.

Athletes also use the hormone erythropoietin, known as EPO, to enhance endurance. Natural erythropoietin is produced by the kidneys and stimulates cells in the bone marrow to differentiate into red blood cells. EPO can enhance endurance by increasing the ability to transport oxygen to the muscles. It therefore increases aerobic capacity and spares glycogen. However, too much EPO can cause production of too many red blood cells, which can lead to excessive blood clotting, heart attacks, and strokes. EPO was banned in 1990, after it was linked to the deaths of more than a dozen cyclists.[50]

Other Supplements

In addition to the supplements discussed thus far, hundreds of other products are marketed to athletes. Most have no effect on performance. For example, brewer's yeast is a source of B vitamins and some minerals but has not been found to have any ergogenic properties. Likewise, there is no evidence to support claims that bee pollen or wheat germ oil enhance performance. Royal jelly is a substance that worker bees produce to help the queen bee grow larger and live longer, but it does not appear to enhance athletic capacity in humans. Supplements of DNA and RNA are marketed to aid in tissue regeneration. DNA and RNA are needed to synthesize proteins, but they are not required in the diet, and supplements do not help replace damaged cells.

Herbal products are also marketed to athletes. Most have not been studied extensively for their ergogenic effects, so the only evidence of their benefits is anecdotal. Many can harm health as well as performance, so athletes should consider the risks before using these products.

CONCEPT CHECK   **STOP**

1. **How** do anabolic steroids affect the production of testosterone?

2. **Why** are creatine supplements beneficial for sprint and strength athletes?

3. **How** does caffeine increase endurance?

Summary

1 Physical Activity, Fitness, and Health 354

- Regular exercise improves **fitness**. How fit an individual is depends on his or her **cardiorespiratory endurance**, **muscle strength**, **muscle endurance**, flexibility, and body composition. Regular **aerobic exercise** improves **aerobic capacity**. **Muscle-strengthening exercise** increases muscle strength and endurance.

- Regular exercise can reduce the risk of chronic diseases such as obesity, heart disease, diabetes, and osteoporosis. It can reduce overall mortality even in obese individuals.

- Exercise helps manage body weight by increasing energy expenditure, as shown in the graph, and by increasing the proportion of body weight that is lean tissue.

Exercise increases energy expenditure • Figure 10.3

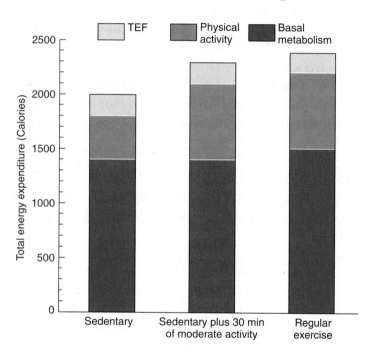

2 Exercise Recommendations 357

- To reduce the risk of chronic disease, a minimum of 30 minutes of moderate-intensity aerobic exercise on most days is recommended, as indicated by the calendar. A well-designed fitness program involves aerobic exercise, stretching, and muscle-strengthening exercises.

Exercise recommendations • Figure 10.4

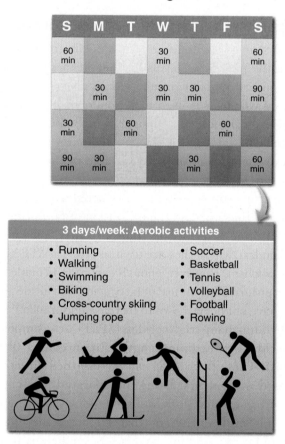

- An exercise program should include activities that are enjoyable, convenient, and safe. Rest is important to allow the body to recover and rebuild. In serious athletes, inadequate rest can lead to **overtraining syndrome**.

3 Fueling Exercise 361

- The graph illustrates that during the first 10 to 15 seconds of exercise, ATP and **creatine phosphate** stored in the muscle provide energy to fuel activity. During the next 2 to 3 minutes, the amount of oxygen at the muscle remains limited, so ATP is generated by the **anaerobic metabolism** of glucose. After a few minutes, the delivery of oxygen at the muscle increases, and ATP can be generated by **aerobic metabolism**. Aerobic metabolism is more efficient than anaerobic metabolism and can utilize glucose, fatty acids, and amino acids as energy sources. The use of protein as an energy source increases when exercise continues for many hours.

Changes in the source of ATP over time • Figure 10.9

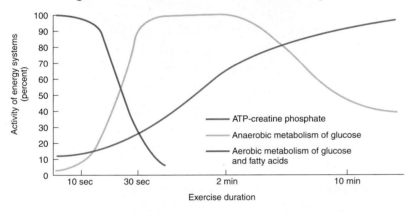

- For short-term, high-intensity activity, ATP is generated primarily from the anaerobic metabolism of glucose from glycogen stores. Anaerobic metabolism uses glucose more rapidly and produces **lactic acid**. Both of these factors are associated with the onset of **fatigue**. For lower-intensity exercise of longer duration, aerobic metabolism predominates, and both glucose and fatty acids are important fuel sources.

- Fitness training causes changes in the cardiovascular system and muscles that improve oxygen delivery and utilization, allowing aerobic exercise to be sustained for longer periods at higher intensity.

4 Energy and Nutrient Needs for Physical Activity 367

- The diet of an active individual should provide sufficient energy to fuel activity. The pressure to compete and maintain a body weight that is optimal for their sport puts some athletes at risk for eating disorders. A com-

bination of excessive exercise and energy restriction puts female athletes at risk for the **female athlete triad**, shown here.

Female athlete triad • Figure 10.15

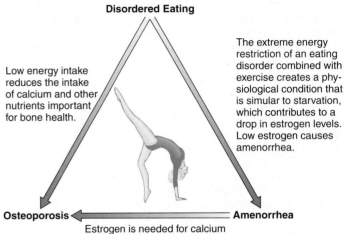

- To maximize glycogen stores, optimize performance, and maintain and repair lean tissue, a diet providing about 60% of energy from carbohydrate, 20 to 25% of energy from fat, and about 15 to 20% of energy from protein is recommended.

- Sufficient vitamins and minerals are needed to generate ATP from macronutrients, to maintain and repair tissues, and to transport oxygen and wastes to and from the cells. Most athletes who consume a varied diet that meets their energy needs also meet their vitamin and mineral needs from their diet alone. Those who restrict their food intake may be at risk for deficiencies. Increased iron needs and greater iron losses due to fitness training put athletes, particularly female athletes, at risk for iron deficiency.

- Water is needed to ensure that the body can be cooled and that nutrients and oxygen can be delivered to body tissues. If water intake is inadequate, dehydration can lead to a decline in exercise performance and increase the risk of **heat-related illness**. Adequate fluid intake before exercise ensures that athletes begin exercise well hydrated. Fluid intake during and after exercise must replace water lost in sweat and from evaporation through the lungs. Plain water is an appropriate fluid to consume for most exercise. Beverages containing carbohydrate and sodium are recommended for exercise lasting more than an hour. Drinking plain water during extended exercise increases the risk of hyponatremia.

- Competitive endurance athletes may benefit from **glycogen supercompensation (carbohydrate loading)**, which maximizes glycogen stores before an event. Meals eaten before competition should help ensure adequate hydration, provide moderate amounts of protein, be high enough in carbohydrate to maximize glycogen stores, be low in fat and fiber to speed gastric emptying, and satisfy the psychological needs of the athlete. During exercise, athletes need beverages and food to replace lost fluid and provide carbohydrate and sodium. Postcompetition meals should replace lost fluids and electrolytes, provide carbohydrate to restore muscle and liver glycogen, and provide protein for muscle protein synthesis and repair.

5 Ergogenic Aids 376

- Many types of **ergogenic aids** are marketed to improve athletic performance. Some are beneficial for certain types of activity, but many offer little or no benefit. An individual risk–benefit analysis should be used to determine whether a supplement is appropriate for you.

- **Anabolic steroids** combined with muscle-strengthening exercise increase muscle size and strength, but these supplements are illegal and have dangerous side effects.

- **Creatine** supplementation increases muscle creatine phosphate levels, as illustrated here, and has been shown to increase muscle mass and improve performance in short-duration, high-intensity exercise. Caffeine use can improve performance in endurance activities, but high doses can cause caffeine toxicity and contribute to dehydration in some athletes.

Creatine boosts creatine phosphate • Figure 10.25

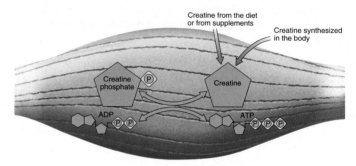

Key Terms

- aerobic capacity 355
- aerobic exercise 355
- aerobic metabolism 361
- aerobic zone 359
- anabolic steroids 379
- anaerobic metabolism 361
- atrophy 354
- cardiorespiratory endurance 355
- creatine 379

- creatine phosphate 362
- endorphins 356
- ergogenic aid 376
- fatigue 365
- female athlete triad 368
- fitness 354
- glycogen supercompensation or carbohydrate loading 373

- heat cramps 371
- heat exhaustion 371
- heat stroke 371
- heat-related illnesses 370
- hypertrophy 354
- lactic acid 361
- maximum heart rate 359
- muscle endurance 355

- muscle strength 355
- muscle-strengthening exercise 355
- overload principle 354
- overtraining syndrome 360
- resting heart rate 355
- sports anemia 370
- steroid precursors 379

Online Resources

- For more information on exercise recommendations, go to www.cdc.gov/physicalactivity/everyone/guidelines/index.html.

- For more information on the health benefits of exercise and how to get started, go to www.mayoclinic.com/health/exercise/HQ01676.

- For more information on eating for athletic competition, go to www.aces.edu/pubs/docs/H/HE-0750/.

- For more information on ergogenic aids, go to http://fnic.nal.usda.gov/nal_display/index.php?info_center=4&tax_level=2&tax_subject=274&topic_id=1329.

- Visit your *WileyPLUS* site for videos, animations, podcasts, self-study, and other media that will aid you in studying and understanding this chapter.

Critical and Creative Thinking Questions

1. On the way to an out-of-town soccer match, Max's team stops at a fast-food restaurant. It is only about an hour before game time. Most of the boys have burgers, fries, and a soft drink. How might this affect their performance in the game? What would you recommend they do differently for the next match?

2. Evaluate your weekly physical activity. Does it meet the current exercise recommendations? Do you include activities to enhance your strength, endurance, and flexibility? Can each of these activities be performed year-round? If not, suggest alternative activities and locations for inclement weather. How could you improve on what you are currently doing?

3. As part of an exercise study, John is asked to ride a stationary bicycle while breathing into a mouthpiece to measure the gases in inhaled and exhaled air. During his ride, the intensity of the exercise is steadily increased. The graph below shows the results of this test. Based on the data in the graph, what is John's aerobic capacity? Explain why?

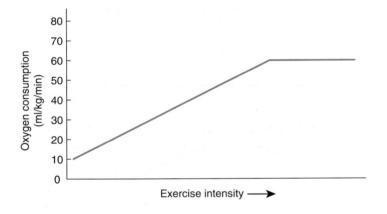

4. Using your knowledge of energy production and body energy stores, explain why during exercise cells rely more on glucose and fat for energy than on protein.

5. Two friends are running a marathon together. One has participated in an intensive training program. The other was too busy and trained only a few hours a week. After about 5 minutes of running the marathon, they have settled into a slow, steady pace and are able to carry on a conversation. After an hour, the well-trained individual is feeling good and so increases her pace. The untrained person tries to keep up but is no longer able to talk, and after about 15 minutes is fatigued and needs to stop. Why does the untrained person tire faster?

6. David is beginning an exercise program. He plans to run before lunch and then play racquetball every night after dinner. When he begins his exercise program, he finds that he feels lethargic and hungry before his late-morning run. After running, he doesn't have much of an appetite, so he saves his lunch until midafternoon. He is still hungry enough to eat dinner at home with his family but finds that he is getting stomach cramps and is too full when he goes to play racquetball. His typical diet is

   > Breakfast: Orange juice, coffee
   >
   > Lunch: Ham and cheese sandwich, potato chips, soft drink, cookies
   >
   > Dinner: Steak, baked potato with sour cream and butter, green beans in butter sauce, salad with Italian dressing, whole milk

   How might David change his diet to make it better suited to his exercise program? Do you think David will be able to stick with this exercise program? Why or why not? Suggest some changes that would make David's exercise program more convenient and more balanced.

7. Do a risk–benefit analysis of an ergogenic aid. (A quick way to do this is to use the Internet to collect information.) List the risks and benefits and then write a conclusion, stating why you would or would not take this substance.

What is happening in this picture?

During competitive events, cyclists often spend six or more hours a day riding their bikes. This rider is collecting water bottles from his team's car. He will carry these ahead and deliver them to the other cyclists on his team.

Think Critically

1. How much might someone need to drink during six hours of cycling?
2. What type of fluid do you think is in the water bottles? Why?
3. What type of food might the riders want to pick up from their team car?

Self-Test

(Check Your Answers In Appendix K.)

1. Which bar on this graph indicates the proportion of energy obtained from glucose, fatty acids, and amino acids that would be used as fuel while studying for an exam?

   a. A   b. B   c. C

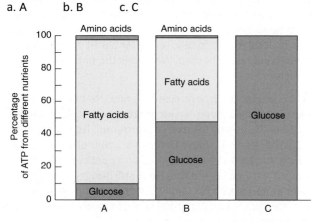

2. Which of the following occurs as a result of aerobic exercise training?

   a. decrease in resting heart rate

   b. increase in the number of red blood cells

   c. more muscle mitochondria

   d. greater glycogen storage

   e. all of the above

3. If an athlete loses a lot of water and salt in sweat but drinks only water, he is at risk for _____.

   a. hypertension   d. hyponatremia

   b. hypodermic   e. dehydration

   c. hyperactivity

4. Which statement is true of the energy system indicated by the arrow?

   a. It provides energy for the first 10 to 15 seconds of activity.

   b. It can use glucose, amino acids, and fatty acids to produce ATP.

   c. It produces ATP rapidly but inefficiently.

   d. It can use only glucose to generate ATP.

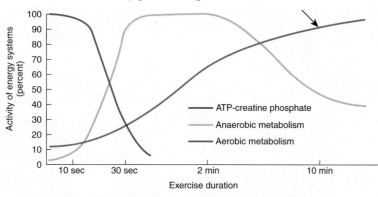

5. Andreas is 30 years old. He would like to exercise at an intensity that ensures he is in his aerobic zone. Use this graph to determine the heart rate range that is appropriate for Andreas.

   a. 114 to 162   d. 87 to 120

   b. 114 to 190   e. 123 to 170

   c. 120 to 170

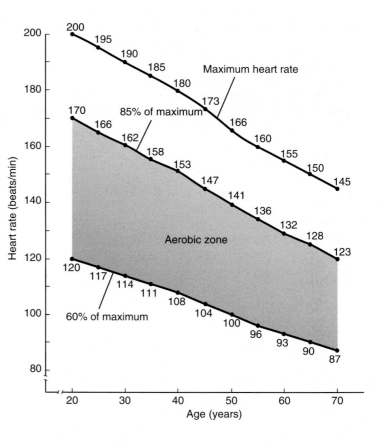

6. The source of fuel in the first few seconds of exercise is _____.

   a. ATP and creatine phosphate

   b. stored glycogen

   c. glucose made by the liver

   d. fatty acids

   e. protein

7. Which nutrient can be used to produce energy in the absence of oxygen?

   a. protein   d. B vitamins

   b. fatty acids   e. lactic acid

   c. glucose

8. The female athlete triad consists of _____.

   a. iron deficiency anemia, disordered eating, and excess menstrual blood loss

   b. disordered eating, amenorrhea, and osteoporosis

   c. dieting, excessive exercise, and folate deficiency

   d. iron, calcium, and zinc deficiency

9. Which of the following statements about carbohydrate loading is false?

   a. It provides a competitive advantage for sprinters and weight lifters.

   b. It causes short-term weight gain.

   c. It involves manipulating diet and activity patterns before an event.

   d. It can enhance endurance.

10. Which of the following is a goal of precompetition meals?

    a. maximize fat stores

    b. increase muscle mass

    c. keep the stomach full

    d. maximize glycogen stores

11. True or false: A fit person will have a higher percentage of lean tissue than an unfit person of the same body weight.

    a. True   b. False

12. The best fluid to consume during a marathon is _____.

    a. plain water

    b. fruit juice

    c. a sports drink containing glucose and sodium

    d. a protein shake

13. How much and how often should athletes drink during exercise?

    a. as much as they can

    b. enough to prevent weight loss

    c. a cup every hour

    d. nothing unless exercise lasts more than 60 minutes

14. Amy lives in Connecticut, where the summer temperature and humidity can vary dramatically from day to day. On Monday, it is 88°F, with a relative humidity of 90%. On Tuesday, the temperature goes up to 96°F, but the humidity drops to 60%. By Wednesday, the temperature has dropped slightly to 92°F, but the humidity has increased to 65%. On Thursday, the temperature drops to 90°F, and the humidity climbs to 85%. Use the table shown here to determine which day has the lowest heat index.

    a. Monday   c. Wednesday

    b. Tuesday   d. Thursday

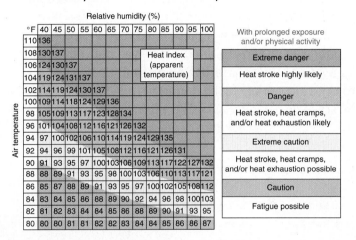

15. Which of the following best describes how creatine supplements enhance performance?

    a. They increase the amount of creatine phosphate in the muscle.

    b. They increase the transport of fatty acids into the mitochondria.

    c. They increase delivery of oxygen to the muscle.

    d. They eliminate free radicals.

THE PLANNER ✓

Review your Chapter Planner on the chapter opener and check off you completed work.

Nutrition During Pregnancy and Infancy

11

"**Y**ou're eating for two now!" Optimal maternal nutrition during pregnancy can help ensure the birth of a healthy baby; too much or too little can compromise fetal health.

Gaining too little weight during pregnancy can produce an undernourished infant who may never catch up with healthy counterparts. Overnutrition poses risks to both mother and child during birth. A fetus may also be subject to dangerous effects from deficiencies or excesses of vitamins and minerals. For example, lack of sufficient iodine during pregnancy has been linked to brain damage in the baby, insufficient iron creates an increased risk of anemia for an infant, and too much vitamin A causes an increased risk of birth defects of the head, face, heart, and brain.

The responsibility of the mother does not stop when the infant is born. The 40 weeks of a pregnancy produce a helpless newborn who requires a lengthy

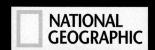

period of care. Breast milk provides optimal nutrition for a growing infant, and a breast-feeding mother's diet continues to affect the nutrition of her child. Infant nutrition can affect both growth in the early years and the potential for developing chronic diseases later in life. Healthier pregnancies yield healthier babies who become healthier children and ultimately healthier adults.

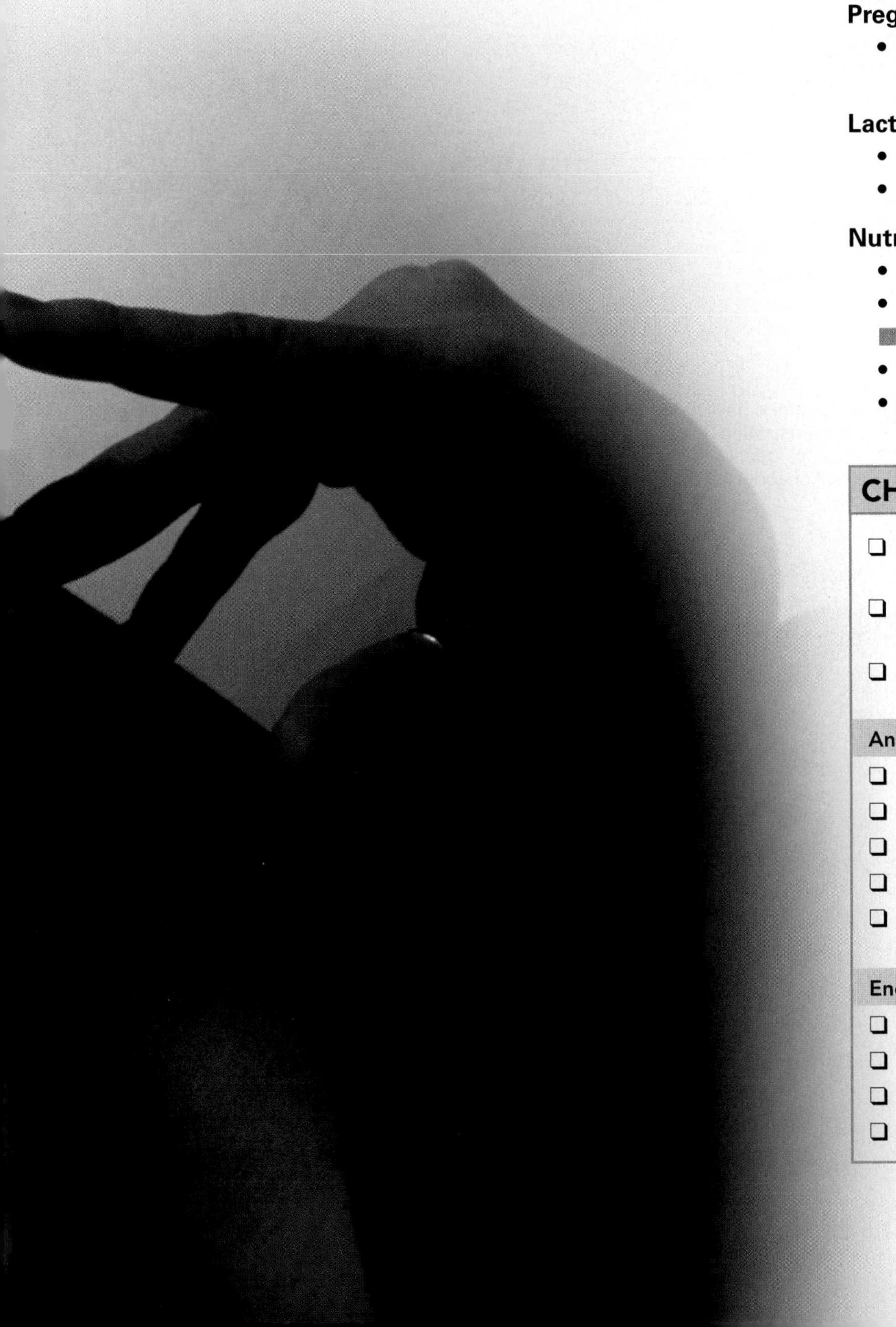

CHAPTER PLANNER ✓

- ❏ Stimulate your interest by reading the opening story and looking at the visual.
- ❏ Scan the Learning Objectives in each section:
  p. 390 ❏   p. 396 ❏   p. 403 ❏   p. 408 ❏   p. 411 ❏
- ❏ Read the text and study all figures and visuals. Answer any questions.

Analyze key features

- ❏ Process Diagram, p. 390 ❏
- ❏ What a Scientist Sees, p. 398 ❏
- ❏ Thinking It Through p. 401 ❏
- ❏ Nutrition InSight, p. 419 ❏
- ❏ Stop: Answer the Concept Checks before you go on:
  p. 395 ❏   p. 402 ❏   p. 408 ❏   p. 410 ❏   p. 419 ❏

End of chapter

- ❏ Review the Summary, Online Resources, and Key Terms.
- ❏ Answer the Critical and Creative Thinking Questions.
- ❏ Answer What is happening in this picture?
- ❏ Complete the Self-Test and check your answers.

Changes in the Body During Pregnancy

LEARNING OBJECTIVES

1. **Describe** how the embryo and fetus are nourished.

2. **Discuss** why appropriate weight gain is important during pregnancy.

3. **Explain** why morning sickness, heartburn, and constipation are common during pregnancy.

4. **Review** the risks associated with the hypertensive disorders of pregnancy and gestational diabetes.

 hether you end up 6 feet 4 inches or 5 ft 3 in. tall, you begin as a single cell that arises from the union of a sperm and an egg. Over the course of 40 weeks, this cell grows and develops into a fully formed human baby. Prenatal growth and development are carefully orchestrated processes that require adequate supplies of all the essential nutrients in order to progress normally.

In the days after **fertilization**, the single cell divides rapidly to form a ball of cells (**Figure 11.1**). The cells then begin to differentiate and move to form

> **fertilization** The union of a sperm and an egg.

PROCESS DIAGRAM

Prenatal development • Figure 11.1

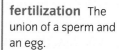 THE PLANNER

This cross section shows the path of the egg and developing embryo from the ovary, where the egg is produced, through the oviduct to the uterus, where most prenatal development occurs.

1 Ovulation releases an egg from the woman's ovary.

2 Fertilization occurs in the oviduct 12 to 24 hours after ovulation.

3 About 30 hours after fertilization, the fertilized egg has completed its first cell division.

4 About 3 or 4 days after fertilization, the developing embryo is a ball of about 100 cells.

5 About 6 days after fertilization, the developing embryo begins to implant itself in the uterine lining. Implantation is complete by 14 days after fertilization.

Oviduct

Ovulation

Ovary

Uterine cavity

Uterus

6 During the embryonic stage of development, from 2 to 8 weeks after fertilization, cells differentiate and arrange themselves in the proper locations to form the major organ systems. The embryo shown here is about 5 to 6 weeks old and less than 3 cm long. The organ systems and external body structures are not fully developed. ▼

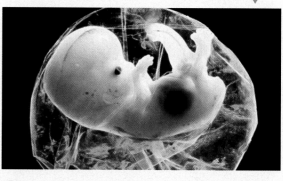

7 The fetal stage of development begins at 9 weeks after fertilization and continues until birth. During this time, the fetus grows, and internal and external body structures continue to develop. This fetus is about 16 weeks old and about 16 cm long. ▼

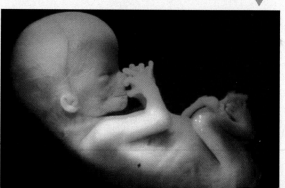

HOW IT WORKS

The placenta • Figure 11.2

The placenta is made up of branchlike projections that extend from the embryo into the uterine lining, placing maternal and fetal blood in close proximity. The placenta allows nutrients and oxygen to pass from maternal blood to fetal blood and waste products to be transferred from fetal blood to maternal blood. Fetal blood travels to and from the placenta via the umbilical cord.

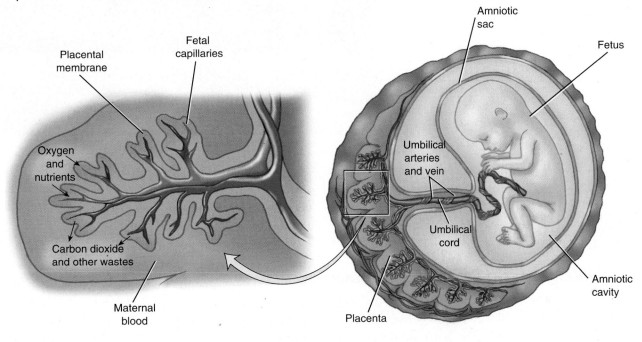

implantation The process through which a developing embryo embeds itself in the uterine lining.

embryo A developing human from two through eight weeks after fertilization.

body structures. During these early steps in development, this ball of cells obtains the nutrients it needs from the fluids around it. About a week after fertilization, the developing embryo begins burrowing into the lining of the uterus; and by two weeks, **implantation** is complete, and the cluster of cells has become an **embryo**.

Nourishing the Embryo and Fetus

The embryonic stage of development lasts until the eighth week after fertilization. During this time, the cells differentiate to form the multitude of specialized cell types that make up the human body. At the end of this stage, the embryo is about 3 centimeters long and has a beating heart. The rudiments of all major external and internal body structures have been formed.

The early embryo gets its nourishment by breaking down the lining of the uterus, but soon this source is inadequate to meet its growing needs. After about five weeks, the **placenta** takes over the role of nourishing the embryo (**Figure 11.2**). The placenta also secretes hormones that are necessary to maintain pregnancy.

From the ninth week on, the developing offspring is a **fetus**. During the fetal period, structures formed during the embryonic period grow and mature. The placenta continues to nourish the fetus until birth. During this time, the length of the fetus increases from about 3 cm to around 50 cm. The fetal period usually ends after 40 weeks, with the birth of an infant weighing 3 to 4 kilograms (6.5 to 9 pounds).[1]

Infants who are born on time but have failed to grow well in the uterus are said to be **small for gestational age**. Those born before 37 weeks of gestation are said to be **preterm**, or **premature**. Whether born too soon or too

placenta An organ produced from maternal and embryonic tissues. It secretes hormones, transfers nutrients and oxygen from the mother's blood to the fetus, and removes metabolic wastes.

fetus A developing human from the ninth week after fertilization to birth.

Low-birth-weight infants • Figure 11.3

Low-birth-weight and very-low-birth-weight infants require special care and a special diet in order to continue to grow and develop. Today, with advances in medical and nutritional care, infants born as early as 25 weeks of gestation and those weighing as little as 1 kg (2.2 lb) can survive.[2]

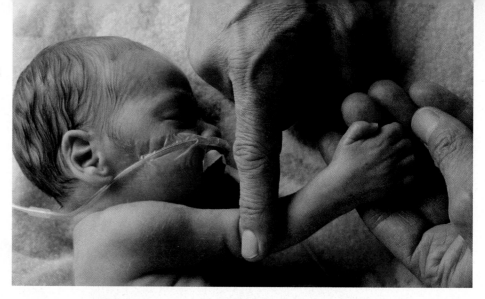

> **low birth weight** A birth weight less than 2.5 kg (5.5 lb).
>
> **very low birth weight** A birth weight less than 1.5 kg (3.3 lb).

small, **low-birth-weight** infants and **very-low-birth-weight** infants are at increased risk for illness and early death (**Figure 11.3**).

Maternal Weight Gain During Pregnancy

During pregnancy, a woman's body undergoes many changes to support the growth and development of her child. Her blood volume increases by 50%. The placenta develops in order to allow nutrients to be delivered to the fetus and produce hormones that orchestrate other changes in the mother's body. The amount of body fat increases to provide the energy needed late in pregnancy. The uterus enlarges, muscles and ligaments relax to accommodate the growing

> **lactation** Production and secretion of milk.

fetus and allow for childbirth, and the breasts develop in preparation for **lactation**. All these changes naturally result in weight gain (**Figure 11.4a**).

A healthy, normal-weight woman should gain 11 to 16 kg (25 to 35 lb) during pregnancy.[1] The rate of weight gain is as important as the amount gained. Little gain is expected in the first 3 months, or **trimester**—usually about 1 to 2 kg (2 to 4 lb). In the second and third trimesters, the recommended maternal weight gain is about 0.5 kg (1 lb)/week. Women who are underweight and women who are overweight or obese at conception should also gain weight at a slow, steady rate, but the total amount of weight gain recommended is higher and lower than for normal-weight women, respectively (**Figure 11.4b**).[1]

Being underweight by 10% or more at the onset of pregnancy or gaining too little weight during pregnancy increases the risk of producing a low-birth-weight baby.[3] Excess weight, whether present before conception or gained during pregnancy, can also compromise pregnancy outcome.

The mother's risks for high blood pressure, diabetes, a difficult delivery, and need for a **cesarean section** are increased by excess weight, as is the risk of having a **large-for-gestational-age** baby.[4] Excessive prenatal weight gain also increases the mother's long-term risk for obesity, and there is evidence that it may increase the risk that the baby will be overweight in childhood.[5,6] However, dieting during pregnancy is not advised, even for obese women. If possible, excess weight should be lost before the pregnancy begins or, alternatively, after the child has been born and weaned.

> **large for gestational age** Weighing more than 4 kg (8.8 lb) at birth.

Physical Activity During Pregnancy

During pregnancy, women gain weight and carry the extra weight in the front of the body, where it can interfere with balance and put stress on bones, joints, and muscles, increasing the risk of exercise-related injury. However, this doesn't mean that a pregnant woman should give up her regular exercise routines. Physical activity during pregnancy can improve digestion; prevent excess weight gain, low back pain, and constipation; reduce the risk of diabetes and high blood pressure; and speed recovery from childbirth. Guidelines for exercise during pregnancy have been developed to maximize the benefits and minimize the risks of injury to mother and fetus. In general, women who were physically active before becoming pregnant can continue a program of about 30 minutes of carefully chosen moderate exercise per day.[3,7] Women who weren't active before pregnancy should slowly add low-intensity, low-impact activities.[7] Because intense exercise can limit the delivery of oxygen and nutrients to the fetus, intense exercise should be limited (**Table 11.1**).

Rate and composition of weight gain during pregnancy • Figure 11.4

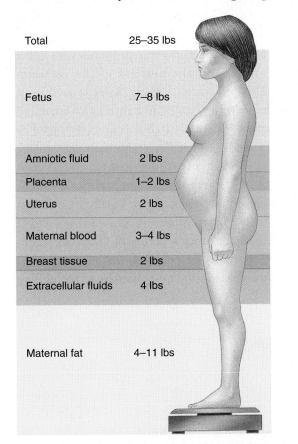

Total	25–35 lbs
Fetus	7–8 lbs
Amniotic fluid	2 lbs
Placenta	1–2 lbs
Uterus	2 lbs
Maternal blood	3–4 lbs
Breast tissue	2 lbs
Extracellular fluids	4 lbs
Maternal fat	4–11 lbs

b. A similar pattern of weight gain is recommended for women who are normal weight, underweight, overweight, or obese at the start of pregnancy, but the recommendations for total weight gain are different.[1] ▼

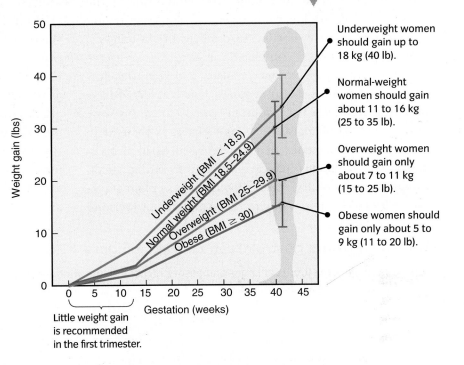

Underweight women should gain up to 18 kg (40 lb).

Normal-weight women should gain about 11 to 16 kg (25 to 35 lb).

Overweight women should gain only about 7 to 11 kg (15 to 25 lb).

Obese women should gain only about 5 to 9 kg (11 to 20 lb).

Little weight gain is recommended in the first trimester.

a. The weight of an infant at birth accounts for about 25% of the mother's weight gain during pregnancy. The placenta, amniotic fluid, and changes in maternal tissues, including enlargement of the uterus and breasts, expansion of the volume of blood and other extracellular fluids, and increased fat stores, account for the rest.

Interpreting Data

How much weight should a woman with a BMI of 27 gain during her pregnancy?

Guidelines for physical activity during pregnancy Table 11.1	
Do . . .	**Don't . . .**
Obtain permission from your health care provider before beginning an exercise program.	Exercise strenuously during the first trimester.
Increase activity gradually if you were inactive before pregnancy.	Exercise strenuously for more than 15 minutes at a time during the second and third trimesters.
Exercise regularly rather than intermittently.	Exercise to the point of exhaustion.
Stop exercising when fatigued.	Exercise lying on your back after the first trimester.
Choose non-weight-bearing activities, such as swimming, that entail minimal risk of falls or abdominal injury.	Scuba dive or engage in activities that entail risk of abdominal trauma, falls, or joint stress.
Drink plenty of fluids before, during, and after exercise.	Exercise in hot or humid environments.

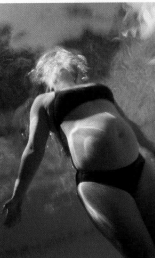

Changes in the Body During Pregnancy 393

Discomforts of Pregnancy

The physiological changes that occur during pregnancy can cause uncomfortable side effects. For example, the expansion in blood volume necessary to nourish the fetus often causes an accumulation of extracellular fluid in the tissues, a condition known as **edema**. Edema can be uncomfortable but does not increase medical risks unless it is accompanied by a rise in blood pressure.

Many women experience nausea and vomiting during the first trimester of pregnancy. This is referred to as **morning sickness**, but symptoms can occur at any time during the day or night. Morning sickness is thought to be related to hormones that are released early in pregnancy. The symptoms may be alleviated by eating small, frequent snacks of dry, starchy foods, such as plain crackers or bread. In most women, the symptoms of morning sickness decrease significantly after the first trimester, but in some they last for the entire pregnancy and, in severe cases, may require intravenous nutrition.

The hormones produced during pregnancy to relax uterine muscles also relax the muscles of the gastrointestinal tract. This relaxation, along with crowding of the organs by the growing baby, can cause heartburn and constipation (**Figure 11.5**). Heartburn can be reduced by limiting high-fat foods, which leave the stomach slowly; avoiding substances, such as caffeine and chocolate, that are known to cause heartburn; eating small, frequent meals; and remaining upright after eating. Constipation can be prevented by maintaining a moderate level of physical activity and consuming plenty of fluids and high-fiber foods. Hemorrhoids are common during pregnancy as a result of both constipation and changes in blood flow.

Crowding of the gastrointestinal tract • Figure 11.5

During pregnancy, the uterus enlarges and pushes higher into the abdominal cavity, exerting pressure on the stomach and intestines.

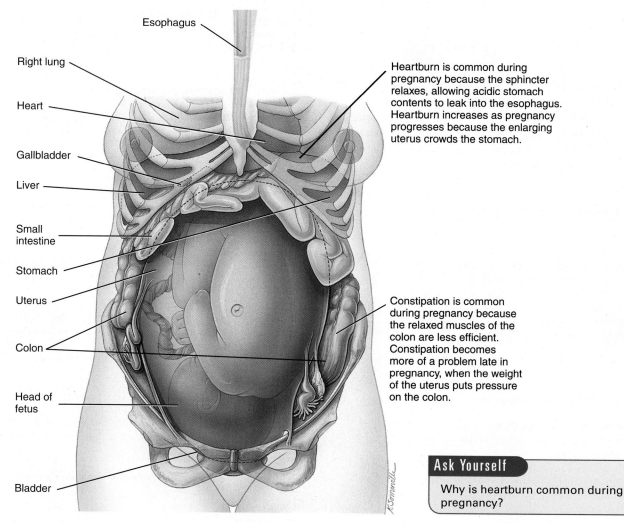

Esophagus

Right lung

Heart

Gallbladder

Liver

Small intestine

Stomach

Uterus

Colon

Head of fetus

Bladder

Heartburn is common during pregnancy because the sphincter relaxes, allowing acidic stomach contents to leak into the esophagus. Heartburn increases as pregnancy progresses because the enlarging uterus crowds the stomach.

Constipation is common during pregnancy because the relaxed muscles of the colon are less efficient. Constipation becomes more of a problem late in pregnancy, when the weight of the uterus puts pressure on the colon.

Ask Yourself

Why is heartburn common during pregnancy?

Complications of Pregnancy

Most of the 4.25 million women who give birth every year in the United States have healthy pregnancies. However, about 12% of babies are born too soon, 8% have low or very low birth weights, and almost 7 out of 1000 of those born alive die in their first year of life.[8] In the United States, about 13 out of every 100,000 women die as a result of childbirth.[9] If complications that occur during pregnancy are caught early, they can usually be managed, resulting in the delivery of a healthy baby.

High blood pressure About 6 to 8% of pregnant women in the United States experience high blood pressure during pregnancy.[10] **Hypertensive disorders of pregnancy** refers to a spectrum of conditions involving elevated blood pressure during pregnancy. It accounts for more than 12% of pregnancy-related maternal deaths in the United States.[11] It is especially common in mothers under 18 and over 35 years of age, low-income mothers, and mothers with chronic hypertension or kidney disease.

About one-third of the hypertensive disorders of pregnancy are due to chronic hypertension that was present before the pregnancy, but the remainder are related to the pregnancy. The least problematic of these is **gestational hypertension**, an abnormal rise in blood pressure that occurs after the 20th week of pregnancy. Gestational hypertension may signal the potential for a more serious condition called **preeclampsia**. Preeclampsia is characterized by high blood pressure along with fluid retention and excretion of protein in the urine; it can result in a weight gain of several pounds within a few days. It is dangerous to the baby because it reduces blood flow to the placenta, and it is dangerous to the mother because it can progress to a more severe condition called **eclampsia**, in which life-threatening seizures occur. Women with preeclampsia require bed rest and careful medical monitoring. The condition usually resolves after delivery.

The causes of hypertension during pregnancy are not fully understood. At one time, low-sodium diets were prescribed to prevent preeclampsia, but studies have not found such diets to be beneficial in lowering blood pressure or preventing this condition.[12] Calcium may play a role in preventing hypertensive disorders of pregnancy. Women with a high intake of calcium have a low incidence of these disorders, and calcium supplements have been found to reduce the risk of preeclampsia in high-risk women.[13] Calcium supplements are not routinely recommended for healthy pregnant women; however, pregnant teens, individuals with inadequate calcium intake, and women who are known to be at risk of developing preeclampsia may benefit from additional dietary calcium.[13]

preeclampsia A condition characterized by elevated blood pressure, a rapid increase in body weight, protein in the urine, and edema. Also called *toxemia*.

eclampsia Convulsions or seizures during or immediately after pregnancy. Untreated, it can lead to coma or death.

Gestational diabetes Diabetes that develops in a pregnant woman is known as **gestational diabetes**. It is common in obese women and those with a family history of type 2 diabetes and occurs more frequently among African American, Hispanic/Latino American, and Native American women than among Caucasian women.[14] Gestational diabetes usually resolves after the birth, but the mother has a 20 to 50% chance of developing diabetes in the next 5 to 10 years.[15] A woman with gestational diabetes requires treatment to normalize maternal blood glucose levels. Because glucose in the mother's blood passes freely across the placenta, when the mother's blood glucose levels are high, the growing fetus receives extra glucose and hence extra calories. The baby grows rapidly and is at risk for being large for gestational age and consequently at increased risk for difficult delivery and abnormal blood glucose levels at birth. Babies born to mothers with gestational diabetes are at increased risk of developing diabetes as adults.[15]

gestational diabetes A condition characterized by high blood glucose levels that develop during pregnancy.

CONCEPT CHECK

1. **How** are nutrients and oxygen transferred from mother to fetus?

2. **How** does a mother's weight gain during pregnancy affect the health of her child?

3. **Why** do heartburn and constipation tend to increase later in pregnancy?

4. **How** does gestational diabetes in a mother affect the baby?

Nutritional Needs During Pregnancy

LEARNING OBJECTIVES

1. **Compare** the energy and protein needs of pregnant and nonpregnant women.
2. **Explain** why pregnancy increases the need for many vitamins and minerals.
3. **Discuss** the need for dietary supplements during pregnancy.

uring pregnancy, the mother's diet must provide all of her nutrients as well as those needed for the baby's growth and development. Because the increase in nutrient needs is greater than the increase in energy needs, a nutrient-dense diet is essential.

Energy and Macronutrient Needs

Although pregnant women are eating for two, they don't need to eat twice as much as they normally do. During the first trimester, energy needs are not increased above levels for nonpregnant women. During the second and third trimesters, an additional 340 and 452 Calories/day, respectively, is recommended (**Figure 11.6**).[16]

Protein needs are increased during pregnancy because protein is needed for the synthesis of new blood cells, formation of the placenta, enlargement of the uterus and breasts, and growth of the baby (see Figure 11.6). An additional 25 grams of protein above the RDA for nonpregnant women, or 1.1 g/kg/day, is recommended for the second and third trimesters of pregnancy.

To ensure sufficient glucose to fuel the fetal and maternal brains during pregnancy, the RDA for carbohydrate is increased by 45 g, to 175 g/day. If this carbohydrate comes from whole grains, fruits, and vegetables, it will also provide the additional 3 g/day of fiber recommended during pregnancy.

Although it is not necessary to increase total fat intake during pregnancy, additional amounts of the essential fatty acids linoleic and α-linolenic acid are recommended because they are incorporated into the placenta and fetal tissues. The long-chain polyunsaturated fatty acids docosahexaenoic acid (DHA) and arachidonic acid (ARA) are important because they not only support maternal health but are essential for development of the eyes and nervous system in the fetus.[17]

Despite increases in the recommended intakes of protein, carbohydrate, and specific fatty acids during pregnancy, the distribution of calories from protein, carbohydrate, and fat should be about the same as that recommended for the general population.

Energy and macronutrient recommendations • Figure 11.6

This graph illustrates the difference between the recommended daily intake of energy, protein, carbohydrate, fiber, essential fatty acids, and water for 25-year-old nonpregnant women and 25-year-old pregnant women during the third trimester.

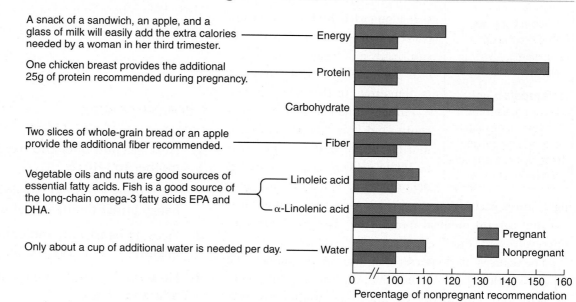

A snack of a sandwich, an apple, and a glass of milk will easily add the extra calories needed by a woman in her third trimester. — Energy

One chicken breast provides the additional 25g of protein recommended during pregnancy. — Protein

— Carbohydrate

Two slices of whole-grain bread or an apple provide the additional fiber recommended. — Fiber

Vegetable oils and nuts are good sources of essential fatty acids. Fish is a good source of the long-chain omega-3 fatty acids EPA and DHA. — Linoleic acid / α-Linolenic acid

Only about a cup of additional water is needed per day. — Water

Pregnant
Nonpregnant

0 100 110 120 130 140 150 160
Percentage of nonpregnant recommendation

Micronutrient needs during pregnancy • Figure 11.7

The graph compares the recommended micronutrient intakes for 25-year-old nonpregnant women and 25-year-old women during the third trimester of pregnancy.

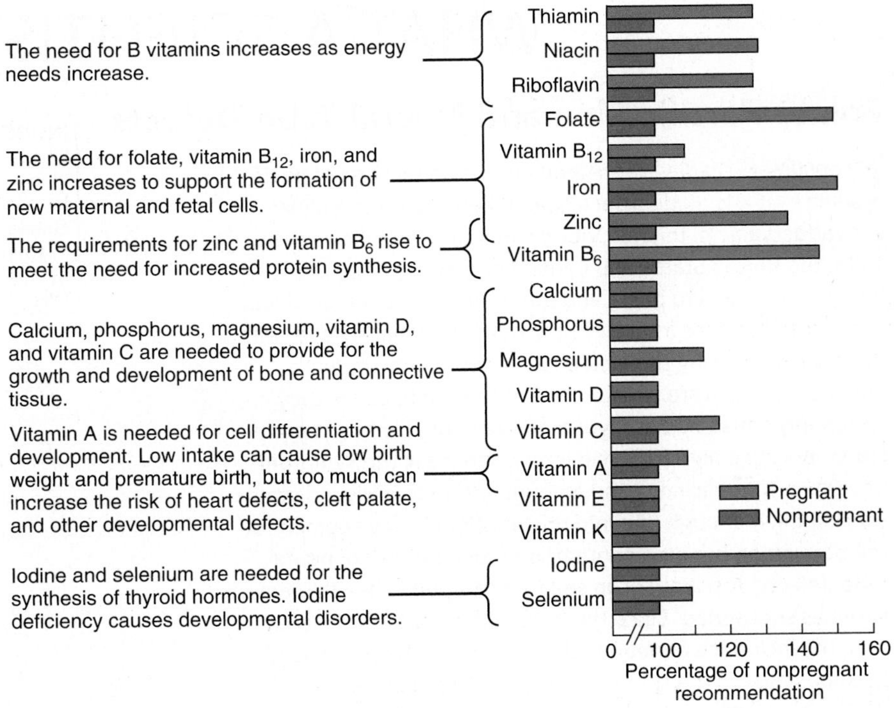

The need for B vitamins increases as energy needs increase.

The need for folate, vitamin B$_{12}$, iron, and zinc increases to support the formation of new maternal and fetal cells.

The requirements for zinc and vitamin B$_6$ rise to meet the need for increased protein synthesis.

Calcium, phosphorus, magnesium, vitamin D, and vitamin C are needed to provide for the growth and development of bone and connective tissue.

Vitamin A is needed for cell differentiation and development. Low intake can cause low birth weight and premature birth, but too much can increase the risk of heart defects, cleft palate, and other developmental defects.

Iodine and selenium are needed for the synthesis of thyroid hormones. Iodine deficiency causes developmental disorders.

WILEY PLUS   Video

Fluid and Electrolyte Needs

During pregnancy, a woman will accumulate 6 to 9 liters of water. Some of this water is intracellular, resulting from the growth of tissues, but most is due to increases in the volume of blood and the fluid between cells. The need for water increases from 2.7 L/day in nonpregnant women to 3 L/day during pregnancy.[18] Despite changes in the amount and distribution of body water during pregnancy, there is no evidence that the requirements for potassium, sodium, and chloride are different for pregnant women than for nonpregnant women.

Vitamin and Mineral Needs

Many vitamins and minerals are needed for the growth of new tissues in both mother and child (**Figure 11.7**). For many of these nutrients, the increased need is easily met with the extra food the mother consumes. For others, the increased need is met because their absorption is increased during pregnancy. For a few, including calcium, vitamin D, folate, vitamin B$_{12}$, iron, and zinc, there is a risk that the woman will not consume adequate amounts without supplementation.

Calcium and vitamin D

During gestation, the fetus accumulates about 30 g of calcium, mostly during the third trimester, when the bones are growing rapidly and the teeth are forming. However, the RDA is not increased during pregnancy because calcium absorption doubles.[19]

The RDA for calcium can be met by consuming three to four servings of dairy products daily. Women who are lactose intolerant can meet their calcium needs with yogurt, cheese, reduced-lactose milk, calcium-rich vegetables, calcium-fortified foods, and calcium supplements. Many pregnant women fail to consume adequate amounts of calcium. Low calcium intake increases the risk that the mother will develop preeclampsia.[13]

Adequate vitamin D is essential to ensure efficient calcium absorption. The RDA for vitamin D during pregnancy is 600 IU (15 µg)/day, the same as it is for nonpregnant women.[19] This is based on the assumption of minimal sun exposure. Vitamin D deficiency is a particular risk for dark-skinned women living at latitudes greater than 40 degrees north or south—for example, farther north than New York City.[20]

Folate and vitamin B$_{12}$

Folate is needed for the synthesis of DNA and hence for cell division. Adequate folate intake before conception and during early pregnancy is crucial because rapid cell division occurs in the first days and weeks of pregnancy.

Low folate levels increase the risk of abnormalities in the formation of the *neural tube*, which forms the baby's brain and spinal cord (see Chapter 7, Figure 7.16). Neural tube closure, a critical step in neural tube development, occurs between 21 and 28 days after conception, often before a woman knows she is pregnant. Therefore, the recommended intake for all women capable of becoming

WHAT A SCIENTIST SEES

THE PLANNER

Folate Fortification and Neural Tube Defects

Consumers reading the ingredient list on this box of pasta see that it is made from a coarse flour called semolina, with added niacin, thiamin, riboflavin, iron, and folic acid. In 1998, the United States and Canada began requiring the addition of folic acid to pasta and other enriched grain products in order to increase intake in women of childbearing age, with the goal of reducing the incidence of neural tube defects. Enriched grains were chosen for fortification because they are commonly consumed in regular amounts by this target population. Because high folic acid intake can mask the symptoms of vitamin B_{12} deficiency, the amount added to enriched grains was kept low enough to avoid this problem in any segment of the population but high enough to reduce the risk of neural tube defects. A scientist can see that this public health measure has succeeded. Since the initiation of folic acid fortification, the incidence of neural tube defects has been reduced by almost 50% in the United States and Canada.[21,22]

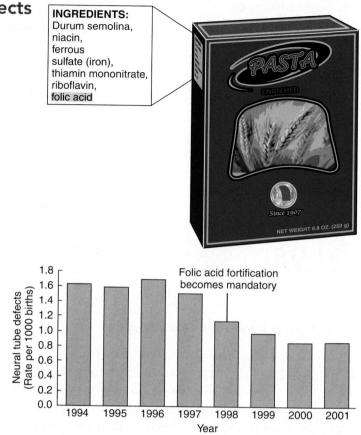

INGREDIENTS:
Durum semolina,
niacin,
ferrous
sulfate (iron),
thiamin mononitrate,
riboflavin,
folic acid

Think Critically Suggest some reasons why fortifying grains with folic acid has not completely eliminated neural tube defects.

pregnant is 400 μg daily of synthetic folic acid from fortified foods, supplements, or a combination of the two, in addition to a varied diet that is rich in natural sources of folate, such as leafy greens, legumes, and orange juice (see *What a Scientist Sees*).

Folate continues to be important even after the neural tube closes. Folate deficiency can cause megaloblastic (macrocytic) anemia in the mother, and inadequate folate intake is associated with premature and low-birth-weight infants and fetal growth retardation.[23] During pregnancy, the RDA is 600 μg/day.[24]

Vitamin B_{12} is essential for the regeneration of active forms of folate. A deficiency of vitamin B_{12} can therefore result in megaloblastic (macrocytic) anemia. Based on the amount of vitamin B_{12} transferred from mother to fetus during pregnancy and on the increased efficiency of vitamin B_{12} absorption during pregnancy, the RDA for pregnancy is set at 2.6 μg/day.[24] This recommendation is easily met by consuming a diet containing even small amounts of animal products. Pregnant women who consume vegan diets must include vitamin B_{12} supplements or foods fortified with vitamin B_{12} to meet their needs as well as those of the fetus.

Iron and zinc Iron needs are high during pregnancy because iron is required for the synthesis of hemoglobin and other iron-containing proteins in both maternal and fetal tissues. The RDA for pregnant women is 27 mg/day, 50% higher than the recommended amount for nonpregnant women.[25] Many women start pregnancy with diminished iron stores and quickly become iron deficient. This occurs even though iron absorption is increased during pregnancy and iron losses decrease because menstruation ceases. Iron deficiency anemia during pregnancy is associated with low birth weight and preterm delivery. Because most of the transfer of iron from mother to fetus occurs during the third trimester, babies who are born prematurely may not have time to accumulate sufficient iron.

Meeting iron needs during pregnancy requires a well-planned diet. Red meat is a good source of the more absorbable heme iron, and leafy green vegetables and fortified cereals are good sources of nonheme iron. Consuming citrus fruit, which is high in vitamin C, or meat, which contains heme iron, along with foods that are good sources of nonheme iron, can enhance iron absorption. Iron supplements are typically recommended during the second and third trimesters, and iron is included in prenatal supplements.

Zinc is involved in the synthesis and function of DNA and RNA and the synthesis of proteins. It is therefore extremely important for growth and development. Zinc deficiency during pregnancy is associated with increased risks of fetal malformations, premature birth, and low birth weight.[26] Because zinc absorption is inhibited by high iron intake, iron supplements may compromise zinc status if the mother's diet is low in zinc. The RDA for zinc is 13 mg/day for pregnant women age 18 and younger and 11 mg/day for pregnant women age 19 and older.[25] As is the case with iron, the zinc in red meat is more absorbable than zinc from other sources.

Meeting Nutrient Needs with Food and Supplements

The energy and nutrient needs of pregnancy can be met by following the MyPlate Daily Food Plans for pregnancy (**Figure 11.8**).

Daily Food Plans for pregnancy • Figure 11.8

This Daily Food Plan for Moms (www.choosemyplate.gov) is for a 26-year-old woman who is 5 ft 4 in. tall, gets 30 to 60 minutes of exercise a day, and weighed 125 lb before she became pregnant. Energy needs are not increased during the first trimester, so the recommended amounts from each group for the first trimester are the same as for a nonpregnant woman.

Ask Yourself

Compared to a nonpregnant woman, how many more cups of milk should a woman in her third trimester be consuming?

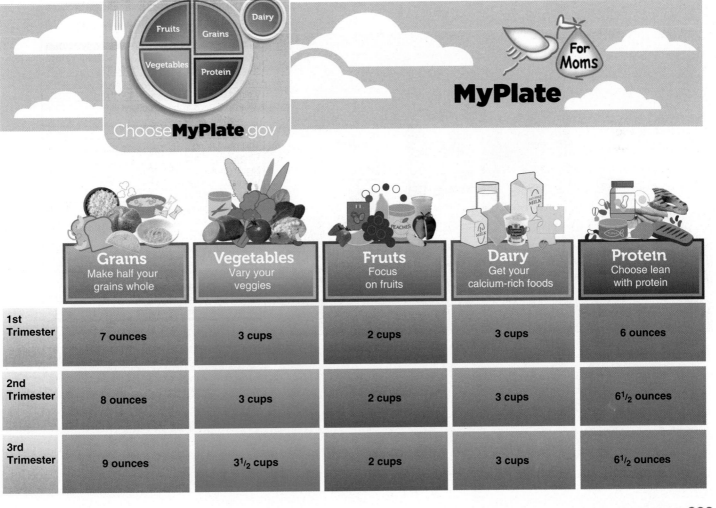

	Grains Make half your grains whole	Vegetables Vary your veggies	Fruits Focus on fruits	Dairy Get your calcium-rich foods	Protein Choose lean with protein
1st Trimester	7 ounces	3 cups	2 cups	3 cups	6 ounces
2nd Trimester	8 ounces	3 cups	2 cups	3 cups	6½ ounces
3rd Trimester	9 ounces	3½ cups	2 cups	3 cups	6½ ounces

Even when a healthy diet is consumed, it is difficult to meet all the vitamin and mineral needs of pregnancy. Therefore, prenatal supplements are generally prescribed for pregnant women. These supplements include the additional folic acid and iron discussed earlier.[1] Prenatal supplements, however, must be taken along with, not in place of, a carefully planned diet (**Figure 11.9**) (see *Thinking It Through*).

Food Cravings and Aversions

Most women experience some food cravings and aversions during pregnancy. The foods most commonly craved are ice cream, sweets, candy, fruit, and fish. Common aversions include coffee, highly seasoned foods, and fried foods. It is not known why women have these cravings and aversions. It has been suggested that hormonal or physiological changes during pregnancy—in particular, changes in taste and smell—may be the cause, but psychological and behavioral factors are also involved.

Usually the foods that pregnant women crave are not harmful and can be safely included in the diet to meet not only nutritional needs but also emotional needs and

Prenatal supplements • Figure 11.9

Prenatal supplements, such as these, typically do not provide enough calcium to meet the needs of pregnant women because to do so, the tablet would have to be very large. They also lack protein needed for tissue synthesis; complex carbohydrates needed for energy; essential fatty acids for brain and nerve tissue development; fiber and fluid to help prevent constipation; and the phytochemicals found in a healthy diet.

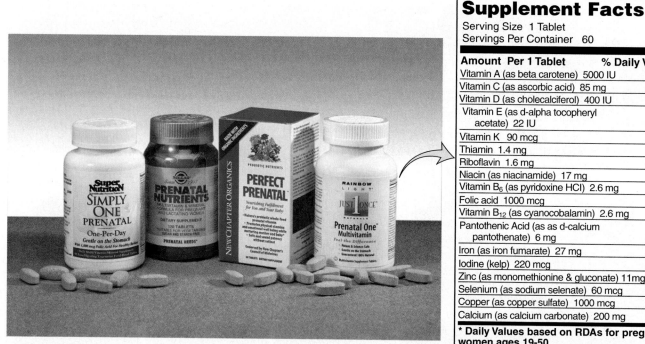

Supplement Facts

Serving Size 1 Tablet
Servings Per Container 60

Amount Per 1 Tablet	% Daily Value
Vitamin A (as beta carotene) 5000 IU	63%
Vitamin C (as ascorbic acid) 85 mg	100%
Vitamin D (as cholecalciferol) 400 IU	200%
Vitamin E (as d-alpha tocopheryl acetate) 22 IU	67%
Vitamin K 90 mcg	100%
Thiamin 1.4 mg	100%
Riboflavin 1.6 mg	100%
Niacin (as niacinamide) 17 mg	100%
Vitamin B_6 (as pyridoxine HCl) 2.6 mg	137%
Folic acid 1000 mcg	167%
Vitamin B_{12} (as cyanocobalamin) 2.6 mg	100%
Pantothenic Acid (as as d-calcium pantothenate) 6 mg	100%
Iron (as iron fumarate) 27 mg	100%
Iodine (kelp) 220 mcg	100%
Zinc (as monomethionine & gluconate) 11mg	100%
Selenium (as sodium selenate) 60 mcg	100%
Copper (as copper sulfate) 1000 mcg	100%
Calcium (as calcium carbonate) 200 mg	20%

* Daily Values based on RDAs for pregnant women ages 19-50
Other ingredients: stearic acid, vegetable stearate, silicon dioxide, croscarmellose sodium, microcrystalline cellulose, natural coating (contains hydroxypropyl methylcellulose, titanium dioxide, riboflavin, polyethylene glycol and polysorbate)

THINKING IT THROUGH

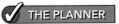

A Case Study on Nutrient Needs for a Successful Pregnancy

Tina is a sedentary 29-year-old at the end of her fourth month of pregnancy. She is 5 ft 6 in. tall and weighed 140 lb at the start of her pregnancy. She is concerned about gaining too much weight because her sister gained 50 lb during her pregnancy and has had difficulty losing the excess weight since her baby was born. Tina's obstetrician recommends that she gain 25 to 35 lb during her pregnancy, but she would like to keep her weight gain to only 15 lb.

Based on the graph below, why would gaining only 15 lb put the baby at risk? Why would gaining 50 lb put the baby at risk?
▼

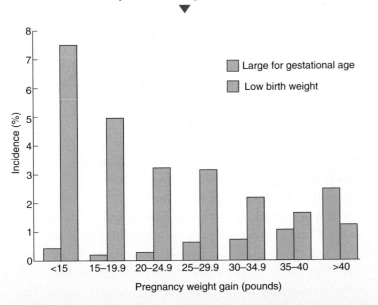

Your answer:

Tina's typical diet provides enough energy for a nonpregnant woman, but during her second and third trimesters, she needs additional calories and nutrients. To decide what to add to her diet, she compares her typical intake to the Daily Food Plan for Moms she finds at ChooseMyPlate.gov. Her current diet includes 8 oz of grains, 1.5 cups of vegetables, 1 cup of fruit, 2 cups of dairy, and 6 oz of protein foods.

How should Tina change the amounts of food she eats from each food group to meet her needs during the second trimester of her pregnancy?
▼

Your answer:

Tina is taking a prenatal supplement but is curious about whether her diet alone can meet her nutrient needs. She analyzes her diet and finds that she is meeting her needs for all nutrients except iron. Her current diet provides only 13.5 mg of iron—significantly less than the RDA of 27 mg for pregnant women.

Use 🔵 iProfile to suggest some foods that Tina could include in her diet in order to obtain an additional 13.5 mg of iron.
▼

Your answer:

Do you think it is reasonable for Tina to consume 27 mg of iron each day from her diet alone? Why or why not?
▼

Your answer:

(Check your answers in Appendix J.)

WHAT SHOULD I EAT?
During Pregnancy

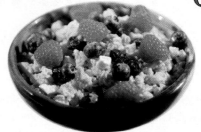

Make nutrient-dense choices
- Have yogurt for a midmorning snack.
- Put some peanut butter on your banana to add some protein to your snack.
- Have a plate of pasta Florentine (with spinach)—it is both a natural and a fortified source of folate.

Drink plenty of fluids
- Have a glass of low-fat milk to boost fluid and calcium intake.
- Keep a bottle of water at your desk or in your car.
- Relax with a cup of tea.

Indulge your cravings, within reason
- Savor some ice cream—it adds calcium and protein.
- Enjoy your cookies with a glass of low-fat milk.

Use iProfile to plan a nutritious 300-Calorie snack for a pregnant woman.

Pica • Figure 11.10

This African American woman in Georgia is eating a white clay called kaolin, which some women crave during pregnancy. Eating kaolin is also a traditional remedy for morning sickness. This example of pica may be related to cultural beliefs and traditions, but pica is also believed to be triggered by nutrient deficiencies, stress, and anxiety. It is most common in African American women, women who live in rural areas, and those with a childhood or family history of pica.[27]

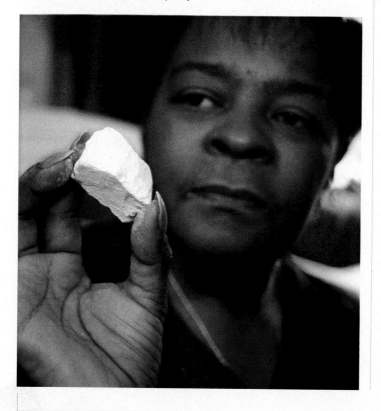

individual preferences (see *What Should I Eat?*). However, **pica** during pregnancy can have serious health consequences. Women with pica commonly consume nonfood substances such as clay, laundry starch, and ashes. Consuming large amounts of these substances can reduce intake of nutrient-dense foods, inhibit nutrient absorption, increase the risk of consuming toxins, and cause intestinal obstructions. Complications of pica include iron-deficiency anemia, lead poisoning, and parasitic infestations.[27] Anemia and high blood pressure are more common in those with pica than among other pregnant women, but it is not clear whether pica is a result of these conditions or a cause. In newborns, anemia and low birth weight are often related to pica in the mother (**Figure 11.10**).

> **pica** An abnormal craving for and ingestion of nonfood substances that have little or no nutritional value.

CONCEPT CHECK

1. **What** snack could a pregnant woman add to her day to meet her increased energy and protein needs?

2. **Why** isn't the recommendation for dietary calcium increased during pregnancy?

3. **Why** are iron supplements recommended during pregnancy?

Factors That Increase the Risks Associated with Pregnancy

LEARNING OBJECTIVES

1. **Discuss** how the critical periods of prenatal development are related to nutrition.

2. **Discuss** how nutritional status can influence the outcome of pregnancy.

3. **Explain** how a pregnant woman's age and health status affect the risks associated with pregnancy.

4. **Describe** the effects of alcohol, mercury, and cocaine on the outcome of pregnancy.

 nything that interferes with embryonic or fetal devlopment can cause a baby to be born too soon or too small or result in birth defects. The embryo and fetus are particularly vulnerable to damage because their cells are dividing rapidly, differentiating, and moving to form organs and other structures. Developmental errors can be caused by deficiencies or excesses in the maternal diet and by harmful substances that are present in the environment, consumed in the diet, or taken as medications or recreational drugs. Any chemical, biological, or physical agent that causes a birth defect is called a **teratogen**. And because each organ system develops at a different time and rate, each has a **critical period** during which exposure to a teratogen is most likely to disrupt development and cause irreversible damage (**Figure 11.11**). Severe damage can result in miscarriage. Some women are at increased risk for complications during pregnancy because of their nutritional status, age, or preexisting health problems. Others are at risk due to exposure to harmful substances.

Critical periods of development • Figure 11.11

The critical periods of development are different for different body systems. Because the majority of cell differentiation occurs during the embryonic period, this is the time when exposure to teratogens can do the most damage, but vital body organs can still be affected during the fetal period. One in every 33 babies born in the United States has a birth defect.[28]

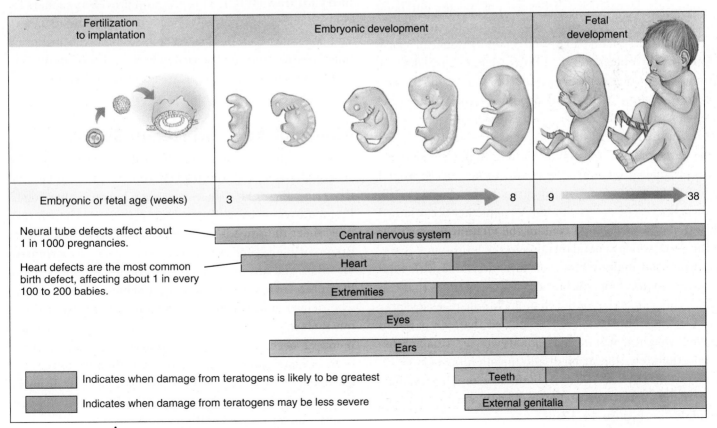

Effects of the Dutch famine • Figure 11.12

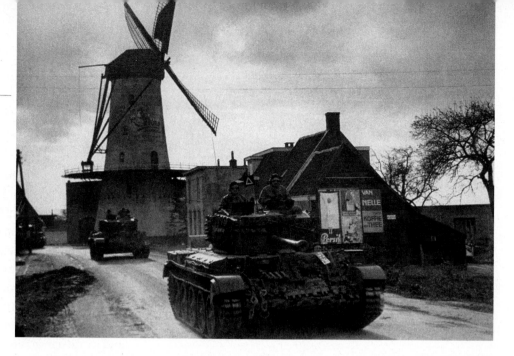

During World War II, an embargo on food transport to the Netherlands in the winter of 1944–1945 caused the average intake per person per day to drop below 1000 Calories. Pregnant women gave birth to smaller babies. In adulthood, the affected babies were more likely than others to have diabetes, heart disease, obesity, and other chronic diseases.[31]

Maternal Nutritional Status

Before pregnancy, proper nutrition is important to allow conception and maximize the likelihood of a healthy pregnancy. Women with reduced body fat due to starvation diets, anorexia nervosa, or excessive exercise may have abnormal hormone levels. When hormone levels are too low, ovulation does not occur, and conception is not possible. Too much body fat can also reduce fertility by altering hormone levels. Deficiencies or excesses of specific nutrients can affect both fertility and the outcome of pregnancy.

During pregnancy, maternal malnutrition can cause fetal growth retardation, low birth weight, birth defects, premature birth, spontaneous abortion, or stillbirth. The effects of malnutrition vary, depending on when during the pregnancy it occurs.[29] As discussed earlier, inadequate folate intake in the first few weeks of pregnancy can affect neural tube development.[24] Too much vitamin A, particularly early in pregnancy, increases the risk of kidney problems and central nervous system abnormalities in the offspring.[25] To reduce the risk of excess vitamin A, supplements consumed during pregnancy should contain the vitamin A precursor β-carotene, which is not damaging to the fetus.

Maternal malnutrition not only interferes with fetal growth and development but also causes changes that can affect the child's risk of developing chronic diseases later in life. Epidemiological studies suggest that compared to normal-weight newborns, individuals who are small or disproportionately thin at birth and during infancy have increased rates of heart disease, high blood pressure, stroke, high blood cholesterol, diabetes, obesity, and osteoporosis in adult life (**Figure 11.12**).[30]

One of the greatest risk factors for poor pregnancy outcome is poverty, which limits access to food, education, and health care. Low-income women are unlikely to receive medical care until late in pregnancy and consequently have a high incidence of low-birth-weight and preterm infants. A federally funded program that addresses the nutritional needs of pregnant women is the **Special Supplemental Nutrition Program for Women, Infants, and Children (WIC)**. This program provides vouchers for the purchase of nutritious foods and referrals to health and other services for low-income women who are pregnant, postpartum, or breast-feeding, and for infants and children up to age 5 who are at risk of malnutrition.

Maternal Age and Health Status

Pregnancy places stresses on the body at any age, but the stresses have a greater impact on women in their teens and those age 35 or older than on women between these ages. Pregnant teens are still growing, so their nutrient intake must meet their needs for growth as well as for pregnancy. Pregnant teenagers are at increased risk of hypertensive disorders and are more likely than pregnant adults to deliver preterm and low-birth-weight babies. Even teenagers who deliver normal-birth-weight infants may stop growing themselves.[32] To produce a healthy baby, a pregnant teenager needs early medical intervention and nutrition counseling (**Figure 11.13**). Although the rate of teenage pregnancy has decreased over the past decade, from 62 babies/1000 teens in 1991 to about 42/1000 in 2008, it remains a major public health problem.[33]

Nutrient needs of pregnant teens • Figure 11.13

Because the nutrient needs of pregnant teens are different from those of pregnant adults, the DRIs include a special set of nutrient recommendations for this age group. This graph illustrates the recommended daily micronutrient intake for 14- to 18-year-old girls during the second and third trimesters of pregnancy compared to the recommendations for 14- to 18-year-old nonpregnant girls.

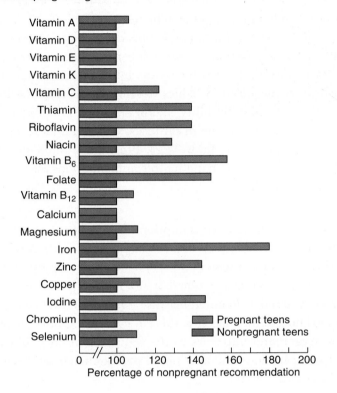

The nutritional requirements for older women during pregnancy are no different from those for women in their 20s, but pregnancy after age 35 carries additional risks. Older women are more likely to already have one or more medical conditions, such as cardiovascular disease, kidney disorders, obesity, or diabetes. These preexisting conditions increase the risks associated with pregnancy. For example, a woman who has preexisting high blood pressure is at increased risk for having a low-birth-weight baby, and a woman who has diabetes is more likely to have a baby who is large for gestational age. Older women are also more likely to develop gestational diabetes, hypertensive disorders of pregnancy, and other complications. They have a higher incidence of low-birth-weight infants. In addition, their infants are more likely to have chromosomal abnormalities, especially **Down syndrome** (Figure 11.14). The frequency of twins and triplets is higher among older mothers in part because of their greater use of fertility treatments. Multiple pregnancies increase nutrient needs and the risk of preterm delivery.

Women with a history of miscarriage or birth defects are also at increased risk. For example, a woman who has had a number of miscarriages is more likely to have another, and a woman who has had one child with a birth defect has an increased risk for defects in subsequent pregnancies. Another factor that increases risks is frequent pregnancies. An interval of less than 18 months between pregnancies increases the risk of delivering a small-for-gestational-age infant. An interval of only 3 months increases the risk of a preterm infant as well as the risk of neonatal death.[35] One reason for these increased risks is that the mother may not have replenished the nutrient stores depleted in the first pregnancy before becoming pregnant again.

Incidence of Down syndrome • Figure 11.14

Down syndrome is caused by a defect during egg or sperm formation that results in extra genetic material in the baby. It causes distinctive facial characteristics, developmental delays, and other health problems. The incidence of Down syndrome rises significantly with maternal age of 35 years or more. However, while older mothers are more likely to conceive a Down syndrome baby, 80% of Down syndrome births are to mothers under age 35, as younger women have more babies overall.[34]

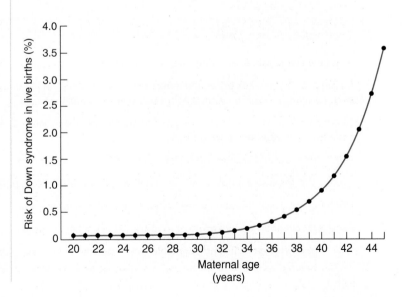

Exposure to Toxic Substances

A pregnant woman's exposure to toxins in food, water, and the environment can affect the developing fetus. Even substances that seem innocuous can be dangerous. For example, herbal remedies, including herbal teas, should be avoided unless their consumption during pregnancy has been determined to be safe.[3]

Caffeine When consumed in excess, coffee and other caffeine-containing beverages have been associated with increased risks of miscarriage or low birth weight.[36] It is recommended that pregnant women limit caffeine consumption to less than 200 mg/day, the amount in 1 or 2 cups of coffee or about two or three 20-ounce caffeinated soft drinks.

Mercury in fish Fish has both benefits and risks for pregnant women. It is a source of lean protein for tissue growth and of omega-3 fatty acids and iodine needed for brain development, but if it is contaminated with mercury, consumption during pregnancy can cause developmental delays and brain damage. Rather than avoid fish, pregnant women should be informed consumers. The 2010 Dietary Guidelines recommend that pregnant women consume 8 to 12 oz/week of seafood from a variety of types of fish and shellfish.[37] Exposure to mercury from fish can be controlled by avoiding varieties that are high in mercury and limiting intake of fish that contain lower amounts of mercury (**Table 11.2**).

Food-borne illness The immune system is weakened during pregnancy, increasing susceptibility to and the severity of certain food-borne illnesses. *Listeria* infections are about 20 times more likely during pregnancy and are especially dangerous for pregnant women, often resulting in miscarriage, premature delivery, stillbirth, or infection of the fetus.[39] About one-quarter of babies born with *Listeria* infections do not survive. The bacteria are commonly found in unpasteurized milk, soft cheeses, and uncooked hot dogs and lunch meats (see Table 11.2).

Toxoplasmosis is an infection caused by a parasite. If a pregnant woman becomes infected, there is about a 40% chance that she will pass the infection to her unborn baby.[40] Some infected babies develop vision and hearing loss, intellectual disability, and/or seizures. The toxoplasmosis parasite is found in cat feces, soil, and undercooked infected meat (see Table 11.2). Pregnant women should follow the safe food-handling recommendations discussed in Chapter 13.

Alcohol Alcohol consumption during pregnancy is one of the leading causes of preventable birth defects. Alcohol is a teratogen that is particularly damaging to the developing nervous system.[41] It also indirectly affects fetal growth and development because it is a toxin that reduces blood flow to the placenta, thereby decreasing the delivery of oxygen and nutrients to the fetus. Use of alcohol can also impair maternal nutritional status, further increasing the risks to the fetus.

Food safety during pregnancy[38] Table 11.2
Don't eat swordfish, shark, king mackerel, or tilefish, which can be high in mercury.
Eat up to 6 oz per week of canned albacore or chunk white tuna and up to 12 oz per week of fish and shellfish that are lower in mercury, such as salmon, shrimp, canned light tuna, pollock, catfish, and cod.
Check local advisories about the safety of fish caught in local waters. If no advice is available, eat up to 6 oz per week but don't consume any other fish during that week.
Don't drink raw (unpasteurized) milk or consume products made with unpasteurized milk, such as certain Mexican-style soft cheeses.
Don't eat refrigerated smoked fish, cold deli salads, or refrigerated pâtés or meat spreads.
Don't eat hot dogs unless they have been reheated to steaming hot.
Don't eat raw or undercooked meat, poultry, fish, shellfish, or eggs.
Don't eat unwashed fruits and vegetables, raw sprouts, or unpasteurized juice.

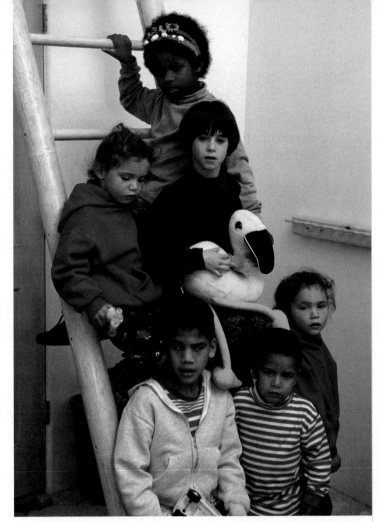

Dangers of alcohol use during pregnancy • Figure 11.15

The facial characteristics shared by children with fetal alcohol syndrome (FAS) include a low nasal bridge, short nose, distinct eyelids, and a thin upper lip. Newborns with FAS may be shaky and irritable, with poor muscle tone. Other problems associated with FAS include heart and urinary tract defects, impaired vision and hearing, and delayed language development. Below-average intellectual function is the most common and most serious effect.

Prenatal exposure to alcohol can cause a spectrum of disorders, depending on the amount, timing, and duration of the exposure. One of the most severe outcomes of alcohol use during pregnancy is delivery of a baby with **fetal alcohol syndrome (FAS)** (**Figure 11.15**). Not all babies who are exposed to alcohol while in the uterus have FAS. The term **fetal alcohol spectrum disorders**

fetal alcohol syndrome (FAS) A characteristic group of physical and mental abnormalities in an infant resulting from maternal alcohol consumption during pregnancy.

(FASDs) is used to refer to all the physical and behavioral disorders or conditions and functional or mental impairments linked to prenatal alcohol exposure.[42] As many as 2 to 5% of young school children in the United States are affected by FASDs.[43] Because alcohol consumption in each trimester has been associated with fetal abnormalities, and there is no level of alcohol consumption that is known to be safe, complete abstinence from alcohol is recommended during pregnancy.

Cigarette smoke If a woman smokes cigarettes during pregnancy, her baby will be affected before birth and throughout life. The carbon monoxide in cigarette smoke binds to hemoglobin in maternal and fetal blood, reducing the amount of oxygen delivered to fetal tissues. The nicotine absorbed from cigarette smoke is a teratogen that can affect brain development.[44] Nicotine also constricts arteries and limits blood flow, reducing the amounts of oxygen and nutrients delivered to the fetus.[45] Cigarette smoking during pregnancy reduces birth weight and increases the risks of stillbirth, preterm delivery, neurobehavioral problems, and early infant death.[3,44] In women who don't smoke, environmental exposure to cigarette smoke has been found to increase the risk of having a low-birth-weight baby. The risks of **sudden infant death syndrome (SIDS)**, or **crib death**, and respiratory problems are also increased in children exposed to cigarette smoke both in the uterus and after birth. The effects of

sudden infant death syndrome (SIDS) or crib death The unexplained death of an infant, usually during sleep.

maternal smoking follow children throughout life; these children are more likely to have frequent colds and develop lung problems later in life.[46]

Drug use Certain drugs—whether over-the-counter, prescribed, or illegal—can affect fetal development. For example, the acne medications Accutane and Retin-A are derivatives of vitamin A that can cause birth defects if used during pregnancy. A woman who is considering becoming pregnant should discuss her plans with her physician in order to determine the risks associated with any medication she is taking.

Substance abuse during pregnancy is a national health issue. It is estimated that 1 to 11% of babies born each year were exposed to drugs during the prenatal period. These percentages include only the use of illegal drugs; they would be much higher if alcohol and nicotine were also included.[47]

Marijuana and cocaine can cross the placenta and enter the fetal blood. There is little evidence that marijuana affects fetal development, but cocaine use creates problems for both the mother and the infant before, during, and after delivery.[48] Cocaine is a central nervous system stimulant, but many of its effects during pregnancy occur because it constricts blood vessels, thereby reducing the delivery of oxygen and nutrients to the fetus. Cocaine use during pregnancy is also associated with an increased risk of miscarriage, fetal growth retardation, premature labor and delivery, low birth weight, and birth defects.[49] Exposure to cocaine and other illegal drugs before birth has also been shown to affect infant behavior and influence learning and attention span during childhood.[50]

CONCEPT CHECK STOP

1. **Why** does the effect of a given teratogen vary, depending on when a pregnant woman is exposed to it?

2. **How** does malnutrition during pregnancy affect the health of the child at birth and later in life?

3. **Why** are the requirements for some nutrients different in pregnant teenage girls than in pregnant adult women?

4. **How** much alcohol can be safely consumed during pregnancy?

Lactation

LEARNING OBJECTIVES

1. **Describe** the events that trigger milk production and let-down.
2. **Discuss** the energy and water needs of lactating women.
3. **Compare** the micronutrient needs of lactating women with those of nonpregnant, nonlactating women.

The need for many nutrients is even greater during lactation than during pregnancy. The milk produced by a breast-feeding mother must meet all the nutrient needs of her baby, who is bigger and more active that he or she was in the womb. To meet these needs, a lactating woman must choose a varied, nutrient-dense diet that follows the MyPlate Daily Food Plans for breast-feeding women.

Milk Production and Let-Down

Lactation involves both the synthesis of milk components—proteins, lactose, and lipids—and the movement

let-down The release of milk from the milk-producing glands and its movement through the ducts and storage sinuses.

of these components through the milk ducts to the nipple (**Figure 11.16**). Milk production and **let-down** are triggered by hormones that are released in response to an infant's suckling. The pituitary

Anatomy of milk production • Figure 11.16

Throughout pregnancy, hormones prepare the breasts for lactation by stimulating the enlargement and development of the milk ducts and milk-producing glands, called *alveoli* (singular *alveolus*). During lactation, milk travels from the alveoli through the ducts to the milk storage sinuses and then to the nipple.

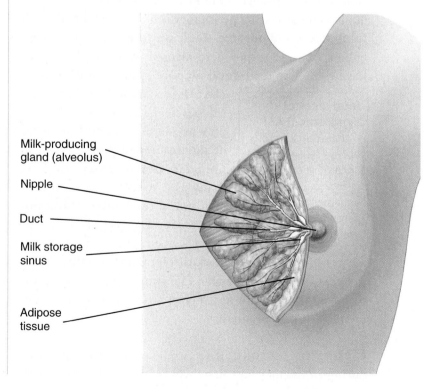

Milk-producing gland (alveolus)

Nipple

Duct

Milk storage sinus

Adipose tissue

This graph compares the energy and macronutrient recommendations for 25-year-old nonpregnant women and 25-year-old women during the third trimester of pregnancy and the first 6 months of lactation.

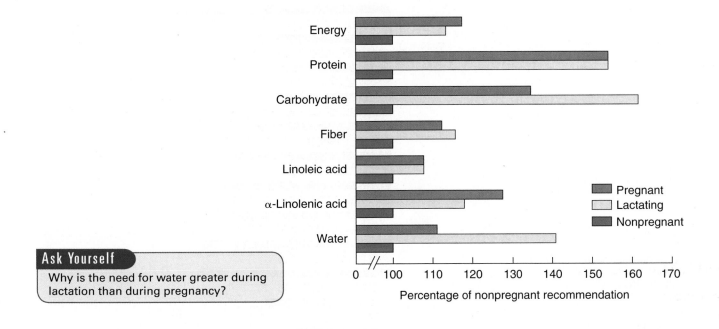

Ask Yourself

Why is the need for water greater during lactation than during pregnancy?

hormone **prolactin** stimulates milk production; the more the infant suckles, the more milk is produced. Let-down is caused by **oxytocin**, another pituitary hormone. Oxytocin release is also stimulated by suckling, but as nursing becomes routine, oxytocin release and let-down may occur in response to just the sight or sound of an infant. Let-down can be inhibited by nervous tension, fatigue, or embarrassment. Because let-down is essential for breast-feeding and makes suckling easier for the child, slow let-down can make feeding difficult.

Energy and Nutrient Needs During Lactation

Human milk contains about 70 Calories/100 milliliters (160 Calories/cup). During the first 6 months of lactation, an average infant consumes 600 to 900 mL (about 2.5 to 4 cups)/day, so approximately 500 Calories are required from the mother each day. Much of this energy must come from the diet, but some can come from maternal fat stores. Because some of the energy for milk production comes from

fat stores, the increase in recommended energy intake is lower during lactation than during pregnancy, even though total energy demands are greater (**Figure 11.17**). An additional 330 Calories/day above nonpregnant, nonlactating needs are recommended during the first 6 months of lactation, and an additional 400 Calories are recommended for the second 6 months. Beginning 1 month after birth, most lactating women lose 0.5 to 1 kg (1 to 2 lb)/month for 6 months. Rapid weight loss is not recommended during lactation because it can decrease milk production.

To ensure adequate protein for milk production, the RDA for lactation is increased by 25 g/day. The recommended intakes of total carbohydrate, fiber, and the essential fatty acids linoleic and α-linolenic acid are also higher during lactation (see Figure 11.17).[16]

To avoid dehydration and ensure adequate milk production, lactating women need to consume about 1 L/day of additional water.[18] Consuming an extra glass of milk, juice, or water at each meal and whenever the infant nurses can help ensure adequate fluid intake. The recommended intakes for several vitamins and minerals are

Micronutrient needs during lactation • Figure 11.18

This graph compares the vitamin and mineral recommendations for 25-year-old nonpregnant women and 25-year-old women during the third trimester of pregnancy and the first 6 months of lactation.

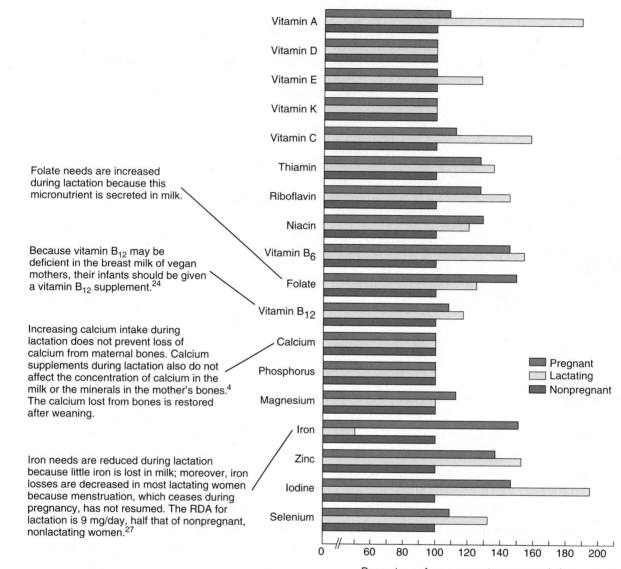

Folate needs are increased during lactation because this micronutrient is secreted in milk.

Because vitamin B_{12} may be deficient in the breast milk of vegan mothers, their infants should be given a vitamin B_{12} supplement.[24]

Increasing calcium intake during lactation does not prevent loss of calcium from maternal bones. Calcium supplements during lactation also do not affect the concentration of calcium in the milk or the minerals in the mother's bones.[4] The calcium lost from bones is restored after weaning.

Iron needs are reduced during lactation because little iron is lost in milk; moreover, iron losses are decreased in most lactating women because menstruation, which ceases during pregnancy, has not resumed. The RDA for lactation is 9 mg/day, half that of nonpregnant, nonlactating women.[27]

increased during lactation to meet the needs for synthesizing milk and to replace the nutrients secreted in the milk (**Figure 11.18**). Maternal intake of vitamins C, B_6, B_{12}, A, and D can affect the composition of milk. For example, low levels of vitamin C in a mother's diet can result in low levels of vitamin C in her milk. For other nutrients, including calcium and folate, levels in the milk are maintained at the expense of maternal stores.

CONCEPT CHECK STOP

1. **What** causes milk let-down?

2. **Where** does the energy for milk production come from?

3. **Why** is the recommended calcium intake for a new mother not increased while she is lactating?

Nutrition for Infants

LEARNING OBJECTIVES

1. **Explain** how growth charts are used to monitor the nutritional well-being of infants.

2. **Contrast** the energy and macronutrient needs of infants and adults.

3. **Compare** the benefits of breast-feeding and formula-feeding.

4. **Discuss** the importance of choosing foods that are appropriate for a child's developmental stage.

After the umbilical cord is cut, a newborn must actively obtain nutrients rather than being passively fed through the placenta. The energy and nutrients an infant consumes must support his or her continuing growth and development, as well as his or her increasing activity level.

Infant Growth and Development

During **infancy**—the first year of life—growth and development are extremely rapid. Infants get bigger and develop physically, intellectually, and socially. Adequate nutrition is essential for achieving growth and developmental milestones.

Healthy infants follow standard patterns of growth—that is, whether a newborn weighs 6 lb or 8 lb at birth, the rate of growth should be approximately the same: rapid initially and slowing slightly as the infant approaches his or her first birthday. A rule of thumb is that an infant's birth weight should double by 4 months of age and triple by 1 year of age. In the first year of life, most infants increase their length by 50%. Growth is the best indicator of adequate nutrition in an infant.

Growth charts can be used to compare an infant's growth with that of other infants of the same age (**Figure 11.19**).[51] The resulting ranking, or percentile, indicates where the

Growth charts • Figure 11.19

This weight-for-age growth chart for boys from birth to 36 months of age can be used to compare a boy's weight at a particular age to standards for the general population. Growth charts for this age group are also available to monitor length for age and head circumference for age in boys and girls.

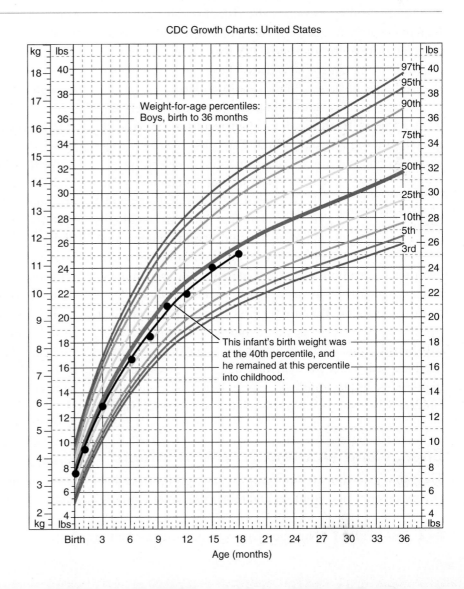

CDC Growth Charts: United States

Weight-for-age percentiles: Boys, birth to 36 months

This infant's birth weight was at the 40th percentile, and he remained at this percentile into childhood.

Interpreting Data

A 24-month-old boy who weighs 30 lb is at the _____ percentile.
a. 25th
b. 50th
c. 75th
d. 90th

infant's growth falls in relationship to population standards. For example, if a newborn boy is at the 20th percentile for weight, 19% of newborn boys weigh less and 80% weigh more. Children usually remain at the same percentile as they grow. For instance, a child who is at the 50th percentile for height and the 25th percentile for weight generally remains close to these percentiles throughout childhood. Small and premature infants often follow a pattern that is parallel to, but below the growth curve for a period of time and then experience catch-up growth that brings them into the same range as children of the same age.

Slight variations in growth rate are normal, but a consistent pattern of not following the established growth curve or a sudden change in growth pattern is cause for concern and could indicate overnutrition or undernutrition. For example, a rapid increase in weight without an increase in height may indicate that the infant is being overfed. Just as there are critical periods in prenatal life, there are critical periods during infancy when nutrition can have permanent effects on growth and development and long-term health. Evidence suggests that accelerated growth due to overfeeding increases the risk of obesity, diabetes, high blood pressure, harmful blood lipid levels, and cardiovascular disease in adulthood.[52] A pattern of accelerated weight increase should be addressed early in life to reduce the likelihood of these chronic conditions later.

Growth that is slower than the predicted pattern indicates **failure to thrive**, a catchall term for any type of growth failure in a young child. The cause may be a congenital condition, disease, poor nutrition, neglect, abuse, or psychosocial problems. The treatment is usually an individualized plan that includes adequate nutrition and careful monitoring by physicians, dietitians, and other health-care professionals. Undernutrition during infancy can permanently affect growth and development as well as health later in life. Because the first year of life is a critical period for brain development, undernutrition interferes with learning and affects behavior. Undernutrition in childhood is a risk factor for diabetes, high blood pressure, and high cholesterol in adulthood, especially in undernourished children who experience rapid weight gain after infancy.[53]

> **failure to thrive**
> Inability of a child's growth to keep up with normal growth curves.

Energy and Nutrient Needs of Infants

The rapid growth rate of infants increases their need for energy, protein, and vitamins and minerals that are impor-tant for growth. Human milk and commercially produced formula are designed to meet infants' nutrient needs. Nevertheless, infants may still be at risk for iron, vitamin D, and vitamin K deficiencies and for suboptimal levels of fluoride.

Energy and macronutrients Infants require more calories and protein per kilogram of body weight than do individuals at any other time of life (**Figure 11.20a**).[16] As infants grow older, their rate of growth slows, but they become more mobile, so the amount of energy they need for activity increases. Because infants change so much during the first year, energy recommendations are made for three age groups—0 to 3 months, 4 to 6 months, and 7 to 12 months—and nutrient recommendations are made for two age groups—0 to 6 months and 7 to 12 months (see inside cover).

The combination of high energy demands and a small stomach means that infants require an energy-dense diet. Healthy infants consume about 55% of their energy as fat during the first 6 months of life and 40% during the second 6 months. These percentages are far higher than the 20 to 35% of energy from fat recommended in the adult diet (**Figure 11.20b**). This energy-dense diet allows the small volume of food that fits in an infant's stomach to provide enough energy to meet the infant's needs.

Fluid needs Infants have a higher proportion of body water than do adults, and they lose proportionately more water in urine and through evaporation. Urine losses are high because the kidneys are not fully developed and hence are unable to reabsorb as much water as adult kidneys. Water losses through evaporation are proportionately higher in infants than in adults because infants have a larger surface area relative to body weight. As a result, they need to consume more water per unit of body weight than do adults. Nevertheless, healthy infants who are exclusively breast-fed do not require additional water.[18] In older infants, some water is obtained from food and from beverages other than milk. When water losses are increased by diarrhea or vomiting, additional fluids may be needed.

Micronutrients at risk Iron is the nutrient that is most commonly deficient in infants who are consuming adequate energy and protein. Iron deficiency usually is not a problem during the first 6 months of life because infants have iron stores at birth and the iron in human

Energy and macronutrient needs • Figure 11.20

a. The total amount of energy required by a newborn is less than the amount needed by an adult. When this amount is expressed as Calories/kg of body weight, however, we see that infants require about three times more energy than an adult male.

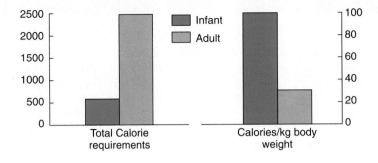

Carbohydrate is a major contributor to an infant's energy intake; most of this comes from lactose.

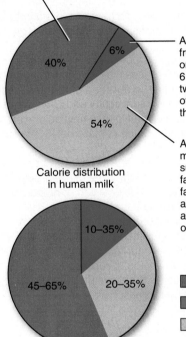

Calorie distribution in human milk

40%
6%
54%

Although the proportion of calories from protein is small, representing only about 9 g/day during the first 6 months, an infant requires almost twice as much protein per kilogram of body weight (1.52 g/kg/day) than an adult (0.8 g/kg/day).

Along with enough dietary fat to meet energy needs, infants need sufficient amounts of the omega-3 fatty acid DHA and the omega-6 fatty acid ARA. These fatty acids are constituents of cell membranes and are important for development of the eyes and nervous system.

b. Comparing the distribution of calories from carbohydrate, fat, and protein in human milk with that recommended for an adult illustrates proportionally how much more fat infants need. As an infant grows and solid foods are introduced into the diet, the percentage of calories from carbohydrate in the diet increases and the percentage from fat decreases.

Recommended calorie distribution for the adult diet

10–35%
45–65%
20–35%

- Carbohydrate
- Protein
- Fat

---

milk, though not abundant, is very well absorbed. The AI for iron from birth to 6 months is 0.27 mg/day. After 4 to 6 months, iron stores are depleted, but iron needs remain high. The RDA for infants 7 to 12 months old increases to 11 mg/day.[25] By this age, the diet of breast-fed infants should contain other sources of iron. Formula-fed infants should be fed iron-fortified formula.

Breast milk is low in vitamin D. Therefore, it is recommended that breast-fed and partially breast-fed infants be supplemented with 400 IU (10 μg)/day of vitamin D beginning in the first few days of life and continuing until they are consuming about 1 L (4 cups) of vitamin D–fortified formula or milk daily.[19,54] Infant formulas contain at least 400 IU (10 μg)/L of vitamin D. Formula-fed infants who consume at least 1 L/day of formula, can meet their vita-

min D needs from the formula alone; those consuming less than 1 L/day should receive a vitamin D supplement of 400 IU (10 μg)/day. The amount of sun exposure necessary to maintain an adequate levels of vitamin D in any given infant at any point in time is not easy to determine. Light-skinned infants are more likely than darker-skinned babies to meet their vitamin D needs from sunlight.[54]

Infants are at risk for vitamin K deficiency because little vitamin K crosses the placenta, and the infant's gut is sterile, so there are no bacteria to synthesize this vitamin. Because lack of vitamin K can cause bleeding, it is recommended that all newborns receive an intramuscular injection containing 0.5 to 1.0 mg of vitamin K, which provides enough of the vitamin to last until the intestines have been colonized with bacteria that synthesize it.[55]

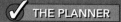

The Issue: The fatty acids docosahexaenoic acid (DHA) and arachidonic acid (ARA) are essential for development of the retina and brain. Some infant formulas in the United States are fortified with DHA and ARA, and advertisements suggest that they provide an advantage for infant development. Will feeding babies these fortified formulas make them smarter and improve their vision?

DHA and ARA are polyunsaturated fatty acids that can be made in the body from the essential omega-3 fatty acid α-linolenic acid and the essential omega-6 fatty acid linoleic acid, respectively. Studies in animals indicate that DHA and ARA are found in high concentrations in the brain and retina and that they are needed for brain development and normal vision.[58] Accumulation of these fatty acids in the brain and retina occurs most rapidly between the third trimester of pregnancy and 24 months of age, so adequate amounts are crucial during this developmental period.

DHA and ARA are found in breast milk, so it seems logical that they should be added to infant formula. But, unlike most other nutrients, the amounts of DHA and ARA in breast milk are variable, depending on maternal diet, so it is unclear what constitutes optimal levels. The amounts of these fatty acids transferred to the fetus by the placenta during the third trimester may be enough to ensure adequate amounts for brain development.[58] Infants born at term are also capable of synthesizing DHA and ARA, so those fed unfortified formula may be able to meet their needs if they have enough α-linolenic acid and linoleic acid in their diet. But there is wide individual variation in the ability to convert α-linolenic acid to DHA, and in some infants conversion may be too low for optimal brain and visual development.[58] Infants born before term cannot synthesize enough of these fatty acids, so DHA and ARA must be included in formula for premature infants.

So will higher intakes of these fatty acids make children smarter? Numerous studies have explored the impact that postnatal intake of these fatty acids has on intelligence and vision. Some have found that higher intakes of DHA increase blood levels of DHA in infants and are associated with improvements in cognitive development or vision compared to infants with lower intakes.[58–60] But not all studies agree. A study of 18-month-old babies found that feeding fortified formulas did not have a significant effect on mental or psychomotor development.[61] A review concluded that feeding infant formulas fortified with DHA and ARA has not been proven to result in benefits with regard to vision or cognition.[62]

There are a number of reasons studies on the effects of fortified formulas are inconsistent. Differences may be due to variations in the DHA content of the formula, the duration of formula-feeding, and the methods used to assess visual acuity and cognitive development. Differences in children's intelligence may be due more to maternal or family characteristics, such as maternal IQ, than to the type of milk they are fed.[63]

When it comes to brain and eye development, no one knows exactly how much DHA or ARA an infant needs. A direct link between use of fortified formula and better vision or higher IQ compared to use of unfortified formula has yet to be established, but fortified formulas are generally recommended.[58,59] They may not make your baby smarter, but published literature has not demonstrated these formulas to be harmful for infants.[64] Breast milk is always best, so the biggest downside to fortified formulas is that advertising may make new mothers believe that they are as good as or better for their babies than breast milk.

Think critically: Why is breast milk still better than these fortified formulas?

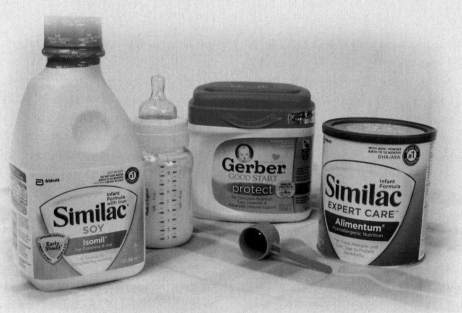

Fluoride is important for tooth development, even before the teeth erupt. Breast milk is low in fluoride, and formula manufacturers use unfluoridated water in preparing liquid formula. Therefore, breast-fed infants, infants who are fed premixed formula, and those who are fed formula mixed with low-fluoride water at home are often given fluoride supplements beginning at 6 months of age. In areas where drinking water is fluoridated, infants who are fed formula reconstituted with tap water should not be given fluoride supplements.

Meeting Needs with Breast Milk or Formula

Because of its health and nutritional benefits, breast-feeding is the recommended choice for the newborn of a healthy, well-nourished mother (see *Debate: DHA-Fortified Infant Formulas*). Health professionals in the United States recommend exclusive breast-feeding for the first 6 months of life and breast-feeding with complementary foods for at least the first year and as long thereafter as mutually desired.[56] As infants begin consuming other foods, their demand for milk is reduced, and milk production decreases, but lactation can continue as long as suckling is maintained.

After the first year, breast-feeding is not necessary to meet the infant's nutrient needs, but in developing nations, where other foods offered to young children are nutrient poor, breast-feeding after the first year helps prevent malnutrition. The World Health Organization recommends breast-feeding for 2 years or more.[57] In both developed and developing nations, breast-feeding after the first year continues to provide nutrition, comfort, and an emotional bond between mother and child.

Whether they are breast-fed or formula-fed, young infants should be fed frequently, on demand. For breast-fed infants, a feeding should last approximately 10 to 15 minutes at each breast. Bottle-fed newborns may consume only a few ounces at each feeding; as the infant grows, the amount consumed will increase to 4 to 8 oz (**Figure 11.21**). A well-fed newborn, whether breast-fed or bottle-fed, should urinate enough to soak six to eight diapers a day and gain about 0.15 to 0.23 kg (0.33 to 0.5 lb)/week.

Nutrients in breast milk and formula Human milk is tailored to meet the needs of human infants. The composition of milk changes continuously to suit the needs of a growing infant. The first milk, called **colostrum**, which is produced by the breast for up to a week after delivery, has beneficial effects

> **colostrum** The first milk, produced by the breast late in pregnancy and for up to a week after delivery. Compared to mature milk, it contains more water, protein, immune factors, minerals, and vitamins and less fat.

Dos and don'ts of formula-feeding • Figure 11.21

a. During bottle feeding, the infant's head should be higher than his or her stomach, and the bottle should be tilted so that there is no air in the nipple. Just as breast-fed infants alternate breasts, bottle-fed infants should be held alternately on the left and right sides to promote equal development of the head and neck muscles.

b. Infants should never be put to bed with a bottle because saliva flow decreases during sleep, and the formula remains in contact with the teeth for many hours. This causes **nursing bottle syndrome**, rapid and serious decay of the upper teeth. Usually the lower teeth are protected by the tongue.

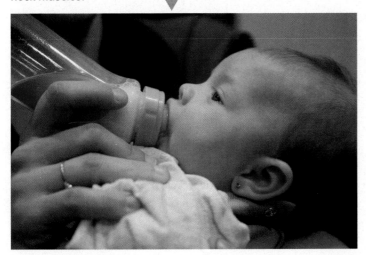

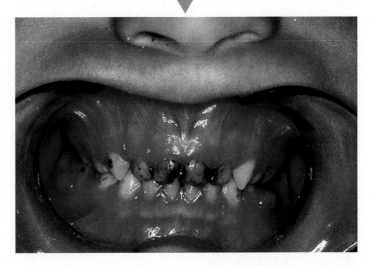

Nutritional composition of breast milk and infant formula   Table 11.3

Nutrient	Amount in breast milk	Amount in formula	Comparisons
Protein	1.8 g/100 mL	1.4 g/100 mL	The relatively low protein content of human milk and formula protects the immature infant kidneys from a too-high load of nitrogen wastes. Alpha-lactalbumin, the predominant protein in human milk, forms a soft, easily digested curd in the infant's stomach. Most formula is made from cow's milk that is modified to mimic the protein concentration and amino acid composition of human milk.
Fat	4 g/100 mL	4.8 g/100 mL	The fat in human milk is easily digested. Human milk is high in cholesterol and the essential fatty acids linoleic acid and α-linolenic acid, as well as their long-chain derivatives ARA and DHA, which are essential for normal brain development, eyesight, and growth. The fat in formula is derived from vegetable oils and provides linoleic and α-linolenic acid. Some formulas are also supplemented with ARA and DHA.
Carbohydrate	7 g/100 mL	7.3 g/100 mL	Lactose, the primary carbohydrate in human milk and most formula, enhances calcium absorption. Because it is digested slowly, it stimulates the growth of beneficial acid-producing bacteria. Oligosaccharides in milk protect against respiratory and gastrointestinal disease.
Sodium	1.3 mg/100 mL	0.7 mg/100 mL	Because breast milk and formula are both low in sodium, the fluid needs of breast-fed and formula-fed infants can be met without an excessive load on the kidneys.
Calcium **Phosphorus**	22 mg/100 mL 14 mg/100 mL	53 mg/100 mL 38 mg/100 mL	The 2:1 ratio of calcium to phosphorus in breast milk and formula enhances calcium absorption.
Iron **Zinc**	0.03 mg/100 mL 3.2 mg/100 mL	0.1 mg/100 mL 5.1 mg/100 mL	Iron and zinc are present in limited amounts in breast milk but are readily absorbed. Most infant formulas are fortified with iron and zinc because the forms present are less absorbable than those in breast milk.
Vitamin D	4 IU/100 mL	41 IU/100 mL	Formulas are fortified with vitamin D, which is present at low levels in breast milk.

on the gastrointestinal tract, acting as a laxative that helps the baby excrete the thick, mucusy stool produced during life in the womb. Colostrum looks watery, but the nutrients it supplies meet the infant's needs until mature milk production begins. Mature breast milk contains an appropriate balance of nutrients in forms that are easily digested and absorbed. Infant formulas try to replicate human milk as closely as possible in order to match the growth, nutrient absorption, and other benefits associated with breast-feeding (**Table 11.3**).

Health benefits of breast-feeding Despite a nutritional profile that is similar, infant formulas can never exactly duplicate the composition of human milk. Antibody proteins and immune-system cells pass from the mother to her child in the breast milk, providing immune protection for the infant. A number of enzymes and other proteins in breast milk prevent the growth of harmful microorganisms, and several of the carbohydrates in breast milk protect against viruses that cause diarrhea. One substance favors the growth of the beneficial bacterium *Lactobacillus bifidus* in the infant's colon; this bacterium inhibits the growth of disease-causing organisms. Growth factors and hormones present in human milk promote maturation of the infant's gut and immune defenses and enhance digestion. In addition to the numerous health benefits that breast-feeding has for infants it has physical, emotional, and financial advantages for the mother (**Figure 11.22**).

Benefits for infants
- Provides optimum nutrition
- Enables strong bonding with mother
- Enhances immune protection
- Reduces allergies
- Decreases ear infections, respiratory illnesses, and asthma
- Reduces the likelihood of constipation, diarrhea, or chronic digestive diseases
- Reduces risk for SIDS
- Lowers risk for obesity, type 1 and 2 diabetes, heart disease, hypertension, high cholesterol, and childhood leukemia
- Aids in the development of the facial muscles, speech development, and correct formation of the teeth
- Lessens the risk of overfeeding because the amount of milk consumed cannot be monitored visually

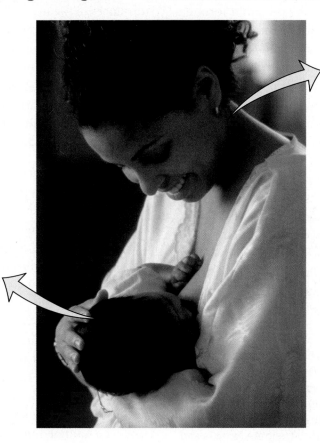

Benefits for mothers
- Provides relaxing, emotionally enjoyable interaction; strengthens bonding with infant
- Reduces financial costs
- Requires less preparation and clean-up time; always available
- Causes uterine contractions that help the uterus return to its normal size more quickly after delivery
- Increases energy expenditure, which may speed return to prepregnancy weight
- Lowers risk of developing type 2 diabetes and breast and ovarian cancers
- Improves bone density and decreases risk of fractures
- Inhibits ovulation, lengthening the time between pregnancies; however, breast-feeding cannot be relied on for birth control
- Decreases the risk of postpartum depression
- Enhances self-esteem in the maternal role

When is formula-feeding better? Despite the benefits of breast milk, formula-feeding may be the best option in some cases. Common illnesses such as colds and skin infections are not passed to the infant in breast milk, but tuberculosis and HIV infection are.[56] Some drugs can also pass from the mother to the baby in breast milk, which means that women who are taking medications should check with their physician about whether they can safely breast-feed while taking their medication. Because alcohol and drugs such as cocaine and marijuana can be passed to a baby in breast milk, alcoholic and drug-addicted mothers are counseled not to breast-feed. Nicotine from cigarette smoke is also rapidly transferred from maternal blood to milk, and heavy smoking may decrease the supply of milk.

Although alcoholic mothers are counseled not to breast-feed, occasional limited alcohol consumption while breast-feeding is probably not harmful if alcohol intake is timed so as to minimize the amount present in milk when the infant is fed. Consuming a single alcoholic drink is safe if the mother then waits at least 4 hours before breast-feeding. Alternatively, milk can be expressed before consuming the drink and fed to the infant later.[37]

Feeding an infant with formula requires more preparation and washing than breast-feeding, but it can give the mother a break because other family members can share the responsibility. For preterm infants and those with genetic abnormalities, formula may be the best option because there are special formulas to meet these infants' unique needs. If an infant is too small or weak to take a bottle, pumped breast milk or formula can be fed through a tube.

Safe Feeding for the First Year

Whether infants are breast-fed or formula-fed, care must be taken to ensure that their needs are met and their food is safe. If proper measurements are not used in preparing formula, the infant can receive an excess or a deficiency of nutrients and an improper ratio of nutrients to fluid

(**Figure 11.23**). If the water and equipment used in preparing formula are not clean or if the prepared formula is left unrefrigerated, food-borne illness may result. Because sanitation is often lacking in developing nations, infections that lead to diarrhea and dehydration occur more frequently in formula-fed infants than in breast-fed infants.

Bacterial contamination is not a concern when a baby is breast-fed, but care must be taken to avoid contamination when milk is pumped from the breast and stored for later feedings. Hands, breast pumps, bottles, and nipples must be washed. Breast milk that is not immediately fed to the baby can be kept refrigerated for 24 to 48 hours. Warming breast milk in a microwave is not recommended because microwaving destroys some of its immune properties and may result in dangerously hot milk. The best way to warm milk is by running warm water over the bottle.

Safe infant feeding • Figure 11.23

To avoid bacterial contamination, wash hands before preparing formula. Clean bottles and nipples by washing them in a dishwasher or placing them in boiling water for five minutes. Boil water for one to two minutes and cool it before using it to mix powdered formula or dilute concentrates. Cover and refrigerate opened cans of ready-to-feed and liquid concentrate formula and use the formula within the period indicated on the can. Prepare formula immediately before a feeding and discard any excess.

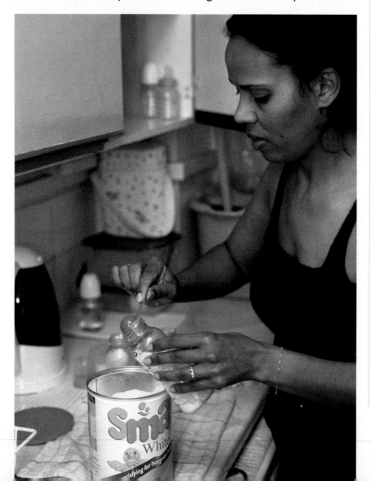

A concern that is unique to feeding breast milk is that substances in the maternal diet may pass into the milk and cause adverse reactions in the infant. For example, caffeine in the mother's diet can make the infant jittery and excitable, so a mother should avoid consuming large amounts of caffeine while breast-feeding. Most of these reactions seem to be unique to a particular mother and child, so as long as a food does not affect the infant's health or response to feeding, it can be included in the mother's diet.

Food allergies Food allergies are common in infants. Because infants' digestive tracts are immature, they allow the absorption of incompletely digested proteins, which triggers a response from the immune system (see Chapters 3 and 6). After about 3 months of age, the risk of developing food allergies is reduced because incompletely digested proteins are less likely to be absorbed. Many children who develop food allergies before age 3 years eventually outgrow them. Allergies that appear after 3 years of age are more likely to be problematic throughout the individual's life.

Exclusive breast-feeding for the first 4 to 6 months reduces an infant's risk of developing a food allergy.[65] If a formula-fed baby becomes allergic to the milk proteins used in the formula, soy formulas should be used. For infants who cannot tolerate milk or soy protein, formulas made from predigested proteins are an option.

Appropriate introduction of solid and semisolid foods can reduce the risk of an infant developing food allergies. The most commonly recommended first food is iron-fortified infant rice cereal mixed with formula or breast milk, because this cereal is easily digested and rarely causes allergic reactions. After rice has been successfully included in the diet, other grains can be introduced, with wheat cereal given last because it is more likely than other cereals to cause an allergic reaction. Each new food should be offered for a few days without the addition of any other new foods. If an allergic reaction occurs, it is then easier to determine that the newly introduced food caused it. Foods that cause symptoms such as rashes, digestive upsets, or respiratory problems should be discontinued, and the symptoms should no longer be present before any other new foods are added.

Developmentally appropriate foods Although most of an infant's nutritional needs are met by breast milk or infant formula, solid and semisolid foods can be gradually introduced into the diet starting at 4 to 6 months of age. By this time, the infant's feeding abilities and gastrointestinal tract are mature enough to handle solid foods. Foods that are offered to infants should be appropriate for their

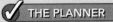

THE PLANNER

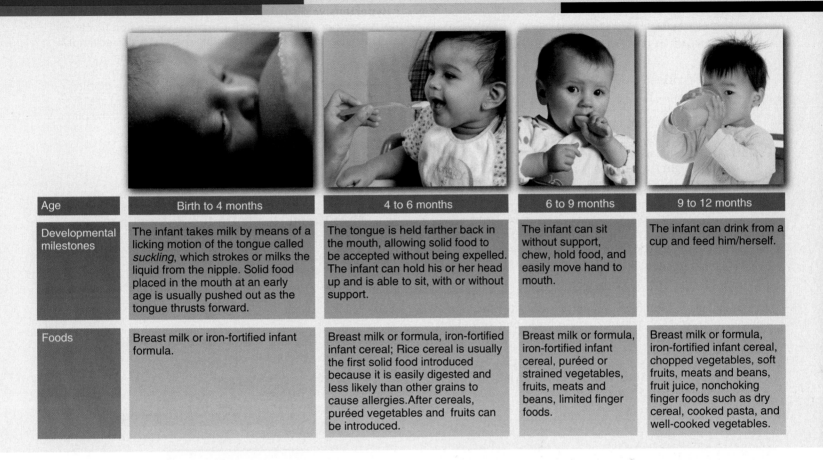

Age	Birth to 4 months	4 to 6 months	6 to 9 months	9 to 12 months
Developmental milestones	The infant takes milk by means of a licking motion of the tongue called *suckling*, which strokes or milks the liquid from the nipple. Solid food placed in the mouth at an early age is usually pushed out as the tongue thrusts forward.	The tongue is held farther back in the mouth, allowing solid food to be accepted without being expelled. The infant can hold his or her head up and is able to sit, with or without support.	The infant can sit without support, chew, hold food, and easily move hand to mouth.	The infant can drink from a cup and feed him/herself.
Foods	Breast milk or iron-fortified infant formula.	Breast milk or formula, iron-fortified infant cereal; Rice cereal is usually the first solid food introduced because it is easily digested and less likely than other grains to cause allergies.After cereals, puréed vegetables and fruits can be introduced.	Breast milk or formula, iron-fortified infant cereal, puréed or strained vegetables, fruits, meats and beans, limited finger foods.	Breast milk or formula, iron-fortified infant cereal, chopped vegetables, soft fruits, meats and beans, fruit juice, nonchoking finger foods such as dry cereal, cooked pasta, and well-cooked vegetables.

digestive and developmental abilities (**Figure 11.24**). Cow's milk should never be fed to infants because it is too high in protein and too low in iron.[66] At 1 year of age, whole cow's milk can be offered; it can be used until 2 years of age, after which reduced-fat or low-fat milk can be used. As a child becomes familiar with more variety, food choices should be made from each of the food groups. To avoid choking, foods that can easily lodge in the throat, such as raw carrots, grapes, and hot dogs, should not be offered to infants or toddlers.

Fruit juice can be fed from a cup when an infant is 9 to 10 months old, but excess quantities of apple and pear juice should be avoided because they contain sorbitol, a poorly absorbed sugar alcohol that can cause diarrhea. The American Academy of Pediatrics recommends that infants not be given juice at bedtime or offered juice from bottles or covered cups that allow them to consume juice easily throughout the day.[67] Added sugars should be offered in moderation to ensure a nutrient-dense diet. Honey should not be fed to children less than 1 year old because it may contain spores of *Clostridium botulinum*, the bacterium that causes botulism poisoning (discussed in Chapter 13). Older children and adults are not at risk from botulism spores because the environment in a mature gastrointestinal tract prevents the bacteria from growing.

CONCEPT CHECK

1. **What** does it mean if a child whose birth weight was in the 50th percentile is now in the 30th percentile for growth?
2. **Why** do infants need more fat than adults?
3. **Why** is breast milk the best choice for healthy mothers and babies?
4. **When** can solid food be introduced into an infant's diet?

Summary

1 Changes in the Body During Pregnancy 390

- During the first 8 weeks of development, all the organ systems necessary for life are formed in the **embryo**. Over the remaining weeks of pregnancy, the **fetus** grows, and organs develop and mature. The **placenta** transfers nutrients and oxygen from maternal blood to fetal blood and removes wastes from the fetus. At birth, a healthy baby weighs 3 to 4 kg (6.5 to 9 lb). **Low-birth-weight** infants and infants who are **large for gestational age** are at increased risk of health problems.

- During pregnancy, the mother's body undergoes many changes to support the pregnancy and prepare for **lactation**. Recommended weight gain during pregnancy is 11 to 16 kg (25 to 35 lb) for normal-weight women. Too little or too much weight gain can place both mother and baby at risk, but weight loss should never be attempted during pregnancy. Normal-weight, underweight, overweight, and obese mothers should gain weight at a steady rate during pregnancy, but as shown here, the total amount of weight gain recommended depends on prepregnancy weight.

Rate and composition of weight gain during pregnancy • Figure 11.4b

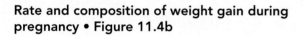
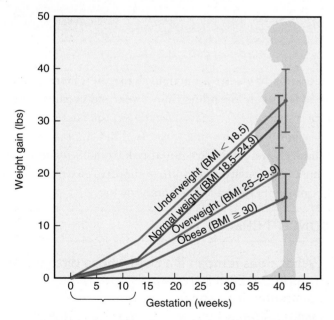

- During healthy pregnancies, moderate-intensity exercise that does not increase the risk of abdominal trauma, falls, or joint stress can be beneficial and safe.

- The hormones that direct changes in maternal physiology and fetal growth and development sometimes cause unwanted side effects, including **edema, morning sickness**, heartburn, constipation, and hemorrhoids.

- **Hypertensive disorders of pregnancy** increase risk for both mother and baby. **Gestational hypertension** involves an increase in blood pressure during pregnancy. **Preeclampsia** is a more severe condition, characterized by edema, weight gain, and protein in the urine, and can progress to life-threatening **eclampsia**. High blood glucose in the mother, called **gestational diabetes**, results in babies who are large for gestational age because extra glucose crosses the placenta from mother to fetus.

2 Nutritional Needs During Pregnancy 396

- During pregnancy, the requirements for energy, protein, carbohydrate, essential fatty acids, and water, shown in the graph, as well as many vitamins and minerals increase above levels for nonpregnant women.

Energy and macronutrient recommendations • Figure 11.6

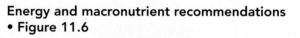
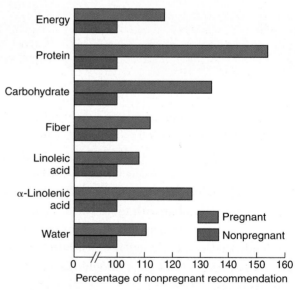

- The RDA for calcium is not increased because the greater need during pregnancy is met by an increase in absorption. Vitamin D deficiency is a concern, particularly for darker-skinned women. Adequate folic acid early in pregnancy reduces the risk of neural tube defects. Iron needs are high, and deficiency is common during pregnancy.

- MyPlate Food Plans for pregnancy can help pregnant women select foods to meet their nutritional needs. A prenatal supplement containing iron and folic acid and other vitamins and minerals is generally prescribed for all pregnant women.

- Food cravings are common during pregnancy. Most are harmless, but **pica** can reduce the intake of nutrient-dense foods, inhibit nutrient absorption, increase the risk of consuming toxins and infectious organisms, and cause intestinal obstructions.

3 Factors That Increase the Risks Associated with Pregnancy   403

- The rapidly developing embryo and fetus are susceptible to damage from poor nutrition and physical, chemical, or other environmental **teratogens**. Malnutrition during pregnancy can cause fetal growth retardation, low infant birth weight, birth defects, premature birth, miscarriage, and stillbirth.

- Pregnant teenagers are at increased risk because they are still growing themselves. Women over age 35 are at increased risk because they are more likely to have preexisting health conditions and to develop hypertensive disorders of pregnancy, gestational diabetes, or other complications during pregnancy.

- Excessive caffeine intake can increase the risk of miscarriage. Following guidelines on fish consumption can minimize exposure to mercury, which can cause brain damage in a fetus. Pregnant women are particularly susceptible to food-borne illness and should follow safe food-handling recommendations. Alcohol consumption during pregnancy is a leading cause of brain damage and other birth defects, such as **fetal alcohol syndrome**, depicted here. Exposure to cigarette smoke causes low birth weight and increases the risk of stillbirth, preterm delivery, and behavioral problems in the baby. The use of illegal drugs, such as, cocaine also increases the risk of low birth weight and birth defects.

Dangers of alcohol use during pregnancy • Figure 11.15

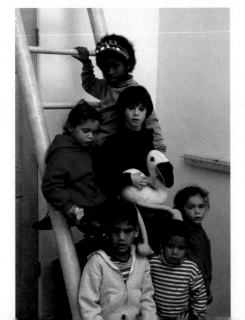

4 Lactation   408

- Milk production and **let-down** are triggered by hormones released in response to the suckling of an infant. During let-down, milk travels from the milk-producing glands shown here to the nipple.

Anatomy of milk production • Figure 11.16

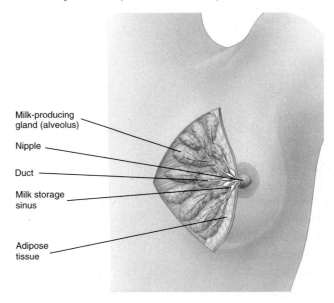

Milk-producing gland (alveolus)
Nipple
Duct
Milk storage sinus
Adipose tissue

- Lactation requires energy and nutrients from the mother to produce adequate milk. The energy for milk production comes from the diet and maternal fat stores. Maternal needs for protein, water, and many vitamins and minerals are even greater during lactation than during pregnancy.

5 Nutrition for Infants   411

- Growth is the best indicator of adequate nutrition in an infant. Healthy infants follow standard patterns of growth. Growth charts can be used to compare an infant's growth with the growth of other infants of the same age. Slow growth indicates **failure to thrive**, whereas excess weight gain may predispose a child to obesity. Undernutrition and overnutrition during infancy can have permanent effects on growth and development and the risk of chronic disease later in life.

- Infants require more calories and protein per kilogram of body weight than do individuals at any other time of life. Fat and fluid needs are also proportionately higher than in adults. Infants are at risk for deficiencies of iron, vitamin D, and vitamin K, as well as low fluoride intake.

- Breast milk is the ideal food for infants. It meets nutrient needs; it is always available; it requires no special equipment, mixing, or sterilization; and it provides immune protection. There are many infant formulas on the market that are patterned after human milk and provide adequate nutrition to a baby. Formula-feeding is the best option when the mother is ill or is taking prescription or illicit drugs, or when the infant has special nutritional needs.

- Introducing solid foods between 4 and 6 months of age, as shown here, adds iron and other nutrients to the diet. Newly introduced foods should be appropriate to the child's stage of development and offered one at a time in order to monitor for food allergies.

Nourishing a developing infant: 4 to 6 months • Figure 11.24

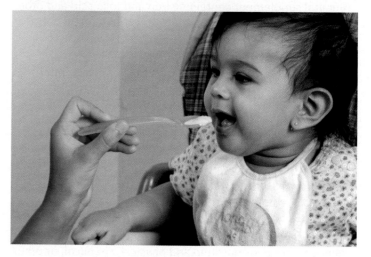

Key Terms

- cesarean section 392
- colostrum 415
- critical period 403
- Down syndrome 405
- eclampsia 395
- edema 394
- embryo 391
- failure to thrive 412
- fertilization 390
- fetal alcohol syndrome (FAS) 407
- fetal alcohol spectrum disorders (FASDs) 407
- fetus 391

- gestational diabetes 395
- gestational hypertension 395
- hypertensive disorders of pregnancy 395
- implantation 391
- infancy 411
- lactation 392
- large for gestational age 392
- let-down 408
- low birth weight 392
- morning sickness 394
- nursing bottle syndrome 415
- oxytocin 409
- pica 402

- placenta 391
- preeclampsia 395
- preterm or premature 391
- prolactin 409
- small for gestational age 391
- Special Supplemental Nutrition Program for Women, Infants, and Children (WIC) 404
- sudden infant death syndrome (SIDS) or crib death 407
- teratogen 403
- trimester 392
- very low birth weight 392

Online Resources

- For information about prenatal care, risks and problems during pregnancy, as well as postnatal care, go to the New York Online Access to Health (NOAH) site, at www.noah-health.org/en/pregnancy/.

- For more information on the health benefits of breast-feeding throughout the world, go to the World Health Organization site, at www.who.int/topics/infant_nutrition/en/.

- For information about how WIC can improve the nutrition of women and children, go to the USDA Food and Nutrition Service site, at www.fns.usda.gov/fns/.

- Visit your *WileyPLUS* site for videos, animations, podcasts, self-study, and other media that will aid you in studying and understanding this chapter.

Critical and Creative Thinking Questions

1. Keep a 3-day diet record. Use 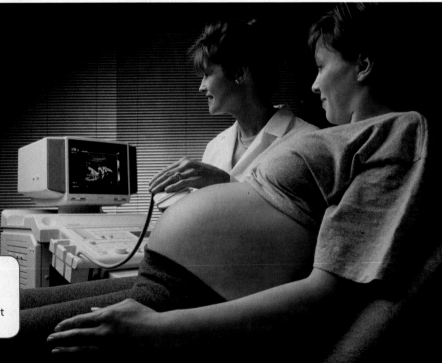 iProfile to analyze the nutrient composition of your diet. Would your diet meet the energy, protein, and micronutrient needs of a 25-year-old pregnant woman who is 5 ft 5 in. tall, weighed 130 lb at the start of her pregnancy, and is now in her second trimester? If not, what foods or supplements would need to be added to meet these needs?

2. Many people object to infant formula manufacturers advertising their products in developing nations. Do you feel it is appropriate to promote the use of formula in developing nations? Why or why not?

3. HIV, the virus that causes AIDS, passes via breast-feeding to one out of seven infants born to HIV-infected mothers, yet in developing countries, some HIV-positive women are advised to breast-feed. Explain why this might be, considering what you know about the benefits of breast-feeding.

4. If an infant is born weighing 6 lb, what should the baby weigh at 4 months of age and at 12 months? Why?

5. Chelsea, a vegan woman, has just found out she is pregnant. What nutrient deficiencies are common for vegans? For pregnant women? What supplements would you recommend that Chelsea take during her pregnancy?

6. Marina, a 16-year-old, is 4 months pregnant. She is 5 ft 4 in. tall and weighed 110 lb before she became pregnant. Her typical diet, which provided 1800 Calories, 60 g of protein, and 15 mg of iron, met her needs before she became pregnant. What changes in the amounts of energy, protein, and iron would you recommend now that Marina is in her second trimester?

What is happening in this picture?

Ultrasound imaging, shown here, uses sound waves to visualize the embryo or fetus in the uterus. It can be used to assess the progress of the pregnancy and identify fetal and maternal health problems.

Think Critically

1. If the baby is larger than expected, what might be the problem?
2. If the baby is smaller than expected, what might be the cause?

Self-Test

(Check your answers in Appendix K.)

1. Which process is indicated by the number 5?

    a. fertilization

    b. implantation

    c. lactation

    d. ovulation

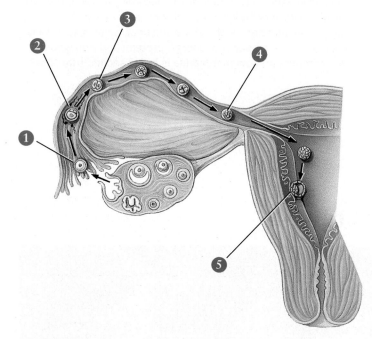

2. The function of the _____ is to transfer nutrients and oxygen from the maternal blood to the fetal blood.

    a. amniotic sac

    b. placenta

    c. uterus

    d. oviduct

3. An infant born at term, weighing 4.5 lb at birth, is considered _____.

    a. large for gestational age

    b. premature

    c. very low birth weight

    d. low birth weight

4. Newborn infants receive an injection of _____ to prevent the possibility of hemorrhage.

    a. iron

    b. folate

    c. vitamin D

    d. vitamin K

5. Use the figure to determine how much of the weight gained during pregnancy is due to an increase in body fluids.

    a. about 4 lb

    b. about 2 lb

    c. as much as 10 lb

    d. less than 4 lb

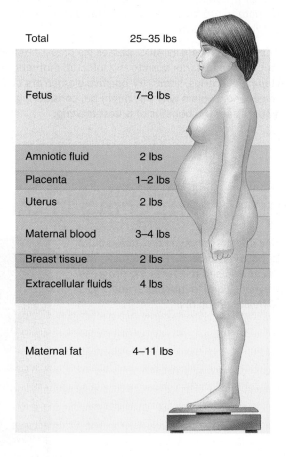

Total	25–35 lbs
Fetus	7–8 lbs
Amniotic fluid	2 lbs
Placenta	1–2 lbs
Uterus	2 lbs
Maternal blood	3–4 lbs
Breast tissue	2 lbs
Extracellular fluids	4 lbs
Maternal fat	4–11 lbs

6. A woman who enters pregnancy with excess weight (BMI > 30) should _____.

    a. lose about 5 to 10 lb during her pregnancy

    b. gain about 11 to 20 lb during her pregnancy

    c. not gain any additional weight during her pregnancy

    d. limit her intake to 1200 Calories/day

7. Which of the following is associated with preeclampsia?

    a. a rise in blood pressure

    b. edema

    c. protein in the urine

    d. all of the above

8. The recommended intake for _____ is the same for non-pregnant and pregnant women.

   a. calcium

   b. iron

   c. protein

   d. zinc

9. During which weeks of development is exposure to a teratogen most likely to result in a heart defect in an embryo or a fetus?

   a. the first 3 weeks

   b. about 3 to 7 weeks

   c. 7 to 8 weeks

   d. any time after 9 weeks

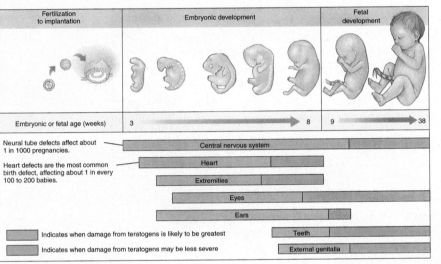

13. According to this growth chart, a 15-month-old infant who weighs 21 lb is at about the _____ percentile for weight.

    a. 5th   c. 25th

    b. 10th   d. 50th

CDC Growth Charts: United States

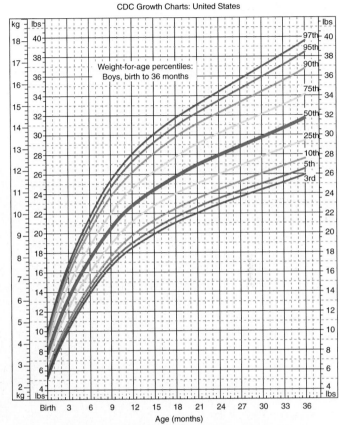

Weight-for-age percentiles:
Boys, birth to 36 months

10. The hormone responsible for the let-down of milk is _____.

    a. estrogen

    b. prolactin

    c. progesterone

    d. oxytocin

11. Solid food should be introduced into an infant's diet _____.

    a. within 2 weeks of birth

    b. around 4 to 6 months of age

    c. at 9 months of age

    d. after 1 year of age

12. The leading cause of preventable birth defects and intellectual disability is _____ during pregnancy.

    a. coffee consumption

    b. tobacco use

    c. alcohol consumption

    d. cocaine use

14. Colostrum is _____.

    a. a type of infant formula that is fortified with omega-3 fatty acids

    b. the first stool passed by the infant after delivery

    c. the first fluid produced by the breast after delivery

    d. the mature milk produced in the later part of a feeding

15. Which of the following statements about breast milk is false?

    a. It contains immune factors that protect the baby from infections.

    b. It provides about 50% of calories from fat.

    c. It contains a high concentration of iron.

    d. The proteins it contains are easily digested.

THE PLANNER ✓

Review your Chapter Planner on the chapter opener and check off your completed work.

Nutrition from 1 to 100

In *As You Like It*, Shakespeare allotted a human life-time seven acts to be played upon the world's stage, beginning with "the infant, mewling and puking in the nurse's arms" and ending in "second childishness . . . sans teeth, sans eyes, sans taste." While our senses and abilities do diminish as we age, with proper nutrition and health maintenance, we may not quite reach the state of helplessness described by the Bard.

For "the whining schoolboy"—and girl—"with . . . shining morning face," nutrition and healthy development go hand in hand. As the adolescent becomes "the lover," then "the soldier" of young adulthood, good nutrition is still necessary to maintain health and build a foundation of well-being for the mature "justice, in fair round belly

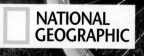

with good capon lin'd"—Shakespeare's archetype of middle age. In his characterization of the closing years of life, "the lean and slipper'd pantaloon . . . a world too wide for his shrunk shank," Shakespeare highlights the muscle withering of old age that, along with other physical, social, and mental changes present a new set of challenges to maintaining nutritional health.

Good nutrition habits adopted in our early years will serve us well through the seven acts of our own "strange eventful history."

CHAPTER OUTLINE

Nutrition for Children 428
- Energy and Nutrient Needs of Children
- Developing Healthy Eating Habits
- ■ What Should I Eat? Childhood
- ■ What a Scientist Sees: Breakfast and School Performance
- Nutrition and Health Concerns in Children
- ■ Thinking It Through: A Case Study on Under- and Overnutrition

Nutrition for Adolescents 438
- Energy and Nutrient Needs of Adolescents
- Meeting Teens' Nutritional Needs
- ■ What Should I Eat? Adolescence
- Special Concerns for Teens

Nutrition for the Adult Years 443
- ■ DEBATE: Can Eating Less Help You Live Longer?
- What Is Aging?
- Nutrition and Health Concerns Throughout Adulthood
- Factors that Increase the Risk of Malnutrition in Older Adults
- Keeping Healthy Throughout the Adult Years
- ■ What Should I Eat? Advancing Age

The Impact of Alcohol Throughout Life 454
- Alcohol Absorption, Transport, and Excretion
- Alcohol Metabolism
- Adverse Effects of Alcohol
- Benefits of Alcohol Consumption

CHAPTER PLANNER ✓

❑ Stimulate your interest by reading the introduction and looking at the visual.
❑ Scan the Learning Objectives in each section:
   p. 428 ❑   p. 438 ❑   p. 443 ❑   p. 454 ❑
❑ Read the text and study all figures and visuals. Answer any questions.

Analyze key features

❑ What a Scientist Sees, p. 431 ❑
❑ Process Diagram, p. 456 ❑
❑ Thinking It Through, p. 436 ❑
❑ Nutrition InSight, p. 434 ❑   p. 438 ❑   p. 448 ❑
❑ Stop: Answer the Concept Checks before you go on:
   p. 437 ❑   p. 442 ❑   p. 453 ❑   p. 458 ❑

End of chapter

❑ Review the Summary, Online Resources, and Key Terms.
❑ Answer the Critical and Creative Thinking Questions.
❑ Answer What is happening in this picture?
❑ Complete the Self-Test and check your answers.

Nutrition for Children

LEARNING OBJECTIVES

1. **Describe** how children's nutrient needs change as they grow.

2. **Discuss** how children's eating habits develop.

3. **Explain** the impact of diet and lifestyle during childhood on the risk of chronic disease.

Nutrient intake during childhood affects health in adulthood. The foods offered to a child must supply the energy and nutrients needed for growth and development as well as for maintenance and activity. They must also be appropriate for the child's stage of physical development and suit his or her developing tastes. A nutritious, well-balanced eating pattern and an active lifestyle allow children to grow to their potential and can prevent or delay the onset of the chronic diseases that plague adults. Therefore, teaching healthy eating and exercise habits will benefit not only today's children but also tomorrow's adults.

Energy and Nutrient Needs of Children

As children grow and become more active, their requirements for energy and most nutrients increase. The average 2-year-old needs about 1000 Calories and 13 grams of protein per day. By age 6, that child needs about 1600 Calories and 19 g of protein per day.[1] The total amount of protein and energy needed continue to increase as children grow into adults; however, the amounts needed per kilogram of body weight decrease (**Figure 12.1**).

The recommended range of carbohydrate intake for children is the same as for adults: 45 to 65% of total energy intake. To provide enough energy to support rapid growth and development, the recommended range of fat intake is higher for children than for adults: 30 to 40% of total energy intake for 1- to 3-year-olds and 25 to 35% for 4- to 18-year-olds. As children grow, the recommended proportion of calories from fat decreases to avoid increasing the risk of developing chronic diseases.

Infants have high water needs, but by 1 year of age, their evaporative losses have decreased and their kidneys have matured, decreasing the loss of water in urine. Therefore, as with adults, in most situations, children can meet their water needs by drinking enough to satisfy thirst.[2] Water needs increase with illness, when the environmental temperature is high, and when activity increases sweat losses.

Because children are smaller than adolescents and adults, the recommended amounts of most micronutrients are also smaller (see inside cover). Recommended intakes do not differ for boys and girls until about age 9, at which time sexual maturation causes differences in nutrient requirements. Like adults, children who consume a varied, nutrient-dense diet can meet all their vitamin and mineral requirements with food. However, in the United States today, diets that frequently include fast-food meals and high-sugar and high-fat snacks put many children at risk for inadequate vitamin and mineral intake.[3] Deficiencies of calcium, vitamin D, and iron are of particular concern.

Calcium, vitamin D, and bone health Calcium intake in school-age children has been declining, primarily due to a decrease in the consumption of dairy products. Adequate calcium intake during childhood is essential for achieving maximum peak bone mass, which is important for preventing osteoporosis later in life (see Chapter 8). The RDA for calcium is 700 mg/day for toddlers (ages 1 to 3) and 1000 mg/day for young children (ages 4 to 8).[4]

Energy needs • Figure 12.1

As children grow, their larger body size causes the total amount of energy they need to increase, but as growth slows, energy needs per kilogram of body weight decline.

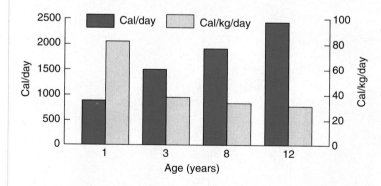

Interpreting Data

How many more Calories per day does a 12-year-old child need than an 8-year-old child?

Vitamin D, which is needed for calcium absorption, is also essential for bone health. Low intakes of milk combined with limited sun exposure may put many children at risk for vitamin D deficiency.[5] The RDA is 600 IU (15 µg)/day for children and adolescents.[4]

Iron and anemia Children's iron needs are high because iron is required for growth. The RDA is 7 mg/day for toddlers and 10 mg/day for young children; the latter recommendation is higher than the RDA for adult men. The high needs and finicky eating habits of young children often lead to iron deficiency anemia, a condition that can impair learning ability and intellectual performance.[6] If anemia is diagnosed, iron supplements are usually prescribed until the child's iron stores have been replenished. These supplements should be kept out of the reach of children to prevent iron toxicity from supplement overdoses (see Chapter 8).

Developing Healthy Eating Habits

Much of what we choose to eat as adults depends on what we learned to eat as children. Caregivers are responsible for deciding what foods should be offered to a child and when and where they should be eaten. The child must then decide whether to eat, what foods to eat, and how much to consume. As children grow older, their choices are increasingly affected by social activities, what they see at school, and what their friends are eating.

What to offer? Children should be offered a balanced and varied diet that is adequate in energy and essential nutrients and is appropriate to their developmental needs. A healthy diet is based on whole grains, vegetables, and fruits; includes adequate milk and other high-protein foods; and contains moderate amounts of fat and sodium. MyPlate can be used as a guide for meeting the dietary goals of preschoolers and older children (**Figure 12.2**).

MyPlate for kids • Figure12.2

MyPlate for kids recommends amounts of food from each group that are appropriate for young children. The recommendations shown here are for a 3-year-old and an 8-year-old who engage in more than 60 minutes of activity daily. Food choices to meet these amounts should be spread throughout the meals and snacks served each day.

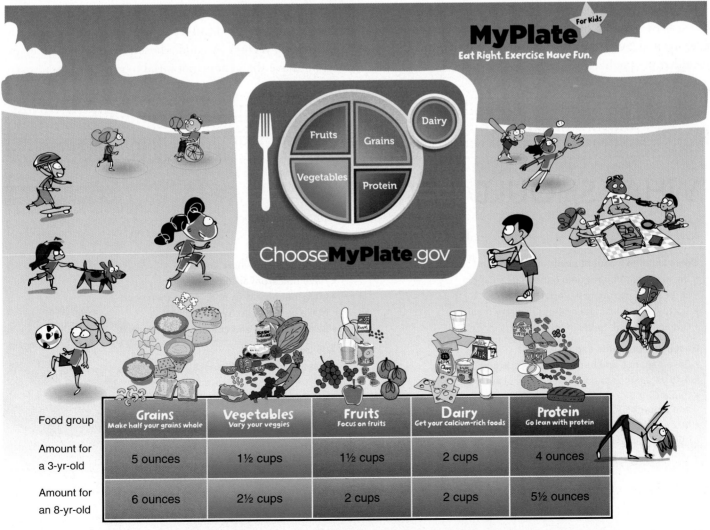

Food group	**Grains** Make half your grains whole	**Vegetables** Vary your veggies	**Fruits** Focus on fruits	**Dairy** Get your calcium-rich foods	**Protein** Go lean with protein
Amount for a 3-yr-old	5 ounces	1½ cups	1½ cups	2 cups	4 ounces
Amount for an 8-yr-old	6 ounces	2½ cups	2 cups	2 cups	5½ ounces

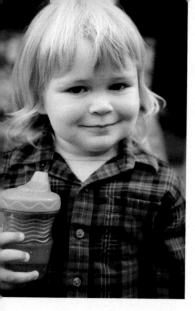

Limiting juice consumption • Figure 12.3

More than half the fruit children consume is as juice rather than whole fruit. Although 100% fruit juice can be part of a healthy diet, too much can cause diarrhea, over- or undernutrition, and dental caries. It is recommended that juice not be offered to children in containers that can be carried around, encouraging continuous sipping.[8,9]

It isn't always easy to persuade a child to eat a variety of foods from all the food groups, as recommended by My-Plate. To increase variety, new foods should be introduced into a child's diet regularly. Children's food preferences are learned through repeated exposure to foods; a new food may need to be offered 8 or 10 times before the child will accept it. Children are also more likely to eat a new food if it is introduced at the beginning of a meal, when the child is hungry, and if the child sees his or her parents or peers eating it. Incorporating healthy foods into familiar dishes can also increase the variety of the diet. Vegetables can be added to soups and casseroles, for example, and lean meats can be added to spaghetti sauce, stews, or pizza. Getting chil-

dren to consume the recommended amount of fruit is usually not difficult, but most servings should come from fruit, with limited amounts from 100% juice, not fruit drinks or juice cocktails. The American Academy of Pediatrics recommends limiting juice to 4 to 6 ounces/day for children ages 1 to 6 and 8 to 12 oz/day for children age 7 and older (**Figure 12.3**).[7]

No matter how erratic children's food intake may be, caregivers should continue to offer a variety of healthy foods at each meal and let children select what and how much they will eat. Children, like adults, tend to eat greater quantities when larger portions are provided.[10] When children are allowed to serve themselves, they eat more appropriate portions than they do when a large portion is put in front of them.

The best indicator that a child is receiving adequate nourishment—neither too little nor too much—is a normal growth pattern. Growth is most rapid in the first year of life, when an infant's length increases by 50%, or about 10 inches. In the second year of life, children generally grow about 5 inches; in the third year, 4 inches; and thereafter, about 2 to 3 inches/year. Although growth often occurs in spurts, growth patterns are predictable and can be monitored by comparing a child's growth pattern with standard patterns shown on growth charts (Appendix B).[11] The stature a child will eventually attain is affected by genetic, environmental, and lifestyle factors. A child whose parents are 5 feet tall may not have the genetic potential to grow to 6 feet.

WHAT SHOULD I EAT?
Childhood

☑ THE PLANNER

Serve children frequent nutritious meals and snacks
- Smear peanut butter on a banana or an apple.
- Offer some carrots with yogurt dip.
- Try to have at least four colors in every meal.
- Cut and arrange foods in interesting shapes.

Sneak in more fruits and vegetables
- Bake bananas and berries into breads and muffins.
- Add vegetables to soups, tacos, and casseroles.
- Blend fruit into shakes and smoothies.
- Mix extra vegetables into spaghetti sauce.

Use iProfile to find snacks that are high in iron.

Include calcium where you can
- Have macaroni and cheese.
- Make oatmeal with milk rather than water.
- Make cream soup by adding milk.
- Serve pudding and custard.

Add iron
- Make your spaghetti sauce with meat.
- Cook your stew in an iron pot.
- Beef up your tacos and burritos.
- Serve iron-fortified breakfast cereal.

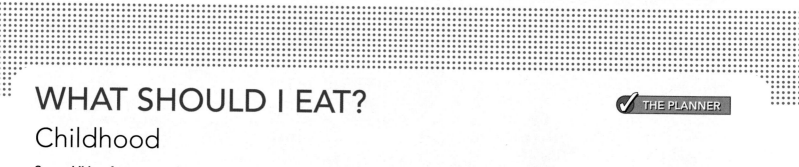

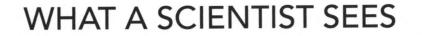

WHAT A SCIENTIST SEES

✓ THE PLANNER

Breakfast and School Performance

This breakfast looks appealing, but regardless of what's on the plate, many children and teens do not make time for breakfast; they are more likely to skip breakfast than to skip any other meal.[12] What a scientist sees is the impact breakfast has on nutritional status and school performance. Skipping breakfast may result in a span of 15 or more hours without food. Because breakfast provides energy and nutrients to the brain, children who skip it are more likely to have academic, emotional, and behavioral problems than those who eat breakfast.[13] Studies have found that compared with nonbreakfast eaters, children who participate in school breakfast programs have better nutrient intakes, and these improvements in nutrient intakes are associated with improvements in academic performance, reductions in hyperactivity, better psychosocial behaviors, and less absence and tardiness (see graph).[14]

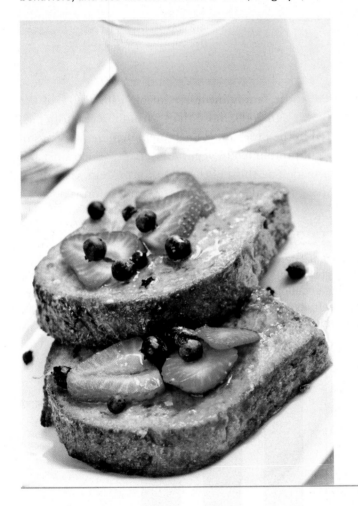

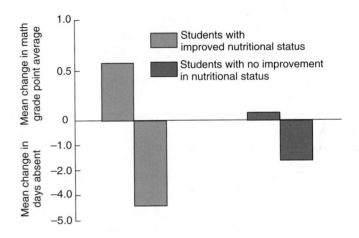

Implementation of a free school breakfast program in the Boston Public Schools improved the nutritional status of many students. Those whose nutritional status improved showed greater improvements in math grades and fewer school absences than students whose nutritional status was not improved.[14]

Think Critically In addition to enhancing learning by fueling the brain after the overnight fast, in what other ways might breakfast contribute to better school performance?

When a child does not get enough to eat, weight gain slows, and if the deficiency continues, growth in height slows. If food intake is excessive, a child is at risk for becoming obese and developing the chronic diseases that are increasingly common in U.S. adults (see *What Should I Eat?*).

When and where to offer meals and snacks

Because children have small stomachs and high nutrient needs, they should consume small, nutrient-dense meals and snacks, ideally every two to three hours throughout the day. Establishing a consistent meal pattern is important because children thrive on routine and feel secure when they know what to expect. Starting the day with a good breakfast is particularly important; children who eat breakfast are more likely than those who do not to meet their daily nutrient needs and do better in school (see *What a Scientist Sees*).[12] Snacks should be as

Typical meal and snack patterns for 3- and 8-year-old children Table 12.1

Food	3-year-old	8-year-old	Food	3-year-old	8-year-old
Breakfast			**Snack**		
Whole grain cereal	1/2 cup	1 cup	Broccoli crowns	4	6
Milk, 2%	1/2 cup	1/2 cup	Ranch salad dressing	1 tsp	2 tsp
Banana	1/2 medium	1 medium	**Dinner**		
Snack			Chicken drumsticks	1	2
Peanut butter	2 Tbsp	2 Tbsp	Baked sweet potato	1/2 cup	1 cup
Whole wheat crackers	5	5	Green beans	1/4 cup	1/2 cup
Milk, 2%	1/2 cup	1 cup	Milk, 2%	1/2 cup	1 cup
Lunch			Graham crackers	1	2
Vegetable soup	1/2 cup	1 cup	**Snack**		
Grilled tuna sandwich	1/2	1	Yogurt	1/2 cup	1 cup
Tomato	1/4 medium	1/2 medium	Berries	1/2 cup	3/4 cup
Orange	1/2 medium	1 medium			
Milk, 2%	1/2 cup	1 cup			

nutritious as meals to ensure that nutrient needs are met (**Table 12.1**).

The setting in which a meal is consumed is also important. Children need companionship, conversation, and a pleasant location at mealtimes. Eating meals together helps children connect with family and culture and is associated with better school performance and decreased risk of unhealthy weight-loss practices and substance abuse. Children learn by example; therefore, the eating patterns, attitudes, and feeding styles of their caregivers influence what they learn to eat. Children whose mothers' eat a healthy diet are more likely to have a healthy diet.[15] Children should be given plenty of time to finish eating. Slow eaters are unlikely to finish eating if they are abandoned by siblings who run off to play and adults who leave to wash dishes. Moreover, if mealtime is to be a nutritious, educational, and enjoyable experience, it should not be a battle zone. Food is not a reward or a punishment: It is simply nutrition.

Meals at day care or school

It is not easy to ensure that meals eaten away from home are nutritious because there is no guarantee that what is served at school or brought from home will be eaten. A packed lunch should contain foods that the child likes and that do not require refrigeration. For children who do not bring meals from home, federal school breakfast and lunch programs provide free or low-cost meals containing age-appropriate foods.

The goals of the **National School Lunch Program** are to improve the dietary intake and nutritional health of children in the United States and to promote nutrition education by teaching children to make appropriate food choices. Meals are provided free or at reduced costs to children whose family income is at or below 130% of the poverty level. In 2009, more than 31 million children participated in the program.[16] Each meal includes servings of milk, high-protein foods, vegetables, fruit, and grains; and must provide one-third of the RDA for protein, vitamin A, vitamin C, iron, calcium, and energy, and contains no more

How good are children's diets? • Figure 12.4

Only a small percentage of children in the United States have "good" diets, based on how well they meet the recommendations of MyPlate. Most American children consume too few fruits and vegetables and whole grains and too much fat, salt, and sugar. As children grow older, their diets worsen.

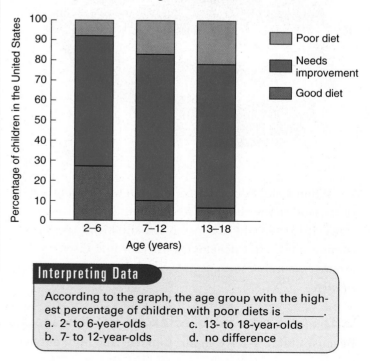

Interpreting Data

According to the graph, the age group with the highest percentage of children with poor diets is _____.
a. 2- to 6-year-olds   c. 13- to 18-year-olds
b. 7- to 12-year-olds   d. no difference

than 30% of energy from fat and 10% from saturated fat. In addition to lunches, federal guidelines regulate foods sold at snack bars and in vending machines that compete with school lunch programs. These must provide at least 5% of the RDA for one or more of the following: protein, vitamin A, vitamin C, niacin, riboflavin, calcium, or iron. An analysis of the foods students chose to eat from the meals offered found that, compared to nonparticipants, students who took part in the school lunch program consumed more vegetables and milk and milk products, fewer salty snacks, and fewer beverages other than milk.[17]

Nutrition and Health Concerns in Children

The diets of U.S. children today are not as healthy as they could be, and as a result, children are not as healthy as they could be (**Figure 12.4**). Some of the nutrition and health concerns affecting children in the United States are related to their dietary and exercise patterns. The high-calorie, high-sugar, high-salt, high-saturated-fat diet and low-activity lifestyle that contribute to obesity and chronic disease in adults are having the same effects in children. Other nutrition-related health concerns in children include dental caries and lead poisoning.

The rising rate of childhood obesity A child's weight is assessed by determining his or her body mass index (BMI) and plotting it on a gender-specific BMI-for-age growth chart to determine his or her percentile (see Chapter 11). The BMI percentile is then used to classify the child as obese, overweight, healthy weight, or underweight (**Figure 12.5**).[18] It is estimated that

BMI-for-age percentiles • Figure 12.5

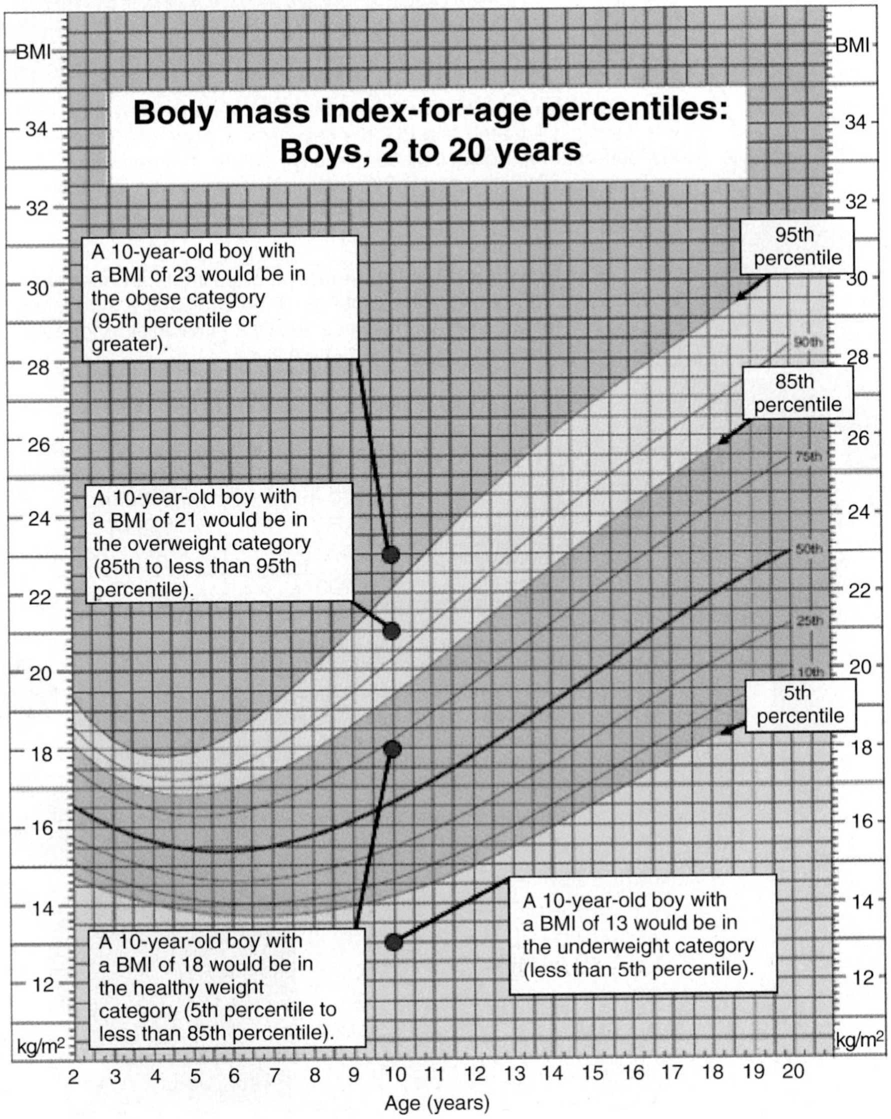

Body mass index-for-age percentiles: Boys, 2 to 20 years

A 10-year-old boy with a BMI of 23 would be in the obese category (95th percentile or greater).

A 10-year-old boy with a BMI of 21 would be in the overweight category (85th to less than 95th percentile).

A 10-year-old boy with a BMI of 18 would be in the healthy weight category (5th percentile to less than 85th percentile).

A 10-year-old boy with a BMI of 13 would be in the underweight category (less than 5th percentile).

This growth chart shows the BMI-for-age percentiles for boys 2 to 20 years of age. The colored areas represent BMI values associated with underweight, healthy weight, overweight, and obesity. A similar growth chart can be used to assess body weight in girls (see Appendix B).

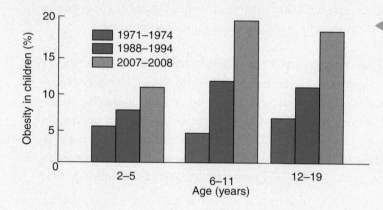

Results from the National Health and Nutrition Examination Surveys illustrate the increase in the percentage of children who are obese over the past 20 years.[19]

Obese children are at risk for depression, unhealthy blood cholesterol levels, high blood pressure, and type 2 diabetes.

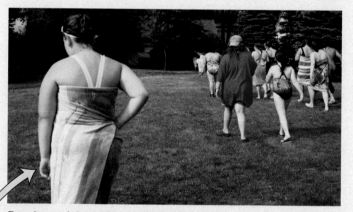

Psychosocial problems: Obese children are more likely than others to be socially isolated and to have depression, poor self-image, and low self-esteem. Social isolation, in turn, results in boredom, depression, inactivity, and withdrawal—all of which can increase eating and decrease activity, worsening the problem.

Elevated blood cholesterol: The American Academy of Pediatrics recommends blood cholesterol monitoring for children and teenagers with a family history of heart disease or high blood cholesterol.[22]

Cholesterol levels in children and adolescents 2 to 19 years old[21]

	Total cholesterol (mg/100 mL)	LDL cholesterol (mg/100 mL)
Acceptable	< 170	< 110
Borderline	170 – 199	110 – 129
High	≥ 200	≥ 130

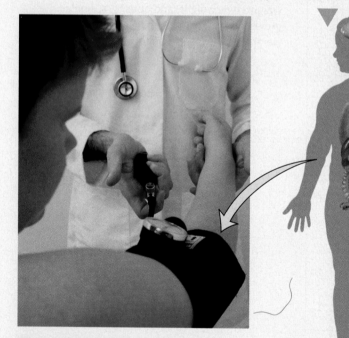

Type 2 diabetes: The longer an individual has diabetes, the greater the risk of complications that can lead to blindness, kidney failure, heart disease or amputations (see Chapter 4).[20]

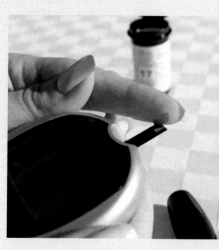

Elevated blood pressure: Children who have blood pressure at the high end of normal are more likely to develop high blood pressure as adults. As with adults, blood pressure can be affected by the amount of body fat, the total pattern of dietary intake, including sodium intake, and activity level.

17% of U.S. children and adolescents ages 2 through 19 are obese.[19] Along with obesity come a number of other chronic conditions, including type 2 diabetes, high blood pressure, and elevated blood cholesterol, as well as social and psychological challenges (**Figure 12.6**).[20]

Addressing the issue of excess weight in children requires changes in both eating and activity patterns. Because children are still growing, weight loss is rarely recommended. Rather, overweight children should be encouraged to slow their weight gain while they continue to grow taller. This allows them to "grow into" their weight. A child who is at the 85th percentile for BMI at age 7 and gains only a few pounds a year can be at the 75th percentile by age 9.

It can be difficult to modify a child's food consumption patterns. Denying food may promote further overeating by making the child feel that he or she will not obtain enough to satisfy hunger. Thus, restrictions on food intake should be relatively mild, and the focus instead should be on offering nutrient-dense foods.

Public health recommendations, including the 2010 Dietary Guidelines, suggest that children be physically active for at least an hour each day. This may be difficult for overweight children, who are often embarrassed by their bodies and shy away from group activities. Increases in physical activity need to be gradual in order to make exercise a positive experience. A good way to start is to limit time spent watching television and playing video and computer games and encourage active games, walks after dinner, bike rides, hikes, swimming, volleyball, and other activities that the whole family can enjoy together. Learning to enjoy sports and exercise in childhood will set the stage for an active lifestyle in adulthood.

Watching television has a major influence on children's energy balance because it affects both food intake and activity level (**Figure 12.7** and *Thinking It Through* on next page). Sitting in front of the television encourages snacking and reduces activity. Television also affects the quality of the diet because commercials introduce children to foods to which they might otherwise not be exposed. Children who view food ads choose those food products more often than children who are not exposed to the ads.[23]

Television affects food intake and activity level • Figure12.7

a. Hours spent watching television are hours when physical activity is at a minimum. Children who watch four or more hours of TV per day are 40% more likely to be overweight than those who watch an hour or less a day.[24]

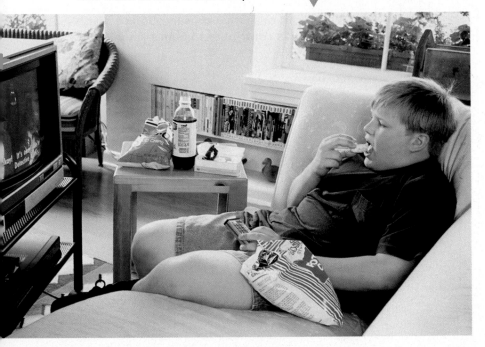

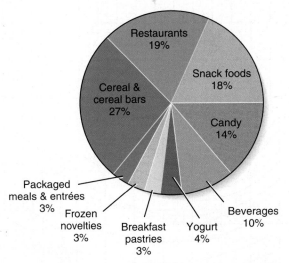

Restaurants 19%
Snack foods 18%
Cereal & cereal bars 27%
Candy 14%
Packaged meals & entrées 3%
Frozen novelties 3%
Breakfast pastries 3%
Yogurt 4%
Beverages 10%

b. During children's television programming, food is the most frequently advertised product category. This chart, which illustrates the types of food advertised on Saturday morning children's television programming, shows that almost half of the commercials advertise candy, snack foods, beverages, and pastries.[25]

THINKING IT THROUGH

✓ **THE PLANNER**

A Case Study on Under- and Overnutrition

Sam is 8 years old and has gained 5 pounds in the past three months. His parents are worried because all Sam wants to do is watch TV. Because Sam's parents are both overweight, they are concerned that he will also have a weight problem, so they take him to see his pediatrician.

Based on this growth chart, how has Sam's BMI percentile changed over the past year?
▼

Your answer:

Reviewing Sam's diet and exercise patterns, the doctor learns that Sam has been watching TV or playing video games for about six hours a day. A recall of his intake shows that he eats donuts and milk for breakfast, gets lunch from the school lunch program, and then snacks so much on chips and candy when he gets home from school that he doesn't really eat dinner. He likes fruit, refuses to eat vegetables, and drinks 5 to 6 cups of whole milk daily.

What nutrients are likely to be excessive or deficient in this dietary pattern?
▼

Your answer:

CDC Growth Charts: United States

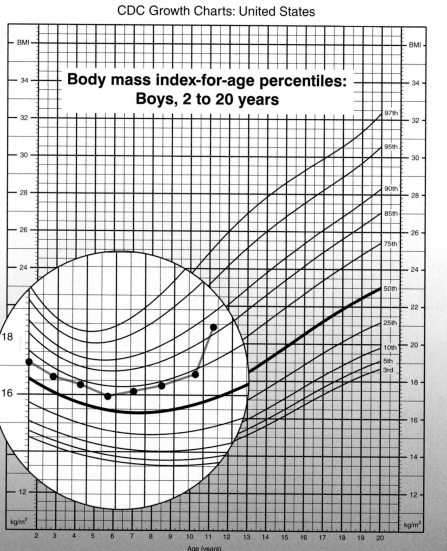

Body mass index-for-age percentiles: Boys, 2 to 20 years

A blood test reveals that Sam has iron deficiency anemia. The pediatrician prescribes an iron supplement and refers Sam and his parents to a dietitian. She recommends that the family switch to 1% milk to reduce Sam's energy and saturated fat intake and to a fortified cereal for breakfast to increase his iron intake. She also recommends that they limit Sam's after-school snacking to fruit so he can eat a better evening meal.

Why might excessive consumption of dairy products contribute to Sam's anemia?
▼

Your answer:

How might Sam's iron deficiency have contributed to his weight gain?
▼

Your answer:

(Check your answers in Appendix J.)

Dental caries A diet that is high in sugary foods promotes the formation of dental caries (see Chapter 4). Because the primary teeth guide the growth of the permanent teeth, maintaining healthy primary teeth is just as important as preserving the permanent ones. Tooth decay is caused by prolonged contact between sugar and bacteria on the surface of the teeth. When soft drinks and other sweetened beverages, which are a major source of added sugar in children's diets, are sipped slowly between meals they, increase the risk of tooth decay.

Hyperactivity Hyperactivity is a problem in 5 to 10% of school-age children, occurring more frequently in boys than in girls. Hyperactivity involves extreme physical activity, excitability, impulsiveness, distractibility, short attention span, and low tolerance for frustration.

> **attention-deficit/ hyperactivity disorder (ADHD)** A condition characterized by a short attention span and a high level of activity, excitability, and distractibility.

Hyperactive children have more difficulty learning but usually are of normal or above-average intelligence. Hyperactivity is now considered part of a larger syndrome known as **attention-deficit/hyperactivity disorder (ADHD)**.

A popular misconception is that hyperactivity is caused by eating sugar, but research on sugar intake and behavior has failed to support this hypothesis.[26, 27] The hyperactive behavior observed after sugar consumption is more likely the result of situational factors. For example, the excitement of a birthday party rather than the sugar in the cake is most likely the cause of hyperactive behavior.

One cause of hyperactive behavior in children is caffeine. Caffeine is a stimulant that causes sleeplessness, restlessness, and irregular heartbeats. Beverages, foods, and medicines containing caffeine are often part of children's diets. For example, caffeinated beverages such as Coke and Mountain Dew are commonly included in children's fast food meals.

Other possible causes of hyperactivity include lack of sleep, overstimulation, desire for more attention, or lack of physical activity. Specific foods and food additives have also been implicated as causes of hyperactivity. Numerous studies have failed to provide sufficient evidence for the efficacy of any dietary treatment for ADHD. However, some children are sensitive to specific additives and may benefit from a diet that eliminates them.[27]

Lead toxicity Lead is an environmental contaminant that can be toxic, especially in children under age 6. Children can be exposed to lead in air pollution, old house paint, lead plumbing, and certain ceramics. Children are at particular risk for lead toxicity because they absorb lead much more efficiently than do adults. It is estimated that infants and young children may absorb as much as 50% of ingested lead.[28] Malnourished children are at particular risk because malnutrition increases lead absorption due to the fact that lead is better absorbed from an empty stomach and when other mineral such as calcium, zinc, and iron are deficient. Once it has been absorbed from the gastrointestinal tract, lead circulates in the bloodstream and then accumulates in the bones and, to a lesser extent, the brain, teeth, and kidneys. Lead disrupts the functioning of neurotransmitters and thus interferes with the functioning of the nervous system.

In young children, lead poisoning can cause learning disabilities and behavior problems. There is evidence that even blood lead levels below 10 μg/100 mL, which were once thought to be safe, may impair IQ in young children.[29] Higher levels of lead can contribute to iron deficiency anemia, changes in kidney function, nervous system changes, and even seizures, coma, and death.

Because of the risks of lead toxicity from environmental contamination, lead is no longer used in house paint, gasoline, or solder. As a result, the number of children ages 1 to 5 with elevated blood lead levels decreased from 77.8% in 1976–1980 to only 1.4% in 1999–2004.[29] Despite these gains, certain groups remain at elevated risk of high blood lead levels. Low-income children are at particular risk. Low-income families are more likely to live in older buildings that still have lead paint and lead plumbing. Typical blood lead levels are also higher for non-Hispanic black children than those for Mexican-American and non-Hispanic white children, in part reflecting differences in socioeconomic status. The effects of lead poisoning are permanent, but if high levels are detected early, the lead can be removed with medical treatment.

CONCEPT CHECK   **STOP**

1. **How** do children's energy and protein requirements change as they age?

2. **What** factors affect children's food choices?

3. **What** health risks are associated with obesity in children?

Nutrition for Adolescents

LEARNING OBJECTIVES

1. **Describe** how puberty affects growth and body composition.

2. **Compare** the energy needs of adolescents with those of children and adults.

3. **Explain** why iron and calcium are of particular concern during the teen years.

4. **Use** MyPlate to plan a day's diet that would appeal to a teenager.

Adolescents are a unique population in many ways, and they have unique nutritional needs. The physical, emotional, mental, and social changes of adolescence transform a child into an adult. Organ systems develop and grow, **puberty** occurs, body composition changes,

> **puberty** A period of rapid growth and physical changes that ends in the attainment of sexual maturity.

and the growth rates and nutritional requirements of boys and girls diverge (**Figure 12.8**). The physiological changes associated with sexual maturation affect nutrient requirements, and social and psychological changes that occur during adolescence influence nutrient intakes.

Nutrition InSight   Adolescent growth • Figure 12.8   ✓ THE PLANNER

The **adolescent growth spurt** is an 18- to 24-month period of peak growth velocity that begins at about ages 10 to 13 in girls and 12 to 15 in boys. During a 1-year growth spurt, girls can gain 3.5 inches in height and boys can gain 4 inches.

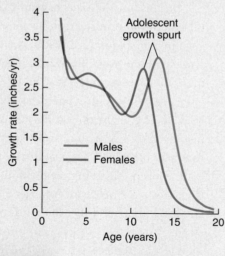

At age 13, some boys are physically still children, while others have matured sexually. Because there are large individual variations in the age at which these growth and developmental changes occur, the stage of maturation is often a better indicator of nutritional requirements than is chronological age.

During the adolescent growth spurt, boys gain some fat but add so much lean mass as muscle and bone that their percentage of body fat actually decreases. Girls gain proportionately more body fat and less lean tissue. By age 20, females have about twice as much adipose tissue as males and about ten percent less lean tissue.

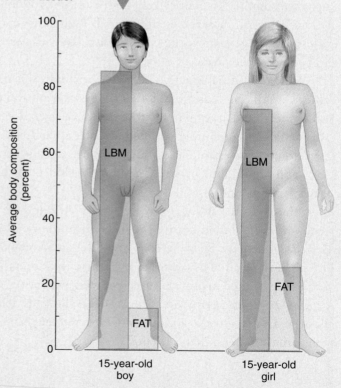

Energy and Nutrient Needs of Adolescents

The DRIs provide recommendations for adolescents in two age groups: 9 through 13 and 14 through 18. Separate recommendations are made for boys and girls because their needs begin to differ during the adolescent years.

Energy and energy-yielding nutrients

The proportions of calories from carbohydrate, fat, and protein recommended for adolescents are similar to those for adults, but the total amount of energy needed by teenagers usually exceeds adult needs. Boys require more energy than girls because they have more muscle and their bodies are larger. Protein requirements per kilogram of body weight are the same for boys and girls, but because boys are generally heavier, they require more total protein than do girls.

Vitamins

The need for most of the vitamins rises to adult levels during adolescence. The requirements for B vitamins, which are involved in energy metabolism, are much higher in adolescence than in childhood because of higher energy needs. The rapid growth of adolescence further increases the need for vitamin B_6, which is important for protein synthesis, and for folate and vitamin B_{12}, which are essential for cell division. The high calorie intakes of teens help them meet most of their vitamin needs, but inadequate intakes of riboflavin and vitamin D put some teens at risk for deficiency. Riboflavin is frequently low in teens' diets, especially in those of girls, possibly due to low milk intake. Vitamin D is important to support the rapid skeletal growth that occurs during adolescence. Low blood levels of vitamin D are problematic due to low intake as well as limited synthesis from sunlight in those with dark skin pigmentation or inadequate exposure to sunlight during the winter months (see Chapter 7).[30]

Iron

The need for iron rises between childhood and adolescence. Iron is needed to synthesize hemoglobin for the expansion of blood volume and myoglobin for the increase in muscle mass. Because growth is more rapid in adolescent boys than in girls, they require more iron for the expansion of blood volume and for tissue synthesis. However, the onset of menstruation in girls increases their iron losses, making total iron needs greater in young women. The RDA is set at 11 mg/day for boys and 15 mg/day for girls ages 14 to 18. Girls are more likely than boys to consume less than the recommended amount because they require more iron, tend to eat fewer iron-rich foods, and consume fewer overall calories. As a result, iron deficiency is common in adolescent females, affecting about 9% of girls ages 12 to 15 and 16% of young women ages 16 to 19.[31]

Calcium

The adolescent growth spurt increases both the length and mass of bones. Adequate calcium is essential for forming healthy bone. The RDA for calcium is 1300 mg/day for everyone between the ages of 9 and 18, but intake is typically below this amount in both sexes.[4] Fewer than 10% of girls and only 25% of boys ages 9 to 13 consume the recommended amount of calcium.[32] This low intake may reduce the level of peak bone mass achieved, increasing the risk of developing osteoporosis later in life.

Because milk and cheese, which are major sources of calcium in teen diets, can be high in saturated fat, adolescents should be encouraged to consume low-fat dairy products, calcium-fortified cereals, and vegetable sources of calcium. One of the contributors to low calcium intake is the use of soda and fruit juices, rather than milk, as a beverage (**Figure 12.9**).

Beverage choices in children and teens[33] • Figure 12.9

Consumption of soft drinks by children and adolescents has increased since the 1970s, and milk consumption has decreased. Today, 46% of their beverage intake by weight is from soft drinks and other sweetened beverages, while only 29% is from milk. This pattern has increased the intake of added sweeteners and decreased the amounts of calcium, magnesium, potassium, protein, riboflavin, vitamin A, and zinc in the diet.

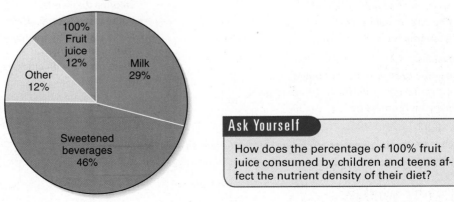

Ask Yourself

How does the percentage of 100% fruit juice consumed by children and teens affect the nutrient density of their diet?

MyPlate recommendations for teens • Figure12.10

The recommendations shown here are for 11- and 18-year-old boys and girls who engage in more than 60 minutes of activity daily. The 10 oz of grains recommended for an active 18-year-old boy may seem like a huge amount. But when spread over the course of a day (in the form of, say, a large bowl of cereal and toast for breakfast, two tacos for lunch, and a dinner that includes spaghetti and garlic bread), it is an amount that is easily consumed by a teenage boy.

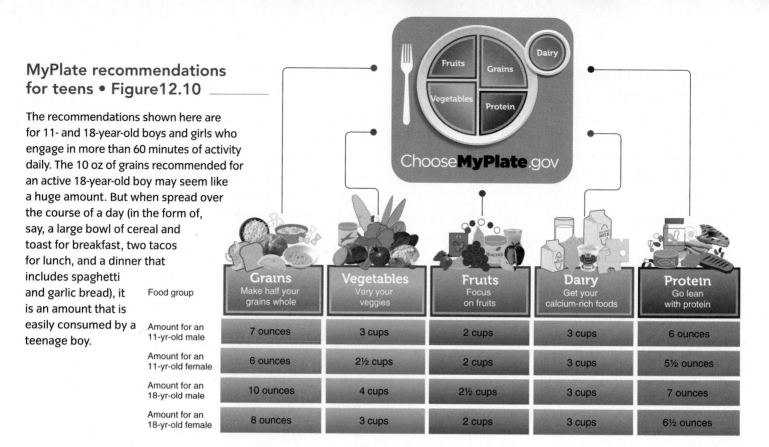

Food group	Grains Make half your grains whole	Vegetables Vary your veggies	Fruits Focus on fruits	Dairy Get your calcium-rich foods	Protein Go lean with protein
Amount for an 11-yr-old male	7 ounces	3 cups	2 cups	3 cups	6 ounces
Amount for an 11-yr-old female	6 ounces	2½ cups	2 cups	3 cups	5½ ounces
Amount for an 18-yr-old male	10 ounces	4 cups	2½ cups	3 cups	7 ounces
Amount for an 18-yr-old female	8 ounces	3 cups	2 cups	3 cups	6½ ounces

Meeting Teens' Nutritional Needs

During adolescence, physiological changes dictate nutritional needs, but peer pressure may dictate food choices. Parents often have little control over what adolescents eat, and skipped meals and meals away from home are common. A food is more likely to be selected because it tastes good, it is easy to grab, or friends are eating it than because it is a healthy choice. No matter when foods are consumed throughout the day, an adolescent's diet should follow the recommendations of MyPlate for the appropriate age, gender, and activity level (see **Figure 12.10** and *What Should I Eat?*). The best indicators of adequate intake are satiety and a growth pattern that follows the curve of the growth charts.

WHAT SHOULD I EAT?

Adolescence

THE PLANNER

Balance unhealthy choices with healthy ones
• Have milk with your burger and fries.
• Eat an extra vegetable with dinner.
• Put peppers on your pizza.
• Try fresh fruit for dessert.

Eat breakfast
• Grab some toast with peanut butter.
• Stick a cereal bar or muffin in your backpack.
• Have a yogurt on the go.

Snack well
• Reach for an apple, a pear, or an orange before the cookies and chips.
• Dip your chips in salsa, guacamole, or hummus.
• Nibble on nuts and seeds.
• Crunch some baby carrots.

Count up your calcium
• Drink milk; low-fat milk has fewer calories than soda.
• Put extra milk on your cereal.
• Make a shake by mixing yogurt and fruit in the blender.
• Have cheese with crackers, on pizza, or in tacos.

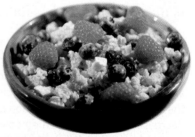

Use iProfile to calculate the calcium content of your favorite fast-food meal.

440

Make healthier fast-food choices   Table 12.2

Instead of . . .	Choose . . .
Double-patty hamburger with cheese, mayonnaise, special sauce, and bacon	Regular single-patty hamburger without mayonnaise, special sauce, and bacon
Breaded and fried chicken sandwich	Grilled chicken sandwich
Chicken nuggets or tenders	Grilled chicken strips
Large french fries	Baked potato, side salad, or small order of fries
Fried chicken wings	Broiled skinless wings
Crispy-shell chicken taco with extra cheese and sour cream	Grilled-chicken soft taco without sour cream
Nachos with cheese sauce	Tortilla chips with bean dip
12-in. meatball sub	6-in. turkey breast sub with lots of vegetables
Thick-crust pizza with extra cheese and meat toppings	Thin-crust pizza with extra veggies
Donut	Cinnamon and raisin bagel with low-fat cream cheese

Making fast food fit There is nothing wrong with an occasional fast-food meal, but a steady diet of burgers, fries, and tacos will likely contribute to an overall unhealthy diet. Fast food is typically high in fat and sodium and low in fruits and vegetables.[34] Most teens in the United States consume more than the recommended amounts of fat and sodium and fewer fruits and vegetables than recommended. The lettuce and tomatoes that garnish a burger or taco are not enough to meet the MyPlate recommendations for vegetables. French fries, which are high in fat and salt, are the most frequently consumed vegetable. To fit fast food into a healthy diet, make more nutrient-dense fast-food choices and make sure other meals and snacks eaten throughout the day supply the nutrients that are not obtained from fast food. Many fast-food franchises now offer fruit, salads, yogurt, and milk. And some of the old standbys are not bad choices. A plain, single-patty hamburger provides a lot less fat and energy than one with two patties and a high-fat sauce. A chicken sandwich can be a healthy choice if it is grilled or barbecued, not breaded and fried (**Table 12.2**).

Keeping vegetarian choices healthy It is not uncommon for a teen to decide to consume a vegetarian diet even if the rest of the family does not. Some give up meat for health reasons or to lose weight, while others give up meat because they are concerned about animals and the environment. A vegetarian diet can be a healthy choice when it is carefully planned to meet nutrient needs, not just to eliminate meat. A poorly planned vegetarian diet will be no healthier than any other poorly planned diet. Adequate protein is generally not a problem, but meatless diets can be low in iron and zinc. Teenage vegans, who consume no animal products, may also be at risk for vitamin B_{12} deficiency and inadequate calcium and vitamin D intake. We generally think of vegetarian diets as being low in fat, but one that relies on high-fat dairy products can be high in total fat, saturated fat, and cholesterol (**Figure 12.11**).

Healthy vegetarian choices • Figure12.11

Cheese pizza and ice cream are high-saturated fat, high-cholesterol vegetarian choices. In contrast, whole-grain pita bread stuffed with chickpeas, corn, spinach, and tomatoes served with reduced-fat milk, is low in saturated fat and cholesterol, high in fiber, and a good source of calcium and iron.

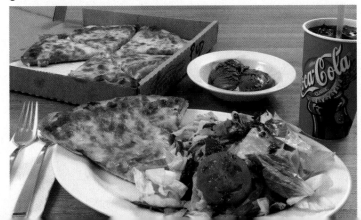
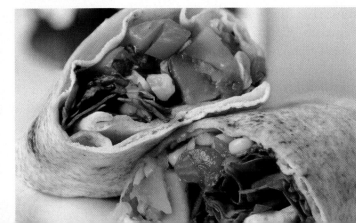

Special Concerns for Teens

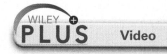

Peer pressure to fit in and concern about physical appearance probably have a greater impact on behavior during adolescence than at any other time in life. Many girls want to lose weight even if they are not overweight, and boys want to gain weight in order to achieve a strong, muscular appearance.

Eating disorders As discussed in Chapter 9, the excessive concern about weight, low self-esteem, and poor body image that are common during the teenage years contribute to the development of eating disorders. These disorders can be fatal, but even in less severe cases, the nutritional consequences of an eating disorder can affect growth and development during adolescence and have a lifelong impact on bone health.

The impact of athletics Participation in competitive sports may affect adolescent nutrient needs and eating patterns. Like adult athletes, teen athletes have increased nutrient needs; they require more water, energy, protein, carbohydrate, and micronutrients than do their less active peers. Individuals involved in sports, such as football, that require the athlete to be large and heavy usually do not have trouble eating enough to meet these additional needs, but they may compromise their health by experimenting with anabolic steroids or other ergogenic supplements in an effort to "bulk up." As discussed in Chapter 10, steroids can stunt growth in adolescence as well as lead to sexual and reproductive disorders, heart disease, liver damage, acne, and aggressive, violent behavior. Teens participating in gymnastics and wrestling may restrict their food intake in order to stay light and lean. Weight restriction at this stage of life may affect nutritional status and maturation and increase the risk of developing an eating disorder. In female athletes, the combination of hard training and weight restriction can lead to the *female athlete triad* (see Chapter 10).

Tobacco use Approximately 20% of high school students in the United States smoke cigarettes.[35] Smoking increases the risk of cardiovascular disease and lung cancer. Smoking can limit appetite, and many teens start smoking in order to control their weight and are afraid to quit because they fear that they will gain weight if they do.[36] Smoking may also impact on nutrient intake; a study of smokers found that they eat more saturated fat and fewer fruits and vegetables than do nonsmokers.[37] This dietary pattern increases the risk of developing heart disease and cancer.

Alcohol use Alcohol is a drug that has short-term effects that occur soon after ingestion and long-term health consequences that are associated with overuse. These effects are discussed in greater depth in the last section of the chapter.

Although it is illegal to sell alcohol to adolescents, alcoholic beverages are commonly available at teen social gatherings, and peer pressure to consume them is strong. Surveys of American youth suggest that approximately 8% of the nation's 8th graders, 24% of 10th graders, and 32% of 12th graders have been drunk during the last month. It is estimated that about 40% of college students "binge" on alcohol at least once during a two-week period.[38] **Binge drinking** involves consumption of five or more drinks in a row for men or four or more in a row for women in about two hours. It often leads to dangerous risk-taking behaviors and blood alcohol levels that are high enough to cause loss of consciousness, coma, and even death.

> **binge drinking**
> A pattern of drinking that brings a person's blood alcohol concentration to 0.08 gram percent (mg/100 mL) or above.

Consumption of alcohol with energy drinks is common among teens and is particularly dangerous. The stimulant effects of the caffeine in the energy drink counters the depressant effects of the alcohol, but judgment and motor function are still impaired. The person is drunk but does not feel drunk. As a result, he or she may drink to the point of alcohol toxicity or think it is safe to get behind the wheel of a car.

CONCEPT CHECK

1. **How** does puberty affect body composition in males and females?

2. **How** do the energy needs of teens compare with those of adults?

3. **What** factors contribute to low calcium intake in teens?

4. **What** could a teen choose at a fast-food restaurant to boost vegetable intake?

Nutrition for the Adult Years

LEARNING OBJECTIVES

1. **Distinguish** life expectancy from healthy life expectancy.

2. **Compare** the energy and nutrient requirements of older and younger adults.

3. **Discuss** how the physical, mental, and social changes of aging increase nutritional risks.

4. **Plan** a diet for a sedentary 80-year-old woman, based on MyPlate recommendations.

 he benefits of a healthy diet do not stop when you stop growing. Good nutrition throughout your adult years can keep you healthy and active into your 80s and beyond. In the United States, **life expectancy** is 77.9 years.[39] However, **healthy life expectancy** is only about 70 years.[40] This means that, on average, the last 8 years of life are restricted by disease and disability.

The goal of successful aging is to increase not only life expectancy but healthy life expectancy. Achieving this goal is particularly important because we live in a nation with an aging population (**Figure 12.12a**). Keeping older adults healthy will benefit not only the aging individuals themselves but also the family members who must find the time and resources to care for them and the public health programs that attempt to meet their needs. Although nutrition is not the key to immortality, a healthy diet can prevent malnutrition and delay the onset of chronic diseases that typically begin in middle age and reduce the quality of life in older adults (**Figure 12.12b**).

> **life expectancy**
> The average length of life for a particular population of individuals.

The number of older adults is rising • Figure 12.12

a. About 12% of the U.S. population is 65 years of age or over; by 2030 this percentage is expected to reach 20%.[41] The **oldest old** (≥ 85 years), one of the fastest-growing age groups, have more activity limitations and chronic conditions and require more public health dollars and services than do younger adults.[42]

b. Chronological age is not always the best indicator of a person's health. A person who is 75 may have the vigor and health of someone who is 55, or vice versa. Some older adults are healthy, independent, and active, while others are chronically ill, dependent, and at high risk for malnutrition.

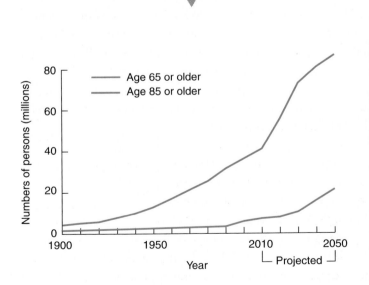

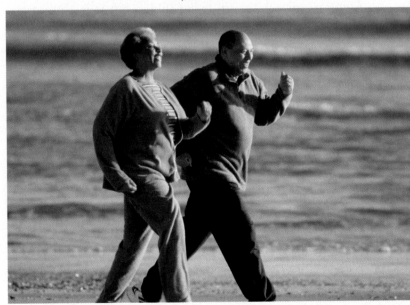

The Issue: Even before Ponce De Leon searched for the fountain of youth in what is now Florida, humans longed for a way to preserve youth. So far, though, the only dietary intervention that has been shown to slow aging and extend life is cutting calorie intake. Is calorie restriction a good way for people to slow aging and extend their lives?

Most of us eat too much. Eating too many calories and too much salt, saturated fat, and sugar shortens life expectancy by increasing the incidence of obesity, high blood pressure, diabetes, heart disease, and cancer. Eliminating dietary excesses can help us live healthier lives, but many argue that eating even less than what is currently recommended will help us live longer and healthier lives.

It has been known since the 1930s that, for many animals, consuming a calorie-restricted diet (20 to 40% less than recommended intake) that meets the need for all essential nutrients will slow aging and increase longevity.[56] There is good evidence that short-lived species such as insects, worms, mice, and other rodents that are fed a calorie-restricted diet live longer—as much as 50% longer—than animals that eat more calories.[57] The calorie-restricted animals have a lower incidence of age-related chronic diseases, better immune function, lower blood glucose, and better overall organ function than do animals whose diets are not calorie restricted.

There is less evidence for the effectiveness of calorie restriction in long-lived animals and humans. One study in rhesus monkeys, begun nearly 25 years ago, suggests that calorie restriction does extend lifespan; the animals have lower body fat and less muscle loss, as well as a lower incidence of cancer, heart disease, and type 2 diabetes.[57] Short-term studies in humans have shown that calorie restriction causes a reduction in body weight, blood pressure, blood cholesterol, blood glucose, and indices of

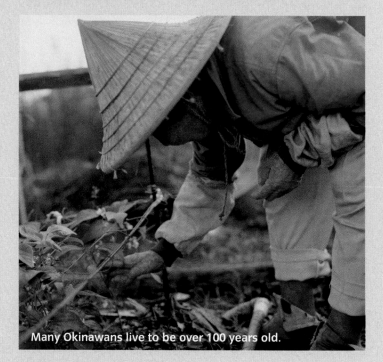

Many Okinawans live to be over 100 years old.

What Is Aging?

Aging is universal to all living things, but it is a process that we still don't fully understand (see *Debate: Can Eating Less Help You Live Longer?*). We know that as organisms grow older, the number of cells in their bodies decreases and the functioning of the remaining cells declines. This loss of cells and cell function occurs throughout life, but the effects are not felt for many years because organisms start out life with more cells and cell function than they need. This reserve capacity allows an organism to continue functioning normally despite a decrease in the number and function of cells. In young adults, the reserve capacity of organs is 4 to 10 times that required to sustain life. As a person ages and reserve

> **aging** The inevitable accumulation of changes associated with and responsible for an ever-increasing susceptibility to disease and death.

capacity decreases, the effects of aging become evident in all body systems. With this loss of function comes a reduction in the ability to repair damage and resist infection, so older people may die from diseases from which they could easily have recovered when they were younger.

The human **life span** is about 120 years, but how long individuals live and the rate at which they age are determined by the genes they inherit, their lifestyle, and the extent to which they are able to avoid accidents, disease, and environmental toxins (**Figure 12.13**). A person with a family history of heart disease who eats a healthy diet and exercises regularly may never be limited by heart disease. In contrast, someone with no family history of heart disease who is inactive, smokes, and eats a poor diet may develop heart problems that lead to disability and death.

> **life span** The maximum age to which members of a species can live.

oxidative stress.[58,59] Long-term evidence of the benefits of calorie restriction comes from epidemiologic studies. The people of Okinawa, a series of islands lying between mainland Japan and Taiwan, enjoy not only the longest life expectancy in the world (81.2 years) but also the longest healthy life expectancy.[60] Traditionally, Okinawans practice calorie restriction by eating until they are only 80% full. In addition, most lead active lives, working as farmers, and consume a nutrient-dense diet that is high in vegetables and fish and low in meat, refined grains, saturated fat, salt, and sugar.[61] They maintain a low BMI and have a lower incidence of chronic diseases than people living in the United States or on mainland Japan (see graph).[61]

The major drawback of calorie restriction is that it is not easy. Calorie restriction would mean a person who eats about 2000 Calories per day could eat only 1200 to 1500 Calories per day. This would cause food cravings, weight loss, a lack of energy, and in some cases psychological consequences. To eat this little while meeting nutrient needs requires carefully planned meals and snacks; a poorly planned diet will lead to malnutrition.

So, is calorie restriction something that we should all practice in order to live longer? In a world in which obesity, diabetes, and other diet-related conditions are limiting our healthy lifetimes, the concept of calorie restriction is intriguing. But it would be challenging to maintain this ascetic lifestyle and meet nutrient needs—far more difficult than drinking from the mythical fountain of youth. The Okinawans consume 40% fewer calories than Americans, yet they live only a few years longer.[59] Would it be worth the sacrifices?

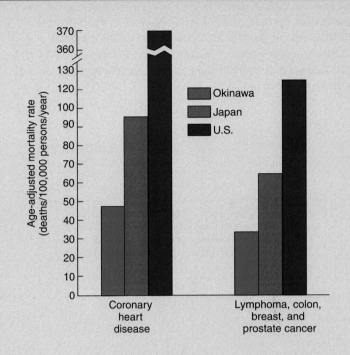

Think critically: Use the graph to compare the incidence of heart disease in Okinawa with that in Japan and the United States. Suggest some possible explanations for these differences.

Factors that affect how fast we age • Figure 12.13

Genes determine the efficiency with which cells are maintained and repaired and also determine our susceptibility to age-related diseases, such as cardiovascular disease and cancer, but lifestyle and environment also affect how fast we age.

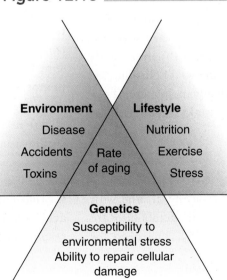

Some of the decline in energy needs in older adults is due to a decrease in muscle mass;[43] the less lean muscle a person has, the lower his or her BMR. The EER for an 80-year-old man is almost 600 Calories less than for a 20-year-old man of the same size and activity level. For women, the difference in EER between an 80- and a 20-year-old of the same height, weight, and physical activity level is about 400 Calories/day.

Think Critically How much daily exercise would an 80-year-old woman need in order to expend about the same number of Calories per day as a sedentary 20-year-old woman of the same height and weight?

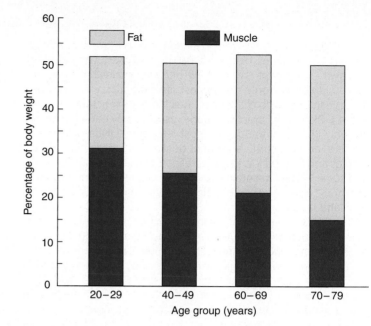

Nutrition and Health Concerns Throughout Adulthood

The physiological and health changes that accompany aging affect energy and nutrient requirements, how some nutrient requirements must be met, and the risk of malnutrition. In order to best recommend nutrient intakes for adults of all ages, the DRIs include four adult age categories: young adulthood (ages 19–30), middle age (ages 31–50), adulthood (ages 51–70), and older adulthood (over age 70). These recommendations are designed to meet the needs of the majority of healthy individuals in each age group. Although the incidence of chronic diseases and disabilities increases with advancing age, these increases are not considered when making general nutrient intake recommendations.

Energy and energy-yielding nutrient recommendations
Adult energy needs typically decline with age, due primarily to decreases in Basal Metabolic Rate (BMR) and activity level (**Figure 12.14**). The need for most nutrients does not change, however, so in order to meet nutrient needs without exceeding energy needs, older adults must consume a nutrient-dense diet. For example, adult protein requirements do not change with age; therefore, older adults must consume a diet that is higher in protein relative to calories than that of younger adults.

The proportions of carbohydrate and fat recommended in the diet also remain the same in older adults as in younger adults. In order to ensure adequate vitamin, mineral, and fiber intake, most dietary carbohydrate should come from unrefined sources. Adequate fiber, when consumed with adequate fluid, helps prevent constipation, hemorrhoids, and diverticulosis—conditions that are common in older adults. High-fiber diets may also be beneficial in the prevention and management of diabetes, cardiovascular disease, and obesity.

Sources of dietary fat should also be chosen with nutrient density in mind. A diet with 20 to 35% of energy from fat that contains adequate amounts of the essential fatty acids and limits saturated fat, *trans* fat, and cholesterol is recommended.

Meeting the water needs of older adults The recommended water intake for older adults is the same as for younger adults, but meeting these needs may be more challenging for older adults. Advanced age brings a reduction in the sense of thirst, which can decrease fluid intake. In addition, older adults are likely to have mobility limitations that reduce their access to beverages. The risk of dehydration is further increased in older adults by greater water losses. The kidneys are no longer as efficient at conserving water as they once were, and many older adults also take medications that increase water loss.

The risk of vitamin and mineral deficiencies in older adults The physiological changes of aging and the decrease in calorie needs put older adults at risk for deficiency of several vitamins and minerals. Recommended intakes are rarely higher than for younger adults, but for a few nutrients, special recommendations are made about how needs should be met.

Intakes of certain B vitamins are a concern for older adults. The RDA for vitamin B_6 is greater in adults ages 51 and older than for younger adults because higher dietary intakes are needed to maintain the same functional levels in the body. Folate intake is a concern because deficiency of folate alone or in combination with vitamin B_{12} and B_6 deficiencies may contribute to the development of cancer, cardiovascular disease, and cognitive dysfunction.

The RDA for vitamin B_{12} is not increased in older adults, but it is recommended that people over 50 meet their RDA for vitamin B_{12} by consuming foods that are fortified with this vitamin or by taking a supplement containing vitamin B_{12}. This is because food-bound vitamin B_{12} is not absorbed efficiently in many older adults due to atrophic gastritis, an inflammation of the stomach lining that causes a reduction in stomach acid (see Chapter 7).[44,45] Reduced secretion of stomach acid also allows microbial overgrowth in the stomach and small intestine, and the greater number of microbes compete for available vitamin B_{12}, further reducing vitamin B_{12} absorption. It is estimated that 10 to 30% of U.S. adults over age 50 and 40% of those in their 80s have atrophic gastritis. The vitamin B_{12} in fortified foods and supplements is not bound to proteins, so it is absorbed even when stomach acid levels are low. Atrophic gastritis may also reduce the absorption of iron, folate, calcium, and vitamin K.

Women over age 50 need less iron than younger women because they no longer lose iron through menstruation. The RDA for women 51 and older is 8 mg, the same as for adult men of all ages. Despite low iron needs, iron deficiency anemia is a concern among women and men in this age group. Common causes are chronic blood loss due to disease and medication and poor iron absorption due to antacid use and low stomach acid.

Calcium status is a problem in elderly people because calcium intake is low and intestinal absorption decreases with age. Without sufficient calcium, bone mass decreases, and the risk of bone fractures due to osteoporosis increases. The reduction in estrogen that occurs with menopause further increases bone loss in women by increasing the rate of bone breakdown and decreasing the absorption of calcium from the intestine. The RDA for adult men 51 years and older is 1000 mg/day. Because of the accelerated bone loss in women during the postmenopausal period, the RDA for women 51 years and older is increased to 1200 mg/day. To reduce age-related bone loss, the RDA for men over 70 years of age is 1200 mg/day.[4]

Vitamin D, which is necessary for adequate calcium absorption, is also a concern in elderly people. Intake is often low, and synthesis in the skin is reduced due to limited exposure to sunlight and because the capacity to synthesize vitamin D in the skin decreases with age. The RDA for people ages 51 to 70 years is 600 IU (15 μg)/day, the same as for younger adults. For individuals over age 70 years, the RDA is increased to 800 IU (20 μg)/day.[4]

Factors That Increase the Risk of Malnutrition in Older Adults

The aging process usually does not cause malnutrition in healthy, active adults, but nutritional health can be compromised by the physical changes that occur with age, the presence of disease, and economic, psychological, and social circumstances.[46] These factors can increase the risk of malnutrition by altering nutrient needs and decreasing the motivation to eat and the ability to acquire and enjoy food. Malnutrition then exacerbates some of these factors, contributing to a downward health spiral from which it is difficult to recover (**Figure 12.15a** on next page).

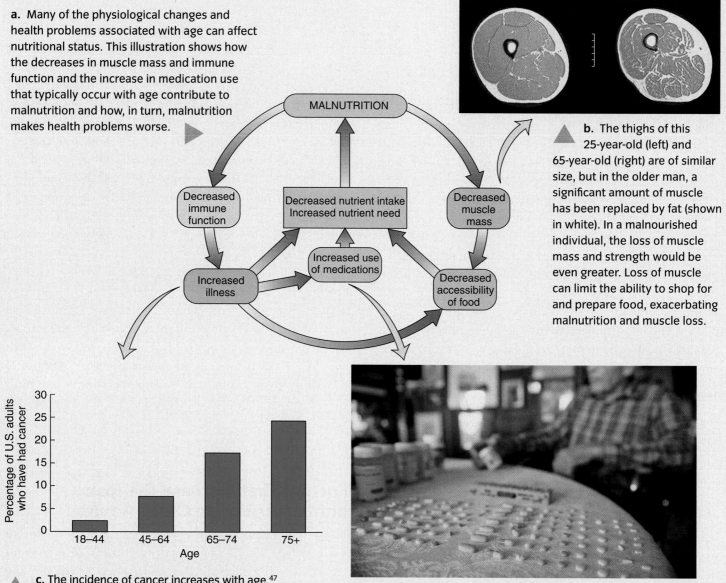

a. Many of the physiological changes and health problems associated with age can affect nutritional status. This illustration shows how the decreases in muscle mass and immune function and the increase in medication use that typically occur with age contribute to malnutrition and how, in turn, malnutrition makes health problems worse. ▶

MALNUTRITION

Decreased immune function

Increased illness

Decreased nutrient intake
Increased nutrient need

Increased use of medications

Decreased muscle mass

Decreased accessibility of food

b. The thighs of this 25-year-old (left) and 65-year-old (right) are of similar size, but in the older man, a significant amount of muscle has been replaced by fat (shown in white). In a malnourished individual, the loss of muscle mass and strength would be even greater. Loss of muscle can limit the ability to shop for and prepare food, exacerbating malnutrition and muscle loss.

c. The incidence of cancer increases with age.[47] One reason for the higher incidence is that the immune system's ability to destroy cancer cells declines. Reduced immune function also increases the frequency of infectious diseases and reduces the ability to recover from these diseases.

d. It is common for older adults to take multiple medications. Shown here are the pills this 73-year-old man takes each week. Medications can affect nutritional status by interfering with taste, chewing, and swallowing; by causing loss of appetite, gastrointestinal upset, constipation, or nausea; and by increasing nutrient losses or decreasing nutrient absorption.

Physiological changes With age comes a decline in muscle size and strength (**Figure 12.15b**). This decline affects both the skeletal muscles needed to move the body and the heart and respiratory muscles needed to deliver oxygen to the tissues. Some of this change is due to changes in hormone levels and muscle protein synthesis, but lack of exercise is also an important contributor.[48] The changes in muscle strength contribute not only to **physical frailty**, which is characterized by general weakness, impaired mobility and balance, and poor endurance, but also to the risk of falls and fractures. In the oldest old, those age 85 years and older, loss of muscle strength is the limiting factor that determines whether they can continue to live independently.

The immune system's ability to fight disease declines with age. With this decline, the incidence of infections, cancers, and autoimmune diseases increases, and the effectiveness of immunizations declines (**Figure 12.15c**). In turn, increases in infections and chronic disease can lead to increased use of medications that affect nutritional status (**Figure 12.15d**). Malnutrition exacerbates the decrease in immune function.[49]

Acute and chronic illness More than 75% of the older population suffers from some form of illness or disability, and the incidence increases with advancing age.[50] These conditions affect the ability to maintain good nutritional health because they can change nutrient requirements, decrease the appeal of food, and impair the ability to obtain and prepare an adequate diet.

Some illnesses change the type of diet that is recommended. For instance, kidney failure reduces the ability to excrete protein waste products, so the diet must be lower in protein. Blood pressure is affected by sodium intake, so a low-sodium diet is recommended for individuals with high blood pressure. Dietary restrictions such as these limit food choices and can affect the palatability of the diet and thereby contribute to malnutrition in elderly people.

Physical disabilities can limit a person's ability to obtain and prepare food. The most common reason for physical disability among older adults is **arthritis**, a condition that causes pain in joints when they are moved (**Figure 12.16**). Arthritis affects more than 45 million Americans.[51] Half of all individuals age 70 and older with arthritis need help with the activities of daily living, including preparing and eating meals.[3]

> **arthritis** A disease characterized by inflammation of the joints, pain, and sometimes changes in structure.

Osteoarthritis • Figure 12.16

Osteoarthritis, the most common form of arthritis, occurs when the cartilage that cushions the joints degenerates, allowing the bones to rub together and cause pain. Anti-inflammatory medications help reduce the pain. Supplements of glucosamine and chondroitin are marketed to improve symptoms and slow the progression of osteoarthritis, but clinical studies have not found the effect of these supplements on pain and function to be significant.[52]

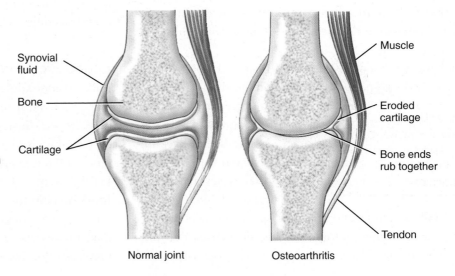

Normal joint   Osteoarthritis

Cataracts • Figure 12.17

A cataract is a clouding of the lens of the eye that impairs vision. When cataracts obscure vision, the affected lens can be removed and replaced with an artificial plastic lens.

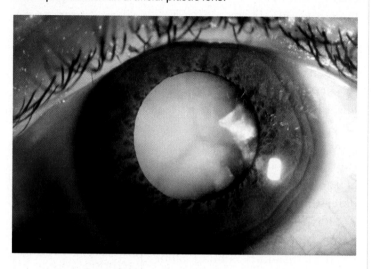

Visual disorders become more common as a person ages. **Macular degeneration** is the most common cause of blindness in older Americans.

macular degeneration Degeneration of a portion of the retina that results in loss of visual detail and eventually blindness.

The **macula** is a small area of the retina of the eye that distinguishes fine detail. If the number of viable cells in the macula is reduced, visual acuity declines, ultimately resulting in blindness. **Cataracts** are another common cause of declining vision (**Figure 12.17**). Oxidative damage is believed to cause both macular degeneration and cataracts. Therefore, a diet that is high in foods containing antioxidant nutrients and phytochemicals might slow or prevent these eye disorders.

Changes in mental status can affect nutrition by interfering with the response to hunger and the ability to eat and

dementia A deterioration of mental state that results in impaired memory, thinking, and/or judgment.

to obtain and prepare food. The incidence of **dementia** increases with age. Dementia involves impairment in memory, thinking, or judgment that is severe enough to cause personality changes and affect daily activities and relationships with others. Causes of dementia include multiple strokes, alcoholism, dehydration, side effects of medication, vitamin B$_{12}$ deficiency, and

Alzheimer's disease. Regardless of the cause, these neurological problems can affect the ability to consume a healthy diet.

Alzheimer's disease A disease that results in a relentless and irreversible loss of mental function.

Another cause of altered mental status in elderly people is depression. Social, psychological, and physical factors all contribute to depression in elderly people. Retirement and the death and relocation of friends and family members can cause social isolation, which contributes to depression. Physical disability causes loss of independence. The inability to engage in normal daily activities, easily visit with friends and family members, and provide for personal needs contributes to depression. Depression can make meals less appetizing and decrease the quantity and quality of foods consumed, thereby increasing the risk of malnutrition.

Use of medications Because elderly people have an increased frequency of acute and chronic illnesses, they are likely to take multiple medications (see Figure 12.15d).[53] Medications can affect nutritional status, and nutritional status can alter the effectiveness of medications. The more medications taken, the greater the chance of side effects that affect nutritional status, such as decreased appetite, changes in taste, and nausea. Diet can also change the effectiveness of medications. For example, vitamin K hinders the action of anticoagulants, which are taken to reduce the risk of blood clots. On the other hand, omega-3 fatty acids, such as those in fish oils, inhibit blood clotting and may intensify the effect of an anticoagulant drug and cause bleeding.

Economic and social issues Approximately 3.4 million older adults live below the poverty level, and many live on a fixed income, making it difficult to afford health care, especially medications, and a healthy diet.[54] Food costs and limited food preparation facilities can reduce the types of foods available. In 2009, 7.5% of households in the United States that included elderly people experienced **food insecurity**,[55] which occurs when the availability of nutritionally adequate, safe food or the ability to acquire food in socially acceptable ways is limited. This in turn increases the risk of malnutrition.

Keeping Healthy Throughout the Adult Years

There is no secret dietary factor that will bestow immortality, but good nutrition and an active lifestyle are major determinants of successful aging. A well-planned, nutritionally adequate diet can extend an individual's years of healthy life by preventing malnutrition and delaying the onset of chronic diseases. Regular exercise can help maintain muscle mass, bone strength, and cardiorespiratory function, helping to prolong independent living. For those with economic, social, or physical limitations, food assistance programs or assisted living can help prevent food insecurity.

Identifying older adults at risk

To address concerns about the nutritional health of elderly individuals, the U.S. Nutrition Screening Initiative promotes screening for nutrition-related problems in older adults. This program is working to increase awareness of nutritional problems among elderly people by involving practitioners and community organizations as well as relatives, friends, and others caring for elderly people in evaluating the nutritional status of the aging population. This program developed the DETERMINE checklist (**Table 12.3**), based on an acronym for the physiological, medical, and socioeconomic situations that increase the risk of malnutrition among elderly people. Older people themselves, as well as family members and caregivers, can use this tool to determine when malnutrition is a potential problem.

Meeting nutrient needs Meeting the nutrient needs of older adults can be challenging (see *What Should I Eat?*). Because energy needs are reduced while most

DETERMINE: A checklist of the warning signs of malnutrition   Table 12.3

Disease	Any disease, illness, or condition that causes changes in eating can predispose a person to malnutrition. Memory loss and depression can also interfere with nutrition if they affect food intake.
Eating poorly	Eating either too little or too much can lead to poor health.
Tooth loss/ mouth pain	Poor health of the mouth, teeth, and gums interferes with the ability to eat.
Economic hardship	Having to, or choosing to, spend less than $25 to $30 per person per week on food interferes with nutrient intake.
Reduced social support	Not having contact with people on a daily basis has a negative effect on morale, well-being, and eating.
Multiple medicines	The more medicines a person takes, the greater the chances of side effects such as weakness, drowsiness, diarrhea, changes in taste and appetite, nausea, and constipation.
Involuntary weight loss or gain	Unintentionally losing or gaining weight is a warning sign that should not be ignored. Being overweight or underweight also increases the risk of malnutrition.
Needs assistance in self-care	Difficulty walking, shopping, and cooking increases the risk of malnutrition.
Elder above age 80	The risks of frailty and health problems increase with increasing age.

WHAT SHOULD I EAT?
Advancing Age

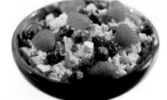

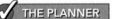
THE PLANNER

Consume plenty of fluids and fiber
- Drink a beverage with every meal.
- Keep a bottle of water handy and sip on it.
- Use whole-wheat bread.
- Bake bran muffins.

Pay attention to vitamin B$_{12}$, calcium, and vitamin D
- Make sure your cereal is fortified with vitamin B$_{12}$.
- Drink milk; it provides both calcium and vitamin D.
- Spend a few minutes in the sun to get some vitamin D with no calories at all.
- Add some canned salmon to a salad for lunch.

Antioxidize
- Have a bowl of strawberries or blueberries.
- Choose colorful vegetables to boost carotenoids.
- Use vegetable oils in cooking to supply vitamin E.
- Eat some nuts, but not too many—they are high in calories.

Work on meals for one
- Ask the grocer to break up larger packages of eggs and meats.
- Buy in bulk and share with a friend.
- Make a whole pot but freeze it in meal-size portions.
- Top a baked potato with leftover vegetables or sauces.

Use iProfile to find foods that are fortified with vitamin B$_{12}$.

micronutrient needs remain the same or increase, food choices must be nutrient dense. In addition, the medical, social, and economic challenges that often accompany aging make it more difficult to meet these needs. Many older adults need supplements of vitamin D, vitamin B_{12}, and calcium to meet their nutrient needs. However, supplements should not take the place of a balanced, nutrient-dense diet that is high in whole grains, fruits, and vegetables (**Figure 12.18**). In addition to essential nutrients, these foods contain phytochemicals and other substances that may protect against disease.

Older adults who have physical limitations need to choose foods that they can easily prepare and consume. For those who have difficulty preparing foods, precooked foods, frozen dinners, and canned soup or dry soup mixes can provide a meal with almost no preparation. Medical nutritional products, such as Ensure or Boost, can also be used to supplement intake.

Physical activity for older adults Regular physical activity can extend years of active, independent life, reduce the risk of disability, and improve the quality of life for older adults. Exercise also allows an increase in food intake without weight gain, so micronutrient needs are met more easily. A physical activity program for older adults should improve endurance, strength, flexibility, and balance.[62] Endurance activities such as walking, biking, and swimming provide protection against chronic disease. Recommendations are the same as for younger adults: a minimum of 150 minutes per week of moderate-intensity aerobic exercise (**Figure 12.19**). Muscle-strengthening exercise is recommended 2 or more days per week to increase strength and lean body mass. Lifting small weights or stretching elastic bands at an intensity that requires some physical effort can provide strength training. Flexibility makes the tasks of everyday life easier. Flexibility exercises should include those that move the muscles through a full range of motion, such as arm circles, as well as those that stretch muscles their full length. Improvements in strength, endurance, and flexibility all enhance balance, which reduces the risk of falls. Specific balance exercises such as backward walking, heel walking, and those practiced in tai chi and yoga can further improve balance.

MyPlate for older adults • Figure 12.18

The MyPlate recommendations shown here are for sedentary 50- and 70-year-old men and women. The MyPlate plan for sedentary 70-year-old women allows only 120 empty Calories/day. To meet this allowance, food choices must be nutrient dense. High-fiber foods are important because fiber is often low in the diets of older adults. Sufficient beverage consumption is important to ensure that water needs are met.

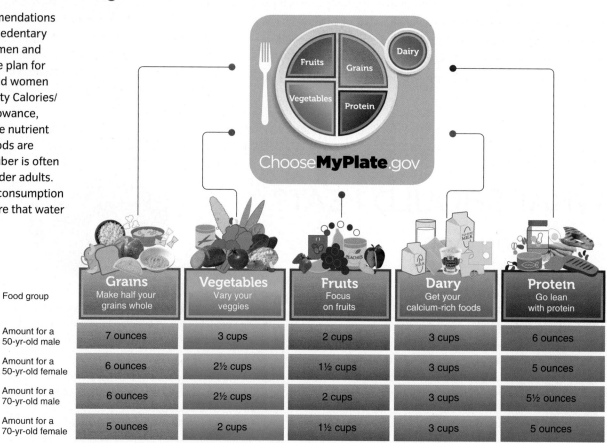

Food group	Grains Make half your grains whole	Vegetables Vary your veggies	Fruits Focus on fruits	Dairy Get your calcium-rich foods	Protein Go lean with protein
Amount for a 50-yr-old male	7 ounces	3 cups	2 cups	3 cups	6 ounces
Amount for a 50-yr-old female	6 ounces	2½ cups	1½ cups	3 cups	5 ounces
Amount for a 70-yr-old male	6 ounces	2½ cups	2 cups	3 cups	5½ ounces
Amount for a 70-yr-old female	5 ounces	2 cups	1½ cups	3 cups	5 ounces

Physical activity for older adults
• Figure 12.19

Exercise classes and other group-based activities can be a good way for older adults to start an exercise program. Water activities, such as water aerobics, and swimming, do not stress the joints and hence can be used to improve endurance in individuals with arthritis or other bone and joint disorders. Some weight-bearing exercise, such as walking, is encouraged to promote bone health.

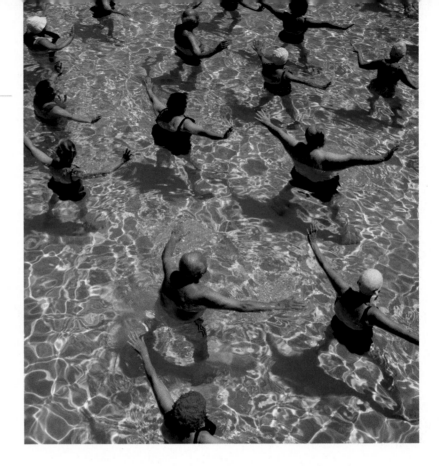

Overcoming economic and social issues

Overcoming economic limitations may involve providing education about economics and food preparation or providing assistance with shopping and food preparation. Options for people with limited incomes include reduced-cost meals at senior centers, federal food assistance programs (discussed in Chapter 14), food banks, and soup kitchens.

Another problem that contributes to poor nutrient intake in older adults is loneliness. Living, cooking, and eating alone can decrease interest in food. Programs that provide nutritious meals in communal settings promote social interaction and can improve nutrient intake. For those who are unable to attend communal meals, home-delivered meals are available. Studies have shown that compared to others, individuals who receive these meals have better-quality diets.[63]

Overcoming physical limitations: Assisted living

The physical and psychological declines associated with aging eventually cause many people to require assistance in everyday living. Assisted living facilities allow individuals to live in their own apartments but provide help, as needed, with activities such as eating, bathing, dressing, housekeeping, and taking medications.

These facilities provide an interim level of care for those who cannot live safely on their own but do not require the total care provided in a nursing home. Eventually, many older adults will need to live in nursing homes. Even though nursing homes provide access to food and medical care, their residents are at increased risk for malnutrition because they are more likely to have medical conditions that increase nutrient needs or interfere with food intake or nutrient absorption; in addition, they are at risk because they are dependent on others to provide for their care. Even when adequate meals are provided, many nursing home residents require assistance in eating and frequently do not consume all the food served, thus increasing their likelihood of developing deficits of energy, water, and other nutrients.[64]

CONCEPT CHECK STOP

1. **What** is the goal of successful aging?
2. **How** do the energy needs of older adults compare to those of younger adults?
3. **Why** are older adults at risk for malnutrition?
4. **How** do the MyPlate recommendations change as adults age?

The Impact of Alcohol Throughout Life

LEARNING OBJECTIVES

1. **Define** moderate alcohol consumption.
2. **Explain** how alcohol is absorbed and metabolized.
3. **Describe** the short- and long-term problems of excess alcohol consumption.
4. **Discuss** the potential benefits of moderate alcohol consumption.

Since the dawn of civilization, almost every human culture has produced and consumed some type of alcoholic beverage. Depending on the times and the culture, alcohol use has been touted, casually accepted, denounced, and even outlawed.

Whether alcohol consumption represents a risk to health or provides some benefits depends on who is drinking and how much is consumed. When consumed by a pregnant woman, alcohol can cause birth defects in the developing child. When consumed during childhood and adolescence, when the brain is still developing and changing, alcohol can cause permanent reductions in learning and memory.[65]

When consumed in excess by anyone, alcohol has medical and social consequences that negatively affect drinkers and those around them. It can reduce nutrient intake and affect the storage, mobilization, activation, and metabolism of nutrients. Its breakdown produces toxic compounds that damage tissues, particularly the liver.

Moderate alcohol consumption by healthy adults, however, provides some health advantages. The Dietary Guidelines define moderate alcohol consumption as no more than one drink per day for women and two drinks per day for men (**Figure 12.20**).[8]

Alcoholic beverages • Figure 12.20

Alcoholic beverages consist primarily of water, ethanol, and carbohydrate, with few other nutrients. A drink, defined as about 5 oz of wine, 12 oz of beer, or 1.5 oz of distilled spirits, contains 12 to 14 g of alcohol. The alcohol provides about 90 Calories (7 Calories/g) and Carbohydrates provide the remaining calories in alcoholic beverages.

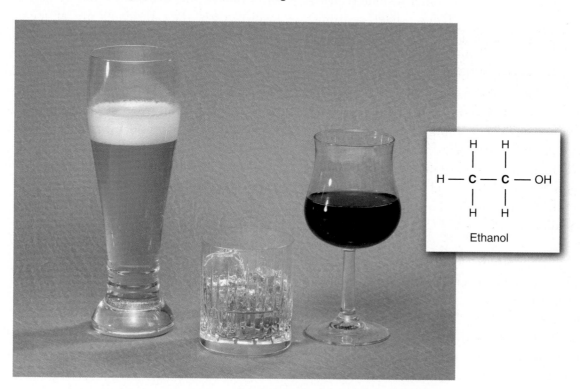

Blood alcohol levels • Figure 12.21

a. Blood alcohol levels are higher in women than in men after consuming the same amount of alcohol. This may be due to lower levels of the enzymes that break down alcohol or to the fact that women have less body water than men, so the alcohol they consume is distributed in a smaller amount of body water.

b. In the lungs, some alcohol diffuses out of the blood, into the air, and is exhaled. The amount of alcohol lost through the lungs is reliable enough to estimate blood alcohol level by using a Breathalyzer test.

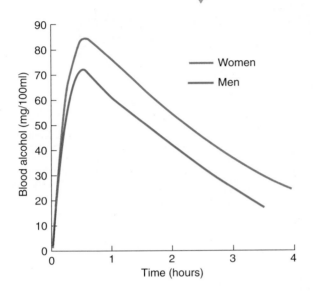

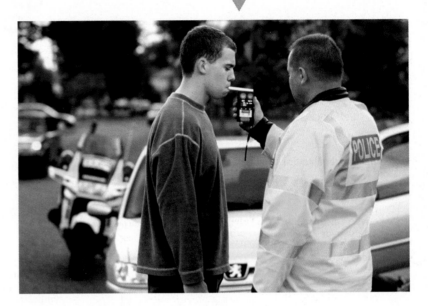

Alcohol Absorption, Transport, and Excretion

Chemically, any molecule that contains an —OH group is an **alcohol**, but we usually use the term to refer to **ethanol** and often to any beverage that contains ethanol (see

> **ethanol** The alcohol in alcoholic beverages; it is produced by yeast fermentation of sugar.

Figure 12.20). Ethanol is a small molecule that is rapidly and almost completely absorbed in the stomach and small intestine. Because some alcohol is absorbed directly from the stomach, its effects are almost immediate, especially when consumed on an empty stomach. If there is food in the stomach, absorption is slowed because food dilutes the alcohol and slows the rate of stomach emptying.

Once it has been absorbed, alcohol enters the bloodstream and is rapidly distributed throughout all body water. Peak blood alcohol concentrations are attained approximately one hour after ingestion. Many variables affect blood alcohol level, including the kind and quantity of alcoholic beverage consumed, the speed at which the beverage is consumed, the food consumed with it, the weight and gender of the consumer, and the activity of alcohol-metabolizing enzymes in the body (**Figure 12.21a**).

Because alcohol is a toxin and cannot be stored in the body, it must be eliminated quickly. Absorbed alcohol travels to the liver, where it is given metabolic priority and is therefore broken down before other molecules. About 90% of the alcohol is metabolized by the liver. The remainder is excreted through the urine or eliminated via the lungs during exhalation (**Figure 12.21b**). The alcohol that reaches the kidney acts as a diuretic, increasing fluid excretion. Therefore, excessive alcohol intake can contribute to dehydration.

Alcohol Metabolism • Figure 12.22

The ADH pathway predominates when small amounts of alcohol are consumed. The MEOS becomes important when larger amounts of alcohol are consumed. The MEOS reaction requires oxygen and the input of energy (ATP) to break down alcohol. It also generates reactive oxygen molecules that can contribute to liver disease.

HOW IT WORKS

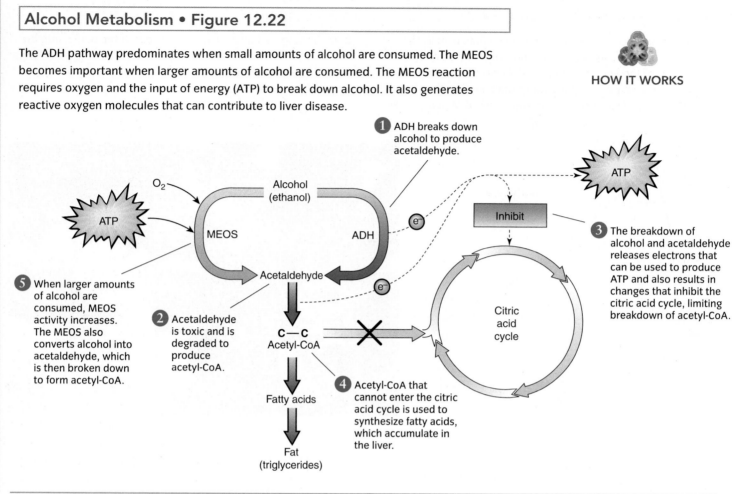

1 ADH breaks down alcohol to produce acetaldehyde.

3 The breakdown of alcohol and acetaldehyde releases electrons that can be used to produce ATP and also results in changes that inhibit the citric acid cycle, limiting breakdown of acetyl-CoA.

5 When larger amounts of alcohol are consumed, MEOS activity increases. The MEOS also converts alcohol into acetaldehyde, which is then broken down to form acetyl-CoA.

2 Acetaldehyde is toxic and is degraded to produce acetyl-CoA.

4 Acetyl-CoA that cannot enter the citric acid cycle is used to synthesize fatty acids, which accumulate in the liver.

Alcohol Metabolism

In people who occasionally consume moderate amounts of alcohol, most of the alcohol is broken down in the liver by the enzyme alcohol dehydrogenase (ADH) (**Figure 12.22**). This enzyme has also been found in all parts of the gastrointestinal tract.[66] When greater amounts of alcohol are consumed, a second pathway in the liver, called the microsomal ethanol-oxidizing system (MEOS), also metabolizes alcohol.[67] The rate at which ADH breaks down alcohol is fairly constant, but MEOS activity increases when more alcohol is consumed. MEOS also metabolizes other drugs, so as activity increases in response to high alcohol intake, it can alter the metabolism of other drugs.

Adverse Effects of Alcohol

The consumption of alcohol has short-term effects that interfere with organ function for several hours after ingestion. Chronic alcohol consumption has long-term effects that cause disease both because the alcohol interferes with nutritional status and because alcohol metabolism produces toxic compounds.

Short-term effects of alcohol When alcohol intake exceeds the liver's ability to break it down, the excess accumulates in the bloodstream. The circulating alcohol acts as a depressant, impairing mental and physical abilities. First, alcohol affects reasoning; if drinking continues, the brain's vision and speech centers are affected. Next, large-muscle control becomes impaired, causing lack of coordination. Finally, if alcohol consumption continues, it can result in **alcohol poisoning**, a serious condition that can slow breathing, heart rate, and the gag reflex, leading to loss of consciousness, choking, coma, and even death. This most frequently occurs in cases of *binge drinking*. Even if an individual does not experience a loss of consciousness, excess drinking may still cause memory loss. Drinking enough alcohol to cause amnesia is called **blackout drinking**. Blackout drinking puts people at risk because they have no memory of events that occurred during the blackout. During alcohol-related memory blackouts, people may engage in risky behaviors such as having unprotected sexual intercourse, vandalizing property, or driving a car—and have no memory of it afterward.

The effects of alcohol on the central nervous system are what make driving while under the influence of alcohol so dangerous. Alcohol affects reaction time, eye-hand coordination, accuracy, and balance. Not only does alcohol impair one's ability to operate a motor vehicle, but it also impairs one's judgment in making the decision to drive. Abuse of alcohol also contributes to domestic violence and is a factor in more than 100,000 deaths per year, including almost 40% of all traffic fatalities.[68]

Alcoholism One risk associated with regular alcohol consumption is the possibility of alcohol addiction, or **alcoholism**. The risk of alcoholism is increased in individuals who begin drinking at a younger age. Alcoholism, like any other drug addiction, is a physiological condition that needs treatment. It is believed to have a genetic component that makes some people more likely to become addicted, but environmental factors also play a significant role.[69] Thus, someone with a genetic predisposition toward alcoholism whose family and peers do not consume alcohol is much less likely to become addicted than someone with the same genes who drinks regularly with friends.

Alcoholic liver disease The most significant physiological effects of chronic alcohol consumption occur in the liver. The metabolism of alcohol by ADH promotes fat synthesis (see Figure 12.22), which leads to the accumulation of fat in the liver. Metabolism by the MEOS generates reactive oxygen molecules, which cause oxidation of lipids, membrane damage, and altered enzyme activities.

Whether alcohol is broken down by ADH or the MEOS, toxic acetaldehyde is formed. Acetaldehyde binds to proteins and inhibits chemical reactions and mitochondrial function, allowing more acetaldehyde to accumulate and causing further liver damage.

Chronic alcohol consumption leads to three types of alcoholic liver disease. **Fatty liver** is the accumulation of fat in liver cells. It occurs in almost all people who drink heavily due to increased synthesis and deposition of fat. If drinking continues, this condition may progress to **alcoholic hepatitis**. Both of these conditions are reversible if alcohol consumption is stopped and good nutritional and health practices are followed. If alcohol consumption continues, **cirrhosis** may develop (**Figure 12.23**).

> **alcoholic hepatitis** Inflammation of the liver caused by alcohol consumption.
>
> **cirrhosis** Chronic and irreversible liver disease characterized by loss of functioning liver cells and accumulation of fibrous connective tissue.

Malnutrition and other health problems Malnutrition is one of the complications of long-term excessive alcohol consumption. Alcohol contributes energy—7 Calories/g—but few nutrients; it may replace more nutrient-dense energy sources in the diet. Alcoholic beverages are also often consumed with high-sugar mixers, which add more empty calories to the diet. In addition to decreasing nutrient intake, alcohol interferes with nutrient absorption. Alcohol causes inflammation of the stomach, pancreas, and intestine, impairing digestion of food and absorption of nutrients into the blood. Deficiency of the B vitamin thiamin is a particular concern related to chronic alcohol consumption. Alcohol also contributes to malnutrition by altering the storage, metabolism, and excretion of other vitamins and some minerals.

Alcoholic cirrhosis • Figure 12.23

The liver on the left is normal. The one on the right has cirrhosis. This is an irreversible condition in which fibrous deposits scar the liver and interfere with its functioning. Because the liver is the primary site of many metabolic reactions, cirrhosis is often fatal.

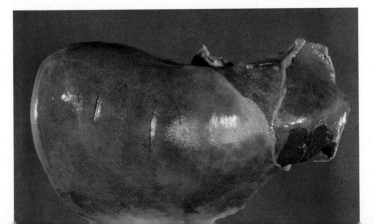
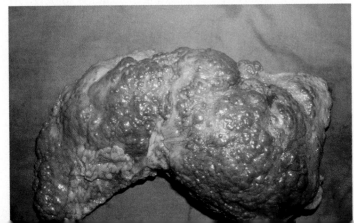

In addition to causing liver disease and malnutrition, heavy drinking is associated with cancer of the oral cavity, pharynx, esophagus, larynx, breast, liver, colon, rectum, and stomach.[70] Even moderate alcohol consumption has been found to increase the risk of certain cancers in women.[71] Alcohol use also increases the risk of hypertension, heart disease, and stroke.[72] Some of this effect is related to the fact that calories consumed as alcohol are more likely to be deposited as fat in the abdominal region, and excess abdominal fat increases the risk of high blood pressure, heart disease, and diabetes.

Benefits of Alcohol Consumption

For some adults, moderate alcohol consumption may be beneficial. Consuming alcoholic beverages can stimulate appetite, improve mood, and enhance social interactions. Light to moderate drinking can also reduce the risk of heart disease and stroke. The primary mechanisms by which alcohol lowers cardiovascular risk are by raising blood levels of HDL cholesterol and by inhibiting the formation of blood clots. The phytochemicals in red wine are thought to make it more cardioprotective than other alcoholic beverages.[73] Moderate alcohol consumption is associated with reduced risk of death among middle-aged and older adults and may help to keep cognitive function intact with age.[8]

Whether or not the benefits of alcohol consumption outweigh the risks, drinking is a personal decision that must take into account medical and social considerations. If you do not drink, you should not begin drinking to reduce cardiovascular risk or achieve other potential health benefits. Even moderate alcohol intake is associated with increased risk of breast cancer, violence, drowning, and injuries from falls and motor vehicle crashes. But anyone who chooses to drink should do so in moderation. Alcohol should be consumed slowly—at a rate of no more than one drink every 1.5 hours. Sipping, not gulping, allows the liver time to break down what has already been consumed. Alternating nonalcoholic and alcoholic drinks will also slow down the rate of alcohol intake and prevent dehydration. Alcohol absorption is most rapid on an empty stomach. Consuming alcohol with meals slows its absorption and may also enhance its protective effects on the cardiovascular system.

CONCEPT CHECK STOP

1. **How** much beer per day constitutes moderate drinking for a man?
2. **How** can alcohol metabolism lead to a fatty liver?
3. **What** are the symptoms of alcohol poisoning?
4. **How** does moderate alcohol intake reduce the risk of cardiovascular disease?

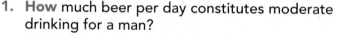

THE PLANNER ✓

Summary

1 Nutrition for Children 428

- A child's diet should meet the needs for growth, development, and activity as well as reduce the risk of chronic disease later in life. Energy and protein needs per kilogram of body weight decrease as children grow, but total needs increase. The acceptable range of fat intake is higher for young children than for adults. Calcium and iron intakes are often low in children's diets, putting them at risk for low bone density and anemia.

- To help children meet their nutrient needs and develop nutritious habits, caregivers should offer a variety of healthy foods at meals and snacks throughout the day. Children can then choose what and how much they consume. The **National School Lunch Program** provides low-cost school lunches designed to meet nutrient needs and promote healthy diets.

- The typical diet of U.S. children contributes to their rising obesity rates, as shown in the graph. Poor diet and obesity

increase the incidence of diabetes, high blood cholesterol, and high blood pressure. Watching television contributes to childhood obesity by promoting the intake of foods that are high in calories, fat, and sugar and by reducing the amount of exercise children get. A diet high in sugary foods can increase the risk of dental caries. Children are at particular risk for lead toxicity. Reductions in the use of lead in paint and gasoline have decreased the incidence of high blood lead levels.

Obesity and the health of America's children • Figure 12.6

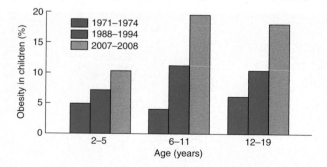

2 Nutrition for Adolescents 438

- During adolescence, the changes associated with **puberty** and the **adolescent growth spurt** have an impact on nutrient requirements. Body composition and the nutritional requirements of boys and girls diverge. Energy and protein requirements are higher in adolescence than in adulthood, and vitamin requirements increase to meet the needs of rapid growth. Calcium intake is often low in the adolescent diet, particularly if more sweetened beverages than milk are consumed, as shown. Iron deficiency anemia is common in adolescent girls due to low intake and iron losses through menstruation.

Beverage choices in children and teens • Figure 12.9

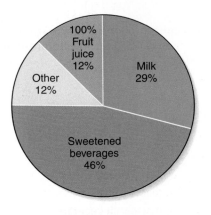

- The food choices of adolescents are usually determined more by social activities, peer pressure, and participation in athletics than by nutrient needs. Teens can improve their diets by making healthier fast-food choices. Poorly planned vegetarian diets can be low in iron, zinc, calcium, vitamin D, and vitamin B$_{12}$ and high in saturated fat and cholesterol.

- Psychological and social changes occurring during the adolescent years make eating disorders more common than at any other time of life. Adolescent nutritional status may also be affected by weight-loss diets, supplements to enhance athletic performance, and the use of cigarettes or alcohol.

3 Nutrition for the Adult Years 443

- As a population, Americans are living longer but not necessarily healthier lives. Increasing **healthy life expectancy** is an important public health goal. The genes people inherit, as well as their diet, lifestyle, and other environmental factors, determine how long they live.

- Energy needs decrease with age, but the needs for protein, water, fiber, and most micronutrients remain the same. Decreases in nutrient intake and absorption and changes in the metabolism or absorption of certain micronutrients, including vitamin B$_{12}$, vitamin D, and calcium, put older adults at risk for deficiency. Iron requirements decrease in women after menopause, but many older adults are at risk for iron deficiency due to poor absorption or blood loss from disease or medications.

- Older adults are at risk for malnutrition due to the physiological changes that accompany **aging**, such as the decline in muscle mass, illustrated here, and immune function. Acute and chronic illnesses, which are more common in elderly people than in younger people, may change nutrient requirements, decrease the appeal of food, and impair a person's ability to obtain and prepare an adequate diet. Medications to treat diseases may also affect nutritional status in older adults. Physical disabilities such as **arthritis** and **macular degeneration**, changes in mental status caused by **dementia** or depression, and social and economic factors increase the risk of **food insecurity**.

Causes and consequences of malnutrition • Figure 12.15b

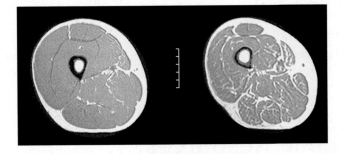

- A nutrient-dense diet and regular exercise can prevent malnutrition, delay the chronic diseases associated with aging, and increase independence in older adults. The DETERMINE checklist helps identify older adults who are at risk for malnutrition. Economic or physical assistance may be required to meet nutritional needs.

4 The Impact of Alcohol Throughout Life   454

- **Alcohol**, which refers to **ethanol**, is absorbed rapidly, causing the blood alcohol level to rise and its effects to be felt almost immediately. Absorption is slowed when there is food in the stomach. Alcohol is metabolized primarily in the liver. Some is excreted in urine and exhaled in expired air.

- Moderate amounts of alcohol are broken down by the enzyme alcohol dehydrogenase (ADH). When greater amounts of alcohol are consumed, a second pathway in the liver, called the microsomal ethanol-oxidizing system (MEOS), also metabolizes alcohol. Alcohol metabolism increases fat synthesis in the liver and generates reactive oxygen molecules that can contribute to liver disease.

- In the short term, excess alcohol consumption causes **alcohol poisoning**, which interferes with brain function. Chronic alcohol consumption can lead to **alcoholism** and can damage the liver, resulting in **fatty liver**, **alcoholic hepatitis**, and eventually **cirrhosis**, shown in the photo. Excess alcohol

consumption also increases the risks of malnutrition and of developing hypertension, heart disease, and stroke, as well as certain types of cancer.

Alcoholic cirrhosis • Figure 12.23

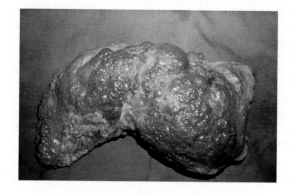

- Moderate alcohol consumption can decrease the risk of heart disease by increasing HDL cholesterol and reducing blood clot formation.

Key Terms

- adolescent growth spurt 438
- aging 444
- alcohol 445
- alcohol poisoning 456
- alcoholic hepatitis 457
- alcoholism 457
- Alzheimer's disease 450
- arthritis 449
- attention-deficit/hyperactivity disorder (ADHD) 437

- binge drinking 442
- blackout drinking 456
- cataracts 450
- cirrhosis 457
- dementia 450
- ethanol 455
- fatty liver 457
- food insecurity 450
- healthy life expectancy 443
- life expectancy 443

- life span 444
- macula 450
- macular degeneration 450
- National School Lunch Program 432
- oldest old 443
- physical frailty 449
- puberty 438

Online Resources

- For more information on weight control in children, go to the National Institute of Diabetes and Digestive and Kidney Disorders site, at www.niddk.nih.gov.

- For more information on food allergies, go to the Food Allergy & Anaphylaxis Network site, at www.foodallergy.org.

- For more information on alcoholism, go to the National Council on Alcoholism and Drug Dependence site, at www.ncadd.org.

- For more information on nutrition and aging go to the National Institute on Aging site, at www.nia.nih.gov/healthinformation/publications/healthyeating.htm.

- Visit your *WileyPLUS* site for videos, animations, podcasts, self-study, and other media that will aid you in studying and understanding this chapter.

Critical and Creative Thinking Questions

1. Use iProfile to look up the nutrient composition of your favorite fast-food meal. What is the percentage of calories from carbohydrate, protein, and fat in the meal? Compare the percentage of calories from carbohydrate, fat, and protein in the meal with the percentages recommended for a 10-year-old boy. Assuming that he exercises for 30 to 60 minutes a day, would he be able to eat this meal and still keep his day's intake within the recommended percentages? Why or why not?

2. Plot these height and weight measurements that were recorded for a girl from age 6 to age 9 on a growth chart and discuss any problems this pattern suggests.

Age	Height (in.)	Weight (lb)
6	45	44
7	48	53
8	50	77
9	52	97

3. Use MyPlate to design a day's menu for a 15-year-old boy who spends two hours a day playing soccer.

4. Use MyPlate to design a day's menu for a sedentary 80-year-old woman who must limit her sodium intake.

5. With age, there is a loss of smell and taste sensation. How might you design meals for a senior center to compensate for this?

6. Jared is 8 years old. He refuses to eat breakfast before leaving for school. What can Jared's parents do to ensure that he has a nutritious meal before school starts?

7. Angela is 55 years old and has a family history of heart disease. She eats a healthy diet that is high in whole grains, fruits, and vegetables, and she does not smoke or consume alcohol. She recently heard that moderate alcohol consumption can help reduce her risk of heart disease. Should she start consuming alcohol? Why or why not?

What is happening in this picture?

Riding your bike makes you thirsty. This boy in Virginia has interrupted his bike ride to purchase a soda.

Think Critically

1. What are the health messages in this photo?
2. What would be a better choice of beverage for quenching the boy's thirst?
3. What could the community do to improve the boy's beverage options?

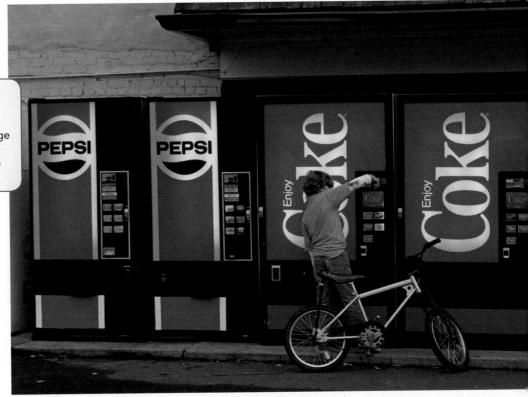

Self-Test

(Check your answers in Appendix K.)

1. Which of the following statements is supported by the graph?

   a. Fewer than 30% of children and teens consume a good diet.

   b. Diet quality gets better as children get older.

   c. The majority of children and teens consume a good diet.

   d. More teenagers ages 13 to 18 eat a good diet than eat a poor diet.

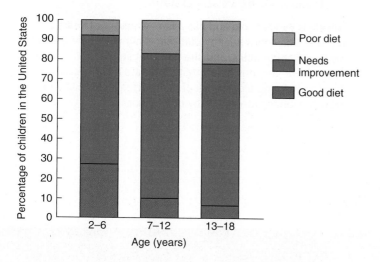

2. Which of the following is not recommended for treating childhood obesity?

   a. skipping breakfast

   b. cutting back on sugary beverages

   c. including 60 minutes or more of moderate-intensity exercise

   d. eating more fruits and vegetables

3. Television affects the nutritional status of children by _____.

   a. exposing them to new snack foods

   b. providing an environment that encourages snacking

   c. reducing the time spent engaged in physical activity

   d. all of the above

4. _____ are likely to be deficient in an adolescent's diet.

   a. Sodium and selenium

   b. Iodine and vitamin A

   c. Iron and calcium

   d. Protein and zinc

5. Which of the following statements about energy requirements is true?

   a. Total energy needs are higher in childhood than at any other time of life.

   b. Energy needs per kilogram of body weight increase as children grow.

   c. Energy needs are the same for adolescent boys and girls.

   d. Energy needs are lower in older adults than in younger adults.

6. The graph shows changes in body composition that occur from _____.

   a. infancy to childhood

   b. childhood to adolescence

   c. young adulthood to older adulthood

   d. moderate to excessive alcohol consumption

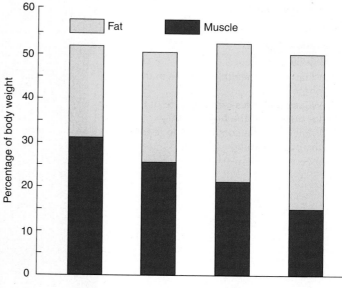

7. Which of the following statements about iron is false?

   a. Iron deficiency is a risk in children, adolescents, and older adults.

   b. The RDA for iron is higher in a 60-year-old women than in a 20-year-old woman.

   c. Iron needs increase in adolescent males due to increases in muscle mass.

   d. Iron needs increase in adolescent females due to menstrual blood losses.

8. Which of the following could contribute to low calcium status in children and teens?

   a. spending too little time outdoors

   b. replacing milk with soda

   c. being lactose intolerant

   d. eating a vegan diet

   e. all of the above

9. Which of the following statements about alcohol is true?

   a. Alcohol is absorbed faster on a full stomach than on an empty stomach.

   b. Alcohol consumption can contribute to malnutrition.

   c. Moderate alcohol consumption lowers HDL cholesterol levels.

   d. Alcohol consumption can reduce the risk of cancer.

10. Life expectancy refers to _____.

    a. the average age to which people in a population live

    b. how long an individual will live

    c. the longest any person can live

    d. how long an individual remains healthy

11. Which of the following statements about vitamin B_{12} is true?

    a. Absorption from food is reduced in individuals with atrophic gastritis.

    b. Older adults are not at risk for vitamin B_{12} deficiency.

    c. It is recommended that older adults meet vitamin B_{12} needs with whole foods.

    d. Vegan diets can easily supply enough vitamin B_{12} to meet needs.

12. For which of the following is the recommended intake lower in older adults than in younger adults?

    a. vitamin D

    b. protein

    c. calories

    d. calcium

13. The DETERMINE checklist is used to _____.

    a. qualify recipients for federal food assistance programs

    b. check for adverse reactions between food and prescription medications

    c. assess the risk of malnutrition in older adults

    d. decide whether an older adult needs assisted living

14. _____ is a type of alcoholic liver disease that results in irreversible scaring.

    a. Fatty liver

    b. Alcohol poisoning

    c. Cirrhosis

    d. Alcoholic hepatitis

15. Which of the following statements about the U.S. population does this graph illustrate?

    a. The number of people who are over age 65 is expected to more than double between 2010 and 2050.

    b. By 2050, 50% of the population will be over 85.

    c. The life expectancy of the population is expected to increase between 2010 and 2050.

    d. The average healthy life expectancy is expected to increase between 2010 and 2050.

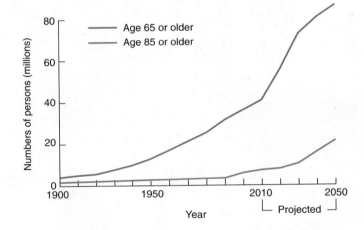

THE PLANNER ✓

Review your Chapter Planner on the chapter opener and check off you completed work.

How Safe Is Our Food Supply?

13

In the summer of 2010, one-half billion eggs distributed by a number of Iowa farms were recalled due to *Salmonella* bacteria contamination. The tainted eggs sickened 2000 people and were found in 14 states. The outbreak lasted from April to August and was probably caused by rodents, contaminated hens, or contaminated feed. Luckily, unlike in a number of other earlier contamination scares, no fatalities were associated with the tainted eggs.

Eggs are now included in the list of foods that have recently sickened or killed a number of Americans: *E. coli* bacteria in Nestlé Toll House cookie dough in 2009; *Salmonella*-tainted jalapeño peppers and peanuts in 2008; *Salmonella* in ground beef and Banquet pot pies in 2007; and *E. coli* in spinach in 2006. Even our water is sometimes threatened: In 2008, residents of a small Colorado town were forced to subsist on bottled and trucked-in water when *Salmonella* was found in the water supply.

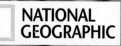

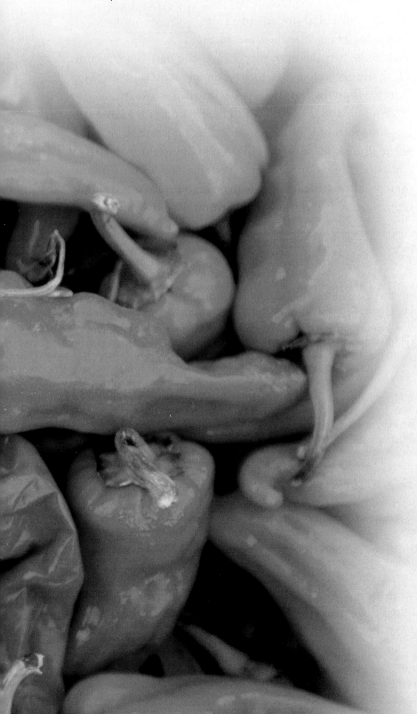

Despite these frightening incidents, most foods arrive in our homes safe and fit to eat, and they remain that way if we handle them properly. The modern U.S. food supply is perhaps the safest in human history, but danger still lurks if adequate food-handling practices are not in place from farm to table.

CHAPTER OUTLINE

CHAPTER PLANNER ✔

- ❑ Stimulate your interest by reading the introduction and looking at the visual.
- ❑ Scan the Learning Objectives in each section:
  p. 466 ❑   p. 470 ❑   p. 481 ❑   p. 489 ❑   p. 494 ❑
- ❑ Read the text and study all figures and visuals. Answer any questions.

Analyze key features

- ❑ Process Diagram, p. 467 ❑   p. 468 ❑   p. 473 ❑ p. 475 ❑   p. 494 ❑
- ❑ Nutrition InSight, p. 471 ❑   p. 478 ❑   p. 495 ❑
- ❑ Thinking it Through, p. 479 ❑
- ❑ What a Scientist Sees, p. 480 ❑
- ❑ Stop: Answer the Concept Checks before you go on: p. 469 ❑   p. 480 ❑   p. 486 ❑   p. 493 ❑   p. 497 ❑

End of chapter

- ❑ Review the Summary, Key Terms, and Online Resources.
- ❑ Answer the Critical and Creative Thinking Questions.
- ❑ Answer What is happening in this picture?
- ❑ Complete the Self-Test and check your answers.

Keeping Food Safe

LEARNING OBJECTIVES

1. **Name** the primary cause of food-borne illness.

2. **Explain** why a contaminated food does not cause illness in everyone who eats it.

3. **Discuss** the roles of the federal agencies responsible for the safety of the U.S. food supply.

4. **Explain** how a HACCP system helps prevent food-borne illness.

 ave you ever had food poisoning? Whether you know it or not, you probably have. Oftentimes what we call the 24-hour flu is actually food poisoning, also called **food-borne illness**. Most food-borne illness is caused by consuming food that has been contaminated by **microbes**; occasionally it is caused by toxic chemicals or other contaminants that find their way into food.

Whether or not you get sick from eating a contaminated food depends on how potent the contaminant is, how much of it you consume, and how often you consume it, as well as on your age, size, and health. Some food contaminants cause harm even when minute amounts are consumed, and almost any substance can be toxic if a large enough amount of it is consumed. How well a substance is absorbed and how it is metabolized by the body affect toxicity. Dietary factors and nutritional status can affect absorption. For example, mercury, which is extremely toxic, is not absorbed well if the diet is high in selenium, and lead absorption is decreased by the presence of iron and calcium in the diet. Contaminants that are stored in the body after being absorbed are more likely to be toxic because they accumulate over time, eventually causing symptoms of toxicity. Contaminants that are easily excreted from the body are less likely to cause toxicity.

An individual's size, overall health and nutritional status, and immune function affect his or her risk of food-borne illness. Infants and children are at greater risk than adults because their immune systems are immature and their small size means that a given amount of contaminant represents a greater amount per unit of body weight than

> **food-borne illness** An illness caused by consumption of contaminated food.
>
> **microbes** Microscopic organisms, or microorganisms, including bacteria, viruses, and fungi.

Agencies that monitor the food supply   Table 13.1

International Organizations

Food and Agriculture Organization of the United Nations (FAO)	Promotes and shares knowledge in all aspects of food quality and safety and in all stages of food production: harvest, post-harvest handling, storage, transport, processing, and distribution.
World Health Organization (WHO)	Develops international food safety policies, food inspection programs, and standards for hygienic food preparation; promotes technologies that improve food safety and consumer education about safe food practices. Works closely with the FAO.

Federal Organizations

U.S. Food and Drug Administration (FDA)	Ensures the safety and quality of all foods sold across state lines with the exception of red meat, poultry, and egg products; inspects food processing plants; inspects imported foods with the exception of red meat, poultry, and egg products; sets standards for food composition; oversees use of drugs and feed in food-producing animals; enforces regulations for food labeling, food and color additives, and food sanitation.
U.S. Department of Agriculture (USDA) Food Safety and Inspection Service (FSIS)	Enforces standards for the wholesomeness and quality of red meat, poultry, and egg products produced in the United States and imported from other countries. If an imported food is suspect, it can be tested for contamination and denied entry into the country.
U.S. Environmental Protection Agency (EPA)	Regulates pesticide levels and must approve all pesticides before they can be sold in the United States; establishes water quality standards.
National Marine Fisheries Service	Oversees the management of fisheries and fish harvesting; operates a voluntary program of inspection and grading of fish products.
National Oceanic and Atmospheric Administration (NOAA)	Oversees fish and seafood products. Its Seafood Inspection Program inspects and certifies fishing vessels, seafood processing plants, and retail facilities for compliance with federal sanitation standards.
Centers for Disease Control and Prevention (CDC)	Monitors and investigates the incidence and causes of food-borne illnesses.

State and Local Governments

Oversee all food within their jurisdiction; also inspect restaurants, grocery stores, and other retail food establishments, as well as dairy farms and milk processing plants, grain mills, and food manufacturing plants within local jurisdictions.	

it would in an adult. Elderly people, people with AIDS, and those receiving chemotherapy or other immunosuppressant drugs are at increased risk because their immune systems may be compromised. Pregnancy weakens the immune system, putting pregnant women and their unborn babies at risk. Poor nutritional status and chronic conditions such as diabetes and kidney disease may decrease the body's ability to detoxify harmful substances.

The Role of Government

Agencies at international, federal, state, and local levels monitor the safety of the food supply (**Table 13.1**). Federal agencies set standards and establish regulations for the safe handling of food and water and for the information included on food labels. They regulate the use of additives, packaging materials, and agricultural chemicals; inspect food processing and storage facilities; monitor domestic and imported foods for contamination; and investigate outbreaks of food-borne illness.

Each year, 1 in 6 Americans, or about 48 million people, get sick, 128,000 are hospitalized, and 3000 die from food-borne illnesses.[1] Media coverage of outbreaks of food-borne illness on cruise ships, of deaths from *E. coli* infection, and of cows infected with mad cow disease have heightened public concern and led to the development of the National Food Safety Initiative. The goal of this initiative is to reduce the incidence of food-borne illness by improving food safety practices and policies throughout the United States. Because food can be contaminated anywhere in the supply chain—from where it is grown to when it is served in your home—the program targets food safety from farm to table (**Figure 13.1**). In 2011, in response to

Keeping food safe from farm to table • Figure 13.1

✔ THE PLANNER

Keeping food safe involves identifying possible points of contamination along a food's journey from the farm to the dinner table and implementing controls to prevent or contain contamination.

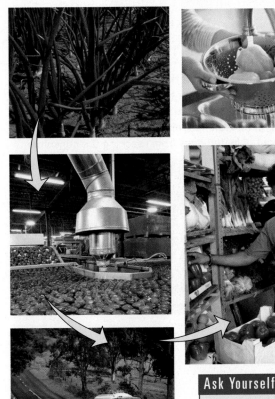
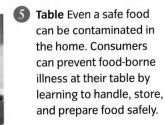

1 **Farm** Crops can be contaminated with bacteria before they are even harvested. Good agricultural practices help minimize contamination during growing, harvesting, sorting, packing, and storage.

2 **Processing** Contamination of processing equipment can transfer microbes to food. To prevent contamination, processors must follow guidelines concerning cleanliness and training of workers; develop a protocol that anticipates how biological, chemical, or physical hazards are most likely to occur; and establish appropriate measures to prevent them from occurring.

3 **Transportation** During transport, poor sanitation and inadequate refrigeration can contaminate food and allow microbes to grow. Clean containers and vehicles, plus refrigeration can prevent the growth of food-borne bacteria.

5 **Table** Even a safe food can be contaminated in the home. Consumers can prevent food-borne illness at their table by learning to handle, store, and prepare food safely.

4 **Retail** Food can become contaminated during handling or storage in grocery stores or during preparation in restaurants. The FDA's Food Code provides recommendations for the handling and service of food in an effort to help owners and employees at retail establishments prevent food-borne illness. Local health inspections ensure cleanliness and proper procedures.

Ask Yourself

Why does contamination that occurs during processing have the potential to make more people sick than contamination that occurs at home?

the continued threat from our food supply, the FDA Food Safety Modernization Act was passed. This legislation focuses on preventing food-borne illness, not just reacting to problems as they occur. It gives the FDA an inspection mandate and new legal powers to ensure that companies are doing their part and to stop potentially unsafe food from entering the marketplace.[2]

The Role of Food Manufacturers and Retailers

The responsibility for providing safe food to the marketplace falls on the shoulders of food manufacturers, processors, and distributors. To meet this responsibility, they must establish and implement a **Hazard Analysis Critical Control Point (HACCP)** system. A HACCP system analyzes food production, processing, and transport, with the goal of identifying potential sources of contamination and points where measures can be taken to control contamination. Then, by monitoring these **critical control points**, contamination can be prevented or eliminated (**Figure 13.2**). Unlike traditional methods of protecting the food supply, which use visual spot checks and random testing to catch contamination after it occurs, HACCP systems are designed to *prevent* contamination.

> **Hazard Analysis Critical Control Point (HACCP)** A food safety system that focuses on identifying and preventing hazards that could cause food-borne illness.

The Role of the Consumer

Although government agencies, manufacturers, and retailers are involved in creating a safe food supply, consumers also need to assume responsibility for their food. Even a food that has been manufactured, packaged, and transported with great care can cause food-borne illness if it is not handled carefully at home. In fact, most cases of food-borne illness are caused by foods prepared at home.[3] Consumers can prevent most food-borne illness through careful food handling, storage, and preparation (discussed in depth later in the chapter). They can also protect themselves and others by reporting incidents involving unsanitary, unsafe, deceptive, or mislabeled food to the appropriate agencies (**Table 13.2**).

PROCESS DIAGRAM

HACCP in liquid egg production • Figure 13.2

The scrambled eggs served in your cafeteria at school or work most likely came out of a carton rather than a shell. To produce this product, eggs are shelled, mixed together in large vats, heated to kill microbial contaminants, packaged, and either refrigerated or frozen. A contaminated batch could sicken hundreds of people. This example shows how a HACCP system might be used to prevent contaminated eggs from reaching the consumer.

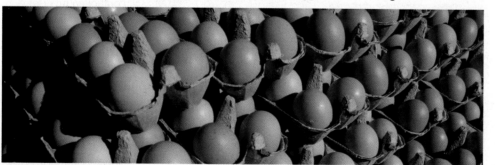

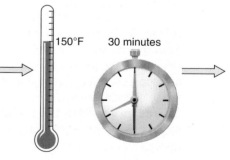

150°F   30 minutes

1 Conduct a hazard analysis
The manufacturer analyzes its processing steps for potential hazards and determines what preventive measures can be taken. In the case of eggs, there is a large potential for contamination with the bacterium *Salmonella*. Adequate heating is a preventive measure that can eliminate this hazard.

2 Identify the critical control points
Critical control points are the steps in a food's processing at which the hazard can be eliminated. In the case of egg processing, the critical control point is heating the shelled egg mixture in a large chamber.

3 Establish critical limits
Critical limits are the parameters that will prevent the hazard. In the case of these eggs, the critical limits are sufficient heating time and temperature to ensure that *Salmonella* bacteria are killed.

How to report food-related issues   Table 13.2

Before reporting a suspected case of food-borne illness, get all the facts. Determine whether you have used the product as intended and according to the manufacturer's instruction. Check to see if the item is past its expiration date. After these steps have been taken, report the incident to the appropriate agency:

- **Problems related to any food except meat and poultry, including adverse reactions:** Report emergencies to the FDA's main emergency number, which is staffed 24 hours a day: 301-443-1240. Nonemergencies can be reported to the FDA consumer complaint coordinator in your area, which you can find at www.fda.gov/Safety/ReportaProblem/default.htm.
- **Issues related to meat and poultry:** Report first to your state department of agriculture and then to the USDA Meat and Poultry Hotline (888-MPHotline or mphotline.fsis@usda.gov).
- **Restaurant food and sanitation problems:** Report directly to your local or state health department.
- **Issues related to alcoholic beverages:** Report to the U.S. Department of the Treasury's Bureau of Alcohol, Tobacco, and Firearms.
- **Pesticide, air, and water pollution:** Report first to your state environmental protection department and then to the U.S. EPA.
- **Products purchased at the grocery store:** Return to the store. Grocery stores are concerned with the safety of the foods they sell, and they will take responsibility for tracking down and correcting the problem. They will either refund your money or replace the product.

CONCEPT CHECK   STOP

1. **What** causes food-borne illness?

2. **Why** might the same food make one person sick and not another person?

3. **Who** is responsible for the safety of the food you eat?

4. **How** does HACCP differ from traditional visual food inspection?

THE PLANNER

Ask Yourself

What is the critical control point for the elimination of *Salmonella* in liquid egg production?

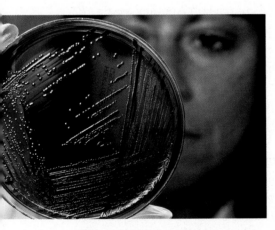

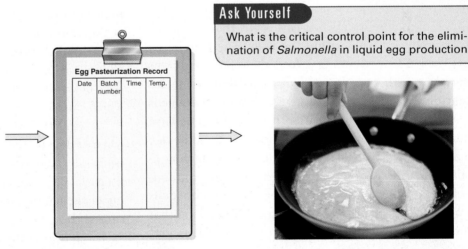

Egg Pasteurization Record

Date	Batch number	Time	Temp.

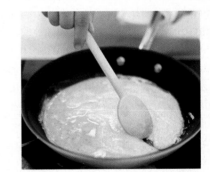

4 Establish monitoring procedures
Procedures need to be in place to continually monitor the critical control points. With egg processing, each batch is tested for the presence of *Salmonella*. If the temperature is not hot enough or the heating is not continued long enough, *Salmonella* can survive, as shown here by the growing bacterial colonies.

5 Establish corrective action
If a critical limit is not met, corrective action is necessary. Batches of eggs that are contaminated with *Salmonella* are discarded, and the temperature of the heat chamber is adjusted to ensure that *Salmonella* in the next batch will be killed.

6 Keep records
Extensive records are kept, documenting the monitoring of critical control points, verification activities, and corrective actions taken. This enables the manufacturer to trace the source of the problem in the event of an outbreak of food-borne illness.

7 Verify procedures
Review of plans and records helps ensure that the HACCP plan is working and only safe eggs are reaching consumers.

Pathogens in Food

LEARNING OBJECTIVES

1. **Distinguish** food-borne infection from food-borne intoxication.

2. **Discuss** three types of bacteria that commonly cause food-borne illness.

3. **Explain** how viruses, molds, and parasites can make us sick.

4. **Describe** how careful food handling can prevent food-borne illness.

Most cases of food-borne illness in the United States are caused by food that has been contaminated with **pathogens**. The pathogens that most commonly affect the food supply include bacteria, viruses, molds, and parasites. A typical case of food-borne illness causes a short bout of flulike symptoms, including abdominal pain, nausea, diarrhea, and vomiting. However, more severe symptoms, such as kidney failure, arthritis, paralysis, miscarriage, and even death, sometimes occur.

> **pathogen** A biological agent that causes disease.

Any food-borne illness caused by pathogens that multiply in the human body is called a **food-borne infection**. Contracting a food-borne infection usually involves consumption of a large number of pathogens that infect the body or produce toxins within the body. Any food-borne illness caused by consuming a food that contains toxins produced by pathogens is referred to as **food-borne intoxication**. Even food that contains only a few pathogens can cause food-borne intoxication if the pathogens have produced enough toxin. Avoiding food-borne illness—both infection and intoxication—requires knowing how to handle and store food in ways that will prevent contamination and prevent or minimize the growth of pathogens that may already be present in the food. Even a food that is contaminated with pathogens can be safe if it is prepared in a manner that destroys any pathogens or toxins that are present.

Bacteria in Food

Bacteria are present in the soil, on our skin, on most surfaces in our homes, and in the food we eat. Most are harmless, some are beneficial, and a few are pathogenic, causing food-borne infection or intoxication.[4]

Bacterial food-borne infection *Salmonella* is the most common cause of food-borne illness in the United States.[4] Contaminated meat, dairy products, seafood, fresh produce, and cereal have caused outbreaks, but poultry and eggs are the foods most commonly contaminated with the bacterium (**Figure 13.3a** and **b**). Because *Salmonella* is killed by heat, foods that are likely to be contaminated should be cooked thoroughly.

Campylobacter jejuni is the leading cause of acute bacterial diarrhea in developed countries.[5] Common sources are undercooked chicken, unpasteurized milk, and untreated water (**Figure 13.3b** and **c**). A sampling of raw chicken from supermarkets found that about 70% of samples were contaminated with *Campylobacter*.[6] This organism grows slowly in cold temperatures and is killed by heat, so careful storage and thorough cooking help prevent infection.

Escherichia coli, commonly called *E. coli*, is a bacterium that inhabits the gastrointestinal tracts of humans and other animals. It comes into contact with food through fecal contamination of water or unsanitary handling of food. Some strains of *E. coli* are harmless, but others can cause serious food-borne infection. One strain of *E. coli*, found in water contaminated by human or animal feces, is the cause of "travelers' diarrhea." Another strain, *E. coli* O157:H7, produces a toxin in the body that causes abdominal pain, bloody diarrhea, and in severe cases a form of kidney failure called **hemolytic-uremic syndrome**, which can be fatal.

E. coli O157:H7 entered the public spotlight in 1993, when it led to the deaths of several children who had consumed undercooked, contaminated hamburgers from a fast-food restaurant (**Figure 13.3d**).[7] Thorough cooking of the hamburgers would have killed the bacteria that caused these deaths. *E. coli* can also contaminate produce such as lettuce, spinach, and green onions and cause illness if the produce is eaten raw (**Figure 13.3e**). In 2010, *E. coli* contamination of lettuce sickened people in five states.[8] In 2011, infected bologna, another food that we don't typically cook, sickened people in five different states.[9] In addition to concerns about *E. coli* O157:H7 in our meat and produce, a new, even more deadly strain of *E. coli* emerged in Europe in 2011, sickening thousands and killing dozens.

How bacteria contaminate our food • Figure 13.3

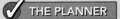 ✓ THE PLANNER

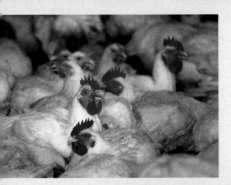

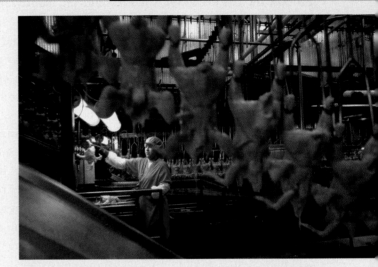

a. Because poultry farms house large numbers of chickens in close proximity, one infected chicken can infect thousands of others. *Salmonella* can infect the ovaries of hens and contaminate the eggs before the shells are formed, so that the bacteria are present inside the shell when the eggs are laid. Therefore, eggs should never be eaten raw.

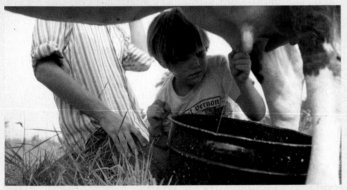

b. In processing plants, *Salmonella* and *Campylobacter* from infected birds can be transferred to the meat of healthy birds. Consumers should always handle raw chicken as if it contains pathogens.

d. *E. coli* O157:H7 can live in the intestines of healthy cattle and contaminate the meat after slaughter. *E. coli*–contaminated meat that comes into contact with a grinder may contaminate hundreds of pounds of ground beef. Ground beef contaminated with *E. coli* O157:H7 is a particular concern because the pathogens are mixed throughout during grinding rather than remaining on the surface, as they do on steaks and chops. The *E. coli* on the outside of the meat are quickly killed during cooking, but those in the interior survive if the meat is not cooked thoroughly.

c. *Campylobacter* are often carried by healthy cattle and by flies on farms. As a result, the bacteria are commonly present in unpasteurized (raw) milk. Unpasteurized milk is also a common source of *Listeria*. During pasteurization, milk is heated to a temperature that is high enough to kill both *Campylobacter* and *Listeria*. Avoiding products made with unpasteurized milk will reduce the risk of *Campylobacter* and *Listeria* infection.

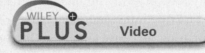
WILEY PLUS Video

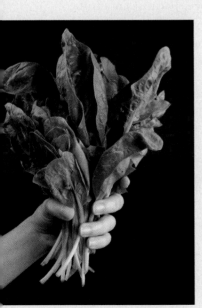

e. *E. coli* and other bacteria can also contaminate fruits and vegetables if they are fertilized with raw or improperly composted manure or irrigated with water containing untreated sewage or manure. Produce may also be contaminated by wash water or through direct or indirect contact with cattle, deer, or sheep. Thoroughly washing fruits and vegetables can reduce the number of pathogens but does not make contaminated produce risk free.

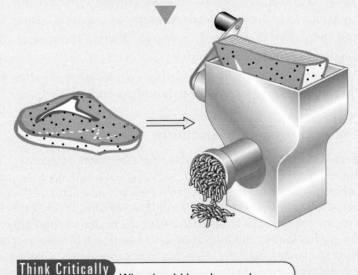

Think Critically Why should hamburger be cooked more thoroughly than steak to prevent *E coli* infection?

Each year in the United States, an estimated 1600 persons become seriously ill due to infection with *Listeria monocytogenes*, and of these, 260 die.[10] In most people, *Listeria* infection just causes flulike symptoms, but in high-risk groups, such as pregnant women, children, elderly people, and people with compromised immune systems, it can be more serious. Pregnant women are at particular risk; *Listeria* infection is 18 times more common in pregnant women than in the general population. Infection during pregnancy is associated with an increased risk of spontaneous abortion and stillbirth, and it can be transmitted to the fetus, causing meningitis and serious blood infections.[11] *Listeria* is ubiquitous in the environment and can survive and grow at refrigerator temperatures. Because it can grow at cool temperatures, this bacterium can infect ready-to-eat foods such as hot dogs and lunch meats, even if they have been kept properly refrigerated. To prevent infection, ready-to-eat meats should be heated to the steaming point, and unpasteurized dairy products should be avoided.

The food-borne infection caused by the bacterium *Vibrio vulnificus* usually causes gastrointestinal upset but can be deadly in people with compromised immune systems. The most common way in which people become infected is by eating raw or undercooked shellfish, particularly oysters. *Vibrio* bacteria grow in warm seawater. The incidence of *Vibrio* infection is higher during the summer months, when warm water favors growth.

Bacterial food-borne intoxication

Staphylococcus aureus is a common cause of bacterial food-borne intoxication. These bacteria live in human nasal passages and can be transferred to food through coughing or sneezing. They can then grow on the food, producing a toxin that causes vomiting soon after ingestion.

Another cause of food-borne intoxication is the bacterium *Clostridium perfringens*. It is often called the *cafeteria germ* because it grows in foods that are stored in large containers like those used in cafeterias. Little oxygen gets to the food at the center of a large container, thus providing an excellent growth environment for bacteria such as these, which thrive in low-oxygen environments. *C. perfringens* are difficult to kill because they form heat-resistant **spores**. Spores are a stage of bacterial life that remains dormant until environmental conditions favor their growth. *C. perfringens* may cause illness through both infection and intoxication.

The deadliest of all bacterial food toxins is produced by *Clostridium botulinum*. Heat-resistant spores of *C. botulinum* are found in soil, water, and the intestinal tracts of animals. The toxin is produced when the spores begin to grow and develop. When consumed, the toxin blocks nerve function, resulting in vomiting, abdominal pain, double vision, and paralysis that leads to respiratory failure. If untreated, **botulism** is often fatal, but modern detection methods and rapid administration of antitoxin have reduced mortality rates. *C. botulinum* grows in low-oxygen, low-acid conditions, so improperly canned foods and foods such as potatoes or stew that are held in large containers where there is little exposure to oxygen provide optimal conditions for botulism spores to germinate (**Figure 13.4**).

Infant botulism is a type of botulism that is seen only in infants. Though rare, it occurs worldwide and is the most common form of botulism in the United States.[12] It is caused by ingestion of botulism spores. When ingested, the spores germinate in the infant's gastrointestinal tract, producing toxin. Some of the toxin is absorbed into the bloodstream, causing weakness, paralysis, and respiratory problems. In the absence of complications, infants generally recover. Only infants are affected, because in adults, competing intestinal microflora prevent spores from germinating. Because honey can be contaminated with botulism spores, it should never be fed to infants under 1 year of age.

Canned foods and botulism • Figure 13.4

Because acid prevents the germination of *Clostridium botulinum* spores, foods that are low in acid, such as green beans, corn, peppers, asparagus, and mushrooms, are more likely to cause botulism than are acidic foods. To avoid botulism, discard bulging cans, as the bulge could indicate the presence of gas produced by the bacteria as they grow. Once it has formed, botulism toxin can be destroyed by boiling for at least 10 minutes, but if the safety of a food is in question, it should be thrown away; even a taste of a food contaminated with botulism toxin can be deadly.

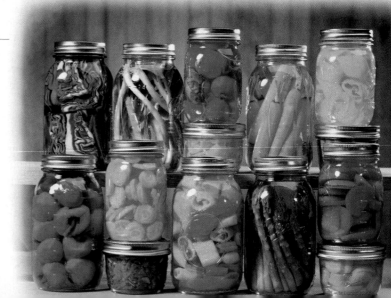

How viruses make us sick • Figure 13.5

Viruses make us sick by reproducing inside our cells. Viruses that cause food-borne illness enter the body through the gastrointestinal (GI) tract. Other types of viruses may enter the body through open cuts, the respiratory tract, or the genital tract.

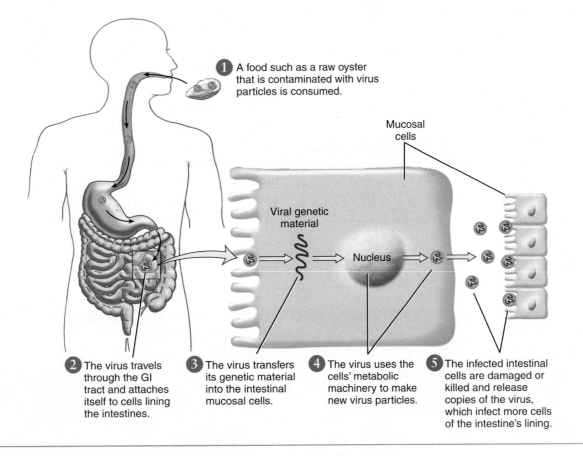

1 A food such as a raw oyster that is contaminated with virus particles is consumed.

Mucosal cells

Viral genetic material

Nucleus

2 The virus travels through the GI tract and attaches itself to cells lining the intestines.

3 The virus transfers its genetic material into the intestinal mucosal cells.

4 The virus uses the cells' metabolic machinery to make new virus particles.

5 The infected intestinal cells are damaged or killed and release copies of the virus, which infect more cells of the intestine's lining.

Viruses in Food

Unlike bacteria, the viruses that cause human diseases cannot grow and reproduce in foods. Human viruses can reproduce only inside human cells. They make us sick by turning our cells into virus-producing factories (**Figure 13.5**).

Noroviruses are a group of viruses that cause gastroenteritis, or what we commonly call "stomach flu." These viruses are believed to be responsible for about 50% of all food-borne gastroenteritis outbreaks in the United States.[13] Norovirus illness is contracted either by eating food that is contaminated with the virus or by touching a contaminated surface and then putting your fingers in your mouth. Shellfish can be contaminated with norovirus if the water in which they live is polluted with human or animal feces. Cooking destroys noroviruses, so uncooked foods and water are the most common causes of norovirus food-borne illness. Norovirus infection can be spread from one infected person to another, so it spreads swiftly where many people congregate in a small area. You may have heard of it as a cause of food-borne illness aboard cruise ships. These outbreaks make headlines, but norovirus outbreaks are just as likely in nursing homes, restaurants, hotels, and dormitories as they are aboard cruise ships.

Hepatitis A is another viral infection that can be contracted from food or water that is contaminated with fecal matter. Hepatitis A infection causes liver inflammation, jaundice, fever, nausea, fatigue, and abdominal pain. The infection can require a recovery period of several months, but it does not require treatment and does not cause permanent liver damage. Hepatitis in drinking water is destroyed by chlorination. Cooking destroys the virus in food, and good sanitation can prevent its spread. A vaccine that protects against hepatitis A infection is available.

Moldy Foods

Many types of **mold** grow on foods such as bread, cheese, and fruit. Under certain conditions, these molds produce toxins (**Figure 13.6**). More than 250 different mold toxins have been

> **mold** Multicellular fungi that form filamentous branching growths.

identified. Cooking and freezing stop mold growth but do not destroy toxins that have already been produced. If a food is moldy, it should be discarded, the area where it was stored should be cleaned, and neighboring foods should be checked to see if they have also become contaminated.

Parasites in Food

Some **parasites** are microscopic single-celled animals, and others are worms large enough to be seen with the naked eye. Parasites that can be transmitted through consumption of contaminated food and water cause food-borne illness. *Giardia lamblia* is a single-celled parasite that is often contracted by hikers who drink untreated water from streams contaminated with animal feces. *Giardia* infection is also becoming a problem in day-care centers where diapers are changed

> **parasite** An organism that lives at the expense of another.

Mold toxin and liver cancer • Figure 13.6

a. The filamentous growths seen in this electron micrograph belong to the mold *Aspergillus flavus*. It produces *aflatoxin*, which is among the most potent carcinogens and mutagens known. This mold commonly grows on corn, rice, wheat, peanuts, almonds, walnuts, sunflower seeds, and spices such as black pepper and coriander. The level of aflatoxin that may be present in foods in the United States is regulated to prevent toxicity. ▼

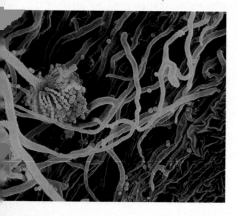

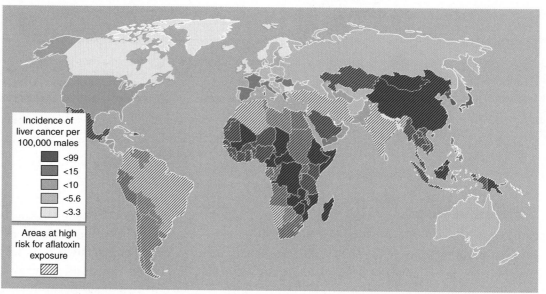

Incidence of liver cancer per 100,000 males
- <99
- <15
- <10
- <5.6
- <3.3

Areas at high risk for aflatoxin exposure

b. Exposure to aflatoxin can lead to liver cancer. Many regions with high rates of liver cancer also have high exposure to aflatoxin.[14]

> **Interpreting Data**
>
> Which continents have the highest incidence of liver cancer? Are these areas also at risk for aflatoxin exposure?

Herring worm • Figure 13.7

The body cavity of this herring contains the larval form of the small roundworm *Anisakis simplex*, also called herring worm. When consumed in raw fish, these parasites invade the stomach and intestinal tract, causing *Anisakis* disease, which is characterized by severe abdominal pain. The fresher the fish when it is eviscerated, the less likely it is to cause this disease because the larvae move from the fish's stomach to its flesh only after the fish dies.

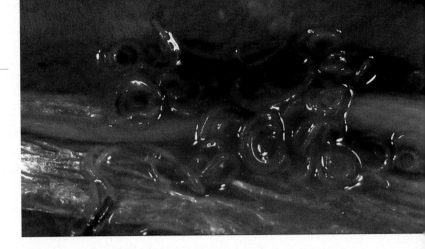

and hands and surfaces are not thoroughly washed.[4] *Cryptosporidium parvum* is another single-celled parasite that is commonly spread by contaminated water, but cases have also been reported in patients who have eaten contaminated raw fruits and vegetables.[15]

Trichinella spiralis is a parasite that is found in raw and undercooked pork and game meats. Once ingested, these small, wormlike organisms find their way to the muscles, where they grow, causing flulike symptoms. Fish are another common source of parasitic infections because they carry the larvae of parasites such as roundworms, flatworms, flukes, and tapeworms (**Figure 13.7**). As the popularity of eating raw fish has increased, so has the incidence of parasitic infections from fish. Parasites, including those in fish, are killed by thorough cooking. When consuming raw fish, parasitic infections can be avoided by eating fish that has been frozen.

Prions in Food

The strangest and scariest yet rarest food-borne illness is caused not by a microbe but by a protein, called a **prion**, that has folded improperly. Abnormal prions are believed to be the cause of mad cow disease, or **bovine spongiform encephalopathy (BSE)**, a deadly degenerative neurological disease that affects cattle. The human form of this disease is **variant Creutzfeldt-Jakob Disease (vCJD)**. People are believed to contract it by eating tissue from a cow infected with BSE (**Figure 13.8**).[16] Symptoms of vCJD begin as mood swings and numbness and within about 14 months progress to dementia and death.

> **prion** A pathogenic protein that is the cause of degenerative brain diseases called spongiform encephalopathies. *Prion* is short for *proteinaceous infectious particle*.

How prions multiply • Figure 13.8

✔ THE PLANNER

The abnormal prions that cause BSE differ from normal proteins in the way they are folded—that is, in their three-dimensional structure. When the improperly folded form of a prion is introduced into the brain after a person has eaten contaminated tissue, it can reproduce by corrupting neighboring proteins, essentially changing their shape so that they, too, become abnormal prions. Because the abnormal prions are not degraded normally, they accumulate and form clumps called plaques. These plaques cause deadly nervous tissue damage.

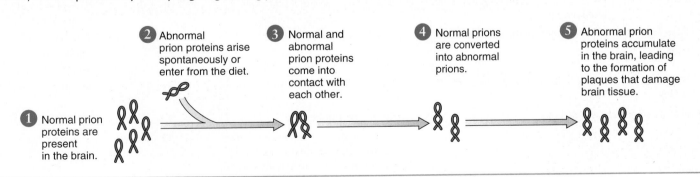

1. Normal prion proteins are present in the brain.

2. Abnormal prion proteins arise spontaneously or enter from the diet.

3. Normal and abnormal prion proteins come into contact with each other.

4. Normal prions are converted into abnormal prions.

5. Abnormal prion proteins accumulate in the brain, leading to the formation of plaques that damage brain tissue.

PROCESS DIAGRAM

Summary of bacterial, viral, and parasitic food-borne illnesses   Table 13.3

Microbe	Sources	Symptoms	Onset (time after consumption)	Duration
Bacteria				
Salmonella	Fecal contamination, raw or undercooked eggs and meat, especially poultry	Nausea, abdominal pain, diarrhea, headache, fever	6–48 hours	1–2 days
Campylobacter jejuni	Unpasteurized milk, untreated water, undercooked meat and poultry	Fever, headache, diarrhea, abdominal pain	2–5 days	1–2 weeks
Listeria monocytogenes	Raw milk products; soft ripened cheeses; deli meats and cold cuts, raw and undercooked poultry; meats; raw and smoked fish; raw vegetables	Fever, headache, stiff neck, chills, nausea, vomiting. May cause spontaneous abortion or stillbirth in pregnant women and menengitis and blood infections in the fetus.	Days to weeks	Days to weeks
Vibrio vulnificus	Raw seafood from contaminated water	Cramps, abdominal pain, weakness, watery diarrhea, fever, chills	15–24 hours	2–4 days
Staphylococcus aureus	Human contamination from coughs and sneezes; eggs, meat, potato, and macaroni salads	Severe nausea, vomiting, diarrhea	2–8 hours	2–3 days
Escherichia coli O157:H7	Fecal contamination, undercooked ground beef	Abdominal pain, bloody diarrhea, kidney failure	5–48 hours	3 days–2 weeks or longer
Clostridium perfringens	Fecal contamination, deep-dish casseroles	Nausea, diarrhea, abdominal pain	8–22 hours	6–24 hours
Clostridium botulinum	Improperly canned foods, deep-dish, casseroles, honey	Lassitude, weakness, vertigo, respiratory failure, paralysis	18–36 hours	10 days or longer (must administer antitoxin)
Shigella	Fecal contamination of water or foods, especially salads such as chicken, tuna, shrimp, and potato salads	Diarrhea, abdominal pain, fever, vomiting	12–50 hours	5–6 days
Yersinia enterocolitica	Pork, dairy products, and produce	Diarrhea, vomiting, fever, abdominal pain; often mistaken for appendicitis	24–48 hours	Weeks
Viruses				
Norovirus	Fecal contamination of water or foods, especially shellfish and salad ingredients	Diarrhea, nausea, vomiting	1–2 days	2–6 days
Hepatitis A	Human fecal contamination of food or water, raw shellfish	Jaundice, liver inflammation, fatigue, fever, nausea, anorexia, abdominal discomfort	10–50 days	1–2 weeks to several months
Parasites				
Giardia lamblia	Fecal contamination of water and uncooked foods	Diarrhea, abdominal pain, gas, anorexia, nausea, vomiting	5–25 days	1–2 weeks, but may be chronic
Cryptosporidium parvum	Fecal contamination of food or water	Severe watery diarrhea	Hours	2–4 days, but sometimes weeks
Trichinella spiralis	Undercooked pork, game meat	Muscle weakness, flulike symptoms	Weeks	Months
Anisakis simplex	Raw fish	Severe abdominal pain	1 hour–2 weeks	3 weeks
Toxoplasma gondii	Meat, primarily pork	Toxoplasmosis (can cause central nervous system disorders, flulike symptoms, and birth defects in the offspring of women exposed during pregnancy, see Chapter 11)	10–23 days	May become chronic

vCJD is believed to be transmitted by consumption of the brain and nervous tissue, intestines, eyes, or tonsils of contaminated animals, but thus far meat (if free of central nervous system tissue) and milk have not been found to transmit either BSE or vCJD.[4] Even though cooking does not destroy prions, the risk of acquiring vCJD is extremely small. Safeguards are in place to prevent cattle in the United States from contracting BSE. These include restrictions on the import of animals and animal products from countries where BSE has occurred, restrictions on what can be included in cattle feed, and testing for BSE before meat is released into the food supply.[17] Several cows with BSE have been identified in the United States, but meat from these animals did not enter the food supply. Thus far there has been no known instance of U.S. beef causing a case of vCJD.

What Bug Has You Down?

There are certainly a wide variety of food-borne pathogens that can make you sick (**Table 13.3**). Recent improvements in governmental outbreak surveillance, attentiveness by health-care professionals, and testing frequency and accuracy have made it possible to identify even more cases of food-borne illness than was possible a few years ago. Given this and the extensive media coverage of outbreaks of food-borne illness and recalls of contaminated foods, one would expect that the incidence of food-borne illness has been rising. In fact, there has been no increase over the past four years.[18] Public awareness of the problem and education on how to handle food safely should make food-borne illness even less frequent in the future.

Preventing Microbial Food-Borne Illness

Microbes in food multiply when they are presented with the right conditions for growth. The first step in preventing microbial food-borne illness is to minimize the presence of microbes by choosing food carefully (**Table 13.4**). Preparing food in a clean kitchen reduces **cross-contamination**. Storing food at refrigerator or freezer temperatures either limits or stops microbial growth. Heating foods to the recommended temperature kills microbes and

cross-contamination The transfer of contaminants from one food or object to another.

Safe grocery choices   Table 13.4

- Purchase food from reputable vendors.

- Make sure jars are closed and seals are unbroken and that safety "buttons" on jar lids have not popped.

- Check to see that cans are not rusted, dented, or bulging.

- Make sure food packaging is secure.

- Select frozen foods from below the frost line in the freezer.

- Make sure frozen foods are solidly frozen and do not contain frost or ice crystals.

- Check voluntary freshness dates and avoid foods with expired dates:

  - **Sell-by or pull-by date:** Used by manufacturers to tell grocers when to remove their product from the shelves. You should buy the product before this date, but if the food has been handled and stored properly, it is usually still safe for consumption after it. For example, milk is usually still good at least a week beyond its sell-by date if it has been properly refrigerated.

  - **Best if used by, use-by, quality assurance, or freshness date:** Used to specify the last date on which the product will retain maximum freshness, flavor, and texture. Beyond this date, the product's quality may diminish, but the food may still be safe if it has been handled and stored properly.

  - **Expiration date:** Used to specify the last day on which a product should be eaten. State governments regulate these dates for perishable items, such as milk and eggs. The FDA regulates only the expiration dates of infant formula.

Ask Yourself

Is the canned pineapple in this photo a safe choice? Why or why not?

Fight Bac! is an educational campaign conducted by the Partnership for Food Safety Education. It is designed to teach food-handling practices that will keep food safe from bacteria and prevent food-borne illness. Fight Bac! recommends that consumers follow four steps—clean, separate, cook, and chill—to prevent food-borne illness (see www.fightbac.org).[19]

Meats and casseroles should be cooked, and leftovers reheated, until they reach the internal temperatures shown here, which will ensure that microbes have been killed. Use a food thermometer to make sure that the food is cooked to a safe internal temperature; color is not a good indicator of safety.

Hands, countertops, cutting boards, and utensils should be washed with warm, soapy water before each step in food preparation.

Foods that are going to be cooked should not be prepared on the same surfaces as foods that are eaten raw.

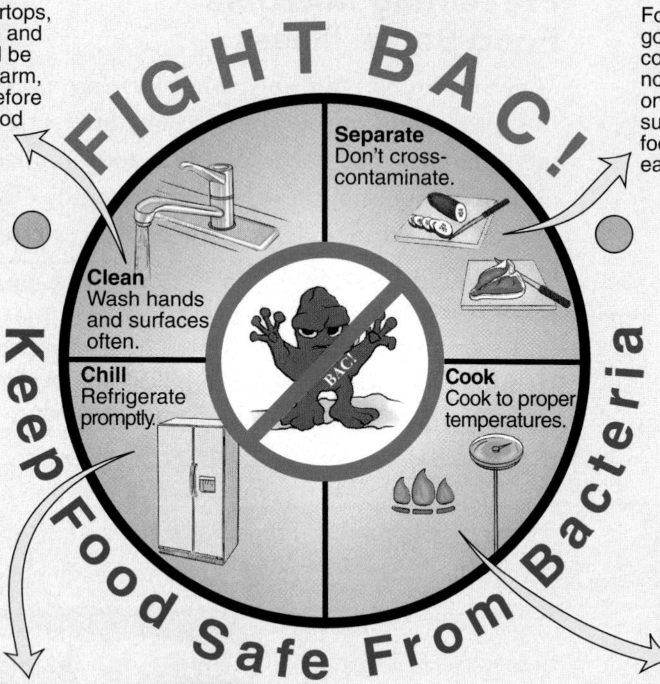

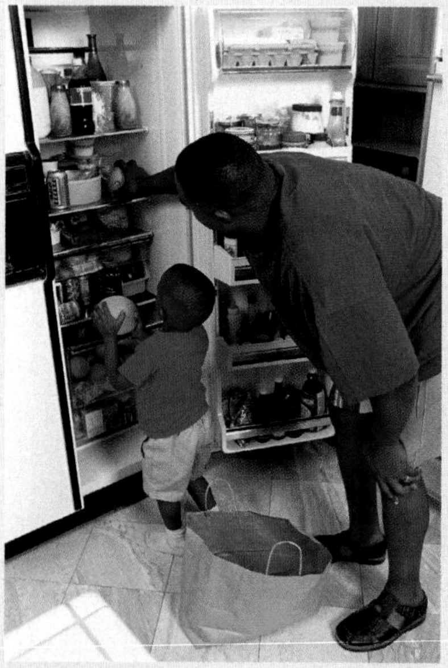

FIGHT BAC!
Keep Food Safe From Bacteria

Separate Don't cross-contaminate.

Clean Wash hands and surfaces often.

Chill Refrigerate promptly.

Cook Cook to proper temperatures.

Safe Cooking Temperatures[19]	
Food item	**Internal temperature (°F) or description**
Beef roasts and steaks	145 (allow meat to rest 3 min before carving or consuming)
Ground meat	160
Pork	145 (allow meat to rest 3 min before carving or consuming)
Poultry	165
Fish	145 or until the flesh is opaque and separates easily with a fork
Eggs	Until the yolk and white are firm, not runny (egg dishes 160)
Leftovers and casseroles	165

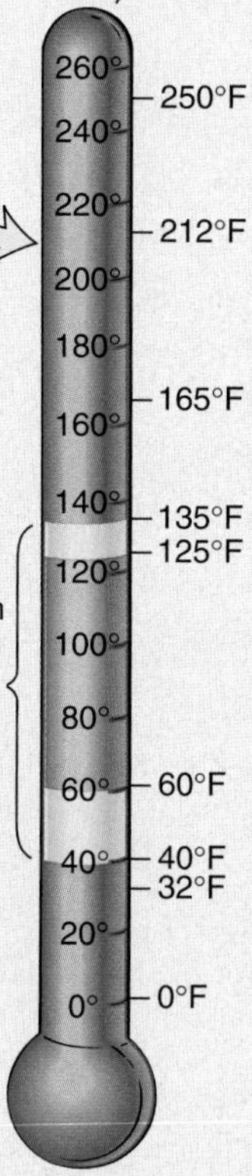

260° — 250°F
240°
220° — 212°F
200°
180°
165°F
160°
140° — 135°F
— 125°F
120°
100°
80°
60° — 60°F
40° — 40°F
— 32°F
20°
0° — 0°F

Canning temperature for low-acid foods in pressure cooker

Range of cooking temperatures to kill most bacteria. The amount of time needed decreases as the temperature increases.

Minimum temperature for reheating foods. Warming temperatures control growth but allow survival of some bacteria.

Some growth may occur: Many bacteria survive.

Danger Zone Temperatures in this zone allow rapid bacterial growth and production of bacterial toxins. Foods should only be allowed to remain in this temperature range for minimal amounts of time.

Some bacterial growth may occur in this zone.

Cold temperatures allow slow growth for a few cold-tolerant organisms but stop the growth of most.

Freezing temperatures prevent bacterial growth but some bacteria are able to survive.

Fresh and frozen foods brought from the store should be refrigerated or frozen immediately. Fresh meat, poultry, and fish should be frozen if it will not be used within a day or two. Processed meats such as hot dogs and bologna should be refrigerated but can be kept longer than fresh meat. Freezers should be set to 0°F and refrigerators to less than 40°F.

Temperature is one of the best weapons consumers have for preventing food-borne illness. Low temperatures slow or stop microbial growth, and high temperatures kill microorganisms.

Think Critically Why is a temperature between 41 and 135°F considered to be the danger zone?

destroys toxins (**Figure 13.9**). Foods that are served cold should be kept cold until they are served. Frozen foods should be kept frozen and then thawed in the refrigerator or microwave before cooking, not thawed at room temperature, which favors microbial growth. Cooked food should be handled with care and kept hot until it is served. When in doubt about the safety of a food, throw it out.

Cross-contamination can occur when uncooked foods containing live microbes come into contact with foods that have already been cooked. Therefore, cooked meat should never be returned to the same dish that held the raw meat, and sauces used to marinate uncooked foods should never be used as sauces on cooked food. Leftover cooked food should be refrigerated as soon as possible after it has been served. The temperature range that is most favorable for microbial growth is the range at which food usually sits between service and storage. Large portions of food should be divided before refrigeration so they will cool quickly. Most leftovers should be kept for only a few days.

Although most food-borne illness in the United States is caused by food prepared in homes, an outbreak in a commercial or institutional establishment usually involves more people and is more likely to be reported (see *Thinking It Through*). Food in retail establishments

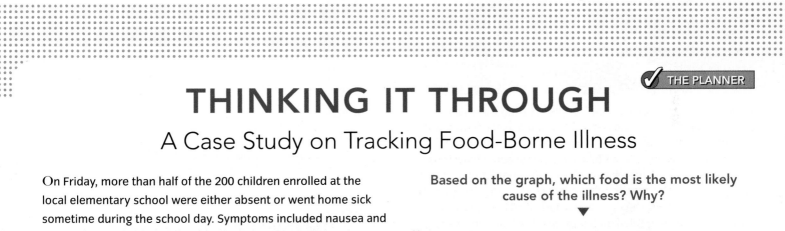

THINKING IT THROUGH ✓ THE PLANNER

A Case Study on Tracking Food-Borne Illness

On Friday, more than half of the 200 children enrolled at the local elementary school were either absent or went home sick sometime during the school day. Symptoms included nausea and vomiting, diarrhea, abdominal pain, and fever. Food-borne illness was suspected, and the local health department was notified. Inspectors were able to trace the source of the outbreak to the Spring Celebration held at the school on Thursday. For this event, the first-graders made cupcakes, the second-graders, cookies; the third-graders, fruit salad, and the fourth-graders, frozen custard. All the children were interviewed about which of these foods they had eaten that day, and the information was used to compile the following graph:

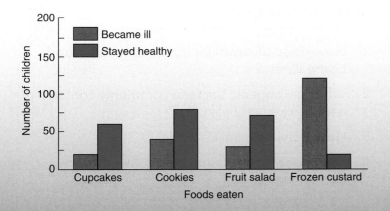

Based on the graph, which food is the most likely cause of the illness? Why?
▼
Your answer:

Physicians saw many of the sick children, and the bacterium *Salmonella enteritidis* was isolated from their stool samples. The health inspectors determined that the fourth-graders had used six grade-A raw eggs to make the frozen custard.

How can eggs become contaminated with *Salmonella*?
▼
Your answer:

The cookie and cupcake recipes also called for eggs. Why are these unlikely to be the cause of the problem?
▼
Your answer:

Suggest a reason why 20 children who consumed the frozen custard did not get ill.
▼
Your answer:

What could the fourth-graders have done to avoid the risk of *Salmonella* in their frozen custard?
▼
Your answer:

(Check your answers in Appendix J.)

WHAT A SCIENTIST SEES

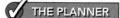

A Picnic for Bacteria

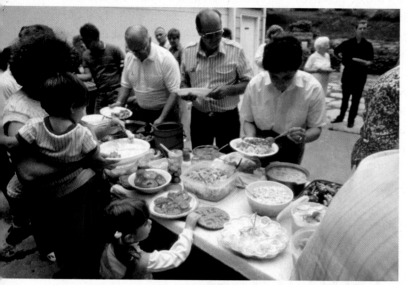

Limiting bacterial growth is a consideration any time food must be carried out of the home. Any food that is transported should be kept cold. Lunches should be transported to and from work or school in a cooler or an insulated bag and refrigerated upon arrival. Perishable foods that are brought home from work or school uneaten should be thrown out and not saved for another day.

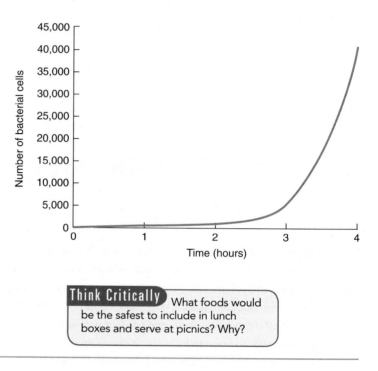

Looks great—lots of food and people together on a warm, sunny day. Most people see lunch, but those concerned with food-borne illness see trouble. If a food is contaminated with pathogenic bacteria, it won't take long before enough bacteria are present to cause food-borne illness. The number of bacterial cells doubles each time the cells divide, resulting in an exponential growth curve like the one shown here. If 10 bacterial cells contaminate the egg salad during preparation and then it sits in the warm sun for 4 hours, during which time the cells divide every 20 minutes, there will be 40,960 bacterial cells in the salad when you scoop a portion of it onto your plate.

Think Critically What foods would be the safest to include in lunch boxes and serve at picnics? Why?

has many opportunities to be contaminated because of the large volume of food handled and the large number of people involved in its preparation. Consumers should choose restaurants with safety in mind. Restaurants should be clean, and cooked foods should be served hot. Cafeteria steam tables should be kept hot enough that the water is steaming and food is kept above 135°F. Cold foods, such as salad bar items, should be kept either refrigerated or on ice to keep the food at 41°F or colder.

Picnics, potluck suppers, and other large events where food is served provide a prime opportunity for bacteria to flourish because food is often left at room temperature or in the sun for long periods before it is consumed. When diners serve themselves, cross-contamination from dirty hands or used plates and utensils is possible. Unlike the food in salad bars at restaurants,

the food at a family picnic is not placed under a sneeze guard to prevent contamination from coughs and sneezes. All food that is served outdoors at a picnic or county fair should be approached with food safety in mind (see *What a Scientist Sees*).

CONCEPT CHECK

1. **How** does *Clostridium botulinum* cause food-borne illness?

2. **What** pathogenic bacteria commonly contaminate chicken and eggs?

3. **How** do viruses make us sick?

4. **How** does refrigeration help prevent food-borne illness?

Agricultural and Industrial Chemicals in Food

LEARNING OBJECTIVES

1. **Illustrate** how contaminants move through the food chain and into our foods.

2. **Compare** the risks and benefits of using pesticides with those of growing food organically.

3. **Describe** how to minimize the risks of exposure to chemical contaminants.

Chemicals used in agricultural production and industrial wastes contaminate the environment and can find their way into the food supply. How harmful these chemicals are depends on whether they persist in the environment and whether they accumulate in the organisms that consume them or can be broken down and excreted by those organisms. Some contaminants are eliminated from the environment quickly because they are broken down by microorganisms or chemical reactions. Others remain in the environment for very long periods, and when taken up by plants and small animals, they are not metabolized or excreted. When these plants or small animals are consumed by larger animals that are in turn eaten by still larger animals, the contaminants accumulate, reaching higher concentrations at each level of the food chain (**Figure 13.10**). This process is called **bioaccumulation**. Because the toxins are not eliminated from the body, the greater the amount consumed, the greater the amount present in the body.

> **bioaccumulation** The process by which compounds accumulate or build up in an organism faster than they can be broken down or excreted.

Contamination throughout the food chain • Figure 13.10

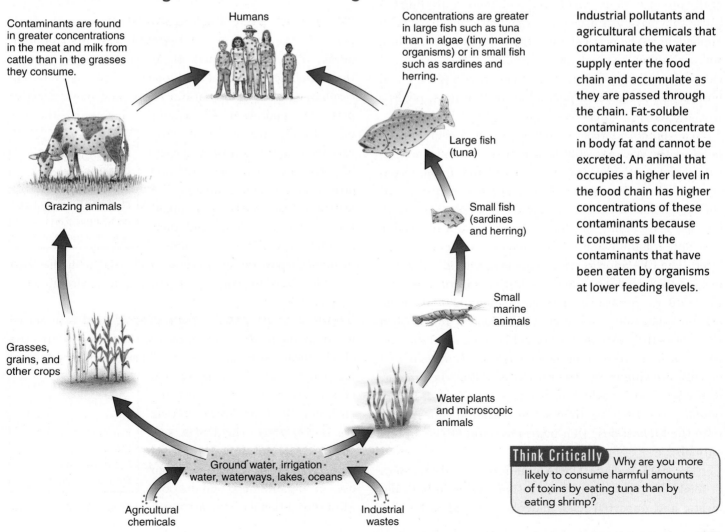

Contaminants are found in greater concentrations in the meat and milk from cattle than in the grasses they consume.

Humans

Grazing animals

Grasses, grains, and other crops

Agricultural chemicals

Ground water, irrigation water, waterways, lakes, oceans

Industrial wastes

Water plants and microscopic animals

Small marine animals

Small fish (sardines and herring)

Large fish (tuna)

Concentrations are greater in large fish such as tuna than in algae (tiny marine organisms) or in small fish such as sardines and herring.

Industrial pollutants and agricultural chemicals that contaminate the water supply enter the food chain and accumulate as they are passed through the chain. Fat-soluble contaminants concentrate in body fat and cannot be excreted. An animal that occupies a higher level in the food chain has higher concentrations of these contaminants because it consumes all the contaminants that have been eaten by organisms at lower feeding levels.

Think Critically Why are you more likely to consume harmful amounts of toxins by eating tuna than by eating shrimp?

As shown in these pie charts from an analysis of samples of domestically produced food and imported food from 100 countries, only a small percentage of foods exceed tolerances.[22] To further reduce pesticide risks and exposure in the United States, more effective, less-toxic chemical pesticides are being developed; the use of older, more toxic products is decreasing; and production methods that result in low-pesticide and pesticide-free produce are being implemented.

Interpreting Data

What percentage of imported food samples was free of pesticide residues?

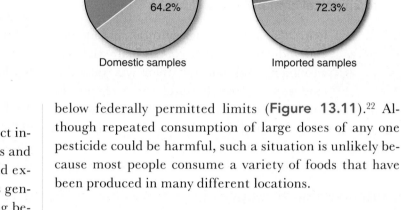

- No residue found
- Residue found but levels are below tolerances
- Residue found that exceeds tolerance or for which no tolerance has been established in the sampled food.

Domestic samples: 0.9%, 34.9%, 64.2%

Imported samples: 4.7%, 23%, 72.3%

Pesticides: Risks and Benefits

Pesticides are used to prevent plant diseases and insect infestations. They are applied both to crops in the fields and to harvested produce in order to prevent spoilage and extend shelf life. Crops that are grown using pesticides generally produce higher yields and look more appealing because they have less insect damage. Once they have been applied, however, pesticides can travel into water supplies, soil, and other parts of the environment. Because pesticides enter the environment, pesticide residues are found not only on the treated plants but also in meat, poultry, fish, and dairy products (see Figure 13.10).

The potential risks of pesticides to consumers depend on the size, age, and health of the person who consumes the pesticides and on the type and amount consumed.[20] To protect public health and the environment, the types of pesticides that may be used on food crops, how often they may be used, and the amount of residue that may remain when foods reach consumers are regulated. The EPA approves and registers pesticides that are used in food production and establishes **tolerances**. Pesticide tolerances are the maximum amounts of pesticide residues that may remain in or on a food.[21] To establish tolerances that are safe for both children and adults, the EPA considers tests done in experimental animals and on cells growing in the laboratory, as well as the amount of the pesticide to which consumers are likely to be exposed. Tolerances are then set at least 100 times lower than the highest dose that has no harmful effects in test animals.

The FDA and the USDA monitor pesticide residues in foods. In general, pesticide residue levels in both domestic and imported foods have been found to be well below federally permitted limits (**Figure 13.11**).[22] Although repeated consumption of large doses of any one pesticide could be harmful, such a situation is unlikely because most people consume a variety of foods that have been produced in many different locations.

Integrated pest management One way to limit pesticide use is through **integrated pest management (IPM)**. IPM is a method of agricultural pest control that combines chemical and nonchemical methods and emphasizes the use of natural toxins and more effective pesticide application. For example, increasing the use of naturally pest-resistant crop varieties that thrive without the use of pesticides can reduce costs and do less environmental damage. IPM programs use information about the life cycles of pests and their interaction with the environment to manage pest damage economically and with the least possible hazard to people, property, and the environment.

> **integrated pest management (IPM)** A method of agricultural pest control that integrates nonchemical and chemical techniques.

Organic food production Organic food is produced using methods that emphasize a reduction in the use of chemical pesticides and fertilizers, the recycling of resources, and the conservation of soil and water to protect the environment (see *Debate: Should You Go Organic?*). The USDA sets standards for substances that can be used in or are prohibited from use in organic food production.

>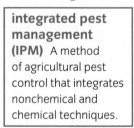
> **organic food** Food that is produced, processed, and handled in accordance with the standards of the USDA National Organic Program.

Most conventional pesticides, fertilizers made with synthetic

Debate   Should You Go Organic?

The Issue: As people become more and more concerned about food safety, nutritional health, and the environment, they are turning to organic food. Is organic food safer, more nutritious, and more environmentally friendly than conventionally produced food?

The sale of organic foods is on the rise. Most of this increase has been from organic fruits and vegetables, which now represent 11.4% of all U.S. fruit and vegetable sales.[24] Do organic production methods make these fruits and vegetables safer than traditional products? If *safer* is defined as containing fewer pesticides, the answer is clear. Organic foods are significantly lower in nitrates and pesticide residues than traditionally grown foods.[25] But, it can be argued that there is little evidence that the current levels of pesticide exposure from conventional produce present risks to human health (see Figure 13.11). And, there are other contamination risks associated with organic foods. Manure is often used for fertilizer. When the manure is not treated properly, it can contain pathogenic bacteria.[26]

Many consumers believe that organically produced food is not only safer but also more nutritious. *Nutritious* can mean that it is more effective at preventing nutrition-related diseases.[27] When consumption of organic food is compared with consumption of conventionally produced foods, the majority of studies do not show organic foods to be beneficial in terms of preventing nutrition-related diseases. Research data on the nutrient content of organically produced food are ambivalent. Some studies report that organically produced foods contain more nutrients than conventionally produced food, and others have found no consistent differences in nutrient content.[28] This confusion is not surprising

because many factors—including growing conditions, season, the fertilizer regime, and the methods used for crop protection (for example, use of pesticides and herbicides)—affect the nutritional composition of fruits and vegetables. Nutrient content is also affected by how the food is stored, transported, and processed prior to consumption.

What about the environment? It is hard to argue that organic farming is not better for the environment. Instead of chemical pesticides and fertilizer, it relies on crop rotation, compost, and cover crops to maintain the soil. The result is preservation of the soil, so crops can be grown far into the future, and reduction in the amounts of chemicals released into the environment. But organic growing still impacts the environment because manure runoff can pollute waterways and because organic food is often shipped long distances. This shipping uses energy and pollutes the environment.

Is a diet based on organic foods safer, more nutritious, and better for the environment? We can assume that both conventional and organic foods sold in the United States are generally safe. Whether organic is more nutritious depends not only on individual foods but on the diet as a whole. If your choices of organic foods are limited by availability or cost, then choosing only organic may limit nutrient intake. Are organic foods better for the environment? They reduce pesticide and fertilizer use, but if organic foods are not available locally the environmental cost of transporting them may outweigh those savings.

Think critically: Are these organic onions that were shipped across the country a better environmental choice than conventionally grown onions from the farm across town?

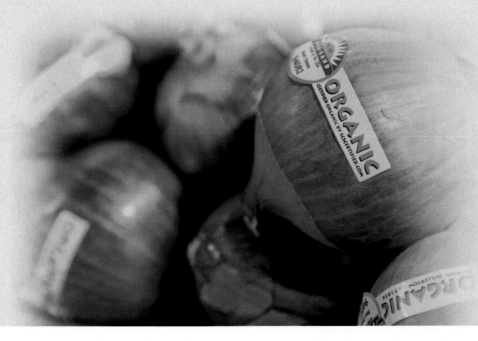

ingredients, sewage sludge, genetically modified ingredients, irradiation, antibiotics, and growth hormones are prohibited from use in organic food production. Before a food can be labeled "organic," the USDA must certify the farming and processing operations that produce and handle the food (**Figure 13.12**).

Organic farming techniques reduce farm workers' exposure to pesticides and decrease the quantity of pesticides introduced into the food supply and the environment. Organic foods, however, are not completely free of synthetic pesticides and other agricultural chemicals not approved for organic use because irrigation water, rain, and a variety of other sources can introduce trace amounts into organically grown foods. The threshold for pesticide residues in organic foods is set at 5% of the EPA's pesticide-residue tolerance.[23] Choosing organic food will reduce pesticide exposure, but it will not make your food risk free.

Industrial Contaminants

Industrial chemicals that contaminate the environment find their way into the food supply. Fish accumulate substances from the water in which they live and feed. Shellfish accumulate contaminants because they feed by passing large volumes of water through their bodies. Pollutants in the water can also contaminate crops and move through the food chain into meat and milk (see Figure 13.10).

One group of carcinogenic compounds that pollutes the environment is **polychlorinated biphenyls (PCBs)**. Prior to the 1970s, these chemicals were used in the manufacture of electrical capacitors and transformers, plasticizers, waxes, and paper. PCBs in runoff from manufacturing plants contaminated water, particularly near the Great Lakes. PCBs are no longer produced, but because they do not degrade, they are still in the environment and accumulate in fish caught in contaminated waters. PCBs are a particular problem for pregnant and lactating women because prenatal exposure to PCBs and consumption of contaminated breast milk can damage the fetal and infant nervous system and cause learning deficits. Pregnant and breastfeeding women should check with their local health department for recommendations regarding fish consumption.

Other contaminants from manufacturing, such as chlordane (used to control termites); radioactive substances such as strontium-90; and toxic metals such as cadmium, lead, arsenic, and mercury, have found their way into fish and shellfish. Cadmium and lead can interfere with the absorption of other minerals. Cadmium can cause kidney damage, and lead can impair brain development. Arsenic is believed to increase the risk of cancer. Mercury, which has been found in large fish, particularly swordfish, king mackerel, tilefish,

Labeling organic foods • Figure 13.12

Products that meet the definition of "100% organic" or "organic" may display the USDA "organic" seal shown here.

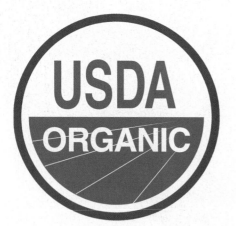

Labeling term	Meaning
100% organic	Contains 100% organically produced raw or processed ingredients.
Organic	Contains at least 95% organically produced raw or processed ingredients.
Made with organic ingredients	Contains at least 70% organically produced ingredients.

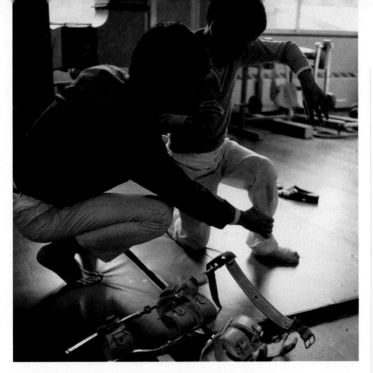

Mercury poisoning • Figure 13.13

This Japanese boy has Minamata disease, a neurological syndrome caused by mercury poisoning. The disease first appeared in Minamata, Japan, in 1956 and was caused by the release of mercury into the water by a local chemical factory. The mercury accumulated in the fat of fish and shellfish that were eaten by the local population.

and shark, damages nerve cells (**Figure 13.13**).[29] Because mercury is especially damaging during prenatal development, pregnant women are advised to avoid certain types of fish and limit their consumption of others (see Chapter 11).

Antibiotics and Hormones

Antibiotics and hormones are administered to animals to improve health, increase growth, or otherwise enhance food production. To prevent these chemicals from being passed on to consumers, both the types of drugs used and when they can be administered are regulated, and animal tissues are monitored for drug residues.[30]

Animals are treated with antibiotics when they are sick, and some animals are also given antibiotics to prevent disease and promote growth. This treatment increases the amount of meat produced and reduces costs, but if it is used improperly, antibiotic residues can remain in the meat. Another concern is the creation of antibiotic-resistant bacteria. When exposed to an antibiotic, bacteria that are resistant to it survive and produce offspring that are also resistant. If these antibiotic-resistant bacteria infect humans, the resulting illness cannot be treated with

that antibiotic. Because nearly half the antibiotics produced in the United States are used to prevent disease in animals, this use is suspected of being a major contributor to the development of antibiotic-resistant strains of bacteria.[31]

Hormones are used to increase weight gain in sheep and cattle and milk production in dairy cows. Some hormones, such as estrogen and testosterone, occur naturally. Generally, these are administered in slow-release form, and their levels are no higher in treated animals than in untreated animals. Before a synthetic hormone can be used, it must be demonstrated that hormone residues in meat from treated animals are within safe limits.

A synthetic hormone that has created public concern is genetically engineered **bovine somatotropin (bST)**. Cows naturally produce bST, which stimulates milk production. Genetically engineered bST is produced by bacteria and injected into cows to further increase milk production (**Figure 13.14**). Milk from cows that have been treated with genetically engineered bST is indistinguishable from other milk.

Bovine somatotropin • Figure 13.14

Consumer groups are concerned that the injection of cows with bST may cause health problems for humans who consume the milk. The FDA has concluded that bST causes no serious long-term health effects, and it does not require milk from bST-treated cows to be specially labeled. Some dairies voluntarily label their products as bST free.

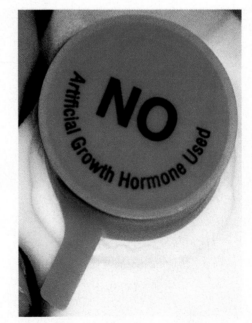

Choosing Wisely to Minimize Agricultural and Industrial Contaminants

Even though individual consumers cannot detect chemical contaminants in food, care in selection and preparation can reduce the amounts consumed. One of the easiest ways to reduce risk is to choose a wide variety of foods, thus avoiding excessive consumption of contaminants that may be present in any one food. To reduce exposure to pesticide residues in fruits and vegetables, consumers can choose organic foods or locally grown produce. Locally grown produce contains fewer pesticides because the pesticides used to prevent spoilage and extend the shelf life of shipped produce are not needed. Exposure to pesticide residues on conventionally grown produce can be minimized by washing and in some cases peeling (**Figure 13.15a**). Pesticides

and other toxins that are ingested by animals concentrate in fat, so intake can be reduced by trimming all fat from meat and removing the skin from poultry.

Intake of pesticides and other chemical pollutants from fish and seafood products can also be minimized by choosing wisely and consuming a variety of fish (**Figure 13.15b**). To minimize consumption of contaminants, remove the skin, fatty material, and dark meat from fish. Use cooking methods such as broiling, poaching, boiling, and baking, which allow contaminants from the fatty portions of fish to drain out. Do not eat the "tomale" in lobster. The tomale, a green paste inside the abdominal cavity of a cooked lobster, serves as the liver and pancreas and is the organ in which toxins accumulate. The analogous organ in blue crabs, called the "mustard" because of its yellow color, should also be avoided (see *What Should I Eat?*).

Reducing exposure to pesticides and pollutants • Figure 13.15

a. Pesticide residues on fruits and vegetables can be removed or reduced by peeling or washing with tap water and scrubbing with a brush, if appropriate. In the case of leafy vegetables such as lettuce and cabbage, the outer leaves can be removed and discarded. Washing apples, cucumbers, eggplant, squash, and tomatoes may not remove all the pesticides because these fruits and vegetables are coated with wax in order to maintain freshness by sealing in moisture, but wax also seals in pesticides. The wax and pesticides can be removed by peeling, but removing the peel also eliminates fiber and some micronutrients.

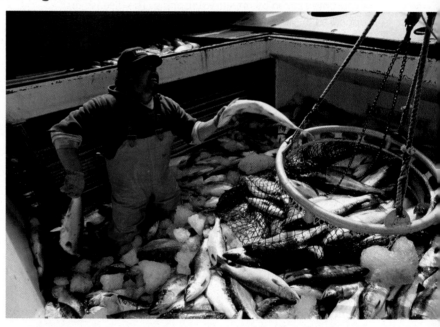

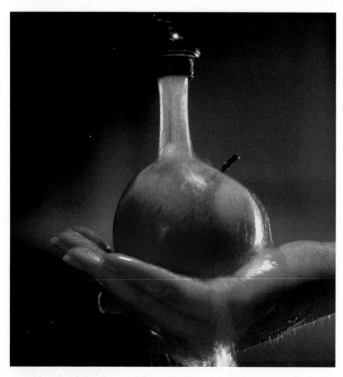

b. Exposure to chemical contaminants can be minimized by choosing saltwater fish caught well offshore, away from polluted coastal waters. Fish that live near the shore or spend part of their life cycle in fresh water are more likely to contain contaminants. Smaller species of fish are safer because they are earlier in the food chain, and smaller fish within a species are safer because they are younger and hence have had less time to accumulate contaminants (see Figure 13.10).

WHAT SHOULD I EAT?
Food Safety

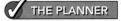

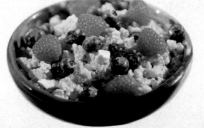

Avoid ingesting pathogenic microbes
- Make sure your burger is well done.
- Skip the runny eggs and have them scrambled.
- Pass on the dough! Treat yourself to chocolate chip cookies only after they come out of the oven.
- Slice up some melon, but make sure the knife, the cutting board, and the skin of the melon are clean before you slice it.

Reduce pesticides and pollutants in your food
- Buy locally grown produce.
- Look for the organic symbol.
- Try the small fish in the pond.
- Make a salad after you have washed the lettuce and peeled off the outer leaves.
- Trim the fat and don't eat the skin of poultry and fish.

Use iProfile to compare the Calories and grams of fat in a chicken breast with and without skin.

CONCEPT CHECK STOP

1. **How** can a pesticide used on broccoli plants end up in milk?

2. **How** can organic food cause food-borne illness?

3. **What** can you do to minimize PCBs in your diet?

Technology for Keeping Food Safe
LEARNING OBJECTIVES

1. **Describe** how temperature is used to prevent food spoilage.

2. **Discuss** how irradiation preserves food.

3. **Explain** how packaging protects food.

4. **Discuss** the risks and benefits of food additives.

ood spoils when its taste, texture, or nutritional value is changed either by enzymes that are naturally present in the food or by microbes that grow on the food. For thousands of years, humans have treated food in order to prevent spoilage. Techniques that preserve food work by destroying enzymes present in the food, by killing microbes, or by slowing microbial growth (**Table 13.5**).

FAT TOM	Table 13.5
The acronym FAT TOM reminds us of the factors that affect microbial growth. Most food preservation techniques modify one or more of these factors to stop or slow microbial growth.	
Food	This is where the bacteria grow.
Acidity	Most bacteria grow best at a pH near neutral. Some food additives, such as citric acid and ascorbic acid (vitamin C), are acids, which prevent microbial growth by lowering the pH of food.
Time	The longer a food sits at an optimum growth temperature, the more bacteria it will contain. Preservation methods such as canning and pasteurization kill microbes by heating food to an appropriate temperature for the right amount of time.
Temperature	The high temperatures of canning, cooking, and pasteurization kill microbes, and the low temperatures of freezing and refrigeration slow or stop microbial growth.
Oxygen	In order to grow, most bacteria need oxygen, so packaging that eliminates oxygen prevents their growth.
Moisture	Bacteria need water to grow, so preservation methods such as drying or use of high concentrations of salt or sugar, which draw water away by osmosis, prevent bacteria from growing.

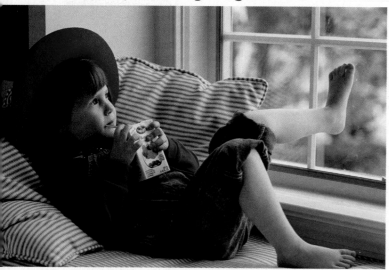

The juice boxes that fit so conveniently into school lunch bags are produced by aseptic processing. This technique heats foods to temperatures that result in sterilization. The sterilized foods are then placed in sterilized packages, using sterilized packaging equipment. If the package remains unopened, juice or milk packaged aseptically can remain free of microbial growth at room temperature for years.

Most of the oldest methods of food preservation—heating, cooling, drying, smoking, and adding substances such as sugar or salt—are still used today. In addition, newer methods, such as irradiation and specialized packaging, have been developed. While all these technologies offer benefits, they can also create risks. Some risk arises when substances find their way into food, either accidentally or as a normal part of the production process. The FDA considers any substance that can be expected to become part of a food a **food additive** and regulates the types and amounts of food additives that may be present in a particular food. Unexpected substances that enter food are considered **accidental contaminants** and are not regulated.

food additive A substance that is intentionally added to or can reasonably be expected to become a component of a food during processing.

accidental contaminant A substance not regulated by the FDA that unexpectedly enters the food supply.

High and Low Temperature

Cooking food is one of the oldest methods of ensuring that food is safe. Cooking kills disease-causing organisms and destroys most toxins. Other preservation techniques that rely on high temperature to kill microbes include **pasteurization**, sterilization, and **aseptic processing** (**Figure 13.16**). Lowering the temperature of food by means of refrigeration or freezing does not kill

pasteurization The process of heating food products in order to kill disease-causing organisms.

aseptic processing The placement of sterilized food in a sterilized package using a sterile process.

microbes but preserves the food and protects consumers because it slows or stops microbial growth.

Preservation techniques that rely on temperature benefit consumers by providing appealing, safe foods, but these foods are not risk free, particularly if they are handled incorrectly. If foods are not heated long enough or to a high enough temperature, or if they are not kept cold enough, they could pose a risk of food-borne illness. In addition, some types of cooking can generate hazardous chemicals. Carcinogenic chemicals produced during the cooking of meats include **polycyclic aromatic hydrocarbons (PAHs)** and **heterocyclic amines (HCAs)**. PAHs are formed when fat drips on a grill and burns. They rise with the smoke and are deposited on the surface of the food. PAH formation can be minimized by selecting lower-fat meat and using a layer of aluminum foil to prevent fat from dripping on the coals. HCAs are produced by the burning of amino acids and other substances in meats and are formed during any type of high-temperature cooking. HCA formation can be reduced by precooking meat, marinating meat before cooking, cooking at lower temperatures, and reducing cooking time by using smaller pieces of meat and avoiding overcooking. The cooking temperatures recommended by the FDA are designed to prevent microbial food-borne illness and minimize the production of PAHs and HCAs. Because PAHs and HCAs are considered accidental contaminants, their amounts in food are not regulated by the FDA.

Another contaminant formed during food preparation is **acrylamide**. It is formed as a result of chemical reactions that occur during high-temperature baking or frying, particularly in carbohydrate-rich foods. The highest levels of acrylamide are found in French fries

Irradiated foods Figure • Figure 13.17

a. Irradiated foods must be labeled with the radura symbol shown here and the statement "treated with radiation" or "treated by irradiation." This symbol is not required on the labels of foods that contain irradiated spices or other irradiated ingredients.

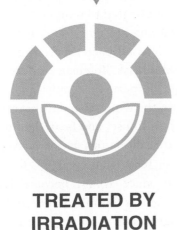

TREATED BY IRRADIATION

NON - IRRADIATED   IRRADIATED

b. Irradiation increases the safety and shelf life of foods and does not compromise nutritional quality or noticeably change food texture, taste, or appearance, as long as it is properly applied to a suitable product. After two weeks in cold storage, the strawberries on the right, which were treated by irradiation, remain free of mold, whereas the untreated strawberries on the left, which were picked at the same time, are covered with mold.

and snack chips. Smaller amounts are found in coffee and in foods made from grains, such as breakfast cereal and cookies. High doses can cause cancer and reproductive problems in experimental animals and act as neurotoxins in humans. Thus far, dietary exposure to acrylamide has not been associated with cancer in humans, and more research is needed to determine whether long-term, low-level exposure has any cumulative effects.[32] Methods for reducing the amounts and potential toxicity of acrylamide in foods are being investigated.[33]

Food Irradiation

Food **irradiation**, also called cold pasteurization, is used in more than 40 countries to treat everything from frog legs to rice. Irradiation exposes food to high doses of X-rays, gamma radiation, or high-energy electrons in order to kill microbes and insects and inactivate enzymes that cause germination and ripening of fruits and vegetables (**Figure 13.17**).[34] Because irradiation produces compounds that are not present in the original

> **irradiation** A process that exposes foods to radiation in order to kill contaminating organisms and retard the ripening and spoilage of fruits and vegetables.

foods, it is treated as a food additive, and the level of radiation that may be used is regulated. At the allowed levels of radiation, the amounts of these compounds produced are almost negligible and have not been found to pose a risk to consumers.[35]

Food irradiation is used relatively infrequently in the United States because of a lack of irradiation facilities and because of public suspicion of the technology. The word *irradiation* fosters the belief that the food becomes radioactive. Opponents of food irradiation claim that it introduces carcinogens, depletes the nutritional value of food, and is used to allow the sale of previously contaminated foods. In fact, irradiated food is not radioactive, and scientific studies conducted over the past 50 years have found that the benefits of irradiation outweigh the potential risks.[36] Irradiation can decrease the amounts of certain nutrients in foods, but these nutrient losses are similar to those that occur with canning or refrigerated storage.[35]

Because irradiation can be used in place of chemical treatments, it reduces consumers' exposure to chemical pesticides and preservatives. It is one of the technologies promoted by the National Food Safety Initiative because of its potential for improving the safety of food and reducing the incidence of food-borne illness.

Food Packaging

Packaging plays an important role in food preservation; it keeps molds and bacteria out, keeps moisture in, and protects food from physical damage. An open package of refrigerated cheddar cheese will be moldy in a few days, but an unopened package will stay fresh for weeks.

Food packaging is continually being improved. In the past two decades, for instance, consumer demand for fresh and easy-to-prepare foods has led manufacturers to offer partially cooked pasta, vegetables, seafood, fresh and cured meats, and dry products such as whole-bean and ground coffee in packaging that, if unopened, will keep perishable food fresh much longer than will conventional packaging. **Modified atmosphere packaging (MAP)** uses plastics or other packaging materials that are impermeable to oxygen. The air inside the package is vacuumed out in order to remove the oxygen. The product can then remain packaged in a vacuum, or the package can be infused with another gas, such as carbon dioxide or nitrogen. The lack of oxygen prevents the growth of aerobic bacteria, slows the ripening of fruits and vegetables, and slows down oxidation reactions, which cause discoloration in fruits and vegetables and rancidity in fats.

> **modified atmosphere packaging (MAP)** A preservation technique used to prolong the shelf life of processed or fresh food by changing the gases surrounding the food in the package.

MAP is often used to package cooked entrées such as pasta primavera or beef teriyaki. The raw ingredients are sealed in a plastic pouch, the air is vacuumed out, and the pouch and its contents are partially precooked and immediately refrigerated. This processing eliminates the need for the extreme cold of freezing or the extreme heat of canning, so flavor and nutrients are better preserved. Because these products are not heated to temperatures high enough to kill all bacteria and are not stored at temperatures low enough to prevent all bacteria from growing, they could pose a food safety risk. To ensure safety, fresh refrigerated foods should be purchased only from reputable vendors, used before the expiration date printed on the package, refrigerated until use, and heated according to the time and temperature directions on the package.

Packaging can protect food from spoilage, but even the best packaging can introduce risk if it becomes part of the food. A variety of substances found in paper and plastic containers and packaging, and even dishes, can leach into food (**Figure 13.18**). Substances that are known to contaminate food are regulated by the EPA and the FDA. However, these regulations apply only to the intended use of the product. When a product is used improperly, substances from its packaging can migrate into food. For instance, some plastics migrate into food when heated in a microwave oven. Thus, only containers designed for microwave cooking should be used for microwaving food.

Bisphenol A from plastics • Figure 13.18

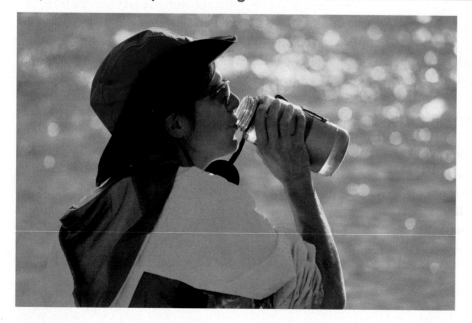

Bisphenol A is a chemical found in polycarbonate plastic used to manufacture hard, transparent water bottles, baby bottles, and food containers as well as the coating inside cans. The transfer of bisphenol A into food and water is a concern for pregnant women and infants. A review by the U.S. National Toxicology Program found that although there is negligible risk of adverse effects in most adults, exposure of pregnant women to bisphenol A could affect fetal brain development, and exposure of infants and children to the chemical could affect the nervous system and accelerate puberty. [37]

To minimize any risk posed by nitrosamines without increasing the risk of bacterial food-borne illness, the FDA limits the amount of nitrate and nitrite that can be added to food and requires the addition of antioxidants such as vitamin C, which reduce nitrosamine formation, to foods that contain these additives. Consumers can reduce nitrosamine exposure by limiting their consumption of cured meat to 3 to 4 ounces per week and maintaining adequate intakes of the antioxidant vitamins C and E.

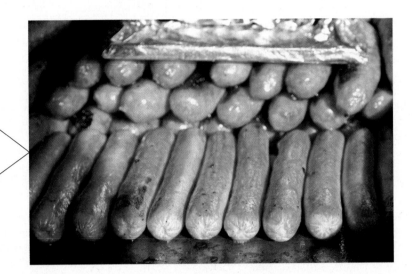

INGREDIENTS: MECHANICALLY SEPARATED CHICKEN, WATER, PORK, MODIFIED CORN STARCH, DEXTROSE, SALT, BEEF, CONTAINS 2% OR LESS OF THE FOLLOWING: CORN SYRUP, FLAVORINGS, SODIUM PHOSPHATES, POTASSIUM LACTATE, SODIUM DIACETATE, SODIUM ASCORBATE (VITAMIN C), OLEO RESIN OF PAPRIKA, SODIUM NITRITE

Food Additives

What keeps bread from molding, gives margarine its yellow color, and keeps Parmesan cheese from clumping in the shaker? The answer to all these questions is food additives. Substances that are intentionally added to foods are called **direct food additives**. Other substances that get into food unintentionally—such as the oil used to lubricate food processing machinery—are referred to as **indirect food additives**. The FDA regulates the amounts and types of direct and indirect food additives in food.

Regulating food additives Food additives improve food quality and help protect us from disease, but if the wrong additive is used or the wrong amount is added, it could do more harm than good. A manufacturer that wants to use a new food additive must submit to the FDA a petition that describes the chemical composition of the additive, how it is manufactured, and how it is detected in food. The manufacturer must prove that the additive will be effective for its intended purpose at the proposed levels, that it is safe for its intended use, and that its use is necessary. Additives may not be used to disguise inferior products or deceive consumers. They cannot be used if they significantly destroy nutrients or if the same effect can be achieved through sound manufacturing processes.

More than 600 chemicals defined as food additives were already in common use when legislation regulating food additives was passed. To accommodate substances that the FDA or the USDA had already determined to be safe, they were designated as **prior-sanctioned substances** and are exempt from regulation. The nitrates and nitrites used to retard the growth of *Clostridium botulinum* in cured meats are prior-sanctioned substances, for instance. However, their use has been controversial because they form carcinogenic **nitrosamines** in the digestive tract. They are still allowed in foods, however, because they prevent botulism, and there is little evidence that they pose a serious risk in the amounts consumed in the human diet (**Figure 13.19**).[38]

direct food additive A substance that is intentionally added to food. Direct food additives are regulated by the FDA.

indirect food additive A substance that is expected to unintentionally enter food during manufacturing or from packaging. Indirect food additives are regulated by the FDA.

Common food additives[40]   Table 13.6

Type of additive	What's on the label	What they do	Where they are used
Preservatives	Ascorbic acid, citric acid, sodium benzoate, calcium propionate, sodium erythorbate, sodium nitrite, calcium sorbate, potassium sorbate, BHA, BHT, EDTA, tocopherols	Maintain freshness; prevent spoilage caused by bacteria, molds, fungi, or yeast; slow or prevent changes in color, flavor, or texture; and delay rancidity	Jellies, beverages, baked goods, cured meats, oils and margarines, cereals, dressings, snack foods, fruits and vegetables
Sweeteners	Sucrose, glucose, fructose, sorbitol, mannitol, corn syrup, high-fructose corn syrup, saccharin, aspartame, sucralose, acesulfame potassium (acesulfame-K), neotame	Add sweetness with or without extra calories	Beverages, baked goods, table-top sweeteners, many processed foods
Color additives	FD&C blue nos. 1 and 2, FD&C green no. 3, FD&C red nos. 3 and 40, FD&C yellow nos. 5 and 6, orange B, citrus red no. 2, annatto extract, beta-carotene, grapeskin extract, cochineal extract or carmine, paprika oleoresin, caramel color, fruit and vegetable juices, saffron, colorings or color added	Prevent color loss due to exposure to light, air, temperature extremes, and moisture; enhance colors; give color to colorless and "fun" foods	Processed foods, candies, snack foods, margarine, cheese, soft drinks, jellies, puddings and pie fillings
Flavors, spices, and flavor enhancers	Natural flavoring, artificial flavor, spices, monosodium glutamate (MSG), hydrolyzed soy protein, autolyzed yeast extract, disodium guanylate or inosinate	Add specific flavors or enhance flavors already present in foods	Many processed foods, puddings and pie fillings, gelatin mixes, cake mixes, salad dressings, candies, soft drinks, ice cream, BBQ sauce
Nutrients	Thiamine hydrochloride, riboflavin (vitamin B_2), niacin, niacinamide, folate or folic acid, beta-carotene, potassium iodide, iron or ferrous sulfate, alpha-tocopherols, ascorbic acid, vitamin D, amino acids (L-tryptophan, L-lysine, L-leucine, L-methionine)	Replace vitamins and minerals lost in processing; add nutrients that may be lacking in the diet	Flour, breads, cereals, rice, pasta, margarine, salt, milk, fruit beverages, energy bars, breakfast drinks
Emulsifiers	Soy lecithin, mono- and diglycerides, egg yolks, polysorbates, sorbitan monostearate	Allow smooth mixing and prevent separation; reduce stickiness; control crystallization; keep ingredients dispersed	Salad dressings, peanut butter, chocolate, margarine, frozen desserts
Stabilizers and thickeners, binders, and texturizers	Gelatin, pectin, guar gum, carrageenan, xanthan gum, whey	Produce uniform texture, improve "mouth-feel"	Frozen desserts, dairy products, cakes, pudding and gelatin mixes, dressings, jams and jellies, sauces
pH control agents and acidulants	Lactic acid, citric acid, ammonium hydroxide, sodium carbonate	Control acidity and alkalinity, prevent spoilage	Beverages, frozen desserts, chocolate, low-acid canned foods, baking powder
Leavening agents	Baking soda, monocalcium phosphate, calcium carbonate	Promote rising of baked goods	Breads and other baked goods
Anti-caking agents	Calcium silicate, iron ammonium citrate, silicon dioxide	Keep powdered foods free-flowing, prevent moisture absorption	Salt, baking powder, confectioners' sugar
Humectants	Glycerin, sorbitol	Retain moisture	Shredded coconut, marshmallows, soft candies, confections

A second category that is not subject to food additive regulation consists of substances **generally recognized as safe (GRAS)**, based either on their history of use in food before 1958 or on published scientific evidence. However, just because a substance is on the GRAS or prior-sanctioned list doesn't mean that it is safe or that it will stay on these lists. If new evidence suggests that a substance in either category is unsafe, the FDA may take action to require that the substance be removed from food products.

> **generally recognized as safe (GRAS)** A group of chemical additives that are considered safe, based on their long-standing presence in the food supply without harmful effects.

Substances that are toxic at some level of consumption may be harmless at a lower level. To ensure that additives are safe, most of those that are allowed in foods can be added only at levels 100 times below the highest level that has been shown to have no harmful effects. This is a greater margin of safety than exists for many vitamins and other naturally occurring substances.

The regulations for substances that cause cancer are far more rigid because of the **Delaney Clause**, part of the 1958 Food Additives Amendment. It states that a substance that induces cancer in either an animal species or humans, at any dosage, may not be added to food. Debate continues regarding whether the Delaney Clause should be liberalized to allow the use of substances that are added at a level so low that they would not represent a significant health risk.

Identifying food additives

Food additives are used to make food safer; maintain palatability and wholesomeness; improve color, flavor, or texture; aid in processing; and enhance nutritional value (**Table 13.6**). Their use ensures the availability of wholesome, appetizing, and affordable foods that meet consumer demands throughout the year. The FDA's database *Everything Added to Food in the United States* lists more than 3000 additives.[39] Many of these, such as sugar and spices, are used in homes every day. Other additives may sound like a chemical soup: calcium propionate in bread, disodium EDTA in kidney beans, and BHA in potato chips. Understanding what these chemicals are used for can help make the ingredient list a source of information rather than a cause for concern.

Sensitivities to additives

Some individuals are allergic or sensitive to certain food additives. For example, the flavor enhancer monosodium glutamate (MSG), commonly used in Chinese food, can cause adverse reactions known as *MSG symptom complex* or *Chinese restaurant syndrome* in sensitive individuals (see Chapter 6). Sulfites can cause symptoms ranging from stomachache and hives to severe asthma. Sulfites are used as preservatives in baked goods, canned foods, condiments, and dried fruits. Sensitive individuals can identify foods that contain sulfites by checking food labels. The forms of sulfites allowed in packaged foods include sulfur dioxide, sodium sulfite, sodium and potassium bisulfite, and sodium and potassium metabisulfite. Foods served in restaurants may also contain sulfites. For example, a potato dish served in a restaurant may be prepared using potatoes that were peeled and soaked in a sulfite solution before cooking.

Color additives can also cause adverse reactions. FD&C yellow no. 5, for instance, listed as tartrazine on medicine labels, may cause itching and hives in sensitive people. It is found in beverages, desserts, and processed vegetables. Color additives are listed in the ingredient list along with other food additives. Colors in foods are classified as certified or exempt. Certified colors are human-made, meet strict specifications for purity, and must be listed by name in the ingredient list. Colors that are exempt from certification include pigments from natural sources such as dehydrated beets and carotenoids; these may be listed collectively in the ingredient list as "artificial color."

CONCEPT CHECK

1. **What** is pasteurization?
2. **How** does irradiation help extend the shelf life of food?
3. **How** does modified atmosphere packaging prevent food spoilage?
4. **Why** are food additives regulated?

Biotechnology

LEARNING OBJECTIVES

1. **Explain** how genetic engineering introduces new traits into plants.

2. **List** ways in which genetic engineering is being used to enhance the food supply.

3. **Discuss** some potential risks associated with genetic engineering.

4. **Describe** how genetically modified foods and crops are regulated to ensure safety.

Biotechnology alters the characteristics of organisms by making selective changes in their DNA. The concept is not new. For centuries, farmers have selected seeds from plants with the most desirable characteristics to plant for the next year's crop, bred the animals that grew fastest or produced the most milk to improve the productivity of the next generation of animals, and crossbred plant varieties to combine the desired traits of each. However, these traditional methods may require many generations to produce the desired results. Biotechnology uses **genetic engineering** to select genes for specific traits. Genetic engineering has significantly sped up the process of modifying the traits of organisms. Like all other new technologies, however, it may introduce new risks.

> **biotechnology** The process of manipulating life forms via genetic engineering in order to provide desirable products for human use.

> **genetic engineering** A set of techniques used to manipulate DNA for the purpose of changing the characteristics of an organism or creating a new product.

> **recombinant DNA** DNA that has been formed by joining DNA from different sources.

How Biotechnology Works

Genetically modified (GM) crops are created through genetic engineering: A piece of DNA containing the gene for a desired characteristic is taken from plant, animal, or bacterial cells and transferred to plant cells (**Figure 13.20**). The DNA is then referred to as **recombinant DNA** because the new DNA is a combination of the DNA from two organisms. The modified cells are then allowed to divide into more and more cells and eventually

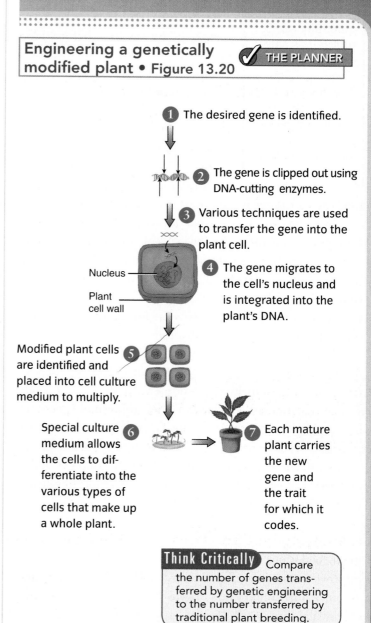

Engineering a genetically modified plant • Figure 13.20 ✓ THE PLANNER

1. The desired gene is identified.
2. The gene is clipped out using DNA-cutting enzymes.
3. Various techniques are used to transfer the gene into the plant cell.
4. The gene migrates to the cell's nucleus and is integrated into the plant's DNA.

Nucleus

Plant cell wall

5. Modified plant cells are identified and placed into cell culture medium to multiply.

6. Special culture medium allows the cells to differentiate into the various types of cells that make up a whole plant.

7. Each mature plant carries the new gene and the trait for which it codes.

Think Critically Compare the number of genes transferred by genetic engineering to the number transferred by traditional plant breeding.

differentiate into the various types of cells that make up a whole plant. The new plant is a **transgenic** organism. Each cell in the new plant contains the transferred gene for the desired trait. This technique is used to introduce characteristics such as disease and drought resistance into plants. Genetic engineering is more difficult in animals because animal cells do

> **transgenic** An organism with a gene or group of genes intentionally transferred from another species or breed.

not take up genes as easily as plant cells do, and making copies of these cells (clones) is also more difficult. However, these techniques have been used to produce cows that yield more milk, cattle and pigs with more meat on them, and sheep that grow more wool.[41]

Applications of Biotechnology

The techniques of biotechnology can be used in a variety of ways in food production to alter quantity, quality, cost, safety, and shelf life. By making plants resistant to herbicides, insects, and various plant diseases, this technology has increased crop yields and reduced damage from insects and plant diseases (**Figure 13.21a** and **b**). By altering enzyme activity and other traits, biotechnology is being used to increase the shelf life of fresh fruits and vegetables and create products that have greater consumer appeal, such as seedless grapes and watermelons.

Biotechnology is also used in food processing. For example, many foods are produced with the help of enzymes. Rennet, an enzyme used in cheese production; enzymes used in the production of high-fructose corn syrup; and the enzyme lactase, used to reduce the lactose content of milk, are now all produced by GM microbes.

Biotechnology also has great potential for addressing the problem of world hunger and malnutrition. Although world hunger is rooted in political, economic, and cultural issues that cannot be resolved by agricultural technology alone, GM crops that target some of the major nutritional deficiencies worldwide are being developed. To address protein deficiency, varieties of corn, soybeans, and sweet potatoes with enhanced levels of essential amino acids are being developed. To address vitamin A deficiency, genes that code for the production of enzymes needed for the synthesis of the vitamin A precursor β-carotene have been inserted into rice (**Figure 13.21c**).[44] To address multiple nutrient deficiencies, the BioCassava Plus program has used biotechnology to develop cassava with increased zinc, iron, protein, and vitamin A levels.[45]

Nutrition InSight   The potential of biotechnology

• **Figure 13.21**

✓ THE PLANNER

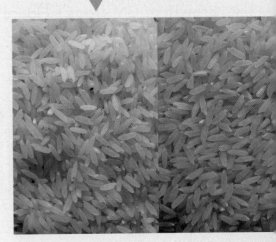

a. Insect-resistant corn is created by inserting a gene from the bacterium *Bacillus thuringiensis* (or Bt). The gene produces a protein called Bt toxin that is toxic to certain insects, such as this European corn borer, but safe for humans and other animals. The presence of the new gene improves the crop yield and also reduces the amounts of chemical pesticides that need to be applied.

c. Half the world's population depends on rice as a dietary staple, but rice is a poor source of vitamin A. Genetically modified rice, called golden rice (seen here compared with white rice) for the color imparted by the β-carotene pigment, has the potential to significantly increase vitamin A intake (discussed further in Chapter 14 *Debate*). One variety contains enough provitamin A in 1/2 cup of dry rice to provide more than 50% of the RDA for a child.[44]

b. In the 1990s the papaya crop in Hawaii was severely diminished by the papaya ring-spot virus (PRSV). In response, researchers developed papaya that is genetically enhanced to resist PRSV. The seeds were released for commercialization in 1998, allowing Hawaiian papaya production to rebound.[42] This was the first genetically enhanced fruit crop on the market. Genes for resistance to various viruses have also been used to create virus-resistant strains of potatoes, squash, cucumbers, and watermelons.[43]

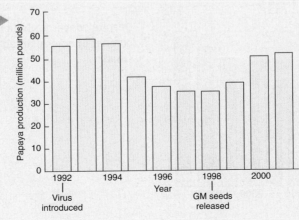

Risks and Regulation of Biotechnology

The rapid advancement of biotechnology during the past decade has created the potential for health problems and environmental damage. Regulations are in place to control the use of genetic engineering and GM products. Despite these precautions, many consumers and scientists believe that the impact of this booming technology has not yet become apparent. They urge that this technology be used with caution to avoid health or environmental impacts that outweigh the benefits.

Consumer concerns Consumer safety concerns related to GM foods include the possibility that the nutrient content of a food may have been negatively affected or that an allergen or a toxin may have inadvertently been introduced into a food that was previously safe. For example, if DNA from fish or nuts—foods that commonly cause allergic reactions—were introduced into soybeans or corn, these foods would then be dangerous to individuals allergic to fish or nuts. To prevent this kind of situation from occurring unintentionally, biotechnology companies have established systems for monitoring the allergenic potential of proteins used for plant genetic engineering. In 1996, allergy testing successfully prevented soybeans containing a gene from a Brazil nut from entering the market.[46]

Environmental concerns An environmental concern about GM crops is that they will be used to the exclusion of other varieties, thereby reducing biodiversity. The ability of populations of organisms to adapt to new conditions, diseases, or other hazards depends on the presence of many different species and varieties that provide a diversity of genes. If farmers plant only GM insect-resistant, high-yielding crops, other species and varieties may eventually become extinct, and the genes for the traits they possess may be lost forever.

Another environmental issue is the possibility that GM crops will create "superweeds." This might occur, for example, if a trait such as increased rate of growth introduced into a domesticated plant species were passed on to a related wild species. This could produce a fast-growing weed, or superweed, that would compete with the domesticated species. As a safeguard, plant developers are avoiding introducing genes for traits that could increase a plant's competitiveness or other undesirable properties in weedy relatives.

There is also concern that crops that have been engineered to produce pesticides will promote the evolution of pesticide-resistant insects. An illustration is the case of insects that feed on plants modified to produce the Bt toxin (see Figure 13.21a). As more and more of the insects' food supply consists of plants that produce this pesticide, only insects that carry genes that make them resistant to Bt toxin survive and reproduce. This increases the number of Bt-resistant insects and therefore reduces the effectiveness of Bt toxin as a method of pest control. Although an important concern when growing GM crops, pesticide-resistant insects may also evolve when pesticides are sprayed on crops.

Regulation of GM food products The most common GM crops are soybeans, corn, cotton, and rapeseed (or canola) (**Figure 13.22**). Therefore, foods produced in the United States that contain corn or high-fructose corn syrup, such as many breakfast cereals, snack foods, and soft drinks; foods made with soybeans and foods made

Growth of GM crops • Figure 13.22

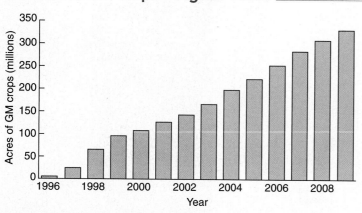

Despite concerns about the impact of GM crops, the number of acres planted with them worldwide has risen steadily.

with cottonseed and canola oils, are likely to contain GM ingredients. You don't recognize these foods as genetically modified because they appear no different from other foods, and food manufacturers are not required to provide special labeling unless the food is known to pose a potential risk.

To ensure that GM plants and foods cause no harm to consumers or to the environment, the FDA, the USDA, and the EPA are all involved in overseeing plant biotechnology. Safety and environmental issues are monitored at all stages of the process. The FDA regulates the safety and labeling of foods containing GM ingredients. Labeling of foods containing GM ingredients is required only if the nutritional composition of the food has been altered; if it contains potentially harmful allergens, toxins, pesticides, or herbicides; if it contains ingredients that are new to the food supply; or if it has been changed significantly enough that its traditional name no longer applies. Premarket approval is required when the new food contains a substance that is not commonly found in foods or when it contains a substance that does not have a history of safe use in foods. To prevent material from a new plant variety intended for food use from inadvertently entering the food supply before its safety has been established, the FDA has asked developers to provide them with information about the safety of the new plants at a relatively early stage of development.[47]

The USDA regulates agricultural products and research concerning the development of new plant varieties, including those developed through genetic engineering. The EPA regulates any pesticides that may be present in foods and sets tolerances for these pesticides. This includes GM plants containing proteins that protect them from insects or disease.

CONCEPT CHECK STOP

1. **Where** does the DNA introduced into GM plants come from?
2. **How** does biotechnology increase crop yields?
3. **Why** might a GM food cause an allergic reaction when the unmodified food does not?
4. **What** types of GM foods carry special labels?

THE PLANNER ✓

Summary

1 Keeping Food Safe 466

- Most **food-borne illness** is caused by food contaminated with disease-causing **microbes**; occasionally, it can be caused by chemical contaminants in food. The harm caused by contaminants in the food supply depends on the type of toxin, dose, length of time over which the contaminant is consumed, how it is metabolized and excreted, and the size, age, and health of the consumer.

- The food supply is monitored for safety by food manufacturers, as shown here, and regulatory agencies at the international, federal, state, and local levels. Federal programs promote the use of **Hazard Analysis Critical Control Point (HACCP)** systems to prevent and eliminate food contamination rather than catch it after it occurs. Consumers can prevent most cases of food-borne illness by following safe food-handling and preparation guidelines.

Keeping food safe from farm to table
• Figure 13.1

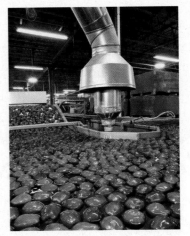

2 Pathogens in Food 470

- The **pathogens** that affect the food supply include bacteria, viruses, molds, parasites, and prions. Some bacteria cause **food-borne infection** because they are able to grow in the gastrointestinal tract when ingested. Others produce toxins in food, and consumption of the toxin causes **food-borne intoxication.**

- Viruses do not grow on food, but when consumed in food, they can reproduce in human cells and cause food-borne illness.

- **Molds** that grow on foods produce toxins that can harm consumers.

- **Parasites** include microscopic single-celled animals, as well as worms that can be seen with the naked eye. They are consumed in contaminated water or food.

- Improperly folded **prion** proteins cause **bovine spongiform encephalopathy (BSE)** in cattle. The risk of acquiring the human form of this deadly degenerative neurological disease is extremely low.

- The risk of food-borne illness can be decreased through proper food selection, preparation, and storage to kill pathogens or minimize their growth. These steps are emphasized by the Fight Bac! campaign illustrated here.

Safe food handling, storage, and preparation • Figure 13.9

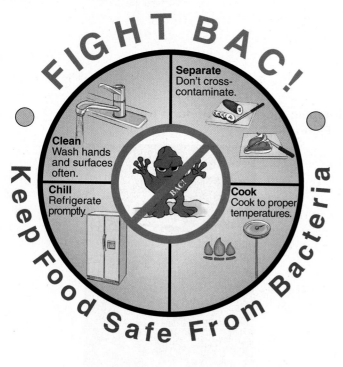

3 Agricultural and Industrial Chemicals in Food 481

- Contaminants in the environment can find their way into the food supply. Those that deposit in the fatty tissue of animals are not eliminated, leading to **bioaccumulation** as they pass through the food chain, as illustrated here.

Contamination throughout the food chain • Figure 13.10

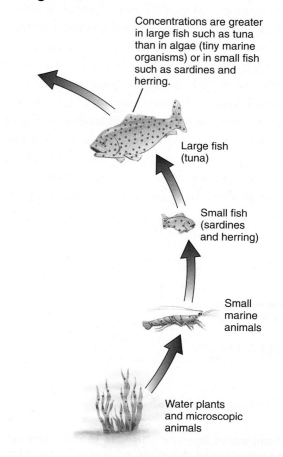

- Pesticides help increase crop yields and the quality of produce. To decrease the risk of pesticide toxicity, **tolerances** are established, and foods are monitored for pesticide residues. Safer pesticides are being developed, and U.S. farmers are reducing the amounts applied by using **integrated pest management (IPM)** and **organic food** production methods.

- Industrial pollutants such as **PCBs** have contaminated some waterways and the fish and shellfish that live in them. Larger, longer-lived fish and those that live in contaminated waters have the highest concentrations.

- Antibiotics and hormones are used in animal food production. The amounts entering the food supply pose little risk, but the use of antibiotics contributes to the development of antibiotic-resistant strains of bacteria.

- Consumers can reduce the amounts of pesticides and other environmental contaminants in food by carefully selecting and handling produce, selecting saltwater varieties of fish caught far offshore in unpolluted waters, and trimming fat from meat, poultry, and fish before cooking.

4 Technology for Keeping Food Safe 487

- Heating foods to high temperatures, cooling them to low temperatures, and altering levels of acidity, moisture, and oxygen prevent food spoilage and lengthen shelf life by killing microbes or slowing their growth.

- **Irradiation** preserves food by exposing it to radiation. This process kills microbes, destroys insects, and slows the germination and ripening of fruits and vegetables. Irradiated foods can be identified by the symbol shown here.

Irradiated foods • Figure 13.17a

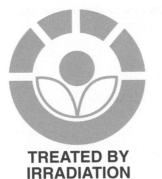

TREATED BY IRRADIATION

- Packaging keeps molds and bacteria out of foods, keeps moisture in, and protects food from physical damage. **Modified atmosphere packaging (MAP)** reduces the oxygen available for microbial growth. The safety of packaging materials must be considered because components of packaging can leach into food.

- **Direct food additives** are used to preserve or enhance the appeal of food. **Indirect food additives** are substances known to find their way into food during cooking, processing, and packaging. Both are FDA regulated. **Accidental contaminants**, which enter food when it is handled or prepared incorrectly, are not regulated by the FDA.

5 Biotechnology 494

- **Biotechnology** produces **genetically modified (GM)** crops by transferring a gene for a desired characteristic from one organism to another, as shown here. The result is a **transgenic** organism.

Engineering a genetically modified plant • Figure 13.20

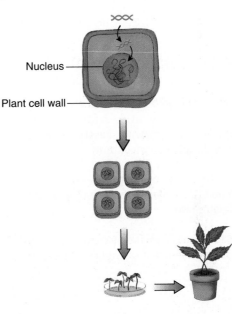

Nucleus

Plant cell wall

- Biotechnology has the potential to improve the volume, safety, and quality of the food supply, but it also has the potential to introduce allergens or toxins into foods or to negatively affect nutrient content. Environmental concerns about the use of GM crops include reduction of biologic diversity, creation of "superweeds," and evolution of pesticide-resistant insects. Regulations are in place to control the use of genetic engineering and GM products.

Key Terms

- accidental contaminant 488
- acrylamide 488
- aseptic processing 488
- bioaccumulation 481
- biotechnology 494
- botulism 472
- bovine somatotropin (bST) 485
- bovine spongiform encephalopathy (BSE) 475
- critical control point 468
- cross-contamination 477
- Delaney Clause 493
- direct food additive 491
- food additive 488
- food-borne illness 466
- food-borne infection 470

- food-borne intoxication 470
- generally recognized as safe (GRAS) 493
- genetic engineering 494
- genetically modified (GM) 494
- Hazard Analysis Critical Control Point (HACCP) 468
- hemolytic-uremic syndrome 470
- heterocyclic amines (HCAs) 488
- indirect food additive 491
- infant botulism 472
- integrated pest management (IPM) 482
- irradiation 489
- microbes 466
- modified atmosphere packaging (MAP) 490
- mold 474

- nitrosamine 491
- organic food 482
- parasite 474
- pasteurization 488
- pathogen 470
- polychlorinated biphenyls (PCBs) 484
- polycyclic aromatic hydrocarbons (PAHs) 488
- prion 475
- prior-sanctioned substance 491
- recombinant DNA 494
- spore 472
- tolerance 482
- transgenic 494
- variant Creutzfeldt-Jakob Disease (vCJD) 475

Online Resources

- For more information on microbial food-borne illness, go to the FDA's Bad Bug Book, at www.fda.gov/Food/FoodSafety/FoodborneIllness/FoodborneIllnessFoodbornePathogensNaturalToxins/BadBugBook/default.htm.

- For more information on pesticides in our foods, go to www.fda.gov/Food/FoodSafety/FoodContaminantsAdulteration/Pesticides/default.htm.

- For more information on food additives, go to www.fda.gov/Food/FoodIngredientsPackaging/ucm115326.htm.

- For more information on biotechnology, go to www.fda.gov/AnimalVeterinary/GuidanceComplianceEnforcement/GuidanceforIndustry/ucm123631.htm.

- Visit your *WileyPLUS* site for videos, animations, podcasts, self-study, and other media that will aid you in studying and understanding this chapter.

Critical and Creative Thinking Questions

1. After 67 people became ill from consuming food at a company picnic, investigators determined that the tossed green salad, the egg salad, and the turkey slices were all contaminated with *Campylobacter*. Invent a scenario that would explain how all three became contaminated.

2. A restaurant decides not to replace an old dishwasher, even though it no longer heats the water to above 135°F. What are the potential risks associated with this decision? How else could the restaurant sanitize the dishes?

3. The chicken Amy brings home from the store is contaminated with *Salmonella*. She prepares a meal by grilling the chicken and making a salad. List the steps in the preparation of this meal that might result in cross-contamination and increase the likelihood of *Salmonella* infection. What steps could Amy take to prevent food-borne illness?

4. A town's voters decide that they can improve their own health and protect the environment by banning the production and sale of all but organically produced foods. What are the risks and benefits of this decision?

5. Fermentation, a process that uses microbes to convert carbohydrates into alcohols or acids, is used to produce alcoholic beverages and yogurt. Explain how fermentation converts milk into yogurt and why yogurt will keep longer than milk.

6. A train crash spills a load of industrial waste into a river that feeds into a local reservoir. Bottled water is provided to the residents of the community. How might this spill impact other segments of the food supply?

7. *Brassica* is a genus of plants that includes cabbage and broccoli, as well as a number of weeds. What risks might be associated with the use of a new genetically engineered variety of *Brassica* that grows faster and produces more seeds than traditional varieties?

What is happening in this picture?

These rye plants are infected with a fungus. When the grain is consumed, the fungal toxins cause a syndrome called ergotism. The symptoms include prickling skin sensations, facial distortions, incomprehensible speech, paralysis, hallucinations, convulsions, and dementia. Ergotism may have caused some of the symptoms exhibited by individuals who were supposedly cursed by the "witches" of 17th-century Salem, Massachusetts.[48]

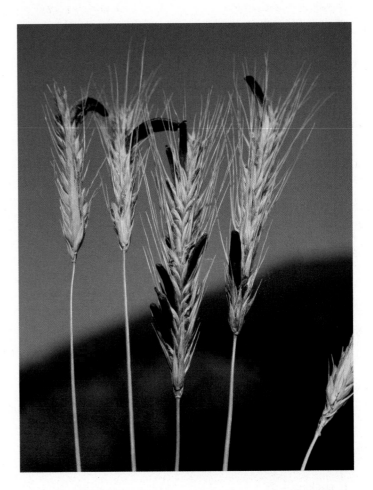

Think Critically

1. How could ergotism cause individuals to appear "bewitched"?
2. Why might moldy rye have been more of a problem in the 17th century than it is today?
3. Why doesn't baking prevent this ailment?

Self-Test

(Check Your Answers in Appendix K.)

1. What is the major cause of food-borne illness in the United States today?

   a. pesticides

   b. microbes

   c. environmental toxins

   d. antibiotics

2. Which factor affects the likelihood that a contaminant will cause food-borne illness in an individual?

   a. body size

   b. immune status

   c. age

   d. dose of toxin

   e. all of the above

3. Foods on the GRAS list _____.

   a. are definitely safe

   b. have been used for years without ill effect

   c. are green

   d. do not need to be listed in an ingredient list

4. Which of the following is not true of a HACCP system?

   a. It relies on visual food inspections.

   b. It identifies steps in food production where contamination can occur or be prevented.

   c. Designing and implementing a HACCP system is the responsibility of a food manufacturer.

   d. It requires extensive record keeping.

   e. It monitors critical points in food production and takes corrective action if criteria are not met.

5. The foods that most frequently cause *Salmonella* infection are _____.

   a. beef and pork

   b. dairy products

   c. eggs and poultry

   d. shellfish

6. Pathogenic bacteria are killed by _____.

   a. freezing

   b. cooking

   c. refrigeration

   d. marinating

7. Below what temperature should food be refrigerated to reduce bacterial growth?

   a. A   b. B   c. C   d. D

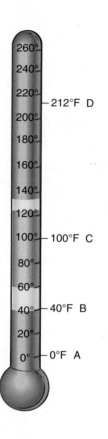

8. Which organism can cause food-borne intoxication and can be present in honey and home-canned foods?

   a. *Escherichia coli*

   b. *Clostridium perfringens*

   c. *Clostridium botulinum*

   d. *Salmonella*

9. Which of the following is most likely to be a concern in hamburger that is cooked to well done on a grill?

   a. polycyclic aromatic hydrocarbons (PAHs)

   b. *Escherichia coli*

   c. *Giardia*

   d. prions

10. Raw hamburger patties are taken to the grill on a platter. After being cooked, they are returned to the unwashed platter and served. This is an example of _____.

    a. efficient use of kitchen equipment

    b. food intoxication

    c. cross-contamination

    d. a HACCP system

11. Glass that enters food from a broken jar is _____.

    a. regulated as an indirect food additive

    b. not regulated

    c. safe because the glass is sterilized

    d. regulated as an accidental contaminant

12. Which organism in this diagram is most likely to contain the highest concentration of industrial contaminants?

    a. A   b. B   c. C   d. D

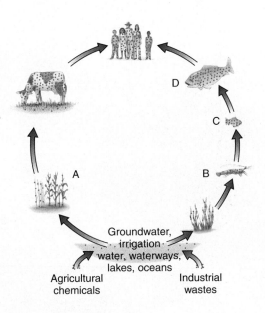

13. The potential benefits of biotechnology include all of the following except _____.

    a. increased biodiversity

    b. enhanced disease resistance

    c. improved crop yields

    d. reduced pesticide use

14. At what step in the process shown here is recombinant DNA formed?

    a. 1

    b. 3

    c. 4

    d. 6

    e. 7

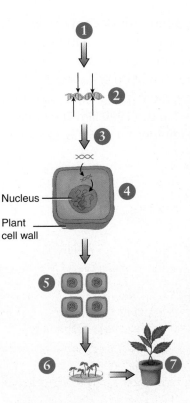

15. The insignia shown here means the food _____.

    a. is not safe to eat

    b. has been irradiated

    c. is radioactive

    d. can safely be stored without refrigeration

THE PLANNER ✓

Review your Chapter Planner on the chapter opener and check off your completed work.

Feeding the World

Fantasists often consider how growing populations will face a world of limited food supplies. In the 1966 novel *Make Room! Make Room!*, New York City's 35 million people subsist on seaweed, oatmeal, rationed water, and soy; meat is a rarity, illegally procured from "meatleggers." In the 1999 film *The Matrix*, a character betrays his comrades for a *virtual* steak dinner.

The 1990s are history, along with the rest of the 20th century, and one may argue that we are not in the dire straits anticipated by these fantasies. Even though disaster has been averted thusfar, the production, distribution, safety, consumption, and sustainability of the world's food and water resources remain matters of great concern to all. A large part of the world's population faces

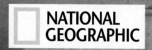

undernutrition and starvation on a daily basis, leading to a plethora of public health issues, another portion faces problems caused by too rich a diet, leading to overnutrition, obesity, and a different—but equally dangerous and costly—set of public health issues.

Governments have historically concerned themselves with adequate food production and distribution for burgeoning populations, but individual self-interest often defeated more altruistic—and sensible—nutrition objectives. Global and national economic and political interests may alleviate or exacerbate world nutrition conditions.

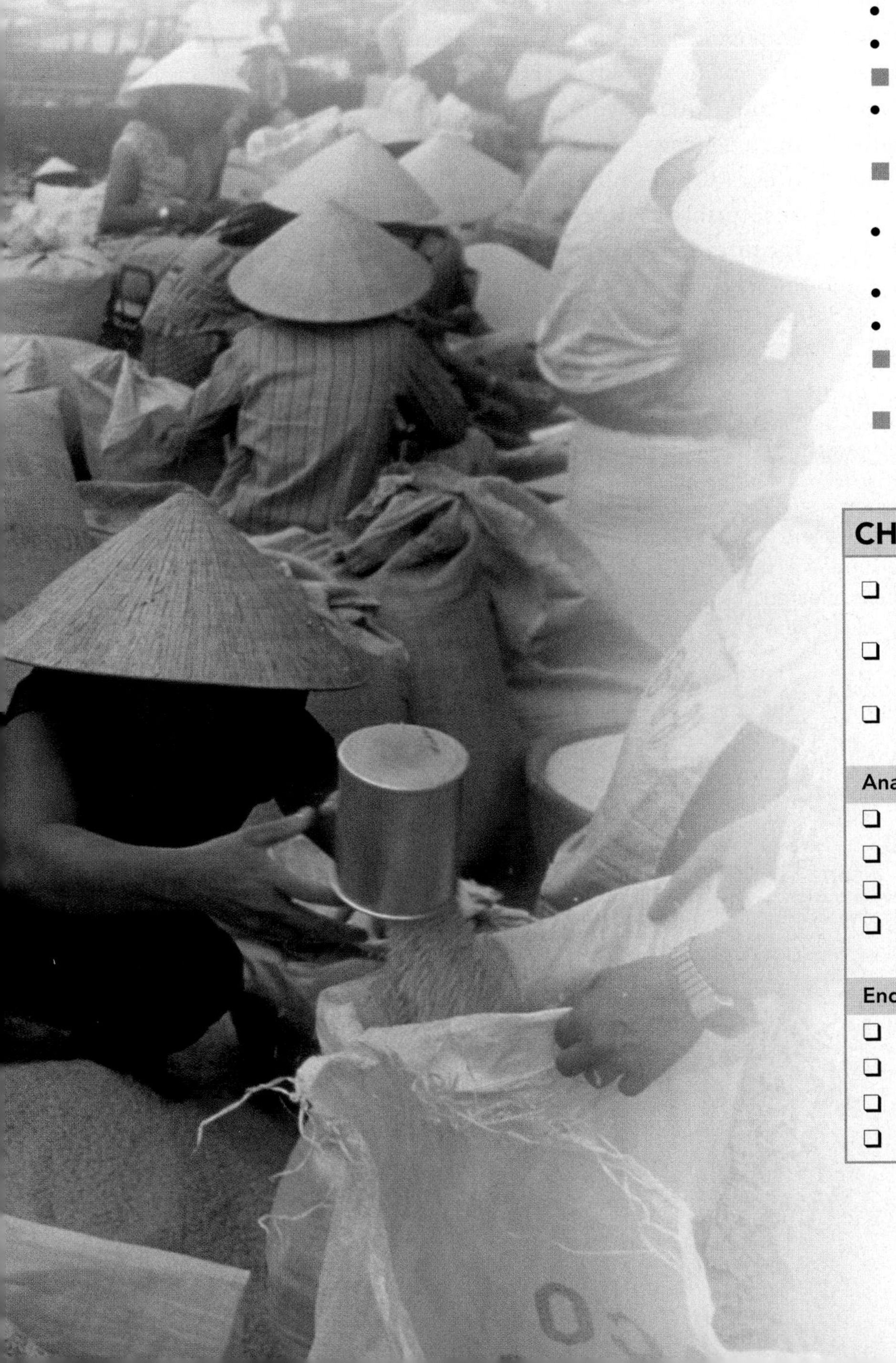

CHAPTER PLANNER ✓

- ❏ Stimulate your interest by reading the introduction and looking at the visual.
- ❏ Scan the Learning Objectives in each section:
  p. 506 ❏   p. 509 ❏   p. 514 ❏   p. 516 ❏
- ❏ Read the text and study all figures and visuals. Answer any questions.

Analyze key features
- ❏ Nutrition InSight, p. 506 ❏   p. 510 ❏
- ❏ What a Scientist Sees, p. 518 ❏
- ❏ Thinking It Through, p. 519 ❏
- ❏ Stop: Answer the Concept Checks before you go on:
  p. 508 ❏   p. 512 ❏   p. 516 ❏   p. 526 ❏

End of chapter
- ❏ Review the Summary, Key Terms, and Online Resources.
- ❏ Answer the Critical and Creative Thinking Questions.
- ❏ Answer What is happening in this picture?
- ❏ Complete the Self-Test and check your answers.

The Two Faces of Malnutrition

LEARNING OBJECTIVES

1. **Compare** the problems of under- and overnutrition in the world today.

2. **Discuss** the impact of undernutrition throughout the life cycle.

3. **Explain** how nutrition transition affects the incidence of obesity.

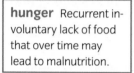

For most of us, the image that comes to mind when we think of malnutrition around the world involves undernutrition: **hunger** and **starvation**. This image is certainly valid because about 925 million people around the world are chronically undernourished, and more than one-third of all deaths in children under age 5 are due to undernutrition.[1,2] At the same time that health organizations are struggling with issues of undernutrition, however, rates of illness related to overnutrition are soaring.[3] The overweight and the undernourished both suffer from malnutrition and experience high levels of sickness and disability, shorter life expectancies, and reduced levels of productivity. These two faces of malnutrition complicate the goal of solving the problem of malnutrition worldwide.

hunger Recurrent involuntary lack of food that over time may lead to malnutrition.

starvation A severe reduction in nutrient and energy intake that impairs health and eventually causes death.

infant mortality rate The number of deaths during the first year of life per 1000 live births.

The Impact of Undernutrition

In populations where hunger is a chronic problem, there is a **cycle of malnutrition** (Figure 14.1a). The cycle begins when women consume a nutrient-deficient diet during pregnancy. These women are more likely than others to give birth to low-birth-weight infants who are susceptible to illness and early death. The **infant mortality rate** and the number of low-birth-weight infants are indicators of a population's health and nutritional status

---

Nutrition InSight | The cycle of malnutrition • Figure 14.1

a. Malnutrition affects the health and productivity of individuals at every stage of life. It often begins in the womb, continues through infancy and childhood, and extends into adolescence and adulthood. Interruption of this cycle of malnutrition at any point can benefit both the individuals affected and their society. Healthy children can then grow into healthy adults, who produce healthy offspring and can contribute fully to society.

b. Low-birth-weight infants are at increased risk for complications, illness, and early death. Survivors often suffer lifelong physical and cognitive disabilities. A higher number of low-birth-weight infants means a higher infant mortality rate. Every year, more than 20 million low-birth-weight babies are born, 95% of them in developing countries.[5]

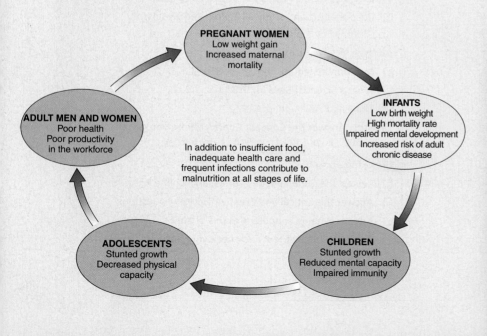

PREGNANT WOMEN
Low weight gain
Increased maternal mortality

INFANTS
Low birth weight
High mortality rate
Impaired mental development
Increased risk of adult chronic disease

In addition to insufficient food, inadequate health care and frequent infections contribute to malnutrition at all stages of life.

CHILDREN
Stunted growth
Reduced mental capacity
Impaired immunity

ADOLESCENTS
Stunted growth
Decreased physical capacity

ADULT MEN AND WOMEN
Poor health
Poor productivity in the workforce

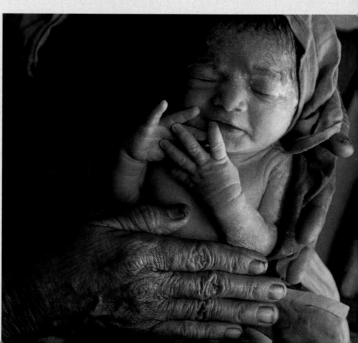

(Figure 14.1b). In most industrialized countries, the infant mortality rate is less than 7 per 1000 live births; in developing countries, the rate is often over 100 per 1000 live births.[4] Low-birth-weight infants who survive require extra nutrients, which usually are not available. Malnutrition in infancy and childhood has a profound effect on growth and development as well as on susceptibility to infectious disease. Infectious diseases are more common in undernourished children, and undernourished children may die of infectious diseases that would not be life threatening in well-nourished children (**Figure 14.1c**).

Malnutrition in children causes **stunting** (**Figure 14.1d**), which is an indicator of undernutrition in a population's children. Stunting in childhood produces smaller adults who have a reduced work capacity and are unable to contribute optimally to their society's economic and social development. Stunted, malnourished women are more likely than others to give birth to low-birth-weight babies. In addition, abdominal obesity in adulthood is more common in those who have experienced lower birth weight and early-childhood stunting.[8]

> **stunting** A decrease in linear growth rate.

Abdominal obesity increases the risk of death from cardiovascular disease, hypertension, and diabetes.

Overnutrition: A World Issue

For the first time in history, with over 1 billion overweight or obese adults worldwide, the number of overnourished people exceeds the number of undernourished people.[9,10] If recent trends continue, by 2030, up to 57.8% of the world's adult population could be either overweight or obese.[11] Because obesity increases the risk of cardiovascular disease, hypertension, stroke, type 2 diabetes, certain cancers, and arthritis, among other conditions, it is a major contributor to the global burden of chronic disease and disability.

The prevalence of overweight and obesity is also growing among children worldwide. According to recent estimates, about 43 million children under age 5 are overweight; 35 million of these children live in developing countries.[9] In some countries, a high prevalence of overweight children now exists alongside a high prevalence of undernourished children. Overweight and obese children are likely to stay obese into adulthood and are more likely to develop diseases such as diabetes and cardiovascular diseases at a younger age.

✓ THE PLANNER

c. Well over half of all deaths in children under 5 years are due to infectious disease. The rate of mortality from infections is increased among malnourished children. It is estimated that 35% of deaths in children under age 5 occur due to the presence of undernutrition.[6] Immunizations against infectious disease are less effective in malnourished children because their immune systems cannot respond normally.

Causes of death in neonates and children under age 5 in the world

- Noncommunicable disease (postneonatal) 4%
- Injuries (postneonatal) 4%
- Other infectious and parasitic diseases 9%
- HIV/AIDS 2%
- Measles 4%
- Malaria 7%
- Neonatal deaths 37%
- Diarrheal diseases (postneonatal) 16%
- Acute respiratory infectious disease (postneonatal) 17%

d. A nurse checks the growth of this child in Indonesia. In developing countries, more than 30% of children under age 5 suffer from stunting.[7] Deficiencies of energy, protein, vitamin A, iodine, iron, and zinc, as well as prolonged infections, have been implicated as causes.

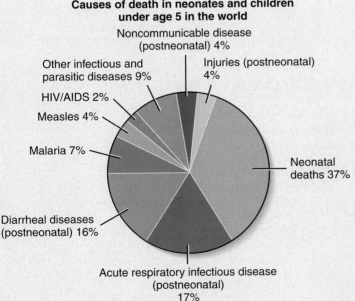

Interpreting Data

Malnutrition increases susceptibility to infections. What percentage of all deaths in children under age 5 is due to infectious diseases?
a. 9%   c. 55%
b. 17%   d. 63%

a. This schematic represents the dietary changes that occur with nutrition transition and the health consequences associated with these changes.[12] The traditional rural diet is often inadequate in energy, protein, or micronutrients. The affluent Western diet meets nutrient needs but is high in fat and sugar and low in fiber. A diet that falls somewhere between these extremes is optimal for health.

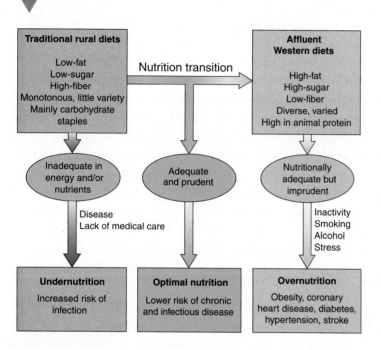

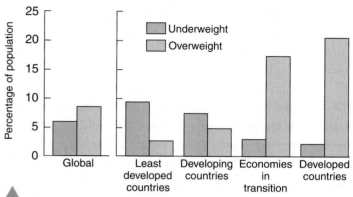

Ask Yourself

Infectious disease is the leading cause of death in developing countries. After a country has undergone nutrition transition, what types of diseases are the leading causes of death?

b. As countries develop economically, they face many of the problems that are common in industrialized countries, including obesity.[10] In Argentina, Colombia, Mexico, Paraguay, Peru, and Uruguay, more than half of the population is overweight or obese.[13] Countries such as China and India, which have historically been plagued by undernutrition, must now also contend with overnutrition.[14] And in parts of Africa, obesity is now considered a major disease, along with AIDS and malnutrition.

Why Do Undernutrition and Overnutrition Exist Side by Side?

We see the problems of undernutrition and overnutrition existing side by side because diets and lifestyles change as economic conditions improve. Traditional diets in developing countries are based on a limited number of foods—primarily starchy grains and root vegetables. As incomes increase and food availability improves, the diet becomes more varied, and energy intake increases with the addition of meat, milk, and other more calorie-dense foods. Along with these dietary changes, there is a decrease in activity due to occupations being less physically demanding, greater access to transportation, more labor-saving technology, and more passive leisure time (**Figure 14.2a**).

Some of the effects of this **nutrition transition** are positive: Life expectancy increases, and the frequencies of low birth weight, infectious diseases, and nutrient deficiencies decrease. However, at the same time, rates of heart disease, cancer, diabetes, obesity, and childhood obesity increase (**Figure 14.2b**).[10] Transition to a diet high in animal protein and refined foods also increases the use of natural resources and in the long term may deplete nonrenewable resources.

nutrition transition A series of changes in diet, physical activity, health, and nutrition that occurs as poor countries become more prosperous.

CONCEPT CHECK

1. **How** prevalent are undernutrition and overnutrition around the world?

2. **What** is the impact of stunting on the health and productivity of a population?

3. **How** does nutrition transition affect a population's health?

Causes of Hunger Around the World

LEARNING OBJECTIVES

1. **Explain** the concept of food insecurity.

2. **Discuss** the factors that cause food shortages for populations and individuals.

3. **Describe** the consequences of three nutrient deficiencies that are common worldwide.

 he specific reasons for hunger and **food insecurity** vary with time and location, but the underlying cause is that the available food is not distributed equitably. This inequitable distribution results in either a shortage of food or the wrong combination of foods to meet nutrient needs. This situation, in turn, results in protein-energy malnutrition and individual nutrient deficiencies.

> **food insecurity** A situation in which people lack adequate physical, social, or economic access to sufficient, safe, nutritious food that meets their dietary needs and food preferences for an active and healthy life.

Food Shortages

The most obvious example of a food shortage is **famine**. Drought, floods, earthquakes, and crop destruction due to diseases or pests are natural causes of famines. Human causes include wars and civil conflicts (**Figure 14.3**).

Food shortages due to famine are very visible because they cause many deaths in an area during a short period, but chronic food shortages take a greater toll. Chronic shortages occur when economic inequities result in lack of money, health care, and education for individuals or populations; when the population outgrows the food supply; when cultural and religious practices limit food choices; or when environmental damage limits the amount of food that can be produced.

> **famine** A widespread lack of access to food due to a disaster that causes a collapse in food production and marketing systems.

Poverty Almost 1.4 billion people around the world live below the international poverty line, earning less than $1.25 per day.[15] Poverty is central to the problem of

---

Famine • Figure 14.3

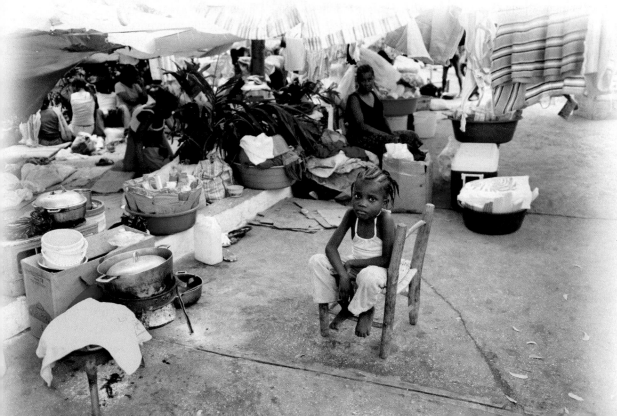

Many survivors of the earthquakes in Haiti live in makeshift camps such as this one. This natural disaster destroyed the infrastructure that once distributed food throughout the country. Regions that have barely enough food to survive under normal conditions are vulnerable to famine. This situation is analogous to a man standing in water up to his nostrils: If all is calm, he can breathe, but if there is a ripple, he will drown. A ripple such as a natural or civil disaster reduces the margin of survival and creates famine.

The regions of the world where poverty is the most prevalent (see map) correspond to the regions where there are the greatest number of undernourished people (see chart). Developing countries, where one in four people subsists on less than $1.25 a day, account for 98% of the world's undernourished people.[1,15] In wealthy countries, hungry people can usually obtain help to get food or money to buy food, but in poor countries, a family that cannot grow enough food or earn enough money to buy food may have nowhere to turn for help. ▼

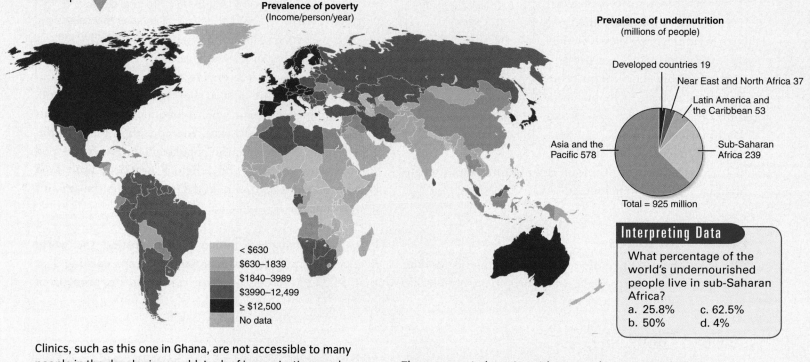

Prevalence of poverty
(Income/person/year)

< $630
$630–1839
$1840–3989
$3990–12,499
≥ $12,500
No data

Prevalence of undernutrition
(millions of people)

Developed countries 19
Near East and North Africa 37
Latin America and the Caribbean 53
Asia and the Pacific 578
Sub-Saharan Africa 239

Total = 925 million

Interpreting Data

What percentage of the world's undernourished people live in sub-Saharan Africa?
a. 25.8%   c. 62.5%
b. 50%   d. 4%

Clinics, such as this one in Ghana, are not accessible to many people in the developing world. Lack of immunizations and treatment for infections and other illnesses results in an increase in infectious disease and a decrease in survival rates from chronic diseases such as cancer. Lack of health care also increases infant ▼ mortality and the incidence of low-birth-weight births.

These young Indonesian girls are working in a textile factory rather than going to school. Lack of education prevents people from escaping poverty and contributes to undernutrition and disease because it leads to inadequate care for infants, children, and pregnant women. ▼

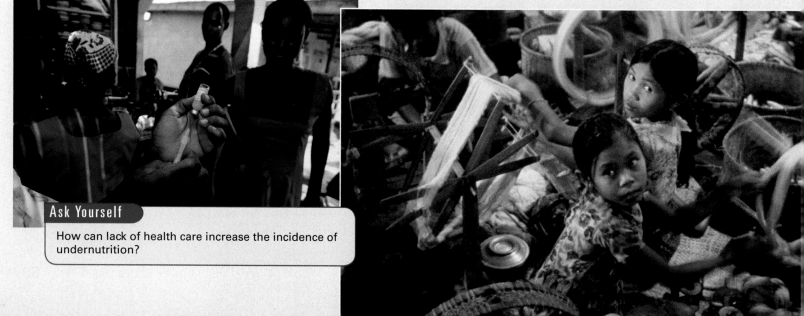

Ask Yourself

How can lack of health care increase the incidence of undernutrition?

hunger and undernutrition (**Figure 14.4**). In addition to creating food insecurity, poverty reduces access to health care, increasing the prevalence of disease and disability. When diseases go untreated, nutrient needs are increased, a situation that further limits the ability to obtain an adequate diet and contributes to malnutrition. Those who are poor also have less access to education, and this lack of access contributes to undernutrition and disease and reduces opportunities to escape poverty. Lack of education about food preparation and storage can affect food safety and the health of the household: Unsanitary food preparation increases the incidence of gastrointestinal diseases, which contribute to malnutrition.

Overpopulation Overpopulation exists when a region has more people than its natural resources can support. A fertile river valley can support more people per acre than can a desert environment. But even in fertile regions of the world, if the number of people increases excessively, resources are overwhelmed, and food shortages occur. At present, enough food is produced throughout the world to prevent hunger if that food is distributed equitably, but demand is rising. The human population is currently growing at a rate of more than 83 million persons per year (**Figure 14.5**).[16] This rate of growth could eventually outstrip the planet's ability to produce enough food to nourish the world's population.

In addition, the demand for grain is increasing as a result of increased consumption of more grain-intensive livestock products and the recent sharp acceleration in the use of grain to produce ethanol to fuel cars.[17] The increased demand has contributed to dramatic increases in food prices, which have made it even more challenging for low- and middle-income families worldwide to obtain enough food. The rising price of grain and fuel oil has also reduced the amount of food aid, widening the gap between the amount of food available and the amount needed to meet nutritional needs.[18]

Cultural practices In some cultures, access to food may be limited for certain individuals in households. For example, because they are viewed as less important, women and girls may receive less food than men and boys. How much food is available to an individual within a household depends on gender, control of income, education, age, birth order, and genetic endowments.

The cultural acceptability or unacceptability of foods also contributes to food shortages and malnutrition. If

World population growth • Figure 14.5

About 90% of the world's population growth is occurring in less-developed countries. Developing countries cannot escape poverty because their economies cannot keep pace with such rapid population growth. Efforts to produce enough food can damage the soil and deplete environmental resources, further reducing the capacity to produce food in the future.

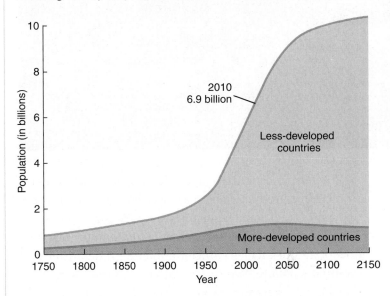

available foods are culturally unacceptable, a food shortage exists unless the population can be educated to accept the new food. For example, insects are eaten in some cultures and are an excellent source of protein, but in other cultures they are unacceptable as food.

Limited environmental resources The land and other resources available to produce food are limited. Some resources, such as minerals and fossil fuels, are present in finite amounts and are nonrenewable—that is, once they have been used, they cannot be replaced within a reasonable amount of time. Others, such as soil and water, are **renewable resources** because they will be available indefinitely if they are used at a rate at which the Earth can restore them. For example, when agricultural land is used wisely—that is, when crops are rotated, erosion is prevented, and contamination is limited—it can be reused almost endlessly. However, if land is not used carefully, damage caused by soil erosion, nutrient depletion, and accumulation of pollutants may reduce the amount of usable land over the long term.

> **renewable resource** A resource that is restored and replaced by natural processes and can therefore be used forever.

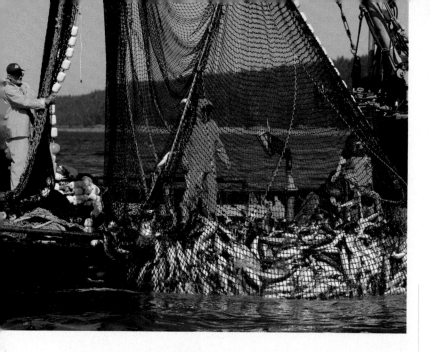

Environmental impact on the oceans
• Figure 14.6

Overfishing has severely reduced the numbers of many marine species. Pollution also threatens the world's fishing grounds. Oil spills and deliberate dumping occur offshore, and sewage, pesticides, organic pollutants, and sediments from erosion wash into coastal waters, where most fish spend at least part of their lives. Even aquaculture, designed to increase fish production, produces wastes that can pollute ocean water and harm other marine organisms.

Modern mechanized agricultural methods have increased food production but use more energy and resources than more traditional labor-intensive farming. Large-scale farming can erode the soil and deplete its nutrients. Fertilizers and pesticides can contaminate groundwater and eventually pollute waterways. And if a product is shipped over long distances, requires refrigeration or freezing, or needs other types of processing, the environmental costs are increased even more.

As more countries undergo nutrition transition, the demand for meat-based diets will increase, as will the use of natural resources and energy. In general, the environmental cost of producing plant-based foods is lower than that of producing animal products.[19] Raising cattle creates both air and water pollution. The animals themselves produce methane, a greenhouse gas, in their gastrointestinal tracts. Large-scale "factory farming" makes the problem worse because more methane is produced when animal sewage is stored in ponds and heaps. In fact, livestock is responsible for a larger percentage of greenhouse gas emissions than all the cars in the world combined. Livestock production also accounts for over 8% of global human water use and releases nutrients, pathogens, and other pollutants into waterways.[20] It is not only the resources of the land that are at risk. Population growth has increased the demand for fish to the point that the Earth's oceans are being depleted (**Figure 14.6**).

Poor-Quality Diets

Even when there is enough food, malnutrition can occur if the quality of the diet is poor. The typical diet in developing countries is based on high-fiber grain products or root

vegetables and has little variety. Adults who are able to consume a relatively large amount of this diet may be able to meet their nutrient needs. But individuals with high nutrient needs because they are ill or pregnant and those with limited capacity to consume this bulky grain diet, such as children and elderly individuals, are at risk for nutrient deficiencies. Deficiencies of protein, iron, iodine, and vitamin A are common with poor-quality diets.[21] The images in **Figure 14.7** will help you recall these common deficiencies that were discussed in greater detail in earlier chapters.

Several other vitamin and mineral deficiencies have recently emerged or reemerged as problems throughout the world. Beriberi, pellagra, and scurvy—diseases caused by deficiencies of thiamin, niacin, and vitamin C, respectively—are rare in the developed world but still occur among extremely poor and underprivileged people and in large refugee populations.[21] In many parts of the world, folate deficiency causes megaloblastic anemia during pregnancy and often compounds existing iron deficiency anemia. Deficiencies of the minerals zinc, selenium, and calcium are also of concern. Zinc deficiency affects about one-third of the world's population and is believed to cause as many deaths as vitamin A deficiency or iron deficiency.[22] Selenium deficiency has been identified in population groups in China, New Zealand, and the Russian Federation. Inadequate calcium intake is a worldwide concern due to its association with osteoporosis.

CONCEPT CHECK

1. **What** causes food insecurity?
2. **How** can environmental damage lead to food shortages?
3. **Why** do children develop protein and micronutrient deficiencies more often than adults?

Protein and micronutrient deficiencies • Figure 14.7

Protein-energy malnutrition is most common in children. When there is a general lack of food, the wasting associated with *marasmus* results, and when the diet is limited to starchy grains and vegetables, *kwashiorkor*, characterized by a bloated belly, can predominate (see Chapter 6). Other factors, such as metabolic changes caused by infection, may also play a role in the development of kwashiorkor.

Think Critically Why are children who consume a starchy, low-protein diet more likely to develop kwashiorkor than adults consuming the same diet?

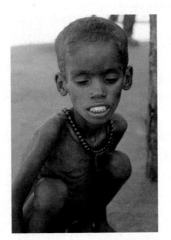

Marasmus   Kwashiorkor

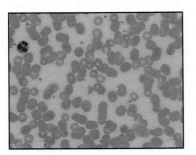
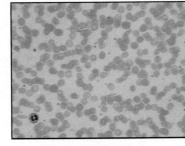

Normal red blood cells   Iron deficiency anemia

More than 2 billion people worldwide suffer from iron deficiency anemia, which is characterized by small, pale red blood cells (see Chapter 8).[23] The lack of iron reduces the amount of hemoglobin produced, and the lack of hemoglobin lowers the blood's ability to deliver oxygen. In developing countries, intestinal parasites, which cause gastrointestinal blood loss, and acute and chronic infections, such as malaria, increase the risk and severity of dietary iron deficiency. Iron deficiency can have a major impact on the health and productivity of a population.

Although goiter, seen here, is a more visible manifestation of iodine deficiency, the more subtle effects of deficiency on mental performance and work capacity may have a greater impact on the population as a whole. Iodine-deficient children have lower IQs and impaired school performance.[24] Iodine deficiency in children and adults is associated with apathy and decreased initiative and decision-making capabilities (see Chapter 8).

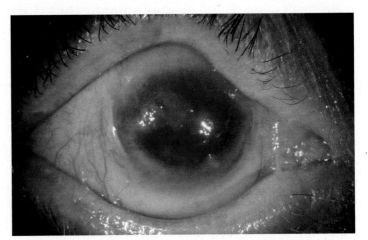

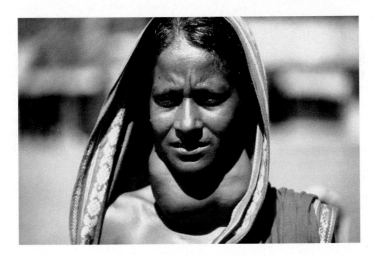

It is estimated that more than 250 million preschool children worldwide suffer from vitamin A deficiency.[25] Vitamin A deficiency leads to *xerophthalmia*, shown here. Vitamin A deficiency is the leading cause of preventable blindness among children. It also depresses immune function, thus increasing the risk of illness and death from infections, particularly measles and diarrheal disease (see Chapter 7).

Causes of Hunger in the United States

LEARNING OBJECTIVES

1. **Discuss** the causes of food insecurity in the United States.

2. **Describe** how lack of access to health care, education, and transportation prevent people from escaping poverty.

3. **List** the population groups that are at greatest risk for undernutrition in the United States.

Most of the nutritional problems in the United States are related to overnutrition.[26] However, about 15% of households in the United States experience food insecurity (**Figure 14.8**).[27] This situation is caused not by a general food shortage but by an inequitable distribution of food and money. The incidence of hunger and food insecurity is highest among women, infants, children, elderly individuals, and those who are poor, homeless, ill, or disabled. However, a sudden decrease in income or increase in living expenses can put anyone at risk for food insecurity.

Poverty and Food Insecurity

In the United States, as elsewhere in the world, poverty is the main cause of food insecurity. Poverty reduces access to food, education, and health care. About 14.3% of Americans (43.6 million people) live at or below the poverty level.[28] These individuals have little money to spend on food and often have limited access to affordable food. Inadequate income also reduces the chances that healthier foods will be consumed. Choosing leaner meats and dairy products and whole grains costs more—about 35 to 40% of low-income consumers' food budgets.[29]

The high price of real estate in cities has driven supermarkets into the suburbs, and because many low-income city families do not own cars, they must shop at small, expensive corner stores or pay cab fares if they wish to take advantage of lower prices at more distant, larger stores. The rural poor may have limited access to food because they live far from grocery stores. High poverty and unemployment rates among Native Americans and Alaska Natives contribute to food insecurity.[30] Migrant workers also have limited access to food because labor camps are in remote locations, and transportation is often unavailable. Low incomes and difficult working and living conditions among migrant workers further limit their ability to purchase food and prepare adequate meals. These conditions have created what is called a **food desert**.[31]

Poverty also limits access to health care, leading to poorer health status. Iron deficiency is more than twice as frequent in low-income children as in children in higher-income families, and the incidence of heart disease, cancer, hypertension, and obesity increases with decreasing income.[32] As in developing nations, poverty is reflected in infant mortality rates. The average infant mortality in the U.S. population is about 6.8 per 1000 live births. However, there are groups within the population that have infant mortality rates as high as those in impoverished nations. Among African Americans, the infant mortality rate is 13.6 per 1000 live births—more than twice that of the general population. This difference may reflect

> **food desert** An area that lacks access to affordable fruits, vegetables, whole grains, low-fat milk, and other foods that make up a healthy diet.

Food insecurity in the United States • Figure 14.8

Current data show that approximately 85% of U.S. households are food secure; the other 15% experienced food insecurity at some point during the year.[27]

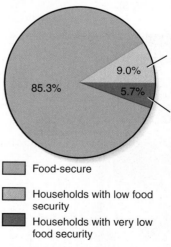

Low food security means that families were able to avoid substantially disrupting their eating patterns or reducing food intake by using coping strategies, such as eating a less varied diet, participating in federal food assistance programs, or getting emergency food from community food pantries.

Very low food security means that the normal eating patterns of one or more household members were disrupted and food intake was reduced at times during the year because families had insufficient money or other resources to use for obtaining food.

85.3%　9.0%　5.7%

- Food-secure
- Households with low food security
- Households with very low food security

Education and poverty • Figure 14.9

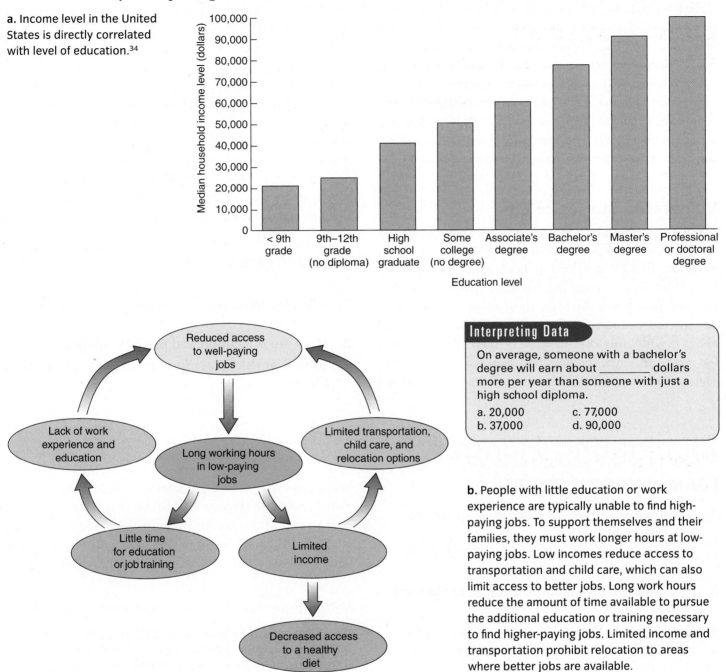

a. Income level in the United States is directly correlated with level of education.[34]

Median household income level (dollars) — Education level: < 9th grade, 9th–12th grade (no diploma), High school graduate, Some college (no degree), Associate's degree, Bachelor's degree, Master's degree, Professional or doctoral degree

Diagram labels:
- Reduced access to well-paying jobs
- Lack of work experience and education
- Long working hours in low-paying jobs
- Limited transportation, child care, and relocation options
- Little time for education or job training
- Limited income
- Decreased access to a healthy diet

Interpreting Data

On average, someone with a bachelor's degree will earn about _____ dollars more per year than someone with just a high school diploma.

a. 20,000   c. 77,000
b. 37,000   d. 90,000

b. People with little education or work experience are typically unable to find high-paying jobs. To support themselves and their families, they must work longer hours at low-paying jobs. Low incomes reduce access to transportation and child care, which can also limit access to better jobs. Long work hours reduce the amount of time available to pursue the additional education or training necessary to find higher-paying jobs. Limited income and transportation prohibit relocation to areas where better jobs are available.

differences in infant mortality risk factors, such as poverty and lack of access to medical care.[33]

Lack of education, which is both a cause and a consequence of poverty, also contributes to food insecurity. For people at or below the poverty level, educational opportunities are fewer and lower in quality than those for people with higher incomes. In the short term, lack of knowledge about food selection, food safety, and home

economics can contribute to malnutrition. Too little food may cause the diet to be deficient in energy or particular nutrients, but poor food choices also allow food insecurity to coexist with obesity. Lack of education about food safety can also increase the incidence of food-borne illness. In the long term, lack of education prevents people from getting the higher-paying jobs that could allow them to escape poverty (**Figure 14.9**).

Poor families must use most of their income to pay for shelter, a situation that seriously reduces the chances that they will be adequately fed. The high cost of housing not only limits food budgets but also contributes to the growing problem of homelessness in the United States. During the course of a year, over 1.5 million Americans rely on an emergency shelter or emergency housing; one-third of these people are members of a homeless family.[35] Homeless people are at high risk of food insecurity because they lack not only money but also cooking and food storage facilities.

Vulnerable Stages of Life

The high nutrient needs of pregnant and lactating women and small children put them at particular risk for undernutrition. Almost one-third of households with children headed by single women live below the poverty line. Poverty and food insecurity place these women and children at risk for malnutrition, and their special nutritional needs magnify this risk. Because of their increased need for some nutrients, malnutrition may occur in pregnant women, infants, and children even when the rest of the household is adequately fed. For example, the amount of iron in the family's diet may be enough to prevent anemia in all the family's members except a pregnant teenager.

Elderly individuals are vulnerable to food insecurity and undernutrition due to the higher frequency of diseases and disabilities in this population group. Disease and disability may limit their ability to purchase, prepare, and consume food. Greater nutritional risk among older adults is associated with more hospital admissions and hence higher health-care costs. The number of individuals over age 85 is expected to triple by 2050; as the number of elderly people increases, so will the number of people at risk for food insecurity.[36]

CONCEPT CHECK STOP

1. **Why** are some Americans hungry in a land of plenty?
2. **How** are education and poverty related?
3. **Who** is at risk for undernutrition in the United States?

Eliminating Hunger

LEARNING OBJECTIVES

1. **Discuss** two strategies that can help reduce population growth.
2. **Discuss** the role of sustainable agriculture in maintaining the food supply.
3. **Explain** how international trade can help eliminate hunger.
4. **Describe** five federal programs designed to alleviate hunger in the United States.

 olving the problem of world hunger is a daunting task. In 1996, the World Food Summit set a goal of cutting world hunger in half by 2015. Unfortunately, despite advances toward this goal in some countries, little progress has been made worldwide. Current estimates put the number of undernourished people in the world at 925 million—82 million more than in the early 1990s.[1]

Solutions to world hunger need to address population growth, ensure that the nutrient needs of a large and diverse population are met with culturally acceptable foods, and increase food production without damaging the global ecosystem (**Figure 14.10**). Meeting these goals will require input from politicians, nutrition scientists, economists, and the food industry. Economic policies, technical advances, education, and legislative measures must put in

Millennium development goals • Figure 14.10

These eight goals, to be achieved by 2015, were adopted by 189 nations during the United Nations (UN) Millennium Summit in September 2000. They correspond to the world's main development challenges. In order to achieve the first goal, stamping out hunger, most of the others must also be addressed.[37]

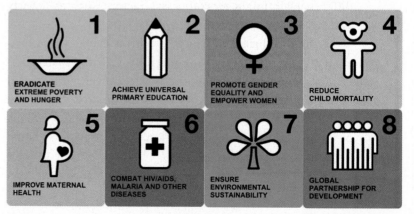

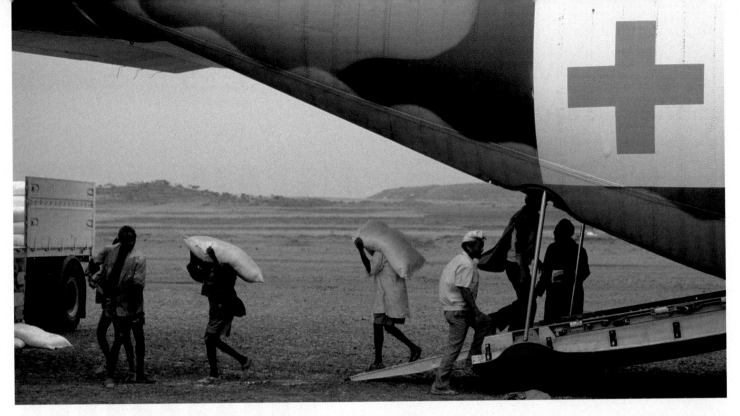

Emergency food relief • Figure 14.11

Many organizations are working to combat world hunger. The American Red Cross and High Commissioner for Refugees of the UN concentrate on famine relief. The Food and Agriculture Organization (FAO) works to improve the production, intake, and distribution of food worldwide. The World Health Organization (WHO) focuses on international health and emphasizes the prevention of nutrition problems, and the UN Children's Fund (UNICEF) targets education and vaccination and responds to crisis situations to improve the lives of children.

place programs and policies to provide food in the short term, and in the long term they must establish sustainable programs to allow the continued production and distribution of acceptable foods.

Providing Short-Term Food Aid

When people are starving, short-term food and medical aid must be provided right away. The standard approach has been to bring food into stricken areas (**Figure 14.11**). This food generally consists of agricultural surpluses from other countries and often is not well planned in terms of its nutrient content. Although this type of relief is necessary for a population to survive an immediate crisis such as famine, it does little to prevent future hunger.

Controlling Population Growth

In the long term, solving the problem of world hunger requires balancing the number of people and the amount of food that can be produced. The world's population has increased dramatically since the middle of the 20th century, but population growth has recently begun to slow. The birth rate worldwide has declined—from 5 children per woman in 1950 to 2.5 in 2010.[38] This downward trend in population growth must continue to ensure that food production and natural resources can support the population. Changes in cultural and economic factors as well as family planning and government policies can be used to influence the birth rate.

Economic and cultural factors that affect birth rate In many cultures, a large family is expected. A major reason for this expectation is high infant and child mortality rates. When infant mortality rates are high, people choose to have many children in order to ensure that some will survive. Higher birth rates in some developing countries are also due to the economic and societal roles of children. Children are needed to work farms, support the elders, and otherwise contribute to the economic survival of families. Programs that foster economic development and ensure access to food, shelter, and medical care have been shown to cause a decline in birth rates because people feel secure having fewer children. Economic development also reduces the need for children as workers.

WHAT A SCIENTIST SEES

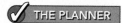

Education and Birth Rate

The large number of children in this impoverished Indonesian family is indicative of the uneven burden of population growth in the developing world. A scientist sees that one of the reasons for the many children in this family is lack of education for women. Education increases the likelihood that women will have control over their fertility and gives them knowledge that can be used to improve the family's health and economic situation. Education builds job skills that allow women to join the workforce, marry later in life, and have fewer children. The graph shows that higher literacy among women is associated with lower birth rates.[40] Women who are better educated have options other than having numerous children.

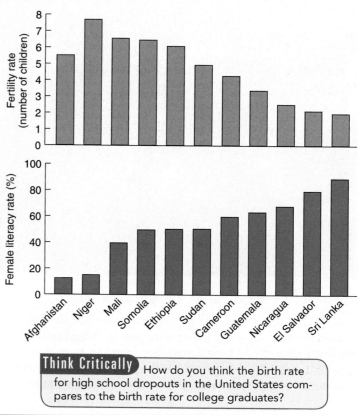

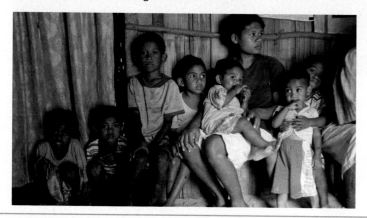

Think Critically How do you think the birth rate for high school dropouts in the United States compares to the birth rate for college graduates?

Another cultural factor that influences birth rate is gender inequality. Girls are often kept at home to work rather than being sent to school. In most developing countries, the literacy rate is lower for women than for men, and fewer women attend primary and secondary school. This lack of education leaves women few options other than remaining home and having children. Providing education for girls has been shown to reduce birth rates (see *What a Scientist Sees*).[39]

Family planning and government policies

Changes in cultural and economic factors may reduce the desire for large families, but reducing birth rate also requires the availability of health and family-planning

Access to birth control • Figure 14.12

a. A birth control vendor explains condoms to women at a market in the Ivory Coast. The birth rate in this West African country declined from nearly 7 children per woman in 1988 to 4 in 2010,[41] due in part to increased use of modern methods of birth control. Increased knowledge and availability of contraceptives is linked to a decrease in birth rate.

b. As seen in the graph, the percentage of women in the least developed countries who are using contraception has been increasing. The availability of contraceptives gives women more control over the number of children they have to support.[42]

services. To be successful, family-planning efforts must be acceptable to the population and compatible with cultural and religious beliefs. Governments around the world have used a number of approaches, such as provision of contraceptives, education, and economic incentives, to decrease population growth (**Figure 14.12**).

Increasing Food Production While Protecting the Environment

Advances in agricultural technology have allowed food production to keep pace with population growth. However, the use of energy-intensive modern agricultural techniques has contributed to serious environmental problems. Commercial inorganic fertilizers and pesticides and modern farm machinery increase food production but at the same time pollute the air and water. Overuse of land causes deterioration of soil quality, which will limit food production in the future. For food production to continue to meet the needs of future generations, we must figure out how to continue to increase food yields and availability while conserving the world's natural resources (see *Thinking It Through*).

THINKING IT THROUGH ✓ THE PLANNER

A Case Study on What One Person Can Do

Keesha is concerned about the problems of hunger and malnutrition and the impact her choices have on the environment. Although she is a college student who cannot afford to make monetary contributions to relief organizations, she would like her everyday choices to have a minimal impact on the environment.

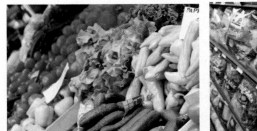 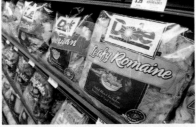

What are the advantages and disadvantages of the salad options above in terms of convenience, food safety, and environmental impact?

▼

Your answer:

Keesha likes fish but has heard that some fish are endangered.

Go to the National Geographic Web site http://ocean.nationalgeographic.com/ocean/take-action/seafood-substitutions/ **to find some ocean-friendly substitutes for her seafood choices.**

▼

Fish	Substitute variety
Atlantic cod	
Chilean sea bass	
Orange roughy	

The following are some inexpensive changes Keesha can make to reduce her impact on the environment.

What are the advantages and disadvantages of each?

▼

Action	Advantages	Disadvantages
Bike instead of drive on short trips around town.		
Buy a canvas bag for carrying groceries.		
Bring juice in a thermos instead of buying a nonrecyclable bottle.		
Compost vegetable scraps.		
Buy locally grown produce.		
Buy organically grown produce.		

(Check your answers in Appendix J.)

A sustainable farm • Figure 14.13

A sustainable farm consists of a total agricultural ecosystem rather than a single crop. It may include field crops, fruit- and nut-bearing trees, herds of livestock, and forests.

Increasing biological diversity in crops and animals protects the farmer, maximizes natural pest control, and minimizes pesticide input.

Wetlands

Sustainable agriculture

Orchard

Certified sustainable timber

Crops

Growing a different crop in a field each year helps keep the soil healthy and minimizes soil erosion. It reduces problems caused by crop diseases, insect pests, and weeds.

Pasture

Having both crops and livestock allows the farmer to recycle crop nutrients by spreading livestock manure on a field. Animals can feed on weeds and crop waste that cannot be used as human food.

---

sustainable agriculture Agricultural methods that maintain soil productivity and a healthy ecological balance while having minimal long-term impacts.

Sustainable agriculture uses food production methods that prevent damage to the environment and allow the land to restore itself so that food can be produced indefinitely. For example, contour plowing and terracing help prevent erosion, keeping the soil available for future crops. Rotating the crops grown in a field prevents the depletion of nutrients in the soil, reducing the need for fertilizers. Sustainable agriculture uses environmentally friendly chemicals that degrade quickly and do not persist as residues in the environment. It also relies on diversification. This approach to farming maximizes natural methods of pest control and fertilization and protects farmers from changes in the marketplace (**Figure 14.13**).

Sustainable agriculture is not a single program but involves choosing options that mesh well with local soil, climate, and farming techniques. In some cases, organic farming, which does not use synthetic pesticides, herbicides, and fertilizers (see Chapter 13), may be a more sustainable option. Organic techniques have a smaller environmental impact because they reduce the use of agricultural chemicals and the release of pollutants into the environment. Organic farming is also advantageous in terms of soil quality and biodiversity, but it has a disadvantage in terms of land use because crop yields are often lower. A combination of organic and conventional

techniques, as is used with integrated pest management (see Chapter 13), might improve land use and protect the environment.

Other sustainable programs include agroforestry, in which techniques from forestry and agriculture are used together to restore degraded areas; natural systems agriculture, which attempts to develop agricultural systems that include many types of plants and therefore function like natural ecosystems; and the technique of reducing fertilizer use by matching nutrient resources with the demands of the particular crop being grown. One modern technology that may be integrated with sustainable systems is genetic engineering. As discussed in Chapter 13, genetic engineering can increase crop yields by inserting genes that improve the efficiency with which plants convert sunlight into food or genes that make plants resistant to herbicides, insects, and plant diseases.

Increasing Food Availability Through Economic Development and Trade

Hunger will exist as long as there is poverty. Even when food is plentiful, the poor do not have access to enough of the right foods to maintain their nutritional health. Economic development that leads to safe and sanitary housing, access to health care and education, and the resources to acquire enough food are essential if hunger is to be eliminated. Government policies can help reduce poverty and improve food security by increasing the population's income, lowering food prices, or funding food programs for those who are poor.

Economic development in the form of industrialization can also help provide food for a county's population by increasing access to international trade. The newly industrialized countries of Asia, such as South Korea, rely on imported food to provide a varied food supply for their populations. In general, countries around the world are becoming more dependent on food imports and on exports of food and other goods to pay for the food they import. This trade can increase the availability of food for the world's population as a whole.

Whether a country's agricultural emphasis is on producing **subsistence crops** or **cash crops** influences the availability of food for its people. Shifting to cash crops improves the country's cash flow but uses local resources to produce crops for export and limits the ability of its people to produce enough food to feed their families. For example, if a large portion of the arable land in a country is used to grow cash crops such as coffee and tea, little agricultural land remains for growing grains and vegetables that nourish the local population. If, however, the cash from the crop is used to purchase nutritious foods from other countries, this decision may help alleviate undernutrition.

> **subsistence crop** A crop that is grown as food for a farmer's family, with little or nothing leftover to sell.
>
> **cash crop** A crop that is grown to be sold for monetary return rather than as food for the local population.

Ensuring a Nutritious Food Supply

To ensure the nutritional health of a population, the foods that are grown or imported must supply both sufficient energy and adequate amounts of all essential nutrients. If the diet does not provide enough of all the essential nutrients, either the dietary pattern must be changed, commonly consumed foods must be fortified, or supplements containing deficient nutrients must be provided. For these changes to be beneficial, consumers must know how to choose foods that provide the needed nutrients and how to handle them safely.

Nutrition education Education can help improve nutrient intake by teaching consumers what foods to grow, which foods to choose, and how to prepare foods safely.

Education is particularly important when introducing a new crop. No matter how nutritious it may be, a new plant variety is not beneficial unless local farmers know how to grow it and the population accepts it as a food source and knows how to prepare it for consumption. For instance, white-fleshed yams are common in some regions but are a poor source of β-carotene, which the body can use to make vitamin A. If the orange-fleshed yam, which is rich in β-carotene, became an acceptable choice, the amount of vitamin A available to the population would increase.

Food safety is also a concern when changing traditional dietary practices. For example, introducing papaya to the diet as a source of vitamin A will not improve nutritional status if it is washed in unsanitary water and causes dysentery among the people it is meant to nourish.

Education to encourage breast-feeding can also improve nutritional status and health (**Figure 14.14**). To achieve optimal growth, development, and health, WHO recommends that infants be exclusively breast fed for the first six months of life. After that, other foods should be offered, while breast-feeding continues for up to two years of age or beyond.[43]

Nutritional and health benefits of breast-feeding • Figure 14.14

Breast milk provides infants with optimal nutrition and immune factors that reduce the risk of infectious diseases. In developing nations, where infant mortality from infectious disease is high, breast-feeding is even recommended for women who are HIV positive if HIV treatment for the mother and a nutritious alternative to breast milk for the infant are not available. In such cases, the risk of the baby dying of malnutrition and other infections outweighs the risk of transmitting the virus in the milk.[44]

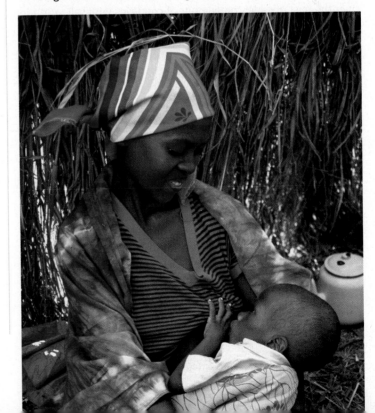

Fortifying the food supply Although food fortification will not provide energy for a hungry population, it can increase the protein quality of the diet and eliminate micronutrient deficiencies. In order to solve a nutritional problem in a population, fortification must be implemented wisely. Fortification works only if vulnerable groups consume centrally processed foods. The foods selected for fortification should be among those that are consistently consumed by the majority of the population so that extensive promotion and reeducation are not needed to encourage their consumption. The nutrient should be added uniformly and in a form that optimizes its utilization.

Fortification has been used successfully in preventing health problems in the United States. Fortification of cow's milk to increase vitamin D intake was a major factor in the elimination of infantile rickets, and enrichment of grains with niacin helped eliminate pellagra. Fortification of salt with iodine is successfully eliminating iodine deficiency diseases in countries around the world (**Figure 14.15**).

An alternative to traditional fortification is biofortification, which uses plant breeding to increase the nutrient content of staple foods. For example, breeders have developed corn that provides higher levels of β-carotene than traditional varieties.[46] The challenge is to get local farmers and consumers to accept biofortified crops. (See *Debate: Combating Vitamin A Deficiency with Golden Rice*.)

Providing supplements Supplementing specific nutrients for at-risk segments of the population can help reduce the prevalence of malnutrition. Of countries where vitamin A deficiency is a public health problem, about three-quarters have policies supporting regular vitamin A supplementation in children. Many have also adopted the WHO's recommendation to provide all breast-feeding women with a high-dose supplement of vitamin A within eight weeks of delivery. This improves maternal vitamin A status and raises the amount of vitamin A that is present in breast milk and is therefore passed to the infant.

Many countries have adopted programs to supplement children older than 6 months with iron and pregnant women with iron and folate.

Eliminating Food Insecurity in the United States

As with world hunger, eliminating hunger in the United States involves improving economic security, keeping food affordable, providing food aid to the hungry, and offering education about healthy diets that will meet nutrient needs and reduce diseases related to overconsumption.

Iodized salt • Figure 14.15

Over the past decade, the number of countries with salt iodization programs has increased dramatically. It is estimated that 70% of households worldwide now have access to iodized salt.[45]

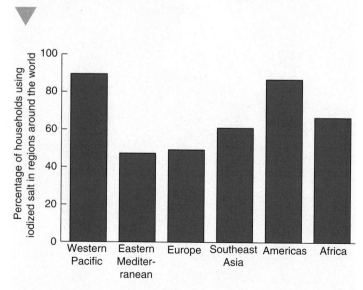

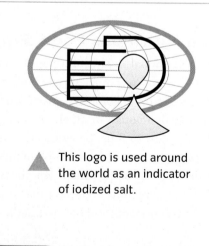

This logo is used around the world as an indicator of iodized salt.

Think Critically The Eastern Mediterranean has the lowest percentage of households with access to iodized salt of any region in the world. Based on your knowledge of dietary sources of iodine, why might this region not have a high incidence of iodine deficiency?

Combating Vitamin A Deficiency with Golden Rice

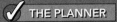

The Issue: Golden Rice is a genetically modified (GM) variety of rice developed to provide vitamin A to populations in which this deficiency is prevalent. Its development has stimulated debate about whether genetic modification is an effective and safe way to help alleviate malnutrition in the developing world.

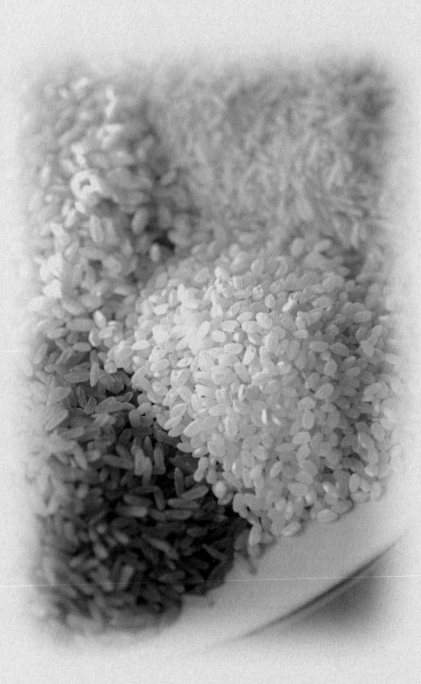

Each year vitamin A deficiency takes the sight and lives of hundreds of thousands of children worldwide. The deficiency is most common in impoverished populations where the dietary staple is deficient in vitamin A. Currently this deficiency is addressed using vitamin A supplementation, fortification of the food supply, and interventions that increase the variety of the diet to include foods that are rich in vitamin A. A more controversial solution is growing rice that has been genetically engineered to synthesize β-carotene, a yellow-orange pigment that is a precursor to vitamin A. If it replaced white rice as a staple, Golden Rice could alleviate vitamin A deficiency. However, the controversy that ensued after it was developed has kept the preventive potential of Golden Rice from even being tested.

Initial concerns about Golden Rice focused on whether it would provide enough vitamin A to alleviate deficiency. The original variety provided so little β-carotene that a 2-year-old child would need to eat 3 kilograms of it each day to get enough vitamin A.[47] A newer variety now provides more than half of the RDA for children in a reasonable serving of ½ cup of rice.[48] But even if children eat Golden Rice, many argue that it may not be a solution to malnutrition. The rice will increase vitamin A intake, but deficient populations typically suffer from other nutrient deficiencies; when protein, fat, or zinc is deficient, the body can't efficiently use vitamin A.[49,50]

So should we continue to spend resources developing Golden Rice? Opponents argue that in the decade since Golden Rice was developed, it has done nothing to prevent vitamin A deficiency, and it has diverted resources from proven programs that address multiple nutrient deficiencies. Proponents contend that the problem is not the rice but rather the regulatory climate that has prevented it from being introduced; Golden Rice was developed in 1999 but will probably not be commercialized until 2012.[51,52] The development costs of Golden Rice have been high, but it is predicted to be cost-effective in the long term because once it is introduced, recurrent costs should be low.[53]

There is also concern that introducing GM rice is not safe for the environment. The worry is that its use will decrease the diversity of rice varieties grown. Reducing diversity increases the risk of crop destruction due to insects and disease.[49] Proponents of GM crops argue that this concern occurs whenever a new crop that is preferred by farmers is introduced.

GM crops such as Golden Rice are not substitutes for traditional solutions to malnutrition but can be used to complement them. Supplementation may be necessary for those in immediate need. Fortification and supplementation may work better in urban settings; Golden Rice may be better at reaching isolated rural populations. In the long term, the goal is to use whatever means are available to solve the problem of vitamin A deficiency and other types of malnutrition.

Think critically: Why is it important to preserve all the varieties of rice that currently exist, even if we do not rely on them as dietary staples?

Programs to prevent undernutrition in the United States Table 14.1

Program	Target population	Goals and methods
Supplemental Nutrition Assistance Program (SNAP)	Low-income individuals	Increases access to food by providing coupons or debit cards that can be used to purchase food at a grocery store
Commodity Supplemental Food Program (CSFP)	Low-income pregnant women, breast-feeding and non-breast-feeding postpartum women, infants and children under age 6, and elderly people	Provides food by distributing U.S. Department of Agriculture (USDA) commodity foods
Special Supplemental Nutrition Program for Women, Infants, and Children (WIC)	Low-income pregnant women, breast-feeding and non-breast-feeding postpartum women, and infants and children under age 5	Provides vouchers for the purchase of foods (including infant formula and infant cereal) high in nutrients that are typically lacking in the program's target population; provides nutrition education and referrals for health care
WIC Farmers' Market Nutrition Program	WIC participants	Increases access to fresh produce by providing vouchers that can be used to purchase produce at authorized local farmers' markets
National School Breakfast Program	Low-income children	Provides free or low-cost breakfasts at school to improve the nutritional status of children
National School Lunch Program	Low-income children	Provides free or low-cost lunches at school to improve the nutritional status of children
Special Milk Program	Low-income children	Provides milk for children in schools, camps, and child-care institutions with no federally supported meal program
Summer Food Service Program	Low-income children	Provides free meals and snacks for children when school is not in session
Child and Adult Care Food Program	Children up to age 12 and elderly and disabled adults	Provides nutritious meals to children and adults in day-care settings
Team Nutrition	School-age children	Provides nutrition education, training and technical assistance, and resources to participating schools, with the goal of improving children's lifelong eating and physical activity habits
Head Start	Low-income preschool children and their families	Provides meals and education, including nutrition education
Nutrition Program for the Elderly	Individuals age 60 and over and their spouses	Provides free congregate meals in churches, schools, senior centers, or other facilities and delivers food to homebound people
Senior Farmers' Market Program	Low-income seniors	Provides coupons that can be exchanged for eligible foods at farmers' markets, roadside stands, and community-supported agricultural programs
Homeless Children Nutrition Program	Preschoolers living in shelters	Reimburses providers for meals served
Emergency Food Assistance Program	Low-income people	Provides commodities to soup kitchens, food banks, and individuals for home use
Healthy People 2020	U.S. population	Sets national health promotion objectives to improve the health of the U.S. population through health-care system and industry involvement, as well as individual actions
Expanded Food and Nutrition Education Program (EFNEP)	Low-income families	Provides education in all aspects of food preparation and nutrition
Temporary Assistance for Needy Families (TANF)	Low-income households	Provides assistance and work opportunities to needy families by granting states federal funds to implement welfare programs
Food Distribution Program on Indian Reservations	Low-income households living on reservations and Native Americans living near reservations	Provides food by distributing USDA commodity foods

The nutrition safety net Federal programs that provide access to affordable food and promote healthy eating have been referred to as a "nutrition safety net" for the American population (**Table 14.1**). The nutrition assistance programs include a combination of general nutrition assistance and specialized programs targeted to groups with particular nutritional risks: children, seniors, infants, women during and after pregnancy, Native Americans living on reservations, people with disabilities, and homeless people.[54] One of every four Americans receives some kind of food assistance, at a total cost of about $79 billion per year.[55]

The largest USDA program designed to make sure that all people have access to an adequate diet is the Supplemental Nutrition Assistance Program (SNAP) (previously known as the Food Stamp Program). SNAP provides monthly benefits in the form of coupons or debit cards that can be used to purchase food, thereby supplementing the food budgets of low-income individuals. Together with SNAP, four other programs that target high-risk populations—the National School Lunch Program; the Special Supplemental Nutrition Program for Women, Infants, and Children (WIC); the Child and Adult Care Food Program; and the National School Breakfast Program—account for 95% of the USDA's expenditure for food assistance.[55]

In addition to federal nutrition assistance programs, church, community, and charitable emergency food shelters provide for the basic nutritional needs of many Americans. In the United States, about 150,000 nonprofit food distribution programs help direct food to those in need.[56] The leading hunger-relief charity in the United States is Feeding America, which provides food assistance to more than 25 million low-income people per year. It includes a network of food banks across the country and supports thousands of local charitable organizations, such as food pantries and soup kitchens, which distribute food directly to hungry Americans.

Virtually all these food distribution programs use food obtained through **food recovery**, which involves collecting food that is wasted in fields, commercial kitchens, restaurants, and grocery stores and distributing it to those in need (**Figure 14.16**). It is estimated that over 25% of America's food—enough to feed 49 million people—goes to waste each year.[57]

Nutrition education People who have more nutrition information and greater awareness of the relationship between diet and health consume healthier diets. Healthy diets not only improve current health by optimizing growth, productivity, and well-being but are essential for preventing chronic diseases. Increasing knowledge about nutrition can reduce medical costs and improve the quality of life.

Field gleaning • Figure 14.16

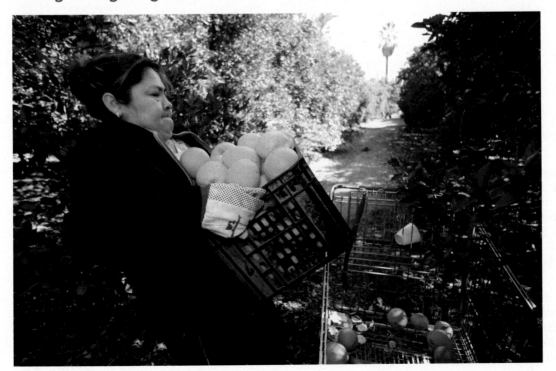

These oranges were harvested in California as part of a local gleaning program. Field gleaning is a type of food recovery that involves collecting crops that are not harvested because it is not economically profitable to harvest them or that remain in fields after mechanical harvesting. The word *gleaning* means "gathering after the harvest" and dates back at least as far as biblical times.

WHAT SHOULD I EAT?
Environmental Impact: Make Your Meals Green

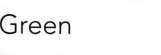

Eat more plants
- Reduce the amount of meat in your meal.
- Eat vegetarian at least some of the time.
- Eat lower on the food chain—more plant foods and small fish.
- Grow and eat some of your own vegetables.

Cut down on pollution
- Buy in bulk in order to cut down on packaging.
- Use reusable bags to take your groceries home.
- Choose locally grown and organically produced foods.
- Cook from scratch—use fewer processed foods.

Use iProfile to compare the nutrients in a vegetarian versus a meat-based meal.

Education can help individuals with lower incomes stretch their limited food dollars by making wise choices at the store and reducing food waste at home. It can promote community gardens to increase the availability of seasonal vegetables. It can teach people how to prepare foods received from commodity distribution programs and food banks. It can explain safe food handling and preparation methods. Knowing which foods to choose and how to handle them safely is as important in preventing malnutrition as having the money to buy enough food. In addition to the programs described in Table 14.1, the *Dietary Guidelines for Americans*, MyPlate, and food labels educate the general public about making wise food choices (see *What Should I Eat?*).

CONCEPT CHECK   STOP

1. **How** does educating women help control population growth?
2. **What** impact does sustainable agriculture have on the world's food supply?
3. **How** can growing cash crops improve a nation's food supply?
4. **What** is the nutrition safety net?

THE PLANNER ✓

Summary

1 The Two Faces of Malnutrition   506

- In poorly nourished populations, a **cycle of malnutrition** exists in which poorly nourished women give birth to low-birth-weight infants at risk for disease and early death. If these children survive, they grow into adults who are physically unable to fully contribute to society. In populations where malnutrition is prevalent, low birth weight, a high **infant mortality rate**, **stunting**, and infections are more common.

- A shown in the graph, overnutrition coexists with **hunger** and **starvation** in both developed and developing nations around the world. As economic conditions improve, **nutrition transition** to more Western diet and lifestyle patterns contribute to the growing problem of overnutrition.

Nutrition transition • Figure 14.2b

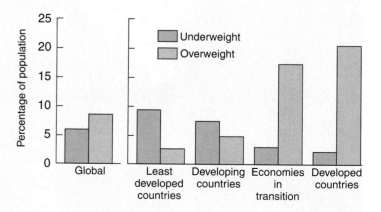

2 Causes of Hunger Around the World 509

- The underlying cause of hunger and **food insecurity** is that the food available in the world is not distributed equitably. **Famine** results from natural and human-caused disasters that temporarily disrupt food production and distribution. Chronic food shortage is most common in the developing world, as shown in the chart. It occurs when economic inequities result in lack of money, health care, and education; when overpopulation and limited natural resources create a situation in which there are more people than food; when cultural practices limit food choices; and when **renewable resources** are misused, limiting the ability to continue to produce food.

The impact of poverty • Figure 14.4

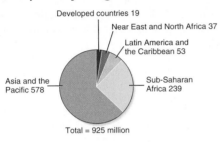

Developed countries 19
Near East and North Africa 37
Latin America and the Caribbean 53
Asia and the Pacific 578
Sub-Saharan Africa 239

Total = 925 million

- Deficiencies of protein, iron, iodine, and vitamin A are common worldwide when the quality of the diet is poor. Pregnant women, children, elderly individuals, and those who are ill may not be able to meet their nutrient needs with the available diet.

3 Causes of Hunger in the United States 514

- Both undernutrition and overnutrition are problems in the United States. As in developing nations, in the United States undernutrition and food insecurity are associated with poverty, which limits education and access to health care and adequate housing, as depicted here.

Education and poverty • Figure 14.9b

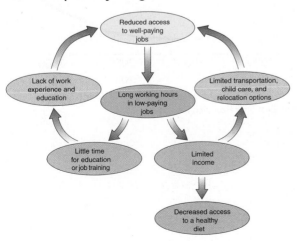

Reduced access to well-paying jobs

Lack of work experience and education

Long working hours in low-paying jobs

Limited transportation, child care, and relocation options

Little time for education or job training

Limited income

Decreased access to a healthy diet

- High nutrient needs increase the risk of malnutrition in women and children, and disease and disability increase risk in elderly individuals.

4 Eliminating Hunger 516

- Short-term solutions to eliminating hunger provide food through relief at local, national, and international levels, as shown here.

Emergency food relief • Figure 14.11

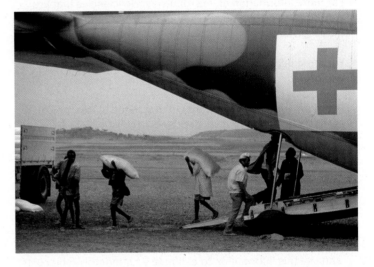

- Eliminating world hunger in the long term requires controlling population growth. This can be addressed by improving economic conditions, providing education, particularly for women, and ensuring access to family planning services.

- **Sustainable agriculture** helps eliminate hunger by allowing food to be produced without damaging the environment.

- Economic development helps prevent hunger by eliminating poverty and ensuring access to health care and education. It also increases access to international trade, which can be used to import food or to export **cash crops** to bring more money into the country.

- Food fortification and dietary supplementation can be used to increase protein quality and eliminate micronutrient deficiencies, improving the overall quality of the diet.

- Nutrition programs in the United States focus on maintaining a nutrition safety net that provides access to affordable food and education to promote healthy eating.

Key Terms

- cash crop 521
- cycle of malnutrition 506
- famine 509
- food desert 514
- food insecurity 509

- food recovery 525
- hunger 506
- infant mortality rate 506
- nutrition transition 508
- renewable resource 511

- starvation 506
- stunting 507
- subsistence crop 521
- sustainable agriculture 520

Online Resources

- For more information on micronutrient deficiencies that are world health issues, go to www.who.int/nutrition/topics/micronutrients/en/.

- For more information on solving world hunger, go to http://usa.wfp.org/advocate/solving-global-hunger.

- For more about food insecurity in the United States, go to www.ers.usda.gov/Briefing/FoodSecurity/.

- For more information on the nutrition safety net in the United States, go to www.fns.usda.gov/fsec/FILES/SafetyNet.pdf.

- Visit your *WileyPLUS* site for videos, animations, podcasts, self-study, and other media that will aid you in studying and understanding this chapter.

Critical and Creative Thinking Questions

1. Keep a record of how much money you spend on food in a day and use this information to estimate your monthly food costs. Would you be able to meet the recommendations of your MyPlate Daily Food Plan on a budget of $3 a day? Which food groups contain the most expensive choices?

2. Compare the cost of a single-serving bottle of orange juice with the same size serving poured from a half-gallon container. Compare the cost of these two products from a large supermarket and from a small corner convenience store. Explain why someone might be forced to buy the higher priced orange juice.

3. Describe the living conditions of people and regions of the world most likely to be affected by undernutrition and the living conditions of people and regions of the world most likely to be affected by overnutrition.

4. The graph below shows the number of bushels of the U.S. corn crop that was used for ethanol (biofuel) production from 1990 to 2010. Why might this impact food insecurity in the United States and around the world?

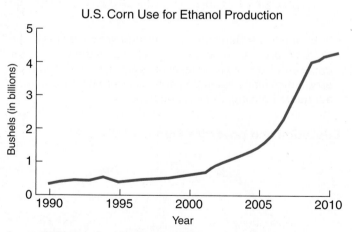

U.S. Corn Use for Ethanol Production

Source: *USDA Agricultural Productions* to 2018, February 2009. USDA Economic Research Service.

5. Discuss which food assistance programs listed in Table 14.1 would benefit homeless people and which would not.

6. The diet in a developing country is deficient in iodine. To solve the problem, the government imports iodized salt, but iodine deficiency continues to be a problem. Why might this be the case?

7. Research one area of the world where hunger and undernutrition are major problems. What are the causes of undernutrition in this area? What solutions are in place or proposed to solve this problem?

What is happening in this picture?

This 250-fold magnification shows the mouth of a hookworm, which it uses to attach to the lining of the small intestine and feed on blood. Hookworm larvae penetrate the skin, infecting people when they walk barefoot in contaminated soil. Hookworm infection affects 740 million people in tropical developing countries.[58]

Think Critically

1. Why is this infection more common in poor tropical and subtropical regions than elsewhere?
2. How would hookworm infection affect iron status? Why?
3. How would hookworm infection affect a population's productivity? Why?

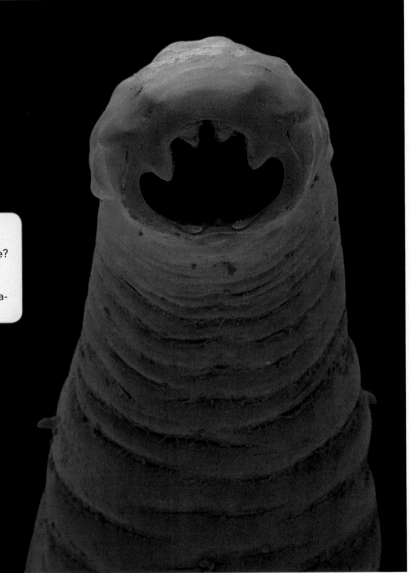

Self-Test

(Check your answers in Appendix K.)

1. The cycle of malnutrition can be broken by _____.
   a. improving health care for children
   b. increasing the availability of nutritious foods for adults
   c. improving health care and nutrition for women during pregnancy
   d. all of the above

2. Which of the following statements about overweight and underweight is supported by the graph?
   a. Underweight is more of a problem in developed countries than in developing countries.
   b. Overweight occurs only in developed countries.
   c. In developed countries, underweight is a problem only among children.
   d. As a country develops economically, the incidence of overweight increases.

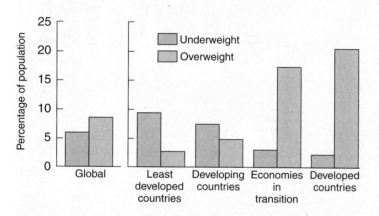

3. Which of the following statements is true of stunting?
   a. It is an indicator of the health and well-being of populations of children.
   b. It is an indicator of the health and well-being of adults.
   c. It is measured with body mass index.
   d. It is highest in well-nourished populations.

4. Which of the following dietary changes is associated with nutrition transition?
   a. consumption of a wider variety of foods
   b. a decrease in the fat and sugar content of the diet
   c. a decrease in the consumption of animal products
   d. an increase in the fiber content of the diet

5. What proportion of the world's undernourished people live in the developing world?
   a. one-half
   b. one-third
   c. more than nine-tenths
   d. less than one-quarter

6. The yellow section of this graph of population growth most likely represents population growth in _____.
   a. developed countries
   b. the entire world
   c. less-developed countries
   d. North America

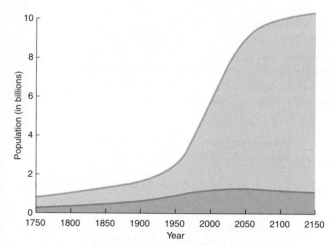

7. What is the largest federal program designed to make sure that all Americans have access to an adequate diet?
   a. Special Supplemental Nutrition Program for Women, Infants, and Children (WIC)
   b. National School Lunch Program
   c. National School Breakfast Program
   d. Supplemental Nutrition Assistance Program (SNAP)

8. Deficiencies of _____ are major world health problems.
   a. vitamins A, K, and C
   b. iodine, vitamin A, and iron
   c. iodine, iron, and chromium
   d. iron, biotin, and vitamin E

9. Crops that are grown to be sold rather than consumed are _____.
   a. sustainable crops
   b. cash crops
   c. subsistence crops
   d. renewable crops

10. Which product is not made from a renewable resource?

    a. paper towels

    b. plastic bags

    c. bread

    d. wooden crates

11. Fortifying _____ will be most likely to eliminate a nutrient deficiency in a country's population.

    a. commonly eaten foods

    b. locally grown foods

    c. foods eaten seasonally

    d. expensive foods

12. Which of the following statements is supported by the information in the pie chart?

    a. In 5.7% of households, food intake was reduced at times during the year.

    b. Food insecurity is highest among women and children.

    c. Food insecurity is a problem for more than 85% of U.S. households.

    d. Food insecurity is high among the homeless.

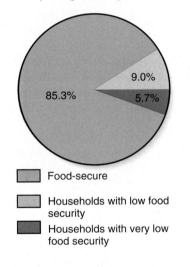

Food-secure

Households with low food security

Households with very low food security

13. Which group in the U.S. population is at risk for undernutrition?

    a. homeless people

    b. children

    c. women

    d. all of the above

14. Which of the following statements about population growth is illustrated in the graphs shown below?

    a. Population growth parallels economic growth.

    b. Education and economic growth increase population growth.

    c. Education decreases population growth.

    d. Economic growth and education do not affect population growth.

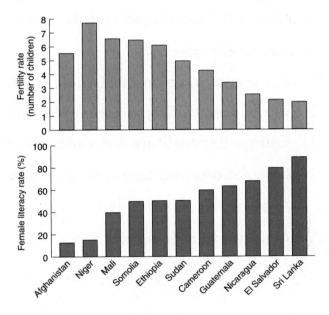

15. Which of the following statements about breast-feeding is true?

    a. It decreases risk of malnutrition in infants.

    b. It is important only for the first 6 months of life.

    c. It is not recommended in poor countries.

    d. It is never recommended for women with HIV

THE PLANNER ✓

Review your Chapter Planner on the chapter opener and check off you completed work.

Appendices

DRI tables for Vitamins and for Minerals are on the front and back covers of this text.

Acceptable Macronutrient Distribution Ranges (AMDR) for Healthy Diets as a Percent of Energy

Age	Carbohydrate	Added Sugars	Total Fat	Linoleic Acid	α- Linolenic Acid	Protein
1–3 y	45–65	≤25	30–40	5–10	0.6–1.2	5–20
4–18 y	45–65	≤25	25–35	5–10	0.6–1.2	10–30
≥19 y	45–65	≤25	20–35	5–10	0.6–1.2	10–35

Source: Institute of Medicine, Food and Nutrition Board. "Dietary Reference Intakes for Energy, Carbohydrate, Fiber, Fat, Fatty Acids, Cholesterol, Protein, and Amino Acids." Washington, D.C.: National Academies Press, 2002, 2005.

Dietary Reference Intakes: Recommended Intakes for Individuals: Carbohydrates, Fiber, Fat, Fatty Acids, Protein, and Water

Life Stage Group	Carbohydrate (g/day)	Fiber (g/day)	Fat (g/day)	Linoleic Acid (g/day)	α-Linolenic Acid (g/day)	Protein (g/kg/day)[a]	Protein (g/day)	Water[b] (L/day)
Infants								
0–6 mo	60*	ND	31*	4.4*†	0.5*‡	1.52*	9.1*	0.7*
6–12 mo	95*	ND	30*	4.6*†	0.5*‡	1.50	11.0	0.8*
Children								
1–3 y	130	19*	ND	7*	0.7*	1.10	13	1.3*
4–8 y	130	25*	ND	10*	0.9*	0.95	19	1.7*
Males								
9–13 y	130	31*	ND	12*	1.2*	0.95	34	2.4*
14–18 y	130	38*	ND	16*	1.6*	0.85	52	3.3*
19–30 y	130	38*	ND	17*	1.6*	0.80	56	3.7*
31–50 y	130	38*	ND	17*	1.6*	0.80	56	3.7*
51–70 y	130	30*	ND	14*	1.6*	0.80	56	3.7*
>70 y	130	30*	ND	14*	1.6*	0.80	56	3.7*
Females								
9–13 y	130	26*	ND	10*	1.0*	0.95	34	
14–18 y	130	26*	ND	11*	1.1*	0.85	46	2.1*
19–30 y	130	25*	ND	12*	1.1*	0.80	46	2.3*
31–50 y	130	25*	ND	12*	1.1*	0.80	46	2.7*
51–70 y	130	21*	ND	11*	1.1*	0.80	46	2.7*
>70 y	130	21*	ND	11*	1.1*	0.80	46	2.7*
Pregnancy	175	28*	ND	13*	1.4*	1.10	71	3.0*
Lactation	210	29*	ND	13*	1.3*	1.10	71	3.8*

ND = not determined. *Values are AI (Adequate Intakes), † Refers to all ω-6 polyunsaturated fatty acids, ‡Refers to all ω-3 polyunsaturated fatty acids.

Source: Institute of Medicine, Food and Nutrition Board. "Dietary Reference Intakes for Energy, Carbohydrate, Fiber, Fat, Fatty Acids, Cholesterol, Protein, and Amino Acids" (2002/2005); "Dietary Reference Intakes for Water, Potassium, Sodium, Chloride, and Sulfate" (2005) Washington, D.C.: National Academies Press.

[a] Based on g protein per kg of body weight for the reference body weight, e.g., for adults 0.8 g/kg body weight for the reference body weight.

[b] Total water includes all water contained in food, beverages, and drinking water.

Dietary Reference Intake Values for Energy: Estimated Energy Requirement (EER) Equations and Values for Active Individuals by Life Stage Group

Life Stage Group	EER Prediction Equation	EER for Active Physical Activity Level (kCal\day)[a]	
		Male	Female
0–3 mo	EER = (89 × weight of infant in kg − 100) + 175	538	493 (2 mo)[c]
4–6 mo	EER = (89 × weight of infant in kg − 100) + 56	606	543 (5 mo)[c]
7–12 mo	EER = (89 × weight of infant in kg − 100) + 22	743	676 (9 mo)[c]
1–2 y	EER = (89 × weight of infant in kg − 100) + 20	1046	992 (2 y)[c]
3–8 y			
Male	EER = 88.5 − (61.9 × Age in yrs) + PA[b][(26.7 × Weight in kg) + (903 × Height in m)] + 20	1742 (6 y)[c]	
Female	EER = 135.3 − (30.8 × Age in yrs) + PA[b][(10.0 × Weight in kg) + (934 × Height in m)] + 20		1642 (6 y)[c]
9–13 y			
Male	EER = 88.5 − (61.9 × Age in yrs) + PA[b][(26.7 × Weight in kg) + (903 × Height in m)] + 25	2279 (11 y)[c]	
Female	EER = 135.3 − (30.8 × Age in yrs) + PA[b][(10.0 × Weight in kg) + (934 × Height in m)] + 25		2071 (11 y)[c]
14–18 y			
Male	EER = 88.5 − (61.9 − Age in yrs) + PA[b][(26.7 × Weight in kg) + (903 × Height in m)] + 25	3152 (16 y)[c]	
Female	EER = 135.3 − (30.8 × Age in yrs) + PA[b][(10.0 × Weight in kg) + (934 × Height in m)] + 25		2368 (16 y)[c]
19 and older			
Males	EER = 662 − (9.53 × Age in yrs) + PA[b][(15.91 × Weight in kg) + (539.6 × Height in m)]	3067 (19 y)[c]	
Females	EER = 354 − (6.91 × Age in yrs) + PA[b][(9.36 × Weight in kg) + (726 × Height in m)]		2403 (19 y)[c]
Pregnancy			
14–18 y			
1st trimester	Adolescent EER + 0		2368 (16 y)[c]
2nd trimester	Adolescent EER + 340		2708 (16 y)[c]
3rd trimester	Adolescent EER + 452		2820 (16 y)[c]
19–50 y			
1st trimester	Adult EER + 0		2403 (19 y)[c]
2nd trimester	Adult EER + 340		2743 (19 y)[c]
3rd trimester	Adult EER + 452		2855 (19 y)[c]
Lactation			
14–18 y			
1st 6 mo	Adolescent EER + 330		2698 (16 y)[c]
2nd 6 mo	Adolescent EER + 400		2768 (16 y)[c]
19–50 y			
1st 6 mo	Adult EER + 330		2733 (19 y)[c]
2nd 6 mo	Adult EER + 400		2803 (19 y)[c]

[a] The intake that meets the average energy expenditure of active individuals at a reference height, weight, and age.

[b] See table entitle "Physical Activity Coefficients (PA Values) for Use in EER Equations" to determine the PA value for various ages, genders, and activity levels.

[c] Value is calculated for an individual at the age in parentheses.

Physical Activity Coefficients (PA Values) for Use in EER Equations

Age and Gender	Sedentary	Low Active	Active	Very Active
3 to 18 y				
Boys	1.00	1.13	1.26	1.42
Girls	1.00	1.16	1.31	1.56
≥19 y				
Men	1.00	1.11	1.25	1.48
Women	1.00	1.12	1.27	1.45

Source: Institute of Medicine, Food and Nutrition Board. "Dietary Reference Intakes for Energy, Carbohydrate, Fiber, Fat, Fatty Acids, Cholesterol, Protein, and Amino Acids." Washington, D.C.: National Academies Press, 2002, 2005.

Dietary Reference Intakes: Tolerable Upper Intake Levels (UL^a): Vitamins

Life Stage Group	Vitamin A (μg/day)^b	Vitamin C (mg/day)	Vitamin D (μg/day)	Vitamin E (mg/day)^c,d	Vitamin K	Thiamin	Riboflavin	Niacin (mg/day)^d	Vitamin B$_6$ (mg/day)	Folate (μg/day)^d	Vitamin B$_{12}$	Pantothenic Acid	Biotin	Choline (g/day)	Carotenoids^e
Infants															
0–6 mo	600	ND^f	25	ND	ND	ND	ND	ND	ND	ND	ND	ND	ND	ND	ND
6–12 mo	600	ND	38	ND	ND	ND	ND	ND	ND	ND	ND	ND	ND	ND	ND
Children															
1–3 y	600	400	63	200	ND	ND	ND	10	30	300	ND	ND	ND	1.0	ND
4–8 y	900	650	75	300	ND	ND	ND	15	40	400	ND	ND	ND	1.0	ND
Males, Females															
9–13 y	1,700	1,200	100	600	ND	ND	ND	20	60	600	ND	ND	ND	2.0	ND
14–18 y	2,800	1,800	100	800	ND	ND	ND	30	80	800	ND	ND	ND	3.0	ND
19–70 y	3,000	2,000	100	1,000	ND	ND	ND	35	100	1,000	ND	ND	ND	3.5	ND
>70 y	3,000	2,000	100	1,000	ND	ND	ND	35	100	1,000	ND	ND	ND	3.5	ND
Pregnancy															
14–18 y	2,800	1,800	100	800	ND	ND	ND	30	80	800	ND	ND	ND	3.0	ND
19–50 y	3,000	2,000	100	1,000	ND	ND	ND	35	100	1,000	ND	ND	ND	3.5	ND
Lactation															
14–18 y	2,800	1,800	100	800	ND	ND	ND	30	80	800	ND	ND	ND	3.0	ND
19–50 y	3,000	2,000	100	1,000	ND	ND	ND	35	100	1,000	ND	ND	ND	3.5	ND

^a UL = The maximum level of daily nutrient intake that is likely to pose no risk of adverse effects. Unless otherwise specified, the UL represents total intake from food, water, and supplements. Due to lack of suitable data, ULs could not be established for vitamin K, thiamin, riboflavin, vitamin B$_{12}$, pantothenic acid, biotin, or carotenoids. In the absence of ULs, extra caution may be warranted in consuming levels above recommended intakes.

^b As preformed vitamin A only.

^c As α-tocopherol; applies to any form of supplemental α-tocopherol.

^d The ULs for vitamin E, niacin, and folate apply to synthetic forms obtained from supplements, fortified foods, or a combination of the two.

^e β-Carotene supplements are advised only to serve as a provitamin A source for individuals at risk of vitamin A deficiency.

^f ND = Not determinable due to lack of data of adverse effects in this age group and concern with regard to lack of ability to handle excess amounts. Source of intakes should be from food only to prevent high levels of intake.

Source: Dietary Reference Intake Tables: The Complete Set. Institute of Medicine, National Academy of Sciences. Available online at www.nap.edu. Reprinted with permission from *Dietary Reference Intakes: The Essential Guide to Nutrient Requirements*, 2006, by the National Academy of Sciences, Washington, D.C. Institute of Medicine, Food and Nutrition Board, Dietary Reference Intakes for Calcium and Vitamin D (2011), National Academies Press, Washington. DC, 2011.

Dietary Reference Intakes: Tolerable Upper Intake Levels (UL[a]): Minerals

Life Stage Group	Arsenic[b]	Boron (mg/day)	Calcium (g/day)	Chromium	Copper (µg/day)	Fluoride (mg/day)	Iodine (µg/day)	Iron (mg/day)	Magnesium (mg/day)[c]	Manganese (mg/day)	Molybdenum (µg/day)	Nickel (mg/day)	Phosphorus (g/day)	Selenium (µg/day)	Silicon[d]	Vanadium (mg/day)[e]	Zinc (mg/day)	Sodium (g/day)	Chloride (g/day)	Potassium
Infants																				
0–6 mo	ND[f]	ND	1.0	ND	ND	0.7	ND	40	ND	ND	ND	ND	ND	45	ND	ND	4	ND	ND	ND
6–12 mo	ND	ND	1.5	ND	ND	0.9	ND	40	ND	ND	ND	ND	ND	60	ND	ND	5	ND	ND	ND
Children																				
1–3 y	ND	3	2.5	ND	1,000	1.3	200	40	65	2	300	0.2	3	90	ND	ND	7	1.5	2.3	ND
4–8 y	ND	6	2.5	ND	3,000	2.2	300	40	110	3	600	0.3	3	150	ND	ND	12	1.9	2.9	ND
Males, Females																				
9–13 y	ND	11	3.0	ND	5,000	10	600	40	350	6	1,100	0.6	4	280	ND	ND	23	2.2	3.4	ND
14–18 y	ND	17	3.0	ND	8,000	10	900	45	350	9	1,700	1.0	4	400	ND	ND	34	2.3	3.6	ND
19–30 y	ND	20	2.5	ND	10,000	10	1,100	45	350	11	2,000	1.0	4	400	ND	1.8	40	2.3	3.6	ND
31–50 y	ND	20	2.5	ND	10,000	10	1,100	45	350	11	2,000	1.0	4	400	ND	1.8	40	2.3	3.6	ND
51–70 y	ND	20	2.0	ND	10,000	10	1,100	45	350	11	2,000	1.0	4	400	ND	1.8	40	2.3	3.6	ND
>70 y	ND	20	2.0	ND	10,000	10	1,100	45	350	11	2,000	1.0	3	400	ND	1.8	40	2.3	3.6	ND
Pregnancy																				
14–18 y	ND	17	3.0	ND	8,000	10	900	45	350	9	1,700	1.0	3.5	400	ND	ND	34	2.3	3.6	ND
19–50 y	ND	20	2.5	ND	10,000	10	1,100	45	350	11	2,000	1.0	3.5	400	ND	ND	40	2.3	3.6	ND
Lactation																				
14–18 y	ND	17	3.0	ND	8,000	10	900	45	350	9	1,700	1.0	4	400	ND	ND	34	2.3	3.6	ND
19–50 y	ND	20	2.5	ND	10,000	10	1,100	45	350	11	2,000	1.0	4	400	ND	ND	40	2.3	3.6	ND

[a]UL = the maximum level of daily nutrient intake that is likely to pose no risk of adverse effects. Unless otherwise specified, the UL represents total intake from food, water, and supplements. Due to lack of suitable data, ULs could not be established for arsenic, chromium, silicon, and potassium. In the absence of ULs, extra caution may be warranted in consuming levels above recommended intakes.

[b]Although the UL was not determined for arsenic, there is no justification for adding arsenic to food or supplements.

[c]The ULs for magnesium represent intake from a pharmacological agent only and do not include intake from food and water.

[d]Although silicon has not been n shown to cause adverse effects in humans, there is no justification for adding silicon to supplements.

[e]Although vanadium in food has not been shown to cause adverse effects in humans, there is no justification for adding vanadium to food and vanadium supplements should be used with caution. The UL is based on adverse effects in laboratory animals and this data could be used to set a UL for adults but not children and adolescents.

[f]ND = Not determinable due to lack of data of adverse effects in this age group and concern with regard to lack of ability to handle excess amounts. Source of intake should be from food only to prevent high levels of intake.

Source: Dietary Reference Intake Tables: The Complete Set. Institute of Medicine, National Academy of Sciences. Available online at www.nap.edu. Reprinted with permission from *Dietary Reference Intakes: The Essential Guide to Nutrient Requirements,* 2006, by the National Academy of Sciences, Washington, D.C. Institute of Medicine, Food and Nutrition Board. Dietary Reference Intakes for Calcium and Vitamin D (2011), National Academies Press, Washington, DC, 2011.

Dietary Reference Intake Values for Energy: Total Energy Expenditure (TEE) Equations for Overweight and Obese Individuals

Life Stage Group	TEE Prediction Equation (Cal/day)	PA Values
Overweight boys aged 3–18 years	TEE = 114 − (50.9 × age in yrs) + PA[(19.5 × weight in kg) + (1161.4 × height in m)]	Sedentary = 1.00 Low active = 1.12 Active = 1.24 Very active = 1.45
Overweight girls aged 3–18 years	TEE = 389 − (41.2 × age in yrs) + PA[(15.0 × weight in kg) + (701.6 × height in m)]	Sedentary = 1.00 Low active = 1.18 Active = 1.35 Very active = 1.60
Overweight and obese men aged 19 years and older	TEE = 1086 − (10.1 × age in yrs) + PA[(13.7 × weight in kg) + (416 × height in m)]	Sedentary = 1.00 Low active = 1.12 Active = 1.29 Very active = 1.59
Overweight and obese women aged 19 years and older	TEE = 448 − (7.95 × age in yrs) + PA[(11.4 × weight in kg) + (619 × height in m)]	Sedentary = 1.00 Low active = 1.16 Active = 1.27 Very active = 1.44

Source: Institute of Medicine, Food and Nutrition Board "Dietary Reference Intakes for Energy, Carbohydrate, Fiber, Fat, Fatty Acids, Cholesterol, Protein, and Amino Acids," Washington, DC: National Academy Press, 2002, 2005.

Body Mass Index (BMI) and Associated Risk

Body mass index (BMI) is the measurement of choice for determining health risks associated with body weight. To use the table, find the appropriate height in the left-hand column. Move across the row to the given weight. The number at the top of the column is the BMI for that height and weight. Use the table below to determine the risks associated with BMI and waist circumference.

BMI (kg/m²)	19	20	21	22	23	24	25	26	27	28	29	30	35	40
Height (in.)	Weight (lb.)													
58	91	96	100	105	110	115	119	124	129	134	138	143	167	191
59	94	99	104	109	114	119	124	128	133	138	143	148	173	198
60	97	102	107	112	118	123	128	133	138	143	148	153	179	204
61	100	106	111	116	122	127	132	137	143	148	153	158	185	211
62	104	109	115	120	126	131	136	142	147	153	158	164	191	218
63	107	113	118	124	130	135	141	146	152	158	163	169	197	225
64	110	116	122	128	134	140	145	151	157	163	169	174	204	232
65	114	120	126	132	138	144	150	156	162	168	174	180	210	240
66	118	124	130	136	142	148	155	161	167	173	179	186	216	247
67	121	127	134	140	146	153	159	166	172	178	185	191	223	255
68	125	131	138	144	151	158	164	171	177	184	190	197	230	262
69	128	135	142	149	155	162	169	176	182	189	196	203	236	270
70	132	139	146	153	160	167	174	181	188	195	202	207	243	278
71	136	143	150	157	165	172	179	186	193	200	208	215	250	286
72	140	147	154	162	169	177	184	191	199	206	213	221	258	294
73	144	151	159	166	174	182	189	197	204	212	219	227	265	302
74	148	155	163	171	179	186	194	202	210	218	225	233	272	311
75	152	160	168	176	184	192	200	208	216	224	232	240	279	319
76	156	164	172	180	189	197	205	213	221	230	238	246	287	328

BMI (kg/m²)		Waist less than or equal to 40 in. (men) or 35 in. (women)	Waist greater than 40 in. (men) or 35 in. (women)
18.5 or less	Underweight	—	N/A
18.5–24.9	Normal	—	N/A
25.0–29.9	Overweight	Increased	High
30.0–34.9	Obese	High	Very High
35.0–39.9	Obese	Very High	Very High
40 or greater	Extremely Obese	Extremely High	Extremely High

Source: Adapted from Partnership for Healthy Weight Management http://www.consumer.gov/weightloss/bmi.htm

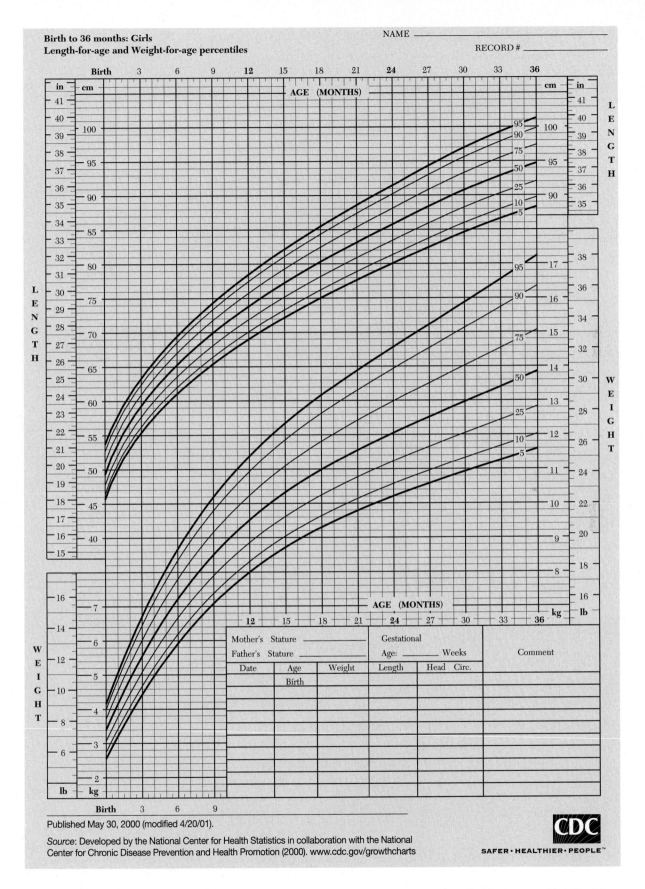

Birth to 36 months: Girls
Length-for-age and Weight-for-age percentiles

NAME

RECORD #

Published May 30, 2000 (modified 4/20/01).

Source: Developed by the National Center for Health Statistics in collaboration with the National Center for Chronic Disease Prevention and Health Promotion (2000). www.cdc.gov/growthcharts

SAFER · HEALTHIER · PEOPLE™

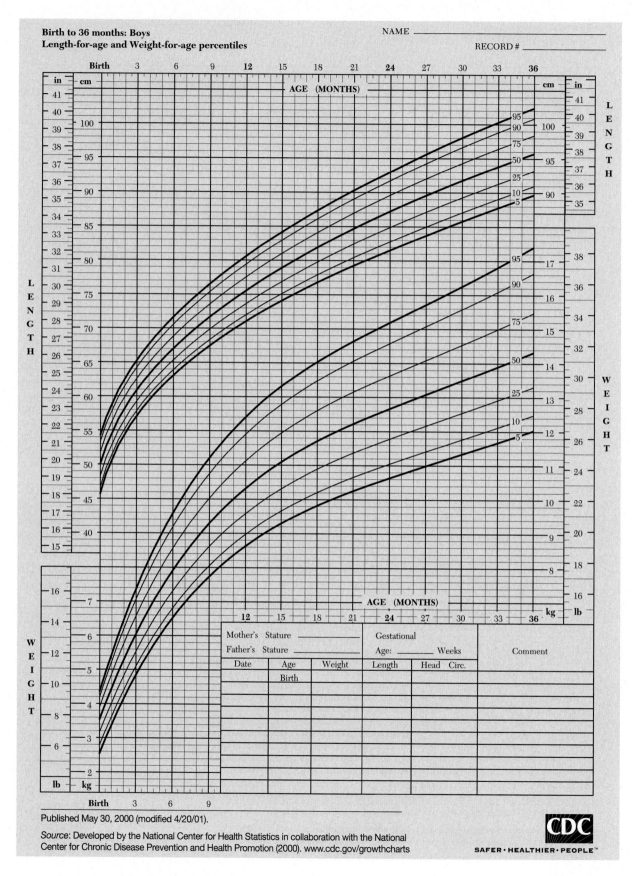

Birth to 36 months: Boys
Length-for-age and Weight-for-age percentiles

NAME _____

RECORD # _____

Published May 30, 2000 (modified 4/20/01).

Source: Developed by the National Center for Health Statistics in collaboration with the National Center for Chronic Disease Prevention and Health Promotion (2000). www.cdc.gov/growthcharts

2 to 20 years: Girls
Body mass index-for-age percentiles

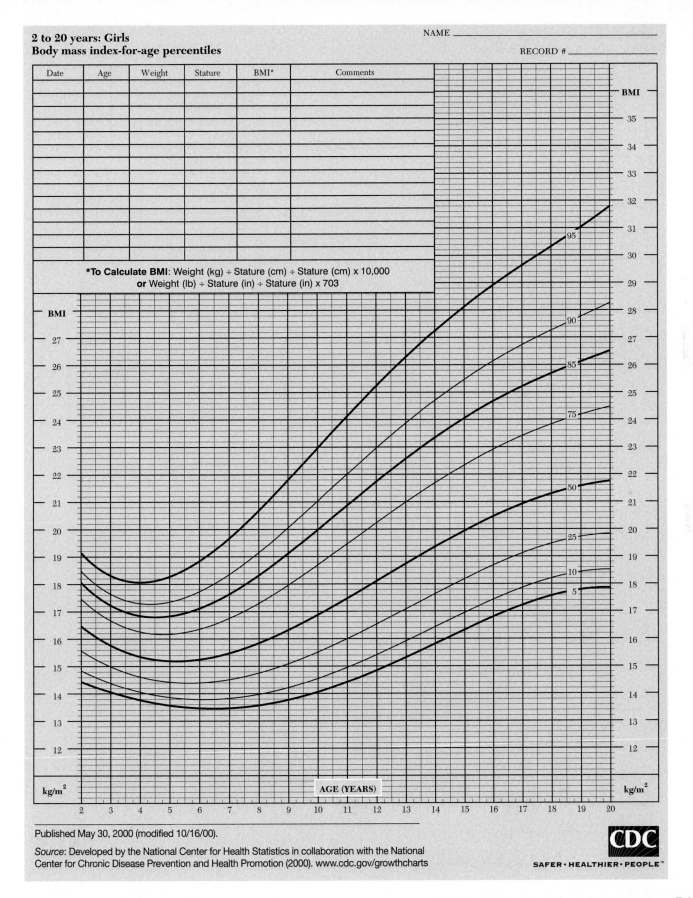

*To Calculate BMI: Weight (kg) ÷ Stature (cm) ÷ Stature (cm) x 10,000
or Weight (lb) ÷ Stature (in) ÷ Stature (in) x 703

AGE (YEARS)

Published May 30, 2000 (modified 10/16/00).

Source: Developed by the National Center for Health Statistics in collaboration with the National Center for Chronic Disease Prevention and Health Promotion (2000). www.cdc.gov/growthcharts

CDC
SAFER · HEALTHIER · PEOPLE™

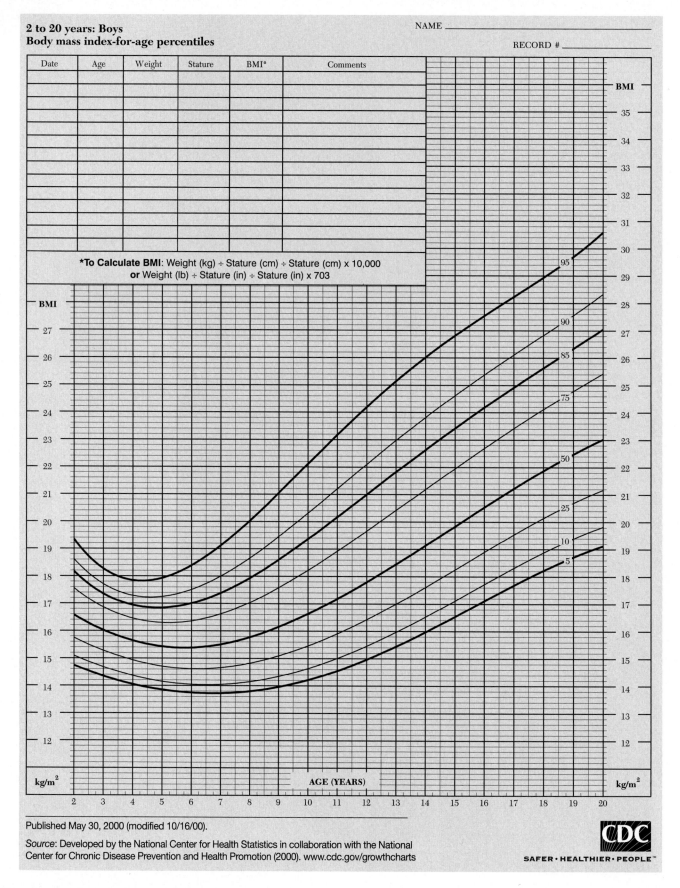

2 to 20 years: Boys
Body mass index-for-age percentiles

NAME _____

RECORD # _____

Date	Age	Weight	Stature	BMI*	Comments

*To Calculate BMI: Weight (kg) ÷ Stature (cm) ÷ Stature (cm) x 10,000
or Weight (lb) ÷ Stature (in) ÷ Stature (in) x 703

BMI

AGE (YEARS)

kg/m²

kg/m²

Published May 30, 2000 (modified 10/16/00).

Source: Developed by the National Center for Health Statistics in collaboration with the National Center for Chronic Disease Prevention and Health Promotion (2000). www.cdc.gov/growthcharts

CDC
SAFER • HEALTHIER • PEOPLE™

Red blood cells	
Men	4.6–6.2 million/mm^3
Women	4.2–5.2 million/mm^3
White blood cells	5,000–10,000/mm^3
Hematocrit	
Men	40–54 ml/100 ml
Women	36–47 ml/100 ml
Children	35–49 ml/100 ml
Hemoglobin	
Men	14–18 g/100 ml
Women	12–16 g/100 ml
Children	11.2–16.5 g/100 ml
Ferritin	
Men	20–300 ng/ml
Women	20–120 ng/ml
Calcium	9–11 mg/100 ml
Iodine	3.8–8 μg/100 ml
Iron	
Men	75–175 μg/100 ml
Women	65–165 μg/100 ml
Zinc	0.75–1.4 μg/ml
Magnesium	1.8–3.0 mg/100 ml
Potassium	3.5–5.0 mEq/liter
Sodium	136–145 mEq/liter
Chloride	100–108 mEq/liter
Vitamin A	20–80 μg/100 ml
Vitamin B_{12}	200–800 pg/100 ml
Vitamin C	0.6–2.0 mg/100 ml
Carotene	48–200 μg/liter
Folate	2–20 ng/ml
pH	7.35–7.45
Total protein	6.6–8.0 g/100 ml
Albumin	3.0–4.0 g/100 ml
Cholesterol	<200 mg/100 ml
Glucose	60–100 mg/100 ml blood, 70–120 mg/100 ml serum

Source: Handbook of Clinical Dietetics, American Dietetic Association, © 1981 by Yale University Press (New Haven, Conn.); and Committee on Dietetics of the Mayo Clinic, Mayo Clinic Diet Manual (Philadelphia: W. B. Saunders Company, 1981), pp. 275–277.

Guidelines for Determining Healthy Lipid Levels

Classification of LDL, Total, and HDL Cholesterol and Triglycerides (mg/dL)

LDL Cholesterol

<100	Optimal*
100–129	Near optimal/above optimal
130–159	Borderline high
160–189	High
≥190	Very high

Total Cholesterol

<200	Desirable
200–239	Borderline high
≥240	High

HDL Cholesterol

<40	Increases risk
≥60	Decreases risk

Triglycerides

<150	Normal
150–190	Borderline high
200–499	High
≥500	Very high

*For very high-risk people, LDL cholesterol should be <70.

Source: National Cholesterol Education Program, ATP III, Quick Reference Guide, 2004 update. Available online at http://www.nhlbi.nih.gov/fuidelines/cholesterol/atglance.pdf

High Blood Pressure (Hypertension) Guidelines

Classification

High	140/90 or above
Prehypertension	120–139 / 80–89
Normal	119/79 or below

Source: Joint National Committee on Prevention, Detection, Evaluation, and Treatment of High Blood Pressure (2003). *The seventh report of the Joint National Committee on Prevention, Detection, Evaluation, and Treatment of High Blood Pressure.* NIH Publication No. 03-5233. Bethesda, MD: U.S. Department of Health and Human Services.

Dietary Guidelines for Americans, 2010

Balancing Calories to Manage Weight

- Prevent and/or reduce overweight and obesity through improved eating and physical activity behaviors.
- Control total calorie intake to manage body weight. For people who are overweight or obese, this will mean consuming fewer calories from foods and beverages.
- Increase physical activity and reduce time spent in sedentary behaviors.
- Maintain appropriate calorie balance during each stage of life-childhood, adolescence, adulthood, pregnancy and breastfeeding, and older age.

Foods and Food Components to Reduce

- Reduce daily sodium intake to less than 2,300 milligrams (mg) and further reduce intake to 1,500 mg among persons who are 51 and older and those of any age who are African American or have hypertension, diabetes, or chronic kidney disease. The 1,500 mg recommendation applies to about half of the U.S. population, including children, and the majority of adults.
- Consume less than 10 percent of calories form saturated fatty acids by replacing them with monounsaturated and polyunsaturated fatty acids.
- Consume less than 300 mg per day of dietary cholesterol.
- Keep *trans* fatty acid consumption as low as possible by limiting foods that contain synthetic sources of *trans* fats, such as partially hydrogenated oils, and by limiting other solid fats.
- Reduce the intake of calories from solid fats and added sugars.
- Limit the consumption of foods that contain refined grains, especially refined grain foods that contain solid fats, added sugars, and sodium.
- If alcohol is consumed it should be consumed in moderation–up to one drink per day for women and two drinks per day for men–and only by adults of legal drinking age.

Foods and Nutrients to Increase

Individuals should meet the following recommendations as part of a healthy eating pattern while staying within their calorie needs.

- Increase vegetable and fruit intake.

- Eat a variety of vegetables, especially dark-green and red and orange vegetables and beans and peas.

- Consume at least half of all grains as whole grains. Increase whole grain intake by replacing refined grains with whole grains.

- Increase intake of fat-free or low-fat milk and milk products, such as milk, yogurt, cheese, or fortified soy beverages.[1]

- Choose a variety of protein foods, which include seafood, lean meat and poultry, eggs, beans and peas, soy products and unsalted nuts and seeds.

- Increase the amount and variety of seafood consumed by choosing seafood in place of some meat and poultry.

- Replace protein foods that are higher in solid fats with choices that are lower in solid fats and calories and/or are sources of oils.

- Use oils to replace solid fats where possible

- Choose foods that provide more potassium, dietary fiber, calcium, and vitamin D, which are nutrients of concern in American diets. These foods include vegetables, fruits, whole grains, and milk and milk products.

Recommendations for Specific Population Groups

Women capable of becoming pregnant [2]

- Choose foods that supply heme iron, which is more readily absorbed by the body, additional iron sources, and enhancers of iron absorption such as vitamin C-rich foods.

- Consume 400 micrograms (mcg) per day of synthetic folic acid (from fortified foods and/or supplements) in addition to food forms of folate from a varied diet.[3]

Women who are pregnant or breastfeeding[2]

- Consume 8 to 12 ounces of seafood per week form a variety of seafood types.

- Due to their high methyl mercury content, limit white (albacore) tuna to 6 ounces per week and do not eat the following four types of fish: tilefish, shark, swordfish, and king mackerel.

- If pregnant, take an iron supplement, as recommended by an obstetrician or other health care provider.

Individuals ages 50 years and older

- Consume foods fortified with vitamin B_{12}, such as fortified cereals, or dietary supplements.

Building Healthy Eating Patterns

- Select an eating pattern that meets nutrient needs over time at an appropriate calorie level.

- Account for all foods and beverages consumed and assess how they fit within a total healthy eating pattern.

- Follow food safety recommendations when preparing and eating foods to reduce the risk of foodborne illnesses.

[1] Fortified soy beverages have been marketed as "soymilk", a product name consumers could see in supermarkets and consumer materials. However, FDA'S regulations do not contain provisions for the use of the term soymilk. Therefore, in this document, the term "fortified soy beverage" includes products that may be marketed as soymilk.

[2] Includes adolescent girls.

[3] "Folic acid" is the synthetic form of the nutrient, whereas, "folate" is the form found naturally in foods.

USDA Food Patterns

For each food group or subgroup,[a] recommended average daily intake amounts[b] at all calorie levels. Recommended intakes from vegetable and protein foods subgroups are per week. For more information an tools for application go to MyPlate.gov

Calorie level of pattern	1,000	1,200	1,400	1,600	1,800	2,000	2,200	2,400	2,600	2,800	3,000	3,200
Fruits	1 c	1 c	1½c	1½ c	1½ c	2 c	2 c	2 c	2 c	2 ½ c	2 ½ c	2 ½ c
Vegetables	1 c	1½ c	1½ c	2 c	2½ c	2 ½ c	3 c	3 c	3 ½ c	3 ½ c	4 c	4 c
Dark-green vegetables	½ c/wk	1 c/wk	1 c/wk	1½ c/wk	1½ c/wk	1½ c/wk	2 c/wk	2 c/wk	2½ c/wk	2½ c/wk	2½ c/wk	2½ c/wk
Red and orange vegetables	2½ c/wk	3 c/wk	3 c/wk	4 c/wk	5½ c/wk	5½ c/wk	6 c/wk	6 c/wk	7 c/wk	7 c/wk	7½ c/wk	7½ c/wk
Beans and peas (legumes)	½ c/wk	½ c/wk	½ c/wk	1 c/wk	1½ c/wk	1½ c/wk	2 c/wk	2 c/wk	2 ½ c/wk	2 ½ c/wk	3 c/wk	3 c/wk
Starchy vegetables	2 c/wk	3 ½ c/wk	3 ½ c/wk	4 c/wk	5 c/wk	5 c/wk	6 c/wk	6 c/wk	7 c/wk	7 c/wk	8 c/wk	8 c/wk
Other vegetables	1½ c/wk	2½ c/wk	2½ c/wk	3½ c/wk	4 c/wk	4 c/wk	5 c/wk	5 c/wk	5½c/wk	5½ c/wk	7 c/wk	7 c/wk
Grains	3 oz-eq	4 oz-eq	5 oz-eq	5 oz-eq	6 oz-eq	6 oz-eq	7 oz-eq	8 oz-eq	9 oz-eq	10 oz-eq	10 oz-eq	10 oz-eq
Whole grains	1 ½ oz-eq	2 oz-eq	2 ½ oz-eq	3 oz-eq	3 oz-eq	3 oz-eq	3 ½ oz-eq	4 oz-eq	4 ½ oz-eq	5 oz-eq	5 oz-eq	5 oz-eq
Enriched grains	1 ½ oz-eq	2 oz-eq	2 ½ oz-eq	2 oz-eq	3 oz-eq	3 oz-eq	3 ½ oz-eq	4 oz-eq	4 ½ oz-eq	5 oz-eq	5 oz-eq	5 oz-eq
Protein foods	2 oz-eq	3 oz-eq	4 oz-eq	5 oz-eq	5 oz-eq	5 ½ oz-eq	6 oz-eq	6 ½ oz-eq	6 ½ oz-eq	7 oz-eq	7 oz-eq	7 oz-eq
Seafood	3 oz/wk	5 oz/wk	6 oz/wk	8 oz/wk	8 oz/wk	8 oz/wk	9 oz/wk	10 oz/wk	10 oz/wk	11 oz/wk	11 oz/wk	11 oz/wk
Meat, poultry, eggs	10 oz/wk	14 oz/wk	19 oz/wk	24 oz/wk	24 oz/wk	26 oz/wk	29 oz/wk	31 oz/wk	31 oz/wk	34 oz/wk	34 oz/wk	34 oz/wk
Nuts, seeds, soy products	1 oz/wk	2 oz/wk	3 oz/wk	4 oz/wk	4 oz/wk	4 oz/wk	4 oz/wk	5 oz/wk	5 oz/wk	5 oz/wk	5 oz/wk	5 oz/wk
Dairy	2 c	2 ½ c	2 ½ c	3 c	3 c	3 c	3 c	3 c	3 c	3 c	3 c	3 c
Oils	15 g	17 g	17 g	22 g	24 g	27 g	29 g	31 g	34 g	36 g	44 g	51 g
Maximum SoFAS[c] **limit, calories (% of calories)**	137 (14%)	121 (10%)	121 (9%)	121 (8%)	161 (9%)	258 (13%)	266 (12%)	330 (14%)	362 (14%)	395 (14%)	459 (15%)	596 (19%)

[a] All foods are assumed to be in nutrient-dense forms, lean or low-fat and prepared without added fats, sugars, or salt. Solid fats and added sugars may be included up to the daily maximum limit identified in the table.

[b] Food group amounts are shown in cup (c) or ounce-equivalents (oz-eq). Oils are shown in grams (g). Quantity equivalents for each food group are:
- Grains, 1 ounce-equivalent is 1 one-ounce slice bread; 1 ounce uncooked pasta or rice: 1/2 cup cooked rice, pasta, or cereal; 1 tortilla (6" diameter); 1 pancake (5" diameter); 1 ounce ready-to-eat cereal (about 1 cup cereal flakes).
- Vegetables and fruits, 1 cup equivalent is: 1 cup raw or cooked vegetable or fruit; 1/2 cup dried vegetable or fruit; 1 cup vegetable or fruit juice; 2 cups leafy salad greens.
- Protein foods, 1 ounce-equivalent is: 1 ounce lean meat, poultry, seafood; 1 egg; 1Tbsp peanut butter; 1/2 ounce nuts or seeds. Also, 1/4 cup cooked beans or peas may also be counted as 1 ounce-equivalent.
- Dairy, 1 cup equivalent is: 1 cup milk, fortified soy beverage, or yogurt; 1 1/2 ounce natural cheese (e.g., cheddar); 2 ounces of processed cheese

[c] SoFAS are calories from solid fats and added sugars. The limit for SoFAS is the remaining amount of calories in each food pattern after selecting the specified amount in each food group in nutrient-dense forms (forms that are fat-free or low-fat and with no added sugars). The number of SoFAS is lower in the 1,200, 1,400, and 1,600 calorie patterns than in the 1,000 calorie pattern. The nutrient goals for the 1,200 to 1,600 calorie patterns are higher and require that more calories be used for nutrient-dense foods from the food groups.

American Institute for Cancer Research Recommendations for Cancer Prevention

Ten recommendations for cancer prevention

1. Be as lean as possible without becoming underweight.
2. Be physically active for at least 30 minutes every day.
3. Avoid sugary drinks. Limit consumption of energy-dense foods.
4. Eat more of a variety of vegetables, fruits, whole grains and legumes such as beans.
5. Limit consumption of red meats (such as beef, pork and lamb) and avoid processed meats.
6. If consumed at all, limit alcoholic drinks to 2 for men and 1 for women a day.
7. Limit consumption of salty foods and foods processed with salt (sodium).
8. Don't use supplements to protect against cancer.
9. It is best for mothers to breastfeed exclusively for up to 6 months and then add other liquids and foods.
10. After treatment, cancer survivors should follow the recommendations for cancer prevention.

And always remember—do not smoke or chew tobacco.

Source: American Institute of Cancer Research. Available online at http://www.aicr.org/reduce-your-cancer-risk. Reprinted with permission from the American Institute for Cancer Research.

Dietary Approaches to Stop Hypertension: DASH Diet Recommendations

Type of food	Daily servings for 1600–3100 Calorie diets	Daily servings for a 2000 Calorie diet
Grains and grain products (include at least 3 whole grain foods each day)	6–12	7–8
Fruits	4–6	4–5
Vegetables	4–6	4–5
Low fat or non fat dairy foods	2–4	2–3
Lean meats, fish, poultry	1.5–2.5	2 or less
Nuts, seeds, and legumes	3–6 per week	4–5 per week
Fats and sweets	2–4	limited

Source: The DASH Diet Eating Plan. Available online at http://dashdiet.org/

Nutrition and Physical Fitness Recommendations from the American Cancer Society

Maintain a healthy weight throughout life.
- Balance calorie intake with physical activity.
- Avoid excessive weight gain throughout life.
- Achieve and maintain a healthy weight if currently overweight or obese.

Adopt a physically active lifestyle.
- **Adults:** Engage in at least 30 minutes of moderate to vigorous physical activity, above usual activities, on 5 or more days of the week; 45 to 60 minutes of intentional physical activity are preferable.
- **Children and adolescents:** Engage in at least 60 minutes per day of moderate to vigorous physical activity at least 5 days per week.

Eat a healthy diet, with an emphasis on plant sources.
- Choose foods and drinks in amounts that help achieve and maintain a healthy weight.
- Eat 5 or more servings of a variety of vegetables and fruits every day.
- Choose whole grains over processed (refined) grains.
- Limit intake of processed and red meats.

If you drink alcoholic beverages, limit your intake.
- Drink no more than 1 drink per day for women or 2 per day for men.

Source: Some adapted from Complete Guide—Nutrition and Physical Activity for Cancer Prevention. Available online at http://www.cancer.org/docroot/PED/content/PED_3_2X_Diet_and_Activity_Factors_That_Affect_Risks.asp?sitearea=PED. Reprinted by the permission of the American Cancer Society, Inc. All rights reserved.

Healthy People 2020

Topics	Indicators	Objectives
Access to care	Proportion of the population with access to healthcare services	1. Increase the proportion of persons with health insurance (AHS 1). 2. Increase proportion of persons with a usual primary care provider (AHS 3). 3. (Developmental) Increase the proportion of persons who receive appropriate evidence-based clinical preventive services (AHS 7).
Healthy Behaviors	Proportion of the population engaged in healthy behaviors	4. Increase the proportion of adults who meet current federal physical activity guidelines for aerobic physical activity and for muscle-strengthing activity (PA 2). 5. Reduce the proportion of children and adolescents who are considered obese (NWS 10). 6. Reduce consumption of calories from solid fats and added sugars in the population aged 2 years and older (NWS 17). 7. Increase the proportion of adults who get sufficient sleep (SH 4).
Chronic Disease	Prevalence and mortality of chronic disease	8. Reduce coronary heart disease deaths (HDS 2). 9. Reduce the proportion of persons in the population with hypertension (HDS 5). 10. Reduce the overall cancer death rate (C 1).
Environmental Determinants	Proportion of the population experiencing a healthy physical environment	11. Reduce the number of days the Air Quality Index (AQI) exceeds 100 (EH 1).
Social Determinants	Proportion of the population experiencing a healthy social environment	12. (Developmental) Improve the health literacy of the population (HC/HIT 1). 13. (Developmental) Increase the proportion of children who are ready for school in all five domains of healthy development: physical development, social-emotional development, approaches to learning, language, and cognitive development (EMC 1). 14. Increase educational achievement of adolescents and young adults (AH 5).
Injury	Proportion of the population that experiences injury	15. Reduce fatal and nonfatal injuries (IVP 1).
Mental Health	Proportion of the population experiencing positive mental health	16. Reduce the proportion of persons who experience major depressive episodes (MDE) (MHMD 4).
Maternal and Infant Health	Proportion of healthy births	17. Reduce low birth weight (LBW) and very low birth weight (VLBW) (MICH 8).
Responsible Sexual Behavior	Proportion of the population engaged in responsible sexual behavior	18. Reduce pregnancy rates among adolescent females (FP 8). 19. Increase the proportion of sexually active persons who use condoms (HIV 17).
Substance Abuse	Proportion of the population engaged in substance abuse	20. Reduce past-month use of illicit substances (SA 13). 21. Reduce the proportion of persons engaging in binge drinking of alcoholic beverages (SA 14).
Tobacco	Proportion of the population using tobacco	22. Reduce tobacco use by adults (TU 1). 23. Reduce the initiation of tobacco use among children, adolescents, and young adults (TU 3).
Quality of Care	Proportion of the population receiving quality health care services	24. Reduce central line-associated blood stream infections (CLABSI) (HA 1).

Strach

Bread	
Food	**Serving Size**
Bagel, large (about 4 oz)	¼ (1 oz)
▽ Biscuit, 2½ inches across	1
Bread	
☺ reduced-calorie	2 slices (1½ oz)
white, whole-grain, pumpernickel, rye, unfrosted raisin	1 slice (1 oz)
Chapatti, small, 6 inches across	1
▽ Cornbread, 1¾ inch cube	1 (1½ oz)
English muffin	½
Hot dog bun or hamburger bun	½ (1 oz)
Naan, 8 inches by 2 inches	¼
Pancake, 4 inches across, ¼ inch thick	1
Pita, 6 inches across	½
Roll, plain, small	1 (1 oz)
▽ Stuffing bread	⅓ cup
▽ Taco shell, 5 inches across	2
Tortilla, corn, 6 inches across	1
Tortilla, corn, 6 inches across	1
Tortilla, flour, 10 inches across	⅓ tortilla
▽ Waffle, 4-inch square or 4 inches across	1

☺ = More than 3 grams of dietary fiber per serving.

▽ = Extra fat, or prepared with added fat. (Count as 1 starch + 1 fat.)

🧂 = 480 milligrams or more of sodium per serving.

Cereals and Grains

Food	Serving Size
Barley, cooked	⅓ cup
Bran, dry	
☺ oat	¼ cup
☺ wheat	½ cup
☺ Bulgur (cooked)	½ cup
Cereals	
☺ bran	½ cup
cooked (oats, oatmeal)	½ cup
puffed	1½ cups
shredded wheat, plain	½ cup
sugar-coated	½ cup
unsweetened, ready-to-eat	¾ cup
Couscous	⅓ cup
Granola	
low-fat	¼ cup
⚠ regular	¼ cup
Grits, cooked	½ cup
Kasha	½ cup
Millet, cooked	⅓ cup
Muesli	¼ cup
Pasta, cooked	⅓ cup
Polenta, cooked	⅓ cup
Quinoa, cooked	⅓ cup
Rice, white or brown, cooked	⅓ cup
Tabbouleh (tabouli), prepared	½ cup
Wheat, germ, dry	3 Tbsp
Wild rice, cooked	½ cup

Starchy Vegetables

Food	Serving Size
Cassava	⅓ cup
Corn	½ cup
on cob, large	½ cup (5 oz)
☺ Hominy, canned	¾ cup
☺ Mixed vegetables with corn, peas, or pasta	1 cup
☺ Parsnips	½ cup
☺ Peas, green	½ cup
Plantain, ripe	⅓ cup
Potato	
baked with skin	¼ large (3 oz)
boiled, all kinds	½ cup or ½ medium (3 oz)
⚠ mashed, with milk and fat	½ cup
French fried (oven-baked)	1 cup (2 oz)
☺ Pumpkin, canned, no sugar added	1 cup
Spaghetti/pasta sauce	½ cup
☺ Squash, winter (acorn, butternut)	1 cup
☺ Succotash	½ cup
Yam, sweet potato, plain	½ cup

Crackers and Snacks

Food	Serving Size
Animal crackers	8
Crackers	
⚠ round-butter type	6
saltine-type	6
⚠ sandwich-style, cheese or peanut butter filling	3
⚠ whole-wheat regular	2–5 (¾ oz)
☺ whole-wheat lower fat or crispbreads	2–5 (¾ oz)
Graham cracker, 2½-inch square	3
Matzoh	¾ oz
Melba toast, about 2-inch by 4-inch piece	4 pieces
Oyster crackers	20
Popcorn	3 cups
⚠☺ with butter	3 cups
☺ no fat added	3 cups
☺ lower fat	3 cups
Pretzels	¾ oz
Rice cakes, 4 inches across	2
Snack chips	
fat-free or baked (tortilla, potato), baked pita chips	15–20 (¾ oz)
⚠ regular (tortilla, potato)	9–13 (¾ oz)

Beans, Peas, and Lentils

The choices on this list count as 1 starch + 1 lean meat.

Food	Serving Size
☺ Baked beans	⅓ cup
☺ Beans, cooked (black, garbanzo, kidney, lima, navy, pinto, white)	½ cup
☺ Lentils, cooked (brown, green, yellow)	½ cup
☺ Peas, cooked (black-eyed, split)	½ cup
ⓢ ☺ Refried beans, canned	½ cup

Fruits

Fruit	
The weight listed includes skin, core, seeds, and rind.	
Food	**Serving Size**
Apple, unpeeled, small	1 (4 oz)
Apples, dried	4 rings
Applesauce, unsweetened	½ cup
Apricots	
canned	½ cup
dried	8 halves
☺ fresh	4 whole (5½ oz)
Banana, extra small	1 (4 oz)
☺ Blackberries	¾ cup
Blueberries	¾ cup
Cantaloupe, small	⅓ melon or 1 cup cubed (11 oz)
Cherries	
sweet, canned	½ cup
sweet fresh	12 (3 oz)
Dates	3
Dried fruits (blueberries, cherries, cranberries, mixed fruit, raisins)	2 Tbsp
Figs	
dried	1½
☺ fresh	1½ large or 2 medium (3½ oz)
Fruit cocktail	½ cup
Grapefruit	
large	½ (11 oz)
sections, canned	¾ cup
Grapes, small	17 (3 oz)
Honeydew melon	1 slice or 1 cup cubed (10 oz)
☺ Kiwi	1 (3½ oz)
Mandarin oranges, canned	¾ cup
Mango, small	1/2 fruit (5½ oz) or ½ cup
Nectarine, small	1 (5 oz)
☺ Orange, small	1 (6½ oz)
Papaya	½ fruit or 1 cup cubed (8 oz)
Peaches	
canned	½ cup
fresh, medium	1 (6 oz)
Pears	
canned	½ cup
fresh, large	½ (4 oz)
Pineapple	
canned	½ cup
fresh	¾ cup
Plums	
canned	½ cup
dried (prunes)	3
small	2 (5 oz)
☺ Raspberries	1 cup
☺ Strawberries	1¼ cup whole berries
☺ Tangerines, small	2 (8 oz)
Watermelon	1 slice or 1¼ cups cubes (13½ oz)

Fruit Juice

Food	Serving Size
Apple juice/cider	½ cup
Fruit juice blends, 100% juice	⅓ cup
Grape juice	⅓ cup
Grapefruit juice	½ cup
Orange juice	½ cup
Pineapple juice	½ cup
Prune juice	⅓ cup

Milk

Milk and Yogurts

Food	Serving Size	Count as
Fat-free or low-fat (1%)		
Milk, buttermilk, acidophilus milk, Lactaid	1 cup	1 fat-free milk
Evaporated milk	½ cup	1 fat-free milk
Yogurt, plain or flavored with an artificial sweetener	⅔ cup (6 oz)	1 fat-free milk
Reduced-fat (2%)		
Milk, acidophilus milk, kefir, Lactaid	1 cup	1 reduced-fat milk
Yogurt, plain	⅔ cup (6 oz)	1 reduced-fat milk
Whole		
Milk, buttermilk, goat's milk	1 cup	1 whole milk
Evaporated milk	½ cup	1 whole milk
Yogurt, plain	8 oz	1 whole milk

Dairy-Like Foods

Food	Serving Size	Count as
Chocolate milk		
fat-free	1 cup	1 fat-free milk + 1 carbohydrate
whole	1 cup	1 whole milk + 1 carbohydrate
Eggnog, whole milk	½ cup	1 carbohydrate + 2 fats
Rice drink		
flavored, low-fat	1 cup	2 carbohydrates
plain, fat-free	1 cup	1 carbohydrate
Smoothies, flavored, regular	10 oz	1 fat-free milk + 2½ carbohydrates
Soy milk		
light	1 cup	1 carbohydrate + ½ fat
regular, plain	1 cup	1 carbohydrate + 1 fat
Yogurt		
and juice blends	1 cup	1 fat-free milk + 1 carbohydrate
low carbohydrate (less than 6 grams carbohydrate per choice)	⅔ cup (6 oz)	½ fat-free milk
with fruit, low-fat	⅔ cup (6 oz)	1 fat-free milk + 1 carbohydrate

Sweets, Desserts, and Other Carbohydrates

Beverages, Soda, and Energy/Sports Drinks

Food	Serving Size	Count as
Cranberry juice cocktail	½ cup	1 carbohydrate
Energy drink	1 can (8.3 oz)	2 carbohydrates
Fruit drink or lemonade	1 cup (8 oz)	2 carbohydrates
Hot chocolate		
regular	1 envelope added to 8 oz water	1 carbohydrate + 1 fat
sugar-free or light	1 envelope added to 8 oz water	1 carbohydrate
Soft drink (soda), regular	1 can (12 oz)	2½ carbohydrates
Sports drink	1 cup (8 oz)	1 carbohydrate

Brownies, Cake, Cookies, Gelatin, Pie, and Pudding

Food	Serving Size	Count as
Brownie, small, unfrosted	1¼-inch square, ⅞ inch high (about 1 oz)	1 carbohydrate + 1 fat
Cake		
angel food, unfrosted	1/12 of cake (about 2 oz)	2 carbohydrates
frosted	2-inch square (about 2 oz)	2 carbohydrates + 1 fat
unfrosted	2-inch square (about 2 oz)	1 carbohydrate + 1 fat
Cookies		
chocolate chip	2 cookies (2¼ inches across)	1 carbohydrate + 2 fats
gingersnap	3 cookies	1 carbohydrate
sandwich, with crème filling	2 small (about ⅔ oz)	1 carbohydrate + 1 fat
sugar-free	3 small or 1 large (¾–1 oz)	1 carbohydrate + 1–2 fats
vanilla wafer	5 cookies	1 carbohydrate + 1 fat
Cupcake, frosted	1 small (about 1¾ oz)	2 carbohydrates + 1–1½ fats
Fruit cobbler	½ cup (3½ oz)	3 carbohydrates + 1 fat
Gelatin, regular	½ cup	1 carbohydrate
Pie		
commercially prepared fruit, 2 crusts	⅙ of 8-inch pie	3 carbohydrates + 2 fats
pumpkin or custard	⅛ of 8-inch pie	1½ carbohydrates + 1½ fats
Pudding		
regular (made with reduced-fat milk)	½ cup	2 carbohydrates
sugar-free or sugar-and fat-free (made with fat-free milk)	½ cup	1 carbohydrate

Candy, Spreads, Sweets, Sweeteners, Syrups, and Toppings

Food	Serving Size	Count as
Candy bar, chocolate/peanut	2 "fun size" bars (1 oz)	1½ carbohydrates + 1½ fats
Candy, hard	3 pieces	1 carbohydrate
Chocolate "kisses"	5 pieces	1 carbohydrate + 1 fat
Coffee creamer		
dry, flavored	4 tsp	½ carbohydrate + ½ fat
liquid, flavored	2 Tbsp	1 carbohydrate
Fruit snacks, chewy (pureed fruit concentrate)	1 roll (¾ oz)	1 carbohydrate
Fruit spreads, 100% fruit	1½ Tbsp	1 carbohydrate
Honey	1 Tbsp	1 carbohydrate
Jam or jelly, regular	1 Tbsp	1 carbohydrate
Sugar	1 Tbsp	1 carbohydrate
Syrup		
chocolate	2 Tbsp	2 carbohydrates
light (pancake type)	2 Tbsp	1 carbohydrate
regular (pancake type)	1 Tbsp	1 carbohydrate

Condiments and Sauces

Food	Serving Size	Count as
Barbeque sauce	3 Tbsp	1 carbohydrate
Cranberry sauce, jellied	¼ cup	1½ carbohydrates
Ⓢ Gravy, canned or bottled	½ cup	½ carbohydrate + ½ fat
Salad dressing, fat-free, low-fat, cream-based	3 Tbsp	1 carbohydrate
Sweet and sour sauce	3 Tbsp	1 carbohydrate

Frozen Bars, Frozen Desserts, Frozen Yogurt, and Ice Cream

Food	Serving Size	Count as
Frozen pops	1	½ carbohydrate
Fruit juice bars, frozen, 100% juice	1 bar (3 oz)	1 carbohydrate
Ice cream		
fat-free	½ cup	1½ carbohydrates
light	½ cup	1 carbohydrate + 1 fat
no sugar added	½ cup	1 carbohydrate + 1 fat
regular	½ cup	1 carbohydrate + 2 fats
Sherbet, sorbet	½ cup	2 carbohydrates
Yogurt, frozen		
fat-free	⅓ cup	1 carbohydrate
regular	½ cup	1 carbohydrate + 0–1 fat

Doughnuts, Muffins, Pastries, and Sweet Breads

Food	Serving Size	Count as
Banana nut bread	1-inch slice (1 oz)	2 carbohydrates + 1 fat
Doughnut		
cake, plain	1 medium (1½ oz)	1½ carbohydrates + 2 fats
yeast type, glazed	3¾ inches across (2 oz)	2 carbohydrates + 2 fats
Muffin (4 oz)	¼ muffin (1 oz)	1 carbohydrate + ½ fat
Sweet roll or Danish	1 (2½ oz)	2½ carbohydrates + 2 fats

Granola Bars, Meal Replacement Bars/Shakes, and Trail Mix

Food	Serving Size	Count as
Granola or snack bar, regular or low-fat	1 bar (1 oz)	1½ carbohydrates
Meal replacement bar	1 bar (1⅓ oz)	1½ carbohydrates + 0–1 fat
Meal replacement bar	1 bar (2 oz)	2 carbohydrates + 1 fat
Meal replacement shake, reduced calorie	1 can (10–11 oz)	1½ carbohydrates + 0–1 fat
Trail mix		
candy/nut-based	1 oz	1 carbohydrate + 2 fats
dried fruit-based	1 oz	1 carbohydrate + 1 fat

Nonstarchy Vegetables

Nonstarchy Vegetables

Amaranth or Chinese spinach
Artichoke
Artichoke hearts
Asparagus
Baby corn
Bamboo shoots
Beans (green, wax, Italian)
Bean sprouts
Beets
ⓢ Borscht
Broccoli
☺ Brussels sprouts
Cabbage (green, bok choy, Chinese)
☺ Carrots
Cauliflower
Celery
☺ Chayote
Coleslaw, packaged, no dressing
Cucumber
Eggplant
Gourds (bitter, bottle, luffa, bitter melon)
Green onions or scallions
Greens (collard, kale, mustard, turnip)
Hearts of palm
Jicama
Kohlrabi

Leeks
Mixed vegetables (without corn, peas, or pasta)
Mung bean sprouts
Mushrooms, all kinds, fresh
Okra
Onions
Oriental radish or daikon
Pea pods
☺ Peppers (all varieties)
Radishes
Rutabaga
ⓢ Sauerkraut
Soybean sprouts
Spinach
Squash (summer, crookneck, zucchini)
Sugar pea snaps
☺ Swiss chard
Tomato
Tomatoes, canned
ⓢ Tomato sauce
ⓢ Tomato/vegetable juice
Turnips
Water chestnuts
Yard-long beans

Meat and Meat Substitutes

Lean Meat and Meat Substitutes

Food	Amount
Beef: Select or Choice grades trimmed of fat: ground round, roast (chuck, rib, rump), round, sirloin, steak (cubed, flank, porterhouse, T-bone), tenderloin	1 oz
ⓢ Beef jerky	1 oz
Cheeses with 3 grams of fat or less per oz	1 oz
Cottage cheese	¼ cup
Egg substitutes, plain	¼ cup
Egg whites	2
Fish, fresh or frozen, plain: catfish, cod, flounder, haddock, halibut, orange roughy, salmon, tilapia, trout, tuna	1 oz
ⓢ Fish, smoked: herring or salmon (lox)	1 oz
Game: buffalo, ostrich, rabbit, venison	1 oz
ⓢ Hot dog with 3 grams of fat or less per oz (8 dogs per 14 oz package) *Note: May be high in carbohydrate.*	1
Lamb: chop, leg, or roast	1 oz
Organ meats: heart, kidney, liver *Note: May be high in cholesterol.*	1 oz
Oysters, fresh or frozen	6 medium
Pork, lean	
ⓢ Canadian bacon	1 oz
rib or loin chop/roast, ham, tenderloin	1 oz

Medium-Fat Meat and Meat Substitutes

Food	Amount
Beef: corned beef, ground beef, meatloaf, Prime grades trimmed of fat (prime rib), short ribs, tongue	1 oz
Cheeses with 4–7 grams of fat per oz: feta, mozzarella, pasteurized processed cheese spread, reduced-fat cheeses, string	1 oz
Egg *Note: High in cholesterol, so limit to 3 per week.*	1
Fish, any fried product	1 oz
Lamb: ground, rib roast	1 oz
Pork: cutlet, shoulder roast	1 oz
Poultry: chicken with skin; dove, pheasant, wild duck, or goose; fried chicken; ground turkey	1 oz
Ricotta cheese	2 oz or ¼ cup
ⓢ Sausage with 4–7 grams of fat per oz	1 oz
Veal, cutlet (no breading)	1 oz
Poultry, without skin: Cornish hen, chicken, domestic duck or goose (well-drained of fat), turkey	1 oz
Processed sandwich meats with 3 grams of fat or less per oz: chipped beef, deli thin-sliced meats, turkey ham, turkey kielbasa, turkey pastrami	1 oz
Salmon, canned	1 oz
Sardines, canned	2 medium
ⓢ Sausage with 3 grams of fat or less per oz	1 oz
Shellfish: clams, crab, imitation shellfish, lobster, scallops, shrimp	1 oz
Tuna, canned in water or oil, drained	1 oz
Veal, lean chop, roast	1 oz

High-Fat Meat and Meat Substitutes

These foods are high in saturated fat, cholesterol, and calories and may raise blood cholesterol levels if eaten on a regular basis. Try to eat 3 or fewer servings from this group per week.

Food	Amount
Bacon	
pork	2 slices (16 slices per lb or 1 oz each, before cooking)
turkey	3 slices (½ oz each before cooking)
Cheese, regular: American, bleu, brie, cheddar, hard goat, Monterey jack, queso, and Swiss	1 oz
Hot dog: beef, pork, or combination (10 per lb-sized package)	1
Hot dog: turkey or chicken (10 per lb-sized package)	1
Pork: ground, sausage, spareribs	1 oz
Processed sandwich meats with 8 grams of fat or more per oz: bologna, pastrami, hard salami	1 oz
Sausage with 8 grams fat or more per oz: bratwurst, chorizo: Italian, knockwurst, Polish, smoked, summer	1 oz

Plant-Based Proteins

Because carbohydrate content varies among plant-based proteins, you should read the food label.

Food	Amount	Count as
"Bacon" strips, soy-based	3 strips	1 medium-fat meat
Baked beans	⅓ cup	1 starch + 1 lean meat
Beans, cooked: black, garbanzo, kidney, lima, navy, pinto, white	½ cup	1 starch + 1 lean meat
"Beef" or "sausage" crumbles, soy-based	2 oz	½ carbohydrate + 1 lean meat
"Chicken" nuggets, soy-based	2 nuggets (1½ oz)	½ carbohydrate + 1 medium-fat meat
Edamame	½ cup	½ carbohydrate + 1 lean meat
Falafel (spiced chickpea and wheat patties)	3 patties (about 2 inches across)	1 carbohydrate + 1 high-fat meat
Hot dog, soy-based	1 (1½ oz)	½ carbohydrate + 1 lean meat
Hummus	⅓ cup	1 carbohydrate + 1 high-fat meat
Lentils, brown, green, or yellow	½ cup	1 carbohydrate + 1 lean meat
Meatless burger, soy-based	3 oz	½ carbohydrate + 2 lean meats
Meatless burger, vegetable- and starch-based	1 patty (about 2½ oz)	1 carbohydrate + 2 lean meats
Nut spreads: almond butter, cashew butter, peanut butter, soy nut butter	1 Tbsp	1 high-fat meat
Peas, cooked: black-eyed and split peas	½ cup	1 starch + 1 lean meat
Refried beans, canned	½ cup	1 starch + 1 lean meat
"Sausage" patties, soy-based	1 (1½ oz)	1 medium-fat meat
Soy nuts, unsalted	¾ oz	½ carbohydrate + 1 medium-fat meat
Tempeh	¼ cup	1 medium-fat meat
Tofu	4 oz (½ cup)	1 medium-fat meat
Tofu, light	4 oz (½ cup)	1 lean meat

Fats

Fats and oils have mixtures of unsaturated (polyunsaturated and monoun-saturated) and saturated fats. Foods on the Fats list are grouped together based on the major type of fat they contain. In general, 1 fat choice equals:

- 1 teaspoon of regular margarine, vegetable oil, or butter
- 1 tablespoon of regular salad dressing

Unsaturated—Monounsaturated Fats

Food	Serving Size
Avocado, medium	2 Tbsp (1 oz)
Nut butters (*trans* fat-free): almond butter, cashew butter, peanut butter (smooth or crunchy)	1½ tsp
Nuts	
almonds	6 nuts
Brazil	2 nuts
cashews	6 nuts
filberts (hazelnuts)	5 nuts
macadamia	3 nuts
mixed (50% peanuts)	6 nuts
peanuts	10 nuts
pecans	4 halves
pistachios	16 nuts
Oil: canola, olive, peanut	1 tsp
Olives	
black (ripe)	8 large
green, stuffed	10 large

Polyunsaturated Fats

Food	Serving Size
Margarine: lower-fat spread (30%–50% vegetable oil, *trans* fat-free)	1 Tbsp
Margarine: stick, tub (*trans* fat-free), or squeeze (*trans* fat-free)	1 tsp
Mayonnaise	
reduced-fat	1 Tbsp
regular	1 tsp
Mayonnaise-style salad dressing	
reduced-fat	1 Tbsp
regular	2 tsp
Nuts	
Pignolia (pine nuts)	1 Tbsp
walnuts, English	4 halves
Oil: corn, cottonseed, flaxseed, grape seed, safflower, soybean, sunflower	1 tsp
Oil: made from soybean and canola oil—Enova	1 tsp
Plant stanol esters	
light	1 Tbsp
regular	2 tsp
Salad dressing	
ⓢ reduced-fat *Note: May be high in carbohydrate.*	2 Tbsp
ⓢ regular	1 Tbsp
Seeds	
flaxseed, whole	1 Tbsp
pumpkin, sunflower	1 Tbsp
sesame seeds	1 Tbsp
Tahini or sesame paste	2 tsp

Saturated Fats

Food	Serving Size
Bacon, cooked, regular or turkey	1 slice
Butter	
reduced-fat	1 Tbsp
stick	1 tsp
whipped	2 tsp
Butter blends made with oil	
reduced-fat or light	1 Tbsp
regular	1½ tsp
Chitterlings, boiled	2 Tbsp (½ oz)
Coconut, sweetened, shredded	2 Tbsp
Coconut milk	
light	⅓ cup
regular	1½ Tbsp
Cream	
half and half	2 Tbsp
heavy	1 Tbsp
light	1½ Tbsp
whipped	2 Tbsp
whipped, pressurized	¼ cup
Cream cheese	
reduced-fat	1½ Tbsp (¾ oz)
regular	1 Tbsp (½ oz)
Lard	1 tsp
Oil: coconut, palm, palm kernel	1 tsp
Salt pork	¼ oz
Shortening, solid	1 tsp
Sour cream	
reduced-fat or light	3 Tbsp
regular	2 Tbsp

Free Foods

A "free" food is any food or drink choice that has less than 20 calories and 5 grams or less of carbohydrate per serving.

Selection Tips

- Most foods on this list should be limited to 3 servings (as listed here) per day. Spread out the servings throughout the day. If you eat all 3 servings at once, it could raise your blood glucose level.
- Food and drink choices listed here without a serving size can be eaten whenever you like.

Low Carbohydrate Foods

Food	*Serving Size*
Cabbage, raw	½ cup
Candy, hard (regular or sugar-free)	1 piece
Carrots, cauliflower, or green beans, cooked	¼ cup
Cranberries, sweetened with sugar substitute	½ cup
Cucumber, sliced	½ cup
Gelatin	
dessert, sugar-free	
unflavored	
Gum	
Jam or jelly, light or no sugar added	2 tsp
Rhubarb, sweetened with sugar substitute	½ cup
Salad greens	
Sugar substitutes (artificial sweeteners)	
Syrup, sugar-free	2 Tbsp

Modified Fat Foods with Carbohydrate

Food	*Serving Size*
Cream cheese, fat-free	1 Tbsp (½ oz)
Creamers	
nondairy, liquid	1 Tbsp
nondairy, powdered	2 tsp
Margarine spread	
fat-free	1 Tbsp
reduced-fat	1 tsp
Mayonnaise	
fat-free	1 Tbsp
reduced-fat	1 tsp
Mayonnaise-style salad dressing	
fat-free	1 Tbsp
reduced-fat	1 tsp
Salad dressing	
fat-free or low-fat	1 Tbsp
fat-free, Italian	2 Tbsp
Sour cream, fat-free or reduced-fat	1 Tbsp
Whipped topping	
light or fat-free	2 Tbsp
regular	1 Tbsp

Condiments

Food	Serving Size
Barbecue sauce	2 tsp
Catsup (ketchup)	1 Tbsp
Honey mustard	1 Tbsp
Horseradish	
Lemon juice	
Miso	1½ tsp
Mustard	
Parmesan cheese, freshly grated	1 Tbsp
Pickle relish	1 Tbsp
Pickles	
ⓢ dill	1½ medium
sweet, bread and butter	2 slices
sweet, gherkin	¾ oz
Salsa	¼ cup
ⓢ Soy sauce, light or regular	1 Tbsp
Sweet and sour sauce	2 tsp
Sweet chili sauce	2 tsp
Taco sauce	1 Tbsp
Vinegar	
Yogurt, any type	2 Tbsp

Drinks/Mixes

Any food on this list—without a serving size listed—can be consumed in any moderate amount.

- ⓢ Bouillon, broth, consomme
- Bouillon or broth, low-sodium
- Carbonated or mineral water
- Club soda
- Cocoa powder, unsweetened (1 Tbsp)
- Coffee, unsweetened or with sugar substitute
- Diet soft drinks, sugar-free
- Drink mixes, sugar-free
- Tea, unsweetened or with sugar substitute
- Tonic water, diet
- Water
- Water, flavored, carbohydrate free

Seasonings

Any food on this list can be consumed in any moderate amount.

- Flavoring extracts (for example, vanilla, almond, peppermint)
- Garlic
- Herbs, fresh or dried
- Nonstick cooking spray
- Pimento
- Spices
- Hot pepper sauce
- Wine, used in cooking
- Worcestershire sauce

Combination Foods

Many of the foods you eat are mixed together in various combinations, such as casseroles. These "combination" foods do not fit into any one choice list. This is a list of choices for some typical combination foods. This list will help you fit these foods into your meal plan. Ask your RD for nutrient information about other combination foods you would like to eat, including your own recipes.

Entrees

Food	Serving Size	Count as
Casserole type (tuna noodle, lasagna, spaghetti with meatballs, chili with beans, macaroni and cheese)	1 cup (8 oz)	2 carbohydrates + 2 medium-fat meats
Stews (beef/other meats and vegetables)	1 cup (8 oz)	1 carbohydrate + 1 medium-fat meat + 0–3 fats
Tuna salad or chicken salad	½ cup (3½ oz)	½ carbohydrate + 2 lean meats + 1 fat

Frozen Meals/Entrees

Food	Serving Size	Count as
Burrito (beef and bean)	1 (5 oz)	3 carbohydrates + 1 lean meat + 2 fats
Dinner-type meal	generally 14–17 oz	3 carbohydrates + 3 medium-fat meats + 3 fats
Entree or meal with less than 340 calories	about 8–11 oz	2–3 carbohydrates + 1–2 lean meats
Pizza		
cheese/vegetarian, thin crust	¼ of a 12 inch (4½–5 oz)	2 carbohydrates + 2 medium-fat meats
meat topping, thin crust	¼ of a 12 inch (5 oz)	2 carbohydrates + 2 medium-fat meats + 1½ fats
Pocket sandwich	1 (4½ oz)	3 carbohydrates + 1 lean meat + 1–2 fats
Pot pie	1 (7 oz)	2½ carbohydrates + 1 medium-fat meat + 3 fats

Salads (Deli-Style)

Food	Serving Size	Count as
Coleslaw	½ cup	1 carbohydrate + 1½ fats
Macaroni/pasta salad	½ cup	2 carbohydrates + 3 fats
Potato salad	½ cup	1½–2 carbohydrates + 1–2 fats

Soups

	Food	Serving Size	Count as
🧂	Bean, lentil, or split pea	1 cup	1 carbohydrate + 1 lean meat
🧂	Chowder (made with milk)	1 cup (8 oz)	1 carbohydrate + 1 lean meat + 1½ fats
🧂	Cream (made with water)	1 cup (8 oz)	1 carbohydrate + 1 fat
🧂	Instant	6 oz prepared	1 carbohydrate
🧂	with beans or lentils	8 oz prepared	2½ carbohydrates + 1 lean meat
🧂	Miso soup	1 cup	½ carbohydrate + 1 fat
🧂	Oriental noodle	1 cup	2 carbohydrates + 2 fats
	Rice (congee)	1 cup	1 carbohydrate
🧂	Tomato (made with water)	1 cup (8 oz)	1 carbohydrate
🧂	Vegetable beef, chicken noodle, or other broth-type	1 cup (8 oz)	1 carbohydrate

Fast Foods

The choices in the **Fast Foods** list are not specific fast food meals or items, but are estimates based on popular foods. You can get specific nutrition information for almost every fast food or restaurant chain. Ask the restaurant or check its website for nutrition information about your favorite fast foots.

Breakfast Sandwiches

	Food	Serving Size	Count as
🧂	Egg, cheese, meat, English muffin	1 sandwich	2 carbohydrates + 2 medium-fat meats
🧂	Sausage biscuit sandwich	1 sandwich	2 carbohydrates + 2 high-fat meats + 3½ fats

Main Dishes/Entrees

	Food	Serving Size	Count as
🧂 ⊕	Burrito (beef and beans)	1 (about 8 oz)	3 carbohydrates + 3 medium-fat meats + 3 fats
🧂	Chicken breast, breaded and fried	1 (about 5 oz)	1 carbohydrate + 4 medium-fat meats
	Chicken drumstick, breaded and fried	1 (about 2 oz)	2 medium-fat meats
🧂	Chicken nuggets	6 (about 3½ oz)	1 carbohydrate + 2 medium-fat meats + 1 fat
🧂	Chicken thigh, breaded and fried	1 (about 4 oz)	½ carbohydrate + 3 medium-fat meats + 1½ fats
🧂	Chicken wings, hot	6 (5 oz)	5 medium-fat meats + 1½ fats

Oriental

	Food	Serving Size	Count as
ⓢ	Beef/chicken/shrimp with vegetables in sauce	1 cup (about 5 oz)	1 carbohydrate + 1 lean meat + 1 fat
ⓢ	Egg roll, meat	1 (about 3 oz)	1 carbohydrate + 1 lean meat + 1 fat
	Fried rice, meatless	½ cup	1½ carbohydrates + 1½ fats
ⓢ	Meat and sweet sauce (orange chicken)	1 cup	3 carbohydrates + 3 medium-fat meats + 2 fats
ⓢ ☺	Noodles and vegetables in sauce (chow mein, lo mein)	1 cup	2 carbohydrates + 1 fat

Pizza

	Food	Serving Size	Count as
	Pizza		
ⓢ	cheese, pepperoni, regular crust	⅛ of a 14 inch (about 4 oz)	2½ carbohydrates + 1 medium-fat meat + 1½ fats
ⓢ	cheese/vegetarian, thin crust	¼ of a 12 inch (about 6 oz)	2½ carbohydrates + 2 medium-fat meats + 1½ fats

Sandwiches

	Food	Serving Size	Count as
ⓢ	Chicken sandwich, grilled	1	3 carbohydrates + 4 lean meats
ⓢ	Chicken sandwich, crispy	1	3½ carbohydrates + 3 medium-fat meats + 1 fat
	Fish sandwich with tartar sauce	1	2½ carbohydrates + 2 medium-fat meats + 2 fats
	Hamburger		
ⓢ	large with cheese	1	2½ carbohydrates + 4 medium-fat meats + 1 fat
	regular	1	2 carbohydrates + 1 medium-fat meat + 1 fat
ⓢ	Hot dog with bun	1	1 carbohydrate + 1 high-fat meat + 1 fat
	Submarine sandwich		
ⓢ	less than 6 grams fat	6-inch sub	3 carbohydrates + 2 lean meats
ⓢ	regular	6-inch sub	3½ carbohydrates + 2 medium-fat meats + 1 fat
	Taco, hard or soft shell (meat and cheese)	1 small	1 carbohydrate + 1 medium-fat meat + 1½ fats

Salads

Food	Serving Size	Count as
Salad, main dish (grilled chicken type, no dressing or croutons)	Salad	1 carbohydrate + 4 lean meats
Salad, side, no dressing or cheese	Small (about 5 oz)	1 vegetable

Sides/Appetizers

Food	Serving Size	Count as
French fries, restaurant style	small	3 carbohydrates + 3 fats
	medium	4 carbohydrates + 4 fats
	large	5 carbohydrates + 6 fats
Nachos with cheese	small (about 4½ oz)	2½ carbohydrates + 4 fats
Onion rings	1 serving (about 3 oz)	2½ carbohydrates + 3 fats

Desserts

Food	Serving Size	Count as
Milkshake, any flavor	12 oz	6 carbohydrates + 2 fats
Soft-serve ice cream cone	1 small	2½ carbohydrates + 1 fat

Alcohol

Nutrition Tips

- In general, 1 alcohol choice (½ oz absolute alcohol) has about 100 calories.

Selection Tips

- If you choose to drink alcohol, you should limit it to 1 drink or less per day for women, and 2 drinks or less per day for men.

- To reduce your risk of low blood glucose (hypoglycemia), especially if you take insulin or a diabetes pill that increases insulin, always drink alcohol with food.

- While alcohol, by itself, does not directly affect blood glucose, be aware of the carbohydrate (for example, in mixed drinks, beer, and wine) that may raise your blood glucose.

- Check with your RD if you would like to fit alcohol into your meal plan.

Alcoholic Beverage	Serving Size	Count as
Beer		
light (4.2%)	12 fl oz	1 alcohol equivalent + ½ carbohydrate
regular (4.9%)	12 fl oz	1 alcohol equivalent + 1 carbohydrate
Distilled spirits: vodka, rum, gin, whiskey 80 or 86 proof	1½ fl oz	1 alcohol equivalent
Liqueur, coffee (53 proof)	1 fl oz	1 alcohol equivalent + 1 carbohydrate
Sake	1 fl oz	½ alcohol equivalent
Wine		
dessert (sherry) dry,	3½ fl oz	1 alcohol equivalent + 1 carbohydrate
red or white (10%)	5 fl oz	1 alcohol equivalent

Sample Food Label for a Granola Bar

Nutrition Facts
Serving Size 1 bar (24g)
Servings Per Container 12

Amount Per Serving

Calories 120	Calories from Fat 45

	% **Daily Value***
Total Fat 5g	8%
Saturated Fat 1g	5%
Trans Fat	0%
Cholesterol 0mg	0%
Sodium 65mg	3%
Total Carbohydrate 17g	6%
Dietary Fiber 1g	4%
Sugars 6g	
Protein 2g	

Vitamin A 0%	•	Vitamin C 0%
Calcium 0%	•	Iron 4%

*Percent Daily Values are based on a 2,000 calorie diet. Your daily values may be higher or lower depending on your calorie needs:

	Calories:	2,000	2,500
Total Fat	Less than	65g	80g
Sat Fat	Less than	20g	25g
Cholesterol	Less than	300mg	300mg
Sodium	Less than	2,400mg	2,400mg
Total Carbohydrate		300g	375g
Dietary Fiber		25g	30g

Caloies per gram
Fat 9 • Carbohydrate 4 • Protein 4

Ingredients: Rolled oats, sugar, sunflower oil, brown sugar syrup, honey, salt, soy lecithin

Daily Reference Values Used to Establish Daily Values

Food Component	Daily Reference Value (2000 Kcal)
Total fat	Less than 65 g (30% of energy)
Saturated fat	Less than 20 g (10% of energy)
Cholesterol	Less than 300 mg
Total carbohydrate	300 g (60% of energy)
Dietary fiber	25 g (11.5 g/1000 Kcal)
Sodium	Less than 2400 mg
Potassium	3500 mg
Protein	50 g (10% of energy)

Source: USDA A Food Labeling Guide Appendix F. Available online at http://www.cfsan.fda.gov/~dms/2lg-xf.html

Sample Supplement Label

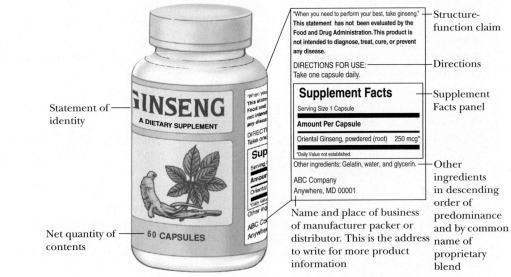

"When you need to perform your best, take ginseng." **This statement has not been evaluated by the Food and Drug Administration. This product is not intended to diagnose, treat, cure, or prevent any disease.** — Structure-function claim

DIRECTIONS FOR USE: — Directions
Take one capsule daily.

Supplement Facts
Serving Size 1 Capsule

Amount Per Capsule

Oriental Ginseng, powdered (root)   250 mcg*

*Daily Value not established.

— Supplement Facts panel

Other ingredients: Gelatin, water, and glycerin. — Other ingredients in descending order of predominance and by common name of proprietary blend

ABC Company
Anywhere, MD 00001

Name and place of business of manufacturer packer or distributor. This is the address to write for more product information

Statement of identity

Net quantity of contents

GINSENG
A DIETARY SUPPLEMENT

60 CAPSULES

Recommended Dietary Intakes (RDIs)* Used to Establish Daily Values

Vitamins and Minerals	Units of Measurement	Adults and Children 4 or more Years of Age	Infants	Children Under 4 Years of Age	Pregnant or Lactating Women
Vitamin A	International Units†	5000 (1000 µg)	1500	2500	8000
Vitamin D	International Units†	400 (10 µg)	400	400	400
Vitamin E	International Units†	30 (10 µg)	5	10	30
Vitamin C	Milligrams	60	35	40	60
Folic acid	Micrograms	400	0.1	0.2	0.8
Thiamin	Milligrams	1.5	0.5	0.7	1.7
Riboflavin	Milligrams	1.7	0.6	0.8	2.0
Niacin	Milligrams	20	8	9	20
Vitamin B_6	Milligrams	2.0	0.4	0.7	2.5
Vitamin B_{12}	Micrograms	6.0	2	3	8
Biotin	Micrograms	300	0.05	0.15	0.30
Pantothenic acid	Milligrams	10	3	5	10
Calcium	Milligrams	1000	0.6	0.8	1.3
Phosphorous	Milligrams	1000	0.5	0.8	1.3
Iodine	Micrograms	150	45	70	150
Iron	Milligrams	18	15	10	18
Magnesium	Milligrams	400	70	200	450
Copper	Milligrams	2.0	0.6	1.0	2.0
Zinc	Milligrams	15	5	8	15
Vitamin K	Micrograms	80	—‡	—‡	—‡
Chromium	Micrograms	120	—	—	—
Selenium	Micrograms	70	—	—	—
Molybdenum	Micrograms	75	—	—	—
Manganese	Milligrams	2	—	—	—
Chloride	Milligrams	3400	—	—	—

*Based on National Academy of Sciences' 1968 Recommended Dietary Allowances.

†The RDIs for fat-soluble vitamins are expressed in International Units (IU). Values that are approximately equivalent in micrograms are given in parentheses.

‡No values yet established for vitamin K, chromium, selenium, molybdenum, manganese, or chloride for this population.

Source: USDA Food Labeling Guide. Available online at http://www.cfsan.fda.gov/~dms/2lg-xf.htm

Health Claims Permitted on Food or Supplement Labels

Health Claims That Meet Significant Scientific Agreement

These are authorized by the FDA based on an extensive review of the scientific literature or information from a scientific body of the U.S. government or the National Academy of Sciences that supports the nutrient/disease relationship.

- Calcium and osteoporosis
- Dietary fat and cancer
- Dietary saturated fat and cholesterol and risk of coronary heart disease
- Dietary non-carcinogenic carbohydrate sweeteners and dental caries
- Fiber-containing grain products, fruits, and vegetables and cancer
- Folic acid and neural tube defects
- Fluoridated water and reduced risk of dental caries
- Fruits, vegetables, and grain products and cancer
- Fruits, vegetables, and grain products that contain fiber, particularly soluble fiber, and risk of coronary heart disease
- Plant sterol/stanol and coronary heart disease
- Potassium and the risk of high blood pressure and stroke
- Saturated fat, cholesterol, and *trans* fat and reduced risk of heart disease
- Sodium and hypertension
- Soluble fiber from certain foods and risk of coronary heart disease
- Soy protein and risk of coronary heart disease
- Stanols/sterols and risk of coronary heart disease
- Whole grain foods and the risk of heart disease and certain cancers

Qualified Health Claims

These are used when there is emerging evidence for a relationship between a food, food component, or dietary supplement and reduced risk of a disease or health-related condition but there is not enough scientific support for the FDA to issue an authorizing regulation.

- Qualified claims about cancer risk: selenium and cancer, antioxidant vitamins and cancer, green tea and cancer, tomatoes and cancer, calcium and colorectal cancer and/recurrent colon rectal polyps.
- Qualified claims about cardiovascular disease risk: nuts and heart disease, walnuts and heart disease, omega-3 fatty acids and coronary heart disease, B vitamins and vascular disease, monounsaturated fatty acids from olive oil and reduced coronary heart disease risk, unsaturated fatty acids from canola oil and coronary heart disease risk, corn oil and coronary heart disease.
- Qualified claims about diabetes: chromium picolinate and diabetes
- Qualified claims about hypertension: calcium and hypertension, pregnancy-indused hypertension and preeclampsia
- Qualified claims about cognitive function: phosphatidylserine and cognitive dysfunction and dementia
- Qualified claims about neural tube birth defects: 0.8 mg folic acid and neural tube birth defects

Source: U.S. Food and Drug Administration. Center for Food Safety and Applied Nutrition. Label Claims. Available online at http://www.cfsan.fda.gov/~dms/2lg-xc.html

Nutrient Content Descriptors Commonly Used on Food Labels

Free	Means that a product contains no amount of, or a trivial amount of, fat, saturated fat, cholesterol, sodium, sugars, or Calories. For example, "sugar free" and "fat free" both mean less than 0.5 g per serving. Synonyms for "free" include "without," "no," and "zero."
Low	Used for foods that can be eaten frequently without exceeding the Daily Value for fat, saturated fat, cholesterol, sodium, or Calories. Specific definitions have been established for each of these nutrients. For example, "low fat" means that the food contains 3 g or less per serving, and "low cholesterol" means that the food contains less than 20 mg of cholesterol per serving. Synonyms for "low" include "little," "few," and "low source of."
Lean and extra lean	Used to describe the fat content of meat, poultry, seafood, and game meats. "Lean" means that the food contains less than 10 g fat, less than 4.5 g saturated fat, and less than 95 mg of cholesterol per serving and per 100 g. "Extra lean" means that the food contains less than 5 g fat, less than 2 g saturated fat, and less than 95 mg of cholesterol per serving and per 100 g.
High	Can be used if a food contains 20% or more of the Daily Value for a particular nutrient. Synonyms for "high" include "rich in" and "excellent source of."
Good source	Means that a food contains 10 to 19% of the Daily Value for a particular nutrient per serving.
Reduced	Means that a nutritionally altered product contains 25% less of a nutrient or of energy than the regular or reference product.
Less	Means that a food, whether altered or not, contains 25% less of a nutrient or of energy than the reference food. For example, pretzels may claim to have "less fat" than potato chips. "Fewer" may be used as a synonym for "less."
Light	May be used in different ways. First, it can be used on a nutritionally altered product that contains one-third fewer kcalories or half the fat of a reference food. Second, it can be used when the sodium content of a low-calorie, low-fat food has been reduced by 50%. The term "light" can be used to describe properties such as texture and color as long as the label explains the intent—for example, "light and fluffy."
More	Means that a serving of food, whether altered or not, contains a nutrient that is at least 10% of the Daily Value more than the reference food. This definition also applies to foods using the terms "fortified," "enriched," or "added."
Healthy	May be used to describe foods that are low in fat and saturated fat and contain no more than 360 mg of sodium and no more than 60 mg of cholesterol per serving and provide at least 10% of the Daily Value for vitamins A or C, or iron, calcium, protein, or fiber.
Fresh	May be used on foods that are raw and have never been frozen or heated and contain no preservatives.

Source: USDA. A food Labeling Guide Appendix A. Available online at
http://www.cfsan.fda.gov/~dms/2lg-xa.html

Ranges of Population Nutrient Intake Goals

Dietary Factor	Goal (% of total energy, unless otherwise stated)
Total fat	15–30%
Saturated fatty acids	<10%
Polyunsaturated fatty acids (PUFAs)	6–10%
n-6 Polyunsaturated fatty acids (PUFAs)	5–8%
n-3 Polyunsaturated fatty acids (PUFAs)	1–2%
Trans fatty acids	<1%
Monounsaturated fatty acids (MUFAs)	By difference[a]
Total carbohydrate	55–75%[b]
Free sugars[c]	<10%
Protein	10–15%[d]
Cholesterol	<300 mg per day
Sodium chloride (sodium)[e]	<5 g per day (<2 g per day)
Fruits and vegetables	≥400 g per day
Total dietary fiber[f]	> 25 g/day
Non-starch polysaccharides (NSP)[f]	> 20 g/day

[a]This is calculated as: total fat − (saturated fatty acids + polyunsaturated fatty acids + trans fatty acids).

[b]The percentage of total energy available after taking into account that consumed as protein and fat, hence the wide range.

[c]The term "free sugars" refers to all monosaccharides and disaccharides added to foods by the manufacturer, cook or consumer, plus sugars naturally present in honey, syrups and fruit juices.

[d]The suggested range should be seen in the light of the Joint WHO/FAO/UNU Expert Consultation on Protein and Amino Acid Requirements in Human Nutrition, held in Geneva from 9 to 16 April 2002 (2).

[e]Salt should be iodized appropriately (6). The need to adjust salt iodization, depending on observed sodium intake and surveillance of iodine status of the population, should be recognized.

[f]The recommended intake of fruits and vegtables and consumption of whole grain foods is likely to provide these amounts.

Source: Diet, nutrition and the prevention of chronic diseases. A report of a Joint WHO/FAO Expert Consultation. © World Health Organization 2003. Available online at http://www.who.int/hpr/NPH/docs/who_fao_expert_report.pdf. Reproduced with permission.

Energy Expenditure for Various Activities

Type of Activity	Calories per Hour (by body weight)				
	100 lb	120 lb	150 lb	180 lb	200 lb
Aerobics (heavy)	363	435	544	653	726
Aerobics (medium)	227	272	340	408	454
Aerobics (light)	136	163	204	245	272
Archery	159	190	238	286	317
Backpacking	408	490	612	735	816
Badminton (doubles)	181	218	272	327	363
Badminton (singles)	231	278	347	416	463
Basketball (nonvigorous)	431	517	646	776	862
Basketball (vigorous)	499	599	748	898	998
Bicycling (6 mph)	159	190	238	286	317
Bicycling (10 mph)	249	299	374	449	499
Bicycling (11 mph)	295	354	442	531	590
Bicycling (12 mph)	340	408	510	612	680
Bicycling (13 mph)	385	463	578	694	771
Billiards	91	109	136	163	181
Bowling	177	212	265	318	354
Boxing—competition	603	724	905	1086	1206
Boxing—sparring	376	452	565	678	753
Calisthenics (heavy)	363	435	544	653	726
Calisthenics (light)	181	218	272	327	363
Canoeing (2.5 mph)	150	180	224	269	299
Canoeing (5 mph)	340	408	510	612	680
Carpentry	227	272	340	408	454
Climbing (mountain)	454	544	680	816	907
Disco dancing	272	327	408	490	544
Ditch digging (hand)	263	316	395	473	526
Fencing	340	408	510	612	680
Fishing (bank/boat)	159	190	238	286	317
Fishing (in waders)	249	299	374	449	499
Football (touch)	340	408	510	612	680
Gardening	145	174	218	261	290
Golf (carry clubs)	227	272	340	408	454
Golf (pull cart)	163	196	245	294	327
Golf (ride in cart)	113	136	170	204	227
Handball (vigorous)	454	544	680	816	907
Hiking (X-country)	249	299	374	449	499
Hiking (mountain)	340	408	510	612	680
Horseback trotting	231	278	347	416	463

(continued)

Energy Expenditure for Various Activities (continued)

Type of Activity	Calories per Hour (by body weight)				
	100 lb	120 lb	150 lb	180 lb	200 lb
Housework	181	218	272	327	363
Hunting (carry load)	272	327	408	490	544
Ice hockey (vigorous)	454	544	680	816	907
Ice skating (10 mph)	263	316	395	473	526
Jazzercise (heavy)	363	435	544	653	726
Jazzercise (medium)	227	272	340	408	454
Jazzercise (light)	136	163	204	245	272
Jog (9 min/mile)	499	599	748	898	998
Jog (10 min/mile)	454	544	680	816	907
Jog (12 min/mile)	385	463	578	694	771
Jog (13 min/mile)	317	381	476	571	635
Jog (14 min/mile)	272	327	408	490	544
Jog (15 min/mile)	227	272	340	408	454
Jog (17 min/mile)	181	218	272	327	363
Lawn mowing (hand)	295	354	442	531	590
Lawn mowing (power)	163	196	245	294	327
Musical instrument playing	113	136	170	204	227
Racquetball (social)	385	463	578	694	771
Racquetball (vigorous)	454	544	680	816	907
Roller skating	231	278	347	416	463
Rowboating (2.5 mph)	200	239	299	359	399
Rowing (11 mph)	590	707	884	1061	1179
Run (5 min/mile)	816	980	1224	1469	1633
Run (6 min/mile)	703	844	1054	1265	1406
Run (7 min/mile)	612	735	918	1102	1224
Run (8 min/mile)	544	653	816	980	1088
Sailing	159	190	238	286	317
Shuffleboard/skeet	136	163	204	245	272
Skiing (X-country)	454	544	680	816	907
Skiing (downhill)	363	435	544	653	726
Square dancing	272	327	407	490	544
Swimming (competitive)	680	816	1020	1224	1361
Swimming (fast)	426	512	639	767	853
Swimming (slow)	349	419	524	629	698
Table tennis	236	283	354	424	472
Tennis (doubles)	227	272	340	408	454
Tennis (singles)	295	354	442	531	590
Tennis (vigorous)	385	463	578	694	771
Volleyball	231	278	347	416	463
Walking (20 min/mile)	159	190	238	286	317
Walking (26 min/mile)	136	163	204	245	272
Water skiing	317	381	476	571	635
Weight lifting (heavy)	408	490	612	735	816
Weight lifting (light)	181	218	272	327	363
Wood chopping (sawing)	295	354	442	531	590

Source: Data reprinted with permission from N-Squared Computing. First Databank Division of the Hearst Corporation.

Weights and Measures

Measure	Abbreviation	Equivalent
1 gram	g	1000 milligrams
1 milligram	mg	1000 micrograms
1 microgram	μg	1/1000000 of a gram
1 nanogram	ng	1/1000000000 of a gram
1 picogram	pg	1/1000000000000 of a gram
1 kilogram	kg	1000 grams
		2.2 lb
1 pound	lb	454 grams
		16 ounces
1 teaspoon	tsp	approximately 5 grams
1 tablespoon	Tbsp	3 teaspoons
1 ounce	oz	28.4 grams
1 cup	c	8 fluid ounces
		16 tablespoons
1 pint	pt	2 cups
		16 fluid ounces
1 quart	qt	2 pints
		32 fluid ounces
1 gallon	gal	128 fluid ounces
		4 quarts
1 liter	l	1.06 quarts
		1000 milliliters
1 milliliter	ml	1000 microliters
1 deciliter	dl	100 milliliters
1 kcalorie	kcal, Cal	1000 calories
		4.167 kilojoules
1 kilojoule	kJ	1000 joules

Converting Vitamin A Units

Form and Source	Amount Equal to 1 µg Retinol
Preformed vitamin A in food or supplements	1 µg
	1 RAE
	1 µg RE
	3.3 IU
β-carotene in foods*	12 µg
	1 RAE
	2 µg RE
	20 IU
α-carotene or β-cryptoxanthin in food	24 µg
	1 RAE
	2 µg RE
	40 IU

*β-carotene in supplements may be better absorbed than β-carotene in food and so provides more vitamin A activity. It is estimated that 2 µg of β-carotene dissolved in oil provides 1 µg of vitamin A activity.

Converting Vitamin E Values into mg α-Tocopherol

To estimate the α-tocopherol intake from foods:

- If values are given as mg α-TEs:

    mg α-TE × 0.8 = mg α-tocopherol

- If values are given in IUs:

    First, determine if the source of the α-tocopherol is natural or synthetic.

- For natural α-tocopherol:

    IU of natural α-tocopherol × 0.67 = mg α-tocopherol

- For synthetic α-tocopherol (dl-α-tocopherol):

    IU of synthetic α-tocopherol × 0.45 = mg α-tocopherol

Source: Institute of Medicine, Food and Nutrition Board, http://www.nap.edu/catalog.php?record_id=9810 *Dietary Reference Intakes for Vitamin C, Vitamin E, Selenium, and Carotenoids* (2000). Available online at http://books.nap.edu/openbook.php?record_id=9810&page=192

Calculating Dietary Folate Equivalents in Fortified Foods

The folate listed on labels of fortified foods is primarily folic acid, which is more available than natural forms of folate. In order to compare the folate content of these foods to recommendations, the amount of folic acid must be converted to dietary folate equivalents, expressed as µg DFE. This calculation assumes that all of the folate in these foods is from added folic acid.

Determine the amount (µg) of folic acid in the fortified food:

- Multiply the Daily Value for folate by the % Daily Values listed on the label.
- Daily Value is 400 µg.

Convert the µg folic acid into µg DFE:

- Multiply the µg folic acid by 1.7.
- Folic acid added to a food in fortification provides 1.7 times more available folate per µg than folate naturally present in foods.

For example:

- A serving of English muffins provides 6% of the Daily Value for folate:

    To find the µg folic acid: 400 µg × 6% = 24 µg folic acid

    To convert to µg DFE: 24 µg folic acid × 1.7 = 41 µg DFE

Source: Institute of Medicine, food and Nutrition Board, http://www.nap.edu/catalog.php?record_id=6015 *Dietary Reference Intakes for Thiamin, Riboflavin, Niacin, Vitamin B6, Folate, Vitamin B12, Pantothenic Acid, Biotin, and Choline* (1998). Available online at http://books.nap.edu/openbook.php?record_id=6015&page=210

Chapter 1: A Case Study on Variety, Balance, and Moderation

What's wrong with Helen's diet? Helen needs to increase the variety in her diet. Not only is she choosing the same foods every day, but she is not choosing foods from all of the food groups. She doesn't eat any fruit, and her only vegetable is broccoli. Increasing the variety of her diet will help ensure she is meeting her nutrient needs as well as getting a variety of phytochemicals. She can still stick with a routine, but have different types of cereal every morning and top them with a variety of fresh and dried fruit. She can have sandwiches for lunch but make them using different types of breads and fillings. For dinner she can try different grains and a variety of vegetables rather than just rice and broccoli.

How does Marty's meal stack up in terms of variety, balance, and moderation? Marty's meal has a lot of variety, with beef, beans, cheese, the tortilla, and lettuce and tomatoes, but the plate is very full. With this much food the meal is short on moderation. If she chooses this large meal she needs to balance it with smaller meals at other times during the day or with added exercise to burn off the extra calories.

Chapter 2: A Case Study on Using Food Labels to Make Healthy Choices

Use the labels shown below to determine which contains more saturated fat and sugars. The old fashioned oats are much lower in saturated fat, providing only 0.5 gram per serving (3% of the Daily Value) and no *trans* fat, compared to 3.5 grams of saturated fat (18% of the Daily Value) and a gram of *trans* fat in the granola. It is recommended that both saturated fat and *trans* fat be limited in the diet. The old fashioned oats are also lower in sugars; 0 gram compared to 16 grams in a serving of granola.

Which choice provides more vitamin C? The orange juice provides more vitamin C: 120% of the Daily Value, compared to 100% of the Daily Value for the juice drink.

Other than water, what is the most abundant ingredient, by weight, in the juice drink? in the orange juice? Added sugar in the form of high fructose corn syrup is the most abundant ingredient (other than water) in the juice drink. In the orange juice it is concentrated orange juice.

The added vitamin C increases the nutrient density of the juice drink, but does that make it a better choice than the orange juice? No. Even through the juice drink is a good source of vitamin C, it contains more total sugar, much of which is added sugar. The sugar in the orange juice is from the oranges used to make the juice and comes with the other nutrients and phytochemicals that are present in these oranges. These nutrients increase the nutrient density of the orange juice. The high fructose corn syrup used to sweeten the juice drink adds calories with few nutrients. Some of the sugar in the juice drink comes from fruit juice concentrates, which do add nutrients, but the fact that this is farther down on the ingredient list tells us that, by weight, they are present in smaller amounts than the high fructose corn syrup.

Chapter 3: A Case Study on How Changes in the GI Tract Affect Health

What effect might this have on his nutrition and health? If he doesn't have enough saliva, he will have difficulty swallowing and tasting his food. This will decrease the appeal of food and may reduce his food intake. Also because saliva helps protect the teeth, the likelihood that he will develop cavities will increase.

How might this affect the digestion and absorption of nutrients contained in the carrots? If she can't chew the carrots well, the enzymes needed to digest them will not have access to all of the carrot. As a result, pieces will remain undigested and pass through the GI tract and the vitamins and minerals they contain will not be available for absorption.

How does this change affect the amount of fluid she needs to consume? Much of the water that enters the large intestine is absorbed there. If most of her large intestine is removed she will lose a lot more water and she will need to consume more fluid than before to prevent dehydration.

What type of foods should he avoid and why? He should avoid fatty foods. Bile is needed for fat absorption. Fat entering the small intestine causes the gallbladder to contract and release bile. A low-fat diet will minimize gallbladder contraction and the pain this causes.

How would this affect nutrient digestion? Enzymes produced in the pancreas aid in the digestion of starches, proteins, and fats. Pancreatic enzyme deficiency can lead to diarrhea from large amounts of these nutrients passing into the large intestine and can lead to malnutrition because without digestion the nutrients can't be absorbed.

Why can't she eat as much food as before? Will the procedure affect nutrient absorption? She can't eat as much food as before because the surgery creates a small stomach pouch that fills up quickly, so she can only consume small amounts of food at any one time. The procedure will not affect nutrient absorption because food still passes through the entire GI tract.

Chapter 4: A Case Study on Healthy Carbohydrates

How does her intake compare with the recommended amounts of carbohydrate and fiber? She consumes about 58% of calories from carbohydrate (320 grams × 4 Cal/g ÷ 2199 Cal), which is within the Acceptable Macronutrient Distribution Range for carbohydrate of 45 to 65% of total calorie intake. However, her fiber intake is only 12 grams; less than half of the AI for women of 25 g/day.

Use iProfile to look up the fiber content of the fruits and vegetables listed below and choose a combination of these that will add at least 13 grams of fiber to Trina's diet. There are many possible answers. For example, a half-cup of beans, a cup of asparagus, and an apple will provide about 14 grams of fiber. A cup of broccoli, 2 kiwis, and an orange provides almost 13 grams.

If Trina replaces the two 20-oz sodas she drinks per day with water, how many calories and how much sugar will this eliminate from her diet? A 20-ounce soda has about 250 Calories and 64 grams of added sugar. If Trina replaces 2 20-ounce sodas with water she will reduce her energy intake by 500 Calories per day and her sugar intake by about 128 grams.

Use the ingredient list to identify the sources of whole grains and added sugars in these two products. The whole grain in the Raisin and Bran cereal comes from whole-grain wheat. Additional bran is added. The Multigrain cereal contains whole-grain corn, oats, barley, wheat, and rice. The added sugar in the Raisin and Bran cereal comes primarily from sugar and high-fructose corn syrup. In the multigrain cereal the added sugar is from sugar and brown sugar syrup.

Based on the amounts of sugars and fiber in each, which one would you recommend? There isn't always a clear choice. The Multigrain cereal has less fiber, 4 grams compared to 5 in the Raisin and Bran cereal, but it has only a third the amount of sugar. Depending on the rest of your diet and nutrition goals, neither is a bad choice; either cereal could easily be part of an overall healthy diet.

Chapter 5: A Case Study on Improving Heart Health

Which of the factors listed here increase Rafael's risk of developing cardiovascular disease? He has a family history of heart disease because his mother had a heart attack before the age of 65. He is a smoker and is inactive, so his lifestyle further increases his risk. His blood pressure is elevated and his total blood cholesterol of 210 mg/100 ml is over the recommended maximum of 200 mg/100 ml. His LDL cholesterol of 160 mg/100 ml is also above the recommended maximum of 100 mg/100 ml and his HDL cholesterol is less than 40 mg/100 mL, which puts him in the high-risk category. His triglycerides are in the healthy range.

What substitutions could Rafael make in his fast-food meal to reduce his intake of saturated fat? He could make sure he orders a plain hamburger, rather than one with a large or double patty and with cheese or sauces. A grilled chicken sandwich would be lower in saturated fat than even a plain hamburger. He can order a smaller order of fries. He could order a salad for lunch instead of the burger and fries. Most fast food restaurants now have a variety of salad options.

Look at the labels from these two granola bars. Based on the amounts of saturated fat, *trans* fat, fiber, and calories in each, explain which one you would recommend. Neither bar has *trans* fat. Granola bar B is lower in saturated fat and higher in fiber than granola bar A so bar B is probably a better choice. Bar A is lower in calories, but since Rafael is trying to add calories to his diet to prevent weight loss he will need to consume about the same number of calories regardless of which bar he chooses. If he ate the same number of calories from the 2 bars, Granola bar A would give him proportionally even more saturated fat, and still not give him as much fiber as Granola bar B.

Chapter 6: A Case Study on Healthy Vegetarian Diets

What is the RDA for protein for someone of Simon's age and weight? The RDA is 0.8 grams per kilogram of body weight. Simon weighs 154 pounds, which is 70 kilograms (154 lbs ÷ 2.2 lbs/kg = 70 kg). Therefore his recommended protein intake is 56 g per day (70 kg × 0.8 g/kg = 56 g).

This is a photo of Simon's typical lunch. Why is it high in saturated fat? Whole-fat dairy products are high in total fat and saturated fat. Cheese provides about 4 grams of saturated fat per ounce. The 2 ounces of cheese on this sandwich would provide about 8 grams of saturated fat. If butter was used to grill the sandwich it adds about 7 grams of saturated fat per tablespoon.

Vegetarian diets are often deficient in calcium, vitamin D, zinc, and iron. Which of these are likely low in Simon's diet? Simon has milk with breakfast and lots of other dairy products throughout the day so he is unlikely to have low intakes of calcium or vitamin D. His breakfast cereal, lasagna noodles, and pizza crust are likely made from enriched grains, which would provide enough iron to meet his needs. He may be low in zinc; it is not included in enriched grains but may be added to his breakfast cereal.

What could Simon have for dinner that would provide less saturated fat and more of the nutrients that are lacking in his diet? A dinner such as a chickpea and vegetable curry with rice would be low in saturated fat and the chickpeas are legumes, which are good sources of both iron and zinc. Serving the curry with a green salad topped with some cranberries and almonds or walnuts would add some additional vegetarian sources of iron, zinc, and calcium.

To reduce his saturated fat intake, Simon wants to try a vegan lunch. Suggest a vegan sandwich Simon could have that makes use of complementary plant proteins. Peanut butter (legumes) and bread (grain) provide complimentary proteins. Another option is hummus, which is made from chickpeas (legume), with bread.

Chapter 7: A Case Study on Vitamin A and Fast Food

Which of the meals shown here is higher in vitamin A? Which ingredients are sources of the vitamin A? The pizza is higher in vitamin A because it has cheese, which is a source of preformed vitamin A and tomato sauce, tomatoes, and peppers, which provide provitamin A. The beef, bun, and fries in the other meal are all poor sources of vitamin A.

What could John add to his breakfast and lunch to provide some good sources of vitamin A? He could boost his provitamin A intake by adding a carotenoid-rich fruit such as cantaloupe, mango, or apricots to his breakfast. He could increase his intake of preformed vitamin A by replacing the soda he has at lunch with a glass of milk. At lunch he could add some dark green or orange vegetables, such as sweet red peppers and spinach, to his sandwich and include a bag of baby carrots.

John also discovers that his diet is low in vitamin C. Suggest one fruit and one vegetable that he could add to his breakfast and/or lunch to increase his intake of vitamin C? Adding strawberries or a glass of orange juice at breakfast and an orange or kiwis at lunch will add vitamin C. Including some sliced sweet peppers or raw broccoli florets with his lunch will provide a vegetable source of vitamin C.

Chapter 8: A Case Study on Iron Deficiency

What factors increase Hanna's risk for iron deficiency anemia? She is a lacto-ovo vegetarian so she does not consume highly absorbable heme iron. She is a menstruating female so her iron losses are high.

What does the blood test reveal about Hanna's iron status? Is she tired due to iron deficiency anemia? Why or why not? The blood test reveals that her iron stores are depleted and iron levels in her plasma are low, but the amount of iron in her red blood cells is still normal so her symptoms are not due to iron deficiency anemia.

Name three dietary factors that put Hanna at risk for iron deficiency. Her overall iron intake is low and she consumes only nonheme iron, which is poorly absorbed. Her diet is high whole grains, which reduce iron absorption because they are high in phytates. She drinks a lot if tea, which is high in tannins, which inhibit iron absorption.

How could Hanna increase her iron intake? She could include more legumes and dark green leafy vegetables in her diet. She could make sure her breakfast cereal is fortified with iron. She could switch to iron cookware; some of the iron leaches into the food.

What could Hanna do to increase the absorption of the nonheme iron in her diet? Include a source of vitamin C, such as an orange, with meals that contain iron.

Chapter 9: A Case Study on Genetics, Lifestyle, and Body Weight

What is her BMI? Is it in the healthy range? Ashya is 64 inches tall and weighs 155 lbs:

Her BMI is equal to $(155 \text{ lbs} \div (64 \text{ in})^2) \times 703 = 26.6 \text{ kg/m}^2$, which is in the overweight range.

What is her EER?

Ashya is 64 inches tall and weighs 155 lbs:

$$64 \text{ in.} \times 0.0254 \text{ m/in.} = 1.63 \text{ m}$$

$$155 \text{ lbs} \div 2.2 \text{ lbs/kg} = 70.4 \text{ kg}$$

Ashya is in the low active activity category, so PA = 1.12

Using the equation in table 9.1 Aysha's EER is equal to:

$$EER = 354 - (6.91 \times 23 \text{ yrs}) + 1.12[(9.36 \times 70.4 \text{ kg}) + (726 \times 1.63 \text{ m})] = 2259 \text{ Calories}$$

Note: This answer uses the EER equations in Table 9.1. Because Ashya is overweight, it is more accurate to use the equations in Appendix A for calculating the total energy expenditure of individuals who are overweight or obese:

$$TEE = 448 - (7.95 \times 23 \text{ yrs}) + 1.16[(11.4 \times 70.4 \text{ kg}) + (619 \times 1.63 \text{ m})] = 2367 \text{ Calories}$$

How does Aysha's EER compare with her intake? Is she in energy balance? She consumes about 2450 Calories per day but is expending only 2259 Calories per day, so she is not in energy balance. She is consuming 191 Calories per day more than she is expending.

How can Meal B have fewer calories even though it looks like more food? Meal A is much higher is fat (9 Calories/gram), making it more energy dense. Meal B includes fruit and vegetables on the sandwich. These are high in fiber and water, which add bulk and volume to the meal, but provide few calories.

Why might Meal B satisfy hunger just as well as or better than Meal A? The high fat content of the meal A provides satiety. In meal B the fiber in the whole grain bread and the fiber and fluid in the apple and vegetables help fill up your stomach and provide satiety.

If Aysha adds an additional 30 minutes of moderate-intensity exercise every day, by how much will her EER increase? This will boost Ashya into the active physical activity category and her EER will increase to:

$$EER = 354 - (6.91 \times 23 \text{ yrs}) + 1.27[(9.36 \times 70.4 \text{ kg}) + (726 \times 1.63 \text{ m})] = 2535 \text{ Calories}$$

Her EER will therefore increase by 276 Calories per day

If the equation from Appendix A for calculating the total energy expenditure of individuals who are overweight or obese is used:

$$TEE = 448 - (7.95 \times 23 \text{ yrs}) + 1.27[(11.4 \times 70.4 \text{ kg}) + (619 \times 1.63 \text{ m}) = 2566 \text{ Calories}$$

An increase of 199 Calories per day

Do you think Aysha is destined to be overweight? Explain your answer. Ashya is not destined to be overweight, but to maintain her weight in a healthy range she probably needs to monitor her energy intake more carefully and exercise more than an individual with no genetic tendency to store excess body fat. If she makes small changes in her diet and exercise patterns that she can stick with, she is more likely to succeed.

Chapter 10: A Case Study on Snacks for Exercise

What are the advantages and disadvantages of energy bars? The biggest advantage of energy bars is their convenience. They are pre-portioned, ready to eat, and transportable. They may also provide a psychological edge if the consumer believes they will enhance performance. A disadvantage is that they are expensive and do not provide everything you get from food. If they take the place of the whole grains, fresh vegetables and fruits, low-fat dairy products, and lean meats or meat substitutes that make up a healthy diet, the overall quality of the diet may suffer. They also don't provide fluid – an essential during any activity. If you choose to use these bars, wash them down with plenty of water. They do provide calories, generally about 200 to 300 per bar. Even though they are eaten to support activity they still add to your overall energy intake and can contribute to weight gain if consumed in excess.

Based on the labels shown here, how do energy bars differ from candy bars? Typically energy bars are lower in total fat, saturated fat, cholesterol, and sugar; higher in fiber and protein; and contain more vitamins and minerals than candy bars.

Suggest a snack for Mark that provides about the same amounts of carbohydrate and calories as an energy bar but less expensive. Granola or cereal bars, fruit-filled cookies, fresh or dried fruit, a sandwich, a bagel, or trail mix.

Chapter 11: A Case Study on Nutrient Needs for a Successful Pregnancy

Based on the graph below, why would gaining only 15 pounds put the baby at risk? Why would gaining 50 pounds put the baby at risk? The graph illustrates that a maternal weight gain of only 15 pounds increases the risk that the baby will have a low birth weight. A weight gain of 50 pounds increases the likelihood that the baby will be large for gestational age. Based on this graph, to minimize having a high- or low-birth-weight baby, Tina should gain between 20 and 35 pounds.

How should Tina change the amounts of food she eats from each food group to meet her needs during the second trimester of her pregnancy? Based on Tina's MyPlate Daily Food Plan for Moms, she should consume 8 ounces of grains, 3 cups of vegetables, 2 cups of fruits, 3 cups of dairy, and 6.5 ounces from the protein group. She would therefore need to add 1.5 cups of vegetables, 1 cup of fruit, 1 cup of milk, and 0.5 ounce of protein foods to her current diet.

Use iProfile to suggest some foods that Tina could include in her diet in order to obtain an additional 13.5 mg of iron. Red meat is the best source of absorbable heme iron, providing about 3 mg in 3 ounces. Good sources of nonheme iron include enriched grains, fortified breakfast cereals, legumes, and leafy greens. A serving of fortified breakfast cereal can provide 25 to 100% of the Daily Value (18 mg); legumes, such as black beans, add about 4 mg/cup; and cooked leafy green vegetables another 1 mg/cup.

Do you think it is reasonable for Tina to consume 27 mg of iron each day from her diet alone? Why or why not? It is only reasonable if she included a highly fortified breakfast cereal everyday. It would be extremely difficult for her to get 27 mg/day of iron from the iron naturally present in foods.

Chapter 12: A Case Study on Under- and Overnutrition

Based on this growth chart, how has Sam's BMI percentile changed over the past year? Sam's BMI has gone from about the 70th percentile to about the 87th percentile in just a few months. The increase in BMI indicates that his weight gain was not accompanied by a corresponding increase in height. This weight gain moves Sam from the healthy weight range into the overweight range.

What nutrients are likely to be excessive or deficient in this dietary pattern? The diet is high in added sugar and fat from the donuts, candy, and chips. The whole milk Sam drinks adds calcium, total fat, saturated fat, and cholesterol. His intake from all the food groups except milk and possibly grains is low so he is likely to consume less than the recommended amounts of vitamin C, vitamin A, and iron.

Why might excessive consumption of dairy products contribute to Sam's anemia? Calcium interferes with iron absorption. Sam seems to have milk with every meal so he is consuming calcium with the iron in his meals and the calcium is reducing iron absorption.

How might Sam's iron deficiency have contributed to his weight gain? Iron deficiency causes fatigue and lethargy, which would have caused a decrease in his activity level, shifting his energy balance toward weight gain.

Chapter 13: A Case Study on Tracking Food-Borne Illness

Based on the graph, which food is the most likely cause of the illness? Why? The frozen custard is most likely to be the cause because a greater number of people who ate the custard because ill than for any of the other foods.

How can eggs become contaminated with *Salmonella*? The outside of the eggs can become contaminated with *Salmonella* when they come in contact with fecal material in the chicken coop. The inside of the egg can be contaminated with *Salmonella* before the shell is formed if the hen is infected with *Salmonella*. Therefore, raw eggs can cause *Salmonella* food-borne illness even if the shell is clean.

The cookie and cupcake recipes also called for eggs. Why are these unlikely to be the cause of the problem? Both of these foods were cooked after the eggs were added. The cooking temperature was high enough to kill the bacteria.

Suggest a reason why 20 children who consumed the frozen custard did not get ill. They may have consumed smaller amounts of custard. They may have been larger children. It takes more bacteria to make a larger person ill than a smaller person.

What could the fourth-graders have done to avoid the risk of *Salmonella* in their frozen custard? They could have made ice cream, which does not call for raw eggs, or used pasteurized liquid eggs instead of whole eggs from the shell.

Chapter 14: A Case Study on What One Person Can You Do

What are the advantages and disadvantages of the salad options above in terms of convenience, food safety, and environmental impact? The prepackaged lettuce in the grocery store is more convenient. It is pre-washed and just needs to be poured into a bowl. The disadvantages are that once open it spoils more quickly, it uses more energy to produce, and it generates plastic waste from the bags. The unpackaged produce requires more washing and cutting to make your salad but uses fewer of the earth's resources.

Go to the National Geographic Web site http://ocean. nationalgeographic.com/ocean/take-action/seafood-substitutions/ to find some ocean-friendly substitutes for her seafood choices.

Fish	Substitute variety
Atlantic cod	Pacific cod, Pacific ling, or Alaskan pollack
Chilean sea bass	Alaskan sablefish
Orange roughy	Tilapi, wreckfish

What are the advantages and disadvantages of each?

Action	Advantages	Disadvantages
Bike instead of drive on short trips around town.	Uses no gas so saves money, reduces fossil fuel use, and reduces pollution, as well as increases your fitness level.	Difficult to carry heavy or bulky items, and requires more time for each errand.
Buy a canvas bag to carry groceries.	Reduces the number of plastic grocery bags that must be disposed of.	Small monetary cost of the bags.
Bring juice in a thermos instead of buying a Non-recyclable bottle.	Reduces the amount of material that ends up in landfills.	Must be washed after each use. This takes time and uses energy to heat water and generates waste water.
Compost vegetable scraps.	Reduces the amount of material that ends up in landfills and generates fertile material that can be added to a garden.	Cost and time needed to set up and maintain a composting bin.
Buy locally grown produce.	Contains fewer pesticides. Likely to be fresher because it is purchased soon after harvest.	Less variety. Not everything is available at all times of the year.
Buy organically grown produce.	Reduces the pesticides on food. Reduces the environmental damage associated with food production.	Costs more. Occasionally has more insect damage.

Chapter 1:

1. b; 2. d; 3. a; 4. b; 5. c; 6. c; 7. d; 8. a; 9. d; 10. d; 11. a; 12. c; 13. c; 14. b; 15. a

Chapter 2:

1. d; 2. c; 3. d; 4. a; 5. b; 6. a; 7. a; 8. d; 9. c; 10. c; 11. e; 12. e; 13. a; 14. b; 15. d

Chapter 3:

1. c; 2. e; 3. a; 4. d; 5. b; 6. c; 7. c; 8. a; 9. c; 10. b; 11. c; 12. c; 13. b; 14. a; 15. b

Chapter 4:

1. c; 2. b; 3. b; 4. a; 5. d; 6. c; 7. b; 8. d; 9. c; 10. c; 11. d; 12. a; 13. a; 14. d; 15. a

Chapter 5:

1. d; 2. a; 3. e; 4. d; 5. b; 6. b; 7. c; 8. e; 9. e; 10. c; 11. b; 12. c; 13. a; 14. c; 15. d

Chapter 6:

1. d; 2. a; 3. d; 4. e; 5. a; 6. b; 7. c; 8. a; 9. b; 10. d; 11. c; 12. b; 13. b; 14. d; 15. a

Chapter 7:

1. d; 2. a; 3. b; 4. c; 5. d; 6. d; 7. c; 8. e; 9. a; 10. c; 11. b; 12. c; 13. e; 14. b; 15. c

Chapter 8:

1. d; 2. e; 3. b; 4. e; 5. b; 6. d; 7. b; 8. a; 9. c; 10. e; 11. b; 12. b; 13. b; 14. a; 15. c

Chapter 9:

1. b; 2. e; 3. a; 4. d; 5. e; 6. d; 7. a; 8. b; 9. a; 10. c; 11. b; 12. c; 13. a; 14. b; 15. b

Chapter 10:

1. a; 2. e; 3. d; 4. b; 5. a; 6. a; 7. c; 8. b; 9. a; 10. d; 11. a; 12. c; 13. b; 14. c; 15. a

Chapter 11:

1. b; 2. b; 3. d; 4. d; 5. c; 6. b; 7. d; 8. a; 9. b; 10. d; 11. b; 12. c; 13. b; 14. c; 15. c

Chapter 12:

1. a; 2. a; 3. d; 4. c; 5. d; 6. c; 7. b; 8. e; 9. b; 10. a; 11. a; 12. c; 13. c; 14. c; 15. a

Chapter 13:

1. b; 2. e; 3. b; 4. a; 5. c; 6. b; 7. b; 8. c; 9. a; 10. c; 11. b; 12. d; 13. a; 14. c; 15. b

Chapter 14:

1. d; 2. d; 3. a; 4. a; 5. c; 6. c; 7. d; 8. b; 9. b; 10. b; 11. a; 12. a; 13. d; 14. c; 15. a.

absorption The process of taking substances from the gastrointestinal tract into the interior of the body.

acceptable daily intake (ADI) The amount of a food additive that can be consumed daily over a lifetime without appreciable health risk to a person on the basis of all the known facts at the time of the evaluation.

Acceptable Macronutrient Distribution Ranges (AMDRs) Healthy ranges of intake for carbohydrate, fat, and protein, expressed as percentages of total energy intake.

accidental contaminant A substance not regulated by the FDA that unexpectedly enters the food supply.

acrylamide A chemical formed in foods when starches and other carbohydrates are overheated (over 120°C or 250°F) during cooking; may be a carcinogen.

active transport The transport of substances across a cell membrane with the aid of a carrier molecule and the expenditure of energy.

adenosine triphosphate (ATP) A high-energy molecule that the body uses to power activities that require energy.

Adequate Intakes (AIs) Nutrient intakes that should be used as a goal when no RDA exists. AI values are an approximation of the nutrient intake that sustains health.

adipocyte A cell that stores fat.

adipose tissue Tissue found under the skin and around body organs that is composed of fat-storing cells.

adjustable gastric banding A surgical procedure in which an adjustable band is placed around the upper portion of the stomach to limit the volume that the stomach can hold and the rate of stomach emptying.

adolescent growth spurt An 18- to 24- month period of peak growth velocity that begins at about ages 10 to 13 in girls and 12 to 15 in boys.

aerobic capacity The maximum amount of oxygen that can be consumed by the tissues during exercise. Also called maximal oxygen consumption, or VO_2 max.

aerobic exercise Endurance exercise that increases heart rate and uses oxygen to provide energy as ATP.

aerobic metabolism Metabolism in the presence of oxygen. It can completely break down glucose to yield carbon dioxide, water, and energy in the form of ATP.

aerobic zone A level of activity that raises the heart rate to between 60 and 85% of maximum heart rate.

age-related bone loss Bone loss that occurs in both men and women as they advance in age.

aging The inevitable accumulation of changes associated with and responsible for an ever-increasing susceptibility to disease and death.

alcohol A molecule that contains 7 Calories per gram and is made by the fermentation of carbohydrates from plant products; the type of alcohol that is consumed in alcoholic beverages is called ethanol.

alcohol poisoning Potentially fatal condition characterized by mental confusion, stupor, vomiting, seizures, slow irregular breathing, and/or hypothermia caused by depression of the central nervous system due to excessive alcohol consumption.

alcoholic hepatitis Inflammation of the liver caused by alcohol consumption.

alcoholism A chronic disorder characterized by dependence on alcohol, with repeated excessive use of alcoholic beverages and development of withdrawal symptoms when alcohol intake is reduced.

aldosterone A hormone secreted by the adrenal glands that increases sodium reabsorption and therefore enhances water reabsorption by the kidney.

allergen A substance that causes an allergic reaction.

alpha-carotene (α-carotene) A carotenoid, some of which can be converted into vitamin A, that is found in leafy green vegetables, carrots, and squash.

alpha-linolenic acid (α-linolenic acid) An 18-carbon omega-3 polyunsaturated fatty acid known to be essential in humans.

alpha-tocopherol (α-tocopherol) The form of tocopherol (vitamin E) active in humans.

Alzheimer's disease A disease that results in a relentless and irreversible loss of mental function.

amenorrhea Delayed onset of menstruation or the absence of three or more consecutive menstrual cycles.

amino acid pool All the amino acids in body tissues and fluids that are available for use by the body.

amino acids The building blocks of proteins. Each contains an amino group, an acid group, and a unique side chain.

anabolic steroids Synthetic fat-soluble hormones that mimic testosterone and are used to increase muscle strength and mass.

anaerobic metabolism Metabolism in the absence of oxygen.

anorexia nervosa An eating disorder characterized by self-starvation, a distorted body image, and abnormally low body weight.

antibody A protein that interacts with and deactivates specific antigens.

antidiuretic hormone (ADH) A hormone secreted by the pituitary gland that increases the amount of water reabsorbed by the kidney and therefore retained in the body.

antigen A foreign substance that, when introduced into the body, stimulates an immune response.

antioxidant A substance that decreases the adverse effects of reactive molecules on normal physiological function.

appetite A desire to consume specific foods that is independent of hunger.

arachidonic acid A 20-carbon omega-6 polyunsaturated fatty acid that can be synthesized from linoleic acid.

arteriole A small artery that carries blood to the capillaries.

artery A blood vessel that carries blood away from the heart.

arthritis A disease characterized by inflammation of the joints, pain, and sometimes changes in structure.

artificial sweetener See nonnutritive sweetener

ascorbic acid The chemical term for vitamin C.

aseptic processing The placement of sterilized food in a sterilized package using a sterile process.

atherosclerosis A type of cardiovascular disease that involves the buildup of fatty material in the artery walls.

atherosclerotic plaque Cholesterol-rich material that is deposited in the arteries of individuals with atherosclerosis. It consists of cholesterol, smooth muscle cells, fibrous tissue, and eventually calcium.

atom The smallest unit of an element that retains the properties of the element.

ATP See adenosine triphosphate

atrophic gastritis An inflammation of the stomach lining that results in reduced secretion of stomach acid, microbial overgrowth, and, in severe cases, a reduction in the production of intrinsic factor.

atrophy Wasting or decrease in the size of a muscle or other tissue caused by lack of use.

attention-deficit/hyperactivity disorder (ADHD) A condition characterized by a short attention span and a high level of activity, excitability, and distractibility.

autoimmune disease A disease that results from immune reactions that destroy normal body cells.

basal metabolic rate (BMR) The rate of energy expenditure under resting conditions. It is measured after 12 hours without food or exercise.

basal metabolism The energy expended to maintain an awake, resting body that is not digesting food.

behavior modification A process that is used to gradually and permanently change habitual behaviors.

beriberi A thiamin deficiency disease that causes weakness, nerve degeneration, and, in some cases, heart changes.

beta-carotene (β-carotene) A carotenoid found in many yellow and red-orange fruits and vegetables that is a precursor of vitamin A. It is also an antioxidant.

beta-cryptoxanthin (β-cryptoxanthin) A carotenoid found in corn, green peppers, and lemons that can provide some vitamin A activity.

bicarbonate A chemical released by the pancreas into the small intestine that neutralizes stomach acid.

bile A digestive fluid made in the liver and stored in the gallbladder that is released into the small intestine, where it aids in fat digestion and absorption.

binge drinking A pattern of drinking that brings a person's blood alcohol concentration to 0.08 gram percent (mg/100 ml) or above.

binge-eating disorder An eating disorder characterized by recurrent episodes of binge eating in the absence of purging behavior.

bioaccumulation The process by which compounds accumulate or build up in an organism faster than they can be broken down or excreted.

bioavailability The extent to which the body can absorb and use a nutrient.

biotechnology The process of manipulating life forms via genetic engineering in order to provide desirable products for human use.

biotin One of the B vitamins, needed in energy production.

blackout drinking Amnesia following a period of excessive alcohol consumption.

blood pressure The amount of force exerted by the blood against the walls of arteries.

body composition The term used to describe the different components (lean versus fat tissues) that when taken together make up an individual's body weight.

body image The way a person perceives and imagines his or her body.

body mass index (BMI) A measure of body weight relative to height that is used to compare body size with a standard.

bolus A ball of chewed food mixed with saliva.

bone remodeling A continuous process in which small amounts of bone are removed and replaced by new bone.

bone resorption The process by which bone is broken down by osteoclasts releasing calcium from bone to the blood.

botulism A severe food-borne intoxication that results from consuming the toxin produced by *Clostridium botulinum*.

bovine somatotropin (bST) A hormone naturally produced by cows that stimulates the production of milk. A synthetic version of this hormone is now being produced by genetic engineering.

bovine spongiform encephalopathy (BSE) A fatal neurological disease that affects cattle (mad cow disease) and may be transmitted to humans by consuming contaminated beef by-products.

bran The protective outer layers of whole grains. It is a concentrated source of dietary fiber.

brush border The microvilli surface of the intestinal mucosa, which contains some digestive enzymes.

bulimia nervosa An eating disorder characterized by the consumption of a large amount of food at one time (binge eating) followed by

purging behaviors such as self-induced vomiting to prevent weight gain.

calcitonin A hormone produced by the thyroid gland that stimulates bone mineralization and inhibits bone breakdown, thus lowering blood calcium levels.

calorie A unit of measure used to express the amount of energy provided by food.

capillary A small, thin-walled blood vessel through which blood and the body's cells exchange gases and nutrients.

carbohydrate loading See glycogen supercompensation

carbohydrates A class of nutrients that includes sugars, starches, and fibers. Chemically, they all contain carbon, along with hydrogen and oxygen, in the same proportions as in water (H_2O).

cardiorespiratory endurance The efficiency with which the body delivers to cells the oxygen and nutrients needed for muscular activity and transports waste products from cells.

cardiovascular disease Any disease affecting the heart and blood vessels.

cardiovascular system The organ system that includes the heart and blood vessels and circulates blood throughout the body.

carotenoids Yellow, orange, and red pigments synthesized by plants and many microorganisms. Some can be converted to vitamin A.

cash crop A crop that is grown to be sold for monetary return rather than as food for the local population.

cataracts A disease of the eye that results in cloudy spots on the lens (and sometimes the cornea), which obscure vision.

celiac disease A disorder that causes damage to the intestines when the protein gluten is eaten.

cell The basic structural and functional unit of living things.

cell differentiation Structural and functional changes that cause cells to mature into specialized cells.

cellular respiration The reactions that break down carbohydrates, fats, and proteins to produce carbon dioxide, water, and energy in the form of ATP.

cellulose An insoluble fiber that is the most prevalent structural material of plant cell walls.

cesarean section The surgical removal of the fetus from the uterus.

Chinese restaurant syndrome See MSG symptom complex

cholesterol A sterol, produced by the liver and consumed in the diet, that is needed to build cell membranes and make hormones and other essential molecules. High blood levels increase the risk of heart disease.

choline A compound needed for the synthesis of the phospholipid phosphatidylcholine and the neurotransmitter acetylcholine. It is important for a number of biochemical reactions, and there is evidence that it is essential in the diet during certain stages of life.

chylomicron A lipoprotein that transports lipids from the mucosal cells of the small intestine and delivers triglycerides to other body cells.

chyme A mixture of partially digested food and stomach secretions.

cirrhosis A chronic and irreversible liver disease characterized by loss of functioning liver cells and accumulation of fibrous connective tissue.

cobalamin The chemical term for vitamin B_{12}.

coenzyme An organic nonprotein substance that binds to an enzyme to promote its activity.

cofactor An inorganic ion or coenzyme that is required for enzyme activity.

collagen The major protein in connective tissue.

colostrum The first milk, produced by the breast late in pregnancy and for up to a week after delivery. Compared to mature milk, it contains more water, protein, immune factors, minerals, and vitamins and less fat.

complete dietary protein See high-quality protein

complex carbohydrates Carbohydrates composed of sugar molecules linked together in straight or branching chains. They include oligosaccharides, starches, and fibers.

conditionally essential amino acids Amino acids that are essential in the diet only under certain conditions or at certain times of life; also called semiessential amino acids.

constipation Infrequent or difficult defecation.

control group In a scientific experiment, the group of participants used as a basis of comparison. They are similar to the participants in the experimental group but do not receive the treatment being tested.

creatine phosphate A compound stored in muscle that can be broken down quickly to make ATP.

creatine A compound that can be converted into creatine phosphate, which replenishes muscle ATP during short bursts of activity. Creatine is a dietary supplement used by athletes to increase muscle mass and delay fatigue during short intense exercise.

cretinism A condition resulting from poor maternal iodine intake during pregnancy that impairs mental development and growth in the offspring.

crib death See sudden infant death syndrome

critical control point A possible point in food production, manufacturing, and transportation where contamination could occur or be prevented or eliminated.

critical period Time in growth and development when an organism is more susceptible to harm from poor nutrition or other environmental factors.

cross-contamination The transfer of contaminants from one food or object to another.

cycle of malnutrition A cycle in which malnutrition is perpetuated by an inability to meet nutrient needs at all life stages.

Daily Value A reference value for the intake of nutrients used on food labels to help consumers see how a given food fits into their overall diet.

DASH (Dietary Approaches to Stop Hypertension) eating plan A dietary pattern recommended to lower blood pressure. It is abundant in fruits and vegetables; includes low-fat dairy products, whole grains, legumes, and nuts; and incorporates moderate amounts of lean meat.

deamination The removal of the amino group from an amino acid.

dehydration A state that occurs when not enough water is present to meet the body's needs.

Delaney Clause A clause added to the 1958 Food Additives Amendment of the Pure Food and Drug Act that prohibits the intentional addition to foods of any compound that has been shown to induce cancer in animals or humans at any dose.

dementia A deterioration of mental state that results in impaired memory, thinking, and/or judgment.

denaturation Alteration of a protein's three-dimensional structure.

dental caries Cavities, or decay of the tooth enamel caused by acid produced when bacteria growing on the teeth metabolize carbohydrate.

designer food or **nutraceutical** A food or supplement thought to have health benefits in addition to its nutritive value.

diabetes mellitus A disease characterized by elevated blood glucose due to either insufficient production of insulin or decreased sensitivity of cells to insulin.

diarrhea An intestinal disorder characterized by frequent or watery stools.

dietary folate equivalent (DFE) The amount of folate equivalent to 1 mg of folate naturally occurring in food, 0.6 mg of synthetic folic acid from fortified food or supplements consumed with food, or 0.5 mg synthetic folic acid consumed on an empty stomach.

Dietary Guidelines for Americans A set of nutrition recommendations designed to promote population-wide dietary changes to reduce the incidence of nutrition-related chronic disease.

Dietary Reference Intakes (DRIs) A set of reference values for the intake of energy, nutrients, and food components that can be used for planning and assessing the diets of healthy people in the United States and Canada.

dietary supplement A product designed to supplement the diet; may include nutrients (vitamins, minerals, amino acids, fatty acids), enzymes, herbs, or other substances.

diet-induced thermogenesis See thermic effect of food

diffusion The movement of molecules from an area of higher concentration to an area of lower concentration without the expenditure of energy.

digestion The process by which food is broken down into components small enough to be absorbed into the body.

dipeptide Two amino acids linked by a peptide bond.

direct food additive A substance intentionally added to food. Direct food additives are regulated by the FDA.

disaccharide A carbohydrate made up of two sugar units.

discretionary calories The calories remaining after an individual has met recommended intake levels with healthy choices from all the food groups.

dispensable amino acid See nonessential amino acid

diuretic A substance that increases the amount of urine passed from the body.

diverticula Sacs or pouches that protrude from the wall of the large intestine.

diverticulitis A condition in which diverticula in the large intestine become inflamed.

diverticulosis A condition in which outpouches (or sacs) form in the wall of the large intestine.

docosahexaenoic acid (DHA) A 22-carbon omega-3 polyunsaturated fatty acid found in fish that may be needed in the diet of newborns. It can be synthesized from α-linolenic acid.

Down syndrome A disorder caused by extra genetic material that results in distinctive facial characteristics, mental impairment, and other abnormalities.

eating disorder A psychological illness characterized by specific abnormal eating behaviors, often intended to control weight.

eating disorders not otherwise specified (EDNOS) A category of eating disorders that do not fit the exact definition of anorexia nervosa or bulimia nervosa.

eclampsia Convulsions or seizures during or immediately after pregnancy. Untreated, it can lead to coma or death.

edema Swelling due to the buildup of extracellular fluid in the tissues.

eicosanoids Regulatory molecules that can be synthesized from omega-3 and omega-6 fatty acids.

eicosapentaenoic acid (EPA) A 20-carbon-omega-3 polyunsaturated fatty acid found in fish that can be synthesized from α-linolenic acid but may be essential in humans under some conditions.

electrolyte A positively or negatively charged ion that conducts an electrical current in solution. Commonly refers to sodium, potassium, and chloride.

element A substance that cannot be broken down into products with different properties.

embryo The developing human from two through eight weeks after fertilization.

empty calories Calories from solid fats and/or added sugars, which add calories to the food but few nutrients.

emulsifier A substance with both water-soluble and fat-soluble portions that can break fat into tiny droplets and suspend it in a watery fluid.

endorphins Compounds that cause a natural euphoria and reduce the perception of pain under certain stressful conditions.

endosperm The largest portion of a kernel of grain. It is primarily starch and serves as a food supply for the sprouting seed.

energy balance The amount of energy consumed in the diet compared with the amount expended by the body over a given period.

energy-yielding nutrients Nutrients that can be metabolized to produce energy in the body. They include carbohydrates, fats, and proteins.

enrichment The addition of specific amounts of thiamin, riboflavin, niacin, and iron to refined grains. Since 1998 folic acid has also been added to enriched grains.

enzyme A protein molecule that accelerates the rate of specific chemical reactions without itself being changed.

epidemiology The branch of science that studies health and disease trends and patterns in populations.

epiglottis A piece of elastic connective tissue that covers the opening to the lungs during swallowing.

ergogenic aid A substance, appliance, or procedure that improves athletic performance.

essential amino acid (also called **indispensable amino acid**) An amino acid that cannot be synthesized by the body in sufficient amounts to meet its needs and therefore must be included in the diet.

essential fatty acid deficiency A condition characterized by dry, scaly skin and poor growth that results when the diet does not supply sufficient amounts of linoleic acid and α-linolenic acid.

essential fatty acid A fatty acid that must be consumed in the diet because it cannot be made by the body or cannot be made in sufficient quantities to meet the body's needs.

essential nutrient A nutrient that must be consumed in the diet because it cannot be made by the body or cannot be made in sufficient quantities to maintain body functions.

Estimated Average Requirements (EARs) Nutrient intakes estimated to meet the needs of 50% of the healthy individuals in a given gender and life-stage group.

Estimated Energy Requirements (EERs) Average energy intake values predicted to maintain body weight in healthy individuals.

ethanol The alcohol in alcoholic beverages; it is produced by yeast fermentation of sugar.

evidence-based practice Using the compiled evidence from all available well-controlled, peer-reviewed studies to develop recommendations and policies regarding nutrition and health care.

Exchange Lists A system of grouping foods based on their carbohydrate, protein, fat, and energy content.

experimental group In a scientific experiment, the group of participants who undergo the treatment being tested.

extreme obesity or **morbid obesity** A body mass index is greater than 40.

facilitated diffusion Assisted diffusion of a substance across the cell membrane.

failure to thrive Inability of a child's growth to keep up with normal growth curves.

famine A widespread lack of access to food due to a disaster that causes a collapse in the food production and marketing systems.

fasting hypoglycemia Low blood sugar that is not related to food intake; often caused by an insulin-secreting tumor.

fatigue Inability to continue an activity at an optimal level.

fat-soluble vitamin A vitamin that does not dissolve in water; includes vitamins A, D, E, and K.

fatty acid A molecule made up of a chain of carbons linked to hydrogens, with an acid group at one end of the chain.

fatty liver The accumulation of fat in the liver. An early symptom of excess alcohol consumption.

feces Body waste, including unabsorbed food residue, bacteria, mucus, and dead cells, which is eliminated from the gastrointestinal tract by way of the anus.

female athlete triad The combination of disordered eating, amenorrhea, and osteoporosis that occurs in some female athletes, particularly those involved in sports in which low body weight and appearance are important.

fertilization The union of a sperm and an egg.

fetal alcohol spectrum disorders (FASDs) A range of physical and behavioral disorders or conditions and functional or mental impairments linked to prenatal alcohol exposure. One of the most severe FASDs is fetal alcohol syndrome.

fetal alcohol syndrome (FAS) A characteristic group of physical and mental abnormalities in an infant resulting from maternal alcohol consumption during pregnancy.

fetus A developing human from the ninth week after fertilization to birth.

fiber A type of carbohydrate that cannot be broken down by human digestive enzymes.

fibrin The protein produced during normal blood clotting that forms an interlacing fibrous network that is essential for formation of the clot.

fitness A set of attributes related to the ability to perform routine physical activities without undue fatigue.

fluorosis A condition caused by chronic overconsumption of fluoride, characterized by black and brown stains and cracking and pitting of the teeth.

foam cell A cholesterol-filled white blood cell.

folate A general term that refers to the many forms of this B vitamin, which is needed for the synthesis of DNA and the metabolism of some amino acids.

folic acid An easily absorbed form of the vitamin folate that is present in dietary supplements and fortified foods.

food additive A substance that is intentionally added to or can reasonably be expected to become a component of a food during processing.

food allergy An adverse immune response to a specific food protein.

food desert An area that lacks access to affordable fruits, vegetables, whole grains, low-fat milk, and other foods that make up a healthy diet.

food guide A food group system that suggests amounts of different types of foods needed to meet nutrient intake recommendations.

food insecurity A situation in which people lack adequate physical, social, or economic access to sufficient, safe, nutritious food that meets their dietary needs and food preferences for an active and healthy life.

food intolerance, or **food sensitivity** An adverse reaction to a food that does not involve the production of antibodies by the immune system.

food recovery The collection of wholesome food for distribution to the poor and hungry, including collection of crops from farmers' fields that have already been mechanically harvested or on fields where it is not economically profitable to harvest.

food sensitivity See food intolerance

food-borne illness An illness caused by consumption of contaminated food.

food-borne infection Illness produced by the ingestion of food containing microorganisms that can multiply inside the body and produce effects that are injurious.

food-borne intoxication Illness caused by consuming a food containing a toxin.

fortification The addition of nutrients to foods.

fortified food A food to which one or more nutrients has been added.

free radical A type of highly reactive atom or molecule that causes oxidative damage.

fructose A monosaccharide found in fruits and honey that is composed of six carbon atoms arranged in a ring structure; commonly called fruit sugar.

functional food A food that has health-promoting properties beyond basic nutritional functions.

galactose A monosaccharide composed of six carbon atoms arranged in a ring structure; when combined with glucose, it forms the disaccharide lactose.

gallstone A stone formed in the gallbladder or bile duct when substances in the bile harden.

gastric banding See adjustable gastric banding

gastric bypass A surgical procedure that reduces the size of the stomach and bypasses a portion of the small intestine.

gastric juice A substance produced by the gastric glands of the stomach that contains an inactive form of pepsin and hydrochloric acid.

gastrin A hormone secreted by the mucosa of the stomach that stimulates the secretion of enzymes and acid in the stomach.

gastroesophageal reflux disease (GERD) A chronic condition in which acidic stomach contents leak into the esophagus, causing pain and damaging the esophagus.

gastrointestinal tract A hollow tube consisting of the mouth, pharynx, esophagus, stomach, small intestine, and large intestine in which digestion of food and absorption of nutrients occur; also called the alimentary canal, GI tract or digestive tract.

gene A length of DNA that contains the information needed to synthesize a polypeptide chain; responsible for inherited traits.

gene expression The events of protein synthesis in which the information coded in a gene is used to synthesize a protein.

generally recognized as safe (GRAS) A group of chemical additives that are considered safe, based on their long-standing presence in the food supply without harmful effects.

genetic engineering A set of techniques used to manipulate DNA for the purpose of changing the characteristics of an organism or creating a new product.

genetically modified (GM) An organism whose genetic material has been altered using genetic engineering techniques; a product containing or produced by genetic modification.

germ The embryo or sprouting portion of a kernel of grain. It contains vegetable oil, vitamins, and minerals.

gestational diabetes A condition characterized by high blood glucose levels that develop during pregnancy.

gestational hypertension (also called pregnancy-induced hypertension) High blood pressure that develops after the 20th week of pregnancy and returns to normal after delivery. It may be an early sign of preeclampsia.

ghrelin A hormone produced by the stomach that affects food intake.

glucagon A hormone made in the pancreas that raises blood glucose levels by stimulating the breakdown of liver glycogen and the synthesis of glucose.

glucose A 6-carbon monosaccharide that is the primary form of carbohydrate used to produce energy in the body. Also known as blood sugar.

glutathione peroxidase A selenium-containing enzyme that protects cells from oxidative damage by neutralizing peroxides.

glycemic index A ranking of the effect that the consumption of a single carbohydrate-containing food has on blood glucose in relation to consumption of a reference carbohydrate such as white bread or glucose.

glycemic load An index of the glycemic response that occurs after eating specific foods. It is calculated by multiplying a food's glycemic index by the amount of available carbohydrate in a serving of the food.

glycemic response The rate, magnitude, and duration of the rise in blood glucose that occurs after food is consumed.

glycogen The storage form of carbohydrate in animals, made up of many glucose molecules linked together in a highly branched structure.

glycogen supercompensation or **carbohydrate loading** A regimen designed to increase muscle glycogen stores beyond their usual level.

glycolysis An anaerobic metabolic pathway that splits glucose into two three-carbon pyruvate molecules; the energy released from one glucose molecule is used to make two molecules of ATP.

goiter An enlargement of the thyroid gland caused by a deficiency of iodine.

goitrogen A substance that interferes with the utilization of iodine or the function of the thyroid gland.

Hazard Analysis Critical Control Point (HACCP) A food safety system that focuses on identifying and preventing hazards that could cause food-borne illness.

health claim A food label claim that describes the relationship between a nutrient or food and a disease or health condition. Only approved health claims may appear on food labels.

healthy life expectancy The amount of time a human can expect to stay healthy.

Healthy People A set of national health promotion and disease prevention objectives for the U.S. population.

heartburn A burning sensation in the chest or throat caused when acidic stomach contents leak back into the esophagus.

heat cramps Muscle cramps caused by an imbalance of sodium and potassium; may result from excessive exercise without adequate fluid and electrolyte replacement.

heat exhaustion Low blood pressure, rapid pulse, fainting, and sweating caused when dehydration decreases blood volume so much that blood can no longer both cool the body and provide oxygen to the muscles.

heat stroke Elevated body temperature as a result of fluid loss and the failure of the temperature regulatory center of the brain.

heat-related illnesses Conditions, including heat cramps, heat exhaustion, and heat stroke, that can occur due to an unfavorable combination of exercise, hydration status, and heat and humidity.

heme iron A readily absorbable form of iron found in meat, fish, and poultry that is chemically associated with certain proteins.

hemochromatosis An inherited disorder that results in increased iron absorption.

hemoglobin An iron-containing protein in red blood cells that binds and transports oxygen through the bloodstream to cells.

hemolytic anemia A condition in which there is an insufficient number of red blood cells because many have burst.

hemolytic-uremic syndrome A disorder, usually in children, that occurs when an infection in the digestive system produces toxic substances that destroy red blood cells causing them to block capillaries, eventually resulting in kidney failure.

hemorrhoid A swollen vein in the anal or rectal area.

hepatic portal vein The vein that transports blood from the gastrointestinal tract to the liver.

heterocyclic amines (HCAs) A class of mutagenic substances produced when there is incomplete combustion of amino acids during the cooking of meats—for example, when meat is charred.

high-density lipoprotein (HDL) A lipoprotein that picks up cholesterol from cells and transports it to the liver so that it can be eliminated from the body.

high quality protein or **complete dietary protein** An easily digestible protein that contains all of the amino acids needed for protein synthesis in amounts similar to those found in body proteins.

hormone A chemical messenger that is produced in one location in the body, released into the blood, and travels to other locations, where it elicits responses.

hunger A desire to consume food that is triggered by internal physiological signals or the recurrent involuntary lack of food that over time may lead to malnutrition.

hydrogenation A process whereby hydrogen atoms are added to the carbon–carbon double bonds of unsaturated fatty acids, making them more saturated.

hydrolyzed protein, or protein hydrolysate A mixture of amino acids or amino acids and polypeptides that results when a protein is completely or partially broken down by treatment with acid or enzymes.

hypercarotenemia A condition caused by the accumulation of carotenoids in the adipose tissue, causing the skin to appear yellow-orange.

hypertension Blood pressure that is consistently elevated to 140/90 mm mercury or greater.

hypertensive disorders of pregnancy A spectrum of conditions involving a rise in blood pressure during pregnancy.

hypertrophy An increase in the size of a muscle or organ.

hypoglycemia Abnormally low blood glucose levels.

hyponatremia Abnormally low concentration of sodium in the blood.

hypothesis A proposed explanation for an observation or a scientific problem that can be tested through experimentation.

implantation The process through which a developing embryo embeds itself in the uterine lining.

incomplete dietary protein A protein that is deficient in one or more of the amino acids required for protein synthesis in humans.

indirect food additive A substance that is expected to unintentionally enter food during manufacturing or from packaging. Indirect food additives are regulated by the FDA.

indispensable amino acid See essential amino acid

infancy The period of early childhood, generally from birth to 1 year of age.

infant botulism A potentially life-threatening disease in which the bacteria *Clostridium botulinum* grows within the baby's gastrointestinal tract.

infant mortality rate The number of deaths during the first year of life per 1000 live births.

inflammation A protective response to injury or destruction of tissues; signs of acute inflammation include pain, heat, redness, swelling and loss of function.

insoluble fiber Fiber that does not dissolve in water and cannot be broken down by bacteria in the large intestine. It includes cellulose, some hemicelluloses, and lignin.

insulin A hormone made in the pancreas that allows glucose to enter cells and stimulates the synthesis of protein, fat, and liver and muscle glycogen.

insulin resistance A condition in which the normal amount of insulin produces a subnormal effect in the body.

integrated pest management (IPM) A method of agricultural pest control that integrates nonchemical and chemical techniques.

intestinal microflora Microorganisms that inhabit the large intestine.

intrinsic factor A protein produced in the stomach that is needed for the absorption of adequate amounts of vitamin B_{12}.

iodized salt Table salt to which a small amount of sodium iodide or potassium iodide has been added in order to supplement the iodine content of the diet.

ion An atom or a group of atoms that carries an electrical charge.

iron deficiency anemia An iron deficiency disease that occurs when the oxygen-carrying capacity of the blood is decreased because there is insufficient iron to make hemoglobin.

iron overload A condition in which iron accumulates in the tissues; characterized by bronzed skin and enlarged liver and diabetes mellitus and abnormalities of the pancreas and the joints.

irradiation A process that exposes foods to radiation in order to kill contaminating organisms and retard the ripening and spoilage of fruits and vegetables.

Keshan disease A heart disease that occurs in an area of China where the soil is very low in selenium.

ketoacidosis A life-threatening condition in which ketone levels in the blood are high enough to increase blood acidity.

ketone or **ketone body** An acidic molecule formed when there is not sufficient carbohydrate to break down acetyl-CoA.

ketone body See ketone

ketosis High levels of ketones in the blood.

kilocalorie (kcal) A unit of heat that is used to express the amount of energy provided by foods. It is the amount of heat required to raise the temperature of 1 kilogram of water 1 degree Celsius (1 kcalorie = 1000 calories. When Calorie is spelled with a capital C it denotes kilocalorie).

kwashiorkor A form of protein-energy malnutrition in which only protein is deficient.

lactation Production and secretion of milk.

lacteal A lymph vessel in the villi of the small intestine that picks up particles containing the products of fat digestion.

lactic acid An end product of anaerobic metabolism and an additive used in food to maintain acidity or form curds.

lactose intolerance The inability to completely digest lactose due to a reduction in the levels of the enzyme lactase.

lactose A disaccharide made of glucose linked to galactose that is found in milk.

large for gestational age Weighing more than 4 kg (8.8 lbs) at birth.

LDL receptor See Low-density lipoprotein receptor.

lean body mass Body mass attributed to nonfat body components such as bone, muscle, and internal organs; also called *fat-free mass*.

lecithin A phosphoglyceride composed of a glycerol backbone, two fatty acids, a phosphate group, and a molecule of choline; often used as an emulsifier in foods.

legume The starchy seed of a plant that produces bean pods; includes peas, peanuts, beans, soybeans, and lentils.

leptin A protein hormone produced by adipocytes that signals information about the amount of body fat.

let-down The release of milk from the milk-producing glands and its movement through the ducts and storage sinuses.

life expectancy The average length of life for a particular population of individuals.

life span The maximum age to which members of a species can live.

limiting amino acid The essential amino acid that is available in the lowest concentration relative to the body's needs.

linoleic acid An omega-6 essential fatty acid with 18 carbons and 2 carbon–carbon double bonds.

lipases Fat-digesting enzymes.

lipid bilayer Two layers of phosphoglyceride molecules oriented so that the fat-soluble fatty acid tails are sandwiched between the water soluble phosphate-containing heads.

lipids A class of nutrients that is commonly called fats. Chemically, they contain carbon, hydrogen, and oxygen, and most of them do not dissolve in water. They include fatty acids, triglycerides, phospholipids, and sterols.

lipoprotein A particle that transports lipids in the blood.

lipoprotein lipase An enzyme that breaks down triglycerides into free fatty acids and glycerol; attached to the outside of the cells that line the blood vessels.

liposuction A procedure that suctions out adipose tissue from under the skin; used to decrease the size of local fat deposits such as on the abdomen or hips.

low birth weight A birth weight less than 2.5 kg (5.5 lbs).

low-density lipoprotein (LDL) A lipoprotein that transports cholesterol to cells.

Low-density lipoprotein receptor A protein on the surface of cells that binds to LDL particles and allows their contents to be taken up for use by the cell.

lumen The inside cavity of a tube, such as the gastrointestinal tract.

lymphatic system The system of lymph vessels and other lymph organs and tissues that drains excess fluid from the space between cells and provides immune function.

lymphocyte A small white blood cell (leukocyte) that plays a large role in defending the body against disease.

macrocytic anemia or **megaloblastic anemia** A reduction in the blood's capacity to carry oxygen that is characterized by abnormally large immature and mature red blood cells.

macronutrients Nutrients needed by the body in large amounts. These include water and the energy-yielding nutrients carbohydrates, lipids, and proteins.

macrophage A type of white blood that ingests foreign material as part of the immune response to foreign invaders such as infectious microorganisms.

macula an oval, yellow-pigmented area on the central retina, that is the central point of sharpest vision.

macular degeneration Degeneration of a portion of the retina that results in loss of visual detail and eventually in blindness.

major mineral A mineral required in the diet in an amount greater than 100 mg/day or present in the body in an amount greater than 0.01% of body weight.

malnutrition A condition resulting from an energy or nutrient intake either above or below that which is optimal.

maltose A disaccharide made of two glucose molecules linked together.

marasmus A form of protein-energy malnutrition in which a deficiency of energy in the diet causes severe body wasting.

maximal oxygen consumption See aerobic capacity

maximum heart rate The maximum number of beats per minute that the heart can attain.

megaloblastic anemia See macrocytic anemia

menopause The time in a woman's life when the menstrual cycle ends.

metabolic pathway A series of chemical reactions inside of a living organism that results in the transformation of one molecule into another.

metabolism The sum of all the chemical reactions that take place in a living organism.

micelle A particle that is formed in the small intestine when the products of fat digestion are surrounded by bile. It facilitates the absorption of lipids.

microbes Microscopic organisms, or microorganisms, including bacteria, viruses, and fungi.

micronutrients Nutrients needed by the body in small amounts. These include vitamins and minerals.

microvillus (plural, **microvilli**) A minute projection on the mucosal cell membrane that increases the absorptive surface area in the small intestine.

mineral In nutrition, an element needed by the body to maintain structure and regulate chemical reactions and body processes.

mitochondrion (plural, *mitochondria*) A cellular organelle that is responsible for generating energy in the form of ATP via aerobic metabolism; the citric acid cycle and electron transport chain are located here.

modified atmosphere packaging (MAP) A preservation technique used to prolong the shelf life of processed or fresh food by changing the gases surrounding the food in the package.

mold Multicellular fungi that form filamentous branching growths.

molecule A group of two or more atoms of the same or different elements bonded together.

monoglyceride A glycerol molecule with one fatty acid attached.

monosaccharide A carbohydrate made up of a single sugar unit.

monosodium glutamate (MSG) An additive used as a flavor enhancer, commonly used in Chinese food; made up of the amino acid glutamate bound to sodium.

monounsaturated fatty acid A fatty acid containing one carbon–carbon double bond.

morbid obesity See extreme obesity

morning sickness Nausea and vomiting that affects many women during the first few months of pregnancy and that in some women can continue throughout the pregnancy.

MSG symptom complex, or **Chinese restaurant syndrome** A group of symptoms including headache, flushing, tingling, burning sensations, and chest pain reported by some individuals after consuming monosodium glutamate (MSG).

mucosa The layer of tissue lining the gastrointestinal tract and other body cavities.

mucosal cell A type of epithelial cell that makes up the lining of the gastrointestinal tract and other body cavities.

mucus A viscous fluid secreted by glands in the digestive tract and other parts of the body. It lubricates, moistens, and protects cells from harsh environments.

muscle endurance The ability of a muscle group to continue muscle movement over time.

muscle strength The amount of force that can be produced by a single contraction of a muscle.

muscle-strengthening exercise Activities that are specifically designed to increase muscle strength, endurance, and size; also called strength-training exercise or resistance-training exercise.

myelin A soft, white fatty substance that covers nerve fibers and aids in nerve transmission.

myoglobin An iron-containing protein in muscle cells that binds oxygen.

MyPlate A plate-shaped food guide released in 2011 that suggests amounts and types of food from five food groups to meet the recommendations of the Dietary Guidelines.

National School Lunch Program A federally funded program designed to provide free or reduced cost lunches to school-age children.

neural tube defect An abnormality in the brain or spinal cord that results from errors that occur during prenatal development.

neurotransmitter A chemical substance produced by a nerve cell that can stimulate or inhibit another cell.

niacin A B vitamin needed in energy metabolism.

niacin equivalent (NE) A unit used to express the amount of niacin present in food, including that which can be made from its precursor, tryptophan. One NE is equal to 1 mg of niacin or 60 mg of tryptophan.

night blindness Inability to see clearly in dim light.

nitrogen balance The amount of nitrogen consumed in the diet compared with the amount excreted over a given period.

nitrosamine A carcinogenic compound produced by reactions between nitrites and amino acids.

nonessential or **dispensable amino acids** Amino acids that can be synthesized by the human body in sufficient amounts to meet needs.

nonexercise activity thermogenesis (NEAT) The energy expended for everything we do other than sleeping, eating, or sports-like exercise.

nonnutritive sweetener or **artificial sweetener** A substance used to sweeten food that provides few or no calories.

nursing bottle syndrome Extreme tooth decay in the upper teeth resulting from putting a child to bed with a bottle containing milk or other sweet liquids.

nutraceutical See designer food

nutrient content claim A claim on food labels used to describe the level of a nutrient in a food. The Nutrition Labeling and Education Act of 1990 defines these terms and regulates the circumstances under which they can be used.

nutrient density A measure of the nutrients provided by a food relative to its calorie content.

nutrients Substances in food that provide energy and structure to the body and regulate body processes.

nutrigenomics See nutritional genomics

Nutrition Facts The portion of a food label that provides information about the nutritional composition of a food and how that food fits into the overall diet.

nutrition transition A series of changes in diet, physical activity, and health that occurs as poor countries become more prosperous.

nutritional genomics or **nutrigenomics** The study of how diet affects our genes and how individual genetic variation can affect the impact of nutrients or other food components on health.

nutritional status An individual's health, as it is influenced by the intake and utilization of nutrients.

obese Having excess body fat. Obesity is defined as having a body mass index (ratio of weight to height squared) of 30 kg/m² or greater.

obesity genes Genes that code for proteins involved in the regulation of body fat. When they are abnormal, the result is abnormal amounts of body fat.

oldest old Individuals 85 years of age and older.

oligosaccharide A carbohydrate made up of 3 to 10 sugar units.

omega-3 fatty acid A fatty acid containing a carbon–carbon double bond between the third and fourth carbons from the omega end; includes α-linolenic acid found in vegetable oils and eicosapentaenoic acid (EPA) and docosahexaenoic acid found in fish oils.

omega-6 fatty acid A fatty acid containing a carbon–carbon double bond between the sixth and seventh carbons from the omega end; includes linoleic and arachidonic acid.

organ A discrete structure composed of more than one tissue that performs a specialized function.

organ system A group of cooperative organs.

organic compound A substance that contains carbon bonded to hydrogen.

organic food Food that is produced, processed, and handled in accordance with the standards of the USDA National Organic Program.

osmosis The unassisted diffusion of water across the cell membrane.

osteomalacia A vitamin D deficiency disease in adults, characterized by loss of minerals from bone, bone pain, muscle aches, and an increase in bone fractures.

osteopenia A reduction in bone density to below normal levels.

osteoporosis A bone disorder characterized by reduced bone mass, increased bone fragility, and increased risk of fractures.

overload principle The concept that the body adapts to the stresses placed on it.

overnutrition Poor nutritional status resulting from a dietary intake in excess of that which is optimal for health.

overtraining syndrome A collection of emotional, behavioral, and physical symptoms that occurs when the amount and intensity of exercise exceeds an athlete's capacity to recover.

overweight Being too heavy for one's height, usually due to an excess of body fat. Overweight is defined as having a body mass index (ratio of weight to height squared) of 25 to 29.9 kilograms/meter² (kg/m²).

oxidative damage Damage caused by highly reactive oxygen molecules that steal electrons from other compounds, causing changes in structure and function.

oxidized LDL cholesterol A substance formed when the cholesterol in LDL particles is oxidized by reactive oxygen molecules. It is key in the development of atherosclerosis because it is taken up by scavenger receptors on white blood cells.

oxytocin A hormone released by the posterior pituitary that stimulates the ejection or let-down of milk during lactation.

pancreatic amylase A starch-digesting enzyme found in pancreatic juice.

pancreatic juice Fluid secreted by the pancreas that contains bicarbonate to neutralize acid and enzymes for the digestion of carbohydrates, fats, and proteins.

pantothenic acid One of the B vitamins, needed in energy metabolism.

parasite An organism that lives at the expense of others.

parathyroid hormone (PTH) A hormone released by the parathyroid gland that acts to increase blood calcium levels.

pasteurization The process of heating food products in order to kill disease-causing organisms.

pathogen A biological agent that causes disease.

peak bone mass The maximum bone density attained at any time in life, usually occurring in young adulthood.

peer-review process The review of the design and validity of a research experiment by experts in the field of study who did not participate in the research.

pellagra A disease resulting from niacin deficiency, which causes dermatitis, diarrhea, dementia, and, if not treated, death.

pepsin A protein-digesting enzyme produced by the stomach. It is secreted in the gastric juice in an inactive form (pepsinogen) and activated by acid in the stomach.

peptic ulcer An open sore in the lining of the stomach, esophagus, or upper small intestine.

peptide Two or more amino acids joined by peptide bonds.

peptide bond The chemical linkage between the amino group of one amino acid and the acid group of another.

peristalsis Coordinated muscular contractions that move material through the GI tract.

pernicious anemia A macrocytic anemia resulting from vitamin B_{12} deficiency that occurs when dietary vitamin B_{12} cannot be absorbed due to a lack of intrinsic factor.

phagocyte A type of white blood cell that engulfs and consumes foreign particles such as bacteria.

pharynx A funnel-shaped opening that connects the nasal passages and mouth to the respiratory passages and esophagus. It is a common passageway for food and air and is responsible for swallowing.

phenylketonuria (PKU) A genetic disease in which the amino acid phenylalanine cannot be metabolized normally, causing it to build up in the blood. If untreated, the condition results in brain damage.

phosphate group A chemical group consisting of one phosphorus atom and four oxygen atoms.

phospholipid A type of lipid whose structure includes a phosphorus atom.

photosynthesis The metabolic process by which plants trap energy from the sun and use it to make sugars from carbon dioxide and water.

physical frailty Impairment in function and reduction in physiologic reserves severe enough to cause limitations in the basic activities of daily living.

phytochemical A substance found in plant foods that is not an essential nutrient but may have health-promoting properties.

pica An abnormal craving for and ingestion of nonfood substances that have little or no nutritional value.

placebo A fake medicine or supplement that is indistinguishable in appearance from the real thing. It is used to disguise the control and experimental groups in an experiment.

placenta An organ produced from maternal and embryonic tissues. It secretes hormones, transfers nutrients and oxygen from the mother's blood to the fetus, and removes metabolic wastes.

plant sterol A compound found in plant cell membranes that resembles cholesterol in structure. It can lower blood cholesterol by competing with cholesterol for absorption in the gastrointestinal tract.

platelets Cell fragments found in blood that are involved in blood clotting.

polychlorinated biphenyls (PCBs) Carcinogenic industrial compounds that have found their way into the environment and, subsequently, the food supply. Repeated exposure causes them to accumulate in biological tissues over time.

polycyclic aromatic hydrocarbons (PAHs) A class of mutagenic substances produced during cooking when there is incomplete combustion of organic materials—for example, when fat drips on a grill.

polypeptide A chain of amino acids linked by peptide bonds that is part of the structure of a protein.

polysaccharide A carbohydrate made up of many sugar units linked together.

polyunsaturated fatty acid A fatty acid that contains two or more carbon–carbon double bonds.

postmenopausal bone loss Accelerated bone loss that occurs in women for about 5 to 10 years surrounding menopause.

prebiotic A substance that pass undigested into the colon and stimulates the growth and/or activity of certain types of bacteria.

prediabetes A consistent elevation of blood glucose levels to between 100 and 125 mg/dl of blood, a level above normal but not high enough to be diagnostic of diabetes but thought to increase the risk of developing diabetes.

preeclampsia A condition characterized by elevated blood pressure, a rapid increase in body weight, protein in the urine, and edema. Also called *toxemia*.

prehypertension Blood pressures of 120 to 139 millimeters of mercury systolic (top number) or 80 to 89 diastolic (bottom number). It increases the risk of developing hypertension as well as the risk of artery damage and heart disease.

premature See preterm

preterm or **premature** An infant born before 37 weeks of gestation.

prion A pathogenic protein that is the cause of degenerative brain diseases called spongiform encephalopathies. *Prion* is short for proteinaceous infectious particle.

prior-sanctioned substance A substance that the FDA or the USDA had determined was safe for use in a specific food prior to the 1958 Food Additives Amendment.

probiotic A product that contains live bacteria, which when consumed temporarily lives in the colon and confers health benefits on the host.

prolactin A hormone released from the anterior pituitary that stimulates the mammary glands to produce milk.

protease A protein-digesting enzyme.

protein A class of nutrients that includes molecules made up of one or more intertwining chains of amino acids. They contain carbon, hydrogen, oxygen, and nitrogen.

protein complementation The process of combining proteins from different sources so that they collectively provide the proportions of amino acids required to meet the body's needs.

protein hydrolysate See hydrolyzed protein

protein quality A measure of how efficiently a protein in the diet can be used to make body proteins.

protein-energy malnutrition (PEM) A condition characterized by loss of muscle and fat mass and an increased susceptibility to infection that results from the long-term consumption of insufficient amounts of energy and/or protein to meet the body's needs.

prothrombin A blood protein required for blood clotting.

provitamin or **vitamin precursor** A compound that can be converted into the active form of a vitamin in the body.

puberty A period of rapid growth and physical changes that ends in the attainment of sexual maturity.

pyridoxal phosphate The major coenzyme form of vitamin B_6 that functions in more than 100 enzymatic reactions, many of which involve amino acid metabolism.

qualified health claim A health claim on a food label that has been approved based on emerging but not well-established evidence of a relationship between a food, food component, or dietary supplement and reduced risk of a disease or health-related condition.

reactive hypoglycemia Low blood sugar that occurs an hour or so after the consumption of high-carbohydrate foods; results from an overproduction of insulin.

recombinant DNA DNA that has been formed by joining DNA from different sources.

Recommended Dietary Allowances (RDAs) Nutrient intakes that are sufficient to meet the needs of almost all healthy people in a specific gender and life-stage group.

refined Refers to foods that have undergone processing to remove the coarse parts of the original food.

renewable resource A resource that is restored and replaced by natural processes and can therefore be used forever.

resistance-training exercise See muscle-strengthening exercise

resistant starch Starch that escapes digestion in the small intestine of healthy people.

resting heart rate The number of times that the heart beats per minute while a person is at rest.

resting metabolic rate (RMR) The rate of energy expenditure at rest. It is measured after 5 to 6 hours without food or exercise.

retinoids The chemical forms of preformed vitamin A: retinol, retinal, and retinoic acid.

retinol activity equivalent *(RAE)* The amount of retinol, α-carotene, β-carotene, or β-crytoxanthin that must be consumed to equal the vitamin A activity of 1 μg of retinol.

retinol-binding protein A protein that is necessary to transport vitamin A from the liver to tissues in need.

rhodopsin A light-sensitive compound found in the retina of the eye that is composed of the protein opsin loosely bound to retinal.

riboflavin A B vitamin needed in energy metabolism.

rickets A vitamin D deficiency disease in children, characterized by poor bone development because of inadequate calcium absorption.

saliva A watery fluid that is produced and secreted into the mouth by the salivary glands. It contains lubricants, enzymes, and other substances.

salivary amylase An enzyme secreted by the salivary glands that breaks down starch into smaller units.

satiety The feeling of fullness and satisfaction caused by food consumption that eliminates the desire to eat.

saturated fat A type of lipid that is most abundant in solid animal fats and is associated with an increased risk of heart disease.

saturated fatty acid A fatty acid in which the carbon atoms are bonded to as many hydrogen atoms as possible; it therefore contains no carbon–carbon double bonds.

scavenger receptor A protein on the surface of macrophages that binds to oxidized LDL cholesterol and allows it to be taken up by the cell.

scientific method The general approach of science that is used to explain observations about the world around us.

scurvy A vitamin C deficiency disease characterized by bleeding gums, tooth loss, joint pain, bleeding into the skin and mucous membranes, and fatigue.

segmentation Rhythmic local constrictions of the intestine that mix food with digestive juices and speed absorption by repeatedly moving the food mass over the intestinal wall.

set point A level at which body fat or body weight seems to resist change despite changes in energy intake or output.

simple carbohydrates Carbohydrates known as sugars that include monosaccharides and disaccharides.

simple diffusion The unassisted diffusion of a substance across the cell membrane.

small for gestational age An infant born at term weighing less than 2.5 kg (5.5 lb).

sodium chloride The chemical formula of table salt.

soluble fiber Fiber that dissolves in water or absorbs water and can be broken down by intestinal microflora. It includes pectins, gums, and some hemicelluloses.

solute A dissolved substance.

solvent A fluid in which one or more substances dissolve.

Special Supplemental Nutrition Program for Women, Infants, and Children (WIC) A program funded by the federal government that provides nutrition education and food vouchers to pregnant and lactating women and their young children.

sphincter A muscular valve that helps control the flow of materials in the gastrointestinal tract.

spina bifida A neural tube defect in which part of the spinal cord is exposed through a gap in the backbone, causing varying degrees of disability.

spore The dormant state of some bacteria that is resistant to heat but can germinate and produce a new organism when environmental conditions are favorable.

sports anemia A temporary decrease in hemoglobin concentration that occurs during exercise training. It occurs as an adaptation to training and does not impair delivery of oxygen to tissues.

starch A carbohydrate found in plants, made up of many glucose molecules linked in straight or branching chains.

starvation A severe reduction in nutrient and energy intake that impairs health and eventually causes death. It is the most extreme form of malnutrition.

steroid precursor An androgenic hormone produced primarily by the adrenal glands and gonads that acts as precursor in the production of testosterone and estrogen.

sterol A type of lipid with a structure composed of multiple chemical rings.

strength-training exercise See muscle-strengthening exercise

structure/function claim A claim on a food label that describes the role of a nutrient or dietary ingredient in maintaining normal structure or function in humans.

stunting A decrease in linear growth rate.

subcutaneous fat Adipose tissue located under the skin, which is not associated with a great increase in the risk of chronic diseases.

subsistence crop A crop that is grown as food for a farmer's family, with little or nothing left to sell.

sucrose A disaccharide commonly known as table sugar that is made of glucose linked to fructose.

sudden infant death syndrome (SIDS, or **crib death)** The unexplained death of an infant, usually during sleep.

sugar unit A sugar molecule that cannot be broken down to yield other sugars.

Supplement Facts The portion of a dietary supplement label that includes information about, serving size, ingredients, amount per serving size (by weight), and percent of Daily Value, if established.

sustainable agriculture Agricultural methods that maintain soil productivity and a healthy ecological balance while having minimal long-term impacts.

teratogen A chemical, biological, or physical agent that causes birth defects.

theory A formal explanation of an observed phenomenon made after a hypothesis has been supported through extensive experimentation.

thermic effect of food (TEF) or **diet-induced thermogenesis** The energy required for the digestion of food and absorption, metabolism, and storage of nutrients.

thiamin A B vitamin needed in energy metabolism.

thirst A sensation of dryness in the mouth and throat associated with a desire for liquids.

thyroid gland A gland located in the neck that produces thyroid hormones and calcitonin.

thyroid hormones Hormones produced by the thyroid gland that regulate metabolic rate.

thyroid-stimulating hormone A hormone that stimulates the synthesis and secretion of thyroid hormones from the thyroid gland.

tissue A collection of similar cells that together carry out a specific function.

tocopherol The chemical name for vitamin E.

Tolerable Upper Intake Levels (ULs) Maximum daily intake levels that are unlikely to pose risks of adverse health effects to almost all individuals in a given gender and life-stage group.

tolerances The maximum amount of pesticide residues that may legally remain in food, set by the EPA.

total energy expenditure The sum of basal energy expenditure, the thermic effect of food, and the energy used in physical activity, regulation of body temperature, deposition of new tissue, and production of milk.

trace mineral A mineral required in the diet in an amount of 100 mg or less per day or present in the body in amounts of 0.01% of body weight or less.

trans **fatty acid** An unsaturated fatty acid in which the hydrogens are on opposite sides of the carbon–carbon double bond.

transamination The process by which an amino group from one amino acid is transferred to a carbon compound to form a new amino acid.

transcription The process of copying the information in DNA to a molecule of mRNA.

transgenic An organism with a gene or group of genes intentionally transferred from another species or breed.

transit time The time between the ingestion of food and the elimination of the solid waste from that food.

translation The process of translating the mRNA code into the amino acid sequence of a protein.

triglyceride The major type of lipid in food and the body, consisting of three fatty acids attached to a glycerol molecule.

trimester A term used to describe each third or three-month period of a pregnancy.

tripeptide Three amino acids linked together by peptide bonds.

tropical oils A term used in the popular press to refer to the saturated plant oils—coconut, palm, and palm kernel oil—that are derived from plants grown in tropical regions.

type 1 diabetes The form of diabetes caused by autoimmune destruction of insulin-producing cells in the pancreas, usually leading to absolute insulin deficiency.

type 2 diabetes The form of diabetes characterized by insulin resistance and relative (rather than absolute) insulin deficiency.

undernutrition Poor nutritional status resulting from a dietary intake below that which meets nutritional needs.

underweight A body mass index of less than 18.5 kg/m^2, or a body weight 10% or more below the desirable body weight standard.

unrefined food A food eaten either just as it is found in nature or with only minimal processing.

unsaturated fat A type of lipid that is most abundant in plant oils and is associated with a reduced risk of heart disease.

unsaturated fatty acid A fatty acid that contains one or more carbon–carbon double bonds; may be either monounsaturated or polyunsaturated.

urea A nitrogen-containing waste product from the breakdown of proteins that is excreted in the urine.

variable A factor or condition that is changed in an experimental setting.

variant Creutzfeldt-Jakob Disease (vCJD) A rare, degenerative, fatal brain disorder in humans. It is believed that the persons who have developed vCJD became infected through their consumption of cattle products contaminated with BSE.

vegan diet A plant-based diet that eliminates all animal products.

vegetarian diet A diet that includes plant-based foods and eliminates some or all foods of animal origin.

vein A vessel that carries blood toward the heart.

venule A small vein that drains blood from capillaries and passes it to larger veins for return to the heart.

very low birth weight A birth weight less than 1.5 kg (3.3 lbs).

very-low-density lipoprotein *(VLDL)* A lipoprotein assembled by the liver that carries lipids from the liver and delivers triglycerides to body cells.

villus (plural, *villi*) A fingerlike protrusion of the lining of the small intestine that participates in the digestion and absorption of foodstuffs.

visceral fat Adipose tissue deposited in the abdominal cavity around the internal organs. High levels are associated with an increased risk of heart disease, high blood pressure, stroke, diabetes, and breast cancer.

vitamin An organic compound needed in the diet in small amounts to promote and regulate the chemical reactions and processes needed for growth, reproduction, and the maintenance of health.

vitamin A A fat-soluble vitamin needed in cell differentiation, reproduction, and vision.

vitamin B$_{12}$ One of the B vitamins, only found in animal foods.

vitamin B$_6$ One of the B vitamins, needed in protein metabolism.

vitamin C A water-soluble vitamin needed for the maintenance of collagen.

vitamin D A fat-soluble vitamin needed for calcium absorption that can be made in the body when there is exposure to sunlight.

vitamin E A fat-soluble vitamin that functions as an antioxidant.

vitamin K A fat-soluble vitamin needed for blood clotting.

vitamin precursor See provitamin

VO$_2$ max See aerobic capacity

water intoxication A condition that occurs when a person drinks enough water to significantly lower the concentration of sodium in the blood.

water-soluble vitamin A vitamin that dissolves in water; includes the B vitamins and vitamin C.

Wernicke-Korsakoff syndrome A form of thiamin deficiency associated with alcohol abuse that is characterized by mental confusion, disorientation, loss of memory, and a staggering gait.

whole-grain product A product made from the entire kernel of a grain including the bran, endosperm, and germ.

xerophthalmia A spectrum of eye conditions resulting from vitamin A deficiency that may lead to blindness.

zoochemical A substance found in animal food (zoo means animal) that is not an essential nutrient but may have health-promoting properties.

Chapter 1

[1] American Dietetic Association. Position of the American Dietetic Association: Fortification and nutritional supplements. *J Am Diet Assoc* 105:1300–1311, 2005.

[2] Galeone, C., Pelucchi, C., Levi, F., et al. Onion and garlic use and human cancer. *Am J Clin Nutr* 84:1027–1032, 2006.

[3] Gullett, N.P., Ruhul Amin, A.R., Bayraktar, S., et al. Cancer prevention with natural compounds. *Semin Oncol* 37:258–281, 2010.

[4] Rice, S., and Whitehead, S.A. Phytoestrogens oestrogen synthesis and breast cancer. *J. Steroid Biochem Mol Biol* 108:186–195, 2008.

[5] Sacks, F.M., Lichtenstein, A., Van Horn, L., et al. Soy protein, isoflavones, and cardiovascular health: An American Heart Association science advisory for professionals from the nutrition committee. *Circulation* 113:1034–1044, 2006.

[6] Cassidy, A., and Hooper, L. Phytoestrogens and cardiovascular disease. *J Br Menopause Soc* 12:49–56, 2006.

[7] Rao, A.V., and Rao, L.G. Carotenoids and human health. *Pharmacol Res* 5:207–216, 2007.

[8] Crozier, A., Jaganath, I.B., and Clifford, M.N. Dietary phenolics: Chemistry, bioavailability and effects on health. *Nat Prod Rep* 26:1001–1043, 2009.

[9] Basu, A., Rhone, M., and Lyons, T.J. Berries: Emerging impact on cardiovascular health. *Nutr Rev* 68:168–177, 2010.

[10] Seeram, N.P. Recent trends and advances in berry health benefits research. *J Agric Food Chem* 58:3869–3870, 2010.

[11] Prasad, K. Flaxseed and cardiovascular health. *J Cardiovasc Pharmacol* 54:369–377, 2009.

[12] Grassi, D., Desideri, G., and Ferri, C. Blood pressure and cardiovascular risk: What about cocoa and chocolate? *Arch Biochem Biophys* 501:112–115, 2010.

[13] Butt, M.S., Sultan, M.T., Butt, M.S., and Iqbal, J. Garlic: Nature's protection against physiological threats. *Crit Rev Food Sci Nutr* 49:538–551, 2009.

[14] Carpentier, S., Knaus, M., and Suh, M. Associations between lutein, zeaxanthin, and age-related macular degeneration: An overview. *Crit Rev Food Sci Nutr* 49:313–326, 2009.

[15] Sanclemente, T., Marques-Lopes, I., Puzo, J., and García-Otín, A.L. Role of naturally-occurring plant sterols on intestinal cholesterol absorption and plasmatic levels. *J Physiol Biochem* 65:87–98, 2009.

[16] Bolling, B.W., McKay, D.L., and Blumberg, J.B. The phytochemical composition and antioxidant actions of tree nuts. *Asia Pac J Clin Nutr* 19:117–123, 2010.

[17] Sadiq Butt, M., Tahir-Nadeem, M., Khan, M.K., et al. Oat: Unique among the cereals. *Eur J Nutr* 47:68–79, 2008.

[18] Manerba, A., Vizzardi, E., Metra, M., and Dei Cas, L. n-3 PUFAs and cardiovascular disease prevention. *Future Cardiol* 6:343–350, 2010.

[19] Lambert, J.D., and Elias, R.J. The antioxidant and pro-oxidant activities of green tea polyphenols: A role in cancer prevention. *Arch Biochem Biophys* 501:65–72, 2010.

[20] Fardet, A. New hypotheses for the health-protective mechanisms of whole-grain cereals: What is beyond fibre? *Nutr Res Rev* 23:65–134, 2010.

[21] Flegal, K.M., Carroll, M.D., Ogden, C.L., and Curtin L.R. Prevalence and trends in obesity among US adults, 1999–2008. *JAMA* 303:235–241, 2010.

[22] U.S. Department of Agriculture and U.S. Department of Health and Human Services. *Dietary Guidelines for Americans, 2010*, 7th Edition, Washington, DC: U.S. Government Printing Office, December 2010.

[23] Mokdad, A.H., Marks, J.S., Stroup, D.F., and Gerberding, J.L. Correction: Actual causes of death in the United States, 2000. *JAMA* 293:293–294, 2005.

[24] Ogden, C.L., Carroll, M.D., Curtin, L.R., et al. Prevalence of high body mass index in US children and adolescents, 2007–2008. *JAMA* 303:242–249, 2010.

[25] Centers for Disease Control and Prevention. Deaths: Final data for 2007. *National Vital Statistics Reports* Vol. 58, No. 19, May 2010. Available online at www.cdc.gov/NCHS/data/nvsr58/nvsr58_19.pdf. Accessed January 17, 2011.

[26] Kaput, J. Nutrigenomics—2006 update. *Clin Chem Lab Med* 45:279–287, 2007.

[27] Division of Nutrition and Physical Activity. Research to Practice Series No. 2: *Portion Size*. Atlanta: Centers for Disease Control and Prevention, 2006. Available online at http://www.cdc.gov/nccdphp/dnpa/nutrition/pdf/portion_size_research.pdf Accessed April 1, 2011.

[28] Cawley, J., and Maclean, J.C., "Report: Unfit for Service: The Implications of Rising Obesity for U.S. Military Recruitment," NBER Working Paper No. 16408, September 2010. Available online at http://www.nber.org/papers/w16408 www.sciencedaily.com/releases/2010/10/101018165430.htm. Accessed March 30, 2011.

[29] Vaitheeswaran, V. Economist Debates Food Policy. *The Economist* December 8, 2009. Available online at http://www.economist.com/debate/days/view/427. Accessed February 3, 2011.

Chapter 2

[1] Davis, C., and Saltos, E. Dietary recommendations and how they have changed over time. In *America's Eating Habits: Changes and Consequences*. Available online at www.ers.usda.gov/publications/aib750/aib750.pdf. Accessed February 26, 2011.

[2] U.S. Department of Agriculture and U.S. Department of Health and Human Services. *Dietary Guidelines for Americans, 2010*. 7th ed., Washington, DC: U.S. Government Printing Office, December 2010.

[3] U.S. Department of Agriculture, Economic Research Service. Major trends in the U.S. food supply, 1909–1999. *Food Review* 23:12, 2000.

[4] Wells, H.F., and Buzby, J.C. Dietary assessment of major trends in U.S. food consumption, 1970–2005. *Economic Information Bulletin* No. 33. Economic Research Service, U.S. Department of Agriculture, March 2008.

[5] U.S. Department of Health and Human Services. *Healthy People*. Available online at www.healthypeople.gov/2020/about/new2020.aspx. Accessed February 20, 2011.

[6] Institute of Medicine, Food and Nutrition Board. *Dietary Reference Intakes for Energy, Carbohydrate, Fiber, Fat, Fatty Acids, Cholesterol, Protein, and Amino Acids*. Washington, DC: National Academies Press, 2002.

[7] Schroder, B.G., Griffin, I., Specker, B.L., and Abrams, S.A. Absorption of calcium from the carbonated dairy soft drink is greater than that from fat-free milk and calcium fortified orange juice in women. *Nutritional Research* 25:737–742, 2005.

[8] He, K. Fish, long-chain omega-3 polyunsaturated fatty acids and prevention of cardiovascular disease—Eat fish or take fish oil supplement? *Prog Cardiovasc Dis* 52:95–114, 2009.

[9] Centers for Disease Control and Prevention. *CDC Estimates of Foodborne Illness in the United States*. Available online at www.cdc.gov/foodborneburden/2011-foodborne-estimates.html Accessed May 25, 2011.

[10] U.S. Food and Drug Administration. *A Key to Choosing Healthful Foods: Using the Nutrition Facts on the Food Label*. Available online at www.fda.gov/Food/ResourcesForYou/Consumers/ucm079449.htm. Accessed February 25, 2011.

[11] U.S. Food and Drug Administration. *New Menu and Vending Machines Labeling Requirements*. Available online at www.fda.gov/Food/LabelingNutrition/ucm217762.htm. Accessed March 1, 2011.

[12] U.S. Food and Drug Administration, Center for Food Safety and Applied

Nutrition. *Guidance for Industry: A Labeling Guide for Restaurants and Other Retail Establishments Selling Away-from-Home Foods*, April 2008. Available online at www.fda.gov/Food/GuidanceComplianceRegulatoryInformation/GuidanceDocuments/FoodLabelingNutrition/ucm053455.htm. Accessed February 26, 2011.

[13] U.S. Food and Drug Administration, Center for Food Safety and Applied Nutrition/Office of Nutrition, Labeling, and Dietary Supplements. *Food Labeling Guide*, April 2008. Available at www.fda.gov/Food/GuidanceComplianceRegulatoryInformation/GuidanceDocuments/FoodLabelingNutrition/FoodLabelingGuide/default.htm. Accessed February 26, 2011.

[14] U.S. Food and Drug Administration, Center for Food Safety and Applied Nutrition/Office of Nutrition, Labeling, and Dietary Supplements. *Dietary Supplement Labeling Guide*, April 2005. Available at www.fda.gov/Food/GuidanceComplianceRegulatoryInformation/GuidanceDocuments/DietarySupplements/DietarySupplementlabelingguide/default.htm. Accessed February 26, 2011.

Chapter 3

[1] Heselmans, M., Reid, G., Akkermans, L.M., et al. Gut flora in health and disease: potential role of probiotics *Curr Issues Intest Microbiol* 6:1–7, 2005.

[2] Johnston, B.C., Supina, A.L., Ospina, M., and Vohra, S. Probiotics for the prevention of pediatric antibiotic-associated diarrhea. *Cochrane Database Syst Rev* 18:CD004827, 2007.

[3] Gill, H., and Prasad, J. Probiotics, immunomodulation, and health benefits. *Adv Exp Med Biol* 606:423–454, 2008.

[4] Isolauri, E., and Salminen, S. Nutrition, Allergy, Mucosal Immunology, and Intestinal Microbiota (NAMI) Research Group Report: Probiotics: Use in allergic disorders: A Nutrition, Allergy, Mucosal Immunology, and Intestinal Microbiota (NAMI) Research Group Report. *J Clin Gastroenterol* 42(Suppl. 2):S91–S96, 2008.

[5] Rescigno, M. The pathogenic role of intestinal flora in IBD and colon cancer. *Curr Drug Targets* 9:395–403, 2008.

[6] Bosscher, D., Breynaert, A., Pieters, L., and Hermans, N. Food-based strategies to modulate the composition of the intestinal microbiota and their associated health effects. *J Physiol Pharmacol* 60(Suppl. 6):5–11, 2009.

[7] Centers for Disease Control and Prevention. *Food Allergies*. Available online at www.cdc.gov/HealthyYouth/foodallergies/. Accessed November 8, 2010.

[8] National Institute of Diabetes, Digestive and Kidney Diseases. *Celiac Disease*. Available online at http://digestive.niddk.nih.gov/ddiseases/pubs/celiac/. Accessed November 8, 2010.

[9] van der Windt, D.A., Jellema, P., Mulder, C.J., et al. Diagnostic testing for celiac disease among patients with abdominal symptoms: a systematic review. *JAMA* 303:1738–1746, 2010.

[10] Vakil, N., Malfertheiner, P., and Chey, W.D. *Helicobacter pylori* infection. *N Engl J Med* 363:595–598, 2010.

[11] The National Digestive Diseases Information Clearinghouse (NDDIC), National Institute of Diabetes and Digestive and Kidney Diseases (NIDDK), and National Institutes of Health of the U.S. Department of Health and Human Services. H. pylori *and Peptic Ulcers*. NIH Publication No. 10–4225, April 2010. Available online at http://digestive.niddk.nih.gov/ddiseases/pubs/hpylori/. Accessed November 8, 2010.

[12] Marieb, E.N., and Hoehn, K. *Human Anatomy and Physiology*, 7th ed. Menlo Park, CA: Benjamin Cummings, 2007.

Chapter 4

[1] Gladwell, M. *Outliers*. London: Allen Lane, 2008.

[2] Marriott, B.P., Olsho, L., Hadden, L., and Connor, P. Intake of added sugars and selected nutrients in the United States, National Health and Nutrition Examination Survey (NHANES) 2003–2006. *Crit Rev Food Sci Nutr* 50:228–258, 2010.

[3] *Lactose Intolerance*. Available online at http://digestive.niddk.nih.gov/ddiseases/pubs/lactoseintolerance/. Accessed December 21, 2010.

[4] Burkitt, D.P., Walker, A.R.P., and Painter, N.S. Dietary fiber and disease. *JAMA* 229:1068–1074, 1974.

[5] Saulnier, D.M., Kolida, S., and Gibson, G.R. Microbiology of the human intestinal tract and approaches for its dietary modulation. *Current Pharmaceutical Design* 15:1403–1414, 2009.

[6] The National Digestive Diseases Information Clearinghouse (NDDIC), National Institute of Diabetes and Digestive and Kidney Diseases (NIDDK). *National Diabetes Statistics, 2011*. Available online at http://diabetes.niddk.nih.gov/dm/pubs/statistics/#7. Accessed May 3, 2011.

[7] American Diabetes Association. Standards of medical care in diabetes—2008. *Diabetes Care* 31:S12–S54, 2008.

[8] American Diabetes Association. Nutrition recommendations and interventions for diabetes. A position statement of the American Diabetes Association. *Diabetes Care* 31:S61–S78, 2008.

[9] Hayes, C., and Kriska, A. Role of physical activity in diabetes management and prevention. *J Am Diet Assoc* 108(4 Suppl. 1): S19–S23, 2008.

[10] Barclay, A.W., Petocz, P., McMillan-Price, J., et al. Glycemic index, glycemic load, and chronic disease risk—A meta-analysis of observational studies. *Am J Clin Nutr* 87:627–637, 2008.

[11] Riccardi, G., Rivellese, A.A., and Giacco, R. Role of glycemic index and glycemic load in the healthy state, in prediabetes, and in diabetes. *Am J Clin Nutr* 87:269S–274S, 2008.

[12] Villegas, R., Liu, S., Gao, Y.T., et al. Prospective study of dietary carbohydrates, glycemic index, glycemic load, and incidence of type 2 diabetes mellitus in middle-aged Chinese women. *Arch Intern Med* 167:2310–2316, 2007.

[13] Krishnan, S., Rosenberg, L., Singer, M., et al. Glycemic index, glycemic load, and cereal fiber intake and risk of type 2 diabetes in US black women. *Arch Intern Med* 167:2304–2309, 2007.

[14] van Dam, R.M., and Seidell, J.C. Carbohydrate intake and obesity. *Eur J Clin Nutr* 61(Suppl. 1):S75–S99, 2007.

[15] Slavin, J.L. Position of the American Dietetic Association: health implications of dietary fiber. *J Am Diet Assoc* 108:1716–1731, 2008. Erratum in *J Am Diet Assoc* 109:350, 2009.

[16] Westman, E.C., Feinman, R.D., and Mavropoulos, J.C. Low-carbohydrate nutrition and metabolism. *Am J Clin Nutr* 86:276–284, 2007.

[17] White, J.S. Straight talk about high-fructose corn syrup: What it is and what it ain't. *Am J Clin Nutr* 88:1716S–1721S, 2008.

[18] Tappy, L., and Lê, K.A. Metabolic effects of fructose and the worldwide increase in obesity. *Physiol Rev* 90:23–46, 2010.

[19] Mellon, M., and Rissler, J. *Environmental Effects of Genetically Modified Food Crops—Recent Experiences*. Available online at www.ucsusa.org/food_and_agriculture/science_and_impacts/impacts_genetic_engineering/environmental-effects-of.html. Accessed January 15, 2011.

[20] Gibson, L., and Benson, G. *Origin, History, and Uses of Corn (Zea mays), 2002*. Available online at www.agron.iastate.edu/courses/agron212/readings/corn_history.htm. Accessed January 16, 2011.

[21] American Dietetic Association. Position of the American Dietetic Association:

Use of nutritive and non-nutritive sweeteners. *J Am Diet Assoc* 104:255–275, 2004.

22 *Stevia Sweetener Gets US FDA Go-ahead*, December 18, 2008. Available online at www.foodnavigator-usa.com/Legislation/Stevia-sweetener-gets-US-FDA-go-ahead. Accessed January 12, 2009.

23 Yang, Q. Gain weight by "going diet"? Artificial sweeteners and the neurobiology of sugar cravings: Neuroscience 2010. *Yale J Biol Med* 83:101–108, 2010.

24 Chong, M.F., Fielding, B.A., and Frayn, K.N. Metabolic interaction of dietary sugars and plasma lipids with a focus on mechanisms and de novo lipogenesis. *Proc Nutr Soc* 66:52–59, 2007.

25 Anderson, J.W., Baird, P., Davis, R.H., Jr., et al. Health benefits of dietary fiber. *Nutr Rev* 67:188–205, 2009.

26 Theuwissen, E., and Mensink, R.P. Water-soluble dietary fibers and cardiovascular disease. *Physiol Behav* 94:285–292, 2008.

27 Anderson, J.W. Whole grains protect against atherosclerotic cardiovascular disease. *Proc Nutr Soc* 62:135–142, 2003.

28 Ryan-Harshman, M., and Aldoori, W. Diet and colorectal cancer: Review of the evidence. *Can Fam Physician* 53:1913–1920, 2007.

29 Key, T.J., and Spencer, E.A. Carbohydrates and cancer: an overview of the epidemiological evidence. *Eur J Clin Nutr* 61(Suppl. 1):S112–S121, 2007.

30 Institute of Medicine, Food and Nutrition Board. *Dietary Reference Intakes for Energy, Carbohydrates, Fiber, Fat, Protein and Amino Acids*. Washington, DC: National Academies Press, 2002.

31 U.S. Department of Agriculture and U.S. Department of Health and Human Services. *Dietary Guidelines for Americans, 2010*, 7th ed., Washington, DC: U.S. Government Printing Office, December 2010.

Chapter 5

1 Popkin, B.M., Siega-Riz, A.M., Haines, P.S., and Jahns, L. Where's the fat? Trends in U.S. diets 1965–1996. *Prev Med* 32:245–254, 2001.

2 Centers for Disease Control and Prevention. Trends in intake of energy and macronutrients—United States, 1971–2000. *MMWR Morb Mortal Wkly Rep* 53:80–82, 2004.

3 U.S. Department of Agriculture, Agricultural Research Service. 2010. Energy Intakes: Percentages of energy from protein, carbohydrate, fat, and alcohol, by gender and age, *What We Eat in America*, NHANES 2007–2008. Available online

at www.ars.usda.gov/ba/bhnrc/fsrg. Accessed April, 16, 2011.

4 Wall, R., Ross, R.P., Fitzgerald, G.F., and Stanton, C. Fatty acids from fish: The anti-inflammatory potential of long-chain omega-3 fatty acids. *Nutr Rev* 68:280–289, 2010.

5 American Heart Association. *Diet and Lifestyle Recommendations*. Available online at www.americanheart.org/presenter.jhtml?identifier=851. Accessed January 7, 2011.

6 Libby, P., Okamoto, Y., Rocha, V.Z., and Folco, E. Inflammation in atherosclerosis: Transition from theory to practice. *Circ J* 74:213–220, 2010.

7 Miller, Y.I., Choi, S.H., Fang, L., and Tsimikas, S. Lipoprotein modification and macrophage uptake: role of pathologic cholesterol transport in atherogenesis. *Subcell Biochem* 51:229–251, 2010.

8 American Heart Association. *Heart Disease and Stroke Statistics: 2008 Update*. Available online at www.americanheart.org/downloadable/heart/1200082005246HS_Stats%202008.final.pdf. Accessed January 7, 2011.

9 Institute of Medicine, Food and Nutrition Board. *Dietary Reference Intakes for Energy, Carbohydrates, Fiber, Fat, Protein, and Amino Acids*. Washington, DC: National Academies Press, 2002.

10 Fernandez, M.L., and Calle, M. Revisiting dietary cholesterol recommendations: Does the evidence support a limit of 300 mg/d? *Curr Atheroscler Rep* 12:377–383, 2010.

11 Kritchevsky, S.B. A review of scientific research and recommendations regarding eggs. *J Am Coll Nutr* 23(6 Suppl):596S–600S, 2004.

12 Djoussé, L., and Gaziano, J.M. Egg consumption and cardiovascular disease and mortality the Physicians' Health Study. *Am J Clin Nutr* 87:964–969, 2008.

13 Djoussé, L., and Gaziano, J.M. Egg consumption and risk of heart failure in the Physicians' Health Study. *Circulation* 117:512–516, 2008.

14 Ratliff, J., Leite, J.O., de Ogburn, R., et al. Consuming eggs for breakfast influences plasma glucose and ghrelin, while reducing energy intake during the next 24 hours in adult men. *Nutr Res*, 30, 96–103, 2010.

15 U.S. Department of Agriculture and U.S. Department of Health and Human Services. *Dietary Guidelines for Americans, 2010*, 7th ed., Washington, DC: U.S. Government Printing Office, December 2010.

16 American Heart Association. *Statistical Fact Sheet—Populations, 2008 Update: African American and Cardiovascular*

Disease—Statistics. Available online at www.americanheart.org/downloadable/heart/1197933296813FS01AF08.pdf. Accessed January 7, 2011.

17 National Cholesterol Education Program. *Adult Treatment Panel III Report, 2001, 2004*. Available online at www.nhlbi.nih.gov/guidelines/cholesterol/atglance.pdf. Accessed April 6, 2011.

18 Fung, T.T., Chiuve, S.E., McCullough, M.L., et al. Adherence to a DASH-style diet and risk of coronary heart disease and stroke in women. *Arch Intern Med* 168:713–720, 2008.

19 Hibbeln, J.R., Nieminen, L.R., Blasbalg, T.L., et al. Healthy intakes of n-3 and n-6 fatty acids: Estimations considering worldwide diversity. *Am J Clin Nutr* 83 (6 Suppl):1483S–1493S, 2006.

20 Kuriyama, S., Shimazu, T., Ohmori, K., et al. Green tea consumption and mortality due to cardiovascular disease, cancer, and all causes in Japan: The Ohsaki study. *JAMA* 296:1255–1265, 2006.

21 Van Horn, L., McCoin, M., Kris-Etherton, P.M., et al. The evidence for dietary prevention and treatment of cardiovascular disease. *J Am Diet Assoc* 108:287–331, 2008.

22 Massaro, M., Scoditti, E., Carluccio, M.A., et al. Omega-3 fatty acids, inflammation and angiogenesis: basic mechanisms behind the cardioprotective effects of fish and fish oils. *Cell Mol Biol* 56:59–82, 2010.

23 Ros, E. Nuts and novel biomarkers of cardiovascular disease. *Am J Clin Nutr* 89:1649S–1656S, 2009.

24 Humphrey, L.L., Fu, R., Rogers, K., et al. Homocysteine level and coronary heart disease incidence: A systematic review and meta-analysis. *Mayo Clin Proc* 83:1203–1212, 2008.

25 Bruckdorfer, K.R. Antioxidants and CVD. *Proc Nutr Soc* 67:214–222, 2008.

26 World Cancer Research Fund/American Institute for Cancer Research (AICR). *Food, Nutrition, Physical Activity, and the Prevention of Cancer: A Global Perspective*. Washington DC: AICR, 2007.

27 Bosetti, C., Pelucchi, C., and La Vecchia, C. Diet and cancer in Mediterranean countries: Carbohydrates and fats. *Public Health Nutr* 12:1595–1600, 2009.

28 Hall, M.N., Chavarro, J.E., Lee, I.M., et al. A 22-year prospective study of fish, n-3 fatty acid intake, and colorectal cancer risk in men. *Cancer Epidemiol Biomarkers Prev* 17:1136–1143, 2008.

29 Gerber, M. Background review paper on total fat, fatty acid intake and cancers. *Ann Nutr Metab* 55:140–161, 2009.

[30] Chajès, V., Thiébaut, A.C.M., Rotival, M., et al. Association between serum trans-monounsaturated fatty acids and breast cancer risk in the E3N-EPIC Study. *Am J Epidemiol* 167:1312–1320, 2008.

[31] Devitt, A.A., and Mattes, R.D. Effects of food unit size and energy density on intake in humans. *Appetite* 42:213–220, 2004.

[32] Ledikwe, J.H., Blanck, H.M., Kettel Khan, L., et al. Dietary energy density is associated with energy intake and weight status in US adults. *Am J Clin Nutr* 83:1362–1368, 2006.

[33] Melanson, E.L., Astrup, A., and Donahoo, W.T. The relationship between dietary fat and fatty acid intake and body weight, diabetes, and the metabolic syndrome. *Ann Nutr Metab* 55:229–243, 2009.

[34] American Dietetic Association. Position of the American Dietetic Association: Fat replacers. *J Am Diet Assoc* 105:266–275, 2005.

[35] Flegal, K.M., Carroll, M.D., Ogden, C.L., and Johnson, C.L. Prevalence and trends in obesity among US adults, 1999–2000. *JAMA* 288:1723–1727, 2002.

[36] Ogden, C.L., Carroll, M.D., Curtin, L.R., et al. Prevalence of overweight and obesity in the United States, 1999–2004. *JAMA* 295:1549–1555, 2006.

Chapter 6

[1] Williams, C.D. Kwashiorkor: Nutritional disease of children associated with maize diet. *Lancet* 2:1151–1154, 1935.

[2] Friedman, A.N. High-protein diets: Potential effects on the kidney in renal health and disease. *Am J Kidney Dis* 44:950–962, 2004.

[3] Heaney, R.P., and Layman, D.K. Amount and type of protein influences bone health. *Am J Clin Nutr* 87:1567S–1570S, 2008.

[4] Darling, A.L., Millward, D.J., Torgerson, D.J., et al. Dietary protein and bone health: A systematic review and meta-analysis. *Am J Clin Nutr* 90:1674–1692, 2009.

[5] Siener, R. Impact of dietary habits on stone incidence. *Urol Res* 34:131–133, 2006.

[6] Gonzalez, C.A., and Riboli, E. Diet and cancer prevention: Contributions from the European Prospective Investigation into Cancer and Nutrition (EPIC) study. *Eur J Cancer* 46:2555–2562, 2010.

[7] Williams, A.N., and Woessner, K.M. Monosodium glutamate "allergy": Menace or myth? *Clin Exp Allergy* 39:640–646, 2009.

[8] National Institute of Diabetes, Digestive and Kidney Diseases. *Celiac Disease*. Available online at http://digestive.niddk.nih.gov/ddiseases/pubs/celiac/. Accessed January 11, 2011.

[9] Fulgoni, V.L. Current protein intake in America: Analysis of the National Health and Nutrition Examination Survey, 2003–2004. *Am J Clin Nutr* 87:1554S–1557S, 2008.

[10] American Dietetic Association. Position of the American Dietetic Association, Dietitians of Canada, and American College of Sports Medicine: Nutrition and athletic performance. *J Am Diet Assoc* 109:509–527, 2009.

[11] Stipanuk, M.H. Protein and amino acid requirements. In Stipanuk, M.H. (ed.), *Biochemical, Physiological and Molecular Aspects of Human Nutrition*, 2nd ed. St. Louis: Saunders Elsevier, 2006, pp. 419–448.

[12] Xiao, C.W. Health effects of soy protein and isoflavones in humans. *J Nutr* 138:1244S–1249S, 2008.

[13] Soyfoods Association of North America. *Soyfood Sales and Trends*. Available online at http://www.soyfoods.org/products/sales-and-trends. Accessed January 14, 2011.

[14] Sacks, F.M., Lichtenstein, A., Van Horn L., et al. Soy protein, isoflavones, and cardiovascular health: An American Heart Association Science Advisory for professionals from the Nutrition Committee. *Circulation* 113:1034–1044, 2006.

[15] Messina, M., and Redmond, G. Effects of soy protein and soybean isoflavones on thyroid function in healthy adults and hypothyroid patients: A review of the relevant literature. *Thyroid* 16:249–258, 2006.

[16] Taku, K., Melby, M.K., Takebayashi, J., et al. Effect of soy isoflavone extract supplements on bone mineral density in menopausal women: Meta-analysis of randomized controlled trials. *Asia Pac J Clin Nutr* 19:33–42, 2010.

[17] Hilakivi-Clarke, L., Andrade, J.E., and Helferich, W. Is soy consumption good or bad for the breast? *J Nutr* 140:2326S–2334S, 2010.

[18] Craig, W.J., Mangels, A.R., and American Dietetic Association. Position of the American Dietetic Association: Vegetarian diets. *J Am Diet Assoc* 109:1266–1282, 2009.

Chapter 7

[1] Miller, D.F. Enrichment programs: Helping mother nature along. *Food Product Development* 12:30–38, 1978.

[2] Butte, N.F., Fox, M.K., Briefel, R.R., et al. Nutrient intakes of US infants, toddlers, and preschoolers meet or exceed dietary reference intakes. *J Am Diet Assoc* 110 (12 Suppl.):S27–S37, 2010.

[3] Institute of Medicine, Food and Nutrition Board. *Dietary Reference Intakes for Vitamin C, Vitamin E, Selenium, and Carotenoids*. Washington, DC: National Academies Press, 2000.

[4] Food and Drug Administration. Food labeling; guidelines for voluntary nutrition labeling of raw fruits, vegetables, and fish. *Fed Regist* 71:42031–42047, July 25, 2006. Available online at www.fda.gov/Food/LabelingNutrition/FoodLabelingGuidanceRegulatoryInformation/RegulationsFederalRegisterDocuments/ucm074884.htm. Accessed January 4, 2009.

[5] Institute of Medicine, Food and Nutrition Board. *Dietary Reference Intakes for Thiamin, Riboflavin, Niacin, Vitamin B-6, Folate, Vitamin B-12, Pantothenic Acid, Biotin, and Choline*. Washington, DC: National Academies Press, 1998.

[6] Saffert, A., Pieper, G., and Jetten, J. Effect of package light transmittance on vitamin content of milk. *Packing Technology and Science* 21:47–55, 2008.

[7] Seal, A.J., Creeke, P.I., Dibari, F., et al. Low and deficient niacin status and pellagra are endemic in postwar Angola. *Am J Clin Nutr* 85:218–242, 2007.

[8] Di Minno, M.N., Tremoli, E., Coppola, A., et al. Homocysteine and arterial thrombosis: Challenge and opportunity. *Thromb Haemost* 103:942–961, 2010.

[9] U.S. Department of Agriculture, Agricultural Research Service, Beltsville Human Nutrition Research Center, Food Surveys Research Group (Beltsville, MD). Continuing Survey of Food Intakes by Individuals 1994-96, 1998 and Diet and Health Knowledge Survey 1994–96. Available online at www.ars.usda.gov/Services/docs.htm?docid=14531.Accessed February 5, 2011.

[10] Piazzini, D.B., Aprile, I., Ferrara, P.E., et al. A systematic review of conservative treatment of carpal tunnel syndrome. *Clin Rehabil* 21:299–314, 2007.

[11] Whelan, A.M., Jurgens, T.M., and Naylor, H. Herbs, vitamins and minerals in the treatment of premenstrual syndrome: a systematic review. *Can J Clin Pharmacol* 16:e407–e429, 2009.

[12] Berry, R.J., Bailey, L., Mulinare, J., Bower, C., and Folic Acid Working Group. Fortification of flour with folic acid. *Food Nutr Bull* 31(1 Suppl.):S22–S35, 2010.

[13] Blencowe, H., Cousens, S., Modell, B., and Lawn, J. Folic acid to reduce neonatal mortality from neural tube disorders. *Int J Epidemiol*. 39(Suppl. 1):i110–i121, 2010.

[14] Hubner, R.A., and Houlston, R.S. Folate and colorectal cancer prevention. *Br J Cancer* 100:233–239, 2009.

[15] Larsson, S.C., Bergkvist, L., and Wolk, A. Folate intake and risk of breast cancer by

estrogen and progesterone receptor status in a Swedish cohort. *Cancer Epidemiol Biomarkers Prev* 17:3444–3449, 2008.

[16] Larsson, S.C., Håkansson, N., Giovannucci, E., and Wolk, A. Folate intake and pancreatic cancer incidence: A prospective study of Swedish women and men. *J Natl Cancer Inst* 98:407–413, 2006.

[17] Craig, W.J., Mangels, A.R., and American Dietetic Association. Position of the American Dietetic Association: Vegetarian diets. *J Am Diet Assoc* 109:1266–1282, 2009.

[18] Heimer, K.A., Hart, A.M., Martin, L.G., and Rubio-Wallace, S. Examining the evidence for the use of vitamin C in the prophylaxis and treatment of the common cold. *J Am Acad Nurse Pract* 21:295–300, 2009.

[19] Zeisel, S.H., and da Costa, K.A. Choline: An essential nutrient for public health. *Nutr Rev* 67:615–623, 2009.

[20] Patterson, K.Y., Bhagwat, S.A., Williams, J.R., et al. *USDA Database for the Choline Content of Common Foods, Release Two, January 2008.* Available online at www.ars.usda.gov/SP2UserFiles/Place/12354500/Data/Choline/Choln02.pdf. Accessed January 25, 2011.

[21] Institute of Medicine, Food and Nutrition Board. *Dietary Reference Intakes: Vitamin A, Vitamin K, Arsenic, Boron, Chromium, Copper, Iodine, Iron, Manganese, Molybdenum, Nickel, Silicon, Vanadium, and Zinc.* Washington, DC: National Academies Press, 2001.

[22] World Health Organization. *Micronutrient Deficiencies: Vitamin A Deficiency: The Challenge.* Available online at www.who.int/nutrition/topics/vad/en/index.html. Accessed January 25, 2011.

[23] Penniston, K.L., and Tanumihardjo, S.A. The acute and chronic toxic effects of vitamin A. *Am J Clin Nutr* 83:191–201, 2006.

[24] Castaño, G., Etchart, C., and Sookoian, S. Vitamin A toxicity in a physical culturist patient: A case report and review of the literature. *Ann Hepatol* 5:293–395, 2006.

[25] Druesne-Pecollo, N., Latino-Martel, P., Norat, T., et al. Beta-carotene supplementation and cancer risk: A systematic review and metaanalysis of randomized controlled trials. *Int J Cancer* 127:172–184, 2010.

[26] Holick, M.F. Vitamin D: Extraskeletal health. *Endocrinol Metab Clin North Am* 39:381–400, 2010.

[27] Institute of Medicine, Food and Nutrition Board. *Dietary Reference Intakes for Calcium and Vitamin D.* Washington, DC: National Academies Press, 2011.

[28] Holick, M.F. Vitamin D deficiency: What a pain it is. *Mayo Clin Proc* 78:1457–1459, 2003.

[29] Holick, M.F., and Chen, T.C. Vitamin D deficiency: A worldwide problem with health consequences. *Am J Clin Nutr* 87(Suppl.):1080S–1086S, 2008.

[30] Sabat, R., Guthmann, F., and Rüstow, B. Formation of reactive oxygen species in lung alveolar cells: Effect of vitamin E deficiency. *Lung* 186:115–122, 2008.

[31] Cordero, Z., Drogan, D., Weikert, C., and Boeing, H. Vitamin E and risk of cardiovascular diseases: A review of epidemiologic and clinical trial studies. *Crit Rev Food Sci Nutr* 50:420–440, 2010.

[32] Galli, F., and Azzi, A. Present trends in vitamin E research. *Biofactors* 36:33–42, 2010.

[33] Maras, J.E., Bermudez, O.I., Qiao, N., et al. Intake of alpha-tocopherol is limited among US adults. *J Am Diet Assoc* 104:567–575, 2004.

[34] Bügel, S. Vitamin K and bone health in adult humans. *Vitam Horm* 78:393–416, 2008.

[35] Prabhoo, R., and Prabhoo, T.R. Vitamin K2: A novel therapy for osteoporosis. *J Indian Med Assoc* 108:253–254, 256–258, 2010.

[36] Council for Responsible Nutrition. *Supplement Usage, Consumer Confidence Remains Steady.* Available online at www.crnusa.org/CRNPR10ConsumerSurvey_Usage+Confidence.html. Accessed January 30, 2011.

[37] American Dietetic Association. Position of the American Dietetic Association: Nutrient supplementation. *J Am Diet Assoc* 109:2073–2085, 2009.

[38] Bruno, R.S., and Traber, M.G. Cigarette smoke alters human vitamin E requirements. *J Nutr* 135:671–674, 2005.

[39] Gershwin, M.E., Borchers, A.T., Keen, C.L., et al. Public safety and dietary supplementation. *Ann N Y Acad Sci* 1190:104–117, 2010.

[40] Ernst, E. The risk–benefit profile of commonly used herbal therapies: Ginkgo, St. John's wort, ginseng, Echinacea, saw palmetto, and kava. *Ann Intern Med* 136:42–53, 2002.

[41] Birks, J., and Grimley Evans, J. Ginkgo biloba for cognitive impairment and dementia. *Cochrane Database Syst Rev* CD003120, 2009.

[42] Gorby, H.E., Brownawell, A.M., and Falk, M.C. Do specific dietary constituents and supplements affect mental energy? Review of the evidence. *Nutr Rev* 68:697–718, 2010.

[43] National Center for Complimentary and Alternative Medicine. *Herbs at a Glance: Ginkgo.* Available online at http://nccam.nih.gov/health/ginkgo/ataglance.htm. Accessed July 5, 2011.

[44] Izzo, A.A., and Ernst, E. Interactions between herbal medicines and prescribed drugs: an updated systematic review. *Drugs* 69:1777–1798, 2009

[45] Linde, K, Berner, M.M., and Kriston, L. St John's wort for major depression. *Cochrane Database Syst Rev* CD000448, 2008.

[46] Xiang, Y.Z., Shang, H.C., Gao, X.M., and Zhang, B.L. A comparison of the ancient use of ginseng in traditional Chinese medicine with modern pharmacological experiments and clinical trials. *Phytother Res* 22:851–858, 2008.

[47] Reinhart, K.M., Talati, R., White, C.M., and Coleman, C.I. The impact of garlic on lipid parameters: A systematic review and meta-analysis. *Nutr Res Rev* 22:39–48, 2009.

[48] Barrett, B., Brown, R., Rakel, D., et al. Echinacea for treating the common cold: A randomized trial. *Ann Intern Med* 153:769–777, 2010.

[49] Gershwin, M.E., Borchers, A.T., Keen, C.L., et al. Public safety and dietary supplementation. *Ann N Y Acad Sci* 1190:104–117, 2010.

[50] Ribnicky, D.M., Poulev, A., Schmidt, B., et al. Evaluation of botanicals for improving human health. *Am J Clin Nutr* 87:472S–475S, 2008.

[51] Food and Drug Administration. *Dietary Supplement Warnings and Safety Information.* Available online at www.fda.gov/Food/DietarySupplements/Alerts/default.htm. Accessed January 21, 2011.

[52] Saper, R.B., Phillips, R.S., Sehgal, A., et al. Lead, mercury, and arsenic in US- and Indian-manufactured Ayurvedic medicines sold via the Internet. *JAMA* 300:915–923, 2008.

[53] Ulbricht, C., Chao, W., Costa, D., et al. Clinical evidence of herb–drug interactions: A systematic review by the natural standard research collaboration. *Curr Drug Metab* 9:1063–1120, 2008.

[54] Food and Drug Administration. Current good manufacturing practice in manufacturing, packaging, labeling, or holding operations for dietary supplements; final rule. *Fed Regist* 72:34751–34958, June 25, 2007.

Chapter 8

[1] World Health Organization and United Nations Children's Fund Joint Monitoring Programme for Water Supply and Sanitation (JMP). *Progress on Drinking Water and Sanitation: Special Focus on Sanitation.* Available online at www.who.int/water_sanitation_health/monitoring/jmp_report_7_10_lores.pdf. Accessed May 25, 2011.

[2] Shen, H.-P. Body fluids and water balance. In Stipanuk, M.H. (ed.). *Biochemical, Physiological, and Molecular Aspects of Human Nutrition*, 2nd ed. St. Louis: Saunders Elsevier, 2006, pp. 973–1000.

[3] Institute of Medicine, Food and Nutrition Board. *Dietary Reference Intakes for Water, Potassium, Sodium, Chloride, and Sulfate*. Washington, DC: National Academies Press, 2004.

[4] International Bottled Water Association. *Bottled Water 2009*. Available online at www.bottledwater.org/files/2009BWstats.pdf. Accessed February 24, 2011.

[5] U.S. Government Accountability Office. *Bottled Water: FDA Safety and Consumer Protections Are Often Less Stringent Than Comparable EPA Protections for Tap Water*, June 2009. Available online at www.gao.gov/new.items/d09610.pdf. Accessed February 24, 2011.

[6] Environmental Working Group. *Bottled Water Quality Investigation: 10 Major Brands, 38 Pollutants*, October 2008. Available online at www.ewg.org/reports/BottledWater/Bottled-Water-Quality-Investigation. Accessed February 24, 2011.

[7] Environmental Working Group. *National Drinking Water Database*. Available online at http://environment.about.com/gi/o.htm?zi=1/XJ&zTi=1&sdn=environment&cdn=newsissues&tm=238&f=20&su=p504.1.336.p_&tt=2&bt=1&bts=0&zu=http%3A//www.ewg.org/tapwater/findings.php. Accessed February 24, 2011.

[8] Sierra Club. *Bottled Water Campaign*. Available online at www.sierraclub.org/committees/cac/water/bottled_water/. Accessed February 24, 2011.

[9] American Heart Association. *High Blood Pressure Statistics*. Available online at http://www.americanheart.org/presenter.jhtml?identifier=4621. Accessed February 14, 2011.

[10] Chobanian, A.V., Bakris, G.L., Black, H.R., et al. Seventh report of the Joint National Committee on Prevention, Detection, Evaluation, and Treatment of High Blood Pressure. Joint National Committee on Prevention, Detection, Evaluation, and Treatment of High Blood Pressure. National Heart, Lung, and Blood Institute. *Hypertension* 42:1206–1252, 2003.

[11] Ostchega, Y., Yoon, S.S., Hughes, J., and Louis, T. *Hypertension Awareness, Treatment, and Control—Continued Disparities in Adults: United States, 2005–2006*. Available online at www.cdc.gov/nchs/data/databriefs/db03.pdf. Accessed February 14, 2011.

[12] American Heart Association. *Understanding Your Risk of Developing HBP*. Available online at www.americanheart.org/presenter.jhtml?identifier=2142. Accessed February 14, 2011.

[13] U.S. Department of Agriculture and U.S. Department of Health and Human Services. *Dietary Guidelines for Americans, 2010*, 7th ed. Washington, DC: U.S. Government Printing Office, December 2010.

[14] Houston, M.C., and Harper, K.J. Potassium, magnesium, and calcium: Their role in both the cause and treatment of hypertension. *J Clin Hypertens (Greenwich)* 10(7 Suppl. 2):3–11, 2008.

[15] Greenland, P. Beating high blood pressure with low sodium DASH. *N Engl J Med* 344:53–55, 2001.

[16] Sacks, F.M., Svetkey, L.P., Vollmer, W.M., et al. Effects on blood pressure of reduced dietary sodium and the Dietary Approaches to Stop Hypertension (DASH) diet. DASH-Sodium Collaborative Research Group. *N Engl J Med* 344:3–10, 2001.

[17] Carvalho, J.J., Baruzzi, R.G., Howard, P.F., et al. Blood pressure in four remote populations in the Intersalt study. *Hypertension* 14:238–246, 1989.

[18] Appel, L.J., Moore, T.J., Obarzanek, E., et al. A clinical trial of the effects of dietary patterns on blood pressure. *N Engl J Med* 336:1117–1124, 1997.

[19] U.S. Department of Health and Human Services and U.S. Department of Agriculture. *Dietary Guidelines for Americans 2005*. Available online at www.healthierus.gov/dietaryguidelines. Accessed May 19, 2005.

[20] Bügel, S. Vitamin K and bone health in adult humans. *Vitam Horm* 78:393–416, 2008.

[21] Looker, A.C., Melton, L.J. III, Harris, T.B., et al. Prevalence and trends in low femur bone density among older US adults: NHANES 2005–2006 compared with NHANES III. *J Bone Miner Res*. 25:64–71, 2010.

[22] U.S. Department of Health and Human Services. *Bone Health and Osteoporosis: A Report of the Surgeon General*. Rockville, MD: US Department of Health and Human Services, Office of the Surgeon General, 2004.

[23] Reid, I.R. Relationships between fat and bone. *Osteoporos Int* 19:595–606, 2008.

[24] Center for Science in the Public Interest. *Liquid Candy: How Soft Drinks Are Harming America's Health*. Available online at www.cspinet.org/new/pdf/liquid_candy_final_w_new_supplement.pdf. Accessed February 15, 2011.

[25] Ilich, J.Z., Brownbill, R.A., and Coster, D.C. Higher habitual sodium intake is not detrimental for bones in older women with adequate calcium intake. *Eur J Appl Physiol* 109:745–755, 2010.

[26] Kerstetter, J.E., O'Brien, K.O., Caseria, D.M., et al. The impact of dietary protein on calcium absorption and kinetic measures of bone turnover in women. *J Clin Endocrinol Metab* 90:26–31, 2005.

[27] Darling, A.L., Millward, D.J., Torgerson, D.J., et al. Dietary protein and bone health: a systematic review and meta-analysis. *Am J Clin Nutr* 90:1674–1692, 2009.

[28] Papapoulos, S.E. Use of bisphosphonates in the management of postmenopausal osteoporosis. *Ann N Y Acad Sci* 1218:15–32, 2011.

[29] Institute of Medicine, Food and Nutrition Board. *Dietary Reference Intakes for Calcium and Vitamin D*. Washington, DC: National Academies Press, 2011.

[30] Nordin, B.E. The effect of calcium supplementation on bone loss in 32 controlled trials in postmenopausal women. *Osteoporos Int* 20:2135–2143, 2009.

[31] Heaney, R.P., Weaver, C.M., and Recker, R.R. Calcium absorption from spinach. *Am J Clin Nutr* 47:707–709, 1988.

[32] Tucker, K.L., Morita, K., Qiao, N., et al. Colas, but not other carbonated beverages, are associated with low bone mineral density in older women: The Framingham Osteoporosis Study. *Am J Clin Nutr* 84:936–942, 2006.

[33] Institute of Medicine, Food and Nutrition Board. *Dietary Reference Intakes for Calcium, Phosphorus, Magnesium, Vitamin D, and Fluoride*. Washington, DC: National Academies Press, 1997.

[34] Nielsen, F.H. Magnesium, inflammation, and obesity in chronic disease. *Nutr Rev* 68:333–340, 2010.

[35] Champagne, C.M. Magnesium in hypertension, cardiovascular disease, metabolic syndrome, and other conditions: a review. *Nutr Clin Pract* 23:142–151, 2008.

[36] Food and Nutrition Board, Institute of Medicine. *Dietary Reference Intakes: Vitamin A, Vitamin K, Arsenic, Boron, Chromium, Copper, Iodine, Iron, Manganese, Molybdenum, Nickel, Silicon, Vanadium, and Zinc*. Washington, DC: National Academies Press, 2001.

[37] Centers for Disease Control and Prevention. Iron deficiency—United States, 1999–2000. *MMWR Morb Mortal Wkly Rep* 51:897–899, 2002. Available online at www.cdc.gov/mmwr/preview/mmwrhtml/mm5140a1.htm. Accessed February 21, 2011.

[38] World Health Organization. *Micronutrient Deficiencies: Iron Deficiency Anemia*. Available online at www.who.int/nutrition/topics/ida/en/index.html. Accessed February 21, 2011.

39 Killip, S., Bennett, J.M., and Chambers, M.D. Iron deficiency anemia. *Am Fam Phys* 75:671–678, 2007.

40 Food and Drug Administration. Iron-Containing Supplements and Drugs; Label Warning Statements and Unit-Dose Packaging Requirements; Removal of Regulations for Unit-Dose Packaging Requirements for Dietary Supplements and Drugs. *Fed Regist* 68:59714–59715, 2003. Available online at www.fda.gov/Food/DietarySupplements/GuidanceComplianceRegulatoryInformation/RegulationsLaws/ucm107400.htm. Accessed March 3, 2011.

41 Camaschella, C., and Poggiali, E. Inherited disorders of iron metabolism. *Curr Opin Pediatr* 23:14–20, 2011.

42 Centers for Disease Control and Prevention. *Hemochromatosis (Iron storage disease) Facts.* Available online at www.cdc.gov/ncbddd/hemochromatosis/facts.html. Accessed February 22, 2011.

43 Maret, W. Metals on the move: Zinc ions in cellular regulation and in the coordination dynamics of zinc proteins. *Biometals* 24:411–418, 2011.

44 Haase, H., and Rink, L. The immune system and the impact of zinc during aging. *Immun Ageing* 6:9, 2009.

45 Prasad, A.S. Zinc: role in immunity, oxidative stress and chronic inflammation. *Curr Opin Clin Nutr Metab Care* 12:646–652, 2009.

46 Brown, K.H., Peerson, J.M., Baker, S.K., and Hess, S.Y. Preventive zinc supplementation among infants, preschoolers, and older prepubertal children. *Food Nutr Bull* 30(1 Suppl.):S12–S40, 2009.

47 Singh, M., and Das, R.R. Zinc for the common cold. *Cochrane Database Syst Rev* 2:CD001364, 2011.

48 Fairweather-Tait, S.J., Bao, Y., Broadley, M.R., et al. Selenium in human health and disease. *Antioxid Redox Signal* 14:1337–1383, 2011.

49 Food and Nutrition Board, Institute of Medicine. *Dietary Reference Intakes for Vitamin C, Vitamin E, Selenium, and Carotenoids.* Washington, DC: National Academies Press, 2000.

50 Clark, L.C., Combs, G.F., Jr., Turnbull, B.W., et al. Effect of selenium supplementation for cancer prevention in patients with carcinoma of the skin. *JAMA* 276:1957–1968, 1996.

51 Novotny, L., Rauko, P., Kombian, S.B., and Edafiogho, I.O. Selenium as a chemoprotective anti-cancer agent: Reality or wishful thinking? *Neoplasma* 57:383–391, 2010.

52 World Health Organization. *Assessment of Iodine Deficiency Disorders and Monitoring Their Elimination.* available online at www.who.int/nutrition/publications/micronutrients/iodine_deficiency/9789241595827/en/index.html. Accessed November 27, 2010.

53 Di Luigi, L. Supplements and the endocrine system in athletes. *Clin Sports Med* 27:131–151, 2008.

54 Vestergaard, P., Jorgensen, N.R., Schwarz, P., and Mosekilde, L. Effects of treatment with fluoride on bone mineral density and fracture risk—A meta-analysis. *Osteoporos Int* 19:257–268, 2008.

55 Populations receiving optimally fluoridated public drinking water—United States, 1992–2006. *MMWR Morb Mortal Wkly Rep* 57:737–741, 2008. Available online at www.cdc.gov/mmwr/preview/mmwrhtml/mm5727a1.htm?s_cid=mm5727a1. Accessed February 23, 2011.

56 Palmer, C., and Wolfe, S.H. Position of the American Dietetic Association: The impact of fluoride on health. *J Am Diet Assoc* 105:1620–1628, 2005.

57 Beltrán-Aguilar, E.D., Barker, L., and Dye, B.A. Prevalence and severity of dental fluorosis in the United States, 1999–2004. *NCHS Data Brief* 53:1–8, 2010. Available online at www.cdc.gov/nchs/data/databriefs/db53.pdf. Accessed February 23, 2011.

Chapter 9

1 Flegal, K.M., Carroll, M.D., Ogden, C.L., and Curtin, L.R. Prevalence and trends in obesity among US adults, 1999–2008. *JAMA* 303:235–241, 2010.

2 World Health Organization. *Obesity and Overweight*, September 2006. Fact sheet no. 311. Available online at www.who.int/mediacentre/factsheets/fs311/en/. Accessed March 13, 2011.

3 Faith, M.S., Butryn, M., Wadden, T.A., et al. Evidence for prospective associations among depression and obesity in population-based studies. *Obes Rev* 12:e438–e453, 2011.

4 Finkelstein, E.A., Trogdon, J.G., Cohen, J.W., and Dietz, W. Annual medical spending attributable to obesity: Payer- and service-specific estimates. *Health Aff* 28:w822–w831, 2009.

5 National Heart, Lung, and Blood Institute. *The Practical Guide: Identification, Evaluation and Treatment of Overweight and Obesity in Adults.* National Institutes of Health publication no. 02-4084. Bethesda, MD: National Institutes of Health, 2000.

6 Flegal, K.M., Graubard, B.I., Williamson, D.F., and Gail, M.H. Excess deaths associated with underweight, overweight, and obesity. *JAMA* 293:1861–1867, 2005.

7 Gallagher, D., Heymsfield, S., Heo, M., et al. Healthy percentage body fat ranges: An approach for developing guidelines based on body mass index. *Am J Clin Nutr* 72:694–701, 2000.

8 Redinger, R.N. The physiology of adiposity. *J Ky Med Assoc* 106:53–62, 2008.

9 Canoy, D., Boekholdt, S.M., and Wareham, N. Body fat distribution and risk of coronary heart disease in men and women in the European Prospective Investigation Into Cancer and Nutrition in Norfolk Cohort: A population-based prospective study. *Circulation* 116:2933–2943, 2007.

10 U.S. Department of Agriculture and U.S. Department of Health and Human Services. *Dietary Guidelines for Americans, 2010*, 7th ed. Washington, DC: U.S. Government Printing Office, December 2010.

11 Bassett, D.R., Schneider, P.L., and Huntington, G.E. Physical activity in an Old Order Amish community. *Med Sci Sports Exerc* 36:79–85, 2004.

12 Ogden, C.L., Carroll, M.D., Curtin, L.R., et al. Prevalence of high body mass index in US children and adolescents, 2007–2008. *JAMA* 303:242–249, 2010.

13 Weinsier, R.L., Nagy, T.R., Hunter, G.R., et al. Do adaptive changes in metabolic rate favor weight regain in weight-reduced individuals? An examination of the set-point theory. *Am J Clin Nutr* 72:1088–1094, 2000.

14 Institute of Medicine, Food and Nutrition Board. *Dietary Reference Intakes for Energy, Carbohydrate, Fiber, Fat, Protein and Amino Acids.* Washington, DC: National Academies Press, 2002.

15 Levine, J.A., Donahoo, W.T., and Melanson, E.L. Cellular and whole-animal energetics. In Stipanuk, M.H. (ed.). *Biochemical, Physiological and Molecular Aspects of Human Nutrition*, 2nd ed. St Louis: Saunders Elsevier, 2006, pp. 593–617.

16 Institute of Medicine, Food and Nutrition Board. *Dietary Reference Intakes for Energy, Carbohydrate, Fiber, Fat, Protein and Amino Acids.* Washington, DC: National Academies Press, 2002.

17 Rankinen, T., Zuberi, A., Chagnon, Y.C., et al. The human obesity gene map: The 2005 update. *Obesity (Silver Spring)* 14:529–644, 2006.

18 Wardle, J., Carnell, S., Haworth, C.M., and Plomin, R. Evidence for a strong genetic influence on childhood adiposity despite the force of the obesogenic environment. *Am J Clin Nutr* 87:398–404, 2008.

[19] Stunkard, A.J., Harris, J.R., Pedersen, N.L., and McClearn, G.E. The body-mass index of twins who have been reared apart. *N Engl J Med* 322:1483–1487, 1990.

[20] Ravussin, E., Valencia, M.E., Esparza, J., et al. Effects of a traditional lifestyle on obesity in Pima Indians. *Diabetes Care* 17:1067–1074, 1994.

[21] Norman, R.A., Thompson, D.B., Foroud, T., et al. Genomewide search for genes influencing percent body fat in Pima Indians: Suggestive linkage at chromosome 11q21-q22. *Am J Human Genet* 60:166–173, 1997.

[22] Esparza, J., Fox, C., Harper, I.T., et al. Daily energy expenditure in Mexican and USA Pima Indians: Low physical activity as a possible cause of obesity. *Int J Obes Relat Metab Disord* 24:55–59, 2000.

[23] Major, G.C., Doucet, E., Trayhurn, P., et al. Clinical significance of adaptive thermogenesis. *Int J Obes (Lond)* 31:204–212, 2007.

[24] Wynne, K., Stanley, S., McGowan, B., and Bloom, S. Appetite control. *J Endocrinol* 184:291–318, 2005.

[25] Moran, T.H. Gut peptides in the control of food intake. *Int J Obes (Lond)* 33(Suppl. 1):S7–S10, 2009

[26] Myers, M.G., Jr,, Leibel, R.L., Seeley, R.J., and Schwartz, M.W. Obesity and leptin resistance: Distinguishing cause from effect. *Trends Endocrinol Metab* 21:643–651, 2010.

[27] Peters, J.C. Control of energy balance. In Stipanuk, M.H. (ed.). *Biochemical and Physiological Aspects of Human Nutrition*, 2nd ed. Philadelphia: W.B. Saunders, 2006, pp. 618–639.

[28] Levine, J.A., Lanningham-Foster, L.M., McCrady, S.K., et al. Interindividual variation in posture allocation: Possible role in human obesity. *Science* 307:584–586, 2005.

[29] Kroke, A., Liese, A.D., Schulz, M., et al. Recent weight changes and weight cycling as predictors of subsequent two year weight change in a middle-aged cohort. *Int J Obes Relat Metab Disord* 26:403–409, 2002.

[30] U.S. Department of Health and Human Services, Office of the Surgeon General. *The Surgeon General's Call to Action to Prevent and Decrease Overweight and Obesity*. Available online at www.surgeongeneral.gov/topics/obesity. Accessed April 6, 2011.

[31] Hill, J.O., Wyatt, H.R., Reed, G.W., and Peters, J.C. Obesity and the environment: Where do we go from here? *Science* 299:853–855, 2003.

[32] Acheson, K.J. Carbohydrate for weight and metabolic control: Where do we stand? *Nutrition*. 26:141–145, 2010.

[33] US Food and Drug Administration. *Beware of Fraudulent Weight-Loss "Dietary Supplements."* Available online at www.fda.gov/ForConsumers/ConsumerUpdates/ucm246742.htm. Accessed April 6, 2011.

[34] Beck, E.J., Tapsell, L.C., Batterham, M.J., et al. Oat beta-glucan supplementation does not enhance the effectiveness of an energy-restricted diet in overweight women. *Br J Nutr* 103:1212–1222, 2010.

[35] Li, J.J., Huang, C.J., and Xie, D. Anti-obesity effects of conjugated linoleic acid, docosahexaenoic acid, and eicosapentaenoic acid. *Mol Nutr Food Res* 52:631–645, 2008.

[36] Saper, R.B., Eisenberg, D.M., and Phillips, R.S. Common dietary supplements for weight loss. *Am Fam Physician* 70:1731–1738, 2004.

[37] Yazaki, Y., Faridi, Z., Ma, Y., et al. A pilot study of chromium picolinate for weight loss. *J Altern Complement Med* 16:291–299, 2010.

[38] Hess, A.M., and Sullivan, D.L. Potential for toxicity with use of bitter orange extract and guarana for weight loss. *Ann Pharmacother* 39:574–575, 2005.

[39] Sarma, D.N., Barrett, M.L., Chavez, M.L., et al. Safety of green tea extracts: A systematic review by the U.S. Pharmacopeia. *Drug Saf* 31:469–484, 2008.

[40] Chan, T.Y. Potential risks associated with the use of herbal anti-obesity products. *Drug Saf* 32:453–456, 2009.

[41] Lautz, D., Goebel-Fabbri, A., Halperin, F., and Goldfien, A.B. The great debate: Medicine or surgery. What is best for the patient with type 2 diabetes? *Diabetes Care* 34:763–770, 2011.

[42] Buchwald, H., Estok, R., Fahrbach, K., et al. Weight and type 2 diabetes after bariatric surgery: Systematic review and meta-analysis. *Am J Med* 122:248–256, 2009.

[43] Pontiroli, A.E., and Morabito, A. Long-term prevention of mortality in morbid obesity through bariatric surgery: A systematic review and meta-analysis of trials performed with gastric banding and gastric bypass. *Ann Surg* 253:484–487, 2011.

[44] McEwen, L.N., Coelho, R.B., Baumann, L.M., et al. The cost, quality of life impact, and cost-utility of bariatric surgery in a managed care population. *Obes Surg*. 20:919–928, 2010.

[45] Mann, D. *Weight Loss Surgery Insurance Coverage*. Consumer Guide to Bariatric Surgery. Available online at www.your-bariatricsurgeryguide.com/insurance/. Accessed May 24, 2011.

[46] Maggard, M.A., Shugarman, L.R., Suttorp, M., et al. Meta-analysis: Surgical treatment of obesity. *Ann Intern Med*. 142:547–559, 2005.

[47] Online Surgery. *Advantages and Disadvantages of Bariatric Surgery*. Available online at www.onlinesurgery.com/article/advantages-and-disadvantages-of-bariatric-surgery.html. Accessed June 17, 2011.

[48] American Dietetic Association. Position of the American Dietetic Association: Nutrition intervention in the treatment of anorexia nervosa, bulimia nervosa, and other eating disorders. *J Am Diet Assoc* 106:2073–2082, 2006.

[49] Stice, E. Sociocultural influences on body weight and eating disturbance. In Fairburn, C.G., and Brownell, K.D. (eds.). *Eating Disorders and Obesity: A Comprehensive Handbook*, 2nd ed. New York: The Guilford Press, 2002, pp. 103–107.

[50] Body image worries hit Zulu women. *BBC News*, April 16, 2004. Available online at http://news.bbc.co.uk/2/hi/health/3631359.stm. Accessed April 5, 2011.

[51] HealthyPlace. *Eating Disorders: Body Image and Advertising*, December 11, 2008. Available online at www.healthyplace.com/eating-disorders/main/eating-disorders-body-image-and-advertising/menu-id-58/. Accessed April 12, 2011.

[52] Spann, N., and Pritchard, M. Disordered eating in men: A look at perceived stress and excessive exercise. *Eat Weight Disord* 13:e25–e27, 2008.

[53] Tozzi, F., Thornton, L.M., Klump, K.L., et al. Symptom fluctuation in eating disorders: Correlates of diagnostic crossover. *Am J Psychiatry* 162:732–740, 2005.

[54] Vandereycken, W. History of anorexia nervosa and bulimia nervosa. In Fairburn, C.G., and Brownell, K.D. (eds.). *Eating Disorders and Obesity: A Comprehensive Handbook*, 2nd ed. New York: The Guilford Press, 2002, pp. 151–154.

[55] Ebeling, H., Tapanainen, P., and Joutsenoja, A. A practice guideline for treatment of eating disorders in children and adolescents. *Ann Med* 35:488–501, 2003.

[56] Healthier You. *Binge Eating Disorder*. Available online at www.healthieryou.com/binge.html. Accessed April 7, 2011.

[57] Sundgot-Borgen, J., and Torstveit, M.K. Prevalence of eating disorders in elite athletes is higher than in the general population. *Clin J Sport Med* 14:25–32, 2004.

Chapter 10

[1] Gallagher, D., Heymsfield, S., Heo, M., et al. Healthy percentage body fat ranges: An approach for developing guidelines based on body mass index. *Am J Clin Nutr* 72:694–701, 2000.

[2] The President's Council on Physical Fitness and Sports. *Physical Activity Protects Against the Health Risks of Obesity*. Available online at www.fitness.gov/digest_dec2000.htm. Accessed March 10, 2011.

[3] aan het Rot, M., Collins, K.A., and Fitterling, H.L. Physical exercise and depression. *Mt Sinai J Med* 76:204–214, 2009.

[4] Institute of Medicine, Food and Nutrition Board. *Dietary Reference Intakes for Energy, Carbohydrates, Fiber, Fat, Protein and Amino Acids*. Washington, DC: National Academies Press, 2002.

[5] Healthy People 2020. *Physical Activity Objectives*. Available online at www.healthypeople.gov/2020/topicsobjectives2020/objectiveslist.aspx?topicid=33. Accessed March 10, 2011.

[6] U.S. Department of Agriculture and U.S. Department of Health and Human Services. *Dietary Guidelines for Americans, 2010*, 7th ed, Washington, DC: U.S. Government Printing Office, December 2010.

[7] U.S. Department of Health and Human Services. *2008 Physical Activity Guidelines for Americans*. Available online at www.health.gov/paguidelines/pdf/paguide.pdf. Accessed March 10, 2011.

[8] Haskell, W.L., Lee, I-M., Pate, R.R., et al. Physical activity and public health: Updated recommendations for adults from the American College of Sports Medicine and the American Heart Association. *Circulation* 116:1081–1093, 2007.

[9] Allen, D.G., Lamb, G.D., and Westerblad, H. Skeletal muscle fatigue: Cellular mechanisms *Physiol Rev* 88:287–332, 2008.

[10] Lambrinoudaki, I., and Papadimitriou, D. Pathophysiology of bone loss in the female athlete. *Ann N Y Acad Sci* 1205:45–50, 2010.

[11] Remick, D., Chancellor, K., Pederson, J., et al. Hyperthermia and dehydration-related deaths associated with intentional rapid weight loss in three collegiate wrestlers—North Carolina, Wisconsin, and Michigan, November–December, 1997. *MMWR Morb Mortal Wkly Rep* 47:105–108, 1998. Available online at www.cdc.gov/mmwr/preview/mmwrhtml/00051388.htm. Accessed March 25, 2009.

[12] American Dietetic Association. Position of the American Dietetic Association, Dietitians of Canada, and American College of Sports Medicine: Nutrition and athletic performance. *J Am Diet Assoc* 109:509–527, 2009.

[13] Tipton, K.D. Efficacy and consequences of very-high-protein diets for athletes and exercisers. *Proc Nutr Soc* 7:1–10, 2011.

[14] Powers, S.K., and Jackson, M.J. Exercise-induced oxidative stress: Cellular mechanisms and impact on muscle force production. *Physiol Rev* 88:1243–1276, 2008.

[15] Margaritis, I., and Rousseau, A.S. Does physical exercise modify antioxidant requirements? *Nutrition Research Reviews* 21:3–12, 2008.

[16] Di Santolo, M., Stel, G., Banfi, G., et al. Anemia and iron status in young fertile non-professional female athletes. *Eur J Appl Physiol* 102:703–709, 2008.

[17] Food and Nutrition Board, Institute of Medicine. *Dietary Reference Intakes: Vitamin A, Vitamin K, Arsenic, Boron, Chromium, Copper, Iodine, Iron, Manganese, Molybdenum, Nickel, Silicon, Vanadium, and Zinc*. Washington, DC: National Academies Press, 2001.

[18] NOAA's National Weather Service. *Heat Index*. Available online at www.weather.gov/os/heat/index.shtml. Accessed June 15, 2011.

[19] Knechtle, B., Gnädinger, M., Knechtle, P., et al. Prevalence of exercise-associated hyponatremia in male ultraendurance athletes. *Clin J Sport Med* 23:226–232, 2011.

[20] Bergstrom, J., Hermansen, L., Hultman, E., and Saltin, B. Diet, muscle glycogen and physical performance. *Acta Physiologica Scandinavica* 71:140–150, 1967.

[21] Burke, L.M. Nutrition strategies for the marathon: Fuel for training and racing. *Sports Med* 37:344–347, 2007.

[22] Bussau, V.A., Fairchild, T.J., Rao, A., et al. Carbohydrate loading in human muscle: An improved 1 day protocol. *Eur J Appl Physiol* 87:290–295, 2002.

[23] Karp, J.R., Johnston, J.D., Tecklenburg, T.D., et al. Chocolate milk as a post-exercise recovery aid. *Int J Sport Nutr Exerc Metab* 16:78–91, 2006.

[24] Beelen, M., Burke, L.M., Gibala, M.J., and van Loon L, J.C. Nutritional strategies to promote postexercise recovery. *Int J Sport Nutr Exerc Metab* 20:515–532, 2010.

[25] Berardi, J.M., Price, T.B., Noreen, E.E., and Lemon, P.W. Postexercise muscle glycogen recovery enhanced with a carbohydrate-protein supplement. *Med Sci Sports Exerc* 38:1106–1113, 2006.

[26] Howarth, K.R., Moreau, N.A., Phillips, S.M., and Gibala, M.J. Coingestion of protein with carbohydrate during recovery from endurance exercise stimulates skeletal muscle protein synthesis in humans. *J Appl Physiol* 106:1394–1402, 2009.

[27] Di Luigi, L. Supplements and the endocrine system in athletes. *Clin Sports Med* 27:131–151, 2008.

[28] Nissen, S.L., and Sharp, R.L. Effect of dietary supplements on lean mass and strength gains with resistance exercise: A meta-analysis. *J Appl Physiol* 94:651–659, 2003.

[29] Birzniece, V., Nelson, A.E., and Ho, K.K. Growth hormone and physical performance. *Trends Endocrinol Metab* 22:171–178, 2011.

[30] Kanaley, J.A. Growth hormone, arginine and exercise. *Curr Opin Clin Nutr Metab Care* 11:50–54, 2008.

[31] Chromiak, J.A., and Antonio, J. Use of amino acids as growth hormone-releasing agents by athletes. *Nutrition* 18:657–661, 2002.

[32] Brown, G.A., Vukovich, M., and King, D.S. Testosterone prohormone supplements. *Med Sci Sports Exerc* 38:1451–1461, 2006.

[33] van Amsterdam, J., Opperhuizen, A., and Hartgens, F. Adverse health effects of anabolic-androgenic steroids. *Regul Toxicol Pharmacol* 57:117–123, 2010.

[34] Tokish, J.M., Kocher, M.S., and Hawkins, R.J. Ergogenic aids: A review of basic science, performance, side effects, and status in sports. *Am J Sports Med* 32:1543–1553, 2004.

[35] NutraBio.com. *Congress Passes Steroid Control Act*. Available online at www.nutrabio.com/News/news.steroid_control_act_2.htm. Accessed June 25, 2008.

[36] Rowlands, D.S., and Thomson, J.S. Effects of beta-hydroxy-beta-methylbutyrate supplementation during resistance training on strength, body composition, and muscle damage in trained and untrained young men: A meta-analysis. *J Strength Cond Res* 23:836–846, 2009.

[37] McNaughton, L.R., Siegler, J., and Midgley, A. Ergogenic effects of sodium bicarbonate. *Curr Sports Med Rep* 7:230–236, 2008.

[38] Tarnopolsky, M.A. Caffeine and creatine use in sport. *Ann Nutr Metab* 57(Suppl. 2): 1–8, 2011.

[39] Volek, J.S., and Rawson, E.S. Scientific basis and practical aspects of creatine supplementation for athletes. *Nutrition* 20:609–614, 2004.

[40] Shao, A., and Hathcock, J.N. Risk assessment for creatine monohydrate. *Regul Toxicol Pharmacol* 45:242–251, 2006.

[41] Smith, W.A., Fry, A.C., Tschume, L.C., and Bloomer, R.J. Effect of glycine propionyl-L-carnitine on aerobic and anaerobic exercise performance. *Int J Sport Nutr Exerc Metab* 18:19–36, 2008.

[42] Clegg, M.E. Medium-chain triglycerides are advantageous in promoting weight loss although not beneficial to exercise performance. *Int J Food Sci Nutr* 61:653–679, 2010.

[43] Sökmen, B., Armstrong, L.E., Kraemer, W.J., et al. Caffeine use in sports: Considerations for the athlete. *J Strength Cond Res* 22:978–986, 2008.

[44] Ganio, M.S., Klau, J.F., Casa, D.J., et al. Effect of caffeine on sport-specific endurance performance: a systematic review. *J Strength Cond Res* 23:315–324, 2009.

[45] Berger, A.J., and Alford, K. Cardiac arrest in a young man following excess consumption of caffeinated "energy drinks" *Med J Aust* 190:41–43, 2009.

[46] Clauson, K.A., Sheilds, K.M, McQueen, C.E., and Persad, N. Safety issues associated with commercially available energy drinks. *J Am Pharm Assoc* 48:e55–e63, 2008.

[47] Ballard, S.L., Wellborn-Kim, J.J., and Clauson, K.A. Effects of commercial energy drink consumption on athletic performance and body composition. *Phys Sportsmen* 38:107–117, 2010.

[48] Higgins, J.P., Tuttle, T.D., and Higgins, C.L. Energy beverages: Content and safety. *Mayo Clin Proc* 85:1033–1041, 2010.

[49] Duchan, E., Patel, N.D., and Feucht, C. Energy drinks: A review of use and safety. *Phys Sportsmed* 38:171–179, 2010.

[50] Birkeland, K.I., Stray-Gundersen, J., Hemmersbach, P., et al. Effect of rhEPO administration on serum levels of sTfR and cycling performance. *Med Sci Sports Exerc* 32:1238–1243, 2000.

Chapter 11

[1] Committee to Reexamine IOM Pregnancy Weight Guidelines, Institute of Medicine, National Research Council. *Weight Gain During Pregnancy: Reexamining the Guidelines.* Washington, DC: National Academies Press, 2009.

[2] Iacovidou, N., Varsami, M., and Syggellou, A. Neonatal outcome of preterm delivery. *Ann N Y Acad Sci* 1205:130–134, 2010.

[3] Kaiser, L., and Allen, L.A. Position of the American Dietetic Association: Nutrition and lifestyle for a healthy pregnancy outcome. *J Am Diet Assoc* 108:553–561, 2008.

[4] American College of Obstetricians and Gynecologists. ACOG Committee Opinion number 315, September 2005. Obesity in pregnancy. *Obstet Gynecol* 106:671–675, 2005.

[5] Mamun, A.A., Kinarivala, M, O'Callaghan, M.J., et al. Associations of excess weight gain during pregnancy with long-term maternal overweight and obesity: evidence from 21 y postpartum follow-up. *Am J Clin Nutr* 91:1336–1341, 2010.

[6] Fraser, A., Tilling, K., Macdonald-Wallis, C., et al. Association of maternal weight gain in pregnancy with offspring obesity and metabolic and vascular traits in childhood. *Circulation* 121:2557–2564, 2010.

[7] U.S. Department of Health and Human Services. *2008 Physical Activity Guidelines for Americans.* Available online at www.health.gov/paguidelines. Accessed September 20, 2011.

[8] National Center for Health Statistics, Centers for Disease Control and Prevention. *Infant Health.* Available online at www.cdc.gov/nchs/fastats/infant_health.htm. Accessed April 4, 2011.

[9] Xu, J.Q., Kochanek, K.D., Murphy, S.L., and Tejada-Vera, B. *Deaths: Final Data for 2007. National Vital Statistics Reports.* Hyattsville, MD: National Center for Health Statistics, 2010.

[10] Leeman, L., and Fontaine, P. Hypertensive disorders of pregnancy. *Am Fam Physician* 78:93–100, 2008.

[11] Berg, C.J., Callaghan, W.M., Syverson, C., and Henderson, Z. Pregnancy-related mortality in the United States, 1998 to 2005. *Obstet Gynecol.* 116:1302–1309, 2010.

[12] Food and Nutrition Board, Institute of Medicine. *Dietary Reference Intakes: Water, Potassium, Sodium, Chloride, and Sulfate.* Washington, DC: National Academies Press, 2004.

[13] Thangaratinam, S., and Langenveld, J., Mol, B.W., and Khan, K.S. Prediction and primary prevention of pre-eclampsia. *Best Pract Res Clin Obstet Gynaecol* 25: 419–433.

[14] Office of Minority Health and Health Disparities, Centers for Disease Control and Prevention. *Eliminate Disparities in Diabetes.* Available online at www.cdc.gov/omhd/amh/factsheets/diabetes.htm. Accessed April 4, 2011.

[15] Damm, P. Future risk of diabetes in mother and child after gestational diabetes mellitus. *Int J Gynaecol Obstet* 104(Suppl. 1):S25–S26, 2009.

[16] Food and Nutrition Board, Institute of Medicine. *Dietary Reference Intakes for Energy, Carbohydrates, Fiber, Fat, Protein and Amino Acids.* Washington, DC: National Academies Press, 2002.

[17] Koletzko, B., Lien, E., Agostoni, C., et al. The roles of long-chain polyunsaturated fatty acids in pregnancy, lactation and infancy: Review of current knowledge and consensus recommendations. *J Perinat Med* 36:5–14, 2008.

[18] Food and Nutrition Board, Institute of Medicine. *Dietary Reference Intakes for Water, Potassium, Sodium, Chloride, and Sulfate.* Washington, DC: National Academies Press, 2004.

[19] Food and Nutrition Board, Institute of Medicine. *Dietary Reference Intakes for Calcium and Vitamin D.* Washington, DC: National Academies Press, 2011.

[20] Holick, M.F. Vitamin D deficiency: What a pain it is. *Mayo Clin Proc* 78:1457–1459, 2003.

[21] Berry, R.J., Bailey, L., Mulinare, J., and Bower, C. Fortification of flour with folic acid. *Food Nutr Bull* 31(1 Suppl.):S22–S35, 2010.

[22] De Wals, P., Tiarou, F., Van Allen, M.I., et al. Reduction in neural-tube defects after folic acid fortification in Canada. *N Engl J Med* 357:135–142, 2007.

[23] Scholl, T.O., and Johnson, W.G. Folic acid: Influence on the outcome of pregnancy. *Am J Clin Nutr* 71(Suppl.):1295S–1303S, 2000.

[24] Food and Nutrition Board, Institute of Medicine. *Dietary Reference Intakes for Thiamin, Riboflavin, Niacin, Vitamin B-6, Folate, Vitamin B-12, Pantothenic Acid, Biotin, and Choline.* Washington, DC: National Academies Press, 1998.

[25] Food and Nutrition Board, Institute of Medicine. *Dietary Reference Intakes for Vitamin A, Vitamin K, Arsenic, Boron, Chromium, Copper, Iodine, Iron, Manganese, Molybdenum, Nickel, Silicon, Vanadium, and Zinc.* Washington, DC: National Academies Press, 2001.

[26] Hess, S.Y., and King, J.C. Effects of maternal zinc supplementation on pregnancy and lactation outcomes. *Food Nutr Bull* 30(1 Suppl.):S60–S78, 2009.

[27] Mills, M.E. Craving more than food: The implications of pica in pregnancy. *Nurs Womens Health* 11:266–273, 2007.

[28] Centers for Disease Control and Prevention. *Birth Defects.* Available online at www.cdc.gov/ncbddd/birthdefects/index.html. Accessed February 3, 2009.

[29] Stein, A.D., Zybert, P.A., van de Bor, M., and Lumey, L.H. Intrauterine famine exposure and body proportions at birth: The Dutch Hunger Winter. *Int J Epidemiol* 33:831–836, 2004.

[30] Gluckman, P.D., Hanson, M.A., Cooper, C., and Thornburg, K.L. Effect of in utero and early-life conditions on adult health and disease. *N Engl J Med* 359:61–73, 2008.

[31] Roseboom, T., de Rooij, S., and Painter, R. The Dutch famine and its long-term consequences for adult health. *Early Hum Dev* 82:485–491, 2006.

[32] Casanueva, E., Roselló-Soberón, M.E., and De-Regil, L.M. Adolescents with adequate birth weight newborns diminish energy expenditure and cease growth. *J Nutr* 136:2498–2501, 2006.

[33] National Center for Health Statistics, Centers for Disease Control and Prevention. *Teen Births.* Available online at www.cdc.gov/nchs/fastats/teenbrth.htm. Accessed April 26, 2011.

34 National Down Syndrome Congress. *Facts About Down Syndrome*. Available online at www.ndsccenter.org/resources/package3.php. Accessed February 4, 2009.

35 Pediatric and Pregnancy Nutrition Surveillance System, Centers for Disease Control and Prevention. *Maternal Health Indicators*. Available online at www.cdc.gov/pednss/what_is/pnss_health_indicators.htm#Maternal%20Health%20Indicators. Accessed April 26, 2011.

36 Weng, X., Odouli, R., and Li, D.K. Maternal caffeine consumption during pregnancy and the risk of miscarriage: A prospective cohort study. *Am J Obstet Gynecol* 198: 279e1–279e8, 2008.

37 U.S. Department of Agriculture and U.S. Department of Health and Human Services. *Dietary Guidelines for Americans, 2010*, 7th ed., Washington, DC: U.S. Government Printing Office, 2010.

38 U.S. Food and Drug Administration, Center for Food Safety and Applied Nutrition. *Food Safety for Moms-to-Be*. Available online at www.cfsan.fda.gov/~pregnant/safeats.html. Accessed April 19, 2009.

39 Delgado, A.R. Listeriosis in pregnancy. *J Midwifery Womens Health* 53:255–259, 2008.

40 Center for the Evaluation of Risks to Human Reproduction (CERHR). *Toxoplasmosis*. Available online at http://cerhr.niehs.nih.gov/common/toxoplasmosis.html. Accessed April 26, 2011.

41 Goodlett, C.R., and Horn, K.H. Mechanisms of alcohol-induced damage to the developing nervous system. *Alcohol Res Health* 25:175–184, 2001. Available online at http://pubs.niaaa.nih.gov/publications/arh25-3/175-184.pdf. Accessed April 20, 2009.

42 Riley, E.P., Infante, M.A., and Warren, K.R. Fetal Alcohol Spectrum Disorders: An Overview. *Neuropsychol Rev* 99:298–302, 2011.

43 May, P.A., Gossage, J.P., Kalberg, W.O., et al. Prevalence and epidemiologic characteristics of FASD from various research methods with an emphasis on recent in-school studies. *Devel Disabil Res Rev* 15:176–192, 2009.

44 Rogers, J.M. Tobacco and pregnancy: Overview of exposures and effects. *Birth Defects Res C Embryo Today* 84:1–15, 2008.

45 Xiao, D., Huang, X., Yang, S., and Zhang, L. Direct effects of nicotine on contractility of the uterine artery in pregnancy. *J Pharmacol Exp Ther* 322: 180–185, 2007.

46 National Center for Chronic Disease Prevention and Health Promotion. *Women and Smoking: A Report of the Surgeon General*, March 2001. Available online at www.surgeongeneral.gov/library/womenandtobacco/. Accessed April 26, 2011.

47 The National Council on Alcoholism and Drug Dependence. *Alcohol- and Other Drug-Related Birth Defects, Facts and Information*. Available online at www.ncadd.org/facts/defects.html. Accessed April 26, 2011.

48 Schempf, A.H. Illicit drug use and neonatal outcomes: A critical review. *Obstet Gynecol Surv* 62:749–757, 2007.

49 Fajemirokun-Odudeyi, O., and Lindow, S.W. Obstetric implications of cocaine use in pregnancy: A literature review. *Eur J Obstet Gynecol Reprod Biol* 112:2–8, 2004.

50 Schiller, C., and Allen, P.J. Follow-up of infants prenatally exposed to cocaine. *Pediatr Nurs* 31:427–436, 2005.

51 National Center for Health Statistics, Centers for Disease Control and Prevention. *2000 CDC Growth Charts: United States*. Available online at www.cdc.gov/growthcharts/. Accessed May 3, 2011.

52 Lanigan, J., and Singhal, A. Early nutrition and long-term health: A practical approach. *Proc Nutr Soc* 68:422–429, 2009.

53 Victora, C.G., Adair, L., Fall, C., et al. Maternal and Child Undernutrition Study Group. Maternal and child undernutrition: consequences for adult health and human capital. *Lancet* 371:340–357, 2008.

54 Wagner, C.L., and Greer, F.R. American Academy of Pediatrics Section on Breastfeeding, American Academy of Pediatrics Committee on Nutrition. Prevention of rickets and vitamin D deficiency in infants, children, and adolescents. *Pediatrics* 122:1142–1152, 2008.

55 American Academy of Pediatrics, policy statement, Committee on Fetus and Newborn. Controversies concerning vitamin K and the newborn. *Pediatrics* 112:191–192, 2003.

56 James. D.C., and Lessen, R. American Dietetic Association. Position of the American Dietetic Association: Promoting and supporting breastfeeding. *J Am Diet Assoc* 109:1926–1942, 2009.

57 World Health Organization, United Nations Children's Fund. *Global Strategy for Infant and Young Child Feeding*. Geneva, Switzerland: World Health Organization, 2003.

58 Guesnet, P., Alessandri, J.M. Docosahexaenoic acid (DHA) and the developing central nervous system (CNS)—Implications for dietary recommendations. *Biochimie* 93:7–12, 2011.

59 Hoffman, D.R., Boettcher, J.A., Diersen-Schade, D.A. Toward optimizing vision and cognition in term infants by dietary docosahexaenoic and arachidonic acid supplementation: A review of randomized controlled trials. *Prostaglandins, Leukot Essent Fatty Acids* 81:151–158, 2009.

60 Birch, E.E., Garfield, S., Castañeda, Y., et al. Visual acuity and cognitive outcomes at 4 years of age in a double-blind, randomized trial of long-chain polyunsaturated fatty acid-supplemented infant formula. *Early Hum Dev* 83:279–284, 2007.

61 Beyerlein, A., Hadders-Algra, M., Kennedy, K., et al. Infant formula supplementation with long-chain polyunsaturated fatty acids has no effect on Bayley developmental scores at 18 months of age—IPD meta-analysis of 4 large clinical trials. *J Pediatr Gastroenterol Nutr* 50:79–84, 2010.

62 Simmer, K., Patole, S.K., Rao, S.C. Longchain polyunsaturated fatty acid supplementation in infants born at term. *Cochrane Database Syst Rev* 23:CD000376, 2008.

63 Gale, C.R., Marriott, L.D., Martyn, C.N., et al. Group for Southampton Women's Survey Study. Breastfeeding, the use of docosahexaenoic acid-fortified formulas in infancy and neuropsychological function in childhood. *Arch Dis Child* 95:174–179, 2009.

64 Makrides, M., Smithers, L.G., and Gibson, R.A. Role of long-chain polyunsaturated fatty acids in neurodevelopment and growth. *Nestle Nutr Workshop Ser Pediatr Program* 65:123–133, 2010.

65 Greer, F.R., Sicherer, S.H., and Burks, A.W. Effects of early nutritional interventions on the development of atopic disease in infants and children: The role of maternal dietary restriction, breastfeeding, timing of introduction of complementary foods, and hydrolyzed formulas. *Pediatrics* 121:183–191, 2008.

66 Ziegler, E.E. Adverse effects of cow's milk in infants. *Nestle Nutr Workshop Ser Pediatr Program* 60:185–196, 2007.

67 American Academy of Pediatrics. The use and misuse of fruit juice in pediatrics. *Pediatrics* 107:1210–1213, 2001.

Chapter 12

1 Institute of Medicine, Food and Nutrition Board. *Dietary Reference Intakes for Energy, Carbohydrate, Fiber, Fat, Protein, and Amino Acids*. Washington, DC: National Academies Press, 2002.

2 Institute of Medicine, Food and Nutrition Board. *Dietary Reference Intakes for Water, Potassium, Sodium, Chloride, and Sulfate*. Washington, DC: National Academies Press, 2004.

3 Nicklas, T.A., and Hayes, D. Position of the American Dietetic Association: Nutrition guidance for healthy children ages 2

to 11 years. *J Am Diet Assoc* 108:1038–1047, 2008.

[4] Food and Nutrition Board, Institute of Medicine. *Dietary Reference Intakes for Calcium and Vitamin D*. Washington, DC: National Academies Press, 2011.

[5] Rovner, A.J., and O'Brien, K.O. Hypovitaminosis D among healthy children in the United States: A review of the current evidence. *Arch Pediatr Adolesc Med* 162:513–519, 2008.

[6] Madan, N., Rusia, U., Sikka, M., et al. Developmental and neurophysiologic deficits in iron deficiency in children. *Indian J Pediatr* 78:58–64, 2011.

[7] American Academy of Pediatrics. The use and misuse of fruit juice in pediatrics. *Pediatrics* 107:1210–1213, 2001.

[8] U.S. Department of Agriculture and U.S. Department of Health and Human Services. *Dietary Guidelines for Americans, 2010*, 7th ed. Washington, DC: U.S. Government Printing Office, 2010.

[9] American Academy of Pediatrics. The use and misuse of fruit juice in pediatrics. *Pediatrics* 107:1210–1213, 2001.

[10] Patrick, H., and Nicklas, T.A. A review of family and social determinants of children's eating patterns and diet quality. *J Am Coll Nutr* 24:83–92, 2005.

[11] U.S. Department of Health and Human Services, Centers for Disease Control and Prevention, National Center for Health Statistics. *Growth Charts*. Available online at www.cdc.gov/growthcharts/. Accessed April 23, 2011.

[12] Rampersaud, G.C., Pereira, M.A., Girard, B.L., et al. Breakfast habits, nutritional status, body weight, and academic performance in children and adolescents. *J Am Diet Assoc* 105:743–760, 2005.

[13] Alaimo, K., Olson, C., and Frongillo, E. Food insufficiency and American school-aged children's cognitive, academic, and psychosocial development. *Pediatrics* 108:44–53, 2001.

[14] Kleinman, R.E., Hall, S., Green, H., et al. Diet, breakfast, and academic performance in children. *Ann Nutr Metab* 46(Suppl. 1):24–30, 2002.

[15] Fisk, C.M., Crozier, S.R., Inskip, H.M., et al. Influences on the quality of young children's diets: The importance of maternal food choices. *Br J Nutr* 105(2):287–296, 2011.

[16] U.S. Department of Agriculture, Food and Nutrition Service. *National School Lunch Program*. Available online at www.fns.usda.gov/cnd/Lunch/AboutLunch/NSLPFactSheet.pdf. Accessed April 23, 2011.

[17] U.S. Department of Agriculture, Food and Nutrition Service. *Diet Quality of American School-Age Children By School Lunch Participation Status: Data from the National Health and Nutrition Examination Survey, July 2008*. Available online at www.fns.usda.gov/ora/MENU/Published/CNP/FILES/NHANES-NSLP.pdf. Accessed May 6, 2011.

[18] Centers for Disease Control and Prevention. *Basics About Childhood Obesity*. Available online at www.cdc.gov/obesity/childhood/defining.html. Accessed April 23, 2011

[19] Ogden, C.L., Carroll, M.D., Curtin, L.R., et al. Prevalence of high body mass index in US children and adolescents, 2007–2008. *JAMA* 303:242–249, 2010.

[20] National Diabetes Information Clearinghouse. *National Diabetes Statistics, 2011*. Available online at http://diabetes.niddk.nih.gov/dm/pubs/statistics/index.htm. Accessed April 23, 2011.

[21] American Heart Association. *Cholesterol and Atherosclerosis in Children*. Available online at www.americanheart.org/presenter.jhtml?identifier=4499. Accessed May 18, 2011.

[22] Academy of Pediatrics, Committee on Nutrition. *Cholesterol in Childhood*. Available online at http://aappolicy.aappublications.org/cgi/content/full/pediatrics;101/1/141. Accessed April 24, 2011.

[23] Coon, K.A., and Tucker, K.L. Television and children's consumption patterns. A review of the literature. *Minerva Pediatr* 54:423–436, 2002.

[24] Eisenmann, J.C., Bartee, R.T., and Wang, M.Q. Physical activity, TV viewing, and weight in U.S. youth: 1999 Youth Risk Behavior Survey. *Obes Res* 10:379–385, 2002.

[25] Batada, A., Seitz, M., Wotan, M., et al. Nine out of ten food advertisements shown during Saturday morning children's television programming are for food high in fat, sodium, or added sugars, or low in nutrients. *J Am Diet Assoc* 108:673–678, 2008.

[26] Cormier, E., and Elder, J.H. Diet and child behavior problems: Fact or fiction? *Pediatr Nurs* 33:138–143, 2007.

[27] Rojas, N.L., and Chan, E. Old and new controversies in the alternative treatment of attention-deficit hyperactivity disorder. *Ment Retard Dev Disabil Res Rev* 11:116–130, 2005.

[28] Farley, D. Dangers of lead still linger. *FDA Consum* 32:16–21, 1998.

[29] Wengrovitz, A.M., and Brown, M.J. Recommendations for blood lead screening of Medicaid-eligible children aged 1–5 years: An updated approach to targeting a group at high risk. *MMWR Morb Mortal Wkly Rep* 58:1–11, 2009. Available online at www.cdc.gov/mmwr/preview/mmwrhtml/rr5809a1.htm. Accessed April 23, 2011.

[30] Weng, F.L., Shults, J., Leonard, M.B., et al. Risk factors for low serum 25-hydroxyvitamin D concentrations in otherwise healthy children and adolescents. *Am J Clin Nutr* 86: 150–158, 2007.

[31] Centers for Disease Control and Prevention. Iron deficiency—United States, 1999–2000. *MMWR Morb Mortal Wkly Rep* 51:897–899, 2002. Available online at www.cdc.gov/MMWR/preview/mmwrhtml/mm5140a1.htm. Accessed April 24, 2011.

[32] National Institute of Child Health & Human Development. *About Milk Matters*. Available online at www.nichd.nih.gov/milk/about/index.cfm. Accessed April 27, 2009.

[33] Risk Factor Monitoring and Methods Branch, National Cancer Institute. *Sources of Beverage Intakes Among the US Population, 2005–06*. Available online at http://riskfactor.cancer.gov/diet/foodsources/beverages/. Accessed May 16, 2011.

[34] USDA/ARC Children's Nutrition Research Center at Baylor College of Medicine. *Survey Tracks Trends in Children's Dietary Habits*. Available online at www.bcm.edu/cnrc/consumer/archives/mealtime.htm. Accessed April 24, 2011.

[35] American Heart Association. *Statistical Fact Sheet—Risk Factors, 2010 Update*. Available online at www.americanheart.org/downloadable/heart/1261004345265FS18TOB10.pdf. Accessed May 6, 2011.

[36] Facchini, M., Rozensztejn, R., and Gonzalez, C. Smoking and weight control behaviors. *Eat Weight Disord* 10:1–7, 2005.

[37] Palaniappan, U., Jacobs Starkey, L., O'Loughlin, J., and Gray-Donald, K. Fruit and vegetable consumption is lower and saturated fat intake is higher among Canadians reporting smoking. *J Nutr* 131:1952–1958, 2001.

[38] National Council on Alcohol and Drug Dependence. *Youth, Alcohol and Other Drugs*. Available online at www.ncadd.org/facts/youthalc.html. Accessed April 20, 2011.

[39] Centers for Disease Control and Prevention. *Deaths and Mortality*. Available online at www.cdc.gov/nchs/fastats/deaths.htm. Accessed April 24, 2011.

[40] World Health Organization. *The World Health Report, 2004—Changing History*. Available online at www.who.int/whr/2004/en/. Accessed April 24, 2011.

[41] Federal Interagency Forum on Aging-Related Statistics. *Older Americans 2008: Key Indicators of Wellbeing, Population*. Available online at www.agingstats.

gov/agingstatsdotnet/Main_Site/Data/Data_2008.aspx. Accessed April 24, 2011.

[42] Fox Wetle, T. The oldest old: Missed public health opportunities *Am J Public Health* 98:1159–1161, 2008.

[43] Cohn, S.H., Vartsky, D., Yasumura, A., et al. Compartmental body composition based on total-body nitrogen, potassium, and calcium. *Am J Physiol* 239:E524–E530, 1980.

[44] Institute of Medicine, Food and Nutrition Board. *Dietary Reference Intakes for Thiamin, Riboflavin, Niacin, Vitamin B6, Folate, Vitamin B12, Pantothenic Acid, Biotin, and Choline*. Washington, DC: National Academies Press, 1998.

[45] National Institutes of Health, Office of Dietary Supplements. *Dietary Supplement Fact Sheet: Vitamin B12*. Available online at http://ods.od.nih.gov/factsheets/vitaminb12.asp. Accessed April 21, 2011

[46] Drewnowski, A. Warren-Mears, V.A. Does aging change nutrition requirements? *J Nutr Health Aging* 5:70–74, 2001.

[47] U.S. Department of Health and Human Services. *Securing the Benefits of Medical Innovation for Seniors: The Role of Prescription Drugs and Drug Coverage*. Available online at http://aspe.hhs.gov/health/Reports/medicalinnovation/. Accessed April 20, 2011.

[48] Sakuma, K., and Yamaguchi, A. Molecular mechanisms in aging and current strategies to counteract sarcopenia. *Curr Aging Sci* 3:90–101, 2010.

[49] Chandra, R.K. Impact of nutritional status and nutrient supplements on immune responses and incidence of infection in older individuals. *Ageing Res Rev* 3:91–104, 2004.

[50] Centers for Disease Control and Prevention. *Health Information for Older Adults*. Available online at www.cdc.gov/Aging/info.htm#2. Accessed April 21, 2011.

[51] Centers for Disease Control and Prevention. *Arthritis*. Available online at www.cdc.gov/nchs/fastats/arthrits.htm. Accessed April 24, 2011.

[52] Wandel, S., Jüni, P., Tendal, B., et al. Effects of glucosamine, chondroitin, or placebo in patients with osteoarthritis of hip or knee: Network meta-analysis. *BMJ* 341:c4675, 2010.

[53] Hajjar, E.R., Cafiero, A.C., and Hanlon, J.T. Polypharmacy in elderly patients. *Am J Geriatr Pharmacother* 5:314–316, 2007.

[54] Administration on Aging. *A Profile of Older Americans: 2007*. Available online at www.agingcarefl.org/aging/AOA-2007profile.pdf. Accessed April 24, 2011.

[55] Nord, M., Coleman-Jensen, A., Andrews, M., and Carlson, S. *Household Food Security in the United States, 2009*. U.S. Department of Agriculture. Economic Research Service. Economic Research Report Number108. November 2010. Available online at www.ers.usda.gov/Publications/ERR108/ERR108.pdf. Accessed May 17, 2011.

[56] Park, H.W. Longevity, aging, and caloric restriction: Clive Maine McCay and the construction of a multidisciplinary research program. *Hist Stud Nat Sci* 40:79–124, 2010.

[57] Kemnitz, J.W. Calorie restriction and aging in nonhuman primates. *ILAR J* 52:66–77, 2011.

[58] Bloomer, R.J., Kabir, M.M., Trepanowski, J.F., et al. 21 day Daniel Fast improves selected biomarkers of antioxidant status and oxidative stress in men and women. *Nutr Metab* 8:17, 2011.

[59] Everitt, A.V., and Le Couteur, D.G. Life extension by calorie restriction in humans. *Ann N Y Acad Sci* 1114:428–433, 2007.

[60] Willcox, B.J., Willcox, D.C., Todoriki, H., et al. Caloric restriction, the traditional Okinawan diet, and healthy aging: The diet of the world's longest-lived people and its potential impact on morbidity and life span. *Ann N Y Acad Sci* 1114:434–455, 2007.

[61] Willcox, D.C., Willcox, B.J., Todoriki, H., and Suzuki, M. The Okinawan diet: health implications of a low-calorie, nutrient-dense, antioxidant-rich dietary pattern low in glycemic load. *J Am Coll Nutr* 28(Suppl.):500S–516S, 2009.

[62] U.S. Department of Health and Human Services. *2008 Physical Activity Guidelines for Americans*. Available online at www.health.gov/paguidelines/. Accessed April 24, 2011.

[63] American Dietetic Association. Position paper of the American Dietetic Association: Nutrition across the spectrum of aging. *J Am Diet Assoc* 105:1203–1210, 2005.

[64] Dorner, B., Friedrich, E.K., and Posthauer, M.E. Position of the American Dietetic Association: Individualized nutrition approaches for older adults in health care communities. *J Am Diet Assoc* 110:1549–1553, 2010.

[65] American Medical Association. *Harmful Consequences of Alcohol Use on the Brains of Children, Adolescents and College Students, 2002*. Available online at www.ama-assn.org/ama1/pub/upload/mm/388/harmful_consequences.pdf. Accessed April 27, 2011.

[66] Bode, C., and Bode, J.C. Effect of alcohol consumption on the gut. *Best Pract Res Clin Gastroenterol* 17:575–592, 2003.

[67] Lieber, C.S. Relationships between nutrition, alcohol use, and liver disease. *Alcohol Res and Health* 27:220–231, 2003.

[68] Yi, H., Chen, C.M., and Williams, G.D. *Surveillance Report #76: Trends in Alcohol-Related Fatal Traffic Crashes, United States, 1982–2004*. Bethesda, MD: National Institute on Alcohol Abuse and Alcoholism, Division of Epidemiology and Prevention Research. Available online at http://pubs.niaaa.nih.gov/publications/surveillance76/FARS04.pdf. Accessed April 24, 2011.

[69] Whitfield, J.B. Alcohol and gene interactions. *Clin Chem Lab Med* 43:480–487, 2005.

[70] Boffetta, P., and Hashibe, M. Alcohol and cancer. *Lancet Oncol* 7:149–156, 2006.

[71] Allen, N.E., Beral, V., and Casabonne, D. Moderate alcohol intake and cancer incidence in women. *J Natl Cancer Inst* 101:296–305, 2009.

[72] Lucas, D.L., Brown, R.A., Wassef, M., and Giles, T.D. Alcohol and the cardiovascular system: Research challenges and opportunities. *J Am Coll Cardiol* 45:1916–1924, 2005.

[73] Saremi, A., and Arora, R. The cardiovascular implications of alcohol and red wine. *Am J Ther* 15:265–277, 2008.

Chapter 13

[1] Centers for Disease Control and Prevention. *CDC Estimates of Foodborne Illness in the United States*. Available online at www.cdc.gov/foodborneburden/2011-foodborne-estimates.html. Accessed May 25, 2011.

[2] Taylor, M.R. *The FDA Food Safety Modernization Act: Putting Ideas into Action*, January 27, 2011. Available online at www.fda.gov/AboutFDA/CentersOffices/OC/OfficeofFoods/ucm241192.htm. Accessed April 29, 2011.

[3] Centers for Disease Control and Prevention. *Foodborne Illness*. Available online at www.cdc.gov/ncidod/dbmd/diseaseinfo/foodborneinfections_g.htm. Accessed April 28, 2011.

[4] U.S. Food and Drug Administration, Center for Food Safety and Nutrition. *Foodborne Pathogenic Microorganisms and Natural Toxins Handbook: The "Bad Bug Book."* Available online at www.fda.gov/Food/FoodSafety/FoodborneIllness/FoodborneIllnessFoodbornePathogensNaturalToxins/BadBugBook/default.htm. Accessed April 29, 2011.

[5] Samuel, M.C., Vugia, D.J., Shallow, S., et al. Epidemiology of sporadic *Campylobacter* infection in the United States and declining trend in incidence, FoodNet

1996–1999. *Clin Infect Dis* 38(Suppl. 3):S165–S174, 2004.

[6] Zhao, C., Ge, B., De Villena, J., et al. Prevalence of *Campylobacter* spp., *Escherichia coli*, and *Salmonella* serovars in retail chicken, turkey, pork, and beef from the greater Washington, D.C., area. *Appl Environ Microbiol* 67:5431–5436, 2001.

[7] Centers for Disease Control and Prevention. Case definitions for infectious conditions under public health surveillance. *MMWR Morb Mortal Wkly Rep* 46:17, 1997.

[8] Centers for Disease Control and Prevention. *Investigation Update: Multistate Outbreak of Human* E. coli *O145 Infections Linked to Shredded Romaine Lettuce from a Single Processing Facility*. Available online at www.cdc.gov/ecoli/2010/ecoli_o145/. Accessed May 25, 2011

[9] Centers for Disease Control and Prevention. *Investigation Announcement: Multistate Outbreak of* E. coli *O157:H7 Infections Associated with Lebanon Bologna*. Available online at www.cdc.gov/ecoli/2011/O157_0311/index.html. Accessed May 25, 2011.

[10] Centers for Disease Control and Prevention, Division of Foodborne, Bacterial, and Mycotic Disease. *Listeriosis*. Available online at www.cdc.gov/nczved/divisions/dfbmd/diseases/listeriosis/. Accessed April 29, 2011.

[11] Lamont, R.F., Sobel, J., Mazaki-Tovi, S., et al. *Listeriosis* in human pregnancy: A systematic review. *J Perinat Med* 39:227–236, 2011.

[12] Koepke, R., Sobel, J., and Arnon, S.S. Global occurrence of infant botulism, 1976–2006. *Pediatrics* 122:73–82, 2008.

[13] Widdowson, M.A., Sulka, A., Bulens, S.N., et al. Norovirus and foodborne disease, United States, 1991–2000. *Emerg Infect Dis* 11:95–102, 2005.

[14] National Institute of Environmental Health Sciences, National Institutes of Health. *Aflatoxin & Liver Cancer*. Available online at www.niehs.nih.gov/health/impacts/aflatoxin.cfm. Accessed April 30, 2011.

[15] Centers for Disease Control and Prevention. Cryptosporidium *Infection*. Available online at www.cdc.gov/ncidod/dpd/parasites/cryptosporidiosis/factsht_cryptosporidiosis.htm. Accessed April 29, 2011.

[16] Centers for Disease Control and Prevention. *vCJD (Variant Creutzfeldt-Jakob Disease)*. Available online at www.cdc.gov/ncidod/dvrd/vcjd/. Accessed April 29, 2011.

[17] Food and Drug Administration. *BSE (Bovine Spongiform Encephalopathy, or Mad Cow Disease)*. Available online at www.cdc.gov/ncidod/dvrd/bse/. Accessed April 29, 2011.

[18] Preliminary Foodnet Data on the Incidence of Infection with Pathogens Transmitted Commonly Through Food—10 States, 2008. *MMWR* 58:333–337, 2009.

[19] Partnership for Food Safety Education. *Cook to Safe Temperature*. Available online at www.fightbac.org. Accessed April 29, 2011.

[20] U.S. Environmental Protection Agency. *Pesticides: Topical & Chemical Fact Sheets*. Available online at www.epa.gov/pesticides/factsheets/index.htm. Accessed April 29, 2011.

[21] U.S. Environmental Protection Agency. *Setting Tolerances for Pesticide Residues in Foods*. Available online at www.epa.gov/pesticides/factsheets/stprf.htm. Accessed April 29, 2011.

[22] U.S. Food and Drug Administration, Center for Food Safety and Applied Nutrition. *Pesticide Monitoring Program FY 2008*. Available online at www.fda.gov/Food/FoodSafety/FoodContaminantsAdulteration/Pesticides/ResidueMonitoringReports/ucm228867.htm#Results_Regulatory_Monitoring. Accessed April 29, 2011.

[23] U.S. Department of Agriculture, Agricultural Marketing Service. *National Organic Program*. Available online at www.ams.usda.gov/AMSv1.0/ams.fetchTemplateData.do?template=TemplateA&navID=NationalOrganicProgram&leftNav=NationalOrganicProgram&page=NOPNationalOrganicProgramHome&acct=AMSPW. Accessed April 29, 2011.

[24] Organic Trade Association. *Industry Statistics and Projected Growth*. Available online at www.ota.com/organic/mt/business.html. Accessed May 1, 2011.

[25] Crinnion, W.J. Organic foods contain higher levels of certain nutrients, lower levels of pesticides, and may provide health benefits for the consumer. *Altern Med Rev* 1:4–12, 2010.

[26] Mukherjee, A., Speh, D., Dyck, E, et al. Preharvest evaluation of coliforms, *Escherichia coli*, *Salmonella*, and *Escherichia coli* O157:H7 in organic and conventional produce grown by Minnesota farmers. *J Food Prot* 67:894–900, 2004.

[27] Dangour, A.D., Lock, K., Hayter, A., et al. Nutrition-related health effects of organic foods: A systematic review. *Am J Clin Nutr* 92:203–210, 2010.

[28] Dangour, A.D., Dodhia, S.K., Hayter, A., et al. Nutritional quality of organic foods: A systematic review. *Am J Clin Nutr* 90:680–685, 2009.

[29] U.S. Department of Health and Human Services and U.S. Environmental Protection Agency. *What You Need to Know About Mercury in Fish and Shellfish*, March 2004.

Available online at www.fda.gov/ResourcesForYou/Consumers/ucm110591.htm. Accessed April 29, 2011.

[30] International Food Information Council. *Fact Sheet: FDA's Approval Process for Food Animal Antibiotics A Focus on Human Food Safety*, April 2011. Available online at www.foodinsight.org/Resources/Detail.aspx?topic=Fact_Sheet_FDA_s_Approval_Process_for_Food_Animal_Antibiotics. Accessed April 29, 2011.

[31] Pew Commission on Industrial Farm Animal Production. *Final Report: Putting Meat on The Table: Industrial Farm Animal Production in America*. Available online at www.ncifap.org. Accessed April 29, 2011.

[32] Tardiff, R.G., Gargas, M.L., Kirman, C.R., et al. Estimation of safe dietary intake levels of acrylamide for humans. *Food Chem Toxicol* 48:658–667, 2010.

[33] Friedman, M., and Levin, C.E. Review of methods for the reduction of dietary content and toxicity of acrylamide. *J Agric Food Chem* 56:6113–6140, 2008.

[34] Morehouse, K.M. *Irradiation of Food and Packaging: An Overview*. Available online at http://www.fda.gov/Food/FoodIngredientsPackaging/IrradiatedFoodPackaging/ucm081050.htm. Accessed April 29, 2011.

[35] U.S. Food and Drug Administration. *Food Irradiation: A Safe Measure*. January 2000. Available online at http://uw-food-irradiation.engr.wisc.edu/materials/irradbro.pdf. Accessed April 29, 2011.

[36] Osterholm, M.T., and Norgan, A.P. The role of irradiation in food safety. *N Engl J Med* 350:1898–1901, 2004.

[37] National Toxicology Program, Center for the Evaluation of Risks to Human Reproduction. *NTP-CERHR Monograph on the Potential Human Reproductive and Developmental Effects of Bisphenol A*. National Institutes of Health publication number 08-5994, September 2008. Available online at http://cerhr.niehs.nih.gov/chemicals/bisphenol/bisphenol.pdf. Accessed April 24, 2011.

[38] Eichholzer, M., and Gutzwiller, F. Dietary nitrates, nitrites, and N-nitroso compounds and cancer risk: A review of the epidemiologic evidence. *Nutr Rev* 56:95–105, 1998.

[39] U.S. Food and Drug Administration, Center for Food Safety and Applied Nutrition. *Everything Added to Food in the United States (EAFUS)*. Available online at www.fda.gov/food/foodingredientspackaging/ucm115326.htm. Accessed April 29, 2011.

[40] International Food Information Council (IFIC) and US Food and Drug Administration (FDA). *Food Ingredients and Colors*. November 2004; revised April 2010 Available Online at www.fda.gov/food/

foodingredientspackaging/ucm094211. htm Accessed June 27, 2011.

[41] Margawati, E.T. *Transgenic Animals: Their Benefits to Human Welfare*. Available online at www.actionbioscience.org/biotech/margawati.html. Accessed March 21, 2009.

[42] Gonsalves, D., and Ferreira, S. *Transgenic Papaya: A Case for Managing Risks of Papaya Ringspot Virus in Hawaii*. Available online at www.plantmanagementnetwork.org/pub/php/review/2003/papaya/. Accessed August 21, 2008.

[43] Smith, N. *Seeds of Opportunity: An Assessment of the Benefits, Safety and Oversight of Plant Genomics and Agricultural Biotechnology*. U.S. House of Representatives report, April 13, 2000. Available online at www.nicksmithconsulting.com/opportunity.pdf. Accessed June 2, 2011.

[44] Paine, J.A., Shipton, C.A., Chaggar, S., et al. Improving the nutritional value of golden rice through increased pro-vitamin A content. *Nat Biotechnol* 23:482–487, 2005.

[45] Sayre, R., Beeching, J.R., Cahoon, E.B., et al. The BioCassava Plus Program: Biofortification of cassava for Sub-Saharan Africa. *Annu Rev Plant Biol* 62:251–272, 2011.

[46] Nordlee, J.A., Taylor, S. L., Townsend, J. A., et al. Identification of a Brazil-nut allergen in transgenic soybeans. *N Engl J Med* 334:688–692, 1996.

[47] U.S. Food and Drug Administration. *Submissions on Bioengineered New Plant Varieties*. Available online at www.fda.gov/Food/Biotechnology/Submissions/default.htm. Accessed May 1, 2011.

[48] Caporael, L.R. Ergotism: The Satan loosed in Salem? *Science* 192:21–26, 1976.

Chapter 14

[1] Food and Agriculture Organization of the United Nations. *The State of Food Insecurity in the World, 2010, Addressing Food Insecurity in Protracted Crisis*. Available online at www.fao.org/docrep/013/i1683e/i1683e.pdf. Accessed November 30, 2010.

[2] Black, R.E., Allen, L.H., Bhutta, Z.A., et al. Maternal and child undernutrition: Global and regional exposures and health consequences. *Lancet* 371:243–260, 2008.

[3] WHO IRIS: 2008–2013 Action Plan for the Global Strategy for the Prevention and Control of Noncommunicable Diseases: Prevent and Control Cardiovascular Diseases, Cancers, Chronic Respiratory Diseases and Diabetes. *WHO/OMS: Extranet Systems*, November 2010. Available online at http://extranet.who.int/iris/handle/123456789/554. Accessed April 26, 2011.

[4] Central Intelligence Agency. Country comparison: Infant mortality rate. *The World Fact Book*. Available online at www.cia.gov/library/publications/the-world-factbook/rankorder/2091rank.html. Accessed December 20, 2010.

[5] World Health Organization. *Low Birth Weight: Country, Regional and Global Estimates*. Available online at http://whqlibdoc.who.int/publications/2004/9280638327.pdf. Accessed November 23, 2010.

[6] World Health Organization. *The Global Burden of Disease: 2004 Update*. Available online at www.who.int/healthinfo/global_burden_disease/2004_report_update/en/index.html. Accessed November 27, 2010.

[7] UNICEF Progress for Children. *A World Fit for Children: Statistical Review*. Available online at www.unicef.org/progressforchildren/2007n6/index_41401.htm. Accessed May 4, 2009.

[8] Corvalán, C., Gregory, C.O., Martorell, R., and Stein, A.D. Size at birth, infant, early and later childhood growth and adult body composition: a prospective study in a stunted population. *Int J Epidemiol* 36:550–557, 2007.

[9] World Health Organization. *Global Strategy on Diet Physical Activity and Health: Obesity and Overweight*. Available online at www.who.int/dietphysicalactivity/childhood_what/en/. Accessed March 12, 2011.

[10] Food and Agricultural Organization of the United Nations. *The Nutrition Transition and Obesity*. Available online at www.fao.org/FOCUS/E/obesity/obes2.htm Accessed November 27, 2010.

[11] Kelly, T., Yang, W., Chen, C.-S., et al. Global burden of obesity in 2005 and projections to 2030. *Int J Obes (Lond)* 32:1431–1437, 2008.

[12] Vorster, H. H., Bourne, L. T., Venter, C. S., and Oosthuizen, W. Contribution of nutrition to the health transition in developing countries: A framework for research and intervention. *Nutr Rev* 57:341–349, 1999.

[13] Eberwine, D. Globesity: A crisis of growing proportions. *Perspectives in Health* 7:12–16, 2002. Available online at www.paho.org/English/DPI/Number15_article2_2.htm. Accessed November 24, 2010.

[14] Cecchini, M., Sassi, F., Lauer, J.A., et al. Tackling of unhealthy diets, physical inactivity, and obesity: Health effects and cost-effectiveness. *Lancet* 376:1775–1784, 2010.

[15] The World Bank. *New Data Show 1.4 Billion Live on Less Than US$1.25 a Day, but Progress Against Poverty Remains Strong*.

Available online at http://web.worldbank.org/WBSITE/EXTERNAL/TOPICS/EXTPOVERTY/0,,contentMDK:21883042~menuPK:2643747~pagePK:64020865~piPK:149114~theSitePK:336992,00.html. Accessed November 30, 2010.

[16] Population Reference Bureau. *2010 World Population Datasheet*. Available online at http://prb.org/pdf10/10wpds_eng.pdf. Accessed November 24, 2010.

[17] Brown, L.R. *World Facing Huge New Challenge on Food Front—Business-as-Usual Not a Viable Option*. April 16, 2008. Available online at www.earthpolicy.org/Updates/2008/Update72.htm. Accessed November 24, 2010.

[18] Rosen, S., and Shapouri, S. Rising food prices intensify food insecurity in developing countries. *Amber Waves* 6(1):16–21, February 2008. Available online at www.ers.usda.gov/AmberWaves/February08/PDF/RisingFood.pdf. Accessed November 24, 2010.

[19] The Pew Charitable Trusts and Johns Hopkins Bloomberg School of Public Health. *Putting Meat on the Table: Industrial Farm Animal Production in America*. Available online at www.pewtrusts.org/uploadedFiles/wwwpewtrustsorg/Reports/Industrial_Agriculture/PCIFAP_FINAL.pdf. Accessed November 24, 2010.

[20] Steinfeld, H., Gerber, P., Wassenaar, T., et al. *Livestock's Long Shadow: Environmental Issues and Options*. 2006. Available online at http://meteo.lcd.lu/globalwarming/FAO/livestocks_long_shadow.pdf. Accessed November 24, 2010.

[21] World Health Organization. *Preventing and Controlling Micronutrient Deficiencies in Populations Affected by an Emergency*. Available online at www.who.int/nutrition/publications/WHO_WFP_UNICEFstatement.pdf. Accessed November 24, 2010.

[22] Lopez, A. Malnutrition and the burden of disease. *Asia Pac J Clin Nutr* 13:S7, 2004.

[23] World Health Organization. *Micronutrient Deficiencies: Iron Deficiency Anemia*. Available online at www.who.int/nutrition/topics/ida/en/index.html. Accessed November 24, 2010.

[24] World Health Organization. *Micronutrient Deficiencies: Iodine Deficiency Disorders*. Available online at www.who.int/nutrition/topics/idd/en/index.html. Accessed November 24, 2010.

[25] World Health Organization. *Micronutrient Deficiencies: Vitamin A Deficiency*. Available online at www.who.int/nutrition/topics/vad/en/index.html. Accessed November 24, 2010.

[26] Centers for Disease Control and Prevention. *Prevalence of Overweight, Obesity, and Extreme Obesity Among Adults: United States,*

Trends 1976–1980 Through 2007–2008. Available online at www.cdc.gov/nchs/data/hestat/obesity_adult_07_08/obesity_adult_07_08.htm. Accessed November 24, 2010.

[27] Nord, M., Andrews, M., and Carlson, S. *Household Food Security in the United States, 2009.* ERR-108, U.S. Department of Agriculture Economic Research Service, November 2010. Available online at www.ers.usda.gov/Publications/Err108/. Accessed December 1, 2010.

[28] U. S. Census Bureau *Income, Poverty, and Health Insurance Coverage in the United States: 2009 Highlights.* Available online at www.census.gov/hhes/www/p60_238sa.pdf. Accessed November 24, 2010.

[29] Kish, S. *Healthy, Low-Calorie Foods Cost More on Average.* Available online at www.csrees.usda.gov/newsroom/impact/2008/nri/03191_food_prices.html. Accessed November 24, 2010.

[30] Companion, M. An Overview of the State of Native American Health: Challenges and Opportunities. Available online at www.ird-dc.org/who/PDFs/Companion%20-%20Indian%20Health%20Report.pdf. Accessed November 24, 2010.

[31] Centers for Disease Control and Prevention. *Food Desert.* Available online at www.cdc.gov/Features/FoodDeserts/. Accessed March 13, 2011.

[32] Hampton, T. Food insecurity harms health, well-being of millions in the United States. *JAMA* 298:1851–1853, 2007.

[33] MacDorman, M.F., and Mathews, T.J. Recent trends in infant mortality in the United States. *NCHS Data Brief*, no. 9. Hyattsville, MD: National Center for Health Statistics, 2008. Available online at www.cdc.gov/nchs/data/databriefs/db09.pdf. Accessed November 24, 2010.

[34] U.S. Census Bureau. Table 676: Money income of households—distribution by income level and selected characteristics: 2007. *The 2010 Statistical Abstract.* Available online at http://www.census.gov/compendia/statab/2010/tables/10s0676.pdf. Accessed November 26, 2010.

[35] U.S. Department of Housing and Urban Development. *The 2009 Annual Homeless Assessment Report to Congress.* June 2010. Available online at www.huduser.org/publications/pdf/5thHomelessAssessmentReport.pdf. Accessed November 26, 2010.

[36] Federal Interagency Forum on Aging Related Statistics. *Older Americans 2010: Key Indicators of Well Being.* Available online at www.agingstats.gov/agingstatsdotnet/Main_Site/Data/2010_Documents/Slides/OA_2010.ppt. Accessed November 26, 2010.

[37] United Nations. *Millennium Development Goals Report 2010.* Available online at www.un.org/millenniumgoals/poverty.shtml. Accessed November 26, 2010.

[38] United Nations. *Population Facts.* August 2010. Available online at www.un.org/esa/population/publications/popfacts/popfacts_2010-5.pdf. Accessed November 27, 2010.

[39] Berg, L.R., Hager, M.C., and Hassenzahl, D.M. *Visualizing Environmental Science*, 3rd ed. Hoboken, NJ: John Wiley & Sons, 2011.

[40] Association of American Geographers. *How Does Education Affect Fertility Rates in Different Places?* Available online at www.aag.org/Education/center/cgge-aag%20site/Population/lesson3_page2.html. Accessed May 5, 2009.

[41] Central Intelligence Agency. Cote d'Ivoire. *The World Fact Book.* Available online at www.cia.gov/library/publications/the-world-factbook/geos/countrytemplate_iv.html. Accessed November 26, 2010.

[42] United Nations. *Millennium Development Goals Report.* 2010. Available online at http://unstats.un.org/unsd/mdg/Resources/Static/Data/2010%20Stat%20Annex.pdf. Accessed December 2, 2010.

[43] World Health Organization. *Global Strategy for Infant and Young Child Feeding.* Available online at www.who.int/nutrition/topics/global_strategy/en/index.html. Accessed November 27, 2010.

[44] World Health Organization. *Guidelines on Breast Feeding and HIV Infection 2010.* Available online at http://whqlibdoc.who.int/publications/2010/9789241599535_eng.pdf. Accessed November 27, 2010.

[45] World Health Organization. *Assessment of Iodine Deficiency Disorders and Monitoring Their Elimination.* Available online at www.who.int/nutrition/publications/micronutrients/iodine_deficiency/9789241595827/en/index.html. Accessed November 27, 2010.

[46] Li, S., Nugroho, A., Rocheford, T., and White, W.S. Vitamin A equivalence of the ß-carotene in ß-carotene-biofortified maize porridge consumed by women. *Am J Clin Nutr* 92:1105–1112, 2010.

[47] Enserink, M. Tough lessons from golden rice. *Science* 320:468–471, 2008.

[48] Tang, G., Qin, J., Dolnikowski, G.G., et al. Golden rice is an effective source of vitamin A. *Am J Clin Nutr* 89:1776–1783, 2009.

[49] Greenpeace International. *Golden Rice's Lack of Luster: Addressing Vitamin A Deficiency Without Genetic Engineering.* November 9, 2010. Available online at www.greenpeace.org/international/en/publications/reports/Golden-rice-report-2010/. Accessed November 27, 2010.

[50] Bienvenido, O. J., *Rice in Human Nutrition.* Available online at www.fao.org/docrep/t0567e/T0567E00.htm#Contents. Accessed March 22, 2011.

[51] Potrykus, I. Lessons from the 'Humanitarian Golden Rice' project: Regulation prevents development of public good genetically engineered crop products. *N Biotechnol* 27:466–472, 2010.

[52] GMO Compass. Golden rice: First field tests in the Philippines. Available online at www.gmo-compass.org/eng/news/358.golden_rice_first_field_tests_philippines.html. Accessed November 28, 2010.

[53] Qaim, M. Benefits of genetically modified crops for the poor: Household income, nutrition, and health. *N Biotechnol* 27:552–557, 2010.

[54] U.S. Department of Agriculture, Food and Nutrition Service. *The National Nutrition Safety Net: Tools for Community Food Security.* Available online at www.fns.usda.gov/fsec/FILES/SafetyNet2003.pdf. Accessed November 27, 2010.

[55] Economic Research Service, U.S. Department of Agriculture. The food assistance landscape: FY 2009 annual report. *Economic Bulletin* 6–7, March 2010. Available online at www.ers.usda.gov/Publications/EIB6-7/EIB6-7.pdf. Accessed November 27, 2010.

[56] Feeding America. *How Our Network Works.* Available online at http://feedingamerica.org/our-network/how-we-work.aspx. Accessed November 27, 2010.

[57] U.S. Department of Agriculture, Food Recovery and Gleaning Initiative. *A Citizen's Guide to Food Recovery.* Available online at www.usda.gov/news/pubs/gleaning/two.htm. Accessed November 27, 2010.

[58] World Health Organization. Initiative for Vaccine Research. *Hookworm Disease.* Available online at www.who.int/vaccine_research/diseases/soa_parasitic/en/index2.html. Accessed December 3, 2010.

Table and Line Art Credits

Chapter 1

Figure 1.1a-b: From *Visualizing Nutrition* by Lori Smolin and Mary Grosvenor, John Wiley & Sons, Inc., Copyright © 2009. Reprinted with permission of John Wiley & Sons, Inc. **Figure 1.5b:** From *Nutrition: Science and Applications* by Lori A. Smolin and Mary B. Grosvenor, John Wiley & Sons, Inc., Copyright © 2008. Reprinted with permission of John Wiley & Sons, Inc. **Figure 1.5d:** From *Visualizing Nutrition* by Lori Smolin and Mary Grosvenor, John Wiley & Sons, Inc., Copyright © 2009. Reprinted with permission of John Wiley & Sons, Inc. **Figure 1.7b:** From *Visualizing Nutrition* by Lori Smolin and Mary Grosvenor, John Wiley & Sons, Inc., Copyright © 2009. Reprinted with permission of John Wiley & Sons, Inc. and National Vital Statistics Reports, Vol. 56, No. 16, June 11, 2008 http://www.cdc.gov/nchs/data/nvsr/nvsr56/nvsr56_16.pdf. **Figure 1.8:** From *Visualizing Nutrition* by Lori Smolin and Mary Grosvenor, John Wiley & Sons, Inc., Copyright © 2009. Reprinted with permission of John Wiley & Sons, Inc. **Figure 1.10:** From *Nutrition: Everyday Choices* by Mary B. Grosvenor and Lori A. Smolin, John Wiley & Sons, Inc., Copyright © 2006. Reprinted with permission of John Wiley & Sons, Inc. **Figure 1.13:** From *Visualizing Nutrition* by Lori Smolin and Mary Grosvenor, John Wiley & Sons, Inc., Copyright © 2009. Reprinted with permission of John Wiley & Sons, Inc. **What a Scientist Sees (left):** From *Nutrition: Everyday Choices* by Mary B. Grosvenor and Lori A. Smolin, John Wiley & Sons, Inc., Copyright © 2006. Reprinted with permission of John Wiley & Sons, Inc. **What a Scientist Sees (right):** From *Visualizing Nutrition* by Lori Smolin and Mary Grosvenor, John Wiley & Sons, Inc., Copyright © 2009, Reprinted with permission of John Wiley & Sons, Inc.

Chapter 2

Table 2.1: U.S. Department of Agriculture. **Table 2.2:** U.S. Food and Drug Administration. **Figure 2.1:** National Agricultural Library, Agricultural Research Service, U. S. Department of Agriculture. **What a Scientist Sees:** U.S. Department of Agriculture. **Figure 2.2 (1):** From *Nutrition: Science and Applications, Fourth Edition* by Lori Smolin and Mary Grosvenor, John Wiley & Sons, Inc., Copyright © 1998. Reprinted with permission of John Wiley & Sons, Inc. **Figure 2.2 (2, 4–5):** From *Visualizing Nutrition* by Lori Smolin and Mary Grosvenor, John Wiley & Sons, Inc., Copyright © 2009. Reprinted with permission of John Wiley & Sons, Inc. **Figure 2.4:** From *Nutrition: Science and Applications* by Lori A. Smolin and Mary B. Grosvenor, John Wiley & Sons, Inc., Copyright © 2008.Reprinted with permission of John Wiley & Sons, Inc. **Figure 2.7a:** Adapted from Dietary Guidelines for Americans, 2010. Figure 5-1. How do typical American diets compare to recommended intake levels or limits? Available online at http://health.gov/dietaryguidelines/dga2010/dietaryguidelines2010.pdf. **Figure 2.7b:** U.S. States Department of Agriculture. **Figures 2.7b, 2.8:** Copyright © 2008 Harvard University. For more information about The Healthy Eating Pyramid, please see The Nutrition Source, Department of Nutrition, Harvard School of Public Health, http://www.thenutritionsource.org, and Eat, Drink, and Be Healthy, by Walter C. Willett, M.D. and Patrick J. Skerrett (2005), Free Press/Simon & Schuster Inc. **Figure 2.9:** From *Nutrition: Science and Applications* by Lori A. Smolin and Mary B. Grosvenor, John Wiley & Sons, Inc., Copyright © 2008. Reprinted with permission of John Wiley & Sons, Inc. **Figure 2.10:** U.S. Department of Agriculture. **Figure 2.11a:** From *Nutrition: Science and Applications* by Lori A. Smolin and Mary B. Grosvenor, John Wiley & Sons, Inc., Copyright © 2008. Reprinted with permission of John Wiley & Sons, Inc. **Figure 2.12a:** From *Nutrition: Everyday Choices* by Mary B. Grosvenor and Lori A. Smolin, John Wiley & Sons, Inc., Copyright © 2006. Reprinted with permission of John Wiley & Sons, Inc. **Thinking It Through:** From *Nutrition: Everyday Choices* by Mary B. Grosvenor and Lori A. Smolin, John Wiley & Sons, Inc., Copyright © 2006. Reprinted with permission of John Wiley & Sons, Inc. **Figure 2.13:** From *Nutrition: Everyday Choices* by Mary B. Grosvenor and Lori A. Smolin, John Wiley & Sons, Inc., Copyright © 2006.Reprinted with permission of John Wiley & Sons, Inc. **Figure 2.14:** From *Nutrition: Science and Applications* by Lori A. Smolin and Mary B. Grosvenor, John Wiley & Sons, Inc., Copyright © 2008. Reprinted with permission of John Wiley & Sons, Inc.

Chapter 3

Table 3.1: From *Principles of Anatomy and Physiology, 12e* by Gerard J. and Bryan H. Derrickson, John Wiley & Sons, Inc., copyright © 2009. Reprinted with permission of John Wiley & Sons, Inc. **Figures 3.1, 3.2:** From *Nutrition: Everyday Choices* by Mary B. Grosvenor and Lori A. Smolin, John Wiley & Sons, Inc., Copyright © 2006. Reprinted with permission of John Wiley & Sons, Inc. **Figure 3.3:** From *Nutrition: Science and Applications* by Lori A. Smolin and Mary B. Grosvenor, John Wiley & Sons, Inc., Copyright © 2008. Reprinted with permission of John Wiley & Sons, Inc. **Figure 3.4:** From *Nutrition: Everyday Choices* by Mary B. Grosvenor and Lori A. Smolin, John Wiley & Sons, Inc., Copyright © 2006. Reprinted with permission of John Wiley & Sons, Inc. **Figures 3.5, 3.6:** From *Nutrition: Science and Applications* by Lori A. Smolin and Mary B. Grosvenor, John Wiley & Sons, Inc., Copyright © 2008. Reprinted with permission of John Wiley & Sons, Inc. **Figure 3.7:** From *Nutrition: Everyday Choices* by Mary B. Grosvenor and Lori A. Smolin, John Wiley & Sons, Inc., Copyright © 2006, and *Visualizing Human Biology, Third Edition* by Kathleen Anne Ireland, John Wiley & Sons, Inc., Copyright © 2011. Reprinted with permission of John Wiley & Sons, Inc. **Figure 3.9:** From *Nutrition: Everyday Choices* by Mary B. Grosvenor and Lori A. Smolin, John Wiley & Sons, Inc., Copyright © 2006. Reprinted with permission of John Wiley & Sons, Inc. **Figure 3.10:** From *Visualizing Nutrition* by Lori Smolin and Mary Grosvenor, John Wiley & Sons, Inc., Copyright © 2009. Reprinted with permission of John Wiley & Sons, Inc. **Figures 3.10, 3.11:** From *Nutrition: Science and Applications* by Lori A. Smolin and Mary B. Grosvenor, John Wiley & Sons, Inc., Copyright © 2008. Reprinted with permission of John Wiley & Sons, Inc. **What a Scientist Sees (b):** From *Visualizing Nutrition* by Lori Smolin and Mary Grosvenor, John Wiley & Sons, Inc., Copyright © 2009. Reprinted with permission of John Wiley & Sons, Inc. **Figure 3.14b:** From *Visualizing Nutrition* by Lori Smolin and Mary Grosvenor, John Wiley & Sons, Inc., Copyright © 2009. Reprinted with permission of John Wiley & Sons, Inc. **Thinking It Through:** From *Visualizing Nutrition* by Lori Smolin and Mary Grosvenor, John Wiley & Sons, Inc., Copyright © 2009. Reprinted with permission of John Wiley & Sons, Inc. **Figure 3.15:** From *Nutrition: Everyday Choices* by Mary B. Grosvenor and Lori A. Smolin, John Wiley & Sons, Inc., Copyright © 2006. Reprinted with permission of John Wiley & Sons, Inc. **Figure 3.16:** From *Visualizing Nutrition* by Lori Smolin and Mary Grosvenor, John Wiley & Sons, Inc., Copyright © 2009. Reprinted with permission of John Wiley & Sons, Inc. **Figure 3.17:** From *Nutrition: Everyday Choices* by Mary B. Grosvenor and Lori A. Smolin, John Wiley & Sons, Inc., Copyright © 2006. Reprinted with permission of John Wiley & Sons, Inc. **Figure 3.18:** From *Nutrition: Science and Applications* by Lori A. Smolin and Mary B. Grosvenor, John Wiley & Sons, Inc., Copyright © 2008. Reprinted with permission of John Wiley & Sons, Inc. **Figure 3.19:** From *Nutrition: Science and Applications, Second Edition* by Lori A. Smolin and Mary B. Grosvenor, John Wiley & Sons, Inc., Copyright © 2010. Reprinted with permission of John Wiley & Sons, Inc.

Chapter 4

Figure 4.2a: From *Nutrition: Everyday Choices* by Mary B. Grosvenor and Lori A. Smolin, John Wiley & Sons, Inc., Copyright © 2006. Reprinted with permission of John Wiley & Sons, Inc. **Figure 4.2b:** Adapted from Oldways Preservation Trust and the Whole Grains

Council www.wholegrainscouncil.org. **Figure 4.3:** From *Visualizing Nutrition* by Lori Smolin and Mary Grosvenor, John Wiley & Sons, Inc., Copyright © 2009. Reprinted with permission of John Wiley & Sons, Inc. **Figures 4.4, 4.5:** From *Nutrition: Everyday Choices* by Mary B. Grosvenor and Lori A. Smolin, John Wiley & Sons, Inc., Copyright © 2006. Reprinted with permission of John Wiley & Sons, Inc. **Figure 4.7:** *Nutrition: From Science to Life* by Mary Grosvenor, John Wiley & Sons, Inc., Copyright © 2001. Reprinted with permission of John Wiley & Sons, Inc. **Figure 4.8:** From *Visualizing Nutrition* by Lori Smolin and Mary Grosvenor, John Wiley & Sons, Inc., Copyright © 2009. Reprinted with permission of John Wiley & Sons, Inc. **Figure 4.9a:** From *Nutrition: Science and Applications* by Lori A. Smolin and Mary B. Grosvenor, John Wiley & Sons, Inc., Copyright © 2008. Reprinted with permission of John Wiley & Sons, Inc. **What a Scientist Sees:** From *Visualizing Nutrition* by Lori Smolin and Mary Grosvenor, John Wiley & Sons, Inc., Copyright © 2009. Reprinted with permission of John Wiley & Sons, Inc. **Figure 4.10:** From *Nutrition: Everyday Choices* by Mary B. Grosvenor and Lori A. Smolin, John Wiley & Sons, Inc., Copyright © 2006. Reprinted with permission of John Wiley & Sons, Inc. Reprinted with permission of John Wiley & Sons, Inc. **Figures 4.11, 4.12:** From *Nutrition: Science and Applications, Second Edition* by Lori Smolin and Mary Grosvenor, John Wiley & Sons, Inc., Copyright © 2010. Reprinted with permission of John Wiley & Sons, Inc. **Figure 4.13:** Copyright 2011 American Diabetes Association From http://www.diabetes.org. Modified with permission from The American Diabetes Association. **Figure 4.13 (line graph):** From *Visualizing Nutrition* by Lori Smolin and Mary Grosvenor, John Wiley & Sons, Inc., Copyright © 2009. Reprinted with permission of John Wiley & Sons, Inc. **Figure 4.14:** Writing Group for the SEARCH for Diabetes in Youth Study Group, Dabelea, D., Bell, R.A., D'Agostino, R.B. Jr., Imperatore, G., Johansen, J.M., Linder, B., Liu, L.L., Loots, B., Marcovina, S., Mayer-Davis, E.J., Pettitt, D.J., Waitzfelder, B. Incidence of diabetes in youth in the United States. JAMA 2007, June 27; 297(24): 2716-24. **Figures 4.19, 4.21:** From *Visualizing Nutrition* by Lori Smolin and Mary Grosvenor, John Wiley & Sons, Inc., Copyright © 2009. Reprinted with permission of John Wiley & Sons, Inc. **Figure 4.22:** From *Nutrition: Everyday Choices* by Mary B. Grosvenor and Lori A. Smolin, John Wiley & Sons, Inc., Copyright © 2006. Reprinted with permission of John Wiley & Sons, Inc.

Chapter 5

Figure 5.2c: From *Visualizing Nutrition* by Lori Smolin and Mary Grosvenor, John Wiley & Sons, Inc., Copyright © 2009. Reprinted with permission of John Wiley & Sons, Inc. and U.S. Department of Agriculture, Agricultural Research Service. 2010. Energy Intakes: Percentages of Energy from Protein, Carbohydrate, Fat, and Alcohol, by Gender and Age, *What We Eat in America*, NHANES 2007-2008. Available: www.ars.usda.gov/ba/bhnrc/fsrg. Accessed November 11, 2010. **Figures 5.3, 5.4a:** From *Nutrition: Science and Applications* by Lori A. Smolin and Mary B. Grosvenor, John Wiley & Sons, Inc., Copyright © 2008. Reprinted with permission of John Wiley & Sons, Inc. **Figures 5.4c, 5.5a:** From *Nutrition: Everyday Choices* by Mary B. Grosvenor and Lori A. Smolin, John Wiley & Sons, Inc., Copyright © 2006. Reprinted with permission of John Wiley & Sons, Inc. **Figure 5.6a:** From *Nutrition: Science and Applications* by Lori A. Smolin and Mary B. Grosvenor, John Wiley & Sons, Inc., Copyright © 2008. Reprinted with permission of John Wiley & Sons, Inc. **Figure 5.6b:** From *Visualizing Nutrition* by Lori Smolin and Mary Grosvenor, John Wiley & Sons, Inc., Copyright © 2009. Reprinted with permission of John Wiley & Sons, Inc. **Figures 5.6c, 5.7:** From *Nutrition: Science and Applications* by Lori A. Smolin and Mary B. Grosvenor, John Wiley & Sons, Inc., Copyright © 2008. Reprinted with permission of John Wiley & Sons, Inc. **Figure 5.8:** From *Nutrition: Everyday Choices* by Mary B. Grosvenor and Lori A. Smolin, John Wiley & Sons, Inc.,

Copyright © 2006. Reprinted with permission of John Wiley & Sons, Inc. **Figures 5.9, 5.10, 5.12:** From *Nutrition: Science and Applications* by Lori A. Smolin and Mary B. Grosvenor, John Wiley & Sons, Inc., Copyright © 2008. Reprinted with permission of John Wiley & Sons, Inc. **Figure 5.13:** From *Nutrition: Science and Applications, Second Edition* by Lori Smolin and Mary Grosvenor, John Wiley & Sons, Inc., Copyright © 2010. Reprinted with permission of John Wiley & Sons, Inc. **Figure 5.14:** From *Nutrition: Everyday Choices* by Mary B. Grosvenor and Lori A. Smolin, John Wiley & Sons, Inc., Copyright © 2006. Reprinted with permission of John Wiley & Sons, Inc. **Figure 5.15:** From *Nutrition: Science and Applications* by Lori A. Smolin and Mary B. Grosvenor, John Wiley & Sons, Inc., Copyright © 2008 and *Visualizing Human Biology, Second Edition* by Kathleen Anne Ireland, John Wiley & Sons, Inc., Copyright © 2010. Reprinted with permission of John Wiley & Sons, Inc. **Figure 5.18:** From *Visualizing Nutrition* by Lori Smolin and Mary Grosvenor, John Wiley & Sons, Inc., Copyright © 2009. Reprinted with permission of John Wiley & Sons, Inc. **Figure 5.19:** From *Visualizing Nutrition* by Lori Smolin and Mary Grosvenor, John Wiley & Sons, Inc., Copyright © 2009. Reprinted with permission of John Wiley & Sons, Inc. **Critical and Creative Thinking Question:** U.S. Department of Agriculture, Agricultural Research Service. 2010. Energy Intakes: Percentages of Energy from Protein, Carbohydrate, Fat, and Alcohol, by Gender and Age, *What We Eat in America*, NHANES 2007-2008. Available: www.ars.usda.gov/ba/bhnrc/fsrg. Accessed November 11, 2010.

Chapter 6

Figure 6.2a-d: From *Nutrition: Everyday Choices* by Mary B. Grosvenor and Lori A. Smolin, John Wiley & Sons, Inc., Copyright © 2006. Reprinted with permission of John Wiley & Sons, Inc. **Figure 6.2e:** From *Visualizing Nutrition* by Lori Smolin and Mary Grosvenor, John Wiley & Sons, Inc., Copyright © 2009. Reprinted with permission of John Wiley & Sons, Inc. **What a Scientist Sees:** From *Visualizing Nutrition* by Lori Smolin and Mary Grosvenor, John Wiley & Sons, Inc., Copyright © 2009. Reprinted with permission of John Wiley & Sons, Inc. **Figure 6.4:** From *Nutrition: Science and Applications* by Lori A. Smolin and Mary B. Grosvenor, John Wiley & Sons, Inc., Copyright © 2008. Reprinted with permission of John Wiley & Sons, Inc. **Figures 6.5, 6.6a-b:** From and *Nutrition: Everyday Choices* by Mary B. Grosvenor and Lori A. Smolin, John Wiley & Sons, Inc., Copyright © 2006. Reprinted with permission of John Wiley & Sons, Inc. **Figure 6.6c:** From *Visualizing Nutrition* by Lori Smolin and Mary Grosvenor, John Wiley & Sons, Inc., Copyright © 2009. Reprinted with permission of John Wiley & Sons, Inc. **Figure 6.7a:** From *Principles of Anatomy and Physiology, 12th Edition* by Gerard J. Tortora and Bryan H. Derrickson, John Wiley & Sons, Inc., Copyright © 2009. Reprinted with permission of John Wiley & Sons, Inc. **Figure 6.7b:** From *Nutrition: Science and Applications* by Lori A. Smolin and Mary B. Grosvenor, John Wiley & Sons, Inc., Copyright © 2008. Reprinted with permission of John Wiley & Sons, Inc. **Figure 6.8:** From *Nutrition: Science and Applications, Second Edition* by Lori Smolin and Mary Grosvenor, John Wiley & Sons, Inc., Copyright © 2010. Reprinted with permission of John Wiley & Sons, Inc. **Figure 6.9c:** Percentage population undernourished world map. Available online at http://commons.wikimedia.org/wiki/File:Percentage_population_undernourished_world_map.PNG. **Figure 6.10:** From *Nutrition: Everyday Choices* by Mary B. Grosvenor and Lori A. Smolin, John Wiley & Sons, Inc., Copyright © 2006. Reprinted with permission of John Wiley & Sons, Inc. **Figure 6.11:** From *Nutrition: Science and Applications* by Lori A. Smolin and Mary B. Grosvenor, John Wiley & Sons, Inc., Copyright © 2008. Reprinted with permission of John Wiley & Sons, Inc. **Figure 6.15a:** From *Nutrition: Everyday Choices* by Mary B. Grosvenor and Lori A. Smolin, John Wiley & Sons, Inc., Copyright © 2006. Reprinted with permission of John Wiley & Sons, Inc. **Figure 6.16:** From *Visualizing Nutrition* by

Lori Smolin and Mary Grosvenor, John Wiley & Sons, Inc., Copyright © 2009. Reprinted with permission of John Wiley & Sons, Inc.

Chapter 7

Figures 7.1, What a Scientist Sees (left): From *Nutrition: Science and Applications* by Lori A. Smolin and Mary B. Grosvenor, John Wiley & Sons, Inc., Copyright © 2008. Reprinted with permission of John Wiley & Sons, Inc. **What a Scientist Sees (right):** Reproduced with permission of United Nations University Press. And *Visualizing Nutrition* by Lori Smolin and Mary Grosvenor, John Wiley & Sons, Inc., Copyright © 2009. Reprinted with permission of John Wiley & Sons, Inc. **Figure 7.3 (left):** From *Nutrition: Science and Applications* by Lori A. Smolin and Mary B. Grosvenor, John Wiley & Sons, Inc., Copyright © 2008. Reprinted with permission of John Wiley & Sons, Inc. **Figure 7.3 (right):** From *Nutrition: Everyday Choices* by Mary B. Grosvenor and Lori A. Smolin, John Wiley & Sons, Inc., Copyright © 2006. Reprinted with permission of John Wiley & Sons, Inc. **Figures 7.5–7.8:** From *Nutrition: Science and Applications* by Lori A. Smolin and Mary B. Grosvenor, John Wiley & Sons, Inc., Copyright © 2008. Reprinted with permission of John Wiley & Sons, Inc. **Figure 7.9a:** From *Visualizing Nutrition* by Lori Smolin and Mary Grosvenor, John Wiley & Sons, Inc., Copyright © 2009. Reprinted with permission of John Wiley & Sons, Inc. **Figures 7.10b, 7.11–7.12:** From *Nutrition: Science and Applications* by Lori A. Smolin and Mary B. Grosvenor, John Wiley & Sons, Inc., Copyright © 2008. Reprinted with permission of John Wiley & Sons, Inc. **Figure 7.14a:** From *Nutrition: Everyday Choices* by Mary B. Grosvenor and Lori A. Smolin, John Wiley & Sons, Inc., Copyright © 2006. Reprinted with permission of John Wiley & Sons, Inc. **Figure 7.14b:** From *Visualizing Human Biology, Second Edition* by Kathleen Anne Ireland, John Wiley & Sons, Inc., Copyright © 2010. Reprinted with permission of John Wiley & Sons, Inc. **Figures 7.14d, 7.15–7.22a, 7.23, 7.24b, 7.25:** From *Nutrition: Science and Applications* by Lori A. Smolin and Mary B. Grosvenor, John Wiley & Sons, Inc., Copyright © 2008. Reprinted with permission of John Wiley & Sons, Inc. **Figure 7.26:** From *Visualizing Nutrition* by Lori Smolin and Mary Grosvenor, John Wiley & Sons, Inc., Copyright © 2009. Reprinted with permission of John Wiley & Sons, Inc. **Figure 7.26 (map):** World Health Organization, Countries categorized by degree of public health importance of Vitamin A deficiency, April 1995. Available online at http://www.who.int/vmnis/vitamina/prevalence/mn_vitamina_map_1995.pdf and from *Visualizing Nutrition* by Lori Smolin and Mary Grosvenor, John Wiley & Sons, Inc., Copyright © 2009. Reprinted with permission of John Wiley & Sons, Inc. **Figure 7.28:** From *Nutrition: Everyday Choices* by Mary B. Grosvenor and Lori A. Smolin, John Wiley & Sons, Inc., Copyright © 2006. Reprinted with permission of John Wiley & Sons, Inc. **Figures 7.30a, 7.31:** From *Nutrition: Science and Applications* by Lori A. Smolin and Mary B. Grosvenor, John Wiley & Sons, Inc., Copyright © 2008. Reprinted with permission of John Wiley & Sons, Inc. **What a Scientist Sees:** From *Visualizing Nutrition* by Lori Smolin and Mary Grosvenor, John Wiley & Sons, Inc., Copyright © 2009. Reprinted with permission of John Wiley & Sons, Inc. **Figures 7.34, 7.36:** From *Nutrition: Science and Applications* by Lori A. Smolin and Mary B. Grosvenor, John Wiley & Sons, Inc., Copyright © 2008. Reprinted with permission of John Wiley & Sons, Inc.

Chapter 8

Figure 8.2: From *Nutrition: Everyday Choices* by Mary B. Grosvenor and Lori A. Smolin, John Wiley & Sons, Inc., Copyright © 2006. Reprinted with permission of John Wiley & Sons, Inc. **Figures 8.3–8.4:** From *Nutrition: Science and Applications* by Lori A. Smolin and Mary B. Grosvenor, John Wiley & Sons, Inc., Copyright © 2008. Reprinted with permission of John Wiley & Sons, Inc. **Figures 8.5–8.6:** From *Visualizing Nutrition* by Lori Smolin and Mary Grosvenor, John Wiley & Sons, Inc., Copyright © 2009. Reprinted with permis-

sion of John Wiley & Sons, Inc. **Debate:** International Bottled Water Association. **Figures 8.8, 8.11:** From *Nutrition: Science and Applications* by Lori A. Smolin and Mary B. Grosvenor, John Wiley & Sons, Inc., Copyright © 2008. Reprinted with permission of John Wiley & Sons, Inc. **Figure 8.12:** From *Visualizing Nutrition* by Lori Smolin and Mary Grosvenor, John Wiley & Sons, Inc., Copyright © 2009. Reprinted with permission of John Wiley & Sons, Inc. **Figure 8.13:** From *Nutrition: Everyday Choices* by Mary B. Grosvenor and Lori A. Smolin, John Wiley & Sons, Inc., Copyright © 2006. Reprinted with permission of John Wiley & Sons, Inc. **Figure 8.14:** From *Nutrition: Science and Applications* by Lori A. Smolin and Mary B. Grosvenor, John Wiley & Sons, Inc., Copyright © 2008. Reprinted with permission of John Wiley & Sons, Inc. **Figure 8.15a:** Republished with permission of the American College of Nutrition, from "Relative contributions of dietary sodium sources," by R.D. Mattes and D. Donnelly, in *the Journal of the American College of Nutrition*, 10:383-393, 1991. Permission conveyed through Copyright Clearance Center, Inc. Also from *Visualizing Nutrition* by Lori Smolin and Mary Grosvenor, John Wiley & Sons, Inc., Copyright © 2009. Reprinted with permission of John Wiley & Sons, Inc. **Figure 8.15b:** From *Nutrition: Science and Applications* by Lori A. Smolin and Mary B. Grosvenor, John Wiley & Sons, Inc., Copyright © 2008. Reprinted with permission of John Wiley & Sons, Inc. **Figure 8.16:** From *Nutrition: Everyday Choices* by Mary B. Grosvenor and Lori A. Smolin, John Wiley & Sons, Inc., Copyright © 2006. Reprinted with permission of John Wiley & Sons, Inc. **Figure 8.17a:** From *Nutrition: Science and Applications* by Lori A. Smolin and Mary B. Grosvenor, John Wiley & Sons, Inc., Copyright © 2008. Reprinted with permission of John Wiley & Sons, Inc. **Figure 8.17c:** From *Visualizing Nutrition* by Lori Smolin and Mary Grosvenor, John Wiley & Sons, Inc., Copyright © 2009. Reprinted with permission of John Wiley & Sons, Inc. **What a Scientist Sees:** From *Nutrition: Science and Applications* by Lori A. Smolin and Mary B. Grosvenor, John Wiley & Sons, Inc., Copyright © 2008. Reprinted with permission of John Wiley & Sons, Inc. **Figure 8.18:** From *Nutrition: Everyday Choices* by Mary B. Grosvenor and Lori A. Smolin, John Wiley & Sons, Inc., Copyright © 2006. Reprinted with permission of John Wiley & Sons, Inc. **Figure 8.19:** From *Nutrition: Science and Applications* by Lori A. Smolin and Mary B. Grosvenor, John Wiley & Sons, Inc., Copyright © 2008. Reprinted with permission of John Wiley & Sons, Inc. **Figure 8.21:** From *Nutrition: Everyday Choices* by Mary B. Grosvenor and Lori A. Smolin, John Wiley & Sons, Inc., Copyright © 2006. Reprinted with permission of John Wiley & Sons, Inc. **Figures 8.22, 8.24:** From *Nutrition: Science and Applications* by Lori A. Smolin and Mary B. Grosvenor, John Wiley & Sons, Inc., Copyright © 2008. Reprinted with permission of John Wiley & Sons, Inc. **Figure 8.25 (middle):** From *Nutrition: Science and Applications* by Lori A. Smolin and Mary B. Grosvenor, John Wiley & Sons, Inc., Copyright © 2008. Reprinted with permission of John Wiley & Sons, Inc. **Figure 8.25 (bottom):** From *Visualizing Nutrition* by Lori Smolin and Mary Grosvenor, John Wiley & Sons, Inc., Copyright © 2009. Reprinted with permission of John Wiley & Sons, Inc. **Thinking It Through:** From *Visualizing Nutrition* by Lori Smolin and Mary Grosvenor, John Wiley & Sons, Inc., Copyright © 2009 and *Nutrition: Science and Applications* by Lori A. Smolin and Mary B. Grosvenor, John Wiley & Sons, Inc., Copyright © 2008. Reprinted with permission of John Wiley & Sons, Inc. **Figures 8.26–8.28:** From *Nutrition: Science and Applications* by Lori A. Smolin and Mary B. Grosvenor, John Wiley & Sons, Inc., Copyright © 2008. Reprinted with permission of John Wiley & Sons, Inc. **Figure 8.29:** Yang, X.E., W.R. Chen, Y. Feng. Improving human micronutrient nutrition through biofortification in the soil-plant system: China as a case study. *Environmental Geochemistry and Health.* 2007 Oct; 29(5):413–28. Epub 2007 Mar 24 © Springer Science+Business Media B.V. 2007. With kind permission of Springer Science and Business Media. There are instances where we have been unable to trace or contact the copyright holder. If notified the publisher will be pleased to rectify any errors or omissions at the earliest opportunity. **Figure 8.30:** From *Nutrition: Science and Applications* by Lori A. Smolin and Mary B. Grosvenor, John Wiley & Sons, Inc., Copyright © 2008. Reprinted with permission of John Wiley & Sons, Inc. **Figure 8.31 (map):** de Benoist, B., et al., eds. Iodine status worldwide. WHO Global Database on Iodine Deficiency. Geneva, World Health Organization, 2004. **Figure 8.33:** Reprinted with permission from Dietary Reference Intakes for Calcium, Phosphorus, Magnesium, Vitamin D and Fluoride. © 1997 by the National Academy of Sciences, Courtesy of the National Academies Press, Washington, D.C.

Chapter 9

Figure 9.1: Centers for Disease Control and Prevention, Percent of Obese (BMI ≥ 30) in U.S. Adults. Available online at http://www.cdc.gov/obesity/data/trends.html. **Figure 9.5a:** From *Visualizing Nutrition* by Lori Smolin and Mary Grosvenor, John Wiley & Sons, Inc., Copyright © 2009. Reprinted with permission of John Wiley & Sons, Inc. **Figure 9.5b:** National Heart, Lung, and Blood Institute as a part of the National Institutes of Health and the U.S. Department of Health and Human Services and *Visualizing Nutrition* by Lori Smolin and Mary Grosvenor, John Wiley & Sons, Inc., Copyright © 2009. Reprinted with permission of John Wiley & Sons, Inc. **Figure 9.6:** Adapted from Nielsen, S.J. and Popkin, B.M. Patterns and trends in food portion sizes, 1977–1998. *JAMA 289*:450–453, 2003. Copyright © 2003, American Medical Association. All rights reserved. **Figure 9.8b:** From *Nutrition: Science and Applications* by Lori A. Smolin and Mary B. Grosvenor, John Wiley & Sons, Inc., Copyright © 2008. Reprinted with permission of John Wiley & Sons, Inc. **Figure 9.8d:** From *Visualizing Nutrition* by Lori Smolin and Mary Grosvenor, John Wiley & Sons, Inc., Copyright © 2009. **Figure 9.8 (scale):** From *Nutrition: Science and Applications* by Lori A. Smolin and Mary B. Grosvenor, John Wiley & Sons, Inc., Copyright © 2008. Reprinted with permission of John Wiley & Sons, Inc. **Figure 9.9:** From *Nutrition: Everyday Choices* by Mary B. Grosvenor and Lori A. Smolin, John Wiley & Sons, Inc., Copyright © 2006. Reprinted with permission of John Wiley & Sons, Inc. **Figures 9.10, 9.12b:** From *Visualizing Nutrition* by Lori Smolin and Mary Grosvenor, John Wiley & Sons, Inc., Copyright © 2009. Reprinted with permission of John Wiley & Sons, Inc. **Figure 9.13** and **What a Scientist Sees:** From *Nutrition: Everyday Choices* by Mary B. Grosvenor and Lori A. Smolin, John Wiley & Sons, Inc., Copyright © 2006. Reprinted with permission of John Wiley & Sons, Inc. **Figure 9.14:** From Levine, James A., Lorraine M. Lanningham-Foster, Shelly K. McCrady, Alisa C. Krizan, Leslie R. Olson, Paul H. Kane, Michael D. Jensen, Matthew M. Clark (2005). Interindividual Variation in Posture Allocation: Possible Role in Human Obesity. Science 307(5709):584–6. Reprinted with permission from AAAS. **Figure 9.15:** From *Visualizing Nutrition* by Lori Smolin and Mary Grosvenor, John Wiley & Sons, Inc., Copyright © 2009. Reprinted with permission of John Wiley & Sons, Inc. **Figure 9.16:** From *Nutrition: Everyday Choices* by Mary B. Grosvenor and Lori A. Smolin, John Wiley & Sons, Inc., Copyright © 2006. Reprinted with permission of John Wiley & Sons, Inc. **Figures 9.17, 9.18a,** and **What a Scientist Sees:** From *Visualizing Nutrition* by Lori Smolin and Mary Grosvenor, John Wiley & Sons, Inc., Copyright © 2009. Reprinted with permission of John Wiley & Sons, Inc. **Figure 9.19a:** From *Nutrition: Science and Applications* by Lori A. Smolin and Mary B. Grosvenor, John Wiley & Sons, Inc., Copyright © 2008. Reprinted with permission of John Wiley & Sons, Inc. **Figure 9.19b:** From *Visualizing Nutrition* by Lori Smolin and Mary Grosvenor, John Wiley & Sons, Inc., Copyright © 2009. Reprinted with permission of John Wiley & Sons, Inc. **Figures 9.20–9.21:** From *Nutrition: Science and Applications* by Lori A. Smolin and Mary B. Grosvenor, John Wiley & Sons, Inc., Copyright © 2008. Reprinted with permission of John Wiley & Sons, Inc. **Figures 9.22–9.24:** From *Nutrition: Everyday Choices* by Mary B. Grosvenor and Lori A. Smolin, John Wiley & Sons, Inc., Copyright © 2006. Reprinted with permission of John Wiley & Sons, Inc.

Chapter 10

Figures 10.1d, 10.3: From *Nutrition: Science and Applications* by Lori A. Smolin and Mary B. Grosvenor, John Wiley & Sons, Inc., Copyright © 2008. Reprinted with permission of John Wiley & Sons, Inc. **Figure 10.4a:** From *Visualizing Nutrition* by Lori Smolin and Mary Grosvenor, John Wiley & Sons, Inc., Copyright © 2009. Reprinted with permission of John Wiley & Sons, Inc. **Figure 10.5a:** From *Nutrition: Science and Applications* by Lori A. Smolin and Mary B. Grosvenor, John Wiley & Sons, Inc., Copyright © 2008. Reprinted with permission of John Wiley & Sons, Inc. **Figure 10.7:** From *Nutrition: Science and Applications 2e* by Lori Smolin and Mary Grosvenor, John Wiley & Sons, Inc., Copyright © 2010. Reprinted with permission of John Wiley & Sons, Inc. **Figures 10.8–10.9:** From *Nutrition: Science and Applications* by Lori A. Smolin and Mary B. Grosvenor, John Wiley & Sons, Inc., Copyright © 2008. Reprinted with permission of John Wiley & Sons, Inc. **Figures 10.10, What a Scientist Sees:** From *Visualizing Nutrition* by Lori Smolin and Mary Grosvenor, John Wiley & Sons, Inc., Copyright © 2009. Reprinted with permission of John Wiley & Sons, Inc. **Figure 10.11:** From *Nutrition: Science and Applications* by Lori A. Smolin and Mary B. Grosvenor, John Wiley & Sons, Inc., Copyright © 2008. Reprinted with permission of John Wiley & Sons, Inc. **Figures 10.13–10.14:** From *Visualizing Nutrition* by Lori Smolin and Mary Grosvenor, John Wiley & Sons, Inc., Copyright © 2009. Reprinted with permission of John Wiley & Sons, Inc. **Figure 10.15:** From *Nutrition: Science and Applications* by Lori A. Smolin and Mary B. Grosvenor, John Wiley & Sons, Inc., Copyright © 2008. Reprinted with permission of John Wiley & Sons, Inc. **Figures 10.17–10.18:** From *Visualizing Nutrition* by Lori Smolin and Mary Grosvenor, John Wiley & Sons, Inc., Copyright © 2009. Reprinted with permission of John Wiley & Sons, Inc. **Figure 10.19:** Adapted from Saltin, B., and Castill, D. I. Fluid and electrolyte balance during prolonged exercise. In *Exercise, Nutrition, and Energy Metabolism*. E. S. Horton, and R. I. Tergung, eds. New York: Macmillan, 1988. Reprinted by permission of The McGraw-Hill Companies, Inc. **Figures 10.20–10.21:** From *Nutrition: Science and Applications* by Lori A. Smolin and Mary B. Grosvenor, John Wiley & Sons, Inc., Copyright © 2008. Reprinted with permission of John Wiley & Sons, Inc. **Figure 10.22:** From Bergstrom, J., L. Hermansen, E. Hultman, and B. Saltin. Diet, muscle glycogen and physical performance. Acta Physiologica Scandinavica 71:140–150, 1967. Wiley-Blackwell Publishers. **Thinking It Through, What a Scientist Sees, Figure 10.25:** From *Visualizing Nutrition* by Lori Smolin and Mary Grosvenor, John Wiley & Sons, Inc., Copyright © 2009. Reprinted with permission of John Wiley & Sons, Inc. **Critical and Creative Thinking Question 3:** From Sports-fitness-advisor.com. There are instances where we have been unable to trace or contact the copyright holder. If notified the publisher will be pleased to rectify any errors or omissions at the earliest opportunity.

Chapter 11

Table 11.2: U.S. Department of Agriculture. **Figure 11.1:** From *Visualizing Human Biology, Second Edition* by Kathleen Anne Ireland, John Wiley & Sons, Inc., Copyright © 2010. Reprinted with permission of John Wiley & Sons, Inc. **Figures 11.2, 11.4:** From *Nutrition: Science and Applications* by Lori A. Smolin and Mary B. Grosvenor, John Wiley & Sons, Inc., Copyright © 2008. Reprinted with permission of John Wiley & Sons, Inc. **Figure 11.5:** From *Visualizing Human Biology, Second Edition* by Kathleen Anne Ireland, John Wiley & Sons, Inc., Copyright © 2010. Reprinted with permission of John Wiley & Sons, Inc. **Figure 11.6:** From *Visualizing Nutrition* by Lori Smolin and Mary Grosvenor, John Wiley & Sons, Inc., Copyright © 2009. Reprinted with permission of John Wiley & Sons, Inc. **Figure 11.7:** From *Nutrition: Science and Applications* by Lori A. Smolin and Mary B. Grosvenor, John Wiley & Sons, Inc., Copyright © 2008. Reprinted with permission of John Wiley & Sons, Inc. **What a Scientist Sees:** From *Visualizing Nutri-*

tion by Lori Smolin and Mary Grosvenor, John Wiley & Sons, Inc., Copyright © 2009. Reprinted with permission of John Wiley & Sons, Inc. **Figure 11.8:** From *Visualizing Nutrition* by Lori Smolin and Mary Grosvenor, John Wiley & Sons, Inc., Copyright © 2009. Reprinted with permission of John Wiley & Sons, Inc. **Figures 11.9, Thinking It Through:** From *Nutrition: Science and Applications* by Lori A. Smolin and Mary B. Grosvenor, John Wiley & Sons, Inc., Copyright © 2008. Reprinted with permission of John Wiley & Sons, Inc. **Figure 11.11:** This figure was published in The Developing Human, 5e, by K. Moore and T. Persaud, copyright Elsevier (1993). **Figure 11.13:** From *Nutrition: Science and Applications* by Lori A. Smolin and Mary B. Grosvenor, John Wiley & Sons, Inc., Copyright © 2008. Reprinted with permission of John Wiley & Sons, Inc. **Figure 11.14:** Reprinted with permission from 'Down Syndrome: Prenatal Risk Assessment and Diagnosis,' August 15, 2000, American Family Physician. copyright © 2000 American Academy of Family Physicians. All Rights Reserved. **Figure 11.16:** From *Nutrition: Science and Applications* by Lori A. Smolin and Mary B. Grosvenor, John Wiley & Sons, Inc., Copyright © 2008. Reprinted with permission of John Wiley & Sons, Inc. **Figure 11.17:** From *Visualizing Nutrition* by Lori Smolin and Mary Grosvenor, John Wiley & Sons, Inc., Copyright © 2009. Reprinted with permission of John Wiley & Sons, Inc. **Figure 11.18:** From *Nutrition: Science and Applications* by Lori A. Smolin and Mary B. Grosvenor, John Wiley & Sons, Inc., Copyright © 2008. Reprinted with permission of John Wiley & Sons, Inc. **Figure 11.19:** Developed by the National Center for Health Statistics in collaboration with the Nation Center for Chronic Disease Prevention and Health Promotion (2000). From *Nutrition: Science and Applications* by Lori A. Smolin and Mary B. Grosvenor, John Wiley & Sons, Inc., Copyright © 2008. Reprinted with permission of John Wiley & Sons, Inc. **Figure 11.20a:** From *Visualizing Nutrition* by Lori Smolin and Mary Grosvenor, John Wiley & Sons, Inc., Copyright © 2009. Reprinted with permission of John Wiley & Sons, Inc. **Figure 11.20b:** From *Nutrition: Everyday Choices* by Mary B. Grosvenor and Lori A. Smolin, John Wiley & Sons, Inc., Copyright © 2006. Reprinted with permission of John Wiley & Sons, Inc. **Figure 11.24:** From *Visualizing Nutrition* by Lori Smolin and Mary Grosvenor, John Wiley & Sons, Inc., Copyright © 2009. Reprinted with permission of John Wiley & Sons, Inc.

Chapter 12

Figure 12.1: From *Visualizing Nutrition* by Lori Smolin and Mary Grosvenor, John Wiley & Sons, Inc., Copyright © 2009. Reprinted with permission of John Wiley & Sons, Inc. **Figure 12.2:** From *Nutrition: Science and Applications* by Lori A. Smolin and Mary B. Grosvenor, John Wiley & Sons, Inc., Copyright © 2008. Reprinted with permission of John Wiley & Sons, Inc. **What a Scientist Sees:** From *Visualizing Nutrition* by Lori Smolin and Mary Grosvenor, John Wiley & Sons, Inc., Copyright © 2009. Reprinted with permission of John Wiley & Sons, Inc. **Figure 12.4:** From *Nutrition: Science and Applications* by Lori A. Smolin and Mary B. Grosvenor, John Wiley & Sons, Inc., Copyright © 2008. Reprinted with permission of John Wiley & Sons, Inc. **Figure 12.5:** From *Nutrition: Science and Applications* by Lori A. Smolin and Mary B. Grosvenor, John Wiley & Sons, Inc., Copyright © 2008. Reprinted with permission of John Wiley & Sons, Inc. Centers for Disease Control. **Figure 12.6a:** From *Nutrition: Science and Applications* by Lori A. Smolin and Mary B. Grosvenor, John Wiley & Sons, Inc., Copyright © 2008. Reprinted with permission of John Wiley & Sons, Inc. **Figure 12.7b:** Reprinted from the Journal of the American Dietetic Association, Vol. 4, Issue 6. Ameena Batada, Maia Dock Seitz, Margo G. Wootan, and Mary Story. Nine out of 10 Food Advertisements Shown During Saturday Morning Children's Television Programming are for Foods High in Fat, Sodium, or Added Sugars, or Low in Nutrients. Pages 673–678, copyright 2008, with permission from Elsevier. http://www.elsevier.com. **Thinking It Through:** From *Nutrition: Science and Applications* by Lori A. Smolin and Mary B. Gros-

venor, John Wiley & Sons, Inc., Copyright © 2008. Reprinted with permission of John Wiley & Sons, Inc. **Figure 12.8 (line graph):** Tanner, J.M., Whitehouse, R.H., Marubini, E., Resele, L.F. (1976). The adolescent growth spurt of boys and girls of the Harpenden growth study. Annals of Human Biology 1976 Mar: 3(2): 109-26. **Figure 12.8 (bar graph):** Adapted from Forbes, G.B. Body Composition. In Present Knowledge in Nutrition, 6th ed. M.L. Brown, ed. Washington, DC: International Life Sciences Institute-Nutrition Foundation, 1990. **Figure 12.9:** Adapted from Figure 3: Distribution of Intake (grams) Across Beverage Types, U.S. Children & Adolescents (2-18 years) 2005–06. Risk Factor Monitoring and Methods Branch Web site. Applied Research Program. National Cancer Institute. http://riskfactor.cancer.gov/diet/foodsources/beverages/figure3.html. Updated December 21, 2010. Accessed May 16, 2011. **Figure 12.10:** From *Nutrition: Science and Applications* by Lori A. Smolin and Mary B. Grosvenor, John Wiley & Sons, Inc., Copyright © 2008. Reprinted with permission of John Wiley & Sons, Inc. **Figures 12.12a, 12.13-12.14, 12.15a:** From *Nutrition: Science and Applications* by Lori A. Smolin and Mary B. Grosvenor, John Wiley & Sons, Inc., Copyright © 2008. Reprinted with permission of John Wiley & Sons, Inc. **Figure 12.15c:** United States Department of Health and Human Services and *Visualizing Nutrition* by Lori Smolin and Mary Grosvenor, John Wiley & Sons, Inc., Copyright © 2009. Reprinted with permission of John Wiley & Sons, Inc. **Figure 12.16:** From *Nutrition: Science and Applications* by Lori A. Smolin and Mary B. Grosvenor, John Wiley & Sons, Inc., Copyright © 2008. Reprinted with permission of John Wiley & Sons, Inc. **Debate:** Willcox BJ, Willcox DC, Todoriki H, et al. Caloric restriction, the traditional Okinawan diet, and healthy aging: the diet of the world's longest-lived people and its potential impact on morbidity and life span. *Ann N Y Acad Sci. 1114*:434–455, 2007. Figure 5. Wiley-Blackwell Publishers. **Figures 12.18, 12.20–12.22:** From *Nutrition: Science and Applications* by Lori A. Smolin and Mary B. Grosvenor, John Wiley & Sons, Inc., Copyright © 2008. Reprinted with permission of John Wiley & Sons, Inc.

Chapter 13

Figures 13.2, 13.3d, 13.5: From *Visualizing Nutrition* by Lori Smolin and Mary Grosvenor, John Wiley & Sons, Inc., Copyright © 2009. Reprinted with permission of John Wiley & Sons, Inc. **Figure 13.6:** National Institute of Environmental Health Sciences. The liver cancer data is from the GLOBOCAN 2002 database, and the aflatoxin data is from Williams et al., Human Aflatoxicosis in Developing Countries, *American Journal of Clinical Nutrition 80*:1106–22, 2004. **Figure 13.8:** From *Visualizing Nutrition* by Lori Smolin and Mary Grosvenor, John Wiley & Sons, Inc., Copyright © 2009. Reprinted with permission of John Wiley & Sons, Inc. **Figure 13.9 (Fight Bac!):** From *Nutrition: Everyday Choices* by Mary B. Grosvenor and Lori A. Smolin, John Wiley & Sons, Inc., Copyright © 2006. Reprinted with permission of John Wiley & Sons, Inc. **Figure 13.9 (thermometer):** From *Nutrition: Science and Applications* by Lori A. Smolin and Mary B. Grosvenor, John Wiley & Sons, Inc., Copyright © 2008. Reprinted with permission of John Wiley & Sons, Inc. **Figures 13.9 (table), Thinking It Through:** From *Visualizing Nutrition* by Lori Smolin and Mary Grosvenor, John Wiley & Sons, Inc., Copyright © 2009. Reprinted with permission of John Wiley & Sons, Inc. **What a Scientist Sees:** From *Nutrition: Science and Applications* by Lori A. Smolin and Mary B. Grosvenor, John Wiley & Sons, Inc., Copyright © 2008. Reprinted with permission of John Wiley & Sons, Inc. **Figure 13.10:** From *Visualizing Nutrition* by Lori Smolin and Mary Grosvenor, John Wiley & Sons, Inc., Copyright © 2009. Reprinted with permission of John Wiley & Sons, Inc. **Figure 13.11:** From *Visualizing Nutrition* by Lori Smolin and Mary Grosvenor, John Wiley & Sons, Inc., Copyright © 2009. Reprinted with permission of John Wiley & Sons, Inc. **Figure 13.12:** From *Nutrition: Science and Applications* by Lori A. Smolin and Mary B. Grosvenor, John Wiley & Sons, Inc., Copyright © 2008. Reprinted with permission of John

Wiley & Sons, Inc. **Figures 13.17a, 13.20:** From *Nutrition: Everyday Choices* by Mary B. Grosvenor and Lori A. Smolin, John Wiley & Sons, Inc., Copyright © 2006. Reprinted with permission of John Wiley & Sons, Inc. **Figure 13.21b:** From *Visualizing Nutrition* by Lori Smolin and Mary Grosvenor, John Wiley & Sons, Inc., Copyright © 2009. Reprinted with permission of John Wiley & Sons, Inc. **Figure 13.22:** James, Clive. 2008. Global Status of Commercialized Biotech/GM Crops: 2008. ISAAA Brief No. 39. ISAAA: Ithaca, NY.

Chapter 14

Figure 14.1a: From *Nutrition: Science and Applications* by Lori A. Smolin and Mary B. Grosvenor, John Wiley & Sons, Inc., Copyright © 2008. Reprinted with permission of John Wiley & Sons, Inc. **Figure 14.1c:** World Health Organization. The Global Burden of Disease: 2004 update, Copyright 2008. Available online at http://www.who.int/healthinfo/global_burden_disease/GBD_report_2004update_full.pdf. **Figure 14.2a:** Adapted from Vorster, H.H., Bourne, L.T., Venter, C.S., and Oosthuizen, W. Contribution of nutrition to the health transition in developing countries: A framework for research and intervention. *Nutr. Rev.* 57:341–349, 1999. Wiley-Blackwell Publishers. **Figure 14.2b:** World Health Organization, 2000. Available online at http://www.fao.org/FOCUS/E/obesity/obes2.htm. **Figure 14.4 (map):** World Bank, 2009. World poverty map. International Fund for Agricultural Development (IFAD). Available online at http://www.ruralpovertyportal.org/web/guest/region. The World Bank: The World Bank authorizes the use of this material subject to the terms and conditions on its website, http://www.worldbank.org/terms. **Figure 14.4 (pie chart):** Food and Agriculture Organization of the United Nations, *The State of Food Insecurity in the World* (2010). Figure 5. Undernourishment in 2010, by region (millions) (page 10). Available online at fao.org/docrep/013/i1683e/i1683e.pdf. **Figure 14.5:** From *Nutrition: Science and Applications* by Lori A. Smolin and Mary B. Grosvenor, John Wiley & Sons, Inc., Copyright © 2008. Reprinted with permission of John Wiley & Sons, Inc. **Figure 14.8:** U.S. Department of Agriculture. **Figure 14.9:** From *Nutrition: Science and Applications* by Lori A. Smolin and Mary B. Grosvenor, John Wiley & Sons, Inc., Copyright © 2008. Reprinted with permission of John Wiley & Sons, Inc. **Figure 14.10:** United Nations Development Programme (UNDP)/Brazil. **What a Scientist Sees:** United Nations Population Fund. 2003. State of World Population. Available on-line from http://www.unfpa.org/publicationsd/index.cfm?filterPub_Type=5. Accessed 7/5/04. **Figure 14.12b:** Millennium Development Goals Report. Statistical Annex 2010, United Nations, New York, 2010. **Figure 14.13:** From *Visualizing Environmental Science, Third Edition* by Linda Berg, Mary Catherine Hager, and Dave Hassenzahl, John Wiley & Sons, Inc., Copyright © 2011. Reprinted with permission of John Wiley & Sons, Inc. **Figure 14.15:** From *Nutrition: Science and Applications* by Lori A. Smolin and Mary B. Grosvenor, John Wiley & Sons, Inc., Copyright © 2008. Reprinted with permission of John Wiley & Sons, Inc. **Critical and Creative Thinking Question 2:** U.S. Department of Agriculture.

Appendices

Appendix A: Page 533 (top). Reprinted with permission from "Dietary Reference Intakes for Energy, Carbohydrates, Fiber, Fat, Protein, and Amino Acids," (2002) by the National Academy of Sciences, Courtesy of the National Academies Press, Washington, D.C. Page 533 (bottom). Reprinted with permission from "Dietary Reference Intakes for Energy, Carbohydrates, Fiber, Fat, Fatty Acids, and Protein" (2002) by the National Academy of Sciences, Courtesy of the National Academies Press, Washington, D.C. Page 534. Reprinted with permission from "Dietary Reference Intakes for Energy, Carbohydrates, Fiber, Fat, Protein, and Amino Acids," (2002) by the National Academy of Sciences, Courtesy of the National Academies

Press, Washington, D.C. Page 535–6. Dietary Reference Intake Tables: The Complete Set. Institute of Medicine, National Academy of Sciences available online at www.nap.edu. Reprinted with permission from Dietary Reference Intakes: The Essential Guide to Nutrient Requirements, 2006, by the National Academy of Sciences, Courtesy of the National Academies Press, Washington, D.C. Page 537. Reprinted with permission from "Dietary Reference Intakes for Energy, Carbohydrates, Fiber, Fat, Protein, and Amino Acids," (2002) by the National Academy of Sciences, Courtesy of the National Academies Press, Washington, D.C. **Appendix C**: Page 543. Handbook of Clinical Dietetics, American Dietetic Association, © 1981 by Yale University Press (New Haven, Conn.). **Appendix D**: Pages 545–7. U.S. Department of Agriculture and U.S. Department of Health and Human Services. Dietary Guidelines for Americans, 2010. 7th Edition, Washington, DC: U.S. Government Printing Office, December 2010. Page 548 (top). American Institute for Cancer Research. Page 548 (bottom). The DASH Diet Action Plan, Pub 2007, Amidon Press, Northbrook, IL. Page 549. Reprinted by the permission of the American Cancer Society, Inc. All rights reserved. Available online at http://www.cancer.org/Healthy/EatHealthyGetActive/ACSGuidelinesonNutritionPhysicalActivityforCancerPrevention/acs-guidelines-on-nutrition-and-physical-activity-for-cancer-prevention-intro. Page 550. U.S. Department of Health and Human Services. Office of Disease Prevention and Health Promotion. Healthy People 2020. Washington, DC. Available at healthypeople.gov. Appendix E: The Exchange Lists are the basis of a meal planning system designed by a committee of the American Diabetes Association and The American Dietetic Association. While designed primarily for people with diabetes and others who must follow special diets, the Exchange Lists are based on principles of good nutrition that apply to everyone. © 2008 by the American Diabetes Association and The American Dietetic Association. **Appendix F**: Page 569, Nutrition labels and illustration. From Nutrition: Science and Applications by Lori A. Smolin and Mary B. Grosvenor, John Wiley & Sons, Inc., Copyright © 2008. Reprinted with permission of John Wiley & Sons, Inc. Page 569 (top right). U.S. Food and Drug Administration. **Appendix G**: Diet, nutrition and the prevention of chronic diseases. A report of a Joint WHO/FAO Expert Consultation. © World Health Organization 2003. Available online at http://www.who.int/hpr/NPH/docs/who_fao_expert_report.pdf. Reproduced with permission. **Appendix I**: Page 577 (top right). Reprinted with permission from "Dietary Reference Intakes for Vitamin C, Vitamin E, Selenium, and Carotenoids," (2000) by the National Academy of Sciences, Courtesy of the National Academies Press, Washington, D.C. Page 577 (bottom) Reprinted with permission from "Dietary Reference Intakes for Thiamin, Riboflavin, Niacin, Vitamin B6, Folate, Vitamin B12, Pantothenic Acid, Biotin, and Choline," (1998) by the National Academy of Sciences, Courtesy of the National Academies Press, Washington, D.C.

Inside Cover Tables

Front Inside Cover: Dietary Reference Intake Tables: The Complete Set. Institute of Medicine, National Academy of Sciences available online at www.nap.edu. Reprinted with permission from Dietary Reference Intakes: The Essential Guide to Nutrient Requirements, 2006, by the National Academy of Sciences, Courtesy of the National Academies Press, Washington, D.C. **Back Inside Cover:** Dietary Reference Intake Tables: The Complete Set. Institute of Medicine, National Academy of Sciences available online at www.nap.edu. Reprinted with permission from Dietary Reference Intakes: The Essential Guide to Nutrient Requirements, 2006, by the National Academy of Sciences, Courtesy of the National Academies Press, Washington, D.C. Institute of Medicine, Food and Nutrition Board Dietary Reference Intakes for Calcium and Vitamin D (2011), National Academies Press, Washington DC, 2011.

Washnik; Page 377: Andy Washnik; Page 378: softservegirl/iStockphoto; Page 380: Tony Cenicola/Redux Pictures.

Chapter 11

Opener: PAUL DAMIEN/NG Image Collection; Page 390: (center) Biophoto Associates/Photo Researchers, (bottom right) © Meitchik/Custom Medical Stock Photo, Inc.; Page 392: Sarah Leen/NG Image Collection; Page 393: HEATHER PERRY/NG Image Collection; Page 400: Andy Washnik; Page 402: (bottom) Michael DiBari, Jr./AP/Wide World Photos; Page 404: Keystone Features/Getty Images, Inc.; Page 407: David-Young Wolff/PhotoEdit; Page 414: Photo Researchers, Inc.; Page 415: (left) Joel Sartore/NG Image Collection, (right) K.L. Boyd, D.D.S./Custom Medical Stock Photo, Inc.; Page 417: Cusp and Flirt/Masterfile; Page 418: Alamy; Page 419: (far left) Raul Touzon/NG Image Collection, (left) Laura Dwight/PhotoEdit, (center) Bubbles Photolibrary/Alamy, (right) Ashok Rodrigues/iStockphoto; Page 421: David-Young Wolff/PhotoEdit; Page 422: Laura Dwight/PhotoEdit; Page 423: Paul Campbell/Getty Images.

Chapter 12

Opener: David McLain/NG Image Collection; Page 430: (top) Tim Laman/NG Image Collection; Page 431: Elena Elisseeva/iStockphoto; Page 434: (top right) Katja Heinemann/Aurora/Getty Images, Inc., (bottom left) Science Photo Library/Photo Researchers, Inc., (bottom right) Bambu Productions/Getty Images; Page 435: Donna Day/Stone/Getty Images, Inc.; Page 438: Sean Murphy/Getty Images; Page 441: (bottom left) Bill Aron/PhotoEdit, (bottom right) Robyn Mackenzie/iStockphoto; Page 443: Purestock/Getty Images, Inc.; Page 444: Ana Nance/Redux Pictures; Page 448: (top right) Courtesy S.A. Jubias and K.E. Conley, University of Washington Medical Center, (bottom right) Joel Sartore/NG Image Collection; Page 450: Western Ophthalmic Hospital/Photo Researchers, Inc.; Page 453: Ira Block/NG Image Collection; Page 454: Andy Washnik; Page 455: Science Photo Library/Photo Researchers, Inc.; Page 457: (left) Martin M. Rotker/Photo Researchers, Inc., (right) Biophoto Associates/Photo Researchers, Inc.; Page 459: Courtesy S.A. Jubias and K.E. Conley, University of Washington Medical Center; Page 460: Biophoto Associates/Photo Researchers, Inc.; Page 461: Bruce Dale/NG Image Collection.

Chapter 13

Opener: Joel Sartore/NG Image Collection; Page 467: (top left and top right) Masterfile, (center left) Thinkstock Images/Getty Images, Inc., (bottom left) David Freund/iStockphoto, (bottom right) Digital Vision/Getty Images, Inc.; Page 468: Keen Press/NG Image Collection; Page 469: (left) Science Photo Library/Photo Researchers, Inc., (right) Dorling Kindersley/Getty Images, Inc.; Page 471: (top left) Pete Ryan/NG Image Collection, (top right) Jim Richardson/NG Image Collection, (center) David Arnold/NG Image Collection, (bottom left) Joel Sartore/NG Image Collection; Page 472: Fuse/Getty Images, Inc.; Page 474: Manfred Kage/Peter Arnold, Inc.; Page 475: Image from http://en.wikipedia.org/wiki/File:Anisakids.jpg; Page 477: Michael P. Gadomski/Photo Researchers, Inc.; Page 478: Reed Kaestner/Alamy Limited; Page 480: James Shaffer/PhotoEdit; Page 483: Drew Rush/NG Image Collection; Page 485: (top) James L. Stanfiled/NG Image Collection, (bottom) Courtesy Lori Smolin; Page 486: (left) Jim Richardson/NG Image Collection, (right) George F. Mobley/NG Image Collection; Page 488: Annie Griffiths Belt/NG Image Collection; Page 489: Council for Agricultural Science and Technology (CAST), 1989. Ionizing Energy in Food Processing and Pest control: II. Applications; Page 490: Alaska Stock Images/NG Image Collection; Page 491: Richard Nowitz/NG Image Collection; Page 495: (center left) Courtesy Marlin E. Rice, (bottom right) Courtesy Golden Rice Humanitarian Board, www.goldenrice.org; Page 497: Thinkstock Images/Getty Images, Inc.; Page 501: H. Reinhard/Peter Arnold, Inc.

Chapter 14

Opener: Steve Raymer/NG Image Collection; Page 506: Karen Kasmauski/NG Image Collection; Page 507: Steve Raymer/NG Image Collection; Page 509: Alison Wright/NG Image Collection; Page 510: (left) RANDY OLSON/NG Image Collection, (right) KENNETH MACLEISH/NG Image Collection; Page 512: Alaska Stock Images/NG Image Collection; Page 513: (top left) Bruce Brander/Photo Researchers, Inc., (top right) ALISON WRIGHT/NG Image Collection, (center left) B &B Photos/Custom Medical Stock Photo, Inc., (center right) Custom Medical Stock Photo, Inc., (bottom left) John Paul Kay/Peter Arnold, Inc., (bottom right) ISM/Phototake; Page 517: Steve Raymer/NG Image Collection; Page 518: (top) ANNIE GRIFFITHS/NG Image Collection, (bottom) Karen Kasmauski/NG Image Collection; Page 519: (left) Waltraud Ingerl/iStockphoto, (right) Justin Sullivan/Getty Images, Inc.; Page 521: Robert Harding Picture LIbrary/Alamy; Page 523: Masterfile; Page 525: Damian Dovarganes/AP/Wide World Photos; Page 527: Steve Raymer/NG Image Collection; Page 529: David Scharf/Peter Arnold, Inc.

Index

623

Proteins *(cont.)*
   structure and regulation and, 176–177
   structure of, 169–171, 170f
   supplements, 185f
   switching to soy and, 186–187
   vegetarian diets and, 190–193, 190t
Provitamins, 204
Psychological issues, eating disorders
      and, 339
Psychosocial problems, childhood obesity
      and, 434f
Puberty, 439
Pyridoxal phosphate, 216

Q

Qualified health claims, 54

R

Rancidity, 138
Reactive hypoglycemia, 116–117
Rebiana, 119t
Recombinant DNA, 494
Recommended Dietary Allowances
      (RDAs), 32, 37, 37f
Red clover, 246t
Reduced-fat products, 159–160, 159f
Refined carbohydrates, 117–119, 117f
Refined foods, 100, 100f
Refined sugar, 101
Registered dietitians, nutritional
      information and, 22
Rehydration, 263, 263f
Renewable resources, food shortages and,
      511–512
Resistant starch, 106
Rest, blood flow at, 87f
Resting heart rate, 355
Resting metabolic rate, 319f
Retin-A, 407
Retinoids, 228–229
Retinol activity equivalents, 229
Retinol-binding protein, 229
Rhodopsin, 230
Riboflavin, 212, 212f
Rickets, 235, 235f
RNA supplements, 381
Royal jelly, 381

S

Saccharin, 119t
Saliva, 71
Salivary amylase, 71
Salmonella, 470
Salt appetite, 271
Satiety, 324
Saturated fatty acids, 136–137, 136f
Saw palmetto, 246t
School meals, 432–433
School performance, breakfast and, 431
Scientific method, nutrition and, 17, 17f
Scurvy, 224, 224f, 572

Secretions, digestive system, 69–70
Selective eating disorder, 344t
Selenium
   cancer and, 295
   deficiency, 572
   glutathione peroxidase and, 295, 295f
   Keshan disease and, 294
   meeting needs of, 295
   soil selenium and health, 294f
Semivegetarian diets, 190t
Senior Farmers' Market Program, 524t
Set point, weight, 324
Short, intense activities, supplements for,
      379–381, 379f
Short-term food aid, 517, 517f
Silicon, 301
Simple carbohydrates, 102f, 103
Skin pigmentation, vitamin D and, 237f
Skinfold thickness, 313f
Small for gestational age, 391
Small intestine, 75–77, 75f
   absorption mechanisms and, 77, 77f
   bicarbonate and, 74
   bile and, 78
   chemical digestion in, 78f
   immune function in, 79, 79f
   lipases and, 78
   lipid transport from, 142
   pancreatic amylase and, 78
   pancreatic juice and, 74
   pancreatic proteases and, 78
   secretions aiding digestion and, 75–77
   segmentation and, 75
Social changes, calorie intake and, 316
Social issues, older adults and, 450, 453
Sociocultural issues, eating disorders and,
      340f, 341
Soda *vs.* milk, 280
Sodium. *See also* Electrolytes
   on food labels, 276f
   food processing and, 274f–275f, 275
   intake of, 275
Sodium chloride, 269
Soluble fiber, 104, 104f, 120, 120f
Solutes, 259
Solvent, water as, 261
Soy, 186–187
Special Milk Program, 524t
Special Supplemental Nutrition Program
      for Women, Infants, and Children
      (WIC), 404, 524t
Sphincter, 72
Spina bifida, 219f
Spores, 472
Sports anemia, 370, 370f
St. John's wort, 245f, 246t
Staphylococcus aureus, 472
Starches, 103, 103f
Starvation, 506
Steroid precursors, 378–379
Sterols, 136, 140, 140f
Stomach
   activity regulation and, 74, 74f

   digestion and, 73–74, 73f
   gastric juice and, 73
Structural proteins, 176
Structure, nutrients and, 10f
Structure/function claims, dietary
      supplement labels and, 54–55
Stunting, 507
Subcutaneous fat, 314f, 315
Subsistence crops, 521
Sucralose, 119t
Sucrose, 102f, 103, 159f
Sudden infant death syndrome (SIDS), 407
Sugar, 101–102
   food labels and, 125f
   recommendations, 122
Sulfites, 493
Sulfur, 286
Summer Food Service Program, 524t
Sun exposure, vitamin D and, 236f–237f
Sunscreens, 237f
Super-fortified foods, 38
Superweeds, 496
Supplement Facts, 54, 54f
Supplemental Nutrition Assistance
      Program (SNAP), 524t
Supplements. *See* Dietary supplements
Sustainable agriculture, 520, 520f
Swallowing, 71, 71f
Sweeteners, 492t

T

Tannins, 267f, 281
Team Nutrition, 524t
Teenage pregnancy, 404–405, 405f
Teens. *See* Adolescent nutrition
Television watching, childhood obesity and,
      435, 435f
Temperature, food, 488–489
Temporary Assistance for Needy Families
      (TANF), 524t
Teratogens, 403
Theory, 17, 17f
Thermic effect of food (TEF), 317
Thiamin, 201–211
   beriberi and, 210–211, 211f
   functioning of, 211f
   meeting needs of, 210f
   neurotransmitter synthesis and, 210
   Wernicke-Korsakoff syndrome and, 211
Thinness, beauty standards and, 340f
Thirst, 260, 270–271
Thyroid gland, iodine and, 295
Thyroid-stimulating hormone, 295
Tissues, 64
Tocopherol, 241
Tolerable Upper Intake Levels (ULs), 37, 38f
Tooth loss, 82f
Toxic substance exposure, pregnancy and,
      406–408
Toxoplasmosis, 406
Trace minerals, 265, 300t–301t
   chromium, 298